Nonhuman Primates in Biomedical Research

Diseases

AMERICAN COLLEGE OF LABORATORY ANIMAL MEDICINE SERIES

Steven H. Weisbroth, Ronald E. Flatt, and Alan L. Kraus, eds.:
The Biology of the Laboratory Rabbit, 1974

Joseph E. Wagner and Patrick J. Manning, eds.:
The Biology of the Guinea Pig, 1976

Edwin J. Andrews, Billy C. Ward, and Norman H. Altman, eds.:
Spontaneous Animal Models of Human Disease, Volume I, 1979;
Volume II, 1979

Henry J. Baker, J. Russell Lindsey, and Steven H. Weisbroth, eds.:
The Laboratory Rat, Volume I: Biology and Diseases, 1979;
Volume II: Research Applications, 1980

Henry L. Foster, J. David Small, and James G. Fox, eds.:
The Mouse in Biomedical Research, Volume I: History,
Genetics, and Wild Mice, 1981; Volume II: Diseases, 1982;
Volume III: Normative Biology, Immunology, and Husbandry, 1983;
Volume IV: Experimental Biology and Oncology, 1982

James G. Fox, Bennett J. Cohen, and Franklin M. Loew, eds.:
Laboratory Animal Medicine, 1984

G. L. Van Hoosier, Jr., and Charles W. McPherson, eds.:
Laboratory Hamsters, 1987

Patrick J. Manning, Daniel H. Ringler, and Christian E. Newcomer, eds.:
The Biology of the Laboratory Rabbit, 2nd Edition, 1994

B. Taylor Bennett, Christian R. Abee, and Roy Henrickson, eds.:
Nonhuman Primates in Biomedical Research: Biology and Management, 1995

Dennis F. Kohn, Sally K. Wixson, William J. White, and G. John Benson, eds.:
Anesthesia and Analgesia in Laboratory Animals, 1997

B. Taylor Bennett, Christian R. Abee, and Roy Henrickson, eds.:
Nonhuman Primates in Biomedical Research: Diseases, 1998

NONHUMAN PRIMATES
IN BIOMEDICAL RESEARCH
DISEASES

EDITED BY

B. Taylor Bennett
Biologic Resources Laboratory
The University of Illinois at Chicago
Chicago, Illinois

Christian R. Abee
Department of Comparative Medicine
University of South Alabama
College of Medicine
Mobile, Alabama

Roy Henrickson
Office of Laboratory Animal Care
University of California, Berkeley
Berkeley, California

ACADEMIC PRESS
San Diego   New York   Boston   London   Sydney   Tokyo   Toronto

Copyright © 1998 by ACADEMIC PRESS

Academic Press
A Division of Harcourt Brace & Company
525 B Street, Suite 1900, San Diego, CA 92101-4495
http://www.apnet.com

Academic Press
24-28 Oval Road, London NW1 7DX
http://www.hbuk.co.uk/ap/

Library of Congress Cataloging-in-Publication Data

Nonhuman primates in biomedical research / edited by B. Taylor
    Bennett, Christian R. Abee, Roy Henrickson.
        p.   cm.
    Includes bibliographical references and index.
    Contents: v. 1. Biology and management
    ISBN 0-12-088665-0 (v. 1)
    1. Primates as laboratory animals.   I. Bennett, B. T. (B. Taylor)
II. Abee, Christian R.   III. Henrickson, Roy.   96-47584
SF407.P7N66   1995   CIP
636.9'8—dc20

PRINTED IN THE UNITED STATES OF AMERICA
98 99 00 01 02 03 MM 9 8 7 6 5 4 3 2 1

Contents

List of Contributors

Numbers in parentheses indicate the pages on which the authors' contributions begin.

MILTON APRIL (245), The Bionetics Corporation, Rockville, Maryland 20850

KATHRYN BAYNE (485), Association for Assessment and Accreditation of Laboratory Animal Care International, Rockville, Maryland 20852-3035

JOSEPH T. BIELITZKI (363), National Aeronautics and Space Administration, Ames Research Center, Moffett Field, California 94035

ALAN G. BRADY (377), Department of Comparative Medicine, University of South Alabama, Mobile, Alabama 36688

P. K. CUSICK (461), Department of Pathology, Division of Drug Safety Evaluation, Abbott Laboratories, Abbott Park, Illinois 60064

MARK L. EBERHARD (111), Division of Parasitic Diseases, Centers for Disease Control and Prevention, Public Health Service, United States Department of Health and Human Services, Atlanta, Georgia 30341-3724

ELIZABETH W. FORD (311), The Scripps Research Institute, La Jolla, California 92037-1093

SUSAN V. GIBSON (59), Department of Comparative Medicine, University of South Alabama, Mobile, Alabama 36688

JAMES C. KEITH, JR. (245), Genetics Institute Research Center, Wyeth Ayerst Pharmaceuticals, Andover, Massachusetts 02140

MATT J. KESSLER (415), Caribbean Primate Research Center, Medical Sciences Campus and Department of Pathology, School of Medicine, University of Puerto Rico, San Juan, Puerto Rico

NORVAL KING (1), New England Regional Primate Research Center, Harvard Medical School, Southborough, Massachusetts 01772

ANN S. LINE (233), Division of Radiology, Wake Forest University, Baptist Medical Center, Winston-Salem, North Carolina 27157

LINDA J. LOWENSTINE (263), School of Veterinary Medicine, University of California, Davis, California 95616

KEITH MANSFIELD (1), New England Regional Primate Research Center, Harvard Medical School, Southborough, Massachusetts 01772

S. J. MORGAN (461), Department of Pathology, Division of Drug Safety Evaluation, Abbott Laboratories, Abbott Park, Illinois 60064

DANIEL G. MORTON (375), Abbott Laboratories, Abbott Park, Illinois 60064-3500

MELINDA NOVAK (485), Department of Psychology, University of Massachusetts, Amherst, Massachusetts 01003

KENT G. OSBORN (263), The Scripps Research Institute, La Jolla, California 92037

KENNETH P. H. PRITZKER (415), Mount Sinai Hospital, University of Toronto, Toronto, Canada M5G 1X5

JEFFREY A. ROBERTS (311), California Primate Research Center, University of California, Davis, California 95616

JANICE L. SOUTHERS (311), Egypt

JOHN D. TOFT, II (111), Battelle Columbus Operations, Columbus, Ohio 43201-2693

RICHARD E. WELLER (207), Pacific Northwest National Laboratory, Richland, Washington 99352

Preface

Nonhuman Primates in Biomedical Research: Diseases represents the first definitive reference source since Ruch published *Diseases of Laboratory Primates* in 1959. In the almost forty years since that classic work was published, the available information on diseases of nonhuman primates has expanded significantly. Although our understanding of how various diseases affect organ systems has also increased, much remains to be learned and documented concerning diseases of nonhuman primates. During the preparation of this volume, we were struck by the paucity of published information on many of the diseases of primates even though much has been learned in the past twenty years about the care of these animals. In spite of this, the authors have been able to review existing knowledge in a way which combines etiologic- and systems-based approaches to produce chapters which will be truly significant contributions to the literature on the diseases of nonhuman primates.

Prior to the development of this book, available information was contained in a multitude of journals and in the minds of a limited number of veterinarians and other scientists specializing in the care of nonhuman primates. In fact, some of the information contained in these chapters represents the experiences of the authors and/or colleagues who work with primates.

This volume is the second one on nonhuman primates sponsored by the American College of Laboratory Animal Medicine as part of the college's collection of published texts. *Nonhuman Primates in Biomedical Research: Biology and Management* provides basic information on husbandry, reproduction, and regulatory issues which must be addressed in caring for captive primate species. It was written to be a general reference for professionals charged with the day-to-day responsibility for the care and use of these animals. This volume addresses the diseases of nonhuman primates with an emphasis on the etiologic factors, clinical signs, diagnostic pathology, therapy, and clinical management. It also serves as a general reference for those who provide care for nonhuman primates and for those who use these animals in biomedical research.

Since the maintenance of large populations of primates for biomedical research is limited to relatively few institutions, those with the prerequisite experience to serve as chapter authors represent a relatively small number of clinical scientists. Additionally, colonies of nonhuman primates available for study are very small compared to those of other commonly used laboratory animal species. The small size of study populations is reflected in the limited number of available publications in some subject areas. This lack of published information presented a formidable challenge in producing this addition to the ACLAM series and served to emphasize the need for consolidating the information in a single reference source. To meet this challenge, it was necessary to seek authors whose areas of expertise spanned a broad range of topics and whose careers had focused on the care and study of primates. Hence, this volume represents the work of a variety of scientists drawn from within our college, from the ranks of other veterinary specialties, and from scientists who have unique knowledge of primate disease conditions. The authors relied heavily on their experience and extrapolation from both the medical and veterinary medical literature. We extend our sincere appreciation to this diverse group of dedicated scientists without whom this text would not have been possible.

While the work of the authors is the heart and soul of this volume, peer review of their work is the conscience. Chapter reviewers have provided an essential critical analysis of the information contained in this text and have served their colleagues by helping to assure high standards of content and subject perspectives. The reviewers are acknowledged by name and affiliation, but we would like to further acknowledge their important role in the development of this volume.

As for all volumes of the ACLAM series, the editors and authors have served without compensation and have donated all publication royalties to the American College of Laboratory Medicine to continue the work for which it was founded in 1957: to encourage education, training, and research in laboratory animal medicine and to recognize veterinary medical specialists in the field by certification and other means. We wish to express our appreciation to the officers and members of the college for their support and assistance during the evolution of this project.

B. Taylor Bennett
Christian R. Abee
Roy Henrickson

List of Reviewers for Chapters in This Volume

Michael R. Adams	Bowman Gray School of Medicine, Winston-Salem, NC
James E. Artwohl	University of Illinois at Chicago, Chicago, IL
Gary B. Baskin	Tulane Regional Primate Research Center, Covington, LA
J. Roger Broderson	University of Georgia, Athens, GA
Joseph D. Burek	Merck Research Laboratories, West Point, PA
Thomas M. Butler	Southwest Foundation for Biomedical Research, San Antonio, TX
Linda C. Cork	Stanford University School of Medicine, Stanford, CA
Judith A. Davis	National Institute of Neurological Diseases and Stroke, Bethesda, MD
W. Richard Dukelow	Michigan State University, East Lansing, MI
Jeffrey D. Fortman	University of Illinois at Chicago, Chicago, IL
James G. Fox	Massachusetts Institute of Technology, Cambridge, MA
Chris H. Gardiner	Registry of Veterinary Pathology, AFIP Field Medical School, Camp Pendleton, CA
Patricia A. Gullett	University of Miami, Miami, FL
Jack R. Harkema	Michigan State University, East Lansing, MI
Michale E. Keeling	University of Texas, M. D. Anderson Cancer Center, Bastrop, TX
R. Wayne Kornegay	University of Tennessee, Knoxville, TN
Arthur S. Hall	Oregon Health Science University, Portland, OR
Thomas E. Hamm, Jr.	North Carolina State University College of Veterinary Medicine, Raleigh, NC
Gene B. Hubbard	Southwest Foundation for Biomedical Research, San Antonio, TX
David E. Lee-Parritz	New England Regional Primate Center, Southborough, MA
David L. Madden	National Institutes of Health, National Center for Research Resources, Bethesda, MD
Preston A. Marx	Aaron Diamond AIDS Research Center, New York University Medical Center-LEMSIP, Tuxedo, NY
Donald H. Maul	Colorado State University, Ft. Collins, CO
Daniel Rosenberg	The Parkinson's Institute, Sunny Vale, CA
Sally Mendoza	California Regional Primate Center, Davis, CA

E. Donald Roberts   Tulane Regional Primate Research Center,
                                        Covington, LA
Sandra Snook   G. D. Searle Co., Skokie, IL
M. Michael Swindle   Medical University of South Carolina,
                                        Charleston, SC
J. Carroll Woodard   University of Florida, College of Veterinary
                                        Medicine, Gainesville, FL

Chapter 1

Viral Diseases

Keith Mansfield and Norval King

I. INTRODUCTION

Viral infections pose a potential threat to the health of (1) laboratory and zoological colonies of nonhuman primates and (2) the personnel involved in their care. This is particularly true at facilities where there is frequent turnover or movement of animals or where animals recently imported from natural habitats are introduced into colonies of highly susceptible colony-born animals.

This chapter discusses those viral diseases of importance to captive primates or to the health of personnel involved in their care by taxonomic family to which the causative agent is classified. The rationale for this is that there is considerable overlap in the clinical and pathologic expression of diseases caused by

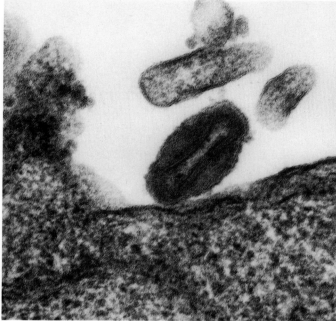

Fig. 1. Vaccinia virus, rhesus macaque (*Macaca mulatta*).

viruses in the same taxonomic family regardless of the species affected. Obvious exceptions exist, but these will be noted.

A doctrine of comparative virology is that infection of the immunocompetent appropriate host often is associated with minimal disease, whereas infection of the inadvertent susceptible host often has devastating consequences. The likelihood of such transmission is increased when changes in the environment, either natural or imposed by humans, place different species in close proximity. An early example of this phenomenon comes from the family Herpesviridae in which infection of the natural reservoir host usually results in minimal clinical disease, whereas infection of other closely related species may result in an acutely lethal cytolytic or neoplastic process.

Because interspecies transmission of viruses may have such devastating consequences, direct contact between different non-human primate species should be prevented. Although isolation of primate species is the norm in well-managed modern facilities, such may not be the case in recently imported animals. Substandard separation of species, coupled with the stress of capture and movement, puts these animals at increased risk. Perhaps of equal importance is the realization that experimental manipulations may inadvertently expose animals to unrecognized pathogens with lethal consequences. Tissue homogenates and cell culture derivatives have transmitted simian immunodeficiency virus (SIV) and simian virus 40 (SV40) in this fashion (Gormus *et al.,* 1989). Moreover, the use of xenografts in both experimental and clinical settings is a potential route by which existing or novel pathogens may be introduced to a new population (Smith, 1993).

II. DISEASES CAUSED BY ENVELOPED DNA VIRUSES

A. Poxviridae

Poxviruses are large (220–450 × 140–260 nm), brick- to ovoid-shaped enveloped viruses. Their envelope is composed of lipid and tubular or globular protein structures that surround one or two lateral bodies and a dumbbell-shaped core containing a single molecule of double-stranded DNA (Fig. 1). Virions contain more than 100 polypeptides, at least one of which has homology with epidermal growth factor. This latter peptide probably accounts for the proliferative epidermal and/or dermal lesions that characterize most poxvirus infections. The core of poxviruses also contains a variety of enzymes involved with transcription and modification of nucleic acids and proteins.

Five members of the poxvirus family belonging to *Orthopoxvirus, Yatapoxvirus,* and *Molluscipoxvirus* genera cause disease in nonhuman primates (Table I).

1. Monkeypox

a. INTRODUCTION. The first reported outbreaks of monkeypox in nonhuman primates occurred in June 1958 at the Statens Seruminstitut in Copenhagen, Denmark, and shortly thereafter at the Biological Development and Control Laboratories of Merck Sharp and Dohme in West Point, Pennsylvania (von Magnus *et al.,* 1959; Sauer *et al.,* 1960; Prier *et al.,* 1960). At that time, both institutes were importing large numbers of macaque monkeys for use in polio vaccine production. In both outbreaks, cynomolgus monkeys (*Macaca fascicularis*) were primarily affected, but at Merck a small number of rhesus monkeys (*Macaca mulatta*) also exhibited signs of the disease. Since then, there have been several additional outbreaks of monkeypox infection involving both New and Old World monkeys and humans (Arita and Henderson, 1968, 1976).

TABLE I
POXVIRIDAE

Genus	Virus
Orthopoxvirus	Variola (smallpox)
	Monkeypox
	Vaccinia
Parapoxvirus	
Avipoxvirus	
Leporipoxvirus	
Yatapoxvirus	Yaba monkey virus
	Tanapox
	Marmosetpoxvirus
Capripoxvirus	
Molluscipoxvirus	Molluscum contagiosum

b. ETIOLOGY. Monkeypox virus is a member of the family Poxviridae, subfamily Chordopoxvirinae, and genus *Orthopoxvirus*. This genus includes variola (smallpox virus), vaccinia (smallpox vaccine virus), cowpox virus, and several other mammalian poxviruses. Immunologically, there is a close antigenic relationship among monkeypox virus, variola, and vaccinia.

c. EPIZOOTIOLOGY. Monkeypox virus exists naturally only in the tropical rain forests of western and central Africa (Brenan *et al.*, 1980; Mutombo *et al.*, 1983) where it causes subclinical endemic infections in several nonhuman primate species and a serious, sometimes fatal, smallpox-like disease in young people in these regions.

Ironically, despite the fact that the original outbreaks of monkeypox were in macaques imported from Malaysia, a subsequent serologic survey of 481 Malaysian monkeys failed to reveal a single animal seropositive to monkeypox virus (Arita *et al.*, 1972). However, African green monkeys (*Cercopithecus aethiops*) have a high prevalence of antibodies to monkeypox virus with no evidence of clinical disease, strongly suggesting that they are the natural host for the virus. Thus it is likely that the macaques involved in the original outbreaks may have been incidentally exposed to infected African green monkeys during shipment from Asia. Monkeypox virus has a relatively broad natural host range that includes humans, anthropoid apes, and Old and New World monkeys. Primates in which spontaneous monkeypox infections occur include cotton-top tamarins (*Saguinus oedipus*), squirrel monkeys (*Saimiri sciureus*), African green monkeys (*Cercopithecus aethiops*), owl-faced monkeys (*C. hamlyni*), rhesus monkeys (*M. mulatta*), cynomolgus monkeys (*M. fascicularis*), hanuman langurs [*Semnopithecus* (*Presbytis*) *entellus*], white-handed gibbons (*Hylobates lar*), orangutans (*Pongo pygmaeus*), gorillas (*Gorilla gorilla*), chimpanzees (*Pan troglodytes*), and human beings (*Homo sapiens*) (Marennikova *et al.*, 1976; Peters, 1966; von Magnus *et al.*, 1959; McConnell *et al.*, 1968). In addition, a variety of rodent species, anteaters, pangolins, and birds from endemic areas of Africa have been shown to have antibodies to the virus.

d. PATHOGENESIS AND PATHOLOGY. In the reported outbreaks of monkeypox, transmission was thought to have occurred via aerosols, although the disease can also be spread by direct contact and by biting insects (Mutombo *et al.*, 1983). Viremia develops 3–4 days following experimental infection, at which time the virus disseminates to multiple sites, including skin, lung, mucous membranes, and spleen. Lesions within the skin initially appear as papules consisting of proliferative acanthocytes and progress to vesicles. Intracytoplasmic eosinophilic inclusions are apparent within acanthocytes. Vesiculation is followed by umbilication to form the classic pock lesion. Progressive dermal changes take place over a 4- to 14-day period. Lesions within the lung are similar, consisting of irregular foci of hemorrhagic necrosis. These may be responsible for more serious clinical sequelae and transmission of the virus by the aerosolized route.

e. CLINICAL FINDINGS. Clinical manifestations of monkeypox vary with the species affected. In general, anthropoid apes are more severely affected than monkeys. A vesicular exanthema appears 6–7 days following experimental inoculation. The skin rash may be accompanied by constitutional signs and in severe cases with respiratory tract involvement. The disease may be fatal.

f. TREATMENT. There is no specific treatment for monkeypox, but supportive therapy may prevent the death of animals with severe systemic disease. Most cases recover spontaneously after several weeks and animals are immune to subsequent infection by the same or related viruses.

g. PREVENTION. Vaccination against smallpox confers immunity to monkeypox infection in most cases (McConnell *et al.*, 1968).

h. ZOONOTIC POTENTIAL. Human beings are susceptible to infection by monkeypox (Arita *et al.*, 1985). The disease is seen sporadically in Africa and is usually not associated with direct nonhuman primate contact. The epidemiology is poorly understood and factors that govern the establishment of infection in humans are unknown. In general, pock lesions are found primarily on the extremities but may disseminate over the entire body. Fatalities have been reported in children.

2. Yaba Virus

a. INTRODUCTION. In 1957 an outbreak of subcutaneous tumors was observed in a group of captive macaques housed in Yaba, Nigeria (Bearcroft and Jamieson, 1958). A viral etiology was subsequently demonstrated and confirmed as a poxvirus. Yaba virus has been shown to naturally infect macaques (*Macaca mulatta, M. fascicularis,* and *M. arctoides*) and baboons (*Papio anubis*) (Downie, 1972). Experimentally, the pig-tailed macaque (*M. nemestrina*), stump-tailed macaque (*M. arctoides*), African green monkey (*Cercopithicus aethiops*), sooty mangabey (*Cerocebus atys*), and the patas monkey (*Erythrocebus patas*) are susceptible (Kupper *et al.*, 1970). Accidental and experimental human infection has been demonstrated. New World primates are resistant.

b. ETIOLOGY. Yaba virus was previously classified in the molluscum contagiosum group. It now is included in a separate genus (*Yatapoxvirus*) with the tanapoxvirus (Downie *et al.*, 1971).

c. EPIZOOTIOLOGY. Relatively few naturally occurring episodes have been documented. Captive-born African monkeys appear susceptible to experimental infection, whereas wild-caught animals are resistant, suggesting that widespread infection with Yaba virus or closely related virus(es) occurs in the wild, conferring life-long immunity to those individuals at an early age. The method of transmission is unknown, but arthropod vectors, tattoo needles, and trauma have been suggested as possible mechanisms.

d. CLINICAL FINDINGS.   The original outbreak of Yaba virus disease in *M. mulatta* was characterized by multiple subcutaneous masses, often on the hands and feet, varying in size from small papules to nodules several centimeters in diameter. Larger masses would occasionally ulcerate and all masses invariably regressed by 6 weeks. Animals often developed new lesions as old lesions regressed. Subsequent cases and outbreaks have had a similar clinical course (Walker *et al.,* 1985; Bruestle *et al.,* 1981; Whittaker and Glaister, 1985). Oral masses have been described in baboons (Bruestle *et al.,* 1981). Intravenous inoculation may produce lesions in many organs, including lung, muscle, heart, and pleura. Because masses spontaneously regress, they are often called "pseudotumors." Aerosol transmission of Yaba virus has been demonstrated experimentally in rhesus and cynomolgus macaques (Wolfe *et al.,* 1968). Inoculated animals developed nasal, pulmonary, and pleural tumors but did not transmit the virus horizontally to cagemates.

e. PATHOGENESIS AND PATHOLOGY.   The characteristic histopathologic lesion consists of large pleomorphic histiocytic cells forming a nonencapsulated and infiltrative mass. These cells have hyperchromatic nuclei and prominent nucleoli. Mitotic figures are frequent. Large eosinophilic intracytoplasmic inclusion bodies may be evident. Regression is associated with erosion, ulceration, and formation of multinucleated cells.

f. ZOONOTIC POTENTIAL.   Both experimentally induced and spontaneous diseases have been recognized in humans. In spontaneous human cases, lesions were most often noted on hands and feet and were associated with lymphadenopathy and fever. As in nonhuman primates, regression occurred within weeks.

3. Tanapox: Benign Epidermal Monkeypox or "Or-Te-Ca" Poxvirus

a. INTRODUCTION.   In 1967 an outbreak of a contagious skin disease of macaques was observed at three primate facilities in Oregon, Texas, and California (Or-Te-Ca) and was traced to a single primate importer (Hall and McNulty, 1967; Crandell *et al.,* 1969; Downie *et al.,* 1971). Affected species in the original outbreak were rhesus macaques (*Macaca mulatta*), pig-tailed macaques (*M. nemestrina*), Japanese macaques (*M. fuscata*), and Sulawesi-black macques (*Macaca nigra*). Tanapox is a relatively benign cutaneous infection of the skin of human beings in East Africa and has been responsible for periodic outbreaks of illness in these regions (Jezek *et al.,* 1985).

b. ETIOLOGY.   Tanapox is classified with the Yaba virus as a *Yatapoxvirus.*

c. EPIZOOTIOLOGY.   The unique circumstances responsible for the initial outbreak of Tanapox infection in macaques are unrecognized. Serologic surveys indicate natural infection of

African but not New World primates (Downie and Espana, 1974; Downie, 1972).

d. PATHOGENESIS AND PATHOLOGY.   Histologically, papules are composed of focally extensive regions of epidermal proliferation and ballooning degeneration and arise after a 4- to 6-day incubation period (Casey *et al.,* 1967; Downie and Espana, 1972). Hair follicles and sebaceous glands may be involved. Eosinophilic, intracytoplasmic viral inclusions may be present. Nuclei are variably distended by large eosinophilic cytoplasmic invaginations. Ultrastructurally mature viral particles are 370×150 μm in size and have an outer coat consisting of seven distinct layers and an inner dumbbell-shaped core. Morphologically, these are indistinguishable from Yaba virus (Casey *et al.,* 1967). Resolution is characterized by necrosis, ulceration, and infiltration of the dermis by a variety of inflammatory cells.

e. CLINICAL FINDINGS.   Following a 4- to 5-day incubation period, small red papules form and progress by 14 days to circular, firm raised foci up to 1 cm in diameter. These lesions may ulcerate and become umbilicated before resolving in 3–4 weeks and are often surrounded by a hyperemic border.

f. TREATMENT.   No treatment is available.

g. PREVENTION.   Previous infection with Tanapox is protective against subsequent challenge. Vaccination with vaccinia did not produce protective immunity.

h. ZOONOTIC POTENTIAL.   Tanapox occurs naturally in regions of Kenya and Zaire. The initial outbreaks in 1957 were associated with flooding of the Zaire River. The definitive host and vector(s) involved in these epidemics are unknown. Transmission from infected monkeys to humans has been documented. In humans, infection is characterized by a short febrile illness accompanied by constitutional signs (McNulty, 1995). As these signs abate, small nodules and papules arise eventually, forming the classic pock lesion.

4. Molluscum Contagiosum

Molluscum contagiosum is a chronic, mildly contagious skin disease of humans characterized by multiple small, pinkish skin tumors from which a waxy material may be extruded. Although it is caused by a pox virus, it is difficult to culture *in vitro* and attempts at experimental infection of a variety of nonhuman primates have been unsuccessful. Histologically, the lesion is composed of a flask-shaped proliferative nodule of epidermal cells in which centrally enlarged acanthocytes contain homogeneous, intracytoplasmic, eosinophilic viral inclusions. These molluscum bodies are shed along with keratin debris through a central pore. A single outbreak with similar clinical and histopathologic findings has been described in chimpanzees (*Pan troglodytes*) (Douglas *et al.,* 1967). It is unknown whether this represented a similar or identical viral agent to that seen in the human disease.

5. Marmosetpoxvirus

A single epizootic of a poxvirus infection occurred in 29 of 80 common marmosets (*Callithrix jacchus* (Gough *et al.,* 1982). The etiologic agent is most closely related to tanapoxvirus and is classified in the *Yatapoxvirus* genus. The disease was characterized clinically by the appearance of erythematous papules that progressed through vesiculation and umbilication over a 4- to 6-week course. Dissemination to internal organs was not noted and deaths were not associated with disease. Pox-like intracytoplasmic inclusions were evident and viral particles characteristic of the genus were found on ultrastructural examination.

B. Herpesviridae

Based on biologic criteria, the family Herpesviridae is divided into three distinct subfamilies: Alphaherpesvirinae, Betaherpesvirinae, and Gammaherpesvirinae (Table II). Although these subfamilies are distinctly different, as a group the herpesviruses do share certain genetic and biologic properties. These include (1) a complex genome encoding a number of enzymes involved in protein processing, DNA synthesis, and nucleic acid metabolism; (2) DNA synthesis and capsid formation in the nucleus; (3) requisite destruction of the host cell to complete the viral replicative process; and (4) viral persistence in a latent form within the host cell.

Alphaherpesvirinae

1. *Herpesvirus simiae*: Herpes B virus

a. INTRODUCTION. Herpes B virus (herpes simiae, Cercopithecine herpesvirus 1) occurs as a common, latent, and asymptomatic infection of Asian macaques and has been demonstrated by viral isolation or serology to occur in rhesus macaques (*Macaca mulatta*), bonnet macaques (*M. radiata*), Japanese macaques (*M. fuscata*), stump-tailed macaques (*M. arctoides*), Formosan rock macaques (*M. cyclopis*), and cynomolgus monkeys (*M. fascicularis*) (Hunt and Blake, 1993a). Although rarely responsible for disease in the natural host, inadvertent infection of humans results in a disseminated viral infection characterized by ascending paralysis and a high case fatality rate. The number of human cases has increased since 1987, spurring renewed interest in the prevention and treatment of this disease. Infection of nonmacaque species, including the patas monkey (*Erythrocebus patas*), black and white colobus (*Colobus abyssinicus*), capuchin monkey (*Cebus appella*), and common marmoset (*Callithrix jacchus*), has reportedly produced

TABLE II

FAMILY HERPESVIRIDAE

Classification	Disease
Alphaherpesvirinae	
Cercopithicine herpesvirus 1	Herpes simiae (B virus)
Cercopithicine herpesvirus 6, 7, 9	Simian varicellovirus
Human herpesvirus 3	Chimpanzee (varicella-zoster-like) herpes
Saimirine herpesvirus 1	Herpes tamarinus (herpes T)
Human herpesvirus 1, 2	Herpes hominis (herpes simplex)
Cercopithicine herpesvirus 2	Herpes papionis (SA8)
Betaherpesvirinae	
Cytomegaloviruses (CMV)	
Cercopithicine herpesvirus 3	SA-6
Cercopithicine herpesvirus 4	SA-15
Cercopithicine herpesvirus 5	African green monkey CMV
Cercopithicine herpesvirus 8	Rhesus monkey CMV
Aotine herpesvirus 1, 3, 4	Herpes aotus types 1, 3, 4
Callitrichine herpesvirus 1, 2	Marmoset CMV
Cebine herpesvirus 1	Capuchin herpes virus (AL-5)
Cebine herpesvirus 2	Capuchin herpesvirus (AL-18)
Gammaherpesvirinae	
Rhadnovirus	
Saimirine herpesvirus 2	Herpes saimiri
Ateline herpesvirus 2, 3	Herpes ateles
Lymphocryptovirus	
Epstein–Barr-like viruses	
Pongine herpesvirus 1	Chimpanzee herpes
Pongine herpesvirus 2	Orangutan herpes
Pongine herpesvirus 3	Gorilla herpes
Cercopithicine herpesvirus 10, 11	Rhesus leukocyte-associated herpes
Cercopithicine herpesvirus 12	Herpes papionis
Cercopithicine herpesvirus 14	African green monkey EBV-like virus

fatal disease (Gay and Holden, 1933; Loomis *et al.,* 1981; Wilson *et al.,* 1990).

b. ETIOLOGY. Herpes B virus is similar to other members of the Alphaherpesviridae. The viral genome is 162 kb in length and encodes approximately 23 major proteins. It shares antigenic determinants with the gD and gB glycoproteins of herpes simplex 1 and 2. Viral replication occurs rapidly, with enveloped capsids present 8–10 hr after infection. In cell culture, syncytial cells and Cowdry-type A inclusions are readily apparent.

c. EPIZOOTIOLOGY. The incidence of infection in immature rhesus macaques is low and increases rapidly with sexual maturity, approaching 80–90% in some colonies by 3–4 years of age (Weigler *et al.,* 1993). The percentage of animals with active oral lesions is much less and in one large study of 14,400 macaques was found to be 2.3% (Keeble, 1960). The virus is transmitted through sexual or biting behavior and by fomites. In overcrowded or unsanitary conditions, animals may become infected at an earlier age and the seropositive rate may be higher. Animals remain infected for life and may periodically shed the virus in oral and genital secretions. The greatest risk of primary infection occurs during the breeding season in sexually adolescent animals 2–3 years of age (Weigler *et al.,* 1990). Disseminated infection in macaques is rare, but when it occurs, it is usually fatal. Viral dissemination to the lung, liver, spleen, bone marrow, and adrenal cortex has been documented (Simon *et al.,* 1993; Wilson *et al.,* 1990).

d. PATHOGENESIS AND PATHOLOGY. The pathogenesis of herpes B infection in macaques is similar to herpes simplex infection in humans. Primary infection results in an initial round of replication at the site of inoculation. Histologically, this is characterized by the ballooning degeneration of keratinocytes with progression to vesiculation. Multinucleated, syncytial cells and eosinophilic to basophilic, intranuclear viral inclusions may be prominent. Immunohistochemistry utilizing antibodies against herpes simplex can be used to demonstrate viral antigen in equivocal lesions. Inflammatory cells may be found within vesicles, epidermis, and subjacent dermis. Endothelial cell necrosis with intranuclear viral inclusions may be seen. In disseminated disease, there is widespread, hemorrhagic necrosis within the liver, lung, brain, and lymphoid organs (Fig. 2) (Espana, 1973; Simon *et al.,* 1993). Herpes B virus should be included in the list of viral agents responsible for multifocal, necrotizing hepatitis in macaques.

Seroconversion occurs soon after primary infection and is associated with the resolution of clinical signs. These antibodies may be detected by enzyme-linked immunosorbent assay (ELISA) and Western blot methods (Ward and Hilliard, 1994). False-negative tests and latently infected immunologically unreactive individuals complicate the interpretation of results on single samples but may be relatively uncommon.

Following initial viral replication, the virus (virion or capsid) is transported by retrograde axonal flow to the sensory ganglion where a latent infection is established for the life of the animal. Centrifugal spread may contribute to the enlargement of lesions or generalization during primary infection. Factors contributing to recrudescence are poorly understood, but stress, fever, ultraviolet light, tissue or nerve damage, and immunosuppression have been identified clinically as contributing factors in the reactivation of herpes simplex in humans and may play a similar role with B virus in macaques. Reactivation of oral lesions has been described in cynomolgus monkeys treated with an immunosuppressive agent (Chellman *et al.,* 1992). Weir *et al.* (1993) found that viral shedding was not commonly associated with the stress of quarantine, parturition, and breeding in single-housed seropositive macaques. Interestingly, reactivation is not commonly recognized in macaques experimentally inoculated with simian immunodeficiency virus (SIV) and dying with acquired immunodeficiency syndrome (AIDS) (Simon *et al.,* 1993).

e. CLINICAL FINDINGS. Infection of Asian macaques is usually mild and self-limiting. Characteristic vesicular lesions occur on oral and genital mucosae, which progress to ulceration and resolve within 10–14 days. As noted, disseminated infection occurs rarely. In these instances, the clinical course may vary from peracute to slowly progressive and B virus is often not suspected as an underlying etiologic agent, thereby increasing the risk of human exposure. During a single epizootic in captive bonnet macaques (*M. radiata*), a respiratory form was recognized in which animals exhibited signs of coryza, rhinorrhea, cough, and conjunctivitis (Espana, 1973). Both morbidity and mortality were high, and hemorrhagic interstitial pneumonia and hepatic necrosis were described at necropsy. Typical B virus lesions of the oral mucosa were lacking.

f. TREATMENT. Animals actively infected and shedding virus should not be treated as this entails considerable risk to the attending personnel. Recommendations for postexposure prophylaxis and treatment of clinical disease in humans have been reviewed and published (Holmes *et al.,* 1995).

g. PREVENTION. Guidelines used to establish B virus specific pathogen-free (SPF) colonies have been published (Ward and Hilliard, 1994). Animals are initially screened by titration ELISA and Western blot. Negative animals should be kept in single cage housing or in small groups and be periodically tested by a modified ELISA for 1 year. Animals that are repeatedly negative by these criteria can then be moved to larger groups. Once in these breeding groups, animals should be periodically tested to screen for seroconversion. Repeated testing during the quarantine period is required because animals may be (1) chronically infected and immunologically unreactive or (2) in the early stages of disease prior to seroconversion. Breaks in the SPF barrier status may occur from introduction of new animals, contact with contaminated fomites, or reactivation of latent infection in seronegative animals. Ideally, SPF colonies should be self-sustaining and not require introduction of new animals. When animals are introduced, appropriate testing and quarantine are required. If non-SPF animals are housed in the same facility, precautions should be taken to prevent transmission of the virus via fomites.

In smaller facilities, the acquisition of seronegative young animals and the subsequent individual housing of those animals have been shown to greatly reduce the occurrence of primary active infections (Di Giamoco and Shah, 1972; Olson *et al.,* 1991). Although inappropriate for large colonies, this method may be adequate for small numbers of animals that are kept for short periods.

Whether the vigorous implementation of such programs can guarantee the B virus-free status of a seronegative colony is unknown and periodic testing is recommended as a component of colony management. It must be remembered that B virus is only one of many potentially dangerous zoonotic agents that macaques may harbor.

h. ZOONOTIC POTENTIAL. Despite the widespread use of macaques and the common occurrence of B virus infection in

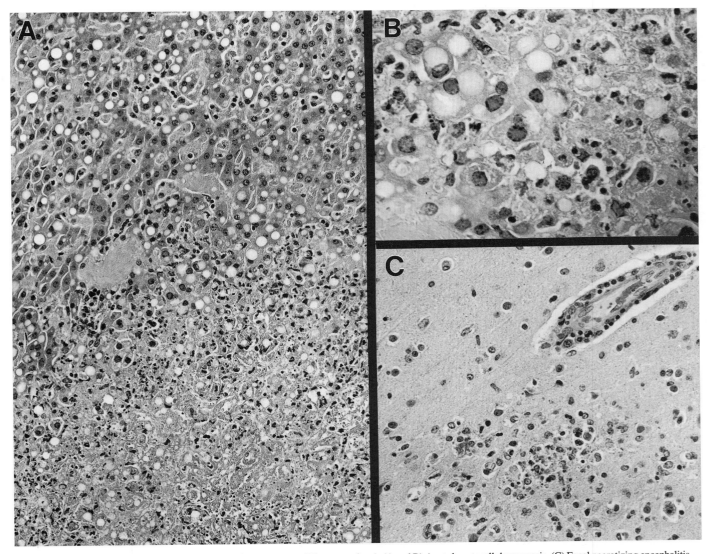

Fig. 2. Disseminated herpes virus B infection in a rhesus macaque (*Macaca mulatta*). (A and B) Acute hepatocellular necrosis. (C) Focal necrotizing encephalitis.

these animals, fewer than 40 documented human cases have been described (Holmes *et al.,* 1995). Early evidence suggested that previous infection by herpes simplex may have had a protective effect against B virus in human subjects (Hull, 1971). However, evidence from recent outbreaks indicates that previous infection with herpes simplex is not protective. The majority of human cases has developed following macaque-induced injury. Rarely has human to human contact, respiratory spread, needle stick injury, laboratory exposure, or unknown exposure been recorded as the method of transmission (Holmes *et al.,* 1990; Weigler, 1992).

In humans, a vesicular dermatitis at the site of inoculation develops as soon as 3–5 days or as late as 24 days postexposure, which is followed by lymphangitis and secondary lymphadenopathy. Pruritus may be intense at the site of inoculation. Neu-

rologic signs appear 3–7 days after the initial cutaneous lesion and are characterized by an ascending myelitis. Fever, paresthesia, muscle weakness, and conjunctivitis may precede these findings. In some cases, premonitory signs and a clinical history of exposure have not been recognized. The case fatality rate in humans is approximately 70%, with death ensuing within 10–14 days (McChesney *et al.,* 1989). Although less frequent, asymptomatic infection and infections characterized by recurrent vesicular rash and respiratory signs have been identified in humans. Evidence suggests that asymptomatic infection is rare (Freifeld *et al.,* 1995). Early recognition of clinical signs is critical as the administration of acyclovir or ganciclovir may be beneficial during the initial stages of infection.

Recommendations for the prevention and treatment of injuries inflicted by macaques have been published (Holmes *et al.,*

1995; Centers for Disease Control and Prevention, 1987). Education of animal care and laboratory personnel in the prevention and risks of herpes B virus infection is critical. An epidemiologic investigation following cases of human herpes B virus infection at a single animal research facility revealed that only 41% of the employees with at least weekly contact with macaques had prior knowledge of herpes B virus (Davenport *et al.*, 1994). Advanced preparation of bite/wound kits and detailed standard operating procedures should be available at all institutions housing macaques and handling their tissues. Following exposure, thorough and vigorous cleansing of the wound with detergent and water for at least 15 min should be initiated, followed by risk assessment by an infectious disease specialist. Because cyclovir and ganciclovir have shown some efficacy when given early in the clinical course of human B virus infection, close clinical follow-up is warranted. The prophylactic use of ganciclovir in high-risk cases is controversial.

2. Varicellovirus: Simian Varicella Virus

a. INTRODUCTION. The simian varicella viruses (SVV) cause a highly contagious viral infection of a variety of Old World nonhuman primates, resulting in high morbidity and mortality. Because of similarities between human varicella-zoster virus (the etiologic agent of chickenpox) and SVV, these viruses have been used as an experimental model to investigate aspects of the pathogenesis and therapy of the human disease.

b. ETIOLOGY. A group of closely related herpesviruses, including Liverpool vervet virus, Patas herpesvirus, Medical Lake macaque virus, and Delta herpesvirus, are antigenically related and cause a similar exanthematous viral disease. Infection of African green monkey (*Cercopithecus aethiops*), patas monkey (*Erythrocebus patas*), pig-tailed macaque (*Macaca nemestrina*), Japanese macaque (*M. fuscata*), cynomolgus monkey (*M. fascicularis*), and Formosan rock macaque (*M. cyclopis*) has been demonstrated. Lesions in these species are typical of an alphaherpesvirus infection (Clarke *et al.*, 1994).

c. EPIZOOTIOLOGY. Between 1966 and 1970, epizootics of SVV occurred at the Liverpool School of Tropical Medicine in *C. aethiops* (Liverpool vervet virus) (Clarkson *et al.*, 1967), at the Delta Regional Primate Research Center in *E. patas* (Delta herpesvirus) (Felsenfeld and Schmidt, 1975), and at the Medical Lake field station of the Washington Regional Primate Research Center in *M. fascicularis, M. fuscata,* and *M. nemestrina* (Medical Lake macaque virus) (Blakely *et al.*, 1973; Wenner *et al.*, 1977). The epizootiology of these outbreaks is poorly understood. In several instances they occurred in recently imported animals. Serologic evidence suggests that the Medical Lake macaque virus may have originated in Malaysia and that epizootics may result from transmission from an unidentified reservoir host to aberrant primate hosts. Neutralizing antibodies have been identified in asymptomatic stump-tailed macaques (*M. arctoides*), suggesting that macaques may play some role in

transmitting the virus to more susceptible species. In *C. aethiops*, latent infection of ganglia with reactivation has been demonstrated, suggesting that as with other alphaherpesviruses, a latent carrier state may play an important role in transmission of the virus (Soike *et al.*, 1984; Mahalingam *et al.*, 1992). Once established within a colony, the virus may spread rapidly, presumably through the respiratory route.

d. CLINICAL FINDINGS. Clinical signs recorded in natural outbreaks and in experimental disease are similar, varying only in the extent of lesions and associated mortality. The disease in macaques may be slightly less severe than in *C. aethopis* and *E. patas*. The clinical course in natural outbreaks was characterized by the eruption of a disseminated, vesicular exanthema with rapid progression to death within 48 hr. The attack and case fatality rates were high.

e. PATHOGENESIS AND PATHOLOGY. Following experimental infection of *C. aethiops*, a vesicular dermatitis appears at 6–8 days postinoculation (Fig. 3) (Dueland *et al.*, 1992; Roberts *et al.*, 1984). Cutaneous lesions are characterized by the formation of multiple vesicles within the epidermis that contain cell debris, erythrocytes, and rarely syncytial cells. Hyperplasia of the basal cell layer is associated with these vesicles. Characteristic eosinophilic, Cowdry-type A, intranuclear inclusions may be found in cells adjacent to the vesicle. A necrotizing vasculitis often exists within the subjacent dermis.

Viral antigen is found widely disseminated by 8 days and may be localized in the liver, lungs, spleen, adrenal gland, kidney, lymph node, skin, and trigeminal ganglion. Within the liver, there is multifocal to coalescing hepatocellular necrosis. Cowdry-type A inclusions may be found within hepatocytes bordering foci of necrosis. Similar necrotizing lesions may be found in the lung and throughout the gastrointestinal tract. Hepatic and pulmonary lesions may be the most severe lesions in affected animals.

f. LABORATORY FINDINGS. Following experimental inoculation, there is marked neutrophilic leukocytosis accompanied by a decrease in platelet numbers, and elevations in alanine aminotransferase, aspartate aminotransferase, and blood urea nitrogen (BUN) levels.

g. TREATMENT. Treatment has not been attempted in natural outbreaks. Acyclovir and interferon have shown some efficacy in experimental models (Soike and Gerone, 1995; Arvin *et al.*, 1983).

h. ZOONOTIC POTENTIAL. Transmission of SVV to human beings has not been documented.

3. Chimpanzee Varicella Herpesvirus

A varicella-zoster-like (chickenpox-like) herpesvirus has been isolated from three juvenile chimpanzees (*Pan troglodytes*) associated with a mild, self-limiting vesicular dermatitis

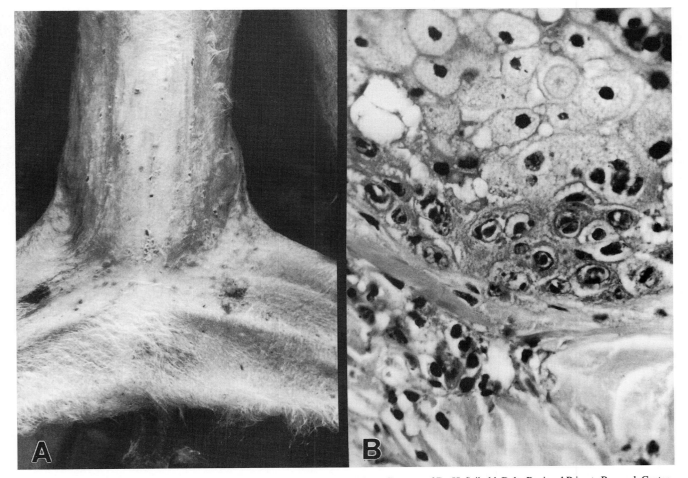

Fig. 3. Simian varicella virus. (A) Vesicular dermatitis. (B) Intranuclear viral inclusions. Courtesy of Dr. H. Seibold, Delta Regional Primate Research Center.

(McClure and Keeling, 1971). Antigenically, this virus is more closely related to human varicella-zoster than to the simian varicella viruses but whether it represents infection by a human varicella-zoster virus or a simian subtype is unknown (Harbour and Caunt, 1979). Additional cases have been reported in gorillas (*Gorilla gorilla*) and orangutans (*Pongo pygmeus*) (White *et al.,* 1972; Heuschele, 1960).

4. *Herpesvirus tamarinus*

a. INTRODUCTION.   *Herpesvirus tamarinus* (Saimirine herpesvirus 1; herpes T; *Herpesvirus platyrrhinae*) infection has many similarities with herpes simplex infection of New World primates. The virus is carried asymptomatically by squirrel monkeys (*Saimiri sciureus*) but induces an acutely lethal disease in owl monkeys (*Aotus* spp.) and several species of marmosets and tamarins (King *et al.,* 1967; Hunt and Melendez, 1966).

b. EPIZOOTIOLOGY.   Squirrel monkeys become affected at an early age and harbor the virus asymptomatically. Viral per-

sistence within sensory ganglia has been documented. Periodic reactivation and shedding of the virus in oral secretions represent the primary reservoir and source of infection. Antibodies to herpes T have been detected in asymptomatic spider monkeys (*Ateles* spp.), capuchin monkeys (*Cebus* spp.), and wooly monkeys (*Lagothrix* spp.) and these animals may represent additional natural reservoir hosts. Initial infection of tamarins, owl monkeys, and marmosets occurs through inadvertent exposure to carrier species. Once established, intraspecies transmission results in an epizootic with high mortality.

c. PATHOGENESIS AND PATHOLOGY.   Following a 7- to 10-day incubation period, viral infection causes a disseminated necrotizing process involving the skin, oral mucosa, and numerous parenchymal organs (Fig. 4). In sections of skin there is full thickness epidermal necrosis. Within these regions a few viable epithelial cells may remain beneath a mass of degenerate eosinophilic material admixed with pyknotic debris. Sebaceous glands, hair follicles, and apocrine glands are relatively spared. There is mild parakeratosis and intercellular edema within the

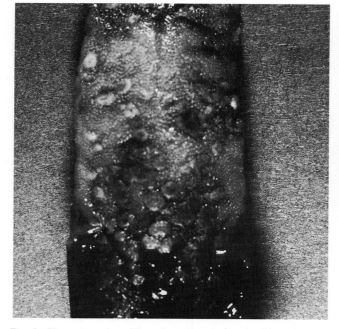

Fig. 4. Herpes tamarinus. Ulcerative and vesicular glossitis, owl monkey (*Aotus trivirgatus*).

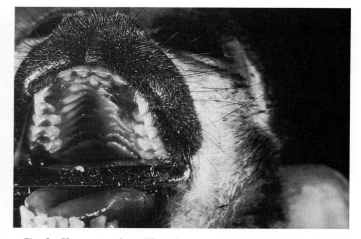

Fig. 5. Herpes tamarinus. Ulcerative stomatitis, squirrel monkey (*Saimiri sciureus*). From Hunt, R. D. and Blake, J. (1993). *Herpesvirus platyrhinae* infection. *In* "Nonhuman Primates." (T. C. Jones, U. Mohr, and R. D. Hunt eds.) Springer-Verlag, New York. With permission.

adjacent epidermis and scattered multinucleated giant cells may be present, often containing intranuclear viral inclusions. Because of the acutely lethal nature of this process, inflammatory reactions within the dermis may be minimal, consisting only of scattered neutrophils.

Foci of full thickness necrosis similar to that present within the skin are found in the mucosa of the oral cavity and in the small and large intestine. Large sections of oral mucosa may develop necrotic plaques and slough (Fig. 5). Multifocal necrosis is noted in the liver, spleen, lung, kidney, and adrenal gland. Hepatic lesions occur multifocally and randomly and are composed of acute hepatocellular necrosis ranging in size from small clusters of two to five cells to large coalescent foci 2–3 mm in diameter. Large numbers of Cowdry-type A intranuclear inclusions may be present in these regions. If present, encephalitis is minimal. The lesions are essentially identical to herpes simplex infection in these species, and viral isolation and characterization are required to distinguish them.

d. CLINICAL FINDINGS. In carrier species (squirrel, spider, capuchin, and wooly monkeys), infection is usually not associated with clinical signs and only rarely are oral vesicles and ulcers present (King *et al.,* 1967). In susceptible species (tamarins, owl monkeys, and marmosets), inadvertent infection results in an epizootic of high mortality with variable oral, labial, and dermal lesions. Clinical signs include pruritus, anorexia, and depression. Progression to death occurs within 24–48 hr.

e. TREATMENT AND PREVENTION. Contact between susceptible and carrier species should be prevented. A live vaccine

that reduces natural infection in owl monkeys has been developed; however, infrequent episodes of vaccine-induced disease have occurred (Daniel *et al.,* 1967), which have been characterized by a rapidly progressive disseminated infection similar to that caused by natural disease. In other instances, a slowly progressive ascending myelitis has been recorded (Asher *et al.,* 1974).

5. *Herpesvirus hominis: Herpesvirus simplex*

a. INTRODUCTION. *Herpesvirus hominis* infection is a common symptomatic infection of humans. Inadvertent infection of gibbons (*Hylobates lar*), gorillas (*Gorilla gorilla*), tree shrews (*Tupaia glis*), and chimpanzees (*Pan* sp.) has been described (McClure *et al.,* 1972, 1980; Marennikova *et al.,* 1973; Emmons and Lennette, 1970; Smith *et al.,* 1969). In these species, infection usually results in mild, self-limiting oral vesicular lesions. Conversely, infection of owl monkeys (*Aotus* sp.) results in a lethal disseminated disease similar to that caused by *H. tamarinus* from which it must be distinguished (Melendez *et al.,* 1969; Hunt and Melendez, 1966). Although natural infection of callithricids has not been reported (Potkay, 1992), intravaginal inoculation of marmosets (*Saguinus oedipus* and *S. fuscicollis*) with herpes simplex 2 resulted in disseminated disease (Felsburg *et al.,* 1973). Experimental inoculation of capuchin monkeys (*Cebus* spp.) produced localized disease (Felsburg *et al.,* 1972).

b. ETIOLOGY. *Herpesvirus hominis* (herpes simplex) is a member of the alphaherpesvirus subfamily. Two distinct subtypes are recognized. Herpes simplex type 1 (HSV-1) is most often responsible for oral lesions and encephalitis in adults, whereas herpes simplex type 2 (HSV-2) is responsible for a sexually transmitted disease causing a genital infection in adults and a disseminated infection in infants. Both types are equally patho-

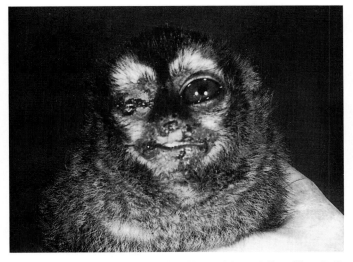

Fig. 6. Herpes simplex, owl monkey (*Aotus trivirgatus*). From Hunt, R. D. (1993). *Herpesvirus simplex* infection. *In* "Nonhuman Primates." (T. C. Jones, U. Mohr, and R. D. Hunt eds.) Springer-Verlag, New York. With permission.

genic in owl monkeys and no difference in the clinical disease has been noted with experimentally inoculated subtypes. An alphaherpesvirus closely related to but antigenically distinct from HSV-2 has been identified by serology in free-ranging mountain gorillas (*Gorilla gorilla beringei*) but as of yet is not associated with clinical signs (Eberle, 1992).

c. EPIZOOTIOLOGY. Nonhuman primates are not naturally infected with herpes simplex in the wild and likely acquire the infection through human contact. Once established within owl monkey colonies the virus spreads rapidly and results in high morbidity and mortality. A natural epizootic in a research colony of gibbons was characterized by a more limited spread.

d. PATHOGENESIS AND PATHOLOGY. The pathogenesis and pathology in owl monkeys are esentially identical to that caused by *H. tamarinus* with the exception that encephalitis may be a more frequent sequela. A multifocal necrotizing and vesicular dermatitis is often most severe on facial skin and is accompanied by blepharitis and stomatitis (Figs. 6 and 7). In gibbons, a multifocal acute meningoencephalitis may be evident in the pons and cerebral cortex. These changes may be accompanied by necrosis, reactive gliosis, and typical Cowdry-type A inclusions.

e. CLINICAL FINDINGS. In gorillas, chimpanzees, and gibbons, infection is usually self-limiting and clinical signs are restricted to vesiculation and ulceration of mucosal surfaces. During one natural outbreak in gibbons, viral encephalitis developed in a minority of animals well after oral lesions healed. Generalized disease in susceptible species is identical to that induced by herpesvirus tamarinus.

f. TREATMENT AND PREVENTION. Protective clothing and face masks should be worn by animal care personnel. A modi-

fied live vaccine has been developed and is protective in owl monkeys (Daniel *et al.,* 1978).

6. *Herpesvirus papionis:* **Simian Agent 8**

a. INTRODUCTION. *Herpesvirus papionis* (SA8) is an alphaherpesvirus originally isolated from an African green monkey (*Cercopithecus aethiops*) neural tissue that is antigenically related to *Herpesvirus simiae* (Malherbe and Harwin, 1958). Subsequent investigation revealed it to be a common infection of baboons that shared many similarities with herpesvirus simplex 2 in humans.

b. EPIZOOTIOLOGY. *Herpesvirus papionis* is a common asymptomatic infection of baboons. As with other alphaherpesvirus infections, the virus may persist latently within sensory ganglia (Kalter *et al.,* 1978). Recrudescence may occur periodically, often associated with exposure to stress, ultraviolet light, or cold. With reactivation, the virus is shed in oral and genital secretions. A single outbreak in baboons suggested that the vi-

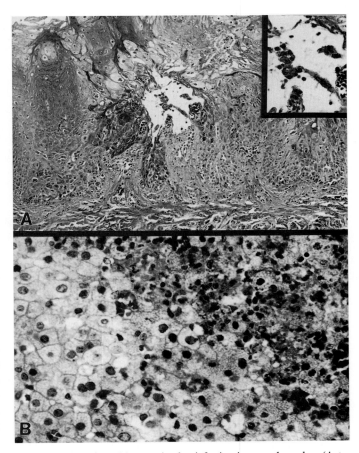

Fig. 7. Disseminated herpes simplex infection in an owl monkey (*Aotus trivigatus*). (A) Vesicular glossitis (inset: syncytial cells). (B) Acute adrenal cortical necrosis with intranuclear viral inclusions.

rus is likely transmitted venerally and as such may represent a model of genital herpesvirus infection (Levin *et al.*, 1988).

c. PATHOGENESIS AND PATHOLOGY.   The pathogenesis of herpesvirus papionis most similar to herpesvirus simplex 2 of humans. Skin lesions include hemorrhagic ulcers, vesicles, and pustules. Following experimental inoculation of infantile baboons, a fibrinonecrotic pulmonary alveolitis developed that was accompanied by multifocal hepatic necrosis. Intranuclear inclusions identical to those described with herpesvirus simiae (herpes B) were noted (Eichberg *et al.*, 1976). Although natural neonatal infection with SA8 has not been described, its occurrence would not be unexpected.

d. CLINICAL FINDINGS.   Many animals carry the virus asymptomatically. During primary infection or recrudescence, small vesicles and pustules may be found on the genital and, less frequently, on oral mucous membranes (Levin *et al.*, 1988). Genital lesions were occasionally severe, involving the vulvar, penile, or perineal tissues, and were accompanied by an inguinal lymphadenopathy. Oral lesions were less severe, although hemorrhagic gingivitis was occasionally noted. Following intravenous inoculation of 1-month-old baboons, an interstitial pneumonia developed within 3–6 days (Eichberg *et al.*, 1976). Lesions on the skin or mucous membranes were not noted.

Betaherpesvirinae

1. Cytomegalovirus

a. INTRODUCTION.   Cytomegalovirus (CMV) is a common asymptomatic infection of humans and many of the nonhuman primates studied to date. Infection of macaques (*Macaca* spp.), capuchin monkeys (*Cebus* spp.), wooly monkeys (*Lagothrix* spp.), squirrel monkeys (*Saimiri sciureus*), chimpanzees (*Pan troglodytes*), baboons (*papio* spp.), white-lipped tamarins (*Saguinus fuscicollis*), and African green monkeys (*Cercopithecus aethiops*) has been demonstrated (Rangan and Chaiban, 1980). Although viruses within this group are generally believed to have a narrow host range, interspecies transmission does occur.

b. ETIOLOGY.   Cytomegaloviruses resemble other herpesviruses ultrastructurally, but differ from alphaherpesviruses in several aspects. They are slowly cytolytic and tend to cause enlargement of the nucleus and cytoplasm (cytomegaly) of infected cells both *in vivo* and *in vitro*. During viral replication, enveloped virions accumulate in large cytoplasmic vacuoles instead of being readily released into intercellular spaces. This feature accounts for their relative cell-associated nature and explains the fact that cytoplasmic inclusion bodies can also be found in infected cells. Cytomegaloviruses also tend to be restricted in terms of their host range, unlike many of the cytolytic herpesviruses. Finally, latent infections tend to persist in glan-

dular tissue, lymphoreticular cells, and kidneys rather than in neurons.

c. EPIZOOTIOLOGY.   Cytomegalovirus infection is common in nonhuman primates. Infection is usually not associated with disease. The virus is spread horizontally in a variety of body secretions, including saliva, blood, urine, milk, and semen (Asher *et al.*, 1974), and may be shed for extended periods (Asher *et al.*, 1974). Macaques become infected within the first year of life (Vogel *et al.*, 1994). Disease occurs in immunocompromised individuals or following intrauterine infection. Rhesus macaques naturally infected with rhesus CMV are susceptible to infection by an antigenically distinct African green monkey CMV and commonly become infected with both strains during captivity (Swack and Hsuing, 1982).

d. CLINICAL FINDINGS.   Infection is usually asymptomatic. Immunosuppressed animals may experience reactivation and dissemination of the virus. In these individuals, clinical signs relate to the anatomic site(s) involved and may include dyspnea, diarrhea, melena, and neurologic signs.

e. PATHOGENESIS AND PATHOLOGY.   Cytomegalovirus persists as a latent infection and may periodically be shed in body secretions. In immunosuppressed macaques, reactivation of the virus may be associated with disseminated lesions in the brain, lymph nodes, liver, spleen, kidney, small intestine, nervous system, and arteries. Disseminated CMV may be initiated by a variety of immunosuppressive events, including viral infection (simian immunodeficiency virus or type D retrovirus) and drug therapy (cyclophosphamide, cortisone, and antithymocyte globulin).

In SIV-infected macaques, reactivation typically occurs as a terminal opportunistic infection associated with severe CD4$^+$ T lymphocyte depletion and is manifest by a necrotizing enteritis, encephalitis, lymphadenitis, and/or pneumonitis (Baskin, 1987). Pulmonary lesions are common and consist of a multifocal to coalescent interstitial pneumonia. The alveolar septa are thickened and lined by hypertrophied type II pneumocytes. Alveolar spaces contain fibrin, alveolar macrophages, and neutrophils. Cytomegaly and large, intranuclear Cowdry-type A inclusion bodies may be evident in alveolar septa and septal lining cells. Similar lesions may be found in the liver, spleen, kidney, and testes (Fig. 8). *In situ* hybridization often reveals many more cells to be infected than would be anticipated on routine stains and may be useful for diagnosis when only equivocal changes (i.e., mild cytomegaly) are present. Smaller amphophilic, intracytoplasmic inclusions are less frequent.

Central nervous system (CNS) lesions are multifocal, involve primarily the leptomeninges and subjacent neuropil, and are characterized by neutrophilic infiltrates with necrosis and fibrinous exudates. These findings are accompanied by characteristic viral inclusions and often by a nonsuppurative, perivascular, meningoencephalitis. In the gastrointestinal tract, hemorrhage, particularly neutrophilic infiltrates, may be prominent. In all

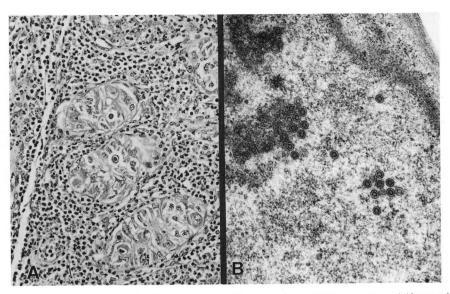

Fig. 8. Cytomegalovirus infection of an immunosuppressed rhesus macaque (*Macaca mulatta*). (A) Degenerate seminiferous tubules containing intranuclear viral inclusions surrounded by the characteristic neutrophilic inflammatory response. (B) Intranuclear virions.

locations, these findings may be accompanied by a necrotizing and proliferative vasculitis. The pathogenesis of CMV infection in SIV inoculated macaques shares many similarities with the disease in human patients with AIDS.

Intrauterine infection of the human fetus may occur if primary infection of the mother coincides with pregnancy. This has been reproduced experimentally in rhesus macaques (London *et al.,* 1986) and squirrel monkeys (Ordy *et al.,* 1981). Association between CMV and accelerated graft vs host rejection of heart and kidney transplants in humans is well established. More controversial is the role of the virus in producing arteriosclerosis in the human population at large.

Gammaherpesvirinae

1. *Lymphocryptovirus*

a. INTRODUCTION. The *Lymphocryptovirus* genus contains a number of species, including Epstein–Barr virus (EBV, herpes virus 4), *Herpesvirus pan, H. pongo, H. papio,* and *H. gorilla* (Gerber *et al.,* 1976, 1977; Falk *et al.,* 1976; Rabin *et al.,* 1980; Levy *et al.,* 1971). These primate viruses share approximately 35–45% homology with each other and EBV (Dillner *et al.,* 1987). In humans infection with EBV is usually asymptomatic but may cause infectious mononucleosis. This illness is characterized by lymphadenopathy, fever, pharyngitis, and circulating atypical lymphocytes in adolescents and young adults. Epstein–Barr virus has been associated with Burkitt's lymphoma, nasopharyngeal carcinoma, and hairy leukoplakia in humans.

b. ETIOLOGY. Lymphocryptoviruses are members of the Gammaherpesvirinae subfamily and, as other herpesviruses, have a complex genome consisting of approximately 170 kb. These viruses apparently lack strict host specificity, as a number of New World species are susceptible to infection with human isolates. In one survey, antibodies to EBV were detected in a large number of captive and wild Old World primate species (Ishida and Yamamoto, 1987). In general, it is accepted that EBV-like viruses are common in Old World primates but not so in New World species and prosimians. Cotton-top tamarins (*Saguinus oedipus*) are susceptible to experimental infection with human EBV and develop multifocal, large cell lymphoma (Niedobitek *et al.,* 1994).

c. EPIZOOTIOLOGY. Epizootiology in Old World primates closely parallels that in human populations. Infection occurs primarily in the young through contact with infected oral secretions and is usually unassociated with clinical signs. In cynomolgus monkeys, infection occurs after the disappearance of maternal immunity but prior to 1 year of age, at which time virtually all animals harbor the virus (Fujimoto and Honjo, 1991). The virus infects B lymphocytes and persists for life, usually in a latent form. Some animals may periodically shed virus. Although a small number of New World species have antibodies to EBV, the significance of these findings is unknown.

d. PATHOGENESIS AND PATHOLOGY. Infection of Old World species is common and usually unassociated with disease. Epstein–Barr-like viruses have been associated with malignant lymphoma in baboons (Deinhardt *et al.,* 1978) and macaques (Rangan *et al.,* 1995). Macaques coinfected with SIV and EBV have been proposed as a model of AIDS-associated

Burkitt's lymphoma (Feichtinger *et al.,* 1992). In New World species (*S. oedipus, S. fuscicollis,* and *C. jacchus*), experimental inoculation of some lymphocryptoviruses produce malignant B-cell lymphomas and death, usually within 1–2 months of inoculation (Miller *et al.,* 1977).

Proliferative squamous epithelial lesions resembling oral hairy leukoplakia have been described in rhesus macaques inoculated with simian immunodeficiency virus and succumbing to AIDS (Baskin *et al.,* 1995). Lesions have been described on the tongue, esophagus, penis, hand, and thorax and are usually not visible grossly. Histologically, focal regions of hyperkeratotic parakeratosis with or without acanthosis or pseudoepitheliomatous hyperplasia are noted. Basophilic intranuclear viral inclusions are present in most cases and are composed of typical herpesvirus virions as observed by electron microscopy.

The molecular pathogenesis of endemic Burkitt's lymphoma in humans has been studied extensively. Briefly, infection of B lymphocytes by EBV results in a sustained polyclonal proliferation of B cells. In conjunction with suppression of B-cell function induced by malarial infection or other cofactors, this expansion leads to c-*myc* protooncogene dysregulation. Most commonly, this entails translocation of the c-*myc* gene from its location on chromosome 8 to chromosome 14 where it is brought into apposition with the immunoglobulin promoting gene. Although EBV induction of lymphoma in New World monkeys may closely parallel Ateline and Saimirine herpesvirus infection (see later) (Cameron *et al.,* 1987), its association with lymphoma in Old World species likely involves a similar translocation of protooncogenes.

Although the molecular events associated with the development of Burkitt's lymphoma in humans are well established, the process of viral latency is less well understood. Critical to the regulation of this state is the expression of EBV-encoded RNAs (EBER-1, and -2), EBV-encoded nuclear antigens (EBNA-1, -2, -3a, -3b, -3c, and -LP), and latent membrane proteins (LMP-1, -2a, and -2b). Factors that govern the relative expression of these viral proteins are largely unknown, but apparently their expression influences the subsequent development of disease.

e. ZOONOTIC POTENTIAL.   Infection of humans with simian EBV-like agents has not been reported.

2. *Rhadinovirus: Herpesvirus ateles and Herpesvirus saimiri*

a. INTRODUCTION.   *Herpesvirus saimiri* and *Herpesvirus ateles* are members of the Gammaherpesvinae subfamily of Herpesviridae. Although a common asymptomatic infection of their natural hosts, inoculation into inappropriate hosts results in the rapid development of malignant lymphoma or leukemia. Evidence of the ability of these viruses to induce disease in naturally infected hosts is more limited (Hunt *et al.,* 1973).

b. ETIOLOGY.   Rhadinoviruses are enveloped, double-stranded DNA viruses containing approximately 170 kb and 20 gene products. As with other herpesviruses, they have an

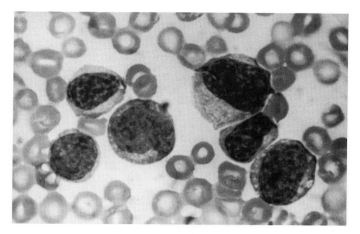

Fig. 9.   Herpes saimiri. Peripheral blood, leukemia.

icosahedral capsid containing 162 capsomers. Recent work has focused on genes encoding the "saimiri transformation-associated protein" (STP) and its ability to acutely transform cells (Jung and Desrosiers, 1992).

c. EPIZOOTIOLOGY.   A large percentage of wild squirrel monkeys (*Saimiri sciureus*) are infected with *H. saimiri* and nearly all animals are seropositive by 1.5–2 years of age. Likewise, approximately 50% of spider monkeys are seropositive for *H. ateles.* Although squirrel and spider monkeys represent the natural reservoir host for their respective viruses, little is known about the natural history and epidemiologic factors that govern transmission in these species.

d. CLINICAL FINDINGS.   Infection of the natural host is not associated with clinical signs. Experimental inoculation of

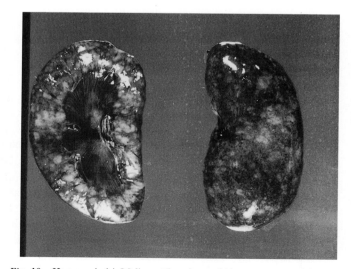

Fig. 10.   Herpes saimiri. Malignant lymphoma, kidney, cotton-topped tamarin (*Saguinus oedipus*).

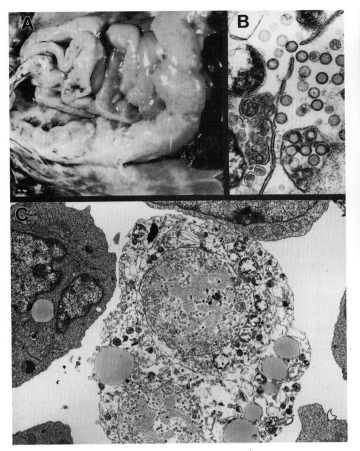

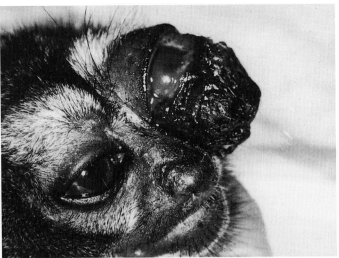

Fig. 12. Herpes saimiri. Retrobulbar malignant lymphoma, owl monkey (*Aotus trivirgatus*). From Hunt, R. D. and Blake, J. (1993). *Herpesvirus saimiri* and *Herpesvirus ateles* infection. *In* "Nonhuman Primates." (T. C. Jones, U. Mohr, and R. D. Hunt eds.) Springer-Verlag, New York. With permission.

Fig. 11. Herpes saimiri. (A) Malignant lymphoma of the gastrointestinal tract and spleen. (B and C) Virions within degenerate lymphoblast in cell culture.

H. saimiri into owl monkeys (*Aotus* sp.), several species of tamarins and marmosets (*Saguinus oedipus, S. fuscicollis, S. nigricollis, S. mystax,* and *Callithrix jacchus*), howler monkeys (*Alouatta carage*), and spider monkeys (*Ateles geoffroyi*) results in lymphoma or lymphocytic leukemia. Following inoculation, the time to development of lymphoma is variable but may be seen as soon as 3 weeks. Generally one of three patterns occurs: (1) survival less than 40 days with development of disseminated lymphoma often associated with extensive necrosis and replacement of vital organs (Figs. 9 and 10), (2) survival from 50 to 150 days with a less aggressive form of lymphocytic lymphoma involving multiple organs and associated with lymphocytic leukemia (Figs. 11 and 12), and (3) survival over 150 days with localized, well-differentiated lymphocytic lymphoma. Limited studies indicate that *H. saimiri* is oncogenic in African green monkeys (*Cercopithecus aethiops*) but not in macaques (*Macaca arctoides* and *M. mulatta*) (Melendez *et al.,* 1970).

Experimental inoculation of *H. ateles* into tamarins, marmosets, and owl monkeys induces lymphoma and leukemia. Although the virus has not been studied as extensively, the oncogenic properties of *H. ateles* are similar to *H. saimiri.*

e. PATHOGENESIS AND PATHOLOGY. Microscopically, cells comprising the neoplastic infiltrate vary considerably in their degree of differentiation. In the most aggressive form the neoplastic cells are large, pleomorphic, and resemble reticulum cells or histiocytes. Many are polygonal to stellate and have a moderate amount of granular cytoplasm. In less aggressive forms the cells are more differentiated, resembling lymphocytes. Neoplastic cells are polyclonal and are of T lymphocyte origin. Ultrastructurally, bizarre convoluted nuclei are seen and viral particles are not visualized. Virus may be recovered in cell culture from tumor explants.

Three different subtypes of Herpes saimiri virus are recognized (A, B, and C) based on homology within the left end of the L-DNA (Jung *et al.,* 1991). A and C types are highly oncogenic and transform peripheral blood lymphocytes of the common marmoset *in vitro.* The STP is encoded in the left terminus of the L-DNA of A and C strains and confers oncogenicity on individual isolates (Jung and Desrosiers, 1991, 1992). It does not share sequence homology with other known viral oncogenes or cellular protooncogenes.

f. TREATMENT AND PREVENTION. The natural infection of callithricids has been reported infrequently. Exposure to tissue or blood products is probably necessary to produce infection in the inappropriate host.

g. ZOONOTIC POTENTIAL. Herpes saimiri virus induces malignant lymphoma when inoculated into a variety of New World primate species and rabbits (Melendez *et al.,* 1970). Its oncogenicity in other species has not been fully explored. Herpes saimiri virus will infect and transform human T lymphocytes *in vitro.*

3. *Herpesvirus aotus*

Several herpesviruses have been isolated from owl monkey cell lines. These tissues originated from healthy monkeys and the animals were asymptomatically and latently infected. *Herpesvirus aotus* type 1 (Aotine herpesvirus 1) and *Herpesvirus aotus* type 3 (Ateline herpesvirus 3) belong to the Beta-herpesvirinae subfamily (Daniel *et al.,* 1973). *Herpesvirus aotus* type 2 (Aotine herpesvirus 2) belongs to the Gammaherpesvirinae subfamily (Barahona *et al.,* 1973). No natural or experimental disease has been associated with them.

4. *Herpesvirus saguinus*

A herpesvirus was isolated from marmoset kidney cell cultures but has not been associated with clinical disease (Melendez *et al.,* 1970).

C. Hepadnaviridae

1. Hepatitis B Virus

a. INTRODUCTION. Hepadnovirus B (hepatitis B virus, HBV) belongs to the genus *Orthohepadnavirus* and is an important cause of viral hepatitis in humans worldwide. Other important viruses within this group are woodchuck hepatitis B virus, duck hepatitis virus, and ground squirrel hepatitis B virus. In nonhuman primates, HBV infection has been described primarily in chimpanzees (*Pan troglodytes*) (Thung *et al.,* 1981; Zuckermann *et al.,* 1978; Maynard *et al.,* 1971) and gorillas (*Gorilla gorilla*) (Linneman *et al.,* 1984) and less frequently in cynomolgus macaques (*Macaca fascicularis*) (Kornegay *et al.,* 1985).

b. ETIOLOGY. Hepatitus B virus is a small (42 nm) enveloped DNA virus with an icosahedral nucleocapsid containing 180 capsomeres. The genome consists of a single strand of circular DNA encoding the complete genome and a shorter incomplete complementary strand. The core consists of a DNA polymerase, the hepatitis B-core antigen (HBVcAG), and the hepatitis B e-antigen (HBVeAG). Detection of these antigens in the peripheral blood of infected human patients occurs in a predictable and sequential fashion and may be used in the diagnosis and staging of clinical disease. In humans, a self-limiting hepatitis, fulminant hepatitis, and chronic carrier state are recognized. Chronic HBV infection is associated with a significant increased risk for the development of chronic active hepatitis and hepatocellular carcinoma.

c. EPIZOOTIOLOGY. Transmission of HBV among humans occurs through intimate contact, blood-borne contamination, or vertical routes. Worldwide vertical transmission from mother to child may represent the most significant route and an estimated 300 million humans are chronically infected carriers of HBV. The epizootiology of nonhuman primate transmission is poorly understood; however, as in humans, mother to infant transmission may play a critical role. Prolonged incubation and a chronic carrier state may be important in propagating the virus in nonhuman primate populations.

d. PATHOGENESIS AND PATHOLOGY. The histopathology of naturally occurring and experimental HBV infection of chimpanzees has been described (Dienstag *et al.,* 1976). The pathology is similar to that described in humans with the exception that chronic active hepatitis and hepatocellular carcinoma have not been recognized as sequelae. Findings vary from essentially normal liver to the occurrence of moderate nonsuppurative inflammatory cell infiltrates centered within portal tracts and extending variably into the hepatic parenchyma. These latter findings are compatible with so-called "chronic persistent infection" of humans and in such specimens the typical ground glass hepatocytes containing viral antigen and scattered hepatocellular necrosis may be evident (Dienstag *et al.,* 1976). Lesions described in cynomolgus monkeys were similar but qualitatively more severe and were accompanied by hepatocellular fatty change and Ito cell proliferation.

e. CLINICAL FINDINGS. Infection of chimpanzees and gorillas demonstrated by serology was not associated with clinical signs. Experimental infection of chimpanzees produces mild anorexia, lethargy, and jaundice. In cynomolgus monkeys, anorexia, lethargy, and hepatomegaly were observed accompanied by elevations in bilirubin and liver enzymes.

f. LABORATORY FINDINGS. Alterations in alanine aminotransferase and the presence of hepatitis B virus surface antigen (HBVsAg), anti-HBVsAg, and anti-HBVcAg have been described following experimental inoculation (Dienstag *et al.,* 1976). In these animals, HBsAg peaked 3 months following infection and coincided with the initial rise in anti-HBsAG and elevations in alanine aminotransferase. It was at this time that the initial histopathologic alterations were seen, which generally resolved with the apparent rise in anti-HBVc between 8 and 12 months.

g. ZOONOTIC POTENTIAL. Viral hepatitis represents a common zoonosis acquired from nonhuman primates (Brack, 1987b). Although the vast majority of cases have resulted from transmission of the hepatitis A virus, the common occurrence of HBV in chimpanzees suggests that the risk of infection should not be underestimated. Bite wounds and needle stick injuries represent possible routes of transmission.

III. NONENVELOPED DNA-CONTAINING VIRUSES

A. Adenoviridae

a. INTRODUCTION. The family Adenoviridae encompasses a large number of ubiquitous viruses that affect a wide range of mammalian and avian species worldwide. The family is divided into two genera, *Mastadenovirus* and *Aviadenovirus,* depending on the host. All mammalian isolates share a common antigen not shared by the avian isolates and vice versa. The family name is derived from the fact that the original isolates were obtained from adenoids (diffuse lymphoid tissue of the nasopharynx) and tonsils of military recruits suffering from acute upper respiratory tract infection and conjunctivitis. At least 27 serotypes of adenoviruses have been isolated from nonhuman primate species, including macaques (*Macaca* spp.), African green monkeys (*Cercopithecus aethiops*), baboons (*Papio cynocephalus*), chimpanzees (*Pan* spp.), squirrel monkeys (*Saimiri sciureus*), and cotton-topped tamarins (*Saguinus oedipus*) (Bullock, 1965; Davis *et al.,* 1992; Eugster *et al.,* 1969; Kim *et al.,* 1967). Although adenoviruses have been confirmed as causing a mild to moderately severe repiratory or enteric disease of monkeys and apes, many isolates have been obtained from oral or anal swabs or from cell cultures derived from clinically healthy animals, suggesting that subclinical infections of these species are common. A more severe disease has been described in animals whose immune systems are compromised either by immunosuppressive drugs or by concomitant infections, such as simian immunodeficiency virus infection, Mason–Pfizer monkey virus, and simian retrovirus (SRV) 1 and 2.

b. ETIOLOGY. Adenoviruses are nonenveloped, iscosahedral viruses, 70–90 nm in diameter with a capsid composed of 252 capsomeres. At the vertices of the icosahedron there are 12 capsomeres that are pentagonal in cross section (pentons) and have long filamentous glycoprotein projections with knobby ends that protrude from their surfaces. The remaining 240 capsomeres are hexagonal in cross section and are referred to as hexons. The adenovirus genome consists of a single linear molecule of double-stranded DNA. Included in the early region of the genome designated E1 are two genes, E1A and E1B, that encode proteins capable of transforming cells *in vitro* and causing neoplasms in hamsters and rats *in vivo.* These proteins have been shown to bind to and presumably inactivate the two well-known tumor suppressor genes, p53 and Rb, thereby causing malignant transformation. Despite the well-recognized ability of certain adenoviruses to experimentally transform cells *in vitro* and *in vivo,* these same agents have not been incriminated as the cause of naturally occurring neoplasia in any species.

c. EPIZOOTIOLOGY. Adenoviruses occur worldwide where they cause sporadic and epidemic forms of disease in human beings and animals. In general, adenoviruses tend to be rather species specific, but closely related species may be infected. Initial infections are generally transmitted through aerosols generated by sneezing and coughing and through oropharyngeal secretions of infected individuals, but the fecal–oral route is also a significant route of transmission due to the persistence of infection in tonsillar tissue and intestinal epithelium long after the clinical illness has subsided. Housing individuals under crowded conditions clearly promotes the spread of infection by these routes. Children and neonatal nonhuman primates are more susceptible to clinically apparent adenovirus infections than adults. The severity of infection varies widely depending on the serotype of the virus, the age and immune status of the patient, and the species infected. As mentioned previously, many such infections remain clinically inapparent even though the patient is shedding large amounts of virus.

d. PATHOGENESIS AND PATHOLOGY. Adenoviruses bind to specific receptors on susceptible cells by the filamentous projections that protrude from the penton capsomeres and are taken into the cell by endocytosis. In endosomes, the filament-bearing penton capsomeres are stripped from the particle, the pH within the endosome drops, and the endosome ruptures, spilling the partially degraded virion into the cytoplasm. These free particle bind to microtubules and are transported to the nuclear pores and the viral DNA is discharged into the nucleus, leaving the capsid in the cytoplasm. During the course of viral replication, cellular DNA and protein synthesis is severely disrupted, as is the normal processing of host messenger RNAs. These processes are incompatible with cell survival. Nuclei of cells containing actively replicating adenovirus develop large, amphophilic to basophilic inclusion bodies that either completely fill the nucleus or are surrounded by a prominent halo. Using electron microscopy, these inclusion bodies show prominent crystalline arrays of virions as well as unassembled viral capsid proteins and unencapsidated viral DNA.

The respiratory airways and lungs are common sites of adenovirus infection (Boyce *et al.,* 1971; Umemura *et al.,* 1985). Grossly, the affected portions of the lungs have patchy areas of firmness and gray–white or red discoloration that do not collapse on opening the thorax. Microscopically, epithelial cells of the trachea, bronchi, bronchioles, and alveoli are variably necrotic and contain basophilic, intranuclear inclusion bodies. These areas of necrosis and associated alveolar spaces typically are infiltrated by variable numbers of neutrophils and macrophages.

The conjunctiva and cornea may also be affected and appear edematous and congested with variable amounts of conjunctival exudate. Microscopically, the conjunctival epithelium contains areas of necrosis and intranuclear inclusion body formation.

The gastrointestinal tract is the second most common organ system affected by adenoviruses. Infection may be associated with diarrhea. Grossly, the mucosa of the stomach and small intestine may appear normal or somewhat congested and edematous. Microscopically, the mucosa contain focal and confluent areas of erosions or ulcerations in which necrotic enterocytes contain typical adenovirus inclusions (Fig. 13) (Baskin and Soike, 1989). There are also several reports of adenovirus pancreatitis in various macaque species (Chandler *et al.,* 1974; McClure *et al.,* 1978; Martin *et al.,* 1991). It would appear from the literature that this lesion occurs most often in young macaques that have been severely immunocompromised by naturally occurring or experimentally induced infections by Mason–Pfizer monkey virus, SRV-1 and 2, and SIVmac (Chandler and McClure, 1982). The pancreas of affected individuals contains

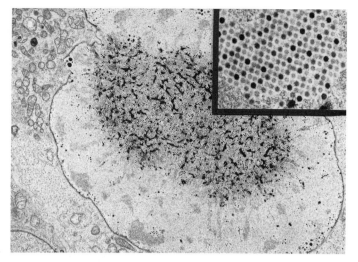

Fig. 13. Adenovirus. Enterocyte with intranuclear virions, rhesus macaque (*Macaca mulatta*).

In human beings, adenoviruses have also been associated with a whooping cough-like syndrome, an acute hemorrhagic cystitis, meningoencephalitis, and intussusceptions.

e. CLINICAL FINDINGS. Monkeys and apes with primary adenovirus infections may appear clinically healthy and asymptomatic or may exhibit a variety of clinical signs, depending on the tropism of the virus. Clinically apparent infections of the respiratory tract are characterized by cough and hyperpnea and, when severe, by dyspnea and cyanosis. There may be an associated keratoconjunctivitis. Most animals, but especially adults, recover within a week to 10 days. Except in neonates, mortality is generally low and is often the result of secondary bacterial infection. Other animals may experience diarrhea as the result of viral replication in the enterocytes of the small intestine. As with the respiratory tract, recovery generally occurs within 2 weeks, but virus may continue to be shed in the feces for many weeks after the animal becomes asymptomatic. This persistent shedding of virus in the feces serves as the source of infection for other susceptible individuals. In rare cases, immunocompromised macaques may experience a severe necrotizing pancreatitis that may be associated with diarrhea and death.

f. LABORATORY FINDINGS. Except for serological tests to detect specific adenovirus serotypes and virus isolation procedures, no routine laboratory tests will confirm the presence of an active adenovirus infection in nonhuman primates. Negative-staining electron microscopy has been used with limited success to detect adenovirus particles in stool samples, but as with virus isolation procedures, clinically healthy animals may yield as many positive samples as animals that are clinically ill.

either white or red foci that correspond to areas of necrosis and hemorrhage microscopically. Histologically, this chronic active pancreatitis is characterized by lobular fibrosis and extensive necrosis often centered on intralobular ducts and infiltrated by large numbers of neutrophils (Fig. 14). These foci are often dispersed among more normal appearing lobules. The acinar and ductal epithelial cells may contain adenovirus inclusions. Necrotizing hepatitis has been described in chimpanzees (*Pan troglodytes*) (Davis *et al.,* 1992).

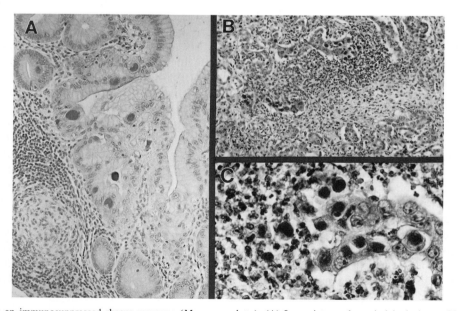

Fig. 14. Adenovirus in an immunosuppressed rhesus macaque (*Macaca mulatta*). (A) Large intranuclear viral inclusions within the gastric epithelium. (B) Chronic fibrosing pancreatitis. (C) Intranuclear viral inclusions within the pancreatic duct epithelium surrounded by degenereate neutrophils.

Viral isolation may be performed on a variety of cell lines, including A549 (human lung carcinoma), Hep-2, HeLa, and KB (epidermoid carcinoma) cells. Typical intranuclear inclusions are a recognized cytopathic change and viral identification by immunofluorescent or immunoperoxidase staining against the common hexon antigen.

g. TREATMENT.   There are no specific antiviral drugs commercially available for adenovirus infection. Consequently, treatment regimens are focused on preventing secondary bacterial infections and dehydration in the case of diarrheal illness. Supportive therapy to maintain caloric intact in animals that are severely anorectic is also beneficial.

h. PREVENTION.   Although adenovirus vaccines have been developed and used by the military to vaccinate new recruits, such vaccines are not commercially available to the civilian public nor do they exist for specific serotypes of nonhuman primate adenoviruses. Accordingly, preventive measures to control or eliminate adenovirus infection in nonhuman primate colonies must be directed toward minimizing the exposure of susceptible populations to potentially infected aerosols or feces. Mixing of animals from different sources during the quarantine period should be avoided so as to reduce the risk of exposure of noninfected animals to those that may have been infected at their previous location. Minimizing overcrowding also reduces the risk of exposure by minimizing the concentration of virus in the environment. Measures to prevent cross-contamination of cages by feces that may contain infectious virus should also be in place.

B. Papovaviridae

Papova is an acronym (pa=papilloma virus, po=polyoma virus, and va=vacuolating agent) and the family Papovaviridae is composed of two genera that share many structural and chemical properties: *Polyomavirus* and *Papillomavirus*. Despite these similarities, the subfamilies are not related genetically or immunologically.

Viruses within the polyomavirus genus have been of considerable scientific interest because of their oncogenic and transforming effects on mammalian cells and because of their ability to induce disease in immunocompromised hosts. These viruses are small (45 nm) and have a naked icosahedral capsid with 72 capsomeres and 420 structural subunits.

Papillomaviruses share this same symmetry but are slightly larger in size (55 nm) and have a more complex genome. Unlike polyomaviruses, these viruses have a propensity to infect skin and mucosal surfaces where they often result in proliferative disorders of keratinocytes. Although for the most part, papillomaviruses have a high degree of species and site specificity, infection of an inappropriate host occasionally results in a more aggressive neoplastic process (e.g., bovine fibropapillomavirus in equine sarcoid).

1. *Polyomavirus macacae:* Simian Virus 40

a. INTRODUCTION.   Simian virus 40 (SV40) is a common latent viral infection of feral and captive Asian monkeys, including rhesus macaques (*Macaca mulatta*), cynomolgus monkeys (*M. fascicularis*), Japanese macaques (*M. fuscata*), and Formosan rock macaque (*M. cyclopis*). Simian virus 40 was originally isolated from normal rhesus and cynomolgus monkey kidney cell cultures and subsequently from cells lines used for the production of killed poliovirus vaccine from 1954 to 1962. Because of its ability to readily transform cells *in vitro* and to produce malignant neoplasms *in vivo*, SV40 is one of the most extensively studied nonhuman primate viruses. Although its capacity to induce neoplasms in suckling hamsters is well established, its association with human disease is controversial.

b. ETIOLOGY.   Simian virus 40 is a double-stranded, DNA-containing virus classified in the polyomavirus genus of the family Papovaviridae. Its genome consists of double-stranded circular DNA approximately 5000 bp in length, encompassing early- and late-coding regions and a noncoding regulatory region. Two DNA-binding proteins coded within the early region are referred to as the large and small T (tumor) antigens and bind to viral regulatory sequences to facilitate the transcription of late viral genes. These genes have been studied extensively and are used in the construction of transgenic animals due to their transcriptional promoting activity. Evidence from macaques suggests that distinct subtypes of SV40 may exist that differ in their genomic sequence and ability to induce disease.

c. EPIZOOTIOLOGY.   Although serologic evidence indicates that infection of macaques with SV40 is common, clinical disease is rare and is usually associated with some immunosuppressive disease. Pathology results from reactivation of latent infection or primary infection during periods of immunosuppression. Concurrent natural or experimental infection with simian immunodeficiency virus (SIV) has been demonstrated in multiple cases and should be considered in others (Horvath *et al.,* 1992).

d. CLINICAL FINDINGS.   The vast majority of animals infected with SV40 do not show clinical signs and harbor the virus asymptomatically. The occurrence of clinical disease should prompt a search for an underlying immunosuppressive agent (most likely SIV). When disease does occur, most animals are in the terminal stages of AIDS with severe depletion of $CD4^+$ T lymphocytes. At this time, clinical signs may relate to a host of other opportunistic infections often present at death.

e. PATHOGENESIS AND PATHOLOGY.   Lesions are confined to the brain, lung, and kidney. The brain lesion consists of multifocal to confluent regions of demyelination scattered throughout the cerebral white matter and subependymal regions. Demyelination results from direct viral injury to oligodendroglial cells. Large basophilic inclusions fill and enlarge nuclei of oligodendrocytes and astrocytes. As the lesion progresses, gitter cells and astrocytes predominate. These lesions resemble progressive multifocal leukoencephalopathy of humans with JC virus reactivation.

Renal lesions are found primarily within the inner cortex and medulla. Collecting tubules are lined by hypertrophic/hyperplastic and occasional dysplastic epithelial cells containing typical viral inclusions (Fig. 15). These inclusions are often found in the desquamated epithelial cells present in tubular casts. Their large size and deep basophilic color often make them visible under the lowest magnification. These findings are accompanied by a chronic nonsuppurative tubulointerstitial nephritis, fibrosis and glomerular sclerosis, and atrophy. It is postulated that renal lesions may predominate in macaques acquiring infection during immunosuppression whereas CNS lesions ae more likely to occur following a recrudescence of latent infection (Horvath et al., 1992). Pulmonary lesions are seen less frequently and consist of a proliferative interstitial pneumonia with intracellular viral inclusions present within hypertrophied type 2 pneumocytes.

A distinct SV40-induced meningoencephalitis without demyelination has been recognized in SIV-inoculated macaques with AIDS (Simon et al., 1995). In these animals, papovavirus infection of astrocytes rather than oligodendrocytes predominates. Sequencing data suggest that this manifestation may be the result of a viral strain of SV40 distinct from that which causes progressive multifocal leukoencephalopathy (PML).

f. LABORATORY FINDINGS. In SIV-infected macaques with renal lesions, clinicopathologic findings included a mild hypochromic microcytic anemia and moderate elevations in BUN and creatinine. Because SV40 is found ubiquitously in macaques, the ability to isolate this virus from tissue is not definitive evidence of its role as a pathogen in an individual animal. The demonstration of papovavirus virions by electron microscopy or papovavirus DNA/RNA by in situ hybridization in typical lesions is diagnostic.

g. ZOONOTIC POTENTIAL. The zoonotic potential of SV40 is controversial (Bergsagel et al., 1992). Although large numbers of individuals have been exposed to SV40 through contaminated poliovirus vaccine, a clear relationship to any human disease has not been demonstrated (Melnick and Butel, 1988). Moreover, although SV40 has been isolated from human neoplasms and cases of PML, the widespread contamination of cell lines by SV40 has interfered with the interpretation of these results.

2. Polyomavirus papionis-1: SA12

SA12 is a papovavirus closely related to, but distinct from, the human papovavirus, BK virus. Natural infection of Chacma baboons (Papio ursinus) as well as vervet monkeys (Cercopithecus pygerythrus) has been demonstrated (Valis et al., 1977). Sera from a small number of rhesus macaques and humans tested were negative. Like SV40, SA12 transforms cells and

has produced neoplasms in hamsters. This virus has not been associated with natural disease and is more closely related to BKV than to JCV or SV40 (Cunningham and Pipas, 1985).

3. Polyomavirus cercopitheci: Lymphotropic Virus

Lymphotropic virus (LPV) is a papovavirus originally isolated from a B-lymphoblastic African green monkey cell line (zur Hazen et al., 1979). It is related to, but distinct from, other primate papovaviruses. Serological surveys indicate that humans and a variety of nonhuman primates are immunoreactive for LPV or an antigenically related virus (Takemoto et al., 1982). This virus does not induce tumors in hamsters and has not been associated with naturally occurring disease.

4. Polyomavirus hominis-2 and Polymomavirus hominis-1: JC Virus and BK Virus

Infection of humans with JCV and BKV is a common occurrence in childhood and while not associated with clinical disease, the virus persists for life. Recrudescence may occur with immunosuppression, leading to viral tubulointerstitial nephritis in the case of BKV and progressive multifocal leukoencephalopathy in the case of JCV. A closely related virus (SV40, see earlier) causes a progressive demyelinating disorder in SIV-inoculated macaques with many clinicopathologic similarities to PML. Despite the fact that a variety of nonhuman primates are susceptible to infection with SV40, there is a paucity of information concerning the occurrence of JCV and BKV in these species. Natural infection of nonhuman primates with these viruses reportedly does not occur (Shah, 1990). Owl monkeys (Aotus spp.) were susceptible to intracerebral inoculation of JCV and developed primitive neural tumors after a prolonged incubation (Major et al., 1987; London et al., 1978).

5. Papillomaviruses

a. INTRODUCTION. Almost 60 different papillomaviruses have been recognized in human beings, many with strict site specificity and different affinities to promote the malignant transformation of keratinocytes. Curiously, far fewer have been recognized in nonhuman primates. It is suspected that more will be identified and that the spectrum of disease with which they are associated will increase. Papillomavirus infection has previously been definitively demonstrated in the Colobus monkey (Colobus guerza), rhesus macaque (Macaca mulatta), chimpanzee (Pan troglodytes), and pygmy chimpanzee (Pan paniscus) (Sundberg et al., 1992; Kloster et al., 1988; Tate et al., 1973). A viral etiology has been suspected in a number of benign and malignant proliferative disorders in a variety of species, including cebus monkeys, other macaque species, baboons, and a squirrel monkey (Sundberg and Reichman, 1993).

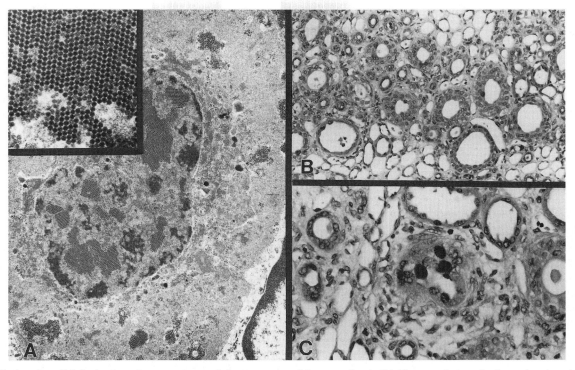

Fig. 15. Simian virus 40 infection in an immunosuppressed rhesus macaque (*Macaca mulatta*). (A) Electron micrograph of cytoplasmic and nuclear viral particles. (B) Chronic interstitial nephritis with viral inclusions and renal tubular epithelial cell hyperplasia. (C) Densely basophilic intranuclear inclusions within karyomegalic cells.

b. ETIOLOGY. Papillomaviruses are spherical, double-stranded DNA viruses 50–55 nm in diameter with a capsid composed of 72 capsomeres. This capsid consists of two proteins: the major capsid protein, which comprises approximately 80% of the total viral protein, and a slightly larger minor capsid protein. Their genome is approximately 8 kb in size and en-

codes 10 open reading frames. Research has focused on trans-regulatory factors (E1 and E2) products and early viral proteins (E6 and E7) and their role in host cell growth dysregulation. Interestingly, papillomaviruses have not been successfully grown in cell culture.

c. EPIZOOTIOLOGY. The epizootiology of papillomavirus infection of nonhuman primates is unknown. In other species, initial infection occurs primarily in the young and is thought to require defects in the superficial layers of the dermis. The virus is spread by fomites, by direct contact, or as a sexually transmitted disease. Lesions may be multiple and generally resolve with the mounting of an effective immune response. It is unknown whether all primate papillomaviruses will be species specific.

d. PATHOGENESIS AND PATHOLOGY. Viral infection of skin or oral mucosa produces an exophytic mass that is often described grossly as "cauliflower like" and may reach 1–2 cm in diameter (Fig. 16). Histologically, there is massive hyperplasia of the stratum spinosum and corneum. Basophilic intranuclear inclusions are occasionally found in the stratum spinosum. Acidophilic intracytoplasmic inclusions likely represent keratohyaline granules. The formation of rete ridges that invest the mass with blood vessels and contain scattered inflammatory cells often accompany epidermal proliferation. Infection with

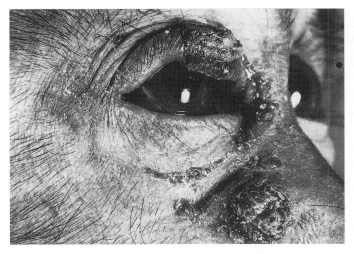

Fig. 16. Multiple papillomas, rhesus macaque (*Macaca mulatta*).

some viruses may induce massive fibroblastic proliferation (fibropapilloma) in which viral antigen may be detected. Genital infection with human papillomavirus (HPV) types 16, 18, and 31 may produce characteristic wart-like growths or more subtle changes characterized by foci of keratinocyte dysplasia.

Specific strains of human papillomavirus (HPV) are associated with an increased risk of cervical carcinoma. Viral DNA in these carcinomas and in viral-induced dysplastic lesions is present in an integrated form. If integration disrupts the E2 open reading frame, the normal control of early viral genes (E6/E7 products) is disrupted. These gene products can promote unregulated cell growth by two mechanisms: E7 protein binds to and deactivates the tumor suppressor protein (pRb) and E6 protein facilitates the degradation of another tumor-suppressing protein (p53). HPV types associated with cervical carcinoma apparently contain early viral proteins with high affinity for pRb and p53 whereas HPV types associated with low cancer risk are not. Other genetic and environmental factors likely act in conjunction with HPV infection to complete carcinogenesis. Papillomavirus DNA was detected in a penile squamous cell carcinoma with lymph node metastasis in a rhesus macaque, indicating that genital infection with this genus of viruses may be carcinogenic for nonhuman primates, as is the case in humans (Kloster *et al.,* 1988).

Focal epithelial hyperplasia has been described as a distinct entity in chimpanzees (*Pan troglodytes*) (Hollander and Van-Noord, 1972; Tate *et al.,* 1973; Glad and Nesland, 1995). Multiple, sessile, well-circumscribed proliferative structures 0.2–0.5 cm in diameter are described within the oral mucosa. These may persist for extended periods and undergo spontaneous regression. Histologically, the most striking feature is marked irregular acanthosis with the formation of anastomosing rete ridges. Typical papillomavirus virions have been demonstrated in some cases.

e. TREATMENT AND PREVENTION. Formalin-inactivated autologous vaccines have been used in the treatment and prevention of papillomavirus infection in cattle and dogs. Their effectiveness is not established.

C. Parvoviridae

1. Simian Parvovirus

a. INTRODUCTION. Parvoviridae represent some of the smallest known vertebrate viruses. They are nonenveloped, measuring 18–22 nm in diameter with icosahedral symmetry and a genome consisting of a single strand of DNA. Although parvovirus infections of cats, dogs, rats, and humans have been well described, parvovirus infection of nonhuman primates has been unrecognized until recently.

b. ETIOLOGY. A new simian parvovirus (SPV) has been described in cynomolgus macaques (*Macaca fascicularis*) concurrently infected with the simian-type D retrovirus (O'Sullivan

et al., 1994). This virus shared 65% homology at the DNA level with human B19 parvovirus within the major capsid protein.

c. EPIZOOTIOLOGY. Infection of a cohort of five cynomolgus monkeys and two additional contacts was demonstrated in an initial report (O'Sullivan *et al.,* 1994). Factors governing the transmission of SPV and the incidence at other primate colonies are unknown. As in human patients with parvovirus B19, it is suspected that infection with SPV is usually asymptomatic and that clinical disease is rarely seen.

d. PATHOGENESIS AND PATHOLOGY. Human infection with parvovirus B19 has been associated with a variety of clinical syndromes, including profound anemia, polyarteritis, fetal loss, and erythema infectiosum (Pattison, 1994). The pathogenesis of these disorders is poorly understood; however, a propensity for the virus to infect rapidly dividing cells likely contributes to clinical manifestations.

Infected cynomolgus monkeys had a variety of gross and microscopic lesions, many of which may have been attributable to underlying immunosuppressive retrovirus infection. Bone marrow revealed marked dyserythropoiesis with a loss of mature erythroid elements and increased numbers of atypical erythroid precursors. Within some animals, large intranuclear inclusion bodies were evident. Typical 24-nm-diameter viral particles were observed ultrastructurally.

e. CLINICAL FINDINGS. Animals clinically affected had concurrent infection with simian retrovirus type D. Clinical signs included diarrhea, dehydration, and moderate to severe anemia. Because these signs are common in macaques infected with simian retrovirus type D infection without concurrent SPV, the specificity of these findings is unknown.

f. LABORATORY FINDINGS. Affected animals had severe, nonregenerative, and normocytic normochromic anemia. In initial reports, parvoviral DNA was demonstrated in the serum of affected animals by dot-blot hybridization using radiolabeled B19 human parvovirus genomic probes. Typical 24-nm parvovirus particles could also be found by electron microscopy within bone marrow.

g. TREATMENT. No treatment is available.

IV. ENVELOPED RNA-CONTAINING VIRUSES

A. Rhabdoviridae

The family Rhabdoviridae encompasses a diverse group of over 100 viruses that infect a number of mammals, plants, reptiles, fish, and crustaceans. They are linked by a common rod-shaped (*Rhabdo*) ultrastructural appearance. Genera *Lyssavirus* and *Vesiculovirus,* respectively, contain the agents of rabies and vesicular stomatitis, the viruses of importance to nonhuman primates.

1. Rabies Virus

a. INTRODUCTION. Rabies has been reported in white-lipped tamarins (*Saguinus nigricollis*), golden lion tamarin (*Leontopithecus rosalia*), squirrel monkeys (*Saimiri sciureus*), capuchin monkeys (*Cebus* spp.), cynomolgus monkeys (*Macaca fascicularis*), rhesus macaques (*M. mulatta*), and chimpanzees (*Pan troglodytes*) (Richardson and Humphrey, 1971; Fiennes, 1972). Given the wide host range of this virus, its occurrence in other nonhuman primate species would not be unexpected.

b. ETIOLOGY The occurrence of rabies in captive-bred nonhuman primates is extraordinarily rare, and present-day housing practices do not facilitate exposure to carrier species. Nonetheless, potential exposures do occur (Smith *et al.,* 1987) and the serious zoonotic potential of this agent dictates that it be considered in sporadic cases of encephalitis. In regions of the world where rabies is endemic, populations of wild nonhuman primates may represent important vectors in the transmission of the virus to domestic species and humans.

c. EPIZOOTIOLOGY. Although nonhuman primates obviously become infected by contact with reservoir or inadvertent host species, the viral strains, vectors, and factors governing this transmission are unknown. Circumstantial evidence suggests that several New World species may have become infected with attenuated vaccine strains during the 1960s (McClure *et al.,* 1972).

d. PATHOGENESIS AND PATHOLOGY. Following experimental infection of rhesus macaques, furious rabies develops in 15–35 days, whereas in the dumb or paralytic form this period may extend to 105 days. The incubation in natural cases is unknown. Evidence in humans suggests that the incubation period may be as long as 6 years or more in unusual cases (Smith *et al.,* 1991).

Following exposure, initial replication of the virus occurs within myocytes at the site of inoculation and the virus is transported through peripheral nerves to the CNS where it spreads rapidly and exclusively infects neurons. Transmission between cells is mediated by the passage of ribonucleoprotein across synaptic junctions and exocytosis of complete virions. Centrifugal spread to peripheral organs occurs near the time of the onset of clinical signs, resulting in widespread dissemination of the virus at the death.

Microscopically, lesions vary from few recognized changes to marked formation of glial nodules, perivascular, nonsuppurative encephalitis, and neuronal degeneration. Negri bodies, which may consist of prominent, eosinophilic intracytoplasmic inclusions within nerve bodies, likely represent the defective assembly of precursor proteins. The changes are qualitatively similar to those seen in other species. Fluorescent antibody testing may be used to confirm the diagnosis on frozen neural tissue.

e. CLINICAL FINDINGS. Both the furious and the paralytic forms of rabies have been recognized in nonhuman primates. Reported clinical signs include self-mutilation, irritability, and paralysis of pharyngeal and pelvic muscles (Bougler, 1966; Fiennes, 1972). These findings are often not suggestive of the diagnosis.

f. PREVENTION. Although nonhuman primates may be vaccinated with killed vaccine, the efficacy of such vaccination is unknown. The use of attenuated vaccines is contraindicated as they have been implicated in the occurrence of vaccine-induced disease (McClure *et al.,* 1972). An inactivated hamster diploid cell vaccine has been used prophylactically in white-handed gibbons potentially exposed to a rabid bat (Smith *et al.,* 1987). A similar protocol might be considered in valuable animals if proper quarantine facilities exist and with the realization that the natural incubation period in primate species is unknown.

g. ZOONOTIC POTENTIAL. Rabies is a significant zoonotic threat, and nonhuman primate to human transmission has been documented.

2. Vesicular Stomatitis Virus

Antibodies to vesicular stomatitis virus have been identified in Geoffroy's marmoset (*Saguinus geoffryi*) in Panama (Srihongse, 1969). No clinical signs were associated with seropositivity. Phlebotomine sandflies may carry the virus, which causes vesicular lesions in the oral mucosa of a variety of mammalian species. The role of New World primates in the arborial cycle of this virus is unknown.

B. Filoviridae

1. Filoviruses

a. INTRODUCTION. In 1967, an outbreak of hemorrhagic fever was identified in Marburg and Frankfurt, Germany, and in Belgrade, Yugoslavia (Smith *et al.,* 1967). The disease was seen in laboratory workers preparing cell lines derived from African green monkey tissue. Twenty-five primary cases with seven deaths were recorded. In addition, the agent spread to an additional six contacts. Reportedly the shipment of African green monkeys from which tissue had been obtained was normal and the source of infection in these animals remains unknown. An interesting account of the management practices concerning the procurement of these animals has been given and suggests that animals were infected in Uganda prior to shipment (Smith, 1982). The first filovirus, Marburg virus, was isolated and characterized from this outbreak. Since that time, isolated and small clusters of cases caused by an antigenically identical virus have been identified in Zimbabwe, Kenya, and Uganda.

The first members of a second group of closely related viruses were identified in 1976 as the etiologic agent of an epidemic of hemorrhagic fever in Zaire and Sudan. During these simultaneous outbreaks, 500 human cases with over 430 deaths were recognized. The virus was named Ebola virus after the

Ebola river in northwest Zaire. As with the Marburg virus, secondary and tertiary cases occurred in contacts. In these contact cases, lower mortality suggested attenuation of the virus. A distinct viral strain, Ebola Côte-d'Ivoire, has been isolated from a 34-year-old female patient with a dengue-like syndrome after she necropsied a chimpanzee (Guenno et al., 1995). More recently, Ebola hemorrhagic fever has been identified in Kikwit, Zaire (Centers for Disease Control and Prevention, 1995).

A distinct filovirus subtype (Ebola Reston) was identified in 1989 and 1990 during an outbreak of hemorrhagic fever in newly imported Asian macaques. The animals originated from the Philippines and were housed at primate quarantine facilities in Virginia, Pennsylvania, and Texas. The virus caused a contagious, hemorrhagic fever with high mortality in cynomolgus monkeys (*Macaca fascicularis*). Although no clinical signs or deaths were recorded in human contacts, inadvertent infection of animal handlers in both United States and Philippine facilities did occur (Centers for Disease Control and Prevention, 1990a, b). In 1992, a similar virus was identified in Siena, Italy, in macaques obtained from the same Philippine source (World Health Organization, 1992).

b. ETIOLOGY.   The family Filoviridae contains one genus (*Filovirus*) with two distinct viruses: Marburg and Ebola. Four subtypes of Ebola virus are recognized (Zaire, Sudan, Reston, and Côte-d'Ivoire). These viruses have a single-stranded antisense RNA genome 12.7 kb in size. Morphologically, the virus forms distinctive filamentous, sometimes branching, structures 800–1000 nm in length and 80 nm in diameter. This structure is surrounded by a closely adherent host membrane in which 10-nm peplomers are found. The virus replicates by budding, and nucleocapsids accumulate in the cytoplasm, forming closely packed arrays of bundled filaments that are visible microscopically as viral inclusions (Fig. 17) (Murphy et al., 1971).

c. EPIZOOTIOLOGY.   Factors that allow filoviruses to become established in primate hosts are unknown and, despite extensive work, a reservoir host has not yet been identified. Once established in the human population, Marburg, Ebola Sudan, and Ebola Zaire viruses were transmitted between close contacts and to medical personnel. The Ebola Reston virus was transmitted between macaques by direct contact, fomites, and aerosolization. The Reston outbreak was associated with concurrent simian hemorrhagic fever virus (SHFV) infection (Dalgard et al., 1992). This infection causes a fatal hemorrhagic fever of macaques, but is carried asymptomatically by a number of African primates, principally the Patas monkey. This suggests that while macaques involved in the Reston outbreak were obtained from the Philippines, they may have become infected by inadvertent contact with African species.

d. PATHOGENESIS AND PATHOLOGY.   The pathogenicity of filoviruses is dependent on the viral strain and species affected. Generally, the African filovirus, Ebola Zaire, is considered the most pathogenic, followed by Ebola Sudan, Marburg, and Ebola Reston (Fischer-Hoch et al., 1992). Macaques are thought to be more susceptible than African green monkeys and humans.

Lesions within the spleen, gastrointestinal tract, lymphoid organs, and kidney are essentially the same as those described in SHFV infection (Dalgard et al., 1992). There is extensive lymphoid necrosis and deposition of fibrin within splenic white pulp. A characteristic lesion present within the liver is scattered hepatocellular necrosis accompanied by a mild, mononuclear inflammatory cell infiltrate (Fig. 17). A similar multifocal ne-

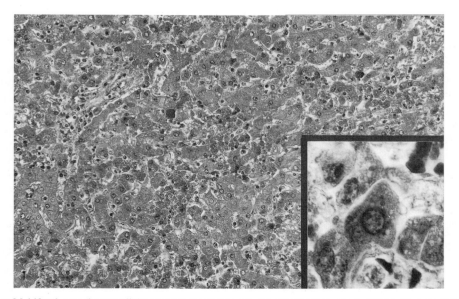

Fig. 17.   Marburg virus. Multifocal, acute hepatocellular necrosis (inset: intracytoplasmic viral inclusions), African green monkey (*Cercopithecus* spp.).

crosis is present within the zona glomerulosa of the adrenal gland. In both locations, large amphophilic to eosinophilic intracytoplasmic inclusions may be evident. Hepatocellular necrosis and necrosis within the adrenal cortex serve to distinguish filovirus infection from SHFV infection. An additional finding described in both Marburg and Ebola Reston viruses is the presence of a mild interstitial pneumonia accompanied by more diffuse evidence of disseminated microvascular thrombosis.

Evidence suggests that an epizootic among chimpanzees in the Tai National Park was responsible for the transmission of Ebola Côte-d'Ivoire to a single human subject (Guenno *et al.,* 1995). This troop experienced episodes of increased mortality in November 1992 and 1994. Although many animals were found in a state of advanced decomposition, tissues examined from one chimpanzee revealed lesions compatible with Ebola hemorrhagic fever, including multifocal necrotizing splenitis and hepatitis. Infrequent acidophilic intracytoplasmic inclusions were identified and were immunoreactive for Ebola-specific antigen.

e. CLINICAL FINDINGS.   Following experimental inoculation with Ebola Reston, there is a variable incubation period of 7–14 days. Once clinical signs appear, progression to death is rapid (<24 hr). Animals become anorexic, lethargic, and hypothermic. Cardiovascular collapse is followed by severe depression and coma. Petechiae are noted on the face, chest, and medial aspects of arms and thighs. A separate study of Ebola Zaire in rhesus macaques indicated prolonged partial thromboplastin time, increased fibrinogen degradation products, and normal prothrombin time (Fischer-Hoch *et al.,* 1983).

Interpretations of clinical signs observed during the occurrence of natural disease in Reston were complicated by the concurrent infection with SHFV. This outbreak was associated with a rapidly progressive and fatal disseminated viral infection. Animals would abruptly become anorexic and lethargic and were often found dead in the morning without premonitory clinical signs.

f. LABORATORY FINDINGS.   Experimental inoculation with filoviruses was associated with significant increases in lactate dehydrogenase (LDH) and aspartate aminotransferase (AST) (Fischer-Hoch *et al.,* 1983). These values peaked earlier following inoculation with African Ebola viruses than with Asian strains and quickly returned to normal in those animals that survived infection. Hematologic changes included thrombocytopenia, neutrophilia, and lymphopenia. A reactive lymphocytosis was noted in survivors.

g. TREATMENT AND PREVENTION.   Because of the serious zoonotic potential associated with filovirus infection, affected animals should be destroyed. Experimental inoculation of animals requires biosafety level 4 conditions and professional expertise. Animals surviving infection with filoviruses may not be protected against subsequent challenge with a heterotypic virus. Recommendations for biocontainment and management of the various hemorrhagic fever-inducing agents have been published by the Centers for Disease Control and Prevention (1988).

h. ZOONOTIC POTENTIAL.   The zoonotic potential with these agents is high. Although the initial outbreak of Marburg virus infection was associated with the handling of infected African green monkey tissue, most other filovirus outbreaks among humans have not been directly linked to contact with infected primates. The single reported case of human Ebola Côte-d'Ivoire virus infection resulted from contact with chimpanzee tissue but was nonlethal and did not spread to secondary contacts. Experience with Ebola Reston indicates that while this virus appears less pathogenic in humans, transmission occurred readily to animal handlers (Centers for Disease Control and Prevention, 1990a,b).

C. Orthomyxoviridae

1. Influenza Viruses

a. INTRODUCTION.   Influenza viruses are an important cause of respiratory illness in humans and occasionally infect nonhuman primates. Worldwide pandemics occurred in 1918, 1957, and 1968, and an estimated 20,000,000 humans died as a result of influenza between 1918 and 1919 (Acha and Szyfres, 1980). Animal infections (swine and fowl) are believed to have played a critical role in the generation of influenza viral strains responsible for these pandemics.

b. ETIOLOGY.   Influenza viruses are 80–120 nm in size with a single-stranded RNA genome encoding 9 to 10 proteins. Based on soluble (S) internal antigens, three types are recognized (A, B, and C). Types B and C infect only humans, have limited antigenic variation, and usually produce only sporadic cases. Type A strains infect a variety of animals species (humans, nonhuman primates, foals, fowl, swine, and seals), are more virulent, and have been responsible for the great pandemics. Two protein subunits within the viral envelope [hemagglutinin (H) antigen and neurominidase (N) antigen] define viral subtypes. The H antigen mediates adhesion of the virion to sialic acid residues on respiratory epithelial cells. The N antigen facilitates viral entrance to the cytosol following fusion and endosome formation.

Infection with a particular strain produces strong immunity, preventing reinfection. Unfortunately, genetic recombination between genes coding for H and N subunits occurs with striking regularity, producing new strains that are unrecognized by the human population. Historically, the emergence of new strains that differ antigenically from existing strains is associated with widespread human infection. Infection of fowl and/or swine is believed to be critical in the production of many of these strains.

c. EPIZOOTIOLOGY.   Evidence shows that gorillas, chimpanzees, orangutans, gibbons, macaques, baboons, African green monkeys, marmosets, tamarins, squirrel monkeys, owl monkeys, and capuchin monkeys are susceptible to infection (Kalter and Heberling, 1978; Kalter *et al.,* 1969, 1974; Murphy *et al.,* 1972; Renegar, 1992). The virus is highly contagious by the aerosolized route and nonhuman primates likely become infected through contact with humans or wildlife species. Once established within a cohort, transmission may occur among nonhuman primate members. Evidence cited from an epizootic in gibbons suggests that adaptation of the virus in a naive population may be associated with increased virulence.

d. PATHOGENESIS AND PATHOLOGY.   In mild cases of upper respiratory tract infection, changes noted grossly may be minimal, consisting of hyperemia of mucous membranes and overproduction of mucoid secretions. Experimental inoculation of gibbons produced a diffuse hemorrhagic alveolitis (Johnsen et al., 1971). Resolution of severe pulmonary involvement is characterized by marked septal thickening and hyperplasia of type II pneumocytes. Natural cases may be complicated by secondary bacterial infection and, in these instances, inflammation may be more purulent. Histologically, a desquamative alveolitis with the formation of hyaline membranes and microvascular thrombi is evident.

e. CLINICAL FINDINGS.   Clinical signs are nonspecific and consist of fever, oculonasal discharge, anorexia, lethargy, and gastrointestinal signs. The incubation period is 1–3 days and the illness may last 3–6 days. Occasionally, nonhuman primate illnesses will coincide with human cases, suggesting a diagnosis.

f. TREATMENT.   No specific treatment is available; however, the prevention of secondary bacterial infections may be beneficial (Johnsen et al., 1971). Demonstration of seroconversion to the S antigen by the hemagglutination–inhibition test is evidence of recent infection. Nasopharyngeal swabs or lung tissue collected at necropsy may be used for viral isolation on primary monkey kidney cell culture or embryonated chicken eggs. CPE is usually not observed and virus is first demonstrated by hemadsorption techniques. Immunofluorescent staining may be used for viral identification.

D. Paramyxoviridae

a. INTRODUCTION.   The family Paramyxoviridae contains two subfamilies known to infect nonhuman primates: Paramyxovirinae and Pneumovirinae (Table III). The former is divided into two genera: *Paramyxovirus,* which includes parainfluenza virus type 1 (Sendai virus), parainfluenza virus type 2 [also known as canine parainfluenza virus, SV (simian virus) 5 and SV41], parainfluenza virus type 3 (also known as simian agent 10), and parainfluenza type 4, and *Morbillivirus,* which includes measles virus. Measles virus is dealt with as a separate entity in this review. The subfamily Pneumovirinae contains only a single genus, *Pneumovirus,* which includes respiratory synctial viruses (chimpanzee coryza agent).

b. ETIOLOGY.   The Paramyxovirinae are pleomorphic, occasionally filamentous, enveloped, RNA-containing viruses with a diameter of 150–200 nm. Their genome consists of a single molecule of single-stranded, mostly negative-sense RNA, but some contain a positive strand. Unenveloped nucleo-

TABLE III

PARAMYXOVIRINAE

Genus	Virus
Morbillivirus	Measles virus
	Paramyxovirus saguinus
Paramyxovirus	Parainfluenza type 1 (sendai virus)
	Parainfluenza type 2 (SV5, SV41, Simian hemadsorbing virus)
	Parainfluenza type 3 (SA10, hemadsorption virus type 1)
	Parainfluenza type 4

capsids consist of long tubular structures and are assembled in the nucleus. These acquire a fuzzy, protein coat once they are released into the cytoplasm. These coated tubular structures then align themselves beneath the cell membrane through which they bud and acquire an envelope. The envelope consists of host cell membrane lipids with inserted viral-encoded proteins and glycoproteins. The latter protrude from the surface of the virions as 8- to 12-nm projections. Members of the genus *Paramyxovirus* contain neuraminidase and a hemagglutinin that agglutinates mammalian and avian erythrocytes. Members of the genus *Morbillivirus* cause agglutination of nonhuman primate but not human erythrocytes and lack neuraminidase. Members of the genus *Pneumovirus,* however, exhibit neither neuraminidase nor hemagglutinin activity. The surface spikes of all paramyxoviruses contain two glycosylated proteins that are responsible for the attachment and fusion of the virus to susceptible cells. The attachment protein also functions as the hemagglutinin in the case of paramyxoviruses and morbilliviruses. The fusion protein is responsible for the fusion of infected cells with noninfected cells to form multinucleated syncytial cells.

c. EPIZOOTIOLOGY.   Parainfluenza viruses have a global distribution where they are highly contagious and responsible for a variety of upper and lower respiratory ailments of a wide variety of species. Serological surveys indicate that most species of monkeys and apes have been infected with one or more paramyxoviruses either in their natural habitats, as in the case of newly imported animals, or after being maintained in laboratory colonies. *Pneumovirus* infections such as the respiratory syncytial virus of chimpanzees, however, appear to occur almost exclusively in apes, particularly gibbons and chimpanzees. Many of these infections are mild and may go clinically undetected. The principal mode of transmission of all members of the family Paramyxoviridae is by aerosols, although direct contact with infected secretions can also be a mode of transmission. Reinfections with the same or related paramyxoviruses occur with some frequency. Members of the paramyxovirus family appear to be less species specific than adenoviruses, as cross-species transmission among nonhuman primates, human beings, rodents, and possibly even dogs and cattle seems likely based on the antigenic relatedness of homologous serotypes isolated from these species.

d. PATHOGENESIS AND PATHOLOGY. Once in the respiratory tract, parainfluenza viruses bind to epithelial cells of the respiratory mucosa in the nasal cavity, nasopharynx, trachea, or bronchi and bronchioles. What determines the predilection of different or even the same serotypes for different regions of the respiratory tract is not known. The virus enters susceptible cells by binding to and fusing with the cell membranes. Its negative-strand RNA is transcribed to form multiple molecules of messenger RNA that code for various viral proteins and as an entire transcript of positive-strand RNA that serves as the template for the synthesis of entire molecules of negative-strand viral progeny RNA. During the replicative process, infected cells develop both intranuclear and intracytoplasmic, eosinophilic viral inclusion bodies corresponding to the naked, intranuclear, tubular nucleocapsid and the fuzzy coated cytoplasmic nucleocapsids, respectively. Infected cells, bearing viral-encoded fusion proteins, often fuse with adjacent noninfected cells to form multinucleated syncytial giant cells. Thus, the hallmark of infection by viruses of the family Paramyxoviridae is the presence of single or multinucleated syncytial cells bearing both intranuclear and intracytoplasmic, eosinophilic inclusion bodies. Infected cells undergo virus-induced lysis and desquamate from the mucosa, thereby predisposing the host to secondary bacterial infection. The disease produced parainfluenza viruses and pneumoviruses vary from a mild upper respiratory infection (coryza) to a rhinotracheobronchitis or croup-like illness to frank pneumonia. Most animals recover from paramyxovirus infections unless secondary bacterial infection results in death. With the exception of measles, most paramyxoviruses do not result in a viremia.

e. CLINICAL FINDINGS. Clinical signs associated with paramyxovirus infections are not specific for any particular genus of virus. Depending on the portion of the respiratory tract most affected, nonhuman primates with active paramyxovirus infection may exhibit no signs of clinical illness or may have nasal discharge and sneezing, wheezing, coughing, and even severe hyperpnea, dyspnea, and cyanosis. Epizootics of parainfluenza type 3 virus have been described in patas monkeys (*Erythrocebus patas*) and gibbons (*Hylobates* spp.) Churchill, 1963; Martin and Kaye, 1983) whereas parainfluenza type 1 (Sendai virus) has resulted in disease in marmosets (Flecknell *et al.,* 1983).

f. LABORATORY FINDINGS. Except for virus isolation procedures, serological tests that demonstrate a rise in antibody titer to a specific viral agent in a convalescent serum are the only practical method to determine which, if any, paramyxovirus is responsible for the respiratory illness. One must be aware, however, that there are numerous viral agents, in addition to paramyxoviruses, that can cause respiratory disease.

g. TREATMENT. As most simians recover naturally from paramyxovirus infections, treatment is largely supportive in nature and is directed toward minimizing the risk of secondary bacterial infection. Parainfluenza 3 virus infection has been shown to predispose to invasive pneumococcal disease in chimpanzees (Jones *et al.,* 1984).

h. PREVENTION. Although there are effective vaccines available commercially for canine parainfluenza virus type 2 and bovine parainfluenza virus type 3, these have not been tested nor are they approved for the prevention of infection by simian isolates of these serotypes. Thus, preventative measures should be similar to those indicated for adenovirus infections, namely the prevention of crowding and minimizing exposure to other species that might harbor similar agents.

MORBILLIVIRUS

The genus *Morbillivirus* contains many viruses of veterinary importance: canine and phocine distmper viruses, Rinderpest virus, virus of Pestes des petites ruminants, measles virus, and the recently documented equine morbillivirus. These agents produce illnesses in a diverse group of animals with remarkable clinical and histopathologic similarities.

1. Measles (Rubeola) Virus

a. INTRODUCTION. Measles virus infection of nonhuman primates is a common viral disease and has been described previously in *Macaca mulatta, M. fascicularis, M. radiata, M. cyclopis, Presbytis cristatus, Cercopithecus aethiiops, Saimiri sciureus, Colobus quereza, Pan troglodytes, Callithrix jacchus, Saguinus oedipus, S. fuscicollis,* and *Aotus trivirgatus* (Albrecht *et al.,* 1980; Scott and Keymer, 1975). Historically, this disease was once widespread in newly imported macaques and responsible for significant morbidity in animals stressed by importation and quarantine procedures. Although serologic surveys indicate that infection is now frequent and generally asymptomatic in this species (Kalter and Heberling, 1990; Mei *et al.,* 1990), Roberts *et al.* (1988) have documented a serious epizootic. Measles virus infection should be considered a serious threat to macaque colonies and appropriate preventative measures should be taken. In addition, infection of several New World species results in significant disease.

b. ETIOLOGY. The measles virus is grouped with the viruses of canine distemper and rinderpest in the genus *Morbillivirus* and family Paramyxoviridae. The virus is spherical to pleomorphic and 120–270 nm in diameter. The core consists of single-stranded negative-sense RNA and virion assembly occurs at the plasma membrane with the formation of spherical particles. Six gene products have been identified: N (nucleoprotein), P (polymerase protein), L (large protein), M (matrix protein), H (hemagglutinin), and F (fusion factor). Neuraminidase, a protein of other Paramyxoviridae, is not present.

c. EPIZOOTIOLOGY. Serological evidence indicates that while measles is a common infection in captive nonhuman primates, it does not occur in their natural habitats. Moreover, seroconversion may occur within weeks of first human contact, which may lead to endemic infection within groups or, if combined with stress of capture, quarantine, or shipping, to epizootics characterized by high morbidity and mortality. Roberts *et al.* (1988) documented an epizootic with high mortality in a group of immunosuppressed macaques inoculated with SIV. In a naive population, the disease spreads rapidly by the aerosolized route. With the prohibition of importation of many primate species and the advent of widespread vaccination, serious epizootics have become less frequent.

d. CLINICAL FINDINGS. Clinical signs vary, depending on the species infected. In macaques the disease is usually mild or asymptomatic unless animals are stressed or immunosuppressed. The incubation period varies from 6 to 10 days and is followed by fever and a maculopapular exanthema (Fig. 18). This rash is most pronounced on the ventral body surface and generally spares plantar and palmar surfaces. It then progresses to a dry or scaly desquamative dermatitis and may continue for up to 2–3 weeks (Hall *et al.*, 1971). While considered pathognomonic, Koplik's spots are present inconsistently. These small, white foci are rimmed by a raised red border and are found within the oral mucosa. In some cases, respiratory signs, including cough and conjunctivitis, may be present. Infected animals may be more susceptible to enteric bacterial infections, such as that caused by *Shigella flexneri,* and these animals may present with primarily gastrointestinal signs (Roberts *et al.,* 1988; McChesney *et al.,* 1989). Such concurrent bacterial infections may adversely impact morbidity and mortality. Abortion and neurologic signs may occur in some individuals (Renne *et al.,* 1973; Steele *et al.,* 1982).

In marmosets and colobines the disease is more severe. In these species the disease is characterized by a rapidly progressive course and a predominance of gastrointestinal signs. The characteristic exanthema is lacking. Edema of the periorbital region may be pronounced. Mortality may approach 100%, and lesions are centered within the gastrointestinal tract.

e. PATHOGENESIS AND PATHOLOGY. The pathogenesis of measles virus infection is similar to that of rinderpest and canine distemper viruses. Following infection by the aerosolized route, there is an initial round of replication within the regional lymph nodes. The resulting viremia leads to dissemination of the virus to lymphoreticular organs and epithelial surfaces. It is in the terminal phases of this viremia that the characteristic skin rash appears. This exanthema coincides with rising neutralizing antibodies and may, in part, represent an Arthus-type (antibody–antigen complex) reaction.

Histologically, there is mild erythema and parakeratotic hyperkeratosis of the skin. Multinucleated syncytial cells may occasionally be found (Hall *et al.,* 1971). Lesions are most pronounced within the hair follicles where follicular necrosis is

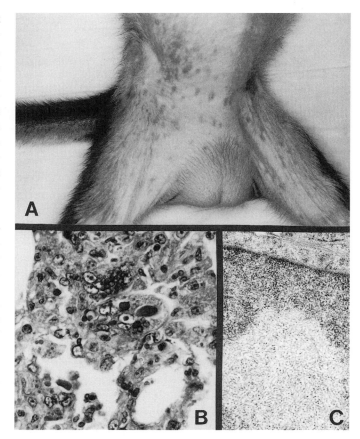

Fig. 18. Measles virus infection of a rhesus macaque (*Macaca mulatta*). (A) Viral exanthema. (B) Multinucleated syncytial cells with nuclear and cytoplasmic viral inclusions within alveoli. (C) Electron micrograph of viral nucleocapsid.

a characteristic change. In more severe cases there is often a proliferative and necrotizing bronchointerstitial pneumonia. Large syncytial cells are often present and careful inspection may reveal intranuclear and intracytoplasmic eosinophilic inclusions present within these cells, as well as type II pneumocytes and histiocytes. A purulent bacterial bronchopneumonia may be superimposed on these findings.

The latter stages of infection may be associated with significant viral-induced immunosuppression which arises from the destructive effect of the virus on thymic tissue, and may predispose animals to bacterial infections of the respiratory and gastrointestinal tracts. Moreover, viral inhibition of interferon-γ-induced upregulation of MHC class II antigen expression may further compromise immunologic function (Leopardi *et al.,* 1993). These effects on the immune system of the host may induce hyporesponsiveness to tuberculin antigen, resulting in a false-negative skin test in sensitized animals. The resolution of infection correlates with the appearance of cytotoxic CD8[+] T lymphocytes.

Giant cells lacking viral inclusions (Warthin–Finkeldey cells) may be found within lymphoid tissue. In the most severe cases, typical viral inclusions may be found in a variety of epithelial surfaces. In marmosets, these changes may be accompanied by a necrotizing gastroenteritis. Ultrastructurally, the virus may be identified in tissues in two forms: (1) nucleocapsids that form tangles of filamentous tubules with a diameter of 20 nm and (2) paracrystalline arrays of filamentous rods 20 nm in diameter surrounded by an outer rim of less electron-dense material, giving the structure an overall diameter of 40–50 nm (Raine *et al.,* 1969). These latter structures can occasionally be found subjacent to the cell membrane in various stages of budding.

A well-characterized postinfectious syndrome in human is subacute sclerosing panencephalitis (SSPE), which occurs in a small minority of patients 5–10 years after primary infection, and is characterized by progressive gliosis, demyelination, and neuronal loss (Tellez-Nagel and Harter, 1966). Intranuclear inclusions composed of viral nucleocapsid are prominent and result from defective viral replication. One or more defects in the M, H, or F antigens prevent the formation of mature virons. Although an acute measles encephalitis in macaques and other species is well recognized (Baringer and Griffith, 1970), it is less clear whether reported cases of SSPE in nonhuman primates critically fulfill all diagnostic requirements of SSPE in humans (Kim *et al.,* 1970; Albrecht *et al.,* 1972).

f. LABORATORY FINDINGS. Presumptive diagnosis may be made on characteristic clinical, histopathologic, and ultrastructural findings. Further support may be gathered by demonstrating seroconversion. Definitive diagnosis requires viral isolation and identification. Isolation is best performed on human or rhesus monkey kidney cells from nasopharyngeal secretions, whole blood, or buffy coat preparations. Cultures should be maintained for 4–6 weeks with weekly transfers of supernatant to fresh cultures. Characteristic CPE include multinucleated syncytial cells and eosinophilic intracytoplasmic and intranuclear viral inclusions.

g. TREATMENT. No specific treatment is available. Epizootics in macaques have been controlled by the infusion of exposed animals with human γ-globulin and vaccination with modified live vaccine (Roberts *et al.,* 1988).

h. PREVENTION. Infant macaques are vaccinated at 3 months of age or older with a modified live vaccine. A second dose given no sooner than 6 weeks produces protective antibody levels. Adult animals in quarantine are vaccinated with a single dose.

i. ZOONOTIC POTENTIAL. A macaque to human transmission has been demonstrated (Roberts *et al.,* 1988).

2. *Paramyxovirus saguinus*

a. INTRODUCTION. A single outbreak of infectious gastroenteritis was diagnosed in cotton-topped tamarins (*Sanguinus oedipus*), red-chested moustached tamarins (*S. labiatus*), black-chested moustached tamarins (*S. mystax*), and common marmosets (*Callithrix jacchus*) at the New England Regional Primate Research Center in 1977 (Fraser *et al.,* 1978).

b. ETIOLOGY. A virus isolated from the spleen of a terminally ill tamarin was identified and used to infect four *S. oedipus* that later developed characteristic lesions and died. The virus was closely related to, but antigenically distinct from, measles virus. Although the exact relationship to measles virus is unknown, the causative agent likely represents a variant of measles virus (Hunt and Blake, 1993b).

c. EPIZOOTIOLOGY. The origin of infection in these animals is unknown. Virus was shed in the feces and a fecal–oral route of transmission seems likely.

d. PATHOGENESIS AND PATHOLOGY. Pathogenesis likely parallels measles virus infection in nonhuman primates. Affected animals had moderate to severe necrotizing colitis and typhilitis with multinucleated syncytial cells present within crypts. Similar syncytial cells were present in pancreatic acini, renal tubules, and hepatic cords. A striking change was the presence of large syncytial cells containing up to 20–25 nuclei and intracytoplasmic viral inclusions within bile duct epithelium. Lymphoid necrosis within germinal centers was evident. No exanthema was recognized, and in contrast to measles virus infection of macaques, lesions were absent in the lungs and brain.

e. CLINICAL FINDINGS. Clinically there was acute onset of anorexia, dehydration, and diarrhea, which progressed rapidly to death. Colony mortality of *S. oedipus* was approximately 10% and approached 100% in *S. mystax* and *S. labiatus* (Hollander and VanNoord, 1972).

f. TREATMENT. No specific treatment is available.

PNEUMOVIRINAE

1. Pneumoviruses: Respiratory Syncytial Virus

a. INTRODUCTION. Respiratory syncytial virus (RSV) was first isolated from a chimpanzee with coryza in 1956 (Morris *et al.,* 1956). Subsequently, this agent has been shown to be an important cause of mild to severe respiratory disease in children worldwide.

b. ETIOLOGY. Respiratory syncytial virus is a single-stranded RNA virus 90–130 nm in diameter. Individual isolates of RSV, in general, have a broad host range.

c. EPIZOOTIOLOGY. The virus is highly contagious and is spread through aerosols. Anti-RSV antibodies are widespread in human and nonhuman primate populations (Richardson-Wyatt *et al.,* 1981). Nonhuman primates likely become infected through human contact.

d. PATHOGENESIS AND PATHOLOGY.   Neutralizing antibodies (IgG) are nonprotective and may predispose individuals to more severe disease through the deposition of immune complexes within pulmonary vessels. Conversely, IgA is protective. The disease is often more severe in children within the first months of life due to the persistence of maternal antibodies (IgG not IgA). Similarly, in a clinical study of children, parenteral inoculation with killed vaccine was found to exacerbate and prolong infection as a consequence of the production of neutralizing antibodies.

In more severe cases, disease is characterized by a necrotizing bronchiolitis to bronchopneumonia. Multinucleated syncytial cells with intracytoplasmic inclusion bodies may be apparent. Lethal episodes are invariably associated with diffuse alveolar damage and microvascular thrombosis, which are characteristic of the acute respiratory distress syndrome (ARDS).

e. CLINICAL FINDINGS.   In nonhuman primates, the disease is mild and is characterized by nonspecific upper respiratory signs, including coughing, sneezing, and mucopurulent oculonasal discharge. A single fatal case has been described in a juvenile chimpanzee associated with an epizootic of mild upper respiratory tract infection in the remaining members of the colony (Clarke *et al.,* 1994).

f. LABORATORY FINDINGS.   Rapid detection of RSV antigen in nasopharyngeal secretions of affected human infants using a direct immunofluorescent test has been described (Choa *et al.,* 1979). Viral isolation may be made on Hep-2 cells or rhesus monkey kidney cells and identified by immunofluorescent staining techniques (Henrickson *et al.,* 1984). CPE is characterized by syncytial formation 1–14 days postinoculation.

g. PREVENTION.   Vaccination by the parenteral route is not recommended because neutralizing antibodies (IgG) may predispose to more severe disease.

E. Togaviridae

Togaviridae are single-stranded, positive-sense RNA viruses that are 70 nm in diameter with a lipid envelope and peplomers composed of a heterodimer of two glycoproteins. The Togaviridae family contains two genera (*Alphavirus* and *Rubivirus*) (Table IV) and numerous human pathogens, including eastern equine encephalitis, western equine encephalitis, Sindbis virus, Chikungunya virus, and rubella virus. *Arterivirus* is a floating genus variably placed in the Togaviridae or Coronaviridae family. Although its exact taxonomic location remains to be determined, it does contain the simian hemorrhagic fever virus, a significant pathogen to nonhuman primates.

ARTERIVIRUS

Arteriviruses represent a new genus of positive-stranded RNA viruses, including simian hemorrhagic fever virus, equine

TABLE IV

Family	Genus	Virus
Togaviridae	*Arterivirus*	Simian hemorrhagic fever virus
	Alphavirus	Chikungunya virus
		Mayaro fever
Flaviridae	*Flavivirus*	Yellow fever virus
		Kyasanur Forest disease virus
		Dengue virus
	Pestivirus	
	Hepatitis C-like viruses	Hepatitis C virus
		GB virus A, B, and C

arteritis virus, lactate dehydrogenase-elevating virus of mice and porcine infertility, and respiratory syndrome virus. Although initially considered a member of the family Togaviridae, this relationship is uncertain and viruses may be more closely related to Coronaviridae.

1. Simian Hemorrhagic Fever Virus

a. INTRODUCTION.   Simian hemorrhagic fever virus (SHFV) is a highly contagious, fatal infectious disease of rhesus macaques. It was first recognized in 1964 simultaneously at the National Institutes of Health (Bethesda, MD) and at the Sukhumi Institute (USSR) (Abildgaard *et al.,* 1975; Palmer *et al.,* 1968; Allen *et al.,* 1968). It must be distinguished from other viruses capable of causing hemorrhagic fevers.

b. ETIOLOGY.   Simian hemorrhagic fever is a single-stranded RNA virus 40–45 nm in diameter. It may be grown on primary macaque macrophage cultures and on the MA-104 embryonic African green monkey kidney cell line (Tauraso *et al.,* 1968). Diagnostic ultrastructural changes become apparent after 24–72 hr in these cells and include the formation of unique lamellar replicative structures.

c. EPIZOOTIOLOGY.   Simian hemorrhagic virus has been shown to naturally infect several African species, including patas monkeys (*Erythrocebus patas*), African green monkeys (*Cercopithecus aethiops*), and baboons (*Papio anubus* and *P. cynocephalus*). Of these, *E. patas* represents the most important reservoir and the greatest risk to macaques. In these species, infection is usually asymptomatic and reportedly animals may be viremic and seronegative (Gravell *et al.,* 1980b). Several strains of SHFV have been identified in Patas monkeys, which vary in their ability to cause clinical disease, persistent infection, and antibody response (Gravell *et al.,* 1986b). Interestingly, *E. patas* monkeys persistently infected and unable to mount an antibody response are able to clear infection when inoculated with a more virulent strain capable of inducing acute disease (Gravell *et al.,* 1986a).

Transmission to Asian macaques results in a fulminant and fatal infection characterized by a bleeding diathesis and rapid progression to death. Initial infection of macaques appears to require parental exposure to infected blood or tissue from carrier species. Once established, the virus is highly contagious and may then be spread from macaque to macaque by aerosolization, direct contact, or fomites (Renquist, 1990).

d. PATHOGENESIS AND PATHOLOGY. *i* Macaques: At necropsy there is striking locally extensive congestion, hemorrhage, and necrosis of the proximal duodenum. Similar foci are found randomly distributed throughout the gastrointestinal tract and in the liver, renal capsule, retrobulbar tissue, subcutis, and lung. The spleen is enlarged two to three times normal and the white pulp may not be visible grossly.

Microscopically, characteristic lesions are found in lymphoid tissue. Extensive lymphoid necrosis and congestion exist within the spleen. Prominent perifollicular hemorrhages are often separated from the subjacent follicular mantle by a fibrinous exudate (Allen *et al.*, 1968). Sinuses may be distended by fibrin and plasma. Necrosis of germinal centers in other lymphoid tissues is prominent. Complete cortical thymic necrosis with sparing of the medulla is reportedly unique to SHF infection (Zack, 1993). Lesions elsewhere are compatible with those associated with disseminated intravascular coagulation and include deposition of fibrin thrombi within glomeruli, hepatic sinusoids, and lung. Lesions within the small intestine consist of extensive hemorrhage within the lamina propria accompanied by intestinal epithelial cell necrosis. As with other arteriviruses, fetal loss is common. A lymphohistiocytic meningoencephalitis is present in a minority of animals. Macrophages represent the principal target cell of SHFV infection, and the unique sensitivity of macaques to this viral infection relates to the propensity of their macrophages to support viral growth (Gravell *et al.*, 1980a).

The absence of hepatic and/or adrenal necrosis in conjunction with the previously described findings is highly suggestive of SHF. Their presence suggests possible infection with Ebola virus, Ebola-like viruses, Marburg virus, or Kyasanur Forest disease virus. Additional distinguishing features of Ebola Reston virus are intracytoplasmic inclusion bodies and patchy interstitial pneumonia.

ii African Monkeys: Simian hemorrhagic fever virus infection of *E. patas, C. aethiops,* and *Papio* spp. is generally asymptomatic. In patas monkeys, the viral strain appears to play a critical role in determining the disease course (Gravell *et al.*, 1986a). Viral strains LVR and P-180, both of which induce lytic infection of patas monkey peritoneal macrophages, may induce an acute and rarely fatal disease in this species. Animals frequently were febrile and showed anorexia, lethargy, facial edema, and dehydration. Small subcutaneous hemorrhages were noted occasionally. These viral strains induced a strong antibody response and did not result in persistent infection. In contrast, viral strains that did not result in lytic infection of patas monkey peritoneal macrophages were more likely to result in asymptomatic infection, poor antibody response, and persistent infection.

e. CLINICAL FINDINGS. Following experimental inoculation of macaques there is an incubation period of 3–7 days. Initially a fever without other clinical signs is recognized followed shortly by a bleeding diathesis (epistaxis, hematuria, melena, ecchymoses and petechiae). In the terminal stages, depression, dehydration, photophobia, and cyanosis are present. The entire clinical course may last from 1 to 7 days (Palmer *et al.*, 1968). Animals may die without obvious clinical signs.

f. LABORATORY FINDINGS. Fibrin degradation products may become elevated as early as 24–48 hr postexperimental inoculation (Abildgaard *et al.*, 1975). There is an increase in aspartate aminotransferase, alanine aminotransferase, and lactate dehydrogenase at the onset of clinical signs. The coagulopathy is characterized by thrombocytopenia and prolonged partial thromboplastin times. Proteinuria and hematuria may be noted on urinalysis.

g. TREATMENT. No treatment is available. A summary of control measures has been published and should be instituted at the first evidence of an epizootic hemorrhagic disease in macaques (Zack, 1993; Gravell *et al.*, 1986b). This multifaceted approach includes (1) elimination of clinically ill and exposed animals, (2) quarantine of remaining animals, (3) disinfection of premises, (4) diagnostic efforts to identify the etiologic agent, (5) notification of appropriate government agencies, and (6) monitoring of human contacts.

h. PREVENTION. Exposure of macaques to African primates and their blood and tissue products should be prevented. When *E. patas* and macaques are housed within the same facility, special precautions should be taken to prevent inadvertent exposure. Serology is reportedly of no value in determining which African primates carry the virus.

i. ZOONOTIC POTENTIAL. There is no evidence that simian hemorrhagic fever virus is a zoonosis. A major concern is that the clinical signs of this disease in macaques mimics several other diseases (Ebola virus, Ebola-like virus, yellow fever virus, Marburg virus, and Kyasanur Forest virus) that may infect human beings with lethal consequences. As such, all macaques exhibiting these clinical signs should be treated as if infected with a potentially lethal zoonotic agent.

F. Flaviviridae

The family Flaviridae (Table IV) encompasses greater than 70 distinct viruses, many of which are important pathogens of humans and animals. In humans, pathogenic flaviviruses characteristically produce meningoencephalitis (e.g., Japanese encephalitis, St. Louis encephalitis) or a hemorrhagic fever syndrome (e.g., yellow fever, dengue). Although many of these viruses are transmitted by arthropod vectors (ticks and mosquitoes), some may be transmitted directly among mammalian hosts. Based on differences within the envelope protein, eight antigenic subgroups and a number of unassigned viruses are recognized. The number of identified flaviviruses is rapidly expanding and the pathogenicity of most for nonhuman primates is unknown. Two novel and distinct Flaviviridae (designated GBV-A and GBVB) have been identified in tamarins inoculated with the serially passaged "GB agent."

1. Yellow Fever Virus

a. INTRODUCTION.   Yellow fever is a devastating viral disease of humans and New World primate species that is transmitted by a variety of mosquito vectors. It is thought that yellow fever virus originated in Africa and was spread to the New World in the 16th and 17th centuries through cross Atlantic trade routes. Once established in native mosquitoes, its introduction was associated with devastating epidemics and epizootics in humans and indigenous nonhuman primates.

b. EPIZOOTIOLOGY.   Yellow fever virus infects forest and bush-living mosquitoes, including *Aedes* spp., *Haemagogus* spp., and *Sabethes* spp., with which it commensally exists. In *A. aegypti* the virus may persist through the dry season by transovarian transmission. The mosquito represents the reservoir host and largely determines the geographic distribution and persistence of the virus in nature.

Yellow fever virus has been shown to infect a variety of primate species. In African species, infection is associated with viremia but few clinical signs and is eliminated with rising neutralizing antibodies generally within 6 days. Wild hosts that support this sylvatic cycle reportedly include baboons (*Papio* sp.), mangabeys (*Cerocebus* sp.), chimpanzees (*Pan* sp.), red colobus monkeys (*Pilocolubus badius*), African green monkeys (*Cercopithecus* spp.), and patas monkeys (*Erythrocebus patas*). Viremia in these animals serves to propagate the virus in vector species and may initiate the urban cycle when transmission to peridomestic mosquitoes such as *A. aegypti* occurs. Once established in mosquito species that feed on humans, epidemics may become established in human populations.

In New World primates, the disease is more severe and epizootics have been described in howler monkeys (*Aloutta* spp.), spider monkeys (*Ateles* spp.), and squirrel monkeys (*Saimiri sciureus*) and may coincide with cases in adjacent human populations. Capuchin monkeys (*Cebus* spp.) and wooly monkeys (*Lagothrix* spp.) may be less susceptible. In tropical South America, human infection generally results from inadvertent exposure of individuals to the sylvatic cycle. With the reduction of *A. aegypti* populations, an urban cycle is currently not recognized.

c. PATHOGENESIS AND PATHOLOGY.   Althogh yellow fever is not found naturally in Asia, experimental inoculation of ma-caques is associated with a rapidly lethal disease that models many of the features present in fatal human cases. As such, much of what is known about the pathogenesis of yellow fever virus infection has been determined in this experimental setting (Klotz and Belt, 1930a,b; Hudson, 1928; Monath *et al.*, 1981).

Following inoculation, initial rounds of replication occur in the regional lymph nodes, with rapid dissemination to multiple organs. While neurotropic and viscerotropic strains are recognized, the viscerotropism of the virus accounts for the cardinal clinical signs. During the initial phase of viremia, virus is visualized first within Kupffer cells and subsequently with hepatocytes. Disseminated intravascular coagulation and depletion of vitamin K-dependent clotting factors contribute to the recognized bleeding diathesis.

Histologically, lesions in the liver are characterized by multifocal hepatocellular necrosis with the formation of Council-man bodies and Torres bodies (Bearcroft, 1960, 1962). These changes are invariably accompanied by the fatty degeneration of the remaining hepatocytes. Lymphoid depletion within germinal centers and splenic arterial sheaths may be prominent. Although not a natural disease of macaques, clinical and pathologic findings following experimental inoculation are remarkably similar to syndromes caused by other hemorrhagic fever agents such as simian hemorrhagic fever virus and Ebola-like viruses.

d. CLINICAL FINDINGS.   Infection of African species is asymptomatic. Natural infection of New World nonhuman primates is generally recognized by an increased mortality in susceptible species and may accompany human cases in the geographical vicinity.

e. PREVENTION.   Yellow fever is primarily a disease of wild nonhuman primates. Because there is a short incubation period and no carrier state is established, the risk of capture and importation of infected animals is relatively low. Nevertheless it should be considered in the differential diagnosis of hemorrhagic fever in endemic regions and in recently imported primates.

2. Kyasanur Forest Disease Virus

Kyasanur Forest disease was first recognized in March of 1957 as a cause of increased mortality in langurs (*Presbytis entellus*) and bonnet macaques (*Macaca radiata*) (Iyer *et al.*, 1959, 1960). Subsequent investigations demonstrated a concurrent illness in adjacent human populations. The virus has been isolated from a variety of ixodid ticks, including *Haemaphysalis spinigera, H. turturis,* and *loxdes petauristae* (Singh *et al.*, 1963). In addition, the virus has been isolated from rodents and bats from the endemic region.

The disease in nonhuman primates is characterized by multifocal hepatocellular necrosis accompanied by hemorrhages within the adrenal gland, brain, kidney, and lung. There is prominent leukopenia, anemia, and thrombocytopenia (Webb and Chatterjea, 1962). In humans, the disease may produce mild nonspecific signs or a fulminant hemorrhagic disease with high mortality.

3. Dengue Viruses; Serotypes 1–4

Dengue viruses are important causes of human hemorrhagic fever in tropical and subtropical regions worldwide. Free-ranging nonhuman primates populations, including cynomolgus monkeys (*Macaca fascicularis*), Toque macaques (*M. sinica*), and brow-ridged langurs [*Trachypithecus (Presbytis) cristatus* and *T. obscura*], may have a high rate of seroreactivity, indicating widespread exposure (Rudnik, 1965; Rodhain, 1991; Peiris *et al.,* 1993). Neutralizing antibodies have been demonstrated in nonhuman primates in association with an epidemic in Nigeria. As with yellow fever, a sylvatic cycle involving *Aedes* spp. mosquitoes and nonhuman primates and an urban cycle in which the disease is spread among the human population are postulated to occur.

Experimental infection of *Macaca* spp., *Cercopithecus* spp., *Cercocebus* spp., and *Papio* spp. produced viremia but was not associated with clinical signs (Halstead, 1981). In experimental settings, vaccination is protective against challenge with homologous virus (Halstead *et al.,* 1973; Halstead and Palumbo, 1973). The significance of dengue virus infection of wild nonhuman primates is unknown.

4. GB Agent Viruses: GBV-A, GBV-B, and GBV-C

Two novel viruses have been identified by subtractive polymerase chain reaction (PCR) in tamarins infected with the serially passaged "GB agent" (Simons *et al.,* 1995; Schlauder *et al.,* 1995a). This agent was first identified in the mid-1960s when serum from a human patient with acute hepatitis was inoculated into four marmosets that subsequently developed a nonsuppurative portal hepatitis (Deinhardt *et al.,* 1967). At the time, investigators questioned whether the agent identified in marmosets represented a human pathogen or reactivation of an indigenous marmoset virus (Parks and Melnick, 1969). These agents are closely related to hepatitis C virus of humans and share similar genomic organization and replication strategies. They are single-stranded, positive-sense RNA viruses with a 9.5-kb genome encoding a single polyprotein that is cleaved by cellular and viral proteaes.

Molecular techniques have identified two distinct viruses (designated GBV-A and GBV-B) in tamarins infected with pooled marmoset plasma from the original studies. Furthermore, a third virus (GBV-C) with close homology to GBV-A has been found in human hepatitis patients. Reactive sera to GBV-C have been identified in intravenous drug abusers and asymptomatic blood donors in the United States; however, the relationship of this virus to clinical disease in humans remains to be determined (Zuckerman, 1995). Moreover, PCR using primers directed against the 5' end of GBV-A has identified GBV-A sequences within tamarins not exposed to the GB agent, suggesting that the virus may be more widespread than origi-

nally thought (Schlauder *et al.,* 1995b). Distinct GBV-A viral sequences have been detected in *Sanguinus labiatus, S. oedipus, S. mystax, Aotus trivirgatus,* and *Callithrix jacchus.* The origin and importance of GBV-like agents to wild and captive marmosets are presently unclear.

G. Arenaviridae

Arenaviruses are pleomorphic, enveloped viruses 110–130 μm in diameter containing two segments of RNA that encode at least three gene products. A characteristic biological feature of arenaviruses is lifelong viral persistence within the definitive rodent host. The persistently infected host sheds the virus in urine and body secretions which then contaminate the environment and play a critical role in the transmission to the inadvertent (primate) host. A number of arenaviruses have been identified, often with restricted geographic distribution (Table V). Although some have been responsible for devastating human epidemics, the factors responsible for these outbreaks are poorly understood.

1. Callithrichid Hepatitis Virus: Lymphocytic Choriomeningitis Virus

a. INTRODUCTION. A rapidly progressive viral hepatitis occurring in zoological collections has been characterized (Montali *et al.,* 1989). Outbreaks have been reported in golden lion tamarins (*Leontopithecus rosalia*), emperor marmosets (*Sanguineous imperator*), common marmosets (*Callithrix jacchus*), cotton-topped tamarins (*Saguinus oedipus*), white-fronted tamarins (*S. nigricollis*), saddle-backed tamarins (*Cebuella pygmaea*), and Goeldi's monkeys (*Calimico goeldi*) (Montali, 1993; Potkay, 1992).

b. ETIOLOGY. The etiologic agent is lymphocytic choriomengingitis virus (LCMV). This arenavirus is pleomorphic and 85–105 nm in diameter and has been identified within cytoplasmic vesicles of affected animals (Montali, 1993). Several hemorrhagic fevers in humans may be caused by similar arenaviruses (Machupo, Junin, and Lassa fever viruses). Although callithrichid hepatitis has been limited to the above species, macaques are susceptible to experimental infection

TABLE V

ARENAVIRIDAE

Complex	Virus
LCM-Lassa	Lymphocytic choriomeningitis virus
	Lassa fever virus
	Mopeia virus
	Mobala virus
Tacaribe	Junin virus (Argentine hemorrhagic fever)
	Machupo virus (Bolivian fever)

with Lassa fever virus and therefore a wider species susceptibility may be anticipated.

c. EPIZOOTIOLOGY.   Animals become infected through ingestion of infected mice. The virus may be introduced to colonies by either wild mice or the intentional feeding of neonatal laboratory mice ("pinkies") (Montali *et al.,* 1995). Clinical disease is limited to those animals that have ingested mice and may become apparent within 1–2 weeks of infection. The attack rate and mortality rate may be high. Serologic evidence of infection of captive marmosets without recognized clinical signs has been demonstrated (Potkay, 1992).

d. CLINICAL FINDINGS.   Clinical signs include dyspnea, anorexia, weakness, and lethargy. Animals may be jaundiced and evidence of coagulopathy may be apparent. In many cases there is sudden death without clinical signs.

e. PATHOGENESIS AND PATHOLOGY.   At necropsy, hepatosplenomegaly, pleural and pericardial effusions, jaundice, and subcutaneous and intramuscular hemorrhages are characteristic (Montali, 1993). Histopathologic lesions within the liver consist of multifocal hepatic necrosis with infiltration by lymphocytes and neutrophils. Acidophilic bodies representing apoptotic hepatocytes are prominent and may be found in hepatic sinusoids or within Kupffer cells (Fig. 19) (Montali, 1993). The LCMV antigen and mRNA have been identified within hepatocytes, suggesting that direct viral infection may be responsible for the observed hepatocellular necrosis (Montali *et al.,* 1995). In addition, necrosis may be evident in the abdominal lymph nodes, adrenal gland, spleen, and gastrointestinal tract (Montali *et al.,* 1989).

f. LABORATORY FINDINGS.   Elevations in liver enzymes, bilirubin, and serum alkaline phosphatase have been demonstrated.

g. TREATMENT.   Treatment directed at correcting hypovolemia and electrolyte disturbances may be of some benefit. Ribavirin therapy in macaques inoculated with the related Junin, Machupo, and Lassa fever viruses has shown some efficacy. The pharmacokinetics and safety of these drugs in marmosets are unknown.

h. PREVENTION.   Screening of food source rodent colonies for LCMV and preventing contact with wild rodents should prevent disease transmission. Biologics of murine origin should be screened for the presence of LCMV before use in tamarins or marmosets.

i. ZOONOTIC POTENTIAL.   Lymphocytic choriomengingitis virus may cause disease in humans. Seroconversion of veterinarians in contact with infected marmosets has been demonstrated (Montali *et al.,* 1995).

2. Bolivian Hemorrhagic Fever Virus: Machupo Virus

Machupo virus is an arenavirus related to the Tacaribe–LCM complex and has been responsible for epidemics of hemor-

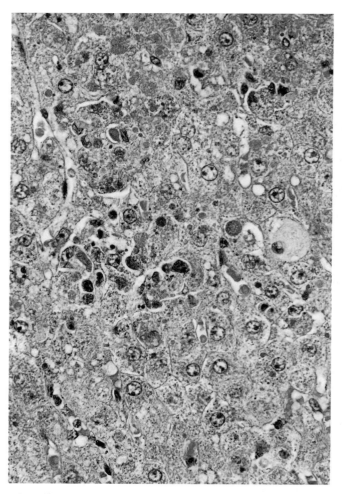

Fig. 19. Lymphocytic choriomeningitis virus. Hepatocellular necrosis (Callitrichid hepatitis).

rhagic fever in Central and South America. The susceptibility and importance of nonhuman primates in natural disease are unknown. Rhesus macques (*Macaca mulatta*), Geoffrey's marmoset (*Saguinus geoffrioy*), and African green monkeys (*Cercopithecus aethiops*) may be experimentally infected with the Machupo virus. In these species it causes a severe, disseminated infection involving the central nervous system, gastrointestinal tract, and lungs. Hemorrhages are found in the skin, liver, oral cavity, and adrenal cortex. The virus has been isolated from rodents within the Muridae and Cricetidae families.

H. Retroviridae

PRIMATE T-CELL LEUKEMIA–BOVINE LEUKEMIA VIRUS GROUP

The primate T-cell leukemia (PTLV)–bovine leukemia virus group is a subgroup of the oncornaviruses that share a common ancestory, genomic organization, and propensity to induce lymphoproliferative disease in the host animal. The association between human T-cell leukemia virus and various disease processes has raised interest in closely related simian viruses. Analysis of a STLV-1 isolate obtained from a pig-tailed macaque (*M. nemestrina*) revealed 90% homology with the env-px-LTR region of HTLV-1 (Watanbe *et al.*, 1985), and analysis of further sequence data from a number of isolates strongly suggests a nonhuman primate origin of HTLV-1 (Sakesena *et al.*, 1994).

1. Simian T-Cell Leukemia Virus

a. INTRODUCTION. Simian T-cell leukemia virus (STLV-1) is a type C retrovirus closely related to human T-cell leukemia virus type 1 (HTLV). Human T-cell leukemia virus type 1 is endemic in Japan and the Caribbean basin and is associated with adult T-cell leukemia/lymphoma (ATLL) and tropical spastic paresis, a demyelinating disorder. As in human patients with HTLV-1, STLV-1 has been associated with lymphoproliferative disease in baboons (*Papio* spp.), gorillas (*Gorilla gorilla*), macaques (*Macaca* spp.), and African green monkeys (*Cercopithecus* spp.) (McCarthy *et al.*, 1990; Traina-Dorge *et al.*, 1992; Lee *et al.*, 1985). Although overt neoplastic disease is an uncommon sequela to infection of some species, STLV-1 agents immortalize T cells *in vitro* and their presence may complicate the interpretation of experimental protocols.

b. ETIOLOGY. Seroreactivity to STLV-1 or STLV-like agents has been demonstrated in at least 33 species of captive and wild African and Asian nonhuman primate species, including *Cercopithecus* spp., *Macaca* spp., Patas monkey (*Erythrocebus patas*), olive baboon (*Papio anubis*), mandrill (*Mandrillis sphinx*), gorilla (*Gorilla gorilla*), and siamang (*Hylobates syndaclytes*) (Ishikawa *et al.*, 1987; Hayami *et al.*, 1984; Sakakibara *et al.*, 1986). Restriction patterns of initial STLV-1 isolates suggested that a number of distinct but related viruses were contained within the STLV grouping. Sequencing data have confirmed the existence of seven clusters or clades. The S1 clade contains Asian STLVs, whereas S2–S7 clades contain African STLV isolates. It is postulated that this diversity is due to repeated cross-species transmission within restricted geographic localities. Moreover, it suggests that STLV-1 has been present in nonhuman primate populations longer than HTLV-1 has been in humans and a possible STLV origin of HTLV-1. The relative species specificity of various isolates and their ability to induce lymphoproliferative disease in the aberrant host are largely unknown.

c. EPIZOOTIOLOGY. Serologic surveys indicate a high rate of infection in many wild and captive African green monkeys, macaques, and baboons. These surveys indicate an increasing prevalence with age and while the mechanism of natural transmission is unknown, parenteral and sexual routes are suspected of being of greater importance than perinatal transmission.

d. PATHOGENESIS AND PATHOLOGY. Although STLV-1 is a common and usually asymptomatic infection, it has been associated with lymphoproliferative disease in several nonhuman primate species. This has perhaps been best characterized in baboons (McCarthy *et al.*, 1990; Voevodin *et al.*, 1985; Hubbard *et al.*, 1993). In this species, STLV-1 infection has been linked to the development of an ATLL-like syndrome characterized by non-Hodgkin's lymphoma and leukemia. Involvement of the lymph nodes, spleen, liver, skin, and especially lung is common. Overt leukemia has been documented in greater than 50% of the cases and is occasionally associated with the presence of circulating multilobulated neoplastic lymphocytes, a clinical feature of ATLL (McCarthy *et al.*, 1990). Unlike human patients with ATLL, hypercalcemia is uncommon. Within the lung, the earliest changes may be present in a perivascular and/or peribronchiolar distribution. Although a variety of cell types have been recognized, most cases have been of T-cell lineage ($CD2^+CD4^+$). Histologically, the infiltrate varies from a monomorphic population of neoplastic lymphocytes to a more pleomorphic population accompanied by multinucleated giant cells, necrosis, and inflammatory cells.

Although STLV-1 is clearly associated with lymphoproliferative disease, the mechanism involved is not completely understood. The *tax* gene product stimulates transcription of viral mRNA by acting on the 5' LTR and is highly conserved among all PTLV isolates, suggesting a fundamental role in viral replication and disease pathogenesis (Sakesena *et al.*, 1994). In addition to stimulating the 5' LTR, *tax* may activate host genes responsible for controlling T-cell proliferation, including c-*fos*, c-*sis*, interleukin-2 (IL-2), IL-2r, and GM-CSF, thereby leading to polyclonal T-cell expansion. It is postulated that secondary events are required for monoclonal neoplastic transformation. Monoclonal integration of STLV-1 has been demonstrated in African green monkeys with non-Hodgkin's lymphoma and preneoplastic lymphoproliferative disease (Tsujimoto *et al.*, 1987). Such integration is considered definitive evidence of the etiologic role of PTLV in lymphomagenesis. Coinfection with other viral agents such as SIV or Epstein–Barr-like viruses may promote neoplastic transformation (Traina-Dorge *et al.*, 1992; Voevodin *et al.*, 1985).

e. CLINICAL FINDINGS. Simian T-cell leukemia virus-associated lymphoma/leukemia in baboons is clinically characterized by depression, anorexia, regional or generalized lymph node enlargement, and hepatosplenomegaly. As in humans with ATLL, radiographic and histologic evidences of pulmonary infiltrates are frequent. Cutaneous involvement, hypercalcemia, and effusions may be noted less commonly. Leukocytosis and multilobulated neoplastic cells within peripheral blood smears are present with the majority but not all cases.

f. PREVENTION. A two-stage testing algorithm to evaluate macaque sera for the presence of antibodies to STLV-I has been published (Lerche *et al.*, 1994). Samples are initially screened by enzyme immunoassay (EIA), and negative results indicate a

TABLE VI
SIMIAN TYPE D RETROVIRUSES

TABLE VI

SIMIAN TYPE D RETROVIRUSES

Classification	Host	Ref.
Endogenous		
Squirrel monkey retrovirus	*S. saimiri*	Heberling *et al.* (1977)
PO-1-Lu	*Presbytis obscurus*	Todaro *et al.* (1978)
Exogenous		
Simian retrovirus type 1 (SRV-1)	*Macaca* sp.	
Simian retrovirus type 2 (SRV-2)	*Macaca* sp.	
Mason–Pfizer monkey virus (SRV-3)	*Macaca* sp.	Chopra and Mason (1970)
Simian retrovirus type 4 (SRV-4)	*Macaca fascicularis*	
Simian retrovirus type 5 (SRV-5)	*Macaca mulatta*	

provisional virus-free status. Positive results are further tested by confirmatory Western blot, and reacting animals are culled or segregated from the colony. The remaining animals are subsequently retested by EIA. Using this technique, seroconversion in the provisional virus-free group was rare (<0.01%), indicating that in this setting the occurrence of seronegative virus-positive animals is uncommon (Lerche *et al.*, 1994).

2. Other Simian T-Cell Leukemia Viruses

A virus closely related to HTLV-II and designated STLV-II has been identified and isolated from a spider monkey (*Ateles fusciceps*) (Chen *et al.*, 1994). This virus, the first STLV-like agent identified in a New World primate, has not yet been linked to disease in this species. Sequence analysis of the px-II region reveals 3% divergence from HTLV-II and its true relationship to this virus is presently unclear.

Two additional STLVs have been isolated from *Papio hamadryas* and *Pan paniscus* and are designated STLVph969 and STLVpan-p, respectively (Goubau *et al.*, 1994). These viruses are highly divergent from STLV-I, HTLV-I, and HTLV-II and are presently not associated with clinical disease in these species, suggesting that additional STLV-like agents may be identified in African primates.

3. Other Type C Retroviruses

Many additional exogenous and endogenous type C retroviruses have been identified in nonhuman primates.

A simian sarcoma virus was isolated from a spontaneous fibrosarcoma of a pet woolly monkey (*Lagothrix* spp.) (Wolfe *et al.*, 1972). Further investigation revealed the isolate to be composed of two agents; a defective transforming virus (simian sarcoma virus, SSV-1) and a replication competent helper virus

(simian sarcoma-associated virus, SSAV-1) (Theilen *et al.*, 1971; Wolfe *et al.*, 1972). When injected intracerebrally into newborn marmosets, animals developed gliomas from which virus could be recovered and identified (Johnson *et al.*, 1975).

Gibbon ape leukemia virus (GALV) has been isolated from a number of captive gibbons (*Hylobates* spp.) with spontaneous hematopoietic neoplasms. Various isolates have been identified (GALV, GALV-1, GALV-SEATO, GBr-1, and Gbr-3) with differing abilities to induce malignant lymphoma and leukemia. Clinical aspects of a spontaneous epizootic in white-handed gibbons (*Hylobates lar*) have been reported and are characterized by a prolonged clinical course, a marked elevation in the peripheral granulocyte count, and involvement of bone marrow, liver, lymph nodes, and spleen (DePaoli *et al.*, 1973). As described later for type D retrovirus infections of macaques, gibbons may not seroconvert following persistent infection with this virus.

TYPE D RETROVIRUSES

a. INTRODUCTION. During the 1960s and 1970s, several regional primate research centers located in the United States experienced epizootics of malignant lymphoma and immunosuppressive disease (Smith *et al.*, 1973; Stowell *et al.*, 1971; King *et al.*, 1983; Hunt *et al.*, 1983; Henrickson *et al.*, 1983). At the time these epizootics were suspected to be the result of an underlying simian viral infection. The issue remained unresolved until the early 1980s, when spurred by a burgeoning epidemic of immunodeficiency in homosexual men, investigators simultaneously identified two agents capable of inducing immunosuppressive disease in macaques. The first virus, a member of the Oncovirinae, was identified and designated simian retrovirus type D (SRV/D) (Marx *et al.*, 1984; Gravell *et al.*, 1984; Daniel *et al.*, 1984). The second, a member of the Lentivirinae, was designated simian immunodeficiency virus of macaques (SIVmac) (Daniel *et al.*, 1985; Letvin *et al.*, 1985). This primate lentivirus is closely related to the etiologic agent of human AIDS and has subsequently been the subject of intensive investigation as an animal model of the human condition. Because the type D retrovirus is more distantly related to the human immunodeficiency viruses than SIVmac, it has received far less attention than its lentivirus cousin. Although SIVmac may be of greater scientific interest as an animal model of human AIDS, SRV/D is clearly of greater significance in the management and care of captive macaques. As experience has shown, not only is SRV/D more difficult to eliminate from macaque colonies, it is also responsible for most cases of spontaneous viral-induced immunodeficiency in captive members of these species.

b. ETIOLOGY. Type D retroviruses are unique to nonhuman primates and exist as both endogenous and exogenous forms (Table VI). Endogenous virus sequences have been recognized in squirrel monkeys and spectacled langurs and are suspected in several species of colobines (Heberling *et al.*, 1977; Todaro

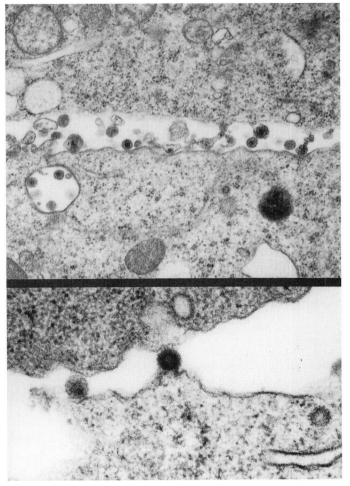

Fig. 20. Simian retrovirus type D.

TABLE VII

CHARACTERISTIC DIFFERENCES OF SIVMAC AND SRV/D INFECTION
OF MACAQUES

Characteristic	SIVmac	SRV/D
Natural host range	Related viruses endemic in several species of African monkeys	Endemic in several species of Asian macaques
Significance as natural disease in captive macaques	Serologic surveys indicate low prevalence	Most significant viral agent of acquired immunodeficiency in captive macaques
Occurrence of seronegative, viral positive infection	Uncommon in natural host	Common
Viral tropism	CD4+ T lymphocytes and macrophages	B and T lymphocytes, macrophages, and epithelial cells
Uniquely associated diseases	Giant cell pneumonia and encephalitis; SIV arteriopathy; lymphoma; *Mycobacterium avium*	Retroperitoneal and subcutaneous fibromatosis; noma

et al., 1978). The original type D retrovirus was isolated in 1970 from the mammary neoplasm of a female rhesus macaque and designated the Mason–Pfizer monkey virus (MPMV) (Chopra and Mason, 1970). Subsequent work indicated that this virus caused a wasting syndrome and thymic atrophy when inoculated into infant rhesus macaques and that approximately 25% of all macaques housed at U.S. regional primate research centers were seroreactive to MPMV or a closely related virus (Fine *et al.,* 1975; Fine and Arthur, 1981). It has since been demonstrated that the prototypic retrovirus, MPMV, is closely related to the more recently discovered SRV/D-1 and SRV/D-2 and that these viruses are the major cause of immunosuppressive disease in captive macaques (Fig. 20).

c. EPIZOOTIOLOGY. In contrast to SIVmac, type D retroviruses appear to be transmitted readily among captive macaques. SRV/D seropositive rates vary widely among colonies and likely relate to past husbandry and housing practices. Investigation of an epizootic of SRV/D in captive Celebes black ma-

caques (*Macaca nigra*) revealed an increase in the seropositive status from 0% to greater than 90% during an 8-year period following the introduction of several infected animals to the colony (Lerche *et al.,* 1986; Shiigi *et al.,* 1989).

SRV-1 may be isolated from the saliva of healthy carrier animals, and biting with inoculation of saliva or blood is the most likely method of horizontal transmission (Lerche *et al.,* 1986). Vertical transmission may play an additional role in the propagation of the virus within macaque colonies. Cesarian-derived infants raised in isolation may be infected (Tsai *et al.,* 1990). Moreover, mother to infant transmission may occur in the perinatal or postnatal period. Of fundamental importance to the design and implementation of control strategies is the fact that animals may be persistently infected, healthy, and shedding virus while seronegative for antibodies against SRV/D. It is these seronegative virus-positive individuals that frustrate control strategies. Evidence suggests that *in utero* infection may be more likely to result in this seronegative, virus-positive status than transmission at other times (Moazed and Thouless, 1993). These animals may play a key role in viral persistence within colonies.

d. PATHOGENESIS AND PATHOLOGY. Superficially there are many similarities between the immunosuppresive diseases induced in macaques by simian type D retroviruses and simian lentiviruses. There are, however, fundamental differences in their molecular biology and genomic organization that impart differences in the resulting clinical syndrome (Table VII). Type D retroviruses have a wider tissue tropism than simian lenti-

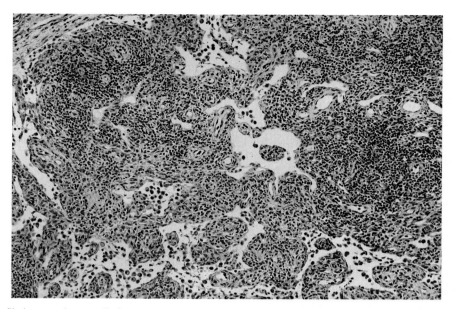

Fig. 21. Simian retrovirus type D. Severe lymphoid depletion, mesenteric lymph node, rhesus macaque (*Macaca mulatta*).

viruses and readily infect T cells (CD4 and CD8), B cells, macrophages, epithelial cells, and cells of the choroid plexus (Maul *et al.,* 1988; Lackner *et al.,* 1989).

The mechanism by which the type D retroviruses produce the severe immunosuppression characteristic of this disease is unknown. Animals may harbor the virus asymptomatically for extended periods with few or no clinical signs. In asymptomatic animals there may be generalized lymphadenopathy characterized by varying proportions of follicular and paracortical lymphocytic hyperplasia consisting of immature CD4$^+$ and CD8$^+$ T lymphocyte subsets. With the onset of severe immunosuppression, eventually the spleen, thymus, and lymph nodes evidence marked lymphoid depletion and complete effacement of normal architecture (Fig. 21). In these nodes the paracortex is often depleted of lymphocytes and plasma cells, which are largely replaced by histiocytes and contain small postreactive follicles with hyalinized arterioles (Osborn *et al.,* 1984). Animals then sucumb to a host of opportunistic infections.

i. Retroperitoneal Fibromatosis: In addition to a syndrome of immunosupressive disease, a unique fibroproliferative lesion has been recognized in association with SRV/D infection since 1976. Retroperitoneal fibromatosis is characteristically a multinodular to coalescent infiltrative process originating from the ileocecal junction and involving the root of the mesentery, mesenteric lymph nodes, and gastrointestinal tract (Fig. 22). It is most frequently associated with SRV/D serotype 2. This lesion rarely infiltrates parenchymal organs but may produce small nodules or plaques disseminated across mesothelial surfaces. In severe cases, the entire gastrointestinal tract may be encased in a large fibrotic mass. A localized subcutaneous fibro-

matosis has also been reported (Tsai *et al.,* 1985b). It is characterized by multiple proliferative nodules within the subcutis and oral cavity, has been described in pig-tailed macaques (*M. nemestrina*), and is most frequently associated with SRV/D serotype 1.

Sclerotic and proliferative patterns of fibromatosis have been recognized and may coexist within the same animal. Histologically, the proliferative lesion is composed of spindle-shaped cells arranged in intersecting fascicles that infiltrate along serosal surfaces and surround normal structures. A variable lymphoplasmacytic inflammatory reaction is usually present. The tissue

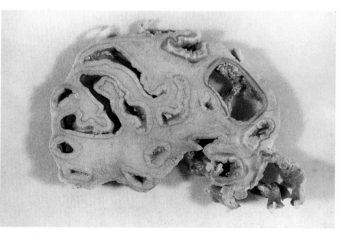

Fig. 22. Simian retrovirus type D. Retroperitoneal fibromatosis with entrapment of small bowel, rhesus macaque (*Macaca mulatta*).

is highly vascular and cells are embedded within a stromal network composed of collagen and reticulin. Absence of nuclear anaplasia and mitotic figures distinguish the lesion from fibrosarcoma. Although viral particles can be visualized by ultrastructural examination in proliferating cells in some lesions, their cell of origin is less clear. These cells are vimentin, desmin, and smooth muscle α-actin positive and reveal variable positivity for the factor VIII-related antigen (Tsai *et al.,* 1995). Currently an origin from vascular smooth muscle (pericyte) is favored.

Simian retrovirus type D-induced retroperitoneal fibromatosis has been suggested as an animal model of Kaposi's sarcoma, a disseminated often cutaneous malignancy in human AIDS patients. Because type D retroviruses and lentiviruses share little homology, this suggests that severe retroviral-induced immunodysregulation may promote the evolution of similar multicentric proliferative disorders, perhaps through alternate initiating events.

ii. Opportunistic Infections: The hallmark of the acquired immunodeficiency in macaques induced by both SRV/D and SIVmac is the occurrence of unusual opportunistic infections. Despite some similarities, there are, for reasons that are presently unclear, differences in the propensity of these viruses to induce disease by specific opportunistic organisms. Simian retrovirus type D-infected animals appear to be more susceptible to infection by pyogenic bacteria and less susceptible to infection by *Mycobacterium avium, Pneumocystis carinii,* SV40, and adenovirus. Moreover, SIV-specific lesions are lacking and the occurrence of overt lymphoma is uncommon in SRV/D-infected animals. Other common opportunistic infections include disseminated CMV, oral and esophageal candidiasis, intestinal cryptosporidiosis, and rapidly progressive necrotizing gingivitis and stomatitis known as noma (cancrum oris) (Lowenstine, 1993).

e. CLINICAL FINDINGS.   Simian retrovirus type D infection of rehsus macaques may be responsible for the induction of several clinical syndromes, including (1) the occurrence of severe immunodeficiency accompanied by viremia with or without an antibody response, (2) the occurrence of a persistent asymptomatic carrier state with or without an antibody response, (3) appropriate antibody response and clearance of infection, (4) retroperitoneal or subcutaneous fibromatosis, and (5) persistent lymphadenopathy (Lowenstine, 1993). These categories are not mutually exclusive and cooccurrence or progression may be seen.

The clinical features and AIDS definition of SRV/D infection are presented in Table VIII. Young animals often present for small body stature and failure to thrive. Body weight may be 40–50% of normal cagemates and these animals are often physically traumatized through intraspecies aggression. Intermittent to chronic gastroenterocolitis is common and results from direct viral infections of mucosal cells or damage induced by a variety of opportunistic organisms. Because the occurrence of an antibody-negative viremia is common in these young animals, diagnosis is best achieved through viral isolation of PCR. Alternatively, in cases in which serum or frozen tissue is not available, the virus may be visualized in formalin-fixed, paraffin-embedded tissue through the use of SRV/D specific probes and *in situ* hybridization. In older animals the illness is more insidious and while wasting may be conspicuous, clinical signs often relate to the specific opportunistic infections present. The occurrence of retroperitoneal fibromatosis is most common in 1- to 2-year-old animals and is rare in those less than 1 year of age (Tsai *et al.,* 1985a).

f. PREVENTION.   The establishment of SRV/D-free macaque colonies is paramount to the continued use of these animals in the many forms of biomedical research. This task has proven difficult primarily because macaques may be seronegative but harbor virus, thus necessitating the use of viral isolation or PCR to confirm virus-free status. Successful algorithms used to establish retrovirus-free breeding colonies have been published (Lerche *et al.,* 1994). This protocol utilizes combined viral isolation and antibody detection (EIA and Western blot) to screen all animals. Once established, colonies should be self-propagating and remain closed with periodic retesting to verify continued virus-free status.

LENTIVIRINAE:
SIMIAN IMMUNODEFICIENCY VIRUSES

a. INTRODUCTION.   Simian immunodeficiency viruses (SIVs) are a group of closely related viruses with the *Lentivirus* genus of the family Retroviridae, which infect a variety of Old World nonhuman primates (Table IX). The striking similarity between SIV-induced disease in macaques and HIV-induced

---

TABLE VIII

CASE DEFINITION OF SIMIAN TYPE D RETROVIRUS-INDUCED SIMIAN AIDS[a]

Generalized lymphadenopathy and/or splenomegaly accompanied by at least four of the following clinical and laboratory findings:

Weight loss (>10%)
Fever (>103°F)
Persistent refractory diarrhea
Chronic infections unresponsive to therapy
Opportunistic infections
Noma (cancrum oris)
Retroperitoneal or subcutaneous fibromatosis
Hematologic abnormalities
   Anemia (PCV<30%)
   Neutropenia (<1700)
   Lymphopenia (<1600)
   Thrombocytopenia (<50,000)
   Pancytopenia
Bone marrow hyperplasia
Characteristic lymph node lesions

[a]From Lackner (1988).

TABLE IX

LENTIVIRUSES OF NONHUMAN PRIMATES

Isolate	Host	Ref.
SIVagm	*Cercopithecus aethiops*	Ohta *et al.* (1987); Daniel *et al.* (1988b); Allan *et al.* (1991)
SIVmac	*Macaca mulatta*	Daniel *et al.* (1985)
SIVcyn	*Macaca fascicularis*	Kestler *et al.* (1988)
SIVstm	*Macaca arctoides*	Lowenstine *et al.* (1992)
SIVsm	*Cercocebus torquatus atys*	Murphey-Corb *et al.* (1986)
SIVsyk	*Cercopithecus mitis*	Emau *et al.* (1991)
SIVmnd	*Mandrillus sphinx*	Tsujimoto *et al.* (1988)
SIVcpz	*Pan troglodytes*	Peeters *et al.* (1989)

disease in humans makes the SIV-infected macaque an extremely valuable model for the study of human HIV infection. Macaques infected with SIV develop many of the same clinical and pathologic abnormalities that occur in AIDS patients and die from the same array of opportunistic infections. Using SIV-infected macaques as a model of human AIDS has produced a volume of research concerning all aspects of lentiviral biology and pathogenesis that cannot begin to be summarized here. The lessons to be reinforced from a standpoint of colony management and conservation are that (1) well-adapted viruses may be carried asymptomatically and silently by one primate species and yet have devastating consequences when introduced into another species and (2) the occurrence of unusual opportunistic infections should spur a vigorous search for an underlying immunosuppressive etiologic agent.

b. ETIOLOGY. The eight different SIV isolates from various species of nonhuman primates have 35–75% sequence homology with two known human lentiviruses, HIV-1 and HIV-2, the etiologic agents of human AIDS. Because of their genetic relationship to HIVs, these nonhuman primate viruses have been designated simian immunodeficiency viruses, even though in reality only four of them have been associated with immunodeficiency disorders (Table IX).

The different SIV isolates are currently designated by a three-letter suffix to indicate the species from which they were originally isolated: SIVmac from rhesus macaques (*Macaca mulatta*) (Daniel *et al.*, 1985), SIVcyn from cynomolgus monkeys (*M. fascicularis*) (Kestler *et al.*, 1988), SIVsm from sooty mangabeys (*Cerocebus atys*) (Fultz *et al.*, 1986), SIVmne from pig-tailed macaques (*M. nemestrina*) (Benveniste *et al.*, 1986), SIVstm from stump-tailed macaques (*M. arctoides*) (Murphey-Corb *et al.*, 1986; Lowenstine *et al.*, 1992), SIVagm from African green monkeys (*Cercopithecus aethiops*) (Ohta *et al.*, 1987), SIVmnd from mandrills (*Mandrillus sphinx*) (Tsujimoto *et al.*, 1988), SIVcmz from chimpanzees (*Pan troglodytes*) (Peeters *et al.*, 1989), and SIVsyk from Syke's monkeys (*C. mitis*) (Emau *et al*, 1991). An extensive summary of seroprevalence of SIV in various nonhuman primate populations

has been published (Hayami *et al.*, 1994). Additional but unconfirmed serologic evidence exists for infection of *Colobus guerza, Miopithecus talapoin,* and *Cercopithecus neglectus* (Lowenstine *et al.*, 1986; Tomonga *et al.*, 1993; Muller *et al.*, 1993). Genetic sequence analysis of the respective polymerase (pol) genes has revealed that the eight different SIVs and the two different HIVs fall into five distinct genetic groupings: (1) HIV-1 and SIVcpz, (2) SIVagm, (3) SIVsyk, (4) SIVmnd, and (5) SIVmac, SIVsm, SIVmne, SIVstm, and HIV-2 (Desrosiers, 1990).

In contrast to the STLVs in which the relatedness of viral isolates correlates with the geographic origin of the host, the relatedness of SIV isolates correlates more closely with speciation of the host (Franchini and Reitz, 1994). This, together with the greater diversity among SIV isolates, suggests that even though interspecies transmission of SIV occurs, it happens with less frequency than with STLV.

The natural lentiviral infection of New World nonhuman primates has not been identified. Common marmosets (*Callithrix jacchus*) and cotton-top tamarins (*Saguinus oedipus*) were susceptible to experimental infection with HIV-2 (McClure *et al.*, 1989). Although animals seroconverted and remained healthy, HIV-specific nucelotide sequences could be demonstrated in tamarin peripheral blood lymphocytes by PCR for extended periods.

c. EPIZOOTIOLOGY. Although the pathobiology following experimental inoculation of macaques with SIVmac has been studied extensively, the epizootiology of SIV infection in natural host populations is poorly understood. In species infected with host-adapted SIV strains, infection likely occurs in both a horizontal and a vertical fashion. Factors contributing to or governing this transmission in nature are largely unknown. Seroprevalence of SIVagm (see Fig. 23) in Ethiopian grivet monkeys (*Cercopithecus aethiops aethiops*) suggests that sexual transmission may be the predominant mode in wild populations (Phillips-Conroy *et al.*, 1994). Likewise, the infection rate increases with sexual maturity in both captive and wild sooty mangabeys, further supporting this route as a major mechanism in the propagation of the virus in nonhuman primate populations (Fultz *et al.*, 1990; Chen *et al.*, 1996b).

As noted earlier, the principal etiologic agent responsible for spontaneous immunosuppressive disease in captive macaques is simian retrovirus type D. Nontheless, retrospective analysis of tissues achieved from outbreaks of opportunistic infections and malignant lymphoma in captive macaques that occurred in the late 1960s and early 1970s demonstrated underlying SIV infection (Lowenstine *et al.*, 1992; Mansfield and Lackner, 1994; Daniel *et al.*, 1988a). Although the source of infection is unknown, the close homology between one of the isolates (SIVstm) and SIVsm suggests a source from sooty mangabeys. In both instances the virus was propagated within the captive populations and resulted in significant morbidity and mortality. Natural mother to offspring transmission was demonstrated in one case (Daniel *et al.*, 1988a).

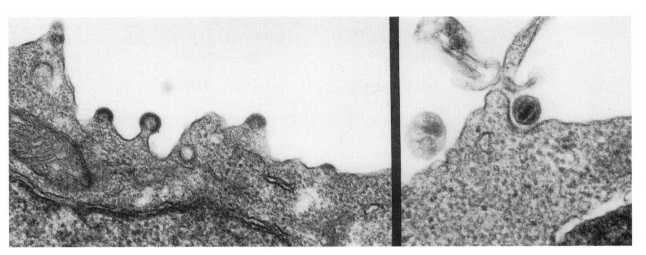

Fig. 23. SIVagm.

In another instance, macaques were inadvertently infected when inoculated with sooty mangabey-derived tissue containing *Mycobacterium leprae* (Gormus *et al.,* 1989). Xenobiotic inoculation or transplantation of tissue carries the risk of introducing unsuspected or unknown agents into the recipient animal. Although such protocols clearly play an important role in biomedical research, they should only be undertaken with the realization of the potential risks involved and recipient animals should be housed in an appropriate fashion to prevent the further transmission of such agents.

d. PATHOGENESIS AND PATHOLOGY. Simian immunodeficiency viruses have marked tropism for cells that express the CD4 molecule on their surface. These cells include the helper–inducer subset of T lymphocytes, monocyte macrophages, and antigen-presenting dendritic cells (Spira *et al.,* 1996). Viruses enter these permissive cells through an interaction between the viral envelope glycoprotein gp120 and the CD4 molecule, which serves as its receptor. Once inside the cell, the single-stranded viral RNA is transcribed via reverse transcriptase into DNA copies of itself, which ultimately become integrated into the host cell DNA. Transcription of this proviral DNA results in the production of progeny virus that bud primarily from the surface of infected lymphocytes. In those species in which the virus causes fatal disease, there is a profound depletion of CD4$^+$ T lymphocytes, leading to severe immune dysfunction and death from opportunistic infection or lymphoma.

The mechanism(s) by which CD4 cells are depleted in these animals is not known but the possibilities include (1) accumulation of toxic quantities of viral nucleic acids or structural proteins in the cytoplasm of infected cells; (2) fusion of infected cells expressing the viral glycoprotein gp120 on their surface with noninfected CD4-bearing cells, resulting in syncytia formation and death; (3) lysis of CD4$^+$ T lymphocytes bearing viral-encoded antigens on their surface by virus-specific CD8$^+$

T cells; (4) lysis of infected CD4$^+$ T lymphocytes by an antibody-dependent cellular cytotoxocity reaction; and (5) enhancement of apoptosis of CD4$^+$ lymphocytes. In contrast, infected macrophages, in which viral assembly occurs primarily within cytoplasmic vacuoles rather than on the surface of infected cells, are seemingly resistant to lysis and in fact may be responsible for dissemination of the virus to nonlymphoid tissue such as the brain.

No microscopic lesions have been described in African green monkeys, sooty mangabeys, Sykes' monkeys, mandrills, or chimpanzees with their respective persistent nonpathogenic SIV infections. In contrast, macaque monkeys dying of naturally acquired or experimentally induced SIVmac, SIVsm, SIVmne, or SIVstm infection have a wide array of microscopic lesions, many of which are associated with the opportunistic infections to which these immunosuppressed animals are predisposed and succumb. Active infection with cytomegalovirus, adenovirus, papovavirus, *Pneumocystis carinii, Mycobacterium avium* complex, *Cryptosporidium* sp., *Cryptococcus neoformans, Toxoplasma gondii,* and *Candidia albicans* have been described in SIV-inoculated macaques. These agents are described elsewhere within this volume.

In addition to these characteristic opportunistic infections, SIVs may induce lesions independent of immunosuppression in a variety of organ systems, including the skin and gastrointestinal, cardiopulmonary, nervous, and lymphoid systems.

i. Lymphoid System: Not unexpectedly lymphoid tissues are a major target of viral infection and six distinct microscopic patterns of change have been recognized: (1) normal morphology, (2) follicular hyperplasia, (3) follicular involution with normal or expanded paracortical regions, (4) depletion of follicular and paracortical regions, (5) distinctive granulomatous (giant cell) lymphadenitis, and (6) a generalized lymphoproliferative syndrome. These morphologic criteria are not mutu-

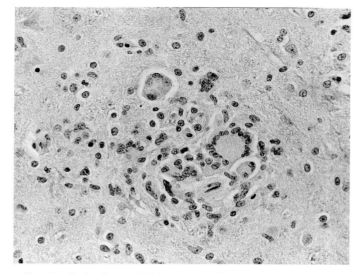

Fig. 24. Simian immunodeficiency virus. Giant cell encephalitis, rhesus macaque (*Macaca mulatta*).

ally exclusive and various patterns may coexist in different lymphoid tissues within the animal at any one time. *In situ* hybridization demonstrates large numbers of infected cells within the first week after experimental inoculation. These positive cells may temporarily disappear with the emergence of an appropriate immunologic response, only to reappear with progressive CD4[+] T lymphocyte depletion and viral destruction of follicular dendritic cells.

ii. Nervous System: Many macaques inoculated with SIV die with a characteristic meningoencephalitis that resembles the encephalopathy that occurs in a high percentage of human patients with AIDS. Simian immunodeficiency virus encephalitis affects the gray and white matter of the spinal cord and brain and is composed of multifocal perivascular aggregates of giant cells and histiocytes with smaller numbers of lymphocytes and rare neutrophils (Fig. 24). Surrounding these foci are evidence of myelin degeneration and the formation of scattered glial nodules. *In situ* hybridization shows that giant cells and histiocytes contain large amounts of replicating virus. Evidence shows that the CNS becomes uniformly infected during primary infection with pathogenic strains of SIVmac and yet only a small percentage of animals develop SIV encephalitis in the chronic phase of the disease (Lackner *et al.,* 1991). The reason for this paradox is unknown, however, alterations in brain endothelium are likely critical because (1) SIV encephalitis is associated with an increased expression of VCAM-1 on brain endothelium (Sasseville *et al.,* 1992, 1994) and (2) inoculation of "endothelial tropic" viral strains accelerate and promote the occurrence of lesions within the CNS (Mankowski *et al.,* 1994).

iii. Gastrointestinal System: Chronic diarrhea and wasting are the most common clinical signs in SIV-infected macaques

(Baskin *et al.,* 1988). Although several opportunistic infections such as *Mycobacterium avium, Cryptosporidium parvum, Entamoeba* spp., and cytomegalovirus may be responsible, in many instances secondary opportunistic agents are lacking and in these cases a direct SIV enteropathy equivalent to AIDS enteropathy in humans is suspected. In fact, experimental evidence indicates that the gastrointestinal tract may represent a major target organ during primary infection due in large part to the number of macrophages and lymphocytes that are normally present in mucosal tissue. A distinct SIV isolate, SIVmacPbj, induces a fulminant necrohemorrhagic gastroenteritis when inoculated into pig-tailed macaques (Fultz and Zack, 1994). Death results within 7–9 days. Similarly, a molecular clone of SIVmac239 (designated SIVmac239YE) produces nearly identical lesions and differs from its parent strain by two amino acids within the *nef* gene product (Zhenjian *et al.,* 1995). These changes apparently affect a tyrosine kinase that indiscriminately causes activation of infected macrophages and lymphocytes and the elaboration of a host of cytokines. The outcome of SIV infection of the gastrointestinal tract (i.e., fulminant, chronic, or asymptomatic infection) likely involves an interplay between host and viral factors, much as is seen in the CNS.

iv. Cardiopulmonary System: Simian immunodeficiency virus arteriopathy is a unique lesion of unknown etiology described in macaques experimentally inoculated with SIVmac (Chalifoux *et al.,* 1992). It is characterized by extensive medial and intimal proliferation of medium- and large-sized pulmonary arteries (Fig. 25). The lesion is often associated with thrombosis of vessels and hemorrhage, consolidation, and infarction of pulmonary parenchyma. The vessels are infiltrated by moderate numbers of CD68 macrophages and rare CD2 lymphocytes. Although CMV antigen can rarely be localized to the lesion, it is unknown whether the arteriopathy is the direct result of SIV infection or another agent. Histologically the lesion resembles a chronic obliterative arteriopathy induced by the virus of malignant catarrhal fever in cattle.

v. Skin: As with many systemic viral infections, a disseminated cutaneous eruption occurs in macaques inoculated with pathogenic strains of SIVmac (Ringler *et al.,* 1987). The rash generally appears within 1–2 weeks following inoculation involving the trunk, groin, medial thighs, and face. Complete resolution is apparent within 1–7 weeks. Histologically the exanthema is characterized by a nondescript, superficial, and perivascular lymphocytic dermatitis with variable swelling and degeneration of the epidermis. Immunohistochemistry has revealed these inflammatory cells to be predominantly CD8[+] lymphocytes and cytotoxic activity directed at epidermal Langerhans cells.

e. PREVENTION AND CONTROL. Epizootics of SIVmac have been controlled by serologic testing of colony members and removal of reactors (Lowenstine *et al.,* 1986). Asian macaques should not be allowed direct contact with African species or

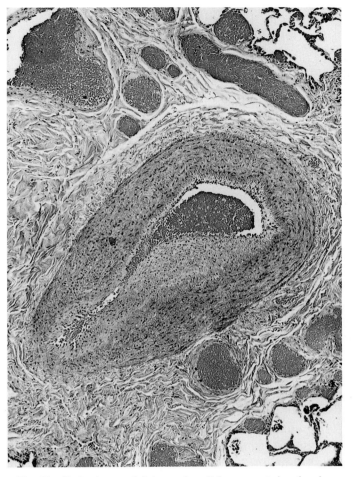

Fig. 25. Simian immunodeficiency virus. Pulmonary arteriopathy, rhesus macaque (*Macaca mulatta*).

TABLE X

SIMIAN FOAMY VIRUSES

Virus	Host	Ref.
SFV-1, 2	*Macaca* sp.	Rustigian *et al.* (1955)
SFV-3	*Macaca* sp.	Stikes *et al.* (1964)
SFV-4	*S. sciureus*	Johnston (1971)
SFV-5	*Galago crassicaudatus*	Johnston (1971)
SFV-6, 7	*P. troglodytes*	Hooks *et al.* (1972)
SFV-8	*Lagothrix* sp.	Hooks *et al.* (1973)
SFV-10	*P. cynocephalus*	Rhodes-Feuillette *et al.* (1987)
FXV	*C. jacchus*	Marczynska *et al.* (1981)
LK-3	*C. aethiops*	Neuman-Haefelin *et al.* (1983)

out gloves while receiving corticosteroids for dermatitis. Whether exposure occurred at this time is unknown. Seroconversion of a laboratory worker was discovered during an anonymous serologic survey (Centers for Disease Control and Prevention, 1992b). Whether this represents a third instance of SIV transmission to a human being or retesting of sera from one of the previously mentioned individuals is unknown. Phylogenetic analysis of HIV-2 from west Africans indicates close homology to SIVsm and suggests that interspecies transmission between feral sooty mangabeys and humans has occurred with some frequency (Chen *et al.*, 1996a). As such, all SIV isolates should be treated as potentially zoonotic.

Guidelines for the prevention of SIV infection of animal care and laboratory personnel have been published (Larimore *et al.*, 1989). Recommendations include biosafety level 2 standard operating procedures, medical surveillance of personnel, and specific training in the handling of primate retroviruses. Although considered optional, collection and storage of sera from personnel have been adopted by several institutions and facilitate investigations following accidental exposure.

their tissue products. It should be reemphasized that SRV/D infection of macaques is presently the most significant viral agent responsible for immunosuppressive disease in colony animals.

Control of host-adapted enzootic SIV strains is more problematic. In contrast to Asian macaques in which natural infection is invariably followed by seroconversion, African species may harbor the virus and not seroconvert.

f. ZOONOTIC POTENTIAL. SIVmac is a known zoonotic agent but has not been associated with disease in humans (Khabbaz *et al.*, 1992, 1994; Centers for Disease Control and Prevention, 1992a,b). In at least two instances, accidental exposure of humans to the virus has resulted in seroconversion and/or infection. Following a needle stick injury, one individual seroconverted but the virus could not be isolated or demonstrated by PCR techniques (Khabbaz *et al.*, 1992). In the second instance, the virus was isolated and could be demonstrated by PCR in a seropositive individual (Khabbaz *et al.*, 1994). This laboratory worker had a history of working with the virus with-

SPUMAVIRINAE: SIMIAN FOAMY VIRUSES

Simian foamy viruses (SFV) are complex retroviruses that have been isolated from a number of Old and New World nonhuman primate species (Table X). Partially characterized isolates include SFV-1 from rhesus macques (Rustigian *et al.*, 1955), SFV-3 from African green monkeys (Stikes *et al.*, 1964), and SFV-6 from chimpanzees (Hooks *et al.*, 1972). These viruses share considerable homology with human foamy viruses (HFV), to which SFV-6 is most closely related.

In cell culture, SFV infection produces CPE characterized by vacuolization of cytoplasm and syncytia formation and superficially may resemble other retroviruses (Fig. 26). Although foamy virus CPE was recognized as early as 1955, a clear association with naturally occurring diseases in humans or nonhuman primates has remained enigmatic. Although HFV has been linked to a number of disorders, including De Quervain's

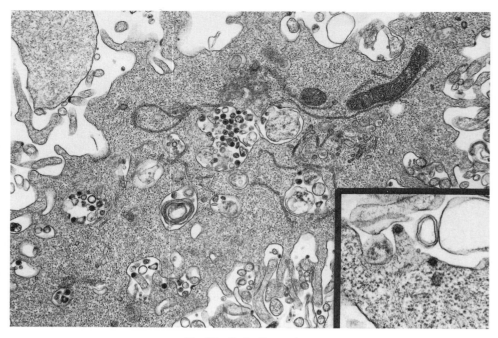

Fig. 26. Simian foamy virus.

thyroiditis, Graves' disease, chronic fatigue syndrome, and amyotrophic lateral sclerosis, definitive proof of a causal relationship is lacking. A severe spongiform encephalopathy has been demonstrated in transgenic mice bearing the human foamy virus *bel* gene (Bothe *et al.,* 1991). Accidental infection of laboratory workers by SFV has been demonstrated (Neuman-Haefelin *et al.,* 1983, 1993).

V. NONENVELOPED RNA-CONTAINING VIRUSES

A. Reoviridae

1. Rotaviruses

a. INTRODUCTION.   Rotaviruses are a common cause of contagious enteritis in young children, piglets, calves, and lambs. Rotaviruses have been isolated from macaques, but their association with disease is less clear.

b. ETIOLOGY.   Rotaviruses are divided into seven groups (A–G) based on antigenic differences within the inner capsid protein VP6. Type A viruses are most often associated with disease in humans. SA11 and rhesus rotavirus are two identified nonhuman primate strains. In addition, colostrum-deprived infant macaques are susceptible to inoculation with human rotavirus isolates (Wyatt *et al.,* 1976). Work documenting the extent and clinical importance of rotavirus infection in nonhuman primates has not been conducted. Experience from other species

suggests that they may be a common cause of mild self-limiting diarrhea during infancy (White *et al.,* 1972).

c. EPIZOOTIOLOGY.   The virus is transmitted by the fecal–oral route. Although no carrier state has been identified, the virus will survive in the environment for extended periods.

d. PATHOGENESIS AND PATHOLOGY.   Unlike other reoviruses, rotaviruses enter the cytoplasm of cells directly by binding of the VP4 capsid protein to specific cellular receptors. This may require trypsin cleavage activation. The virus replicates in the epithelium of the distal one-third of the villus tip, resulting in epithelial cell necrosis and villous atrophy. Defects caused by epithelial cell loss are closed within hours by reconstitution; however, full repair may take several days and require maturation of newly formed enterocytes. Villous atrophy is associated with diarrhea, which peaks 72 hr after infection. Rhesus rotavirus may induce hepatic disease in inappropriate murine hosts (Uhno *et al.,* 1990).

e. CLINICAL FINDINGS.   Following a short incubation period of 24–48 hr, viral infection causes profuse watery diarrhea, which persists for several days. Infection is usually self-limiting and usually does not require clinical attention.

f. LABORATORY FINDINGS.   Although antibodies to SA11 were demonstrated in 15 of 16 species of New and Old World nonhuman primates studied (Kalter *et al.,* 1982), electron microscopy did not reveal SA11 viral particles in 123 random fecal samples from baboons (*Papio* spp.), macaques (*Macaca* spp.), squirrel monkeys (*Saimiri sciureus*), and capuchin mon-

TABLE XI

PICORNAVIRIDAE

Genus	Virus
Hepatovirus	Hepatovirus A
Cardiovirus	Encephalomyocarditis virus
Enterovirus	Poliovirus
	Coxsackie virus A and B
	Simian enterovirus
	Echovirus

keys (*Cebus* spp.) (Kalter *et al.*, 1979). The virus may be identified in diarrheic stool following ultracentrifugation by negative staining electron microscopy. Commercially available ELISA and latex agglutination kits can also be used to detect type A rotaviruses within stool samples. Immunoelectron microscopy techniques utilizing antisera against rotaviruses will increase the sensitivity of viral visualization considerably.

g. TREATMENT AND PREVENTION. The ubiquitous nature of rotaviruses makes their prevention difficult. Therapy in most cases is not required.

B. Picornaviridae

Picornaviruses (pico=small, rna=ribonucleic acid) are small, single-stranded, nonenveloped RNA-containing viruses. The family Picornaviridae contains many viruses of medical importance, including *Hepatovirus, Enterovirus, Rhinovirus, Apthovirus,* and *Cardiovirus* genera (Table XI).

HEPATOVIRUS

1. Jeotos A Virus Group

a. INTRODUCTION. Hepatitis A virus (HAV) is variably classified as an enterovirus or as a separate subgroup within the family Picornaviridae. It is responsible for approximately 10–25% of all cases of viral hepatitis in human beings and may be transmitted by the fecal–oral route during acute infection or by the ingestion of uncooked contaminated shellfish. It is well accepted that chimpanzees, tamarins (*Saguinus* sp.), cynomolgus macaques (*Macaca fascicularis*), and owl monkeys (*Aotus trivirgatus*) are susceptible to HAV. Serologic evidence exists for the infection of *M. mulatta, M. arctoides, Papio* sp., *Cercopithecus aethiops, Cebus albifrons, Callithrix jacchus, Cynopithecus niger, Ateles geoffroyi, Hylobates lar, Mandrillus sphinx,* and *Erythrocebus patas* with the same or similar viruses (Eichberg and Kalter, 1980; Potkay, 1992; Brack, 1987a; Burke and Graham, 1981; Lankas and Jensen, 1987; Shevstsova *et al.*, 1988).

b. ETIOLOGY. The hepatitis A virus is a small, 25- to 30-nm-diameter RNA virus with a dodecahedral configuration composed of 12 pentamers. The 7.4-kb genome consists of a single open reading frame encoding a large polypeptide that is cleaved into 11 functional proteins posttranslationally. Although a variety of nonhuman primates may be infected experimentally with human HAV isolates, the relationship of these isolates to those obtained from spontaneous nonhuman primate cases is less clear. Isolates from naturally occurring cases in *Aotus* sp., *M. fascicularis,* and *C. aethiops* have been shown to differ substantially from clinical human isolates, suggesting that despite antigenic similarities, HAV may represent a more heterogeneous group than originally appreciated (Tsarev *et al.*, 1991; Lemon *et al.*, 1987; Nainan *et al.*, 1991). A great wealth of information exists on the experimental infection of tamarins. These animals have served as an important animal model of the human disease and were critical in the initial characterization of the virus and subsequent vaccine development.

c. EPIZOOTIOLOGY. Transmission likely occurs by the fecal–oral route. Serologic evidence of infection has been demonstrated in both wild-caught and captive nonhuman primates. In several instances, seroconversion has occurred during the initial period of captivity, suggesting that the combination of stress and environmental factors at this time may promote transmission of the virus. Most experimental work indicates that animals shed virus and are contagious for only short periods (Cohen *et al.*, 1989). A single report suggests that under some circumstances animals may remain viremic and shed virus for extended periods (Lapin and Shevtsova, 1990).

d. PATHOGENESIS AND PATHOLOGY. Pathogenesis and histopathology are similar in all species studied to date. Following fecal–oral transmission there is a prolonged incubation of 20–50 days. Abnormalities of liver enzymes may be noted at this time. Virus is shed in feces for 10–30 days and onset of this shedding usually precedes detectable clinicopathologic alterations.

Hepatocellular injury is mediated by cytotoxic CD8$^+$ T lymphocytes and is not the direct cytolytic effect of the virus itself. Characteristic histopathologic changes are the activation of sinusoidal cells, focal hepatocellular necrosis, and portal, nonsuppurative inflammatory cell infiltrates. Hyperplasia of bile ducts and bile duct epithelial cell necrosis have been described in chimpanzees. The occurrence of these findings closely parallels elevations in liver enzymes (Dienstag *et al.*, 1976).

e. CLINICAL FINDINGS. Clinical signs are uncommon and nonspecific. Anorexia and diarrhea have been noted in some chimpanzees infected with HAV (Brack, 1987a).

f. LABORATORY FINDINGS. Elevations of alanine aminotransferase and aspartate aminotransferase 2 to 10 times above normal, as well as mild increases in bilirubin, have been documented and coincide with the development of humoral and cellular immunity. Anti-HAV IgM and anti-HAV IgG increase and may be used to confirm infection. Although the disease associated with HAV is often mild, infection with this virus in several instances has interfered with the interpretation of clinicopathologic data collected during toxicology studies (Slighter *et al.,* 1988; Lankas and Jensen, 1987).

The hepatitis A virus is difficult to grow in cell culture and serologic evidence is often utilized in clinical diagnosis. Commercially available immunoassays have been used in a number of Old and New World primate species (Eichberg and Kalter, 1980; Lankas and Jensen, 1987) and may demonstrate acute-phase IgM or convalescent-phase IgG anti-HAV antibodies.

g. TREATMENT.   In most nonhuman primates, infection is usually self-limiting. Previous infection with HAV is protective.

h. ZOONOTIC POTENTIAL.   Numerous cases of human HAV infection contracted from nonhuman primates have been documented (Brack, 1987a). The vast majority of these cases have been transmitted from chimpanzees. Hepatitis A virus infection of human beings is usually asymptomatic or associated with minimal clinical signs. Fulminant fatal hepatitis is a rare outcome. In contrast to HBV, chronic infection and carrier states are not seen.

CARDIOVIRUS

1. Encephalomyocarditis Viruses

a. INTRODUCTION.   Encephalomyocarditis viruses are a group of closely related viruses 30 nm in diameter with a genome characteristic of Picornaviridae. Five strains are identified by hemagglutinin assays: Mengo-, MM-, Columbia-SK-, murine encephalomyelitis (ME), and encephalomyocarditis viruses. As with other members of the Picornaviridae, they are relatively resistant to a number of environmental factors, including desiccation and freezing.

b. EPIZOOTIOLOGY.   Encephalomyocarditis viruses infect a variety of wild rodents and have been infrequently implicated in causing disease in rhesus macaques, owl monkeys, squirrel monkeys, and chimpanzees (Blanchard *et al.,* 1987; Gainer, 1967; Baskin, 1993). Several epizootics have been recognized in baboons, suggesting a unique susceptibility (Hubbard *et al.,* 1992). Animals likely become infected when rodents contaminate food or other surfaces with feces. Although mice represent the natural reservoir host, rats are often implicated in transmission of the virus to nonhuman primates and swine. Horizontal intraspecies transmission has been documented in swine and rodents and such transmission in primates is suspected.

c. PATHOGENESIS AND PATHOLOGY.   Clinical disease is due primarily to the destructive effect of viral replication and host immunologic response within the myocardium. Ultrastructurally, viral particles may be found within myocytes and endothelium. At necropsy, pulmonary congestion, pericardial effusion, and mottling of the myocardium may be noted. Histologically,

there is a multifocal to coalescing, necrotizing, nonsuppurative myocarditis (Tesh and Wallace, 1978; Hubbard *et al.,* 1992).

Pathologic findings may be suggestive, but definitive diagnosis requires viral isolation. Differential diagnosis should include other agents such as coxsackie virus and toxoplasmosis and trypanosomiasis (Chagas' disease).

d. CLINICAL FINDINGS.   Affected nonhuman primates are usually found dead with no premonitory clinical signs. Following experimental inoculation, time to death in squirrel and African green monkeys was highly variable, ranging from 4 to 41 days (Blanchard *et al.,* 1987). In less peracute cases, tachypnea, dyspnea, and frothing from the nostrils have been recorded. In a large biomedical research colony, increased fetal loss was suspected.

e. TREATMENT AND PREVENTION.   No treatment is available. Prevention and control should center on the elimination of reservoir rodent hosts. This may be difficult in outdoor gang housing, and the virus may persist in the environment for extended periods.

ENTEROVIRUS

The genus *Enterovirus* contains a large number of viruses pathogenic for humans. Since 1969, all isolates from humans have been designated as enteroviruses and numbered sequentially. As a group, these viruses are resistant to a variety of chemical disinfectants, including ammonia compounds and deoxycholate. They are, however, susceptible to UV light and dehydration. The pathogenesis of all enterovirus infections share certain features: (1) entry through the gastrointestinal tract, (2) a brief period of viremia associated with minimal clinical disease in the majority of those infected, (3) gastrointestinal shedding of the virus, (4) frequent antigenic mutation, and (5) infrequent dissemination of virus from the gastrointestinal tract to distant target organs. In humans, enteroviruses are associated with a number of clinical entities, including encephalomyelitis, meningitis, myocarditis, cutaneous exanthemas, respiratory disease, congenital malformations, acute hemorrhagic conjunctivitis, and diabetes mellitus. These serious sequelae are rare and, in general, the vast majority of human beings infected have minimal clinical signs.

Because of the widespread nature of enteroviruses and the frequent asymptomatic infection of most individuals, it is often difficult to establish an etiologic relationship between a specific enterovirus and disease occurrence. The following criteria have been recommended: (1) a high rate of viral isolation from individuals with disease versus individuals without disease, (2) seroconversion during the course of illness, (3) a lack of evidence of concurrent infectious agent, and (4) virus present in significant concentrations in body fluids.

Subgroups of enteroviruses are clearly associated with disease (polioviruses and coxsackieviruses) in nonhuman primates. Eighteen different "simian" enterovirus serotypes have also been identified; however, their association with disease is less clear. While polioviruses, coxsackieviruses, and echoviruses isolated prior to 1969 have retained their initial designation, separation of these viruses from remaining enteroviruses is somewhat artificial.

1. Simian Enteroviruses 1–18

A large number of enteroviruses have been isolated from nonhuman primates and are distinguished by specific antisera (Kalter, 1982). Affected species include chimpanzees, macaques, vervet monkeys, African green monkeys, baboons, langurs, and marmosets. Many isolates have been made from animals with no clinical signs or mild diarrhea and their association with specific disease entities is unclear. Some isolates apparently lack strict species specificity, and the possibility that infection of an inappropriate host (including humans) may be associated with a more virulent disease should be considered.

A single outbreak of myocarditis and meningoencephalitis occurred in the fall of 1970 at the Lawrenceville facility of the Centers of Disease Control (Kaufmann *et al.,* 1973). This outbreak was associated with high morbidity and mortality in rhesus macaques (*Macaca mulatta*) and African green monkeys (*Cercopithecus aethiops*). Most of the rhesus macaques were found dead without clinical signs whereas others had dysentery and experienced convulsions on handling. Lesions in these animals were inconsistent and composed of increased numbers of mononuclear cells within the cerebrospinal fluid (CSF) and scattered perivascular hemorrhages. An enterovirus (simian agent 16) was cultured from 4 of 10 brains. African green monkeys died with chronic-active myocarditis and a nonsuppurative encephalitis. Simian agent 16 is a common isolate from macaques, and this virus did not produce clinical disease when inoculated into rhesus monkeys. Its association with virulent disease at the Lawrenceville facility is therefore unusual and illustrates the difficulty in making the association between disease and an enteroviral agent.

2. Poliovirus

a. INTRODUCTION. The epidemic form of human poliomyelitis has occurred since antiquity. Asian macaques have served as an important experimental model of this disease and have been critical in vaccine development and safety testing (Sabin, 1985). The experimental susceptibility of macaques was first demonstrated in 1908, and in the 1950s approximately 200,000 nonhuman primates were imported annually to support this research (Vickers, 1986). Despite the overall success of human vaccination programs, more than 200,000 cases of poliomyelitis per year are reported, mostly from third world African and Asian countries.

b. ETIOLOGY. Three distinct serotypes of wild-type poliovirus are recognized (Brunhilde, Lancing, Leon). Individual isolates may vary in their virulence and invasiveness.

c. EPIZOOTIOLOGY. Natural infection of the chimpanzee (*Pan troglodytes*), gorilla (*Gorilla gorilla*), orangutan (*Pongo pygmeus*), and rhesus macaque (*Macaca mulatta*) has been demonstrated. These occurrences have been rare in North America since the advent of widespread vaccination of the human population, but may be expected to continue in regions of the world where poliovirus is endemic. The gastrointestinal tract becomes infected and animals may shed virus in feces.

d. PATHOGENESIS AND PATHOLOGY. Prior to the vaccine era, polio was a disease of the young and immunosuppressed. The poliovirus infects specialized enterocytes (M cells) and initially replicates in gut-associated lymphoid tissue. In the face of an appropriate immune response or maternally acquired neutralizing antibodies, infection is eliminated or limited to the gastrointestinal tract. In cases in which the immune response is deficient, the virus disseminates to the central nervous system and is capable of infecting and destroying neurons.

Lesions are found scattered throughout the gray matter of the central nervous system with a propensity to affect the spinal cord, cerebellar nuclei, and diencephalon (Fig. 27). The initial inflammatory response consists of polymorphonuclear cells that are rapidly replaced by lymphocytes and plasma cells forming perivascular aggregates and infiltrating the meninges. Neuronal necrosis and glial nodules may be evident.

e. CLINICAL FINDINGS. In many cases, no clinical signs are evident. Disseminated infection to the spinal cord may lead to paresis, paraplegia, and death. Skeletal biometric changes have been documented in Gombe chimpanzees as a long-term sequela to poliomyelitis and deinnervation atrophy of skeletal muscle.

f. ZOONOTIC POTENTIAL. Although possible, transmission from nonhuman primates to humans has not been demonstrated.

g. PREVENTION. The Sabin live virus oral polio vaccine has reportedly been used to vaccinate and protect Gombe chimpanzees and a variety of great apes (Morbeck *et al.,* 1991; Allmond *et al.,* 1967). Caution is advised in using any modified-live vaccine in species in which proper testing of efficacy and biosafety have not been conducted.

C. Caliciviridae

1. Primate *Calicivirus Pan paniscus* type 1: PCV-Pan 1

A calicivirus has been isolated from a Pygmy chimpanzee (*Pan paniscus*) with a mild vesicular stomatitis resembling herpes simplex infection (Smith *et al.,* 1983). The virus was antigenically distinct from other known caliciviruses but had characteristic morphologic features ultrastructurally. The virus

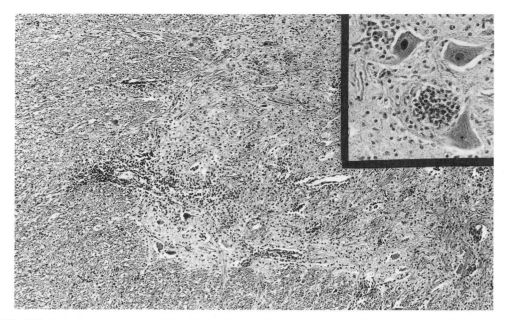

Fig. 27. Poliovirus. Nonsuppurative myelitis of the ventral horn (inset: neuronal necrosis), rhesus macaque (*Macaca mulatta*).

was isolated on two separate occasions 6 months apart and while contact chimpanzees were seropositive, none showed clinical signs.

2. Hepatitis E Virus

a. INTRODUCTION.   The hepatitis E virus (HEV) is an important etiologic agent of epidemic hepatitis (non-A,non-B) in third world countries. Outbreaks usually occur following heavy rainfall and have been associated with sewage contamination of drinking water.

b. ETIOLOGY.   The agent is a single-stranded RNA virus tentatively assigned to the *Calicivirus* genus. It is 37–34 nm in diameter and has a genome of approximately 7.2 kb in length.

c. EPIZOOTIOLOGY.   Humans become infected by the fecal–oral route. Natural infection of nonhuman primates has not been identified. Following experimental inoculation, a number of species appear susceptible, including owl monkeys (*Aotus trivirgatus*), cynomolgus monkeys (*Macaca fascicularis*), rhesus macaques (*M. mulatta*), moustached tamarins (*Saguinus mystax*), African green monkeys (*Cercopithecus aethiops*), and chimpanzees (*Pan troglodytes*) (Ticehurst *et al.,* 1992; Bradley *et al.,* 1987; Potkay, 1992).

d. PATHOGENESIS AND PATHOLOGY.   Cynomolgus monkeys appear to be the most susceptible to experimental inoculation. Similar to HAV infection in this species, minimal clinical signs were associated with infection with HEV. Viral antigen was detected in the liver 30–37 days postinoculation and was associated with elevations in liver enzymes, a mild nonsuppur-

ative portal hepatitis, and the appearance of an antibody response. Virus was shed in the feces through bile and was identified by electron microscopy.

e. TREATMENT AND PREVENTION.   As of yet, HEV has not been identified as an etiologic agent of hepatitis following natural infection in nonhuman primates. The widespread occurrence of HEV in humans and the susceptibility of a variety of nonhuman primates suggest that such infection is possible.

ACKNOWLEDGMENTS

This work was supported by NHI Grants RR00128 and RR07000. The authors thank Drs. R. D. Hunt and A. Lackner for case material, J. MacKey for use of electron micrographs, and Alison Hampson and June Armstrong for photographic assistance.

REFERENCES

Abildgaard, C., Harrison, J., Espana, C., Spangler, W., and Gribble, D. (1975). Simian hemorrhagic fever: Studies of coagulation and pathology. *Am. J. Trop. Med. Hyg.* **24,** 537–544.

Acha, P. N., and Szyfres, B. (1980). Influenza. *In* "Communicable Diseases Common to Man and Animals". World Health Organization, Washington, DC.

Albrecht, P., Shabo, A. L., Burns, G. R., and Tauraso, N. M. (1972). Experimental measles encephalitis in normal and cyclophosphamide-treated rhesus monkeys. *J. Infect. Dis.* **126,** 154–161.

Albrecht, P., Lorenz, D., Klutch, M. J., Vickers, J. H., and Ennis, F. A. (1980). Fatal measles infection in marmosets pathogenesis and prophylaxis. *Infect. Immun.* **27,** 969–978.

Allan, J. S., Short, M., Taylor, M. E., Su, S., Hirsch, V. M., Johnson, P. R., Shaw, G. M., and Hahn, B. H. (1991). Species-specific diversity among simian immunodeficiency viruses from African green monkeys. *J. Virol.* **65**, 2816–2828.

Allen, A. M., Palmer, A. E., Tauraso, N. M., and Shelokov, A. (1968). Simian hemorrhagic fever. II. Studies in pathology. *Am. J. Trop. Med. Hyg.* **17**, 413–421.

Allmond, B. W., Froeschle, J. E., and Guilloud, N. B. (1967). Paralytic poliomyelitis in large laboratory primates: Virologic investigation and report on the use of oral poliomyelitis virus (OPV). *Am. J. Epidemiol.* **85**, 229–239.

Arita, I., and Henderson, D. A. (1968). Smallpox and monkeypox in nonhuman primates. *Bull. W.H.O.* **39**, 347–353.

Arita, I., and Henderson, D. A. (1976). Monkeypox and whitepox viruses in West and Central Africa. *Bull. W.H.O.* **53**, 347–353.

Arita, I., Gispen, R., Kalter, S. S., Wah, L. T., Marrenikova, S. S., Netter, R., and Pagaya, I. (1972). Outbreaks of monkeypox and serological surveys in nonhuman primates. *Bull. W.H.O.* **46**, 625–631.

Arita, I., Jezek, Z., Khodakevich, L., and Kalisa-Ruti, J. (1985). Human monkeypox: A newly emerged orthopoxvirus zoonosis in the tropical rainforests of Africa. *Am. J. Trop. Med. Hyg.* **34**, 781–789.

Arvin, A. M., Martin, D. P., Gard, E. A., and Merigan, T. C. (1983). Interferon prophylaxis against simian varicella in *Erythrocebus patas* monkeys. *J. Infect. Dis.* **147**, 149–154.

Asher, D. M., Gibbs, C. J., Lang, D. J., and Gajdusek, D. C. (1974). Persistent shedding of cytomegalovirus in the urine of healthy rhesus monkeys. *Proc. Soc. Exp. Biol. Med.* **145**, 794–801.

Barahona, H. H., Melendez, L. V., King, N. W., Daniel, M. D., Fraser, C. E. O., and Preville, A. C. (1973). Herpesvirus aotus type 2: A new viral agent from owl monkeys *(Aotus trivirgatus). J. Infect. Dis.* **127**, 171–178.

Baringer, J. R., and Griffith, J. F. (1970). Experimental measles virus encephalitis. *Lab. Invest.* **23**, 355–346.

Baskin, G. B. (1987). Disseminated cytomegalovirus infection in immunodeficient rhesus monkeys. *Am. J. Pathol.* **129**, 345–352.

Baskin, G. B. (1993). Encephalomyocarditis virus infection, nonhuman primates. *In* "Monographs on the Pathology of Laboratory Animals: Nonhuman Primates" (T. C. Jones, U. Mohr, and R. D. Hunt, eds.), Vol. 2, pp. 104–107. Springer-Verlag, Berlin and New York.

Baskin, G. B., and Soike, K. F. (1989). Adenovirus enteritis in SIV infected rhesus monkeys. *J. Infect. Dis.* **160**, 905–907.

Baskin, G. B., Murphey-Corb, M., Watson, E. A., and Martin, L. N. (1988). Necropsy findings in rhesus monkeys experimentally infected with cultured simian immunodeficiency virus (SIV)/delta. *Vet. Pathol.* **25**, 456–467.

Baskin, G. B., Roberts, E. D., Kuebler, D., Martin, L. N., Blauw, B., Heeney, J., and Zurcher, C. (1995). Squamous epithelial proliferative lesions associated with rhesus Epstein-Barr virus in simian immunodeficiency virus-infected rhesus macaques. *J. Infect. Dis.* **172**, 535–538.

Bearcroft, W. G. (1960). Cytological and cytochemical studies on the liver cells of yellow fever infected rhesus monkeys. *J. Pathol. Bacteriol.* **80**, 19–31.

Bearcroft, W. G. (1962). Studies on the livers of yellow fever infected monkeys. *J. Pathol. Bacteriol.* **83**, 49–58.

Bearcroft, W. G., and Jamieson, M. F. (1958). An outbreak of subcutaneous tumours in rhesus monkeys. *Nature (London)* **182**, 195–194.

Benveniste, R. E., Arthur, L. O., Tsai, C., Sowder, R., Copeland, T. D., Henderson, L. E., and Oroszlan, S. (1986). Isolation of a lentivirus from a macaque with lymphoma: Comparison with HTLV-III/LAV and other lentiviruses. *J. Virol.* **60**, 483–490.

Bergsagel, D. J., Finegold, M. J., Butel, J. S., Kupsky, W. J., and Garcea, R. L. (1992). DNA sequences similar to those of simian virus 40 in ependymomas and choroid plexus tumors of childhood. *N. Engl. J. Med.* **326**, 988–993.

Blakely, G. A., Lourie, B., and Morton, W. G. (1973). A varicella-like disease in macaque monkeys. *J. Infect. Dis.* **127**, 617–625.

Blanchard, J. L., Soike, K., and Baskin, G. B. (1987). Encephalomyocarditis virus infection in African green monkeys: Comparison of pathologic effects. *Lab. Anim. Sci.* **37**, 635–639.

Bothe, K., Aguzzi, A., Lassmann, H., Rethwilm, A., and Horak, I. (1991). Progressive encephalopathy and myopathy in transgenic mice expressing human foamy virus genes. *Science* **253**, 555–557.

Bougler, L. R. (1966). Natural rabies in a laboratory monkey. *Lancet* **1**, 941–943.

Boyce, J. T., Giddens, W. E., and Valerio, M. (1971). Simian adenoviral pneumonia. *Am. J. Pathol.* **91**, 259–276.

Brack, M. (1987a). Viruses. *In* "Agents Transmissible from Simians to Man" (M. Brack, ed.), pp. 1–90. Springer-Verlag, New York.

Brack, M. (1987b). Hepatitis viruses. *In* "Agents Transmissible from Simians to Man" (M. Brack, ed.), pp. 83–89. Springer-Verlag, New York.

Bradley, D. W., Krawczynski, K., Cook, E. H., McCaustland, K. A., Humphrey, C. D., Spelbring, J. E., Myint, H., and Maynard, J. E. (1987). Enterically transmitted non-A non-B hepatitis: Serial passage of disease in cynomolgus macaques and tamarins and recovery of disease associated 27- to 34-nm, viruslike particles. *Proc. Natl. Acad. Sci. U.S.A.* **84**, 6277–6281.

Brenan, J. G., Kalisa-Ruti, J., Steniowsoski, M., Zanotto, E., Gromoyko, A. I., and Arita, I. (1980). Human monkeypox 1970–1979. *Bull. W.H.O.* **58**, 165–182.

Bruestle, M. E., Golden, J. G., Hall, A., and Banknieder, A. R. (1981). Naturally occurring Yaba tumor in a baboon *(Papio papio). Lab. Anim. Sci.* **31**, 292–294.

Bullock, G. (1965). An association between adenoviruses isolated from simian tonsils and episodes of illness in captive monkeys. *J. Hyg.* **63**, 383–387.

Burke, D. S., and Graham, R. R. (1981). Hepatitis A virus in primates outside of captivity. *Lancet* **2**, 928.

Cameron, K. R., Stamminger, T., Craxton, M., Bodemer, W., Honess, R. W., and Fleckenstein, B. (1987). The 160,000-Mr protein encoded at the right end of the herpesvirus saimiri genome is homologous to the 140,000-Mr membrane antigen encoded at the left end of EBV genome. *J. Virol.* **61**, 2063–2070.

Casey, H. W., Woodruff, J. M., and Butcher, W. I. (1967). Electron microscopy of benign epidermal pox disease of rhesus monkeys. *Am. J. Pathol.* **51**, 431–446.

Centers for Disease Control and Prevention (1987). Guidelines for prevention of Herpesvirus simiae (B virus) infection in monkey handlers. *Morbid. Mortal. Wkly. Rep.* **36**, 680–689.

Centers for Disease Control and Prevention (1988). Management of patients with suspected viral hemorrhagic fever. *Morbid. Mortal. Wkly. Rep.* **37**, Suppl. S-3, 1–16.

Centers for Disease Control and Prevention (1990a). Update: Evidence of filovirus infection in animal caretakers in research service facility. *Morbid. Mortal. Wkly. Rep.* **32**, 296.

Centers for Disease Control and Prevention (1990b). Update: Filovirus infection in animal handlers. *Morbid. Mortal. Wkly. Rep.* **39**, 221.

Centers for Disease Control and Prevention (1992a). Seroconversion to simian immunodeficiency virus in two laboratory workers. *Morbid. Mortal. Wkly. Rep.* **41**, 678–681.

Centers for Disease Control and Prevention (1992b). Anonymous survey for simian immunodeficiency virus seropositivity in SIV-laboratory researchers-United States. *Morbid. Mortal. Wkly. Rep.* **41**, 814–815.

Centers for Disease Control and Prevention (1995). Outbreak of Ebola viral hemorrhagic fever-Zaire. *Morbid. Mortal. Wkly. Rep.* **44**, 381–382.

Chalifoux, L. V., Simon, M. A., Pauley, D. R., MacKey, J. J., Wyand, M. S., and Ringler, D. J. (1992). Arteriopathy in macaques infected with simian immunodeficiency virus. *Lab. Invest.* **67**, 338–349.

Chandler, F. W. and McClure, H. M. (1982). Adenoviral pancreatitis in rhesus monkeys: Current knowledge. *Vet. Pathol.* **19**, Suppl. 7, 171–180.

Chandler, F. W., Callaway, C. S., and Adams, S. R. (1974). Pancreatitis associated with an adenovirus in a rhesus monkey. *Vet. Pathol.* **11**, 165–171.

Chellman, G. J., Lukas, V. S., Eugui, E. M., Altera, K. P., Almquist, S. J., and Hilliard, J. K. (1992). Activation of B virus (*Herpesvirus simiae*) in chronically immunosuppressed cynomolgus monkeys. *Lab. Anim. Sci.* **42**, 146–151.

Chen, Y. A., Jang, Y., Kanki, P. J., Yu, Q., Wang, J., Montali, R. J., Samuel, K. P., and Papas, T. S. (1994). Isolation and characterization of simian T-cell leukemia virus type II from new world monkeys. *J. Virol.* **68,** 1149–1157.

Chen, Z., Telfer, P., Gettie, A., Reed, P., Zhang, L., Ho, D. D., and Marx, P. A. (1996a). Genetic characterization of new west african SIVsm: Genetically diverse viruses from a single feral sooty mangabey troop and geographic clustering of household-derived SIV strains with HIV-2 subtypes. *J. Virol.* **70,** 3617–3627.

Chen, Z., Telfer, P., Reed, P., Zhang, L., Gettie, A., Ho, D. D., and Marx, P. A. (1996b). Isolation and characterization of the first simian immunodeficiency virus from a feral sooty mangabey (*Cercocebus atys*) in West Africa. *J. Med. Primatol.* **24,** 108–115.

Choa, R. K., Fishaut, M., Schwartzman, J. D., and McIntosh, K. (1979). Detection of respiratory syncytial virus in nasal secretion from infants by enzyme-linked immunosorbent assay. *J. Infect. Dis.* **139,** 483–486.

Chopra, H. C., and Mason, M. M. (1970). A new virus in a spontaneous mammary tumor of a rhesus monkey. *Cancer Res.* **30,** 2081–2086.

Churchill, A. E. (1963). The iolation of parainfluenza 3 virus from fatal cases of pneumonia in *Erythrocebus patas* monkeys. *Br. J. Exp. Pathol.* **44,** 529–537.

Clarke, C. J., Watt, N. J., Meredith, A., McIntyre, N., and Burns, S. M. (1994). Respiratory syncytial virus-associated bronchopneumonia in a young chimpanzee. *J. Comp. Pathol.* **110,** 207–212.

Clarkson, M. J., Thorpe, E., and McCarthy, K. (1967). A virus disease of captive vervet monkeys (*Cercopithecus aethiops*) caused by a new herpesvirus. *Arch. Gesamte Virusforsch.* **22,** 219–234.

Cohen, J. I., Feinstone, S., and Purcell, R. H. (1989). Hepatitis A virus infection in a chimpanzee: Duration of viremia and detection of virus in saliva and throat swabs. *J. Infect. Dis.* **160,** 887–890.

Crandell, R. A., Casey, H. W., and Brumlow, W. B. (1969). Studies of a newly recognized poxvirus of monkeys. *J. Infect. Dis.* **119,** 80–88.

Cunningham, T. P., and Pipas, J. M. (1985). Simian agent 12 is a BK virus-like papovavirus which replicates in monkey cells. *J. Virol.* **54,** 483–492.

Dalgard, D. W., Hardy, R. J., Pearson, S. L., Pucak, G. J., Quander, R. V., Zack, P. M., Peters, C. J., and Jahrling, P. B. (1992). Combined simian hemorrhagic fever and Ebola virus infection in cynomolgus monkeys. *Lab. Anim. Sci.* **42,** 152–157.

Daniel, M. D., Karpas, A., Melendez, L. V., King, N. W., and Hunt, R. D. (1967). Isolation of Herpes T virus from spontaneous disease in squirrel monkeys (*Saimiri sciureus*). *Arch. Gesamte Virusforsch.* **22,** 324–331.

Daniel, M. D., Melendez, L. V., King, N. W., Barahona, H. H., Fraser, C. E. O., Garcia, F. G., and Silva, D. (1973). Isolation and characterization of a new virus from owl monkeys: Herpesvirus aotus type 3. *Am. J. Phys. Anthropol.* **38,** 497–500.

Daniel, M. D., Barahona, H., Melendez, L. V., Hunt, R. D., Sehgal, P., Marshall, B., Ingalls, J., and Forbes, M. (1978). Prevention of fatal herpes infections in owl and marmoset monkeys by vaccination. *In* "Recent Advances in Primatology" (D. J. Chivers and E. H. R. Ford, eds.), Vol. 4, pp. 67–69. Academic, New York.

Daniel, M. D., King, N. W., Letvin, N. L., Hunt, R. D., Sehgal, P. K., and Desrosiers, R. C. (1984). A new type D retrovirus isolated from macaques with an immunodeficiency syndrome. *Science* **223,** 602.

Daniel, M. D., Letvin, N. L., King, N. W., Kannagi, M., Sehgal, P. K., and Hunt, R. D. (1985). Isolation of T-cell tropic HTLV-III-like retrovirus from macaques. *Science* **228,** 1201–1204.

Daniel, M. D., Letvin, N. L., Sehgal, P. K., Schmidt, D. K., Silva, D. P., Solomon, K. R., Hodi, F. S., Jr., Ringler, D. J., Hunt, R. D., King, N. W., and Desrosiers, R. C. (1988a). Prevalence of antibodies to 3 retroviruses in a captive colony of macaque monkeys. *Int. J. Cancer* **41,** 601–608.

Daniel, M. D., Li, Y., Naidu, M., Durda, P. J., Schmidt, D. K., Troup, C. D., Silva, D. P., MacKey, J. J., Kestler, H. W., Sehgal, P. K., King, N. W., Ohta, Y., Hayami, M., and Desrosiers, R. C. (1988b). Simian immunodeficiency virus from African green monkeys. *J. Virol.* **62,** 4123–4128.

Davenport, D. S., Johnson, D. R., Holmes, G. P., Jewett, D. A., Ross, S., and Hilliard, J. K. (1994). Diagnosis and management of human B virus (herpes simiae) infections in Michigan. *Clin. Infect. Dis.* **19,** 33–41.

Davis, K. J., Hubbard, G. B., Soike, K. F., and Butler, T. M. (1992). Fatal necrotizing adenoviral hepatitis in a chimpanzee (*Pan troglodytes*) with disseminated cytomegalovirus infection. *Vet. Pathol.* **29,** 547–549.

Dienhardt, F., Holmes, A. W., and Capps, R. B. (1967). Studies on the transmission of human viral hepatitis to marmoset monkeys. I. Transmission of disease, serial passage and description of liver lesions. *J. Exp. Med.* **125,** 673–688.

Deinhardt, F., Falk, L. G., Wolfe, A., Schudel, A., Nonyama, M., Lai, P., Lapin, B., and Yakovleva, L. (1978). Susceptibility of marmosets to Epstein-Barr virus-like baboon herpesviruses. *Primate Med.* **10,** 163–170.

DePaoli, A., Johnsen, D. O., and Noll, M. D. (1973). Granulocytic leukemia in white handed gibbons. *J. Am. Vet. Med. Assoc.* **163,** 624–628.

Desrosiers, R. C. (1990). HIV-1 origins, a finger on the missing link. *Nature (London)* **345,** 288–289.

Dienstag, J. L., Popper, H., and Purcell, R. H. (1976). The pathology of viral hepatitis types A and B in chimpanzees. *Am. J. Pathol.* **85,** 131–148.

Di Giamoco, R. F., and Shah, K. V. (1972). Virtual absence of infection with herpesvirus simiae in colony reared rhesus monkeys (*Macaca mulatta*), with a literature review on antibody prevelance in natural and laboratory rhesus populations. *Lab. Anim. Sci.* **22,** 61–67.

Dillner, J., Rabin, H., Letvin, N., Henle, W., Henle, G., and Klein, G. (1987). Nuclear DNA binding proteins determined by the Epstein-Barr virus related simian lymphotropic herpesviruses *H. gorilla, H. pan, H. pongo,* and *H. papio. J. Gen. Virol.* **68,** 1587–1596.

Douglas, J. D., Tanner, K. N., Prine, J. R., Van Riper, D. C., and Derwelis, S. K. (1967). Molluscum contagiosum in chimpanzees. *J. Am. Vet. Med. Assoc.* **151,** 901–903.

Downie, A. W. (1972). Serologic evidence of infection with Tana and Yaba pox viruses among several species of monkeys. *J. Hyg.* **72,** 245–250.

Downie, A. W., and Espana, C. (1972). Comparison of tanapox virus and Yaba-like viruses causing epidermic disease in monkeys. *J. Hyg.* **70,** 23–33.

Downie, A. W., and Espana, C. (1974). Serologic evidence of infection with tanapox and Yaba virus. *J. Hyg.* **72,** 245–250.

Downie, A. W., Taylor-Robinson, C. H., Caunt, A. E., Nelson, G. S., and Mansohn-Bahr, P. E. C. (1971). Tanapox: A new disease caused by a pox virus. *Br. Med. J.* **1,** 363–368.

Dueland, A. N., Martin, J. R., Devlin, M. E., Wellish, M., Mahalingam, R., Cohrs, R., Soike, K. F., and Gilden, D. H. (1992). Acute simian varicella infection: Clinical laboratory, pathologic and virologic features. *Lab. Invest.* **66,** 762–773.

Eberle, R. (1992). Evidence for an alphaherpesvirus indigenous to mountain gorillas. *J. Med. Primatol.* **21,** 246–251.

Eichberg, J. W., and Kalter, S. S. (1980). Hepatitis A and B: Serologic survey of human and nonhuman primate sera. *Lab. Anim. Sci.* **30,** 541–543.

Eichberg, J. W., McCullough, B., Kalter, S. S., Thor, D. E., and Rodriguez, A. R. (1976). Clinical, virological and pathological features of herpesvirus SA8 infection in conventional and gnotobiotic infant baboons (*Papio cynocephalus*). *Arch. Virol.* **50,** 255–270.

Emau, P., McClure, H. M., Isahakai, M., Else, J. G., and Fultz, P. N. (1991). Isolation from African Sykes' monkeys (*Cercopithecus mitis*) of a lentivirus related to human and simian immunodeficiency viruses. *J. Virol.* **65,** 2134–2140.

Emmons, R. W., and Lennette, E. H. (1970). Natural herpesvirus hominis infection of a gibbon (*Hylobates lar*). *Arch. Gesamte Virusforsch.* **31,** 215–218.

Espana, C. (1973). Herpes simiae infection in *Macaca radiata. Am. J. Phys. Anthropol.* **38,** 447–454.

Eugster, A. K., Kalter, S. S., Kim, C. S., and Pinkerton, M. E. (1969). Isolation of adenoviruses from baboons (*Papio* sp.) with respiratory and enteric infections. *Arch. Gesamte Virusforsch.* **26,** 260–270.

Falk, L., Deinhardt, F., Nonoyama, M., Wolfe, L. G., Berholz, C., Lapin, B., Yakovleva, L., Agrba, V., Henle, G., and Henle, W. (1976). Properties of a baboon lymphotropic herpes virus related to Epstein-Barr virus. *Int. J. Cancer* **18**, 798–807.

Feichtinger, H., Li, S., Kaaya, E., Putkonen, P., Grunewald, K., Weyrer, K., Bottiger, D., Ernberg, I., Linde, A., Biberfeld, G., and Biberfeld, P. (1992). A monkey model of Epstein-Barr virus associated lymphomagenesis in human acquired immunodeficiency syndrome. *J. Exp. Med.* **176**, 281–286.

Felsburg, P. J., Heberling, R. L., and Kalter, S. S. (1972). Experimental genital infection of cebus monkeys with oral and genital isolates of herpesvirus hominis types 1 and 2. *Arch. Gesamte Virusforsch.* **39**, 223–227.

Felsburg, P. J., Heberling, R. L., Brack, M., and Kalter, S. S. (1973). Experimental genital infection of the marmoset. *J. Med. Primatol.* **2**, 50–60.

Felsenfeld, A. D., and Schmidt, N. J. (1975). Immunological relationship between Delta herpes virus of patas monkeys and varicella-zoster virus of humans. *Infect. Immun.* **12**, 261–266.

Fiennes, R. N. (1972). Rabies. *In* "Pathology of Simian Primates" (R. N. T. W. Fiennes, ed.), pp. 646–662. Karger, London.

Fine, D. L., and Arthur, L. O. (1981). Expression of natural antibodies against endogenous and horizontally transmitted macaque retroviruses in captive macaques. *Virology* **112**, 49–61.

Fine, D. L., Landon, J. C., Pienta, R. J., Kubicek, M. T., Valerio, M. G., and Chopra, H. C. (1975). Responses of infant rhesus monkeys to innoculation with Mason-Pfizer monkey virus materials. *J. Natl. Cancer Inst. (U.S.)* **54**, 651–658.

Fischer-Hoch, S. P., Platt, G. S., Lloyd, G., and Simpson, D. I. H. (1983). Haemotological and biochemical monitoring of Ebola infection in rhesus monkeys: Implications for patient management. *Lancet* **1**, 1055–1058.

Fischer-Hoch, S. P., Brammer, T. L., Trappier, S. G., Hutwagner, L. C., Farrar, B. B., Ruo, S. L., Brown, B. G., Hermann, I. M., Perez-Oronoz, G. I., Goldsmith, C. S., Hanes, M. A., and McCormick, J. B. (1992). Pathogenic potential of filoviruses: Role of geographic origin of primate host and virus strain. *J. Infect. Dis.* **166**, 753–763.

Flecknell, P. A., Parry, R., Needham, J. R., Ridley, R. M., Baker, H. F., and Bowes, H. F. (1983). Respiratory disease associated with parainfluenza virus type I (Sendai) virus in a colony of marmosets (*Callithrix jacchus*). *Lab. Anim.* **17**, 111–113.

Franchini, G., and Reitz, M. S. (1994). Phylogenesis and genetic complexity of nonhuman primate retroviridae. *AIDS Res. Hum. Retroviruses* **10**, 1047–1060.

Fraser, C. E. O., Chalifoux, L., Sehgal, P., Hunt, R. D., and King, N. W. (1978). A paramyxovirus causing fatal gastroenteritis in marmoset monkeys. *In* "Primates in Medicine" (E. I. Goldsmith and J. Moor-Jankowski, eds.), pp. 261–270. Karger, Basel.

Freifeld, A. G., Hilliard, J., Southers, J., Murray, M., Savarese, B., Schmitt, J. M., and Strauss, S. E. (1995). A controlled seroprevalence survey of primate handlers for evidence of asymptomatic herpes B virus infection. *J. Infect. Dis.* **171**, 1031–1034.

Fujimoto, K., and Honjo, S. (1991). Presence of antibody to Cyno-EBV in domestically bred cynomolgus monkeys (*Macaca fascicularis*). *J. Med. Primatol.* **20**, 42–45.

Fultz, P. N., and Zack, P. M. (1994). Unique lentivirus-host interactions: SIVsmmPBj14 infection of macaques. *Virus Res.* **32**, 205–225.

Fultz, P. N., McClure, H. M., Anderson, D. C., Swenson, R. B., Anad, R., and Srinivasan, A. (1986). Isolation of a T lymphotropic retrovirus from naturally infected sooty mangabey monkeys (*Cerocebus atys*). *Proc. Natl. Acad. Sci. U.S.A.* **83**, 5286–5290.

Fultz, P. N., Gordon, R. P., Anderson, D. C., and McClure, H. M. (1990). Prevalence of natural infection with SIVsmm and STLV-1 in a breeding colony of sooty mangabeys. *AIDS* **4**, 619–625.

Gainer, J. H. (1967). Encephalomyocarditis virus infections in Florida, 1960–1966. *J. Am. Vet. Med. Assoc.* **151**, 421–425.

Gay, F. P., and Holden, M. (1933). The herpes encephalitis problem. *J. Infect. Dis.* **53**, 287–303.

Gerber, P., Prichett, R. F., and Kieff, E. D. (1976). Antigens and DNA of a chimpanzee agent related to Epstein-Barr virus. *J. Virol.* **19**, 1090–1099.

Gerber, P., Kalter, S. S., Schildlovsky, G., Peterson, W. D., and Daniel, M. D. (1977). Biologic and antigenic characteristics of Epstein-Barr related herpesviruses of chimpanzees and baboons. *Int. J. Cancer* **20**, 448–459.

Glad, W. R., and Nesland, J. M. (1995). Focal epithelial hyperplasia of the oral mucosa in two chimpanzees (*Pan troglodytes*). *Am. J. Primatol.* **10**, 83–89.

Gormus, B. J., Murphey-Corb, M., Martin, L. N., Zhang, J., Baskin, G. B., Trygg, C. B., Walsh, G. P., and Meyers, W. M. (1989). Interactions between Simian immunodeficiency virus and *Mycobacterium leprae* in experimentally innoculated rhesus monkeys. *J. Infect. Dis.* **160**, 405–413.

Goubau, P., Van Brussel, M., Vandamme, A. M., Lui, H. F., and Desmuyter, J. (1994). A primate T-lymphotropic virus (PTLV-L) different from HTLV-I and II in a wild caught baboon. *Proc. Natl. Acad. Sci. U.S.A.* **91**, 2848–2852.

Gough, A. W., Barsoum, N. J., Gracon, S. I., Mitchell, L., and Sturgess, J. M. (1982). Poxvirus infection in a colony of common marmosets (*Callithrix jacchus*). *Lab. Anim. Sci.* **32**, 87–90.

Gravell, M., London, W. T., Rodriguez, M., Palmer, A. E., Hamilton, R. S., and Curfman, B. L. (1980a). Studies on hemorrhagic fever virus infection of patas monkeys. I. Serology. *In* "The Comparative Pathology of Zoo Animals" (R. J. Montali and G. Migaki, eds.), pp. 167–170. Smithsonian Institution Press, Washington, DC.

Gravell, M., Palmer, A. E., Rodriguez, M., London, W. T., and Hamilton, R. S. (1980b). Method to detect asymptomatic carriers of simian hemorrhagic fever virus. *Lab. Anim. Sci.* **30**, 988–991.

Gravell, M., London, W. T., Houff, S. A., Hamilton, R. S., Sever, J. L., Kapaikian, A. Z., Murti, G., Arthur, L. O., Gilden, R. V., Osborn, K. G., Marx, P. A., Henrickson, R. V., and Gardern, M. B. (1984). Transmission of simian AIDS with a type D retrovirus isolate. *Lancet* **1**, 334–335.

Gravell, M., London, W. T., Leon, M. E., and Hamilton, R. S. (1986a). Differences among isolates of simian hemorrhagic fever (SHF) virus. *Proc. Soc. Exp. Biol. Med.* **181**, 112–119.

Gravell, M., London, W. T., Leon, M., Palmer, A. E., and Hamilton, R. S. (1986b). Elimination of persistent simian hemorrhagic fever (SHF) virus infection in patas monkeys. *Proc. Soc. Exp. Biol. Med.* **181**, 219–225.

Guenno, B. L., Formentry, P., Wyers, M., Gounon, P., Walker, F., and Boesch, C. (1995). Isolation and partial characterization of a new strain of Ebola virus. *Lancet* **345**, 1271–1274.

Hall, A. S., and McNulty, W. P. (1967). A contagious pox disease in monkeys. *J. Am. Vet. Med. Assoc.* **151**, 833–838.

Hall, W. C., Kovatch, R. M., Herman, P. H., and Fox, J. G. (1971). Pathology of measles virus infection. *Vet. Pathol.* **8**, 307–319.

Halstead, S. B. (1981). Dengue and dengue hemorrhagic fever. *In* "Section B: Viral Zoonoses" (G. W. Beran, ed.), pp. 421–435. CRC Press, Boca Raton, FL.

Halstead, S. B., and Palumbo, N. E. (1973). Studies of the immunization of monkeys against denge: II. Protection following inoculation of combinations of viruses. *Am. J. Trop. Med. Hyg.* **22**, 375.

Halstead, S. B., Casals, J., Shotwell, H., and Palumbo, N. (1973). Studies on the immunization of monkeys against dengue: I. Protection derived from single and sequential virus infections. *Am. J. Trop. Med. Hyg.* **22**, 365.

Harbour, D. A., and Caunt, A. E. (1979). The serological relationship of varicella-zoster virus to other primate herpesviruses. *J. Gen. Virol.* **45**, 469–477.

Hayami, M., Komuro, A., Nozawa, K., Shotake, T., Ishikawa, K. I., Yamamoto, K., Ishida, T., Honjo, S., and Hinuma, Y. (1984). Prevalence of antibody to adult T-cell leukemia virus associated antigens (ATLA) in Japanese monkeys and other nonhuman primates. *Int. J. Cancer* **33**, 179–183.

Hayami, M., Ido, E., and Miura, T. (1994). Survey of simian immunodeficiency virus among nonhuman primate populations. *Cur. Top. Microbiol. Immunol.* **188**, 1–20.

Heberling, R. L., Baker, S. T., Kalter, S. S., Smith, G. C., and Helmke, R. J. (1977). Oncornavirus isolated from a squirrel monkey (*Saimiri sciureus*) lung culture. *Science* **195**, 289–292.

Henrickson, R. V., Maul, D. H., Osborn, K. G., Sever, J. L., Madden, D. L., Ellingsworth, L. R., Anderson, J. H., Lowenstine, L. J., and Gardner, M. B.

(1983). Epidemic of acquired immunodeficiency in rhesus monkeys. *Lancet* **1**, 338–390.

Henrickson, R. V., Maul, D. H., Lerche, N. W., Osborn, K. G., Lowenstine, L. J., Prahalada, S., Sever, J. L., and Gardner, M. B. (1984). Clinical features of simian acquired immunodeficiency syndrome (SAIDS) in rhesus monkeys. *Lab. Anim. Sci* **34**, 140–145.

Heuschele, W. P. (1960). Varicella (Chicken pox): In three young anthropoid apes. *J. Am. Vet. Med. Assoc.* **136**, 256–257.

Hollander, C. F., and VanNoord, M. J. (1972). Focal epithelial hyperplasia: A virus induced oral mucosal lesion in the chimpanzee. *Oral Surg.* **33**, 220–226.

Holmes, G. P., Chapman, L. E., Stewart, J. A., Straus, J. A., Straus, S. E., Hilliard, J. K., and Davenport, D. S. (1995). Guidelines for the prevention and treatment of B-virus infections in exposed persons. *Clin. Infect. Dis.* **20**, 421–439.

Holmes, G. P., Hilliard, J. K., Klontz, K. C., Rupert, A. H., Schindler, C. M., Parrish, E., Griffin, G., Ward, G. S., Bernstein, N. D., Bean, T. W., Ball, M. R., Brady, J. A., and Wilder, M. H. (1990). B virus (*Herpesvirus simiae*) infection in humans: Epidemiologic investigation of a cluster. *Ann. Intern. Med.* **112**, 833–839.

Hooks, J. J., Gibbs, C. J., Cutchins, E. C., Rogers, N. G., Lampert, P., and Gajdusek, D. V. (1972). Characterization and distribution of two foamy viruses isolated from chimpanzees. *Arch. Gesamte Virusforsch.* **38**, 38–55.

Horvath, C. J., Simon, M. A., Bergsagel, D. J., Pauley, D. R., King, N. W., Garcea, R. L., and Ringler, D. J. (1992). Simian virus 40-induced disease in rhesus monkeys with simian acquired immunodeficiency syndrome. *Am. J. Pathol.* **140**, 1431–1440.

Hubbard, G. B., Soike, K. F., Butler, T. M., Carey, K. D., Davis, H., Butcher, W. I., and Gauntt, C. J. (1992). An encephalomyocarditis virus epizootic in a baboon colony. *Lab. Anim. Sci.* **42**, 233–239.

Hubbard, G. B., Mone, J. P., Alan, J. S., Davis, K. J., Leland, M. M., Banks, P. M., and Smir, B. (1993). Spontaneously generated non-hodgkin's lymphoma in twenty-seven simian T-cell leukemia virus type 1 antibody positive baboons (*Papio* sp.). *Lab. Anim. Sci.* **43**, 301–309.

Hudson, N. P. (1928). The pathology of experimental yellow fever in the *macacus rhesus:* II. Microscopic pathology. *Am. J. Pathol.* **4**, 407–418.

Hull, R. N. (1971). B virus vaccine. *Lab. Anim. Sci.* **21**, 1068–1071.

Hunt, R. D., and Blake, B. J. (1993a). Herpesvirus B infection. *In* "Monographs on the Pathology of Laboratory Animals: Nonhuman Primates" (T. C. Jones, U. Mohr, and R. D. Hunt, eds.), Vol. 1, pp. 78–81. Springer-Verlag, Berlin and New York.

Hunt, R. D., and Blake, B. J. (1993b). Gastroenteritis due to paramyxovirus. *In* "Monographs on the Pathology of Laboratory Animals: Nonhuman Primates" (T. C. Jones, U. Mohr, and R. D. Hunt, eds.), Vol. 2, pp. 32–37. Springer-Verlag, Berlin and New York.

Hunt, R. D., and Melendez, L. V. (1966). Spontaneous herpes-T infection in the owl monkey (*Aotus trivirgatus*). *Vet. Pathol.* **3**, 1–26.

Hunt, R. D., Garcia, F. G. Barahona, N. H., King, N. W., Fraser, C. E. O., and Melendez, L. V. (1973). Spontaneous herpesvirus saimiri lymphoma in an owl monkey. *J. Infect. Dis.* **127**, 723–725.

Hunt, R. D., Blake, B. J., Chalifoux, L. V., Sehgal, P. K., King, N. W., and Letvin, N. L. (1983). Transmission of naturally occurring lymphoma in macaque monkeys. *Proc. Natl. Acad. Sci. U.S.A.* **80**, 5085–5089.

Ishida, T., and Yamamoto, K. (1987). Survey of nonhuman primates for antibodies reactive with Epstein-Barr virus (EBV) antigens and susceptibility of their lymphocytes for immortalization with EBV. *J. Med. Primatol.* **16**, 359–371.

Ishikawa, K. I., Fukasawa, M., Tsujimoto, H., Else, J. G., Isahakai, M., Ubhi, N. K., Ishida, T., Takenaka, O., Kawamoto, Y., Spriatna, Y., Abe, K., and Yamamoto, K. (1987). Serological survey and virus isolation of simian T-cell leukemia in their native countries. *Int. J. Cancer* **40**, 233–239.

Iyer, C. G., Laxmana, R., Work, T. H., and Narasimha Murthy, D. P. (1959). Kyasanur forest disease VI: Pathologic findings in three human cases of Kyasanur forest disease. *Indian J. Med. Sci.* **13**, 1011–1022.

Iyer, C. G. S., Work, T. H., Narasimha Murthy, D. P., Trapido, H., and Rajagopalan, P. K. (1960). Pathologic findings in monkeys, *Presbytis entellus* and *Macaca radiata* found dead in the forest. *Indian J. Med. Res.* **48**, 276–286.

Jezek, Z., Arita, I., Szczeniowski, M., Paluku, K. M., Ruti, K., and Nakano, J. H. (1985). Human tanapox in Zaire: Clinical and epidemiological observations on cases confirmed by laboratory studies. *Bull. W.H.O.* **63**, 1027–1035.

Johnson, L., Wolffe, L. G., Whisler, W. W., Norton, T., Thakkar, B., and Deinhardt, F. (1975). Induction of gliomas in marmosets by simian sarcoma virus type 1 (SSV-1). *Proc. Am. Assoc. Cancer Res.* **16**, 119 (abstr.).

Jones, E. E., Alford, P. L., Reingold, A. L., Russel, H., Keeling, M. E., and Broome, C. V. (1984). Predisposition to invasive pneumococcal illness following parainfluenza 3 virus infection in chimpanzees. *J. Am. Vet. Med. Assoc.* **185**, 1351–1353.

Johnsen, D. O., Wooding, W. L., Tanticharoenyos, P., and Karnjanaprakorn, C. (1971). An epizootic of A2/Hong Kong/68 influenza in Gibbons. *J. Infect. Dis.* **123**, 365–369.

Jung, J. U., and Desrosiers, R. C. (1991). Identification and characterization of the Herpesvirus saimiri oncoprotein STP-C488. *J. Virol.* **65**, 6953–6960.

Jung, J. U., and Desrosiers, R. C. (1992). Herpesvirus saimiri oncogene STP-488 encodes a phospholipoprotein. *J. Virol.* **66**, 1777–1780.

Jung, J. U., Trimble, H. J., King, N. W., Biesinger, B., Fleckenstein, B. W., and Desrosiers, R. C. (1991). Identification of transforming genes of subgroup A and C strains of herpesvirus saimiri. *Proc. Natl. Acad. Sci. U.S.A.* **88**, 7051–7055.

Kalter, S. S. (1982). Enteric diseases of nonhuman primates. *Vet. Pathol.* **19**, Suppl. 7, 33–43.

Kalter, S. S., and Heberling, R. L. (1978). Serologic response of primates to influenza viruses. *Proc. Soc. Exp. Biol. Med.* **159**, 414–417.

Kalter, S. S., and Heberling, R. L. (1990). Viral battery testing in nonhuman primate colony management. *Lab. Anim. Sci.* **40**, 21–23.

Kalter, S. S., Heberling, T. E., Vice, T. E., Lief, F. S., and Rodriguez, A. R. (1969). Influenza (A2/Hong Kong/68) in the baboon (*Papio* sp). *Proc. Soc. Exp. Biol. Med.* **132**, 357–361.

Kalter, S. S., Heberling, R. L., and Cooper, R. W. (1974). Serologic testing of various primate species maintained in a single outdoor breeding colony. *Lab. Anim. Sci.* **24**, 636–645.

Kalter, S. S., Weiss, S. A., Heberling, R. L., Guajardo, J. E., and Smith, G. C. (1978). The isolation of herpesvirus from trigeminal ganglia of normal baboons (*Papio cynocephalus*). *Lab. Anim. Sci.* **28**, 705–709.

Kalter, S. S., Smith, G. C., and Heberling, R. L. (1979). Electron microscopic examination of primate feces for rotavirus. *Lab. Anim. Sci.* **29**, 516–518.

Kalter, S. S., Rodriguez, A. R., and Heberling, R. L. (1982). Rotavirus (SA11) antibody in nonhuman primates. *Lab. Anim. Sci.* **32**, 291–293.

Kaufmann, A. F., Gary, G. W., Broderson, J. R., Perl, D. P., Quist, K. D., and Kissling, R. E. (1973). Simian virus 16 associated with an epizootic of obscure neurologic disease. *Lab. Anim. Sci.* **23**, 812–818.

Keeble, S. A. (1960). B virus infection in monkeys. *Ann. N. Y. Acad. Sci.* **85**, 960–969.

Kestler, H. W., Li, Y., Naidu, Y. M., Butler, C. V., Ochs, M. F., Jaenel, G., King, N. W., Daniel, M. D., and Desrosiers, R. C. (1988). Comparison of simian immunodeficiency isolates. *Nature (London)* **331**, 619–621.

Khabbaz, R. F., Rowe, T., Murphey-Corb, M., Heneine, W. M., Schable, C. A., George, J. R., Pau, C. P., Parekh, B. S., Lairomore, M. D., Curran, J. W., Kaplan, J. E., and Schochetman, G. (1992). Simian immunodeficiency virus needlestick accident in a laboratory worker. *Lancet* **340**, 271–273.

Khabbaz, R. F., Heneine, W., George, J. G., Paarekh, B., Rowe, T., Woods, T., Switzer, W. M., McClure, H. M., Murphey-Corb, M., and Folks, T. M. (1994). Brief report: Infection of a laboratory worker with simian immunodeficiency virus. *N. Engl. J. Med.* **330**, 172–177.

Kim, C. S., Sueltenfuss, E. A., and Kalter, S. S. (1967). Isolation and characterization of simian adenoviruses isolated in association with an outbreak of pneumoenteritis in vervet monkeys (*Cercopithecus aethiops*). *J. Infect. Dis.* **117**, 239–300.

Kim, C. S., Kriewaldt, F. H., Hagino, N., and Kalter, S. S. (1970). Subacute sclerosing panencephalitis-like syndrome in the adult baboon. *J. Am. Vet. Med. Assoc.* **157,** 730–735.

King, N. W., Hunt, R. D., Daniel, M. D., and Melendez, L. V. (1967). Overt herpes-T infection in squirrel monkeys (*Saimiri sciureus*). *Lab. Anim. Care* **17,** 413–423.

King, N. W., Hunt, R. D., and Letvin, N. L. (1983). Histopathologic changes in macaques with an acquired immunodeficiency syndrome (AIDS). *Am. J. Pathol.* **113,** 382–388.

Kloster, B. E., Manias, D. A., Ostrow, R. S., Shaver, M. K., McPherson, S. W., Rangen, S. R. S., Uno, H., and Faras, A. J. (1988). Molecular cloning and characterization of the DNA of two papillomaviruses from monkeys. *Virology* **166,** 30–40.

Klotz, O. and Belt, T. H. (1930a). The pathology of the spleen in yellow fever. *Am. J. Pathol.* **6,** 655–662.

Klotz, O. and Belt, T. H. (1930b). The pathology of the liver in yellow fever. *Am. J. Pathol.* **6,** 663–687.

Kornegay, R. W., Giddens, W. E., Van Hoosier, G. L., and Morton, W. R. (1985). Subacute nonsuppurative hepatitis associated with hepatitis B infection in two cynomolgus monkeys. *Lab. Anim. Sci.* **35,** 400–404.

Kupper, J. L., Casey, H. W., and Johnson, D. K. (1970). Experimental Yaba and benign epidermal monkey pox in rhesus monkeys. *Lab. Anim. Care* **20,** 979–988.

Lackner, A. A. (1988). Tissue distribution of simian AIDS retrovirus serotype 1 and its relationship to the pathogenesis of simian AIDS. University of California at Davis.

Lackner, A. A., Schiodt, M., Armitage, G. C., Moore, P. F., Munn, R. J., Marx, P. A., Gardner, M. B., and Lowenstine, L. J. (1989). Mucosal epithelial cells and langerhans cells are targets for infection by immunosuppressive the type D retrovirus Simian AIDS retrovirus serotype 1. *J. Med. Primatol.* **18,** 195–207.

Lackner, A. A., Smith, M. O., Munn, R. J., Martfeld, D. J., Gardner, M. B., Marx, P. A., and Dandekar, S. (1991). Localization of simian immunodeficiency virus in the central nervous system of rhesus monkeys. *Am. J. Pathol.* **139,** 609–621.

Lankas, G. R., and Jensen, R. D. (1987). Evidence of hepatitis A infection in immature rhesus monkeys. *Vet. Pathol.* **20,** 340–344.

Lapin, B. A., and Shevtsova, Z. V. (1990). Persistence of spontaneous and experimental hepatitis A in rhesus macaques. *Exp. Pathol.* **39,** 59–60.

Larimore, M. D., Kaplan, J. E., Daniel, M. D., Lerche, N. W., Nara, P. L., McClure, H. M., McVivar, J. W., McKinney, R. W., Hendry, M., Gerone, P., Rayfield, M., Allan, J., Ribas, J. L. Klein, H. J., Jahrling, P. B., and Brown, B. (1989). Guidelines for the prevention of simian immunodeficiency virus infection in laboratory workers and handlers. *J. Med. Primatol.* **18,** 167–174.

Lee, R. V., Prowten, A. W., Satchidanand, S., and Srivastava, B. I. S. (1985). Non-Hodgkins lymphoma and HTLV-I antibodies in a gorilla. *N. Engl. J. Med.* **312,** 118–119.

Lemon, S. M., Choa, S., Jansen, R. W., Binn, L. N., and Leduc, J. W. (1987). Genomic heterogenicity among human and nonhuman strains of hepatitis A virus. *J. Virol.* **61,** 735–742.

Leopardi, R., Ilonen, J., Mattila, L., and Salmi, A. A. (1993). Effect of measles virus infection of MHC class II expression and antigen expression in human monocytes. *Cell. Immunol.* **147,** 338–396.

Lerche, N. W., Osborn, K. G., Marx, P. A., Prahalda, S., Maul, D. H., Lowenstine, L. J., Munn, R. J., Bryant, M. L., Henrickson, R. V., Arthur, L. O., Gilden, R. V., Barker, C. S., Hunter, E., and Gardner, M. B. (1986). Inapparent carriers of simian AIDS type D retrovirus and disease transmission with saliva. *J. Natl. Cancer Inst.* **77,** 489–496.

Lerche, N. W., Yee, J. L., and Jennings, M. B. (1994). Establishing specific retrovirus-free breeding colonies of macaques: An approach to primary screening and surveillance. *Lab. Anim. Sci.* **44,** 217–221.

Letvin, N. L., Daniel, M. D., Sehgal, P. K., Desrosiers, R. C., Hunt, R. D., Waldron, L. M., MacKey, J. J., Schmidt, D. K., Chalifoux, L. V., and King,

N. W. (1985). Induction of AIDS-like disease in macaque monkeys with T-cell tropic retrovirus STLV-III. *Science* **230,** 71–73.

Levin, J. L., Hilliard, J. K., Lipper, S. L., Butler, T. M., and Goodwin, W. J. (1988). A naturally occurring epizootic of simian agent 8 in the baboon. *Lab. Anim. Sci.* **38,** 394–397.

Levy, J. A., Levy, S. B., Hirshaut, Y., Kafuko, G., and Prince, A. (1971). Presence of EBV antibodies in sera from wild chimpanzees. *Nature (London)* **233,** 559–560.

Linneman, C. C., Kramer, L. W., and Askey, P. A. (1984). Familial clustering of hepatitis B infection in gorillas. *Am. J. Epidemiol.* **119,** 424–430.

London, W. T., Houff, S. A., Madden, D. L., Fuccillo, D. A., Gravel, M., Wallen, W. C., Palmer, A. E., and Sever, J. L. (1978). Brain tumors in owl monkeys inoculated with a human polyomavirus (JC virus). *Science* **201,** 1246–1249.

London, W. T., Martinez, A. J., Houff, S. A., Wallen, W. C., Curfman, B. L., Traub, R. G., and Sever, J. L. (1986). Experimental congenital disease with simian cytomegalovirus in rhesus monkeys. *Teratology* **33,** 323–331.

Loomis, M. R., O'Neill, T., Bush, M., and Montali, R. J. (1981). Fatal herpesvirus infection in Patas monkeys and a black and white colobus monkey. *J. Am. Vet. Med. Assoc.* **179,** 1236–1239.

Lowenstine, L. J. (1993). Typer D retrovirus infection, macaques. *In* "Monographs on the Pathology of Laboratory Animals: Nonhuman Primates" (T. C. Jones, U. Mohr, and R. D. Hunt, eds.), Vol. 1, pp. 20–32. Springer-Verlag, Berlin and New York.

Lowenstine, L. J., Pedersen, N. C., Higgins, J., Pallis, K. C., Uyeda, A., Marx, P., Lerche, N. W., Munn, R. J., and Gardner, M. B. (1986). Seroepidemiologic survey of captive Old-World primates for antibodies to human and simian retroviruses and isolation of a lentivirus from sooty mangabeys (*Cercocebus atys*). *Int. J. Cancer* **38,** 563–574.

Lowenstine, L. J., Lerche, N. W., Yee, J. L., Uyeda, A., Jennings, M. B., Munn, R. J., McClure, H. M., Anderson, D. C., Fultz, P. N., and Gardner, M. B. (1992). Evidence for a lentiviral etiology in an epizootic of immune deficiency and lymphoma in stump-tailed macaques (*Macaca arctoides*). *J. Med. Primatol.* **21,** 1–14.

Mahalingam, R., Clarke, P., Wellish, M., Dueland, A. N., Soike, K. F., Gilden, D. H., and Cohrs, R. (1992). Prevalence and distribution of latent simian varicella virus DNA in monkey ganglia. *Virology* **188,** 193–197.

Major, E. O., Vacante, D. A., Traub, R. G., London, W. T., and Siever, J. L. (1987). Owl monkey astrocytoma cells in culture spontaneously produce infectious JC virus which demonstrates altered biologic properties. *J. Virol.* **61,** 1435–1441.

Malherbe, H., and Harwin, R. (1958). Neurotropic virus in African monkeys. *Lancet* **2,** 530.

Mankowski, J. L., Spelman, H. G., Strandberg, J. D., Laterra, J., Carter, D. L., Clements, J. E., and Zink, M. C. (1994). Neurovirulent simian immunodeficiency virus replicates productively in endothelial cells of the central nervous system in vivo and in vitro. *J. Virol.* **68,** 8202–8208.

Mansfield, K. G., and Lackner, A. (1994). SIV infection in macaques at the NERPRC during 1970–72. *J. Med. Primatol.* **23,** 244 (abstr).

Marennikova, S. S., Maltseva, V. I., Shelukhina, E. M., Shenkman, L. S., and Korneeva, V. I. (1973). A generalized herpetic infection simulating small pox in a gorilla. *Intervirology* **2,** 280–286.

Marennikova, S. S., Shelukhina, E. M., Maltseva, V. I., and Ladnnyj, I. D. (1976). Poxviruses isolated from clinically ill and asymptomatically infected monkeys and a chimpanzee. *Bull. W.H.O.* **46,** 613–620.

Martin, B. J., Dysko, R. C., and Chrisp, C. E. (1991). Pancreatitis associated with simian adenovirus 23 in a rhesus monkey. *Lab. Anim. Sci.* **41,** 382–384.

Martin, D. P., and Kaye, H. S. (1983). Epizootic of parainfluenza-3 virus infections in gibbons. *J. Am. Vet. Med. Assoc.* **183,** 1185–1187.

Marx, P. A., Maul, D. H., Osborn, K. G., Lerche, N. W., Moody, P., Lowenstine, L. J., Henrickson, R. V., Arthur, L. O., Gilden, R. V., Gravell, M., London, W. T., Sever, J. L., Levy, J. A., Munn, R. J., and Gardner, M. B. (1984). Simian AIDS: Isolation of a type D retrovirus and transmission of the disease. *Science* **223,** 1083–1086.

Maul, D. H., Zaiss, C. P., Mackenzie, M. R., Shigi, S. M., Marx, P. A., and Gardner, M. B. (1988). Simian retrovirus D serotype 1 has a broad cellular tropism for lymphoid and nonlymphoid cells. *J. Virol.* **62**, 1768–1773.

Maynard, J. E., Hartwell, W. V., and Berquist, K. R. (1971). Hepatitis-associated antigen in chimpanzees. *J. Infect. dis.* **126**, 660–664.

McCarthy, T. J., Kennnedy, J. L., Blakeslee, J. R., and Bennet, B. T. (1990). Spontaneous malignant lymphoma and leukemia in a simian T-lymphotropic virus type 1 (STLV-1) antibody positive olive baboon. *Lab. Anim. Sci.* **40**, 79–81.

McChesney, M. B., Fujinami, R. S., Lerche, N. W., Marx, P. A., and Oldstone, M. B. (1989). Virus-induced immunosuppression: Infection of peripheral blood mononuclear cells and suppression of immunoglobulin synthesis during natural measles virus infection of rhesus monkeys. *J. Infect. Dis.* **159**, 757–760.

McClure, H. M., and Keeling, M. E. (1971). Viral diseases noted at the Yerkes Primate center colony. *Lab. Anim. Sci.* **21**, 1002–1010.

McClure, H. M., Keeling, M. E., Olberling, B., Hunt, R. D., and Melendez, L. V. (1972). Natural herpesvirus hominis infection of tree shrews *(Tupia glis). Lab. Anim. Sci.* **22**, 517–521.

McClure, H. M., Chandler, F. W., and Hierholzer, J. C. (1978). Necrotizing pancreatitis due to simian adenovirus type 31 in a rhesus monkey. *Arch. Pathol. Lab. Med.* **102**, 150–153.

McClure, H. M., Swenson, R. B., Kalter, S. S., and Lester, T. L. (1980). Natural genital herpes virus hominis infection in chimpanzees. *Lab. Anim. Sci.* **30**, 895–901.

McClure, M. O., Schulz, T. F., Tedder, R. S., Gow, J., McKeating, J. A., Weiss, R. A., and Baskerville, A. (1989). Inoculation of new world primates with human immunodeficiency virus. *J. Med. Primatol.* **18**, 329–335.

McConnell, S. J., Hickman, R. L., Wooding, W. L., and Huxsoll, D. L. (1968). Monkey-pox: Experimental infection in chimpanzees and immunization with vaccinia virus. *Am. J. Vet. Res.* **29**, 1675–1680.

McNulty, W. P. (1972). Pox diseases in primates. *In* "Pathology of Simian Primates" (R. N. T.-W. Fiennes, ed.), pp. 612–645. Karger, New York.

Mei, Z., Meng, Y., Shufan, C., Jingyn, X., and Ping, S. (1990). Virological survey of rhesus monkeys in China. *Lab. Anim. Sci.* **40**, 29–32.

Melendez, L. V., Espana, C., Hunt, R. D., and Daniel, M. D. (1969). Natural herpes simplex infection in the owl monkey *(Aotus trivirgatus). Lab. Anim. Care* **19**, 38–45.

Melendez, L. V., Hunt, R. D., Daniel, M. D., and Trum, B. F. (1970). New world monkeys, herpes viruses, and cancer. *In* "Infections and Immunosuppression in Subhuman Primates" (H. Balner and W. J. B. Beveridge, eds.), pp. 111–117. Munksgaard, Copenhagen.

Melnick, J. L., and Butel, J. S. (1988). Neurologic tumors in offspring after inoculation of mothers with killed-poliovirus vaccine. *N. Engl. J. Med.* **318**, 1226.

Miller, G., Shope, T., Coope, D., Waters, L., Pagano, J., Bornkamm, G. W., and Henle, W. (1977). Lymphoma in cotton-topped marmosets after inoculation with Epstein-Barr virus: Tumor incidence, histologic spectrum, antibody responses, demonstration of viral DNA and characterization of virus. *J. Exp. Med.* **145**, 948–967.

Moazed, T. C., and Thouless, M. E. (1993). Viral persistence of simian type D retrovirus (SRV-2/W) in naturally infected pigtailed macaques *(Macaca nemestrina). J. Med. Primatol.* **22**, 382–389.

Monath, T. P., Brinker, K. R., Chamdler, F. W., Kemp, G. E., and Cropp, C. B. (1981). Pathophysiologic correlations in a rhesus monkey model of yellow fever. *Am. J. Trop. Med. Hyg.* **30**, 431–443.

Montali, R. J. (1993). Callitrichid hepatitis. *In* "Monographs on the Pathology of Laboratory Animals: Nonhuman Primates" (T. C. Jones, U. Mohr, and R. D. Hunt, eds.), Vol. 2, pp. 61–62. Springer-Verlag, Berlin and New York.

Montali, R. J., Ramsay, E. C., Stephensen, C. B., Worley, M., Davis, J. A., and Holmes, K. V. (1989). A new transmissible viral hepatitis of marmosets and tamarins. *J. Infect. Dis.* **160**, 759–765.

Montali, R. J., Scanga, C. A., Pernikoff, D., Wessner, D. R., Ward, R., and Holmes, K. V. (1995). A common source outbreak of callitrichid hepatitis in captive tamarins and marmosets. *J. Infect. Dis.* **167**, 946–950.

Morbeck, M. E., Zihlman, A. L., Summner, D. R., and Galloway, A. (1991). Poliomyelitis and skeletal asymmetry in Gombe chimpanzees. *Primates* **32**, 77–91.

Morris, J. A., Blount, R. E., and Savage, R. E. (1956). Recovery of cytopathogenic agent from chimpanzees with coryza. *Proc. Soc. Exp. Biol. Med.* **92**, 544–549.

Muller, M. C., Saksena, N. K., Nerrienet, E., Chappey, C., Herve, V. M. A., Durand, J. P., Legal-Compodonico, P., Lang, M. C., Digoutte, J. P., Georges, J. P., Georges-Courbot, M. C., Sonigo, P., and Barre-Sinousii, F. (1993). Simian immunodeficiency viruses from central and western Africa. *J. Virol.* **67**, 1227–1235.

Murphey-Corb, M., Martin, L. N., Rangan, S. S., Baskin, G. B., Gormus, B. J., Wolf, R. H., Andes, W. A., West, M., and Montelaro, R. C. (1986). Isolation of an HTLV-III-related retrovirus from macaques with simian AIDS and its possible origin in asymptomatic mangabeys. *Nature (London)* **321**, 435–437.

Murphy, B. L., Maynard, J. E., Krushak, D. H., and Berquist, K. R. (1972). Microbial flora of imported marmosets: Viruses and enteric bacteria. *Lab. Anim. Sci.* **22**, 339–343.

Murphy, F. A., Simpson, D. I. H., Whitfield, S. G., Zlotnik, I., and Carter, G. B. (1971). Marburgvirus infection in monkeys. *Lab. Invest.* **24**, 279–291.

Mutombo, W. M., Arita, I., and Jezek, Z. (1983). Human monkey pox transmitted by a chimpanzee in a tropical rainforest area of Zaire. *Lancet* **1**, 735–737.

Nainan, O. V., Margolis, H. S., Robertson, B. H., Balayan, M., and Brinton, M. A. (1991). Sequence analysis of a new hepatitis virus naturally infecting cynomolgus macaques *(Macaca fascicularis). J. Gen. Virol.* **72**, 1685–1689.

Neuman-Haefelin, D., Rethwilm, A., Bauer, G., Gudat, F., and Hausen, H. (1983). Characterization of a foamy virus isolated from *Cercopithecus aethiops* lymphoblastoid cells. *Med. Microbiol. Immunol.* **172**, 75–86.

Neuman-Haefelin, D., Fleps, U., Renne, R., and Schweizer, M. (1993). Foamy viruses. *Intervirology* **35**, 196–207.

Niedobitek, G., Agathanggelou, A., Finerty, S., Tierney, R., Watkins, P., Jones, E. L., Morgan, A., Young, L. S., and Rooney, N. (1994). Latent Epstein-Barr virus infection in cottontop tamarins. *Am. J. Pathol.* **145**, 969–978.

Ohta, Y., Masuda, T., Tsujimoto, H., Ishikawa, K. I., Kodoma, T., Morikawa, S., Nakai, M., Honjo, S., and Hayami, M. (1987). Isolation of simian immunodeficiency virus from African green monkeys and seroepidemiologic survey of the virus from various non-human primates. *Int. J. Cancer* **41**, 115–122.

Olson, L. C., Pryor, W. H., and Thomas, J. M. (1991). Persistent reduction of B virus *(Herpesvirus simiae)* seropositivity in rhesus macaques acquired for a study of renal allograft tolerance. *Lab. Anim. Sci.* **41**, 540–544.

Ordy, J. M., Rangan, S. R. S., Wolf, R. H., Knight, C., and Dunlap, W. P. (1981). Congenital cytomegalovirus effects on postnatal neurologic development of squirrel monkey *(Saimiri sciureus)* offspring. *Exp. Neurol.* **74**, 728–747.

Osborn, K. G., Prahalda, S., Lowenstine, L. J., Gardner, M. B., Maul, D. H., and Henrickson, R. V. (1984). The pathology of an epizootic of acquired immunodeficiency in rhesus macaques. *Am. J. Pathol.* **114**, 94–103.

O'Sullivan, M. G., Anderson, D. C., Fikes, J. D., Bain, F. T., Carlson, C. S., Green, S. W., Young, N. S., and Brown, K. E. (1994). Identification of a novel simian parvovirus in cynomolgus monkeys with severe anemia. *J. Clin. Invest.* **93**, 1571–1576.

Palmer, A. E., Allen, A. M., Tauraso, N. M., and Shelokov, A. (1968). Simian hemorrhagic fever. I. Clinical and epizootic aspects of an outbreak among quarantined monkeys. *Am. J. Trop. Med. Hyg.* **17**, 404–412.

Parks, W. P., and Melnick, J. L. (1969). Attempted isolation of hepatitis viruses in marmosets. *J. Infect. Dis.* **120**, 539–547.

Pattison, J. R. (1994). A new parvovirus: Similarities between monkeys and humans. *J. Clin. Invest.* **93**, 1354.

Peeters, M., Honore, C., Huet, T., Bedjabaga, L., Ossari, S., Bussi, P., Cooper, R. W., and Delaporte, E. (1989). Isolation and partial characterization of an HIV related virus occurring naturally in chimpanzees in Gabon. *AIDS* **3**, 625–630.

Peiris, J. S. M., Dittus, W. P. J., and Ratnayake, C. B. (1993). Seroepidemiology of dengue and other arboviruses in a natural population of toque macaques *(Macaca sinica)* at Polonnaruwa Sri Lanka. *J. Med. Primatol.* **22,** 240–245.

Peters, J. C. (1966). An epizootic of monkey-pox at Rotterdam Zoo. *Int. Zool. Yearb.* **6,** 274–275.

Phillips-Conroy, J. E., Jolly, C. J., Petros, B., Allan, J. S., and Desrosiers, R. C. (1994). Sexual transmission of SIVagm in wild grivet monkeys. *J. Med. Primatol.* **23,** 1–7.

Potkay, S. (1992). Diseases of Callitrichidae: A review. *J. Med. Primatol.* **21,** 189–236.

Prier, J. E., Sauer, R. M., Malsberger, R. G., and Sillaman, J. M. (1960). Studies on a pox disease of monkeys. II. Isolation of the etiologic agent. *Am. J. Vet. Res.* **21,** 381–384.

Rabin, H., Strnad, B. C., Neubauer, R. H., Brown, A. M., Hopkins, R. F., and Mazur, R. A. (1980). Comparisons of nuclear antigens of Epstein-Barr virus (EBV) and EBV like simian viruses. *J. Gen. Virol.* **48,** 265–272.

Raine, C. S., Feldman, L. A., Sheppard, R. D., and Bornstein, M. B. (1969). Ultrastructure of measles virus in cultures of hamster cerebellum. *J. Virol.* **4,** 169–181.

Rangan, S. R. S., and Chaiban, J. (1980). Isolation and characterization of a cytomegalovirus from the salivary gland of a squirrel monkey *(Saimiri sciureus)*. *Lab. Anim. Sci.* **30,** 532–540.

Rangan, S. R. S., Martin, L. N., Bozelka, B. E., Wang, N., and Gomus, B. J. (1995). Epstein-Barr virus-related herpesvirus from a rhesus monkey *(Macaca mulatta)* with malignant lymphoma. *Int. J. Cancer* **38,** 425–432.

Renegar, K. B. (1992). Influenza virus infections and immunity: A review of human and animal models. *Lab. Anim. Sci.* **42,** 222–232.

Renne, R. A., McLaughlin, R., and Jenson, A. B. (1973). Measles virus-associated endometritus, cervicitis and abortion in a rhesus monkey. *J. Am. Vet. Med. Assoc.* **163,** 639–641.

Renquist, D. (1990). Outbreak of simian hemorrhagic fever. *J. Med. Primatol.* **19,** 77–80.

Richardson, J. H. and Humphrey, G. L. (1971). Rabies in imported nonhuman primates. *Lab. Anim. Sci.* **21,** 1082–1803.

Richardson-Wyatt, L. S., Belshe, R. B., London, W. T., Sly, D. L., Camargo, E., and Chanock, R. M. (1981). Respiratory syncytial virus antibodies in nonhuman primates and domestic animals. *Lab. Anim. Sci.* **31,** 413–415.

Ringler, D., Hancock, W. W., King, N. W., Letvin, N. L., Daniel, M. D., Desrosiers, R. C., and Murphy, G. F. (1987). Immunophenotypic characterization of the cutaneous exanthema of SIV-infected rhesus monkeys. *Am. J. Pathol.* **126,** 199–207.

Roberts, E. D., Baskin, G. B., Soike, K., and Gibson, S. V. (1984). Pathologic changes of experimental simian varicella (Delta herpes) infection in African green monkeys *(Cercopithecus aethiops)*. *Am. J. Vet. Res.* **45,** 523–530.

Roberts, J. A., Lerche, N. W., Markovits, J. E., and Maul, D. H. (1988). Epizootic measles at the CRPRC. *Lab. Anim. Sci.* **38,** 492 (abstr.).

Rodhain, F. (1991). The role of monkeys in the biology of dengue and yellow fever. *Comp. Immunol. Microbiol. Infect. Dis.* **14,** 9–19.

Rudnik, A. (1965). Studies of the ecology of Dengue in Malaysia. A preliminary report. *J. Med. Entomol.* **2,** 203–208.

Rustigian, R., Johnston, P., and Reihart, H. (1955). Infection of monkey kidney tissue cultures with virus-like agents. *Proc. Soc. Exp. Biol. Med.* **88,** 8–16.

Sabin, A. B. (1985). Oral poliovirus vaccine: History of its development and use and current challenge to eliminate poliomyelitis from the world. *J. Infect. Dis.* **151,** 420–436.

Sakakibara, I., Sugimoto, Y., Sasawa, A., Honjo, S., Tsujimoto, H., Nakamura, H., and Hayami, M. (1986). Spontaneous malignant lymphoma in an African green monkey naturally infected with STLV-1. *J. Med. Primatol.* **15,** 311–318.

Sakesena, N. K., Herve, V., Durand, J. P., Leguenno, B., Diop, O. M., Digoutte, J. P., Mathiot, C., Muller, M. C., Love, J. L., Dube, S., Sherman, M. P., Benz, P. M., Erensoy, S., Galat-Luong, A., Galat, G., Paul, B., Dube, D. K., Barre-Sinoussi, F., and Poiesz, B. J. (1994). Seroepidemiologic, molecular and phylogenetic analyses of STLV-I from various naturally infected monkey species from central and western Africa. *J. Virol.* **198,** 297–310.

Sasseville, V. G., Newman, W. A., Lackner, A. A., Smith, M. O., Lausen, N. C. G., Beall, D., and Ringler, D. J. (1992). Elevated vascular cell adhesion molecule-1 in AIDS encephalitis induced by simian immunodeficiency virus. *Am. J. Pathol.* **141,** 1021–1030.

Sasseville, V. G., Newman, W., Brodie, S. J., Hesterberg, P., Pauley, D. R., and Ringler, D. J. (1994). Monocyte adhesion to endothelium in simian immunodeficiency virus-induced AIDS encephalitis is mediated by vascular cell adhesion molecule-1/a4b1 integrin interactions. *Am. J. Pathol.* **144,** 1–13.

Sauer, R. M., Prier, J. E., Buchanan, R. S., Creamer, A. A., and Fegley, H. C. (1960). Studies of a pox disease of monkeys. *Am. J. Vet. Res.* **21,** 377–380.

Schlauder, G. G., Dawson, G. J., and Simons, J. N. (1995a). Molecular and serologic analysis in the transmission of the GB hepatitis agents. *J. Med. Virol.* **46,** 81–90.

Schlauder, G. G., Pilot-Matais, T. J., Gretchen, S. G., Simons, J. N., Muerhoff, A. S., and Dawson, G. J. (1995b). Origin of GB-hepatitis viruses. *Lancet* **346,** 447–448.

Scott, G. B. D., and Keymer, I. F. (1975). The pathology of measles in Abyssinian colobus monkeys *(Colobus guereza)*: A description of an outbreak. *J. Pathol.* **117,** 229–233.

Shah, K. V. (1990). Polyomaviruses. *In* "Virology" (B. N. Fields and D. M. Knipe, eds.), 2nd ed. pp. 1609–1623. Raven Press, New York.

Shevstsova, Z. V., Lapin, B. A., Doroshenko, N. V., Krilova, R. I., Korzaja, L. I., Lomovskaya, I. B., Dzhelieva, Z. N., Zairov, G. G., Stahkanova, V. M., Belova, E. G., and Sazhchenko, L. A. (1988). Spontaneous and experimental hepatitis A in old world monkeys. *J. Med. Primatol.* **17,** 177–194.

Shiigi, S., Wilson, B., Leo, G., MacDonald, N., Toyooka, D., Hallick, L., Karty, R., Belozer, M. L., McNulty, W., Wolff, J., van Bueren, A., Howard, C., and Axthelm, M. (1989). Serologic and virologic analysis of type D simian retrovirus infection in a colony of celebes black macaques *(Macaca nigra)*. *J. Med. Primatol.* **18,** 183–185.

Simon, M. A., Daniel, M. D., Lee-Parritz, D., King, N. W., and Ringler, D. J. (1993). Disseminated B virus infection in a cynomolgus monkey. *Lab. Anim. Sci.* **43,** 545–550.

Simon, M. A., Ilyinskii, P. O., Veazey, R., Baskin, G. B., Young, H., Pauley, D., Daniel, M., and Lackner, A. (1995). Association of SV40 with a CNS lesion distinct from PML in macaques with AIDS. *Vet. Pathol.* **32,** 576 (abstr.).

Simons, J. N., Pilot-Matias, T. J., and Leary, T. P. (1995). Identification of two flavivirus-like genomes in the GB hepatitis agent. *Proc. Natl. Acad. Sci. U.S.A.* **92,** 3401–3405.

Singh, K. R., Pavris, K., and Anderson, C. R. (1963). Experimental transovarian transmission of Kyasanur forest disease virus in *Haemsphysalis spinigera*. *Nature (London)* **199,** 513.

Slighter, R. G., Kimball, J. P., Barbolt, A. D., and Drobeck, H. P. (1988). Enzootic hepatitis A infection in cynomolgus monkeys *(Macaca fascicularis)*. *Am. J. Primatol.* **14,** 73–81.

Smith, A. W., Skilling, D. E., Ensley, P. K., Bernirschke, K., and Lester, T. L. (1983). Calcivirus isolation and persistence in a pygmy chimpanzee *(Pan paniscus)*. *Science* **221,** 79–81.

Smith, C. E. G., Simpson, D. I. H., Bowen, E. T. W., and Zlotnick, E. T. (1967). Fatal human disease from Vervet monkeys. *Lancet* **2,** 1119–1112.

Smith, D. M. (1993). Endogenous retroviruses in xenografts. *N. Engl. J. Med.* **328,** 142.

Smith, E. K., Hunt, R. D., Garcia, F. G., Fraser, C. E., Merkal, R. S., and Karlson, A. G. (1973). Avian tuberculosis in monkeys. *Am. Rev. Respir. Dis.* **107,** 469–471.

Smith, J. S., Fishbein, D. B., Rupprecht, C. E., and Clark, K. (1991). Unexplained rabies in three immigrants in the United States: A virologic investigation. *N. Engl. J. Med.* **324,** 205–210.

Smith, M. W. (1982). Field aspects of the Marburg virus outbreak: 1967. *Primate Supply* **7,** 11–15.

Smith, P. C., Yuill, T. M., Buchanan, R. D., Stanton, J. S., and Chaicumpa, V. (1969). The gibbon *(Hylobates lar)*; a new primate host for Herpesvirus hominis. I. A natural epizootic in a laboratory a colony. *J. Infect. Dis.* **120,** 292–297.

Smith, R. E., Pirie, G. J., and England, J. J. (1987). Rabies vaccination of captive white handed gibbons potentially exposed to wild rabies virus. *Lab. Anim. Sci.* **37,** 668–669.

Soike, K. F., and Gerone, P. J. (1995). Acyclovir in the treatment of simian varicella infection of the African green monkey. *Am. J. Med.* **73,** 112–117.

Soike, K. F., Rangan, S. R. S., and Gerone, P. J. (1984). Viral disease models of primates. *Adv. Vet. Sci. Comp. Med.* **28,** 151–191.

Spira, A. I., Marx, P. A., Patterson, B. K., Mahoney, J., Koup, R. A., Wolinsky, S. M., and Ho, D. D. (1996). Cellular targets of infection and route of viral dissemination after an intravaginal inoculation of simian immunodeficiency virus into rhesus macaques. *J. Exp. Med.* **183,** 215–225.

Srihongse, S. (1969). Vesicular stomatitis virus in panamanian primates and other vertebrates. *Am. J. Epidemiol.* **90,** 69–76.

Steele, M. D., Giddens, W. E., Valerio, M., Sumi, S. M., and Stetzer, E. R. (1982). Spontaneous paramyxoviral encephalitis in nonhuman primates *(M. mulatta and M. nemestrina). Vet. Pathol.* **19,** 132–139.

Stikes, G. E., Bittle, J. L., and Cabasso, V. J. (1964). Comparison of simian foamy virus strains including a new serologic type. *Nature (London)* **201,** 1350–1351.

Stowell, R. E., Smith, E. K., Espana, C., and Nelson, V. G. (1971). Outbreak of malignant lymphoma in rhesus monkeys. *Lab. Invest.* **25,** 476–479.

Sundberg, J. P., and Reichman, M. E. (1993). Papillomavirus infections. *In* "Monographs on the Pathology of Laboratory Animals: Nonhuman Primates" (T. C. Jones, U. Mohr, and R. D. Hunt, eds.), Vol. 2, pp. 1–8. Springer-Verlag, Berlin and New York.

Sundberg, J. P., Shima, A. L., and Adkison, D. L. (1992). Oral papillomavirus infection in a pygmy chimpanzee *(Pan paniscus). J. Vet. Diag. Invest.* **4,** 70–74.

Swack, N. S., and Hsuing, G. D. (1982). Natural and experimental simian cytomegalovirus infections at a primate center. *J. Med. Primatol.* **11,** 169–177.

Takemoto, K. K., Furuno, A., Kato, K., and Yoshike, K. (1982). Biological and biochemical studies of African green monkey lymphotropic papovavirus. *J. Virol.* **42,** 502–509.

Tate, C. L., Conti, P. A., and Nero, E. P. (1973). Epithelial hyperplasia in the oral mucosa of a chimpanzee. *J. Am. Vet. Med. Assoc.* **163,** 619–621.

Tauraso, N. M., Shelokov, A., Palmer, A. E., and Allen, A. M. (1968). Simian hemorrhagic fever. III. Isolation and characterization of a viral agent. *Am. J. Trop. Med. Hyg.* **17,** 422–431.

Tellez-Nagel, I., and Harter, D. H. (1966). Subacute sclerosing leukoencephalitis: Ultrastructure of intranuclear and intracytoplasmic inclusions. *Science* **154,** 899–901.

Tesh, R. B., and Wallace, G. D. (1978). Observations on the natural history of encephalomyocarditis virus. *Am. J. Trop. Med. Hyg.* **27,** 133–143.

Theilen, G. H., Gould, D., Fowler, M., and Dungworth, D. L. (1971). C-type virus in tumor tissue of a wooly monkey *(Lagothrix* sp.). *J. Natl. Cancer Inst. (U.S.)* **47,** 881–889.

Thung, S. N., Gerber, M. A., Purcell, R. H., London, W. T., Mihalik, K. B., and Popper, H. (1981). Chimpanzee carriers of hepatitis B virus. *Am. J. Pathol.* **105,** 328–332.

Ticehurst, J., Rhodes, L. L., Krawczynski, K., Asher, L. V. S., Engler, W. F., Mensing, T. L., Caudill, J. D., Sjoren, M. H., Hoke, C. H., Leduc, J. W., Bradley, D. W., and Binn, L. N. (1992). Infection of owl monkeys *(Aotus)* and cynomolgus monkeys *(Macaca fascicularis)* with hepatitis E virus from Mexico. *J. Infect. Dis.* **165,** 835–845.

Todaro, G. J., Benveniste, R. E., Sherr, C. J., Scholm, J., Schidlovsky, G., and Stephenson, J. R. (1978). Isolation and characterization of a new type D retrovirus from the Asian primate, *Presbytis obscurus* (spectacled langur). *Virology* **84,** 189–194.

Tomonga, K., Katahira, J., Fukasawa, M., Hassan, M. A., Akari, H., Miura, T., Goto, T., Nakai, M., Suleman, M., Isahakia, M., and Hayami, M. (1993). Isolation and characterization of a simian immunodeficiency virus from African white-crowned mangabey monkeys *(Cercocebus torquatas lunulatas). Arch. Virol.* **129,** 77–92.

Traina-Dorge, V., Blanchard, J., Martin, L., and Murphey-Corb, M. (1992). Immunodeficiency and lymphoproliferative disease in an African green

monkey dually infected with SIV and STLV-1. *AIDS Res. Hum. Retroviruses* **8,** 97–100.

Tsai, C.-C., Giddens, W. E., Morton, W. R., Rosenkranz, S. L., Ochs, H. D., and Benveniste, R. E. (1985a). Retroperitoneal fibromatosis and acquired immunodeficiency syndrome in macaques: Epidemiologic studies. *Lab. Anim. Sci.* **35,** 460–464.

Tsai, C.-C., Warner, T. F. C. S., Uno, H., Giddens, W. E., and Ochs, H. (1985b). Subcutaneous fibromatosis associated with an acquired immune deficiency syndrome in pig-tailed macaques. *Am. J. Pathol.* **120,** 30–37.

Tsai, C.-C., Follis, K. E., Synder, K., Windsor, S., Thouless, M. E., Kuller, L., and Morton, W. R. (1990). Maternal transmission of type D simian retrovirus (SRV-2) in pigtailed macaques. *J. Med. Primatol.* **19,** 203–216.

Tsai, C.-C., Wu, H., and Meng, F. (1995). Immunocytochemistry of Kaposi's sarcoma-like tumor cells from macaques with simian AIDS. *J. Med. Entomol.* **24,** 43–48.

Tsarev, S. A., Emerson, S. U., Balayan, M. S., Ticehurst, J., and Purcell, R. H. (1991). Simian hepatitis A virus (HAV) strain AGM-27: Comparison of genome structure and growth in cell culture with other HAV strains. *J. Gen. Virol.* **72,** 1677–1683.

Tsujimoto, H., Noda, Y., Ishikawa, K. I., Nakamura, H., Fukasawa, M., Sakakibara, I., Honjo, S., and Hayami, M. (1987). Development of adult T-cell leukemia disease in African green monkey associated with clonal integration of simian T-cell leukemia virus type 1. *Cancer Res.* **47,** 269–274.

Tsujimoto, H., Cooper, R. W., Kodoma, T., Fukasawa, M., Miura, T., Ohta, Y., Ishikawa, K. I., Nakai, M., Frost, E., Roelants, G. E., Roffi, J., and Hayami, M. (1988). Isolation and characterization of simian immunodeficiency virus from mandrills in Africa and its relationship to other human and simian immunodeficiency viruses. *J. Virol.* **62,** 4044–4050.

Uhno, I., Riepenhoff-Talty, M., Dharakul, T., Chegas, P., Fischer, J. E., Greenberg, H. B., and Ogra, P. L. (1990). Extramucosal spread and development of hepatitis in immunodeficient and normal mice infected with rhesus rotavirus. *J. Virol.* **64,** 361–368.

Umemura, T., Inagaki, H., Goryo, M., and Itakura, C. (1985). Aspiration pneumonia with adenovirus infection in a Japanese macaque *(Macaca fuscata fuscata). Lab. Anim.* **19,** 39–41.

Valis, J. D., Newell, N., Reissig, M., Malherbe, H., Kaschula, V. R., and Shah, K. V. (1977). Characterization of SA12 as a simian virus-40-related papovavirus of Chacma baboons. *Infect. Immun.* **17,** 247–252.

Vickers, J. H. (1986). Approaches to determining colony infections and improving colony health. *In* "Primates: The Road to Self-Sustaining Populations" (J. Bernischke, ed.), pp. 521–530. Springer-Verlag, Berlin and New York.

Voevodin, A. F., Lapin, B. A., Yakovleva, L. A., Ponomaryena, T. I., Oganyan, T. E., and Razmadze, E. N. (1985). Antibodies reacting with human T-lymphotropic retrovirus (HTLV-1) or related antigens in lymphomatous and healthy hamadryas baboons. *Int. J. Cancer* **36,** 579–584.

Vogel, P., Weigler, B. J., Kerr, H., Hendrick, A. G., and Barry, P. A. (1994). Seroepidemiologic studies of CMV infection in a breeding population of rhesus macaques. *Lab. Anim. Sci.* **44,** 25–30.

von Magnus, P., Andersen, E. K., Petersen, K. B., and Birch-Anderson, A. (1959). A pox like disease in cynomolgus monkeys. *Acta Pathol. Microbiol. Scand.* **46,** 156–176.

Walker, D. H., Voelker, F. A., and Nakano, J. H. (1985). Diagnostic exercise: Tumors in a baboon. *Lab. Anim. Sci.* **35,** 627–628.

Ward, J. A., and Hilliard, J. K. (1994). B virus-specific pathogen-free (SPF) breeding colonies of macaques: Issues, surveillance, and results in 1992. *Lab. Anim. Sci.* **44,** 222–228.

Watanabe, T., Seiki, M., Tsujimoto, H., Miyoshi, I., Hayami, M., and Yoshida, M. (1985). Sequence homology of the simian retrovirus genome with human T-cell leukemia virus type 1. *Virology* **144,** 59–65.

Webb, H. E., and Chatterjea, J. B. (1962). Clinicopathologic observations on monkeys infected with Kyasanur forest disease virus with special reference to the hematopoietic system. *Bri. J. Haematol.* **8,** 401–413.

Weigler, B. J. (1992). Biology of B virus in macaque and human hosts: A review. *Clin. Infect. Dis.* **14,** 555–567.

Weigler, B. J., Robert, J. A., Hird, D. W., Lerche, N. W., and Hilliard, J. K. (1990). A cross sectional survey for B virus antibody in a colony of group housed rhesus macaques. *Lab. Anim. Sci.* **40,** 257–261.

Weigler, B. J., Hird, D. W., Hilliard, J. K., Lerche, N. W., Roberts, J. A., and Scott, L. M. (1993). Epidemiology of Cercopithecine herpesvirus 1 (B virus) infection and shedding in a large breeding cohort of rhesus macaques. *J. Infect. Dis.* **167,** 257–263.

Weir, E. C., Bhatt, P. N., Jacoby, R. O., Hilliard, J. K., and Morgenstern, S. (1993). Infrequent shedding and transmission of herpesvirus simiae from seropositive macaques. *Lab. Anim. Sci.* **43,** 541.

Wenner, H. A., Abel, D., Barrick, S., and Seshumurty, P. (1977). Clinical and pathologenetic studies of medical lake virus infections in cynomolgus monkeys (simian varicella). *J. Infect. Dis.* **135,** 611–622.

White, R. J., Simmons, L., and Wilson, R. B. (1972). Chickenpox in young anthropoid apes: Clinical and laboratory findings. *J. Am. Vet. Med. Assoc.* **161,** 690–692.

Whittaker, D., and Glaister, J. R. (1985). A Yaba-like condition in a young baboon *(Papio anubis)*. *Lab. Anim.* **19,** 177–179.

Wilson, R. B., Holscher, M. A., Chang, T., and Hodges, J. R. (1990). Fatal herpesvirus simiae B (B virus) infection in a patas monkey *(Erythrocebus patas)*. *J. Vet. Diagn. Invest.* **2,** 242–244.

Wolfe, L. G., Griesemer, R. A., and Farrell, R. L. (1968). Experimental aerosol transmission of Yaba virus in monkeys. *J. Natl. Cancer Inst. (U.S.)* **41,** 1175–1195.

Wolfe, L. G., Smith, R. K., and Deinhardt, F. (1972). Simian sarcoma virus type I *(lagothrix)*: Focus assay and demonstration of nontransforming associated virus. *J. Natl. Cancer Inst. (U.S.)* **48,** 1905–1908.

World Health Organization (1992). Viral hemorrhagic fever in imported monkeys. *Wkly. Epidemiol. Rec.* **67,** 142–143.

Wyatt, R. G., Sly, D. L., London, W. T., Palmer, A. E., Kalica, A. R., Kirk, D. H., Chanock, R. M., and Kapikian, A. Z. (1976). Induction of diarrhea in colostrum deprived newborn rhesus monkeys with the human reovirus-like agent in infantile gastroenteritis. *Arch. Virol.* **50,** 17–27.

Zack, P. M. (1993). Simian hemorrhagic fever. *In* "Monographs on the Pathology of Laboratory Animals: Nonhuman Primates" (T. C. Jones, U. Mohr, and R. D. Hunt, eds.), Vol. 1. Springer-Verlag, Berlin and New York, 118–131.

Zhenjian, D., Lang, S., Sasseville, V. G., Lackner, A., Ilynski, P. O., Daniel, M. D., Jung, J. U., and Descrosiers, R. C. (1995). Identification of a nef allele that causes lymphocytic activation and acute disease in macaque monkeys. *Cell (Cambridge, Mass.)* **82,** 665–674.

Zuckerman, A. J. (1995). The GB hepatitis viruses. *Lancet* **345,** 1453–1454.

Zuckermann, A. J., Thorton, A., Howard, C. R., Tsiquaye, K. N., Jones, D. M., and Brambell, M. R. (1978). Hepatitis B outbreak among chimpanzees at the London zoo. *Lancet* **2,** 652–654.

zur Hausen, H. L., Gissmann, A., Mincheva, A., and Bocker, J. F., (1979). Lymphotropic papoviruses isolated from African green monkey and human cells. *Med. Microbiol. Immunol.* **167,** 137–153.

Chapter 2

Bacterial and Mycotic Diseases

Susan V. Gibson

I. INTRODUCTION

Bacterial diseases can be significant causes of morbidity and mortality in nonhuman primate colonies. They may affect large numbers of primates, as in the case of shigellosis, campylobacteriosis, or leptospirosis, or just one individual, as may be seen with opportunistic infections with *Staphylococcus aureus* and *Pseudomonas* spp. Diagnosis requires culture and identification through a battery of biochemical or serologic tests. Effective treatment depends on accurate diagnosis and knowledge of the antibiotic sensitivities of bacterial isolates from the specific animal populations being treated. This chapter presents common and some uncommon bacterial diseases of nonhuman primates. Where possible, reported effective treatment regimens have been given; however, these regimens should not replace those based on historical antibiograms of isolates from primates at your facilities. Bacteria are presented in the general order of gram-positive, gram-negative, and acid-fast organisms.

Mycotic diseases occur less frequently than bacterial diseases in nonhuman primates. With the exception of the dermatophytoses, *Candida,* and *Histoplasma capsulatum* var. *duboisii,* most mycotic infections in nonhuman primates are diagnosed postmortem and therefore are not subject to treatment. Because of the importance of histopathology in diagnosis, the mycotic diseases are presented and organized here based on histologic appearance of the agent in tissues.

New and more sensitive methods of diagnosis of bacterial and fungal diseases are rapidly being developed using molecular diagnostic techniques. As these techniques become standardized and readily available, diagnosis and epidemiologic studies of these diseases will be greatly enhanced.

II. BACTERIAL DISEASES

A. *Streptococcus*

Streptococci are gram-positive coccoid bacteria, approximately 1 μm in diameter, which characteristically grow in chains in broth culture. Streptococci are divided in the Lancefield system into 18 distinct antigenic groups based on serologic differences of the cell wall carbohydrates. Streptococci are also differentiated by their ability to produce hemolysis on blood agar; most pathogenic streptococci (groups A, B, C, and G) produce complete or β hemolysis on blood agar. There are six general categories of streptococci recognized: pyogenic, oral, enterococci, lactic, anaerobic, and other. In nonhuman primates, the primary streptococcal pathogens reported are *Streptococcus pneumoniae* and group A, B, and C streptococci.

1. *Streptococcus pneumoniae*

Streptococcus pneumoniae (*Diplococcus pneumoniae, Pneumococcus pneumoniae*) is a gram-positive, encapsulated coccoid bacterium that produces α hemolysis on blood agar. The organism normally occurs in pairs, hence the designation *Diplococcus*. It is distinguished from other α hemolytic streptococci by its sensitivity to growth inhibition by optochin.

Infections are acquired by aerosol by way of the upper respiratory tract, middle ear, or orally (Graczyk *et al.,* 1995). *Streptococcus pneumoniae* has been isolated from the nasal passages and throats of healthy macaques (Good and May, 1971; Lund and Petersen, 1959). Cell wall proteins facilitate attachment to mucosal membranes and subsequent invasion. Stress-related factors, including capture, transportation, and quarantine (Kaufmann and Quist, 1969a; Fox and Wikse, 1971); viral infection (Brendt *et al.,* 1974; Jones *et al.,* 1984); and decreased immunocompetence in neonates due to waning passive immunity (Graczyk *et al.,* 1995) have been reported to predispose nonhuman primates to *S. pneumoniae* infection and disease. Experimental infection in stump-tailed macaques, in which *S. pneumoniae* was inoculated intracisternally, was rapidly progressive with bacteremia and death within 14–24 hr of inoculation (Mellins *et al.,* 1972).

Streptococcus pneumoniae is the primary cause of bacterial meningitis in nonhuman primates. It is a disease of low morbidity but high mortality. Pneumonia and septicemia (Jones *et al.,* 1984; Padovan and Cantrell, 1983), purulent conjunctivitis and panophthalmitis (Herman and Fox, 1971), and peritonitis (Kaufmann and Quist, 1969a) have also been reported. Disease was usually rapidly progressive and death could occur without prodromal clinical signs (Kaufmann and Quist, 1969a; Fox and Wikse, 1971; Graczyk *et al.,* 1995). A typical case of fulminating streptococcal meningitis was presented by Gilbert *et al.* (1987) in which a normally active 4-year-old cynomolgus monkey withdrew to the back of the cage and was observed to be lethargic and uncoordinated. Clinical evaluation revealed depression of the placing and extensor thrust reflexes. The monkey became ataxic, head pressed, and developed nuchal rigidity. Hypotension and coma followed, and the monkey died within 8 hr of development of clinical signs (Gilbert *et al.,* 1987). Other clinical presentations reported in macaques include generalized muscle tremors and incoordination, flaccid paralysis of the legs, circling, clonic seizures, convulsions, constricted pupils or delayed light reflexes, nystagmus, and head pressing (Kaufmann and Quist, 1969a; Fox and Wikse, 1971; Herman and Fox, 1971). Duration of illness when present ranged from less than 1 to 3 days (Fox and Wikse, 1971).

Clinical presentation of streptococcal meningitis in chimpanzees began with preliminary signs of upper respiratory tract infection: slight coughing and a seromucoid to mucopurulent nasal discharge (Solleveld *et al.,* 1984). Chimpanzees were predisposed to pneumococcal illness following upper respiratory tract infection with parainfluenza 3 virus (Jones *et al.,* 1984). Lethargy, vestibular signs, purulent conjunctivitis, head holding, cervical rigidity, lip droop, seizures, nystagmus, blindness, hemiparesis, dysphagia, and pyrexia developed as the disease progressed (Keeling and McClure, 1974; Solleveld *et al.,* 1984). Duration of clinical illness ranged from 2 to 14 days.

Due to the rapid progression of streptococcal meningitis, prompt diagnosis and initiation of treatment are critical. Macaques have been reported to present as hypothermic (Gilbert *et al.*, 1987) with moderate to marked leukocytosis due to neutrophilia and a left shift (Fox and Wikse, 1971; Gilbert *et al.*, 1987). In chimpanzees, streptococcal meningitis was characterized by rectal temperature exceeding 40°C, marked peripheral leukocytosis (40×10^3 WBC /μl), neutrophilia with a left shift, and elevated white blood cell (WBC) count and protein levels in the cerebral spinal fluid (Keeling and McClure, 1974; Solleveld *et al.*, 1984). Presence of free or phagocytized encapsulated gram-positive diplococci in smears of the cerebrospinal fluid (CSF) provided a presumptive diagnosis of pneumococcal meningitis (Keeling and McClure, 1974; Solleveld *et al.*, 1984).

Precise diagnosis may be made from recovery of *S. pneumoniae* from the blood, spinal fluid, upper respiratory tract, or lesioned organs at necropsy. *Streptococcus pneumoniae* grows well on 5% sheep blood agar or brain heart infusion broth. Identification can be made from appearance with Gram stain, sensitivity to optochin, and characteristic α hemolysis on blood agar. Commercial kits are available for the identification of streptococci, and specific strains of *S. pneumonia* may be differentiated by serotyping. Serotypes 2, 3, 6, 14, 18, and 19 have been isolated from infections in nonhuman primates (Kaufmann and Quist, 1969a; Keeling and McClure, 1974; Jones *et al.*, 1984; Graczyk *et al.*, 1995). Differential diagnoses include bacteria that are commonly associated with meningitis in nonhuman primates such as *Klebsiella pneumoniae*, and *Pasteurella multocida* and bacteria which are commonly associated with meningitis in humans, *Hemophilus influenza*, and *Neisseria meningitides*.

Grossly, mild to marked engorgement of the meningeal vasculature of the cerebrum and/or cerebellum (Fig. 1) has been reported in macaques (Kaufmann and Quist, 1969a; Fox and Wikse, 1971) and chimpanzees (Solleveld *et al.*, 1984). The leptomeninges may appear dull, thickened, and opaque (Fox and Wikse, 1971; Solleveld *et al.*, 1984; Gilbert *et al.*, 1987). *Streptococcus pneumoniae* meningitis has also been characterized by white, yellow, or gray-yellow purulent exudate filling the subarachnoid space, covering the cortex, and filling the sulci and/or the ventricles (Kaufmann and Quist, 1969a; Fox and Wikse, 1971; Gilbert *et al.*, 1987; Solleveld *et al.*, 1984; Graczyk *et al.*, 1995). Petechiae have been observed in the meninges and white and gray matter in severe cases of meningoencephalitis (Fox and Wikse, 1971). Lesions may extend to the spinal cord. In individual chimpanzees with a more chronic progression of disease, asymmetry of the cerebral hemispheres and severe malacia of the ventral frontal lobes of the brain have been reported (Solleveld *et al.*, 1984).

Lesions were not confined to the central nervous system (CNS). Congestion of the lungs, pulmonary edema, acute purulent bronchopneumonia, and gray hepatization of the ventral lung lobes were reported in macaques (Kaufmann and Quist, 1969a; Fox and Wikse, 1971; Herman and Fox, 1971). Diffuse suppurative peritonitis with adhesions, suppurative arthritis

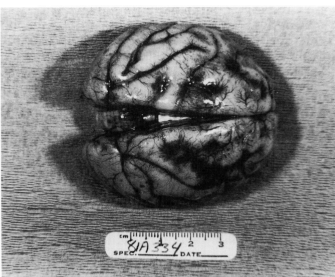

Fig. 1. Brain from a rhesus monkey with vascular congestion due to streptococcal meningitis.

(Fox and Wikse, 1971), and panophthalmitis also occurred (Herman and Fox, 1971). Multifocal hemorrhage may be observed as the result of *S. pneumoniae* septicemia. In chimpanzees, gross lesions included purulent otitis interna, sinusitis, and tonsillitis (Solleveld *et al.*, 1984).

Microscopically, *S. pneumoniae* meningoencephalitis was characterized by severe fibrinopurulent leptomeningitis extending into the cerebral and cerebellar cortices (Kaufmann and Quist, 1969a; Fox and Wikse, 1971; Solleveld *et al.*, 1984; Graczyk *et al.*, 1995). The cellular infiltrate in the meninges predominated in neutrophils with lesser numbers of mononuclear cells. Necrotizing vasculitis and thrombosis due to fibrin deposition were common. Encephalitis involving the cerebral and cerebellar cortices consisted of foci of hemorrhage, malacia, and leukocyte infiltration and accumulations of neutrophils and macrophages in the Virchow–Robbins spaces. As in the meninges, necrotizing vasculitis and thrombosis were common in both gray and white matter. Ischemic necrosis of adjacent parenchyma occurred in areas with vascular thrombosis. In chimpanzees in which the duration of disease was more chronic, polioencephalomalacia, astrocytosis, and multifocal hemorrhage in the cerebral and cerebellar cortices occurred. Multifocal neuronal necrosis and mineralization were also seen. The cellular infiltrate was predominately lymphocytes (Solleveld *et al.*, 1984).

Lung lesions ranged from acute serous inflammation with hyperemic congestion to exudative bronchopneumonia (Kaufmann and Quist, 1969a; Fox and Wikse, 1971). In monkeys with concomitant septicemia there was multifocal acute purulent inflammation in the lung, heart, or kidney (Herman and Fox, 1971). Acute fibrinopurulent peritonitis and thromboembolic lymphadenitis were reported in one macaque (Kaufmann and Quist, 1969a). Severe renal cortical necrosis with fibrinoid degeneration of renal afferent arterioles, multifocal myocardial necrosis, and diffuse suppurative panophthalmitis occurred as sequelae to *S. pneumoniae* septicemia in a young rhesus monkey (Herman and Fox, 1971).

Treatment of pneumococcal meningitis has had limited success, probably due to the fulminating nature of the disease. Reports of treatment success were limited to chimpanzees. A chimpanzee recovered from *S. pneumoniae* meningitis following aggressive treatment with a combination of intramuscular and intravenous penicillin (8×10^6 units/day) and ampicillin at 4 g/day for 11 days (Keeling and McClure, 1974). Another drug combination consisting of sodium penicillin G (2×10^5 IU), ampicillin (200–400 mg), and chloramphenicol (25 mg) per kg body weight given three times daily was also effective in treating chimpanzees (Solleveld *et al.*, 1984). Pernikoff and Orkin (1991) recommended ceftriaxone, 50–100 mg/kg body weight for great apes, to be administered once or twice daily for 7–10 days. Ceftriaxone has a long half-life with excellent penetration into and rapid sterilization of the CSF. The drug is effective in other bacterial meningitides in humans and can be administered intramuscularly (Pernikoff and Orkin, 1991). Supportive therapy in chimpanzees consisted of intravenous fluids and electrolytes and diazepam (20–30 mg/day) to modulate seizure activity (Solleveld *et al.*, 1984).

Prophylactic antibiotic administration was recommended for macaques during quarantine (Fox and Wikse, 1971). Change of cleaning procedures to reduce aerosols, reduction of population density, and vaccination with a human polyvalent vaccine were successful in preventing further cases of pneumococcal meningitis in a colony of chimpanzees (Solleveld *et al.*, 1984). Use of a polyvalent pneumococcal vaccine was ineffective in preventing pneumococcal pneumonia, septicemia, and meningitis in a colony of chimpanzees (Jones *et al.*, 1984).

2. Other *Streptococcus* spp.

Streptococcus zooepidemicus is a group C, pyogenic, β hemolytic streptococcus associated with fatal cervical lymphadenitis in guinea pigs (Harkness and Wagner, 1988) and cervicitis, metritis, mastitis, arthritis, and septicemia in mares, cows, and swine (Cole, 1990). In one report, *S. zooepidemicus* septicemia caused the death of red-bellied tamarins and Goeldii monkeys in a zoo (Schiller *et al.*, 1989). Clinical signs included pyrexia, diarrhea, submandibular swelling, and abdominal distension. The white blood cell count was elevated. Gross lesions consisted of suppurative submandibular and retropharyngeal lymphadenitis, similar to the disease in guinea pigs, and suppurative hepatitis and splenitis. *Streptococcus zooepidemicus* was recovered from multiple organs, ascitic fluid, and blood in affected monkeys. The source of the infection was horse meat fed to armadillos that also occupied the exhibit (Schiller *et al.*, 1989).

Metritis, fetal sepsis, and neonatal meningoencephalitis have occurred in baboons and cynomolgus monkeys infected with β hemolytic streptococci (Brack *et al.*, 1975; Wagner *et al.*, 1992), and ascending uterine infections in rhesus monkeys have been attributed to α hemolytic streptococci (Swindle *et al.*, 1982). In baboons, streptococcal infection was associated with abortion (Karasek, 1969) and meningoencephalitis with concomitant septic arthritis, skin abscesses, and pneumonia in neonates (Brack *et al.*, 1975). Neonatal baboons died with no clinical signs. Streptococcal infections in neonatal baboons were distinguished from *Escherichia coli* infections by the presence of septic arthritis in multiple joints, including the hips, knees, shoulders, elbows, and ankles (Brack *et al.*, 1975). Hemorrhagic suppurative leptomeningitis extending into the cortices was observed microscopically.

Group A streptococcal metritis and hemolytic uremic syndrome were diagnosed in a cynomolgus macaque with gestational diabetes mellitus (Wagner *et al.*, 1992). The dam died shortly after delivering a large stillborn fetus; group A, β hemolytic streptococci were isolated from fetal brain and maternal uterus. Multifocal periportal hepatic necrosis was found in the fetus with gram-positive cocci observed in the liver and myocardium. Multifocal necrosis, villar microthrombi, and bacterial colonization were found in the placenta. The dam had severe suppurative bacterial metritis with ulceration and erosion of the endometrium and bacterial colonization between the necrotic fibrils of the myometrium. The microscopic renal lesions of mild to moderate glomerular hypercellularity, increased mesangial matrices, and fibrin deposition within capillary loops were considered indicative of hemolytic uremic syndrome (Wagner *et al.*, 1992).

An unusually high incidence of abortions and stillbirths in a harem breeding colony of rhesus monkeys was associated with an α hemolytic streptococcus that was part of the normal vaginal flora (Swindle *et al.*, 1982). Antibiotic treatment of female rhesus monkeys with histories of repeated reproductive failure and a positive cervical culture for α hemolytic streptococcus resulted in improved reproductive outcomes.

B. *Staphylococcus*

Bacteria of the genus *Staphylococcus* are aerobic and facultatively anaerobic, catalase positive, nonsporing, nonmotile, and fermentative gram-positive cocci. These bacteria generally form clusters or pairs, but may be seen as short chains in smears from fluid culture media. The organisms are uniformly spherical, 1 μm in diameter. *Staphylococcus aureus,* one of the species frequently associated with disease conditions, is further characterized by pigmented colonies with zones of β hemolysis and the production of coagulase. Staphylococci are ubiquitous inhabitants of the environment, as well as the skin and upper respiratory tract of humans and animals. These organisms tolerate prolonged drying and ordinary disinfectants and are among the most resistant of nonsporulating bacteria.

The pathogenicity of staphylococci is related to a variety of factors, including the formation of extracellular toxins; a cell wall mucopeptide in encapsulated strains that inhibits host defenses; and staphylococcal hypersensitivity. Staphylococcal hypersensitivity is due to a nonspecific interaction of host immunoglobulins with protein A, a cell wall protein, that leads to activation of both humoral and cellular inflammatory processes. Extracellular toxins include coagulase, exfoliatin, hemolysins, staphylokinase, and enterotoxins.

Both coagulase-positive staphylococci (16%) and coagulase-negative staphylococci (28%) were recovered from throat cultures of tamarins, *Saguinus oedipus,* and *S. fusicollis* after importation (J. B. Deinhardt *et al.,* 1967). The incidence of colonization decreased to 12 and 19%, respectively, following acclimatization. Coagulase-positive staphylococci were isolated from the oropharynx of 45% of owl monkeys received over a 1-year period (Weller, 1994).

Various staphylococci were recovered from abscesses, ascitic fluid, ocular discharges, fistulas, heart, nasal cavity, and trachea of clinically ill owl monkeys (Weller, 1994). *Staphylococcus aureus* was one of the most common bacterial pathogens isolated during a 2-year retrospective study of clinical vaginitis in macaques (Doyle *et al.,* 1991). At Yerkes Primate Center, *S. aureus* was the most frequent isolate from bacterial cultures of external wounds and joint specimens from monkeys with arthritis and was a frequent isolate of blood cultures from clinical cases or necropsies of a variety of nonhuman primate species over a 5-year period (McClure *et al.,* 1986).

Individual infections due to staphylococci have been reported in nonhuman primates. A tamarin died of bronchopneumonia from which *Staphylococcus* spp. was isolated (F. Deinhardt *et al.,* 1967). *Staphylococcus aureus* was associated with a retrobulbar abscess in a rhesus infant. The 24-day-old infant presented with exophthalmos and downward deviation of the left eye. Leukocytosis with neutrophilia was the primary hematologic alteration. Treatment consisted of aspiration of exudate from the retrobulbar area, systemic oxacillin at 50 mg/kg divided TID, and temporary tarsorrhaphy (Rosenberg and Blouin, 1979). *Staphylococcus aureus* and *Actinomyces* spp. were isolated as the probable causative organisms in a case of pyometra in a rhesus monkey that had been bred 2 months earlier (Lang and Benjamin, 1969). This monkey presented comatose with abdominal distension and hemopurulent vaginal discharge. Hematology revealed a leukocytosis with neutrophilia and a left shift and anemia. Initial treatment with chloramphenicol followed with oxytetracycline, and electrolyte solutions were effective.

There are two reports of staphylococcal infection in great apes. *Staphylococcus aureus* was isolated from a 12-day-old orangutan with oral ulcers and white necrotic plaques on the tongue and lower gingiva (Hoopes *et al.,* 1978). Initial treatment with a variety of antibiotics and topical medications for the ulcers led to healing of the oral lesions; however, the infection progressed as a septicemia, and subsequently the infant developed suppurative arthritis of the coxofemoral and radiohumeral joints. Intensive treatment with aspiration of synovial exudate, installation of indwelling drains, oral chloramphenicol

(30 mg/kg, QID), and joint infusion with lincomycin (90 mg, BID) was unsuccessful. The infant developed pyrexia and loss of appetite. Subsequent therapy with cephalexin (60 mg/kg, QID) given subcutaneously, oral acetaminophen (60 mg/kg, TID) for fever, and arthrotomy to drain the joints resulted in recovery. Staphylococcal meningitis was diagnosed by CSF culture in a 3.5-year-old chimpanzee with a history of mild flu-like symptoms for 2 days that had progressed to depression, social isolation, dehydration, and neckache evidenced by uplifted shoulders and a reluctance to move her head (Pernikoff and Orkin, 1991).

C. *Corynebacterium*

Corynebacteria are small, $0.5 \times 3–5$ μm, gram-positive pleomorphic nonsporing rods, many of which occur widely in nature or as commensal organisms on the skin or mucous membranes of animals. There are few reports of naturally occurring disease resulting from corynebacterial infection in nonhuman primates.

Corynebacterium ulcerans has been isolated from bite wounds in a macaque and a langur; from nasal swabs and focal abscesses in necrotic, consolidated lungs in macaques; from a case of pneumonia in an infant macaque (May, 1972); and from mastitis in a bonnet macaque. The monkey with mastitis had a swollen, firm, discolored breast and expressed milk contained purulent debris. Treatment with kanamycin (30 mg BID) administered intramuscularly for 7 days was effective (Fox and Frost, 1974). *Corynebacterium equi* was recovered from a large pulmonary abscess in a cotton-top tamarin following a short illness characterized by anorexia, dyspnea, general unthriftiness, and weight loss (Stein and Scott, 1979). Pyogranulomatous bronchopneumonia, necrotic pleuritis, fibrinopurulent epicarditis, and pyogranulomatous pancreatic serositis were the microscopic lesions. *Corynebacterium pseudotuberculosis* was isolated from a chimpanzee with interstitial nephritis (Kim, 1976) and from three monkeys with pneumonia and septicemia (McClure *et al.,* 1986).

D. *Listeria*

Listeria monocytogenes is a small, 0.5-2 μm, weakly gram-positive, nonspore-forming pleomorphic coccobacillus. It is motile and has peritrichous flagella. *Listeria monocytogenes* is facultatively aerobic and produces small round colonies on blood agar with a narrow zone of β hemolysis. Cold enrichment may be necessary for isolation of this organism.

Listeria monocytogenes is ubiquitous in nature and infects a variety of hosts. A lipid component of the cell wall that produces delayed hypersensitivity and a hemolytic toxin that produces damage to tissue contribute to the pathogenicity of this organism.

Listeriosis is reported infrequently in nonhuman primates; most cases involve reproductive failure evidenced by abortion

(Vetési *et al.,* 1972), stillbirth (McClure, 1980; Paul-Murphy *et al.,* 1990), neonatal death due to septicemia (McClure and Strozier, 1975; Chalifoux and Hajema, 1981; Paul-Murphy *et al.,* 1990), or infection of the dam (McClure *et al.,* 1986). Most reports have originated from a colony of Celebes black apes, *Macaca maura,* with a history of poor reproductive performance (McClure, 1980; McClure *et al.,* 1986). Gross lesions in stillbirths and neonates included focal hepatic necrosis and splenomegaly with multifocal necrosis. Common microscopic lesions consisted of diffusely scattered multifocal hepatic and splenic necrosis with varying degrees of inflammation and fibrinopurulent placentitis. Small gram-positive rods were identified in foci of necrosis within these organs (McClure, 1980; McClure *et al.,* 1986).

Diagnosis was based on the clinical history of reproductive failure, characteristic microscopic lesions, and recovery of the organism from the placenta, abortus, or infant (McClure *et al.,* 1986; Paul-Murphy *et al.,* 1990). There was poor response to antibiotic therapy.

E. *Erysipelothrix*

Erysipelas is a systemic disease affecting a variety of wild and domestic animals and humans. The causative agent, *Erysipelothrix rhusiopathiae,* is a small, 0.3–2.5 μm, pleomorphic, facultative anaerobe, nonmotile, nonspore-forming, grampositive bacillus. The organism forms small round, α hemolytic colonies on blood agar with sparse growth at 24 hr and readily apparent colonies at 48 hr postinoculation. The organism survives and proliferates in soil and manure, preferring alkaline conditions.

There are two reports of erysipelas in nonhuman primates: septicemia in a black and red tamarin, *Saguinus nigricollis* (Hirsh *et al.,* 1975), and in two diana monkeys, *Cercopithecus diana* (Wallach, 1977). The tamarin presented with depression, dehydration, weakness, hypothermia, and bradycardia and died within 10 hr following supportive treatment. The clinical signs of the diana monkeys included depression, a soft cough, pyrexia, and icterus. They also died within a few hours of presentation.

There were no gross lesions in the tamarin (Hirsh *et al.,* 1975). Microscopic examination of tamarin tissues revealed numerous, large gram-positive rods in skeletal muscle, heart, kidneys, lymph nodes, and salivary glands. The diana monkeys had paintbrush hemorrhages and petechiae on the serosa of the small intestine and the stomach, hepatomegaly, splenomegaly, hemorrhagic lymph nodes, and icterus (Wallach, 1977). No tissues were collected for histopathology.

Diagnosis in both reports was made by isolation of *E. rhusiopathiae* from the kidneys (Hirsh *et al.,* 1975) or blood, spleen, and liver (Wallach, 1977). Small dew drop colonies with α hemolysis were produced on blood agar 12–48 hr postinoculation. Morphologically the bacterium was a gram-positive pleomorphic rod.

F. *Clostridium*

Bacteria of the genus *Clostridium* are large, 0.6 × 4-8 μm, gram-positive, spore-forming, usually motile, and anaerobic bacilli with peritrichous flagella. Many are encapsulated and most produce potent extracellular toxins. These bacteria are normally found in the soil or as flora of the gastrointestinal tract. Four species of clostridia have been associated with disease in nonhuman primates: *C. tetani, C. perfringens, C. botulinum,* and *C. piliforme.* All may be difficult to isolate from cases of clinical disease, and diagnosis is frequently based on clinical signs or characteristic gross pathology.

1. *Clostridium tetani:* Tetanus

Clostridium tetani is a gram-positive, nonencapsulated, obligate anaerobe that produces round terminal end spores in broth culture. The spores are found in the environment, particularly the soil, and in human and animal feces.

Tetanus is caused by a powerful neurotoxin produced by *C. tetani* during vegetative growth in the body. Spores are introduced by wounds or penetrating injuries, and vegetative growth occurs under anaerobic conditions. Germination is enhanced by the presence of a foreign body, tissue necrosis, or concomitant microbial infection with other organisms. Tetanospasmin, a 13 amino acid peptide, is a potent neuroexotoxin that migrates retrograde from axons of motor nerves in the vicinity of the active infection to the neuronal cell body in the spinal cord (Greene, 1984). The toxin inhibits the function of Renshaw cells that control duration and intensity of motoneuron impulses, resulting in the continuous stimulation of skeletal muscles. Other toxins produced by *C. tetani,* including tetanolysin, which causes lysis of erythrocytes and peripherally nonspasmodic toxin, contribute little to clinical signs.

Tetanus has been a significant cause of mortality in freeranging or outdoor-housed monkeys (DiGiacomo and Missakian, 1972; Kessler and Brown, 1979; Rawlins and Kessler, 1982; Goodwin *et al.,* 1987). The source of infection was soil contamination of fight wounds or postpartum infection in rhesus macaques (DiGiacomo and Missakian, 1972; Rawlins and Kessler, 1982), external wounds due to bites or other trauma in squirrel monkeys (Kessler and Brown, 1979), and frostbite lesions in the tail of baboons (Goodwin *et al.,* 1987). Most cases in free-ranging rhesus monkeys occurred during the breeding season, with additional cases during the birthing season (Rawlins and Kessler, 1982).

Clinical signs in rhesus monkeys have been well documented. Affected monkeys became torporus, were reluctant to interact with other monkeys, were unable to prehend food, and exhibited excessive thirst and difficulty swallowing. The rhesus monkeys developed progressive stiffness and adduction of the pectoral limbs. The gait was altered to bipedal hopping and running. As the disease advanced, piloerection (Fig. 2) and the classic triad of human lesions—trismus, opisthotonos, and

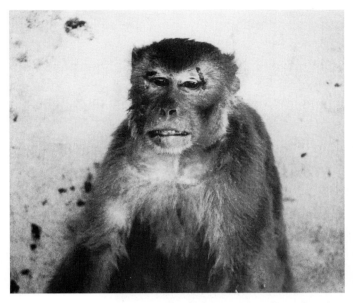

Fig. 2. Adult male rhesus monkey with tetanus. Note piloerection, abrasions, and facial grimace. (Photo from Matt Kessler.) Courtesy of the Carribean Primate Center.

status epilepticus—were observed. Older monkeys had an increased mortality rate. Obese monkeys were more likely to survive, presumably because of increased nutritional reserves. The clinical course of the disease in fatal cases ranged from 1 to 10 days (Rawlins and Kessler, 1982). Rhesus monkeys may have more than one episode of tetanus; previous *C. tetani* infection was not protective.

The initial stage of tetanus in squirrel monkeys was characterized by the development of a slow, deliberate, stiff gain (Kessler and Brown, 1979). Squirrel monkeys were reluctant to cross the pen floor; occasionally an affected monkey would take a few steps and fall into lateral recumbency. The disease rapidly progressed to trismus, extensor rigidity, and opisthotonos. Death resulted from respiratory paralysis or exhaustion within 24 hr of onset (Kessler and Brown, 1979). Baboons with frostbite lesions were found moribund with trismus and extensor rigidity (Goodwin *et al.,* 1987).

Tetanus was diagnosed by clinical signs in most cases. Most monkeys had an external wound or history of recent parturition (Kessler and Brown, 1979; Rawlins and Kessler, 1982; Goodwin *et al.,* 1987). Culture of *C. tetani* can be difficult because organisms are present in the wounds in low numbers. In one case report, *C. tetani* was recovered from a domesticated rhesus monkey from swabs of a deep neck wound and from skeletal muscle collected at necropsy (Sharma *et al.,* 1990). The cultures were inoculated into cooked meat medium and incubated anaerobically for 72 hr at 37°C. Gram-positive, nonencapsulated thin rods with terminal spores typical of *C. tetani* were observed (Sharma *et al.,* 1990). Identification may be made from cultural

characteristics, biochemical reactions, or animal bioassay for tetanospasmin.

Treatment in baboons consisted of 1500 units of veterinary tetanus antitoxin and supportive therapy for 5–11 weeks (Goodwin *et al.,* 1987). Acepromazine (3–5 mg QID for 3 weeks) and Valium (1.5 mg QID for 10 days) were given to relieve tetany. Intensive therapy for a squirrel monkey with tetanus, including tetanus antitoxin, tetanus toxoid, penicillin, and supportive care, was ineffective (Kessler and Brown, 1979). Tetanus toxoid administered IM followed by a single booster was protective for rhesus macaques and baboons (Kessler *et al.,* 1988; Goodwin *et al.,* 1987). Immunization with tetanus toxoid is advised for populations at risk.

2. *Clostridium perfringens:* Acute Gastric Dilatation

Clostridium perfringens is a nonmotile clostridium associated with wound infections, mastitis, dysentery, and enterotoxemia in sheep, cattle, and swine. The organism produces smooth, round glistening colonies surrounded by a wide zone of incomplete hemolysis with a narrow zone of complete hemolysis on blood agar. The organisms are short and spores are rarely seen. Five types of *C. perfringens,* A–E, have been recognized based on the extracellular production of lethal necrotic toxins.

Acute gastric dilatation or bloat in nonhuman primates has been associated with gastric proliferation of *C. perfringens* (Newton *et al.,* 1971; Bennett *et al.,* 1980; Stein *et al.,* 1981), although a definitive causal relationship has not been proven. Bloat has been reported to develop in nonhuman primates following overeating and drinking, alteration of gastric flora from antimicrobial therapy, or following anesthesia, transportation, or other changes in routine (Chapman, 1967; Newton *et al.,* 1971; Soave, 1978; Stein *et al.,* 1981). In one review of 24 cases of acute gastric dilatation, Bennett *et al.* (1980) reported that none of the monkeys involved had a disruption in schedule nor had they been recently anesthetized or tranquilized. *Clostridium perfringens* was isolated from gastric contents of 21 of the 24 monkeys and from monkey diet biscuits fed to the animals (Bennett *et al.,* 1980). Individual monkeys had a predisposition for developing acute gastric dilatation and experienced multiple episodes (Soave, 1978).

Early clinical signs of bloat included discomfort, as indicated by frequent grimacing and reduction in activity (Soave, 1978). Monkeys with more advanced disease would be found in a crouched position or lying prone in the cage (Newton *et al.,* 1971; Soave, 1978). Marked abdominal distension, shallow labored respiration, and coma occurred terminally (Newton *et al.,* 1971; Soave, 1978). Frequently monkeys were found dead with no clinical signs.

Diagnosis of acute gastric dilatation was based on clinical signs when present, radiographs (B. T. Bennett, personal communication, 1997), and gross necropsy results. Note the marked gaseous distension of the stomach in the radiograph in Fig. 3.

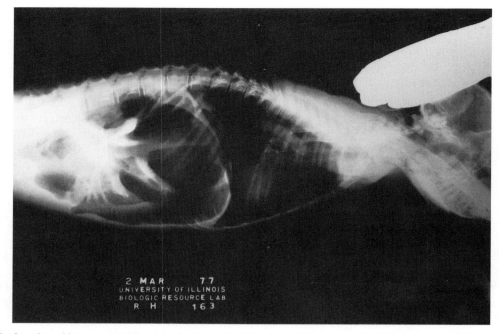

Fig. 3. Radiograph of monkey with acute gastric dilatation. (Photo from B. Taylor Bennett.) Courtesy of the Biologic Resources Laboratory, University of Illinois at Chicago.

In some cases, culture of stomach contents and blood resulted in recovery of *C. perfringens* (Soave, 1978; Bennett *et al.*, 1980; Stein *et al.*, 1981). Gastric distension due to gastric volvulus, blockage, or overconsumption of food and water should be considered as alternative diagnoses.

Acute gastric dilatation is a medical emergency and must be treated promptly. Soave (1978) reported the following procedures for treatment of bloat in macaques: sedation with ketamine hydrochloride (10–15 mg/kg body weight IM), gastric intubation to relieve intragastric pressure, administration of an antigassing agent to control gas formation, oral administration of ampicillin (30,000 IU/kg), intravenous administration of lactated Ringers solution (20–30 ml/kg), and cortisone (1 mg/kg) administered IV or IM to counter shock. Gas and fluid should be removed slowly to minimize vascular collapse following release of gastric pressure.

The primary lesion at necropsy was marked abdominal distension due to severe distension of the stomach and small intestines with large amounts of gas and brownish fluid (Newton *et al.*, 1971; Bennett *et al.*, 1980; Stein *et al.*, 1981). In some cases there was subcutaneous emphysema due to gas migration (Newton *et al.*, 1971; Bennett *et al.*, 1980; Stein *et al.*, 1981). Antemortem rupture of the stomach or intestine occurred rarely (Newton *et al.*, 1971; Bennett *et al.*, 1980). Mucosal hyperemia of the small and large intestine was also reported (Newton *et al.*, 1971; Stein *et al.*, 1981).

The most common microscopic lesions were hyperemia, hemorrhage, and necrosis of the mucosa of the small or large intestine (Newton *et al.*, 1971; Stein *et al.*, 1981). Thinning of

the gastric and intestinal wall was reported by Bennett *et al.* (1980). Acute tubular necrosis and congestion of the kidneys, hepatocellular hydropic degeneration, lymphoid and erythrocyte depletion in the spleen, and adrenal congestion and hemorrhage were found (Newton *et al.*, 1971; Bennett *et al.*, 1980).

3. *Clostridium botulinum:* Botulism

Botulism is an intoxication caused by a neurotoxin produced by *C. botulinum.* There are seven antigenically distinct neurotoxins (A–G) used to type *C. botulinum.* Botulism results from ingestion of one of the toxins that are produced during vegetative growth of the organism. Botulinal toxin acts at the neuromuscular junction of cholinergic nerve fibers to prevent synaptic release of acetylcholine.

Botulism associated with the feeding of cooked chicken has been reported in squirrel monkeys and capuchins (Smart *et al.*, 1980). Clinical signs included motor dysfunction of the eye, facial, and tongue muscles; progressive paralysis; and death within 24–72 hr of development of clinical signs. There were no gross or microscopic lesions. Type C botulinum toxin was recovered from the blood, stomach contents, and chicken.

4. *Clostridium piliforme:* Tyzzer's Disease

Clostridium piliforme, formerly *Bacillus piliformis* (Duncan *et al.*, 1993), an obligate intracellular, spore-forming bacteria, has been isolated from many species of domestic and wild animals with hepatic and intestinal disease (Harkness and Wagner,

1988). *Clostridium piliforme* infection has been reported incidently in a rhesus monkey with diarrhea (Niven, 1968) and in nursery deaths in cotton-top tamarin infants (Snook *et al.,* 1992).

G. *Neisseria*

Neisseria menigitidis is a gram-negative, oxidase-positive, catalase-positive coccus. Group A causes fulminating meningitis in humans. Group C has been isolated from blood culture of a chimpanzee and from an ocular discharge of a chimpanzee with purulent conjunctivitis (McClure *et al.,* 1986).

Experimental meningococcal infection in stump-tail monkeys was characterized by a fall in cardiovascular output, decreased renal blood flow, and increased systemic resistance (Mellins *et al.,* 1972). Systemic arterial and central venous pressure remained normal. Bacteremia and death occurred 5–15 hr postinoculation. Intravascular fibrin thrombi were the characteristic microscopic lesion (Mellins *et al.,* 1972).

H. *Branhamella*

Branhamella catarrhalis is a gram-negative, oxidase-positive, and catalase-positive diplococcus that was once considered normal flora of the human upper respiratory tract. More recently, this bacterium has been implicated in upper respiratory tract infections in humans during the winter months. It has been isolated from calves with pneumonia. It has also been associated with epistaxis and nasal discharge in cynomolgus macaques (VandeWoude and Luzarraga, 1991). Clinical signs in the cynomolgus included sneezing, epistaxis, and mucohemorrhagic nasal discharge, with two monkeys developing periorbital swelling. Affected monkeys had white blood cells, erythrocytes, and large diplococcal organisms in nasal cytologic preparations. A mild leukocytosis and neutrophilia were associated with infection. *Branhamella catarrhalis* was isolated from 64% of the monkeys with epistaxis. Bacteria produced small, convex, gray-white, nonhemolytic colonies on blood agar. Low environmental humidity (<45%) occurred during outbreaks. Treatment with long-acting penicillin cleared the infection and eliminated clinical disease (VandeWoude and Luzarraga, 1991). Differential diagnoses for epistaxis in macaques include simian hemorrhagic fever and Ebola Reston infection.

I. *Escherichia*

Escherichia coli is a ubiquitous aerobic to facultatively anaerobic gram-negative rod. There is great variation within the species, especially in terms of virulence. *Escherichia coli* are serotyped by O, K, and H (if motile) antigens. *Escherichia coli* is a frequent normal fecal flora isolate in nonhuman primates. Mucoid and hemolytic colony types have been associated with increased pathogenicity. Enterotoxin production, invasion of intestinal cells, or effacement of luminal epithelial cells are the three mechanisms of disease production by *E. coli.* A thermoregulated, contact hemolysin has been associated with the ability of invasive *E. coli* to destroy the phagosome membrane vacuole once transported inside the cell (Haider *et al.,* 1991).

Clinical signs of infection with a pathogenic *E. coli* varied with the primate species and the bacterial serotype. A bacteriological survey of laboratory animals revealed that asymptomatic rhesus macaques were infected with a variety of *E. coli* serotypes, all of which had been associated with gastroenteritis in humans, calves, pigs, or rabbits (Schiff *et al.,* 1972). Young chimpanzees and an orangutan with pathogenic *E. coli* infection had mild to moderately severe watery diarrhea for 2–10 days (McClure *et al.,* 1972). The stool was occasionally mucoid, and in one case contained small amounts of blood. The orangutan became dehydrated and developed a left shift in the leukocyte differential. Peracute disease developed in two chimpanzees, resulting in death within a few hours. In one chimpanzee, lethargy and dysentery were noted in the afternoon before ensuing death the following morning, whereas in the second chimpanzee, marked dehydration and dysentery were noted a few hours prior to death (McClure *et al.,* 1972). Serotypes 0119:B14, 055:B5, and 026:B6 were isolated from affected apes. In squirrel monkey infants, death with no clinical signs occurred in infections with *E. coli* serotype 0-13 (Scimeca and Brady, 1990). Tamarins infected with a hemolytic *E. coli* developed a watery diarrhea (Potkay, 1992).

Gross lesions in the apes included diffuse mucosal hemorrhage in the gastrointestinal tract, splenomegaly, congested and slightly enlarged mesenteric lymph nodes, and pulmonary hemorrhages and edema (McClure *et al.,* 1972). Microscopic lesions in the apes consisted of hemorrhage and necrosis of the gastrointestinal mucosa and pulmonary hemorrhage and edema. There was extensive mucosal hemorrhage, necrosis, and acute inflammation in the colon. Gross lesions in the squirrel monkey infants were confined to congestion of the liver, spleen, and adrenal glands (Scimeca and Brady, 1990). Invasive colitis or typhlocolitis and septic meningitis were the microscopic lesions in squirrel monkeys. Tamarins with diarrhea had congestion, edema, and necrosis of the mucosa of the ileum and colon (Potkay, 1992).

J. *Salmonella*

Salmonella are gram-negative, motile, facultatively anaerobic bacteria. Members of this genus are pathogens infecting humans, mammals, reptiles, birds, and insects. *Salmonella* have been classified on both biochemical and serologic differences, leading to many taxonomic changes. Those species of pathogenic significance to humans and animals include *S. choleraesuis, S. arizonae, S. enteritidis,* and *S. typhimurium. Salmonella enteritidis* has been further subdivided into bioserotypes, each with a distinguishing name. A variety of *Salmonella* species have been isolated from nonhuman primates; the most frequently reported isolates include *S. typhimurium, S. choleraesuis, S. anatum, S. stanley, S. derby,* and *S. oranienburg* (Galton *et al.,* 1948; Good *et al.,* 1969; McClure, 1980; Potkay, 1992). The last four species are bioserotypes of *S. enteritidis.*

Salmonella infection usually occurs from fecal–oral transmission. Infection can result from ingestion of contaminated food, water, or fomites; airborne infection is rare but can occur as the organism can survive dried on airborne particles in the absence of organic material. Insects have served as mechanical vectors. Salmonellae can survive and multiply for relatively long periods in the environment.

The pathogenesis of experimenal *Salmonella* infection has been described in the rhesus monkey. Eighty percent of rhesus monkeys inoculated orally with *S. typhimurium* developed diarrhea, which peaked in severity at 48 to 72 hr postinoculation (Rout *et al.,* 1974). Mild morphologic changes occurred in the jejunum in animals with diarrhea, including shortening of villi, villar edema, mild elongation of crypts, reduction of mucus content in goblet cells, and an increase of mononuclear cells in the epithelium. Alterations in the ileum and colon were more severe and corresponded to the severity of the diarrhea. The ileum from monkeys with severe diarrhea had flattened villi with elongated crypts, numerous crypt microabscesses, marked edema, and dense polymorphonuclear cell infiltrates in the lamina propria; a decrease in mucus content of crypts and surface epithelial cells; and attenuation and disorganization of the surface epithelium. Similar changes occurred in the colon with multifocal areas of microabscess formation, disruption and attenuation of the surface epithelium, and edema and marked polymorphonuclear cell infiltration in the lamina propria. *Salmonella* were observed invading both epithelial cells and the lamina propria of the ileum and colon. Alterations in intestinal water and electrolyte transport correlated with intraluminal *Salmonella* concentration and changes in intestinal morphology in the ileum and colon (Rout *et al.,* 1974). Changes in sodium and chloride transport coincided with changes in water transport and were similar in magnitude and direction. All monkeys with diarrhea had severe colitis with either marked inhibition of colonic water absorption or net colonic secretion. Monkeys with mild diarrhea had severely impaired jejunal and moderately impaired ileal transport; monkeys with severe diarrhea had net water secretion into the jejunum, ileum, and colon. Failure of the colon to reabsorb excess fluid secreted by the small intestine was believed to be the mechanism for mild diarrhea following *Salmonella* infection. Severe diarrhea was the result of profound transport abnormalities in both small and large intestines (Rout *et al.,* 1974). Subsequent studies revealed that secretion of water and electrolytes was not due to altered intestinal permeability (Kinsey *et al.,* 1976), but the result of activation of adenylate cyclase subsequent to penetration of *Salmonella* into the intestinal epithelium (Gianella *et al.,* 1975).

A survey of intestinal flora of wild rhesus monkeys 15 days after capture revealed that none of the 63 monkeys was infected with *Salmonella* (Agarwal and Chakravarti, 1969), suggesting that *Salmonella* infection may be acquired and not a normal component of the intestinal flora of wild monkeys. A survey of 5076 primates of 10 species, including macaques, vervets, owl monkeys, and langurs, imported from 1964 to 1966 revealed that 12% were infected with *Salmonella,* usually *S. anatum* or *S. stanley* (Good *et al,* 1969). In 1967, examination of 1570 primates imported by the same facility revealed a 3% incidence of *Salmonella* infections. During the 1964–1966 period, approximately 20% of *Presbytis entellus* were infected with *Salmonella* spp. Infection in any primate was rarely associated with clinical disease (Good *et al.,* 1969). In another survey, *Salmonella* was isolated from 2.7% of imported cynomolgus monkeys with diarrhea during quarantine, 0.6% of cynomolgus monkeys with diarrhea after quarantine, and 0.2% of normal cynomolgus monkeys (Tribe and Fleming, 1983). Isolation of *Salmonella* from feces of newly imported tamarins ranged from 19 (J. B. Deinhardt *et al.,* 1967) to 3% (Murphy *et al.,* 1972). *Salmonella* infection and diarrhea were reported in newly imported cynomolgus monkeys (Takasaka *et al.,* 1988).

Reports of *Salmonella* infection and disease within established primate colonies are rare. A mild to severe diarrheal disease associated with infection with either *S. miami* or *S. oranienburg* occurred in chimpanzees (Galton *et al.,* 1948). They were coinfected with *Shigella* and intestinal parasites. *Salmonella* was isolated from 23 of 379 enteric cultures from nonhuman primates with diarrhea at a primate research center (McClure, 1980); 21 of the isolates were *S. derby.* Most of the isolates were recovered from rhesus infants during an outbreak in the nursery (McClure, 1980). Clinical signs of enteric salmonellosis included watery diarrhea, sometimes with hemorrhage or mucus. Pyrexia commonly occurred with infection (Paul-Murphy, 1993). Extraintestinal infections have included neonatal septicemia, abortion, osteomyelitis, pyelonephritis, and a gluteal abscess (Thurman *et al.,* 1983; Klumpp *et al.,* 1986; Duncan *et al.,* 1994). Depression and marked hemorrhage from the vulva were noted in the gibbon with septic abortion due to *S. heidelberg* (Thurman *et al.,* 1983). The rhesus monkey with osteomyelitis initially presented with severe, watery diarrhea, hypothermia, lethargy, and dehydration. Blood and serum chemistry evaluation revealed a degenerative left shift, azotemia, and hypoproteinemia (Klumpp *et al.,* 1986). Forty-two days after the initial illness, the left leg was swollen and the monkey was pyrexic. The swelling was fluctuant and purulent exudate was collected. Radiographs revealed a pathologic fracture of the distal femur, sequestrum, and were considered diagnostic of chronic active osteoymelitis (Klumpp *et al.,* 1986). Response to antibiotic therapy was poor and the monkey was euthanized.

Diagnosis of salmonellosis requires isolation of the organism from a rectal swab, stool culture, or lesion site. Optimally, a recently passed, uncontaminated stool sample of 1–2 g is rapidly placed in gram-negative or selenite broth and incubated at 37°C. Cultures should be taken during the acute phase of illness if possible. If transported prior to inoculation of culture media, the sample should be refrigerated. Cultures of organs at necropsy should include liver, spleen, lung, intestinal tract, lymph nodes, and placenta, uterus, and fetus if septic abortion is suspected. Primary cultures may also be inoculated on blood, MacConkey, brilliant green, and *Salmonella/Shigella* agars for isolation and identification. Colonies of *Salmonella* are lactose negative and appear as clear round colonies on MacConkey agar. The organism is motile, which can be confirmed by microscopic examination of a hanging drop or wet mount or by inoculation of motility media. Serotyping has been useful in epidemiologic investigations due to the large number of *Salmonella* serovars.

Spontaneous, clinical enteric salmonellosis was characterized by edema, hyperemia, and rare mucosal ulceration in the ileum and colon. The mesenteric lymph nodes were enlarged occasionally. The spleen may be enlarged and congested. Hyperplasia and erosion of the mucosal epithelium in the colon with accumulation of necrotic debris in the lumen and inflammatory infiltrate in the lamina propria were the primary microscopic lesions. Microabscesses were rarely found in colonic lymphoid tissue. In cases of septicemia, areas of focal necrosis were found in the liver and spleen (Kent *et al.,* 1966; Potkay, 1992). Focal clusters of gram-negative rods were observed in the lungs of an aborted gibbon fetus (Thurman *et al.,* 1983). Emaciation, enlargement of the left leg to twice the normal size, draining sinus tracts, granulation tissue, and fibrosis were noted along the affected femur (Klumpp *et al.,* 1986). The lymph nodes draining the area were enlarged. Mild colitis, hepatic microgranulomas, and mold tubulointerstitial nephritis were noted microscopically (Klumpp *et al.,* 1986).

Treatment for *Salmonella* infections required an antibiotic to which the organism was known to be sensitive and supportive care to compensate for fluid loss, electrolytes, and acid–base imbalance resulting from diarrhea. Many isolates had multiple antibiotic resistance. Antibiotic resistance is usually plasmid mediated. Antibiotic therapy should be reserved for animals with severe diarrhea or septicemia to reduce the likelihood that a carrier state may develop. The zoonotic potential of *Salmonella* and the difficulty in eliminating the carrier state may necessitate culling of carrier animals.

K. *Shigella*

Shigella are gram-negative, nonmotile, aerobic, and facultatively anaerobic bacteria. The organism grows well on standard laboratory media, including blood and MacConkey agars, at 37°C. *Shigella* are divided into four serogroups on the basis of biochemical and serologic properties: *S. dysenteriae, S. flexneri,*

S. boydii, and *S. sonnei.* Serogroups are further divided into subserotypes of varying pathogenicity. *Shigella* are not as environmentally resistant as Salmonellae, being susceptible to inactivation by sunlight, acid pH, temperatures of 55°C for 1 hr, and 1% phenol for 30 min. *Shigella* will survive for a few days in nonacidic stools in the dark. Thus, the carrier animal is important in maintaining the organism in nature.

Shigella is and has been one of the most common enteric pathogens recovered from captive nonhuman primates, occurring in a variety of species, including marmosets, tamarins, spider monkeys, cebus, macaques, baboons, and apes (Galton *et al.,* 1948; Pinkerton, 1968; Mannheimer and Rubin, 1969; Mulder, 1971; Cooper and Needham, 1976; McClure *et al.,* 1976a). *Shigella flexneri* was the most frequent isolate, including serotypes 1a, 2a, 3, 4, 5, 6, and 15 (Russell and DeTolla, 1993). As with *Campylobacter* infections, shigellosis appears to be a disease acquired by primates in captivity from their association with humans. Endemic infections within colonies are maintained by asymptomatic carriers and potentially by rodent reservoirs (Banish *et al.,* 1993b; Russell and DeTolla, 1993). Infection is spread by the fecal–oral route among primates within the same group, by movement of primates between groups, and through importation of new primates into the colony. Infection and disease with subsequent antibody production do not provide immunity and animals may be chronically reinfected (Banish *et al.,* 1993a). Overt disease, diarrhea, or dysentery may not occur in endemically infected animals without a stressor, such as social group formation or transport to a new facility.

Development of clinical shigellosis is dependent on bacterial invasion and intracellular replication within the colonic epithelium and mucosa. Expression of both chromosomal- and plasmid-encoded genes are required for virulence; temperature and osmolarity regulate virulence genes (Maurelli and Sansonetti, 1988; Bernadini *et al.,* 1990). The genes for cellular invasion, *pInv,* and intracellular and extracellular replication, *virG,* are carried on large plasmids. The invasion plasmid antigens are large polypeptides that are coordinately expressed and are necessary for bacterial entry into the cell. Chromosomally encoded virulence factors such as *purE,* which regulates the plasmid gene *virG* determining intra- and extracellular spread, are needed for full virulence expression (Russell and DeTolla, 1993). *Shigella* enter the cell through a phagosome; once within the cell, bacteria replicate in and lyse the phagocytic vacuole. A thermoregulated, contact hemolysin has been associated with the ability of the bacteria to destroy the phagosome membrane vacuole (Haider *et al.,* 1991). Bacteria then multiply within the cytoplasm and spread between cells by pseudopods (Pal *et al.,* 1989). Intracellular bacterial movement is facilitated by host cell F-actin microfilaments (Russell and DeTolla, 1993). Toxins in varying levels are also produced by Shigellae. Shiga toxin from *S. dysenteriae* is highly cytotoxic and causes fluid accumulation in rabbit ileal loops. The A subunit of Shiga toxin inhibits protein synthesis in the target cell (O'Brien and Holmes, 1987).

The pathophysiology of experimental shigellosis has been described in rhesus monkeys (Rout *et al.*, 1975). The monkeys were infected orally with 5×10^{10} *S. flexneri* 2a bacteria. Those monkeys that developed only dysentery had decreased colonic absorption or a net colonic secretion of water and electrolytes. Monkeys with dysentery and diarrhea or diarrhea alone had net jejunal secretion and defective colonic absorption. Ileal transport was normal in all monkeys. All monkeys with clinical disease had severe colitis with intramucosal bacteria; there were minimal morphologic changes in the small intestine and bacterial invasion was not seen in the small intestine (Rout *et al.*, 1975).

The frequency of *Shigella* isolation from primates on capture, importation, and during quarantine varies with the species imported and with the reporting institution. Surveys of wild or recently captured rhesus or cynomolgus monkeys have revealed no *Shigella* infections (Takasaka *et al.*, 1964; Carpenter and Cooke, 1965; Agarwal and Chakravarti, 1969). Subsequent screening of recently acquired cynomolgus revealed 13.2% of the previously culture negative monkeys were culture positive in the dealer's compound and 20.1% were infected with *Shigella* on arrival in quarantine (Takasaka *et al.*, 1964). A cultural survey of Shigellae in wild, newly imported, and captive in residence baboons revealed a 3% incidence of infection in wild animals and 37.8 and 35% incidence in newly imported and resident baboons, respectively (Pinkerton, 1968). Among 10 species of 6646 newly imported monkeys surveyed from 1964 to 1967, 12% were infected with *Shigella* and 75% of the isolates were *S. flexneri* 4 (Good *et al.*, 1969). Thirty-two percent of rhesus macaques in quarantine in India were infected with *S. flexneri*, and 97% of these monkeys had diarrhea or blood and mucus in the stool (Arya *et al.*, 1973). *Shigella flexneri* was isolated from 23% of imported rhesus monkeys with diarrhea; peak incidence of diarrhea and cultural recovery occurred 3 weeks into quarantine (Lindsey *et al.*, 1971). *Shigella* infection in rhesus and cynomolgus macaques imported into Great Britain was 5.5% within 48 hr of arrival and 2.5% 14 days later (Hartley, 1975), and *Shigella* was isolated from 8.7% of imported cynomolgus with diarrhea during the first month of quarantine (Tribe and Fleming, 1983).

Clinical signs of shigellosis included diarrhea with mucus, frank blood, and/or mucosal fragments in the stool. Affected monkeys were weak, moderately to severely dehydrated, and suffered from weight loss. Macaques would sit forward in a hunched posture with their head between the legs; they had a drawn appearance and occasionally experienced edema of the face and neck (Mulder, 1971). Depression, diarrhea with blood and leukocyte exudate, and leukocytosis with a left shift were characteristic of cases of *Shigella* dysentery in long-tailed macaques (Line *et al.*, 1992). In an infected spider monkey with concomitant rickets, clinical signs included vomiting, gingivitis, bilateral nystagmus, and hypothermia (Mannheimer and Rubin, 1969). An adult cebus monkey developed nystagmus,

muscle tremors, and diarrhea, whereas a cebus infant became inappetant, lost interest in her surroundings, and produced frothy, pasty feces covered with mucus (Mannheimer and Rubin, 1969). Shigellosis in marmosets and tamarins was characterized by lethargy, depression, and dehydration (Cooper and Needham, 1976). The animals sat hunched, became hypothermic, and had dried blood around the anus. Buccal membranes were pale; one monkey developed facial edema and one a head tilt (Cooper and Needham, 1976). Feces beneath the cages were blood stained. Pig-tailed macaque infants raised in the nursery developed watery diarrhea with *Shigella* infection (Russell and DeTolla, 1993). Gibbons and spider monkeys with chronic recurrent infection experienced episodes of consistently loose stools or diarrhea of several days duration and weight loss (Banish *et al.*, 1993a).

Nonenteric *Shigella* infections have been reported (McClure *et al.*, 1976a), including gingivitis, abortion, and air sac infection. Rhesus monkeys with gingivitis had swollen, hyperemic gums with scattered yellow-white foci of necrosis. The lesions were most severe around the premolar and molar teeth. Severely affected monkeys had gingival recession and root exposure with accumulation of tartar and exudate. The monkeys with gingivitis were anorectic; two had concomitant diarrhea. One rhesus monkey had a septic abortion following 1 day of severe diarrhea. The adult orangutan with acute *Shigella* air sac infection presented with lethargy, anorexia, vomiting, and distension of the submandibular air sac (McClure *et al.*, 1976a).

Definitive diagnosis of enteric *Shigella* infection requires culture of the organism from a rectal swab or fresh stool specimen; a 1- to 2-g fresh, uncontaminated stool specimen is preferred. For nonenteric infections, the affected site should be cultured. The sample should be transported rapidly to the laboratory for immediate culture to optimize conditions for isolation (Dow *et al.*, 1989). Samples should be protected from direct sunlight. Repeated cultures may be required to isolate *Shigella*. Inoculation of specimens may be made in or on a variety of media, including gram-negative broth, selenite broth, and blood, MacConkey, brilliant green, and *Salmonella/Shigella* agars and incubated at 37°C. *Shigella* colonies are clear or whitish on MacConkey agar or *Salmonella/Shigella* agar and pink with a red halo on brilliant green agar. Speciation may be performed by a battery of biochemical tests.

Lesions of enteric shigellosis occurred primarily in the cecum and colon. The colon and cecal walls were thick and edematous with hyperemic congestion and swollen rugae. In acute cases, lesions were most severe in the cecum and ascending colon. Luminal contents varied from fluid mucous with fibrin and cellular debris to frank hemorrhage and mucus in the lumen (Lindsey *et al.*, 1971; Mulder, 1971). Multifocal ulcers penetrating through the cecal and colonic mucosa were observed in some monkeys. In areas of severe ulceration, hemorrhage and fibronecrotic material adhered to the mucosa forming a pseudodiphtheritic membrane. Intussusception of the small intestine and rectal prolapse were found in some cases. Spelnic enlargement with subcapsular, petechial hemorrhages was reported in infected rhesus monkeys (Mulder, 1971). Mesenteric lymph nodes were enlarged, congested, and edematous (Russell and DeTolla, 1993; Cooper and Needham, 1976). Gross lesions in marmosets and tamarins were confined to the cecum and colon (Cooper and Needham, 1976), consisting of multifocal ulcers from 0.5 to 3.0 mm and pinpoint hemorrhages in the cecal mucosa and small erosions and petechia in the colon of some monkeys. Blood and fluid feces were found throughout the large bowel.

The primary microscopic mucosal lesion was erosion or ulceration with peripheral hemorrhage and necrotic debris in the center of the ulcer (Cooper and Needham, 1976). The lamina propria was infiltrated with neutrophils and mononuclear cells; the mucosa and submucosa were edematous with a neutrophilic infiltrate. Fibrin thrombi occurred in serosal and submucosal vessels. Diphtheritic colitis was characterized by the presence of a pseudomembrane containing fibrin, erythrocytes, inflammatory cells, bacteria, and dead epithelial cells overlying eroded and ulcerated areas of the intestinal wall (Russell and DeTolla, 1993). *Shigella* were detected with specific antibodies on the surface of the mucous membrane, within surface epithelium and crypt lumina and occasionally in the lamina propria (Ogawa *et al.*, 1966; Mulder, 1971). Large numbers of *Shigella* were observed in crypt abscesses and ulcerations; in deep ulcerative lesions, bacteria were found in the lamina propria and lymphoid tissue (Ogawa *et al.*, 1964). Microscopic examination of biopsies from monkeys with gingivitis revealed scattered areas of intense neutrophil inflammation in the mucosa and submucosa with prominent mononuclear cell infiltrates in the submucosa (McClure *et al.*, 1976a).

Treatment for shigellosis should include antibiotic therapy based on sensitivity testing and aggressive correction of deficits in hydration, acid/base balance, and electrolytes. Empirical antibiotic therapy may be necessary in acute cases based on colony history. *Shigella* rapidly develop antibiotic resistance and many species have multiple drug resistance. Antibiotics reported to be successful in treating *Shigella* infections include enrofloxacin, 5 mg/kg body weight once a day (Line *et al.*, 1992; Banish *et al.*, 1993b), and combination therapy with oral trimethoprim sulfamethoxazole, erythromycin, and tetracycline (Olsen *et al.*, 1986). *Shigella* was eliminated from a marmoset and tamarin colony by initiation of quarantine procedures and administration of neomycin in the drinking water for 10 days (Cooper and Needham, 1976).

Treatment of an infected colony and thorough cleaning of the premises may be a more successful strategy instead of treating individual animals. Development of multiply-resistant strains of *Shigella* can occur rapidly (Lindsey *et al.*, 1971). Elimination of the *Shigella* carrier state has been reported in research and commercial macaque colonies (Pucak *et al.*, 1977; Olsen *et al.*, 1986; Line *et al.*, 1992) and in a primate collection in a zoo (Banish *et al.*, 1993b). An eradication program should include identification and isolation of carrier animals through repeated

culturing, followed by treatment with an antibiotic to which the organism has been found to be susceptible (Banish *et al.*, 1993b). Multiple posttreatment culturing of carrier animals and retreatment or culling of persistent *Shigella* carriers should follow the initial antibiotic therapy. Potential environmental sources of infection must be eliminated by concomitant disinfection and thorough cleaning of primate housing areas.

Shigellosis is a zoonotic disease and has been transmitted from monkeys to children and to animal caretakers (Mulder, 1971; Tribe and Flemming, 1983), from asymptomatic pet spider monkeys to their owners (Fox, 1975), and to technical assistants in a primate research unit (Kennedy *et al.*, 1993). Severe dysentery resulted from infection and, in one instance, death occurred (Fox, 1975).

L. *Yersinia*

Bacteria of the genus *Yersinia* are gram-negative, pleomorphic coccobacilli that are facultatively anaerobic. *Yersinia* have peritrichous flagella, are motile, and do not have a capsule. There are two species of medical significance for nonhuman primates: *Y. enterocolitica* and *Y. pseudotuberculosis*. These two species differ biochemically in that *Y. enterocolitica* produces acid in sucrose and is ornithine decarboxylase positive whereas *Y. pseudotuberculosis* produces acid in rhamnose and is ornithine decarboxylase negative. Both species grow at a wide range of temperatures from 4 to 43°C on a standard laboratory media.

Both *Yersinia* spp. share a common pathogenesis. Infections are acquired by the fecal–oral route. The bacteria adhere to the cell membrane of intestinal epithelial cells and are subsequently ingested by bacterial endocytosis with vacuole formation. Dissolution of the vacuolar membrane allows the bacteria to migrate through the cytoplasm. The bacteria penetrate the lamina propria and multiply, particularly in lymph follicles and Peyer's patches, eliciting a marked inflammatory response of neutrophils and macrophages. Virulent strains resist phagocytosis by neutrophils and intracellular killing by macrophages. The bacteria subsequently drain into the mesenteric lymph nodes and eventually become systemic. Virulence is encoded by both chromosomal and plasmid genes. Endocytosis in intestinal epithelial cells is encoded on the bacterial chromosome. Resistance to phagocytosis and intracellular killing is determined by a 70-kb plasmid. The role of the heat-sensitive endotoxin produced by *Y. enterocolitica* is unknown (Cornelius *et al.*, 1987).

Yersinia enterocolitica has a worldwide distribution and infects humans and a variety of animal species. *Yersinia enterocolitica* infections have been reported in galagos, lemurs, marmosets, owl monkeys, patas, vervets, and mangabeys (Giorgi *et al.*, 1969; Mair *et al.*, 1970; McClure *et al.*, 1971b; Baggs *et al.*, 1976; Bresnahan *et al.*, 1984; Skavlen *et al.*, 1985). Clinical signs varied with the species infected. Galagos displayed listlessness and severe diarrhea soon followed by death (Mair *et al.,* 1970). Lemurs were anoretic and lethargic with diarrhea; abdominal pain, hyperpyrexia, and decreased peristaltic sounds occurred in some animals (Bresnahan *et al.,* 1984). Hematological results varied among affected lemurs, ranging from mild to moderate neutrophilia and monocytosis, with a degenerative left shift reported for one animal. Affected lemurs consistently had lymphopenia and eosinopenia. Serum chemistry abnormalities included hyperglycemia in all lemurs and elevated lactate dehydrogenase and alanine transaminase activities in one animal (Bresnahan *et al.,* 1984). One vervet presented with emaciation, abdominal distension, and peripheral lymphadenopathy and another with anorexia and lethargy progressing to a semicomatose state (McClure *et al.,* 1971b). The second vervet had a marked leukocytosis of 27,400 with 91% neutrophils. Yersiniosis in a male mangabey, *Cercocebus torquatus,* presented as bloody diarrhea with death occurring the next day (McClure *et al.,* 1971b). The clinical signs of *Y. enterocolitica* septicemia in two patas monkeys included anorexia, depression, weakness, dehydration, and hypothermia (temperature <95°F); jaundice of the skin, sclera, and mucous membranes was reported in one monkey (Skavlen *et al.,* 1985). Clinical pathology abnormalities included leukopenia, WBC = 1761–3996 cells/mm³, and elevated aspartate aminotransferase activity, 315–715 U/liter (Skavlen *et al.,* 1985).

Yersinia pseudotuberculosis infections have been reported in ring-tailed lemurs, slow loris, bushbabies, common marmosets, talapoins, squirrel monkeys, patas monkeys, African green monkeys, mangabeys, and macaques (Bronson *et al.,* 1972; Hirai *et al.,* 1974; Chang *et al.,* 1980; Rosenberg *et al.,* 1980; Buhles *et al.,* 1981; MacArthur and Wood, 1983; Parsons, 1991; Brack and Hosefelder, 1992; Plesker and Claros, 1992). Clinical signs in bushbabies included lethargy, dehydration, diarrhea, dyspnea, and pyrexia (Chang *et al.,* 1980). Squirrel monkeys displayed nonspecific clinical signs such as inactivity; weakness and failure to cling to the dam; and cervical lymph node enlargement (Plesker and Claros, 1992). Depression and anorexia 1–2 days prior to death were reported in patas monkeys (Hirai *et al.,* 1974), and depression, severe weakness, and apathy were observed in an infected African green monkey (Plesker and Claros, 1992). Depression and diarrhea were reported for macaques with *Y. pseudotuberculosis* infections by Bronson *et al.* (1972). Vomiting, severe abdominal pain, mild dehydration, and blood-stained feces were observed in infected cynomolgus monkeys by MacArthur and Wood (1983). Rosenberg *et al.* (1980) reported diarrhea, moderate dehydration, abortions, and stillbirths in a troop of cynomolgus monkeys with *Y. pseudotuberculosis* infections. Leukocytosis due to neutrophilia, hyponatremia, hypochloremia, prerenal azotemia, and moderate hyperfibrinogenemia were noted in affected monkeys (Rosenberg *et al.,* 1980).

Presumptive diagnosis of *Yersinia* infection was made from clinical presentation and lesions at necropsy. Impression smears from necrotic foci in liver, spleen, or lymph nodes have revealed numerous, pleomorphic, gram-negative rods with bipolar staining (McClure *et al.,* 1971b). *Yersinia* can be recovered by rectal culture of monkeys presenting with diarrhea or from lesioned organs at necropsy. The organism grows well on a variety of media when it is the sole isolate; however, it may be slow growing at standard bacterial isolation temperatures of 37°C and thus overgrown by more rapidly growing bacteria in mixed cultures. Cold enrichment of samples at 4–7°C may be necessary for recovery and isolation.

Yersinia infections in nonhuman primates usually present with a triad of lesions at necropsy: multifocal hepatic and splenic necrosis or abscess formation, mesenteric lymphadenopathy, and ulcerative enterocolitis. In galagos, severe enterocolitis, congestion of the liver and spleen, and multiple 1-mm foci of necrosis in the spleen were noted at necropsy (Shive *et al.,* 1969). Multifocal mucosal ulceration of the ileum, cecum, and colon; congestion of abdominal viscera; and fine white mottling on the liver were reported for a lemur with *Y. enterocolitica* infection (Bresnahan *et al.,* 1984). Another animal from the same group had primary pulmonary disease with diffuse yellow to red-gray consolidation of the lung and a large 20-cm abscess in the right lung lobe. Multiple liver abscesses occurred in common marmosets and black-tufted-ear marmosets, *C. penicillata* (Giorgi *et al.,* 1969). Multiple, pinpoint to 2 cm, foci of necrosis in the spleen and liver were found in affected owl monkeys as well as multiple, irregular, raised, white foci with peripheral zones of hyperemia or hemorrhage in the mucosa of the terminal ileum, cecum, and colon (Baggs *et al.,* 1976). Hepatomegaly, splenomegaly, mesenteric lymphadenopathy, abdominal and/or thoracic exudation, and mesenteric and thoracic adhesions were noted in patas monkeys (Skavlen *et al.,* 1985). Numerous spherical yellow foci of necrosis, 1 mm to 3 cm in diameter, were observed in the liver and spleen, and one patas monkey had multifocal mucosal ulcerations 1–4 mm in diameter throughout the cecum and colon. Similar lesions to those reported for the patas monkeys occurred in one vervet monkey; the other vervet had extensive mucosal ulceration throughout the gastrointestinal tract with diffuse small foci of necrosis in the liver (McClure *et al.,* 1971b). The mangabey had extensive mucosal ulceration in the entire small intestine and large intestine as well as extensive cecocolic serosal hemorrhage (McClure *et al.,* 1971b).

Galagos with fatal *Y. pseudotuberculosis* infection had marked splenomegaly and pneumonitis as well as ulcerative enterocolitis, multifocal splenic and hepatic necrosis, and mesenteric lymphadenopathy and edema (Chang *et al.,* 1980). Squirrel monkeys infected with *Y. pseudotuberculosis* had an unusual presentation in that cervical lymph nodes, as well as mesenteric lymph nodes, were markedly enlarged (Plesker and Claros, 1992). Emaciation; severe ulcerative, necrotizing enterocolitis with diphtheroid membrane formation; multiple necrotic foci in the spleen and liver; and necrotizing pharyngitis, esophagitis, and gastritis were also noted in affected squirrel monkeys. Cynomolgus monkeys had enlarged and edematous mesenteric lymph nodes, enterocolitis, and miliary necrosis of the liver and spleen in one report (MacArthur and Wood, 1983) and acute ulcerative enterocolitis in another (Rosenberg et al., 1980). A similar pattern of lesions was reported for patas monkeys (Hirai et al., 1974). In an Y. pseudotuberculosis outbreak involving M. cynomolgus, M. radiata, M. nemestrina, and Cercocebus fulliginosus, ulcerative gastritis and enterocolitis with diphtheritic membrane formation; multiple white foci, 1–3 mm, in the liver and spleen; and mild mesenteric lymph node enlargement were the primary necropsy findings (Bronson et al., 1972).

Multifocal, purulent and necrotizing hepatitis, splenitis, lymphadenitis, and ulcerative gastroenterocolitis were the characteristic microscopic lesions of Yersinia infection in nonhuman primates. Hepatic and splenic lesions consisted of randomly distributed, sometimes spherical, areas of necrosis and inflammation (McClure et al., 1971b; Baggs et al., 1976; MacArthur and Wood, 1983; Bresnahan et al., 1984; Skavlen et al., 1985). Frequently, one or more bacterial colonies to large masses of bacteria were located within the central core of the lesion, encased by necrotic debris and a peripheral border of mononuclear cells and neutrophils (Bronson et al., 1972; Hirai et al., 1974; Chang et al., 1980). Similar lesions were observed less frequently in the lymph nodes, kidney, lung, and uterus (McClure et al., 1971b; Baggs et al., 1976; Bresnahan et al., 1984). Intestinal lesions ranged from focal mucosal necrosis with bacterial colonization to full thickness mucosal necrosis with adherent intestinal contents, cellular debris, and bacteria (McClure et al., 1971b; Baggs et al., 1976). Ulcerative lesions frequently overlay gut-associated lymphoid tissue (Bronson et al., 1972). Lymphatic hyperplasia with few giant cells was observed microscopically in the intestine of infected squirrel monkeys (Plesker and Claros, 1992). In lemurs, ulcerative typhlocolitis with submucosal edema, marked hyperemia of the lamina propria, and large discrete masses of bacteria in the mucosa, submucosa, and serosa was observed (Bresnahan et al., 1984). Inflammatory infiltrates ranged from acute to chronic, with macrophages and neutrophils usually noted within intestinal lesions (McClure et al., 1971b; Baggs et al., 1976; Bresnahan et al., 1984). Acute suppurative pneumonia with edema occurred in one lemur (Bresnahan et al., 1984) and multifocal nonsuppurative pneumonitis was reported for bushbabies (Chang et al., 1980). A squirrel monkey had nonsuppurative meningoencephalitis (Plesker and Claros, 1992).

In many advanced cases of yersiniosis, treatment was ineffective. Oral neomycin sulfate at 25 mg/kg body weight for 2 days and 100 mg of tetracycline/liter of drinking water for 10 days were used to successfully treat and eliminate Y. enterocolitica infection in asymptomatic and mildly ill lemurs (Bresnahan et al., 1984). Chloramphenicol, electrolyte fluids, and atropine were used to successfully treat a lemur with more advanced disease. Chloramphenicol administered IM at 100 mg/kg body weight, divided TID, in conjunction with intravenous and oral rehydration with electrolyte solutions was moderately successful in treating cynomolgus monkeys infected with Y. pseudo-

tuberculosis (Rosenberg et al., 1980). Oral ampicillin was used to treat affected galagos (Mair et al., 1970).

M. Klebsiella

Klebsiella pneumoniae is a gram-negative, aerobic, nonmotile rod-shaped, encapsulated bacterium. Nonpathogenic strains are widely distributed in nature as free living forms in the soil and water or as commensals in the intestinal tract of humans and animals. This bacterium constitutes normal fecal and oral flora in many nonhuman primates. Pathogenic K. pneumoniae strains associated with the upper respiratory tract are usually heavily encapsulated. Many pathogenic strains possess fimbriae, which act as adhesins, a virulence factor, that permit colonization of mucosal surfaces. Some strains have pili, which also serve as adhesins and inhibit phagocytosis and intracellular killing of Klebsiella. The capsule also serves as a virulence factor by inhibiting phagocytosis.

Klebsiella infections cause significant morbidity and mortality in nonhuman primates. Disease has been associated with shipping, quarantine, and overcrowding. Klebsiella was isolated from the throats of 64% of newly arrived, feral tamarins and from cases of pneumonia, septicemia, and enteritis (F. Deinhardt et al., 1967). Klebsiellosis in infant squirrel monkeys has been associated with trauma, maternal neglect, and failure of hand-rearing (Moisson and Gysin, 1994). Klebsiella infection occurred primarily in young chimpanzees (Schmidt and Butler, 1971) and was one of the primary causes of respiratory disease deaths within a chimpanzee colony (Hubbard et al., 1991a).

Klebsiella pneumoniae has been associated with peritonitis, septicemia, air sac infections, pneumonia, and meningitis in New and Old World primate species and in apes. Antemortem diagnosis was frequently not made due to the acute course of the disease. Purulent peritonitis and hepatic and pulmonary abscesses were reported in moustached tamarins, Saguinus mystax, that died with no clinical signs (Gozalo and Montoya, 1991b). Thirteen percent of a breeding colony of common marmosets in Brazil died with Klebsiella infection (Campos et al., 1981). Young animals were affected more frequently than adults; diarrhea and hypothermia were the primary clinical signs (Campos et al., 1981). Acute peritonitis, septicemia, and pyothorax occurred in owl monkeys, tamarins, and one squirrel monkey in an animal colony in Peru (Gozalo and Montoya, 1991a). Clinical signs, including diarrhea, prostration, and anorexia, were observed in a few monkeys prior to death. Owl monkeys had pyrexia with fever to 106°F and distended painful abdomens (Gozalo and Montoya, 1991a). Klebsiella infections have been a significant cause of mortality in some owl monkey colonies with an incidence of 25–29% at necropsy (Snyder et al., 1970). Monkeys with peracute septicemia died without signs of disease. Intermittent anorexia and serous nasal discharge were observed in owl monkeys with acute septicemia, 1 to 5 days prior to death.

Anorexia, dyspnea, and serous to mucous nasal discharge were reported for owl monkeys with pneumonia (Snyder *et al.,* 1970). *Klebsiella* air sacculitis in owl monkeys frequently was undiagnosed antemortem (Giles *et al.,* 1974). Two owl monkeys had purulent nasal discharge and swelling of the cervical mandibular area. Other owl monkeys exhibited anorexia, depression, and listlessness for a few days prior to death. Pneumonia and septicemia due to *K. pneumoniae* were the primary causes of morbidity and mortality in a colony of Guyanese squirrel monkeys with mortality rates approaching 100% for young monkeys (Moisson and Gysin, 1994). Young squirrel monkeys with septicemia frequently had external abscesses often located on the throat.

Clinical signs of pneumonia and meningitis in rhesus monkeys included anorexia, adipsia, listlessness, reluctance to move, and droopy eyelids (Fox and Rohovsky, 1975). Bilateral rales were heard in one monkey with pneumonia on auscultation. Clinical pathology revealed leukocytosis, WBC of 17,700, due to neutrophilia (Fox and Rohovsky, 1975). Respiratory signs, including coughing, clear to purulent nasal discharge, and pulmonary congestion, were reported in chimpanzees (Schmidt and Butler, 1971; Hubbard *et al.,* 1991a).

Diagnosis of *Klebsiella* infection depends on isolation of the organism from clinical specimens or at necropsy. *Klebsiella* spp. grow well at 37°C on standard bacterial media, including sheep blood and MacConkey agars. Colonies of *Klebsiella* are large, mucoid, and have a viscous consistency due to the large amount of polysaccharide material within the capsule.

Purulent peritonitis and mesenteric lymphadenopathy were the primary lesions reported in tamarins with *Klebsiella* infection (Gozalo and Montoya, 1991a,b). Fibrinous lobar pneumonia was the primary finding in one colony of common marmosets (Chalmers *et al.,* 1983). Gaseous distension and congestion of the small intestine and hepatic enlargement with multifocal areas of yellow discoloration were the gross findings in another colony of common marmosets (Campos *et al.,* 1981). Gross lesions of *Klebsiella* septicemia in owl monkeys included hyperemic congestion of mesenteric vasculature, serosal and mucosal hemorrhage, and peritonitis (Snyder *et al.,* 1970; Gozalo and Montoya, 1991a). Purulent meningitis and consolidating pneumonia were also reported for owl monkeys (Snyder *et al.,* 1970; Gozalo and Montoya, 1991a). Owl monkeys with acute air sacculitis had diffuse hyperemia of the air sac mucosa and thickening and edema of the adventitia (Giles *et al.,* 1974). Subacute infections were characterized by purulent exudate within the air sac and exudate covering the surfaces of the salivary glands, trachea, and larynx. In some cases, severe distension of the air sac led to rupture into the thoracic cavity (Giles *et al.,* 1974). In addition to air sacculitis, suppurative sialitis, suppurative cervical lymphadenitis, and bronchopneumonia were occasionally seen. Gross necropsy findings in rhesus monkeys included exudative bronchopneumonia and hemopurulent meningitis (Good and May, 1971; Fox and Rohovsky, 1975).

Chimpanzees had firm, inflated, red-purple lung lobes with yellow-white foci throughout the parenchyma (Schmidt and Butler, 1971).

Microscopic lesions varied with the extent, severity, and stage of the disease. Intense congestion with infiltrates of mononuclear and polymorphonuclear leukocytes was found in lesioned organs in common marmosets (Campos *et al.,* 1981). Inflammation and suppuration of Peyer's patches and cecal lymphoid tissue were observed in owl monkeys with *Klebsiella* septicemia (Gozalo and Montoya, 1991a). The most striking lesion observed in acute air sacculitis in owl monkeys was thromboembolism of the subepithelial vasculature of the air sac (Giles *et al.,* 1974). Numerous gram-negative organisms were observed within the thrombi. Concomitant lesions included vasculitis, hemorrhage, and edema in the subepithelial region and adventitia, with very mild inflammation of the adventitia. Severe, necrotizing suppurative air sacculitis occurred in owl monkeys with subacute infections (Giles *et al.,* 1974). There was loss of air sac epithelium and accumulation of polymorphonuclear cells and necrotic debris. Suppurative inflammation extended frequently into the adjacent adipose tissue and perilaryngeal skeletal muscle and in one instance involved a salivary gland and cervical lymph node.

Diffuse fibrinopurulent bronchopneumonia, suppurative bronchitis, and pleuritis were observed in rhesus monkeys with *Klebsiella* pneumonia (Fox and Rohovsky, 1975). Alveoli contained fibrin and hemorrhage. Gram-negative bacteria were associated with multifocal necrosis and exudation within the lung. Fibrinopurulent meningitis with numerous gram-negative organisms within the exudate, vasculitis, and thrombosis of meningeal vessels were characteristic of *Klebsiella* meningitis in rhesus monkeys (Fox and Rohovsky, 1975). Thickening and collapse of alveolar septae, congestion, alveolar hemorrhage, and edema with mononuclear and neutrophilic inflammatory cell infiltrates characterized pneumonia in the chimpanzees (Schmidt and Butler, 1971). Multifocal microabscesses and filling of bronchioles with necrotic debris and inflammatory cells were described.

Treatment of *Klebsiella* infections has been difficult due to the fulminating course of disease and the high incidence of multiple drug resistance (Fox and Rohovsky, 1975). Intensive antibiotic therapy was successful in controlling an outbreak in a rhesus monkey colony; however, during bacterial isolation and determination of antibiotic sensitivity, 12 monkeys died (Hunt *et al.,* 1968). Administration of tetracycline, 55 mg/kg body weight, in the drinking water for 5 consecutive days was effective in controlling an outbreak in a colony of tamarins and owl monkeys (Gozalo and Montoya, 1991a). Improvement of colony hygiene and treatment with kanamycin, chloramphenicol, and cephalosporin–aminoglycoside for 8–12 days halted an outbreak in a colony of common marmosets (Campos *et al.,* 1981). Screening of the oropharynx or feces of a monkey population to determine the number of asymptomatic carriers and drug sensitivity of the isolate may help in determining therapeutic regimens prior to occurrence of disease.

Prevention of infection by the use of a killed, whole *K. pneumoniae* aluminum hydroxide-adsorbed bacterin in owl monkeys (Obaldia, 1991) and a capsular polysaccharide vaccine in squirrel monkeys (Postal *et al.,* 1988) has been effective in reducing morbidity and mortality in the respective colonies. Autogenous vaccination has also been used in a breeding colony of common marmosets (Chalmers *et al.,* 1983). Infant and adult owl monkeys were vaccinated with two doses of bacterin administered subcutaneously at 1-month intervals (Obaldia, 1991). Seroconversion was 90% after the second dose. Mortality due to *K. pneumoniae* infections dropped from 20–22% to 3–4% following vaccination of the owl monkey colony. Drawbacks to vaccination included the development of small, 0.5- to 1-cm granulomas with fistulous tract at the inoculation site and the death of two owl monkey infants less than 1 month of age from bacterin-associated endotoxemia (Obaldia, 1991). The use of the capsular polysaccharide vaccine was similarly successfully in the squirrel monkey colony, reducing total infant mortality from 45 to 20% (Postal *et al.,* 1988). There were no side effects associated with vaccination in squirrel monkeys.

N. *Bordetella*

Bordetella bronchiseptica are pleomorphic, gram-negative, minute, coccobacilli. These bacteria are strictly aerobic, motile, produce urease, and use citrate. *Bordetella bronchiseptica* have pili that facilitate attachment to the ciliated epithelium of the respiratory tract. These bacteria actively attach to cilia and can produce significant ciliostasis within 5 min of contact (Bemis *et al.,* 1977).

The organism is carried as a commensal by many monkeys within the nasopharynx. Disease has historically been associated with recent shipping, quarantine, poor condition, and overcrowding (Seibold *et al.,* 1970; Pinkerton, 1972). Outbreaks have occurred in established colonies of common marmosets in which the initiating factor was unknown (Baskerville *et al.,* 1983; Chalmers *et al.,* 1983).

Clinical signs in affected common marmosets, *Callithrix jacchus,* included bilateral mucopurulent nasal discharge, dyspnea during handling, and pyrexia. Affected marmosets usually remained bright and alert. Death occurred in marmosets less than 1 year of age; adults survived. Titi monkeys, *Callicebus* sp., developed bilateral mucoid or mucopurulent nasal discharge that then formed occlusive crusts (Seibold *et al.,* 1970). Open mouth breathing, dyspnea, tachypnea, anorexia, and lethargy were observed as the disease progressed. Survival after onset of clinical disease ranged from 1 to 33 days (Seibold *et al.,* 1970). An infected African green monkey presented with hypothermia, poor peripheral circulation, dehydration, dyspnea, and bradycardia (Graves, 1968). The African green monkey had marked

hypoglycemia, a mild electrolyte imbalance, and leukopenia. One of three lesser bushbabies, *Galago senegalensis,* that died from *B. bronchiseptica* infection experienced seizures and torticollis (Kohn and Haines, 1977). Seizures were characterized by bilateral nystagmus, pupillary dilatation, and grand mal seizure lasting 15–30 sec. The other two bushbabies succumbed without clinical disease.

Diagnosis of *B. bronchiseptica* infection was based on isolation of the organism from clinical specimens, such as nasal or oropharyngeal swabs, or from lesioned tissues at necropsy. *Bordetella bronchiseptica* can be cultured on standard laboratory media, including blood and MacConkey agars at 37°C. After 24–48 hr of growth, convex smooth colorless colonies that may be hemolytic will form on blood agar. The organism may be difficult to recover if there is heavy contamination with other bacteria.

Bronchopneumonia affecting all lung lobes was the primary gross lesion in common marmosets, titi monkeys, and an African green monkey (Graves, 1968; Pinkerton, 1972; Seibold *et al.,* 1970; Baskerville *et al.,* 1983; Chalmers *et al.,* 1983). Common marmosets were in good condition with gross lesions limited to the respiratory tract (Baskerville *et al.,* 1983). The right and accessory lung lobes were consistently the worse affected; variable areas of consolidation and congestion were observed in all lung lobes (Baskerville *et al.,* 1983). Some marmosets had thickened pericardia and fibrinopurulent visceral pleurisy. In titi monkeys the pattern of consolidation ranged from small multifocal areas, to patchy and diffuse patterns within different lung lobes, to diffuse consolidation within all lobes (Seibold *et al.,* 1970). Otitis media occurred in the bushbaby with seizures; fibrinopurulent pleuritis, pericarditis, extensive pulmonary consolidation, and localized consolidative pneumonia in a diaphragmatic lobe were reported for the other bushbabies (Kohn and Haines, 1977).

The typical microscopic pulmonary lesion was purulent bronchopneumonia. In common marmosets, multifocal necrosis of the bronchiolar epithelium and filling of bronchioles with basophilic necrotic cellular debris, polymorphonuclear cells, and macrophagess occurred. Exudate extended continuously through branches of bronchioles, alveolar ducts, and alveoli, and occasionally small bronchioles were obliterated by exudate and cellular debris. Bronchial lymph nodes were edematous and reactive. Mild rhinitis, necrotizing laryngitis, and fibrinopurulent pericarditis were observed less frequently (Baskerville *et al.,* 1983). In titi monkeys, there was dense cellular and fibrinocellular exudate in and around bronchioles. Acute hemorrhage was frequently observed in areas bordering the inflammatory cell infiltrates. Confluence of some brochopneumonia areas occurred with diffuse uniform exudation into alveoli (Seibold *et al.,* 1970). In monkeys with a prolonged clinical course, thickening of alveolar walls and proliferation of alveolar lining cells were found. Pneumonic lesions in lesser bushbabies were interstitial in distribution and consisted of mononuclear and neutrophilic cell infiltrates (Kohn and Haines, 1977). The bushbaby with seizures had thrombosis of meningeal veins and multifocal hemorrhagic infarctions in the cerebral cortex secondary to thrombosed vessels. The tympanic bullae were filled with necrotic debris and leukocytes (Kohn and Haines, 1977).

Pinkerton (1972) reported that prophylactic administration of penicillin to African green monkeys prior to shipment prevented the development of *B. bronchiseptica* pneumonia on arrival. Treatment of adult common marmosets with intramuscular oxytetracycline for 8 days resolved clinical disease, but did not eliminate the organism from the nasal passages (Baskerville *et al.,* 1983). Use of an autogenous bacterin in *C. jacchus* colonies has been reported, but its efficacy was not discussed (Chalmers *et al.,* 1983).

O. *Pasteurella*

Pasteurella multocida are gram-negative, nonmotile, encapsulated, pleomorphic, bipolar-staining coccobacilli. *Pasteurella multocida* has limited growth on MacConkey agar and does not produce hemolysis on blood agar. Smooth colonies have increased virulence.

There are limited reports of pasteurellosis in nonhuman primates. In most cases, disease has been associated with recent shipment (Greenstein *et al.,* 1965; Benjamin and Lang, 1971; Pinkerton, 1972), and affected monkeys have been in poor condition (Benjamin and Lang, 1971). In addition to those cases, baboons developed *Pasteurella* infections secondary to surgical procedures, chair restraint, or chronic catheterization (Bronsdon and DiGiacomo, 1993).

A shipment of 20 squirrel monkeys arrived with 1 dead monkey (Greenstein *et al.,* 1965). In the next 10 days, the remainder of the shipment and additional monkeys with which they had been housed died. Clinical signs included unsteady gait, ocular and head nystagmus, head tilt, circling in one direction, edema of the eyelids, and serosanguinous discharge from the ears. Conjunctivitis with petechial hemorrhages, hemorrhages in the kidney, skeletal muscles, and intestinal serosa, cardiac enlargement, and cloudy cerebrospinal fluid were the primary gross lesions. Microscopic lesions in tissues from two squirrel monkeys included acute suppurative myocarditis and endocarditis, otitis media, meningitis, and lymphadenitis (Greenstein *et al.,* 1965). *Pasteurella multocida* was isolated from an eyelid, a brain and spinal cord suspension and cerebrospinal fluid.

Three of four juvenile owl monkeys died 3–6 days after receipt from a commercial supplier (Benjamin and Lang, 1971). The owl monkeys were lethargic, anorectic, and in poor condition. Pneumonia, pneumonia and pleuritis, congestion of the meninges, and cloudy cerebrospinal fluid were observed at necropsy. Two monkeys had necrotizing, fibrinopurulent pneumonia with thrombosis of small blood vessels. Gram-negative, bipolar bacilli were observed within alveolar macrophages. Severe, acute interstitial pneumonia with multifocal necrosis of

alveolar septae was also found in two monkeys. All monkeys had purulent enterocolitis with focal mucosal necrosis. Bacterial emboli were found in the liver, kidney, heart, and endometrium. One monkey had severe, diffuse suppurative meningoencephalitis. *Pasteurella multocida* was isolated from pleural fluid and lung.

Pasteurella multocida air sac infection was reported as a postsurgical complication in baboons (Bronsdon and DiGiacomo, 1993). Baboons also developed abscesses in the neck or femoral region secondary to chair restraint or chronic catheterization. *Pasteurella multocida* was part of the commensal pharyngeal flora in healthy wild-born adult baboons (Bronsdon and DiGiacomo, 1993).

Pasteurella hemolytica was recovered from a Goeldie's monkey that died suddenly (Gozalo *et al.,* 1992). The monkey was thin. Multiple small white foci were observed on the liver surface. Hepatic foci were composed of mixed inflammatory cells predominating in neutrophils with a central area of necrosis and clusters of bacteria. Birds were believed to be the source of the infection. *Pasteurella haemolytica* was recovered from liver samples cultured on blood agar and MacConkey agar. Unlike *P. multocida, P. haemolytica* can produce hemolysis on blood agar.

P. *Francisella*

Francisella tularensis is a pleomorphic, nonmotile, gramnegative bacterium that requires cystine-enriched media for growth. The bacterium is widespread, infecting more than 50 species of mammals, birds, and reptiles in North America alone, with rabbits, hares, muskrats, and squirrels serving as reservoirs. Infection can be acquired orally, via the respiratory route, from bites of infected vertebrates, from an arthropod vector, or from direct contact with infected tissues. There are few reports of naturally acquired tularemia in nonhuman primates.

There have been two reports of tularemia in squirrel monkeys. One was a pet animal that became irritable, anorectic, and aggressive (Emmons *et al.,* 1970). The affected monkey bit its owner; the monkey died 5 days later. Only the brain was submitted for laboratory testing, primarily for rabies examination. *Francisella tularensis* was recovered from the brain following mouse inoculation and culture of mouse brain and liver suspensions on blood and chocolate agars. The owner developed tenderness in the axilla and was treated with penicillin. The origin of the infection was not determined. In another case, a colony-raised squirrel monkey became moribund with extensive cutaneous petechiation. Gross lesions were consistent with disseminated intravascular coagulation and sepsis. *Francisella tularensis* was cultured from the liver.

Tularemia has been reported in black and red tamarins, *S. nigricollis,* and talapoins, *Cercocebus talapoin,* in a zoologic park (Nayar *et al.,* 1979). The tamarins collapsed acutely and were hypothermic. One talapoin died following a day of anorexia. The second talapoin had profuse salivation, nasal and ocular discharges, and severe ulceration of the tongue. Treatment with fluids, vitamins, and oxytetracycline was ameliorative; however, 2 weeks later the monkey had abscesses in the tongue and submandibular region. The monkey recovered when treated with oral ampicillin and parenteral B vitamins for 10 days. The source of the infection was wild ground squirrels within the park.

Necropsy lesions were similar in the tamarins and talapoin (Nayar *et al.,* 1979). Multiple tiny white foci were scattered throughout the liver and spleen; the spleen was enlarged; and there was slight excess abdominal fluid. Fibrinous peritonitis and marked mesenteric lymphadenopathy and edema were seen. Multifocal caseous necrosis was found in the liver and spleen microscopically. Pneumonitis, acute glomerulitis, enteritis, and lymphadenitis of varying severity were found in each monkey. *Francisella tularensis* was recovered from lung, liver, and spleen and from the tongue abscess of the talapoin that recovered. *Francisella tularensis* was isolated from the liver and spleen of a ground squirrel and from fleas infesting the squirrel. Cultures grew on chocolate agar and Eugon agar maintained at 37°C both aerobically and in 5–10% CO_2 environments.

The veterinarian treating the monkeys was bitten on the hand by an infected tamarin and developed axillary lymph node enlargement, malaise, fever, and diarrhea. The lesions resolved without treatment, but recurred. Serologic testing revealed a rising titer to *F. tularensis* (Nayar *et al.,* 1979).

Q. *Pseudomonas*

1. *Pseudomonas aeruginosa*

Pseudomonas aeruginosa is an ubiquitous, gram-negative bacterium that inhabits freshwater and marine environments, soil, plants, and animals. It is a opportunistic pathogen. *Pseudomonas aeruginosa* grows well on blood, tryptose, and trypicase agars, producing large gray colonies with irregular spreading margins. Colonies are frequently β hemolytic on blood agar, may have a metallic sheen, and sometimes have a distinctive "grape" or fruit-like odor.

In common with other gram-negative bacteria, *Pseudomonas* spp. produce pathogenic endotoxins: leukocidin, which impairs neutrophils and macrophages, and adenosine diphosphate-ribosyl transferase or endotoxin A. One of the primary factors contributing to the virulence of *P. aeruginosa* is the ability of the bacterium to form adherent, exopolysaccharide-enclosed microcolonies within the blood vessels of the host (Peterson, 1980). These protected microcolonies limit the defense response of the host and sequester the bacteria from circulating antibiotics.

Pseudomonas sp., including *P. aeruginosa*, were isolated from 12% of monkeys with diarrhea and were isolated frequently from external wounds, blood cultures, and air sac infections in nonhuman primates at the Yerkes Primate Center (McClure, 1980). *Pseudomonas* sp. were isolated from 23% of

rectal swabs and 11% of throat swabs from recently imported *Saguinus* sp. (F. Deinhardt *et al.,* 1967). *Pseudomonas* sp. were associated with bronchopneumonia, empyema, vegetative endocarditis, pancarditis, and septicemia in Callithricidae (J. B. Deinhardt *et al.,* 1967; Cicmanec, 1977). *Pseudomonas aeruginosa* has been isolated from squirrel monkeys with meningitis, pododermatitis and cellulitis (Lausen *et al.,* 1986), necrotizing cellulitis (Line *et al.,* 1984), and a maxillofacial abscess (Langner *et al.,* 1986); an African green monkey with bacterial myocarditis and pneumonia (Stills *et al.,* 1979); and from a chimpanzee with suppurative nephritis (Migaki *et al.,* 1979).

The squirrel monkey with meningitis developed nystagmus, involuntary head movements, severe CNS depression, and coma while being treated for diarrhea. The monkey was tachycardic and had ectopic ventricular contractions. Clinical pathology findings included leukopenia with a mild left shift, uremia, an elevated serum creatinine, and elevated serum alanine aminotransferase and alkaline phosphatase activity. Another animal in the same colony had a chronic ulcer on the plantar surface of its foot that progressed into fulminant pododermatitis with cellulitis, edema of the entire leg, and severe lytic osteomyelitis of the bones of the foot and ankle. On initial presentation this monkey was depressed, had fever, and had an elevated WBC of 16,500; subsequently, during treatment, the monkey became anemic, PCV of 28%, and the white blood cell count normalized (Lausen *et al.,* 1986). A squirrel monkey presenting with a 1-cm bite wound on the ventral thorax and depression had severe neutropenia and lymphopenia (<1000 cells/μl) (Line *et al.,* 1984). Extensive skin necrosis and serosanguinous discharge were found at the bite wound site the next day. Bacterial myocarditis and pneumonia in the African green monkey presented as an acute illness during quarantine, characterized by dehydration, hypothermia, cyanosis, and dyspnea (Stills *et al.,* 1979). The chimpanzee presented with lethargy and poor appetite, turgid skin, pale dry, mucous membranes, and tenderness in the lower abdomen (Migaki *et al.,* 1979). Laboratory results included uremia, marked elevation of serum phosphorus, reduced serum calcium, and markedly reduced total protein (1.2 g/100ml).

Gross necropsy lesions in the squirrel monkey that died with CNS signs included swelling and softening of the brain, distorted calvarial sutures, and hemorrhagic foci throughout the cerebral parenchyma. The stomach had multiple areas of mucosal hemorrhage and there were multifocal serosal petechia. Microscopic lesions in the squirrel monkey included multifocal necrosis and hemorrhage with a primarily neutrophilic infiltrate in the brain and leptomeninges and multifocal mucosal and submucosal hemorrhages with necrosis in the stomach (Lausen *et al.,* 1986). Numerous gram-negative bacteria were observed around and within the cerebral vessels with minimal inflammation. Small pale raised nodules on the left ventricular endocardium and myocardium and consolidation of the right middle and caudal lung lobes were noted in the African green monkey

(Stills *et al.*, 1979). Acute bacterial myocarditis with focal liquefactive necrosis and abscess formation, acute necrotizing bronchopneumonia, and focal hemorrhagic encephalitis were the microscopic diagnoses. Small kidneys with many yellow 1- to 2-mm nodules, excessive peritoneal fluid, and a slight increase in pericardial fluid were noted in the chimpanzee (Migaki *et al.*, 1979). Renal lesions included multiple foci of neutrophilic inflammation and necrosis containing gram-negative bacteria that extended from the subcapsular cortex through the medulla, interstitial fibrosis, and distention of collecting tubules with neutrophils and cellular debris. Lesions were indicative of a hematogenous infection (Migaki *et al.*, 1979).

Treatment in all cases involved aggressive antibiotic therapy. Successful antibiotic regimens included gentamicin (1.25 mg/kg, every 12 hr) and procaine penicillin (50,000 units/kg every 12 hr) intramuscularly and polymyxin B (12,500 IU/kg, intramuscular every 12 hr) (Line *et al.*, 1984; Lausen *et al.*, 1986). The monkey with pododermatitis and osteomyelitis required amputation of the foot (Lausen *et al.*, 1986). Necrotizing cellulitis from the bite wound responded to surgical debridement and antibiotic therapy; split skin thickness grafts were performed after *P. aeruginosa* infection had cleared (Line *et al.*, 1984). Enucleation, povidone iodine lavage of the orbit, and oral antibiotic therapy for 10 days successfully eliminated *Pseudomonas* infection from a squirrel monkey with a maxillofacial abscess (Langner *et al.*, 1986).

2. *Pseudomonas pseudomallei*: Melioidosis

Pseudomonas pseudomallei is a small, gram-negative, bipolar staining, pleomorphic bacillus. The bacterium grows well on standard laboratory media and is obligately aerobic, nonspore-forming, and motile. *Pseudomonas pseudomallei* is a tropical or subtropical saprophytic organism commonly found in soil and water. Endemic human disease has been documented in southeast Asia and Australia, and less frequently on the Indian subcontinent, portions of Central and South America, Africa, and the Middle East (Dance, 1991). The organism commonly enters through skin abrasions, but can also be transmitted by ingestion or inhalation. Infected animals can be imported and escape detection during quarantine because *P. pseudomallei* may remain latent for several years.

The attributes of *P. pseudomallei* that contribute to its pathogenicity are poorly understood. The long periods of latency in some cases of melioidosis suggest that this organism is capable of intracellular survival, possibly in macrophages, although this theory has not been proven (Dance, 1990). *Pseudomonas pseudomallei* has a classical endotoxin, produces a heat-labile, lethal exotoxin, and produces several extracellular enzymes with the potential to damage tissue (Dance, 1990). The organism usually acts as an opportunistic pathogen, causing disease in people with underlying chronic diseases, such as diabetes mellitus, urinary tract calculi, and other renal disease, or in persons immu-

nosuppressed through drug therapy, tuberculosis, or cirrhosis (Dance, 1990). However, melioidosis has occurred in people without any of these predisposing factors.

Naturally acquired melioidosis has been reported in a banded leaf-monkey, *Presbytis melaphos*, macaques, and great apes (Retnasabapathy and Joseph, 1966; Strauss *et al.*, 1969; Kaufmann *et al.*, 1970; Butler *et al.*, 1971; Smith and Damit, 1982; Mutalib *et al.*, 1984; Fritz *et al.*, 1986). Several of the affected nonhuman primates had histories of experimental surgery or fight wound trauma (Strauss *et al.*, 1969; Kaufmann *et al.*, 1970; Butler *et al.*, 1971; Fritz *et al.*, 1986) prior to the development of melioidosis. All animals were imported from endemic areas with the exception of a chimpanzee that was thought to have acquired the infection in the laboratory (Kaufmann *et al.*, 1970). Incubation time to development of overt disease ranged from 3 months to 10 years (Kaufmann *et al.*, 1970; Fritz *et al.*, 1986).

Clinical signs were nonspecific and varied with the primary system involved. Serous nasal discharge and sneezing consistent with an upper respiratory tract infection progressed to listlessness, depression, and increased lung sounds on auscultation in an orangutan with pneumonia (Smith and Damit, 1982). Nasal crusts, anorexia, and hard feces were noted in a leaf monkey that developed *P. pseudomallei* bronchopneumonia (Mutalib *et al.*, 1984). Weakness and paraplegia occurred in macaques with vertebral osetomyelitis (Strauss *et al.*, 1969; Fritz *et al.*, 1986). Subcutaneous abscesses, peripheral lymphadenopathy, and swelling of carpal joints were reported (Strauss *et al.*, 1969; Kaufmann *et al.*, 1970; Butler *et al.*, 1971). In some animals, exudation at sites of experimental implants (Kaufmann *et al.*, 1970; Butler *et al.*, 1971) or abscess formation along a surgical scar (Kaufmann *et al.*, 1970) were the first indication of *P. pseudomallei* infection.

Clinical pathology data were sporadic. Moderate to marked leukocytosis was reported for two macaques with vertebral osteomyelitis and a chimpanzee with an infected implant (Strauss *et al.*, 1969; Butler *et al.*, 1971; Fritz *et al.*, 1986) and one macaque had an elevated erythrocyte sedimentation rate (Strauss *et al.*, 1969). Pale green discoloration of serum samples was noted in macaques and a chimpanzee with melioidosis (Kaufmann *et al.*, 1970). Radiographs documented vertebral osteomyelitis, paravertebral abscess formation, and vertebral fusion at L3 and L4 in one paraplegic macaque (Strauss *et al.*, 1969); scoliosis of the spine at T10 through T13 was observed in the other (Fritz *et al.*, 1986).

Diagnosis was based on history of origin from an endemic area and culture of *P. pseudomallei* from antemortem or postmortem lesions. *Pseudomonas pseudomallei* grows readily on most routine laboratory media, but may be overgrown by commensals in specimens with a mixed bacterial flora. A sweet, earthy to pungent smell has been associated with fresh cultures of the organism (Dance, 1991). Identification is achieved by a battery of chemical tests or use of specific antisera (Dance,

1991). Laboratory-acquired infections have occurred, so careful handling of specimens and cultures is necessary. Serum hemagglutination titers were also used to try to determine exposure and infection in recently imported macaques (Kaufmann *et al.*, 1970). Serum titers 1:320 or greater were considered to be highly suggestive of active disease.

Gross necropsy lesions included bronchopneumonia with profuse yellow watery bronchial exudate (Smith and Damit, 1982) and pulmonary congestion and consolidation with multifocal abscesses ranging from miliary to 2.5 cm in diameter (Retnasabapathy and Joseph, 1966; Butler *et al.*, 1971; Mutalib *et al.*, 1984). Multifocal abscesses in the liver, spleen, trachea, and stomach were observed in many cases (Kaufmann *et al.*, 1970; Butler *et al.*, 1971; Mutalib *et al.*, 1984). Subcutaneous abscesses and abscessed peripheral lymph nodes were noted in macaques (Kaufmann *et al.*, 1970). Swollen metacarpal joints containing exudate and peripheral lymphadenopathy with edema occurred in a chimpanzee (Butler *et al.*, 1971). Exudation was noted around surgical implants (Kaufmann *et al.*, 1970; Butler *et al.*, 1971). The scoliotic lesion at T10–T13 in the paraplegic rhesus monkey was associated with spinal cord compression, mild exudation in the vertebral canal, and fibrosis of vertebral bodies (Fritz *et al.*, 1986).

Multifocal microabscesses in the lung, liver, spleen, stomach, lymph nodes, and/or trachea were the primary microscopic lesion (Retnasabapathy and Joseph, 1966; Kaufmann *et al.*, 1970; Butler *et al.*, 1971; Mutalib *et al.*, 1984). Gram-negative bacteria could be visualized in the necrotic centers of the abscesses in some cases (Kaufmann *et al.*, 1970). Acute suppurative bronchopneumonia was characterized by neutrophilic infiltration within and around bronchioles (Butler *et al.*, 1971; Mutalib *et al.*, 1984). Suppurative inflammation extended into surrounding alveoli, and the alveolar septae were thickened. Acute and chronic osteomyelitis occurred in affected thoracic vertebrae and metacarpal bones (Butler *et al.*, 1971; Fritz *et al.*, 1986).

In no case was antibiotic therapy successful. One monkey experienced spontaneous remission of disease (Strauss *et al.*, 1969). *Pseudomonas pseudomallei* is resistant to many antibiotics, including penicillin, ampicillin, colistin, and polymyxin, aminoglycosides, and first and second generation cephalosporins (Dance, 1990). *Pseudomonas pseudomallei* also develops antibiotic resistance rapidly during the course of treatment (Dance, 1990).

R. *Aeromonas*

Aeromonas hydrophila are gram-negative, pleomorphic bacilli with a single polar flagellum. They are nonsporing, fermentative, oxidase positive, facultative aerobes frequently found in fresh water and sewage. They are easy to grow on standard laboratory media and produce β hemolysis on blood agar. Usually considered a pathogen of fish and amphibians, *Aeromonas*

spp. have been implicated in diarrheal disease in humans (Altwegg and Geiss, 1989).

In a 5-year survey of nonhuman primates with diarrheal disease, *A. hydrophilia* was isolated from 47 cases and was the sole enteric pathogen in 26 of the cases (McClure *et al.*, 1986). *Aeromonas hydrophila* was isolated from 14 nonhuman primates with septicemia or bacteremia, multifocal hepatic necrosis with bacterial colonization, pneumonia, or enterocolitis over a 12-year period (Chalifoux *et al.*, 1993). Cases were sporadic and occurred more frequently in New World monkeys than in Old World species. *Aeromonas hydrophila* infection was diagnosed in a cotton-top tamarin with peritonitis. The tamarin had a history of chronic weight loss and intermittent diarrhea; it presented with abdominal bloating and weakness. A complete blood count revealed anemia, thrombocytopenia, and a left shift with a normal neutrophil count. Cloudy amber fluid was recovered from the thorax and abdomen at necropsy. Fibrinous peritonitis and colonic perforation were found. The tamarin had metastatic colonic adenocarcinoma. *Aeromonas hydrophila* was isolated from the colon; gram-negative bacilli were seen in multiple tissues (Chalifoux *et al.*, 1993).

S. *Campylobacter*

Campylobacter are slender, curved, motile, microaerophilic bacteria. The bacteria as a group grow at 37°C; thermophilic strains associated with diarrheal disease in hymans and nonhuman primates prefer 42°C. The two most frequent isolates from nonhuman primates are *C. jejuni* and *C. coli*, with *C. fetus, C. laridis, C. sputorum,* and *C. hyointestinalis* found less frequently (Russell, 1992; Paul-Murphy, 1993). Both *C. jejuni* and *C. coli* are oxidase and catalase positive; they can be distinguished by their ability to hydrolyze hippurate: *C. jejuni* is hippurate positive. *Campylobacter* are widely distributed throughout the world. Infection usually occurs by the fecal–oral route.

Although *C. jejuni* has been isolated frequently from humans and animals with diarrhea, the pathogenic properties of this bacterium have not been well described. Isolates from people with bloody invasive-type diarrhea or watery secretory diarrhea were compared; the invasive strains produced a cytotoxin and the secretory diarrheal strains produced an enterotoxin (Klipstein *et al.*, 1985). The toxins were not found in *Campylobacter* strains isolated from asymptomatic infections. The role of cellular invasion in the pathogenesis of *C. jejuni* colitis was investigated following oral inoculation of infant pig-tailed macaques (Russell *et al.*, 1993). The infants developed diarrhea 32 hr postinoculation. *Campylobacter* were found penetrating the apex of columnar epithelial cells in the colon. As the bacteria penetrated the cell, dense accumulations of microfilaments formed in the apical cytoplasm. The bacterium initially was localized in a membrane-bound cytoplasmic vacuole; subsequently, there was cytoplasmic swelling, rounding of the cell, and blunting of the microvilli as the bacteria became free within the cytoplasm. The damaged cells were exfoliated into the colonic lumen (Russell *et al.*, 1993). *Campylobacter jejuni* apparently accelerates apoptosis, damaging the superficial colonic epithelium and thus initiating degenerative changes, resulting in mucosal damage and diarrhea (Russell *et al.*, 1993).

Some experimental infections of *C. jejuni* in rhesus monkeys and pig-tailed macaques have induced colitis and clinical diarrhea similar to that reported for naturally infected humans (Fitzgeorge *et al.*, 1981; Russell *et al.*, 1989). Young rhesus monkeys infected with *C. jejuni* developed mild disease with inappetence and diarrhea of short duration; however, intermittent excretion of *C. jejuni* in the feces was prolonged (Fitzgeorge *et al.*, 1981). There were no gross lesions attributable to *C. jejuni* at necropsy (Fitzgeorge *et al.*, 1981). Inoculation of young pig-tailed macaques resulted in clinical diarrhea 24–32 hr postinfection (Russell *et al.*, 1989). Microscopic lesions in the colon were characterized by a moderate inflammatory cell infiltrate, including neutrophils and mononuclear cells, with necrosis and loss of columnar epithelium at 48–72 hr postinfection (Russell *et al.*, 1989).

Oral inoculation of infant rhesus macaques 3.5 to 4.5 months of age with *C. jejuni* caused acute diarrhea 24–36 hr after administration (Russell, 1992). Diarrhea progressed from semiformed feces to fluid and watery feces. The diarrheal illness was self-limiting, with an average duration of 9 days. Organisms were shed in the feces for 15–21 days postinoculation. Inoculation of *C. jejuni* in 6-month-old cynomolgus monkeys did not cause diarrhea; the organism was shed in the feces for 20–35 days postinoculation. Challenge of previously infected pig-tailed macaque infants with another oral inoculation of *C. jejuni* did not cause diarrhea, and *C. jejuni* was recovered from feces 7–9 days postinfection (Russell, 1992). These experiments indicate that *C. jejuni* infections in nonhuman primates are self-limiting and that reexposure is unlikely to cause disease.

Campylobacter jejuni and *C. coli* were the most frequent fecal bacterial isolates from both asymptomatic and clinically affected nonhuman primates (Tribe *et al.*, 1979; Tribe and Fleming, 1983; McClure *et al.*, 1986; Russell *et al.*, 1987). Prevalence of infection varied greatly, with some colonies reporting a 100% infection rate (Russell *et al.*, 1988). Isolates from monkeys with no clinical disease comprised up to 81% of the total (Taylor *et al.*, 1989). A survey of recently trapped tamarins revealed that 22.2% of *S. mystax* and 37.5% of *S. labiatus* were infected with *C. coli* (Gozalo *et al.*, 1991). Tamarins that had been in the colony for 1 year had a much lower prevalence of infection, 14.8% of *S. mystax* and 13.3% of *S. labiatus*. There was no correlation between *C. coli* infection and diarrheal disease (Gozalo *et al.*, 1991). *Campylobacter jejuni* was isolated from 46% of lion tamarins in a Brazil zoo; half were asymptomatic (Pinheiro *et al.*, 1993). *Saguinus oedipus* infants experienced diarrhea with their initial infection with *C. jejuni;* subsequent infections with *C. jejuni* or *C. coli* usually

were not associated with diarrhea (Russell, 1992). In one study of primates in a zoo, *C. jejuni* was isolated more frequently from animals with diarrhea than from animals with normal feces (Leuchtefeld *et al.*, 1981). *Campylobacter jejuni* infection in macaques was not acquired naturally in the wild, but was probably the result of exposure to contaminated water and foodstuffs after capture (Morton *et al.*, 1983). Prevalence of infection increased (36 to 77%) as time in captivity increased.

Clinically, diarrheal disease associated with *Campylobacter* infection tends to present as watery diarrhea, although mucohemorrhagic diarrhea also has been reported (Paul-Murphy, 1993). Hemorrhagic diarrhea and weight loss were reported for a baboon with *Vibrio fetus* infection (Bonck *et al.*, 1972). Mucohemorrhagic diarrhea occurred in outdoor-housed *Callithrix penicillata* (Carvalho *et al.*, 1987). Chronic, intermittent, or persistent diarrhea with or without melena was observed in patas monkeys with *C. jejuni* infection (Bryant *et al.*, 1983). Chronic diarrhea was reported for baboons (Tribe *et al.*, 1979) and persistent, recurring diarrhea in orangutans (Pazzaglia *et al.*, 1994) infected with *Campylobacter. Campylobacter* spp. were isolated from a Celebes macaque and from two pale-faced Saki monkeys with histories of chronic intermittent diarrhea (Leuchtefeld *et al.*, 1981). White blood counts in primates with diarrhea and *Campylobacter* infection vary from normal leukocyte counts to leukocytosis with a left shift (Paul-Murphy, 1993). Severe electrolyte abnormalities, including hyponatremia, hypochloremia, acidosis, and high anion gap, were found in rhesus monkeys with diarrhea and infection with *C. jejuni* or *C. coli* (George and Lerche, 1990). Serum sodium concentrations <132 mEq/liter and serum Cl concentrations <93 mEq/liter were found consistently in monkeys with *Campylobacter* infection (George and Lerche, 1990).

Diagnosis of infection with *C. jejuni* or *C. coli* is based on recovery of the organism from feces, rectal swabs, or intestinal biopsies or intestinal lesions at necropsy. Both organisms grow best on a Skirrows media with 5–7% lysed horse blood, Butzler's medium composed of thioglycolate agar with 15% sheep blood, or BAP, a commercially available *Brucella* agar plate. All media contain selected antibiotics to prevent commensal overgrowth. Plates should be incubated at 42°C in a 5–10% oxygen, 5–10% CO_2 environment for 2–3 days. The gas environment can be created by using an anaerobe jar or plastic pouch with a commercially available gas-generating envelope or an appropriate gas mixture may be purchased. Colonies are raised, round, and translucent and sometimes have a spreading mucoid appearance. Definitive identification can be made from a series of biochemical tests. *Campylobacter* spp. can be identified by their characteristic comma or spiral shapes when gram stained. *Campylobacter* have a characteristic darting motality when viewed using dark-field or phase-contrast microscopy of a wet drop mount from culture or fresh feces. Serologic testing for immunoglobulin G (IgG) and IgM antibodies may be a useful tool for the diagnosis of *Campylobacter* infection in young primates (Russell, 1992). The titers rise 10 days postinfection and remain elevated for up to 4 weeks. Fluorescent antibody or avidin–biotin antibody staining of intestinal biopsy or necropsy specimens can provide confirmation of *Campylobacter* infection when only tissue samples are available.

Gross lesions of *C. jejuni* or *C. coli* infection in imported cynomolgus monkeys were reported as thinning of the bowel wall, distension of the bowel with pasty-to-fluid yellow-gray feces, and wasting of the carcass (Tribe and Fleming, 1983). Gross lesions seen in patas monkeys during surgical biopsy included thickening and rigidity of the terminal ileum, cecum, and proximal colon (Bryant *et al.*, 1983). The mucosal surface of biopsy specimens from the ileocecal junction and colon was covered with blood and mucus. Mesenteric and celiac lymph nodes were enlarged and there was a slight serosanguinous transudate in the abdominal cavity (Bryant *et al.*, 1983).

Microscopic lesions in the small intestine of patas monkeys infected with *C. jejuni* included thickening and shortening of the villi, dilated lacteals, and infiltration of the lamina propria with macrophages, lymphocytes, and necrotic debris (Bryant *et al.*, 1983). The mucosal epithelium was low columnar to cuboidal. In the large intestine, lesions varied among animals and included mild to moderate hyperplasia of the epithelium, edema of the lamina propria or submucosa, and multifocal crypt abscesses (Bryant *et al.*, 1983). Spiral or comma-shaped bacteria were observed on the epithelial surface and in the lamina propria of the small and large intestine stained with Warthin–Starry silver stain.

Based on the electrolyte imbalances reported for rhesus monkeys with diarrhea and *Campylobacter* infection, rehydration and replacement of electrolytes using normonatremic fluids such as lactated Ringer's solution or normal saline should be considered (George and Lerche, 1990). As many infections were self-limiting and reinfection was frequent (Russell *et al.*, 1987), the efficacy of using of antibiotics to treat *Campylobacter* diarrhea is debatable and should probably be determined on a case by case basis. Erythromycin has been the antibiotic of choice; however, resistant *Campylobacter* strains have been reported (Tribe and Fleming, 1983). Oral erythromycin administered at 30–50 mg/kg body weight/day for 7 days was successful in eliminating *Campylobacter* infection and diarrhea in a group of orangutans (Pazzaglia *et al.*, 1994). Oral dosing of erythromycin at 25 mg/animal/day, once a day, for 8 days was effective in lion tamarins with *C. jejuni* infection and diarrhea (Pinheiro *et al.*, 1993). Patas monkeys treated with either oral erythromycin (250 mg/animal twice daily for 10 days) or oxytetracycline (900 mg/liter) in the drinking water for 10 days had clinical resolution of diarrheal disease and became culture negative for *C. jejuni* (Bryant *et al.*, 1983).

T. *Helicobacter*

1. *Helicobacter pylori*

Helicobacter pylori, formerly *Campylobacter pylori*, is a gram-negative, spiral or curved, flagellated bacterium found in the gastric mucosa of humans and some nonhuman primates. *Helicobacter pylori* is implicated as a causative agent of gastritis (Blaser, 1990) and duodenal ulcer disease (Graham *et al.*, 1992) and is a risk factor for adenocarcinoma and lymphoma of the stomach in humans (Isaacson and Spencer, 1993; Hu *et al.*, 1994). *Helicobacter pylori* has been isolated from rhesus monkeys and baboons (Curry *et al.*, 1987; Dubois *et al.*, 1991) and a distantly related organism, *H. nemestrinae*, from pig-tailed macaques (Bronsdon *et al.*, 1991). As in humans *H. pylori* infection in rhesus monkeys was associated with gastritis (Dubois *et al.*, 1991, 1994). *Helicobacter finelliae* and *H. cinaededi* have been transmitted to monkeys experimentally.

Helicobacter pylori live within the mucus layer overlaying the gastric epithelium. Infection in humans and probably nonhuman primates persists for years once acquired. Several properties contribute to the development of persistent infection and virulence of *H. pylori*. *Helicobacter pylori* possesses strong urease activity, which enables the breakdown of urea in gastric juice and the production of bicarbonate and ammonia around the bacterium, effectively neutralizing gastric acidity (Marshall, 1994). The spiral shape and flagella allow motility within the mucus and provide resistance to peristalsis (Blaser, 1993). The ability to survive in a microaerobic environment allows the bacterium to reside in the mucus layer and adhesion production promotes stability (Hazell *et al.*, 1986; Blaser, 1993). The amonia byproduct of urease activity is toxic to epithelial cells (Mobley *et al.*, 1991), and urease itself elicits a strong immune response contributing to gastric inflammation. The bacterium produces superoxide dismutase and catalase, which protect it from being killed in neutrophil phagosomes (Marshall, 1994). Two independent virulence factors, cagA and vacA, are associated with most clinical isolates in humans. CagA, cytotoxin associated gene A, is strongly correlated with duodenal ulceration, and vacA, vacuolating cytotoxin, is associated with polymorphonuclear leukocyte infiltrates in the gastric mucosa (Phadnis *et al.*, 1994; Telford *et al.*, 1994). Inoculation with vacA alone can produce gastric ulceration in mice (Xiang *et al.*, 1995).

Naturally acquired infections in nonhuman primates have not caused clinical disease. Diagnosis of *H. pylori* infection was based on gastric endoscopy and biopsy or necropsy, with detection of urease activity within gastric tissue, culture of the biopsy or necropsy specimen, and serology. Microscopic gastric lesions ranged from mild mononuclear mucosal inflammation to marked mononuclear cell infiltrates within the gastric mucosa, polymorphonuclear leukocytes within the glands, and surface erosions (Dubois *et al.*, 1994). *Helicobacter pylori* were identified by light microscopy in gastric pits or crypts, in close contact with the epithelial surface, in the corpus and antrum of the stomach. Elevated plasma IgG to *H. pylori* was detected in infected monkeys (Dubois *et al.*, 1994). Tissue homogenates from gastric biopsies were cultured on Müeller–Hinton agar supplemented with 5% sheep blood, Columbia blood agar with 5% horse blood, or agar maintained in a microaerophilic environment at 37°C for 5 to 7 days (Drazek *et al.*, 1994; Dubois *et al.,* 1994). The microaerophilic environment was prepared using a gas atmosphere of 90% N_2, 5% O_2, and 5% CO_2. *Helicobacter pylori* colonies were pinpoint, "waterspray" type that were urease, oxidase, and catalase positive.

Attempts to eliminate *H. pylori* infection in rhesus monkeys with oral ampicillin, metronidazole, and bismuth subsalicylate administered in Tang were unsuccessful (Dubois *et al.,* 1994).

2. *Helicobacter*-like Organisms

Large, 8 μm long by 0.7 μm wide, spiral bacteria with bipolar flagella have been reported in the stomach of clinically normal rhesus monkeys and baboons (Sato and Takeuchi, 1982; Curry *et al.,* 1987; Dubois *et al.,* 1991). The organisms are gram-negative, urease-positive, tightly coiled spirilla morphologically identical to *Helicobacter heilmanii* (formerly *Gastrospirillum hominis*) by light and electron microscopy (Curry *et al.,* 1987; Dubois *et al.,* 1991). The bacteria were concentrated in gastric glands in the isthmus of the stomach, occurred less frequently in the neck and base, and were absent from the gastric lumen (Sato and Takeuchi, 1982). Gastric spirilla were closely associated with and penetrated parietal cells (Sato and Takeuchi, 1982; Dubois *et al.,* 1991). No inflammatory response or changes in host cytocomponents were observed in response to the spirilla in some rhesus monkeys (Sato and Takeuchi, 1982). The organisms were associated with mild gastritis or no gastritis in other studies in rhesus monkeys (Dubois *et al.,* 1991, 1994). These bacteria have not been cultured *in vitro.* They present a potential complicating factor when rhesus macaques or baboons are used for experimental studies of *Helicobacter* infection (Hazell *et al.,* 1992). Diagnosis was made by gastric biopsy, anatomic location, urease activity of biopsy specimens, and morphology (Dubois *et al.,* 1994).

U. *Arcobacter*

Arcobacter butzleri is an aerotolerant bacterium associated with diarrhea in humans and animals, originally assigned to the genus *Campylobacter* (Kiehlbauch *et al.,* 1991). The bacterium grows at a wide range of temperatures (15–42°C) on both MacConkey and agars under aerobic and anaerobic conditions. Most isolates are catalase negative or weakly positive, have no or intermediate resistance to nalidixic acid, and are strongly oxidase positive (Kiehlbauch *et al.,* 1991). *Arcobacter butzleri* has been isolated from pig-tailed macaque nursery infants with no clinical disease (Russell, 1992) and from adult and juvenile macaques, rhesus, cynomolgus, pig-tailed, and stump-tailed species, with diarrhea at another facility (Anderson *et al.,* 1993). The monkeys with diarrheal disease were greater than 6 months of age. Mild to moderately severe chronic active colitis was diagnosed in three monkeys from which *A. butzleri* was cultured at necropsy (Anderson *et al.,* 1993). *Arcobacter butz-*

leri was not isolated from normal monkey feces (Anderson *et al.,* 1993).

V. *Leptospira*

Leptospira are gram-negative, tightly coiled, spiral-shaped bacteria, 0.1 by 6 to 20 μm long. Genera include aquatic and saprophytic species that have adapted to a pathogenic existence. Many have adapted to reservoir hosts that shed bacteria in the urine for long periods of time. Infection can occur through direct contact with an infected animal, by ingestion of infected meat, by venereal or placental transfer, or by bite wounds. Indirect transmission occurs through exposure of susceptible animals to contaminated soil, vegetation, water, food, bedding, or other fomites.

Leptospires can penetrate mucous membranes without causing local inflammation and they multiply rapidly upon entering the blood. Bacteremia occurs from 4 to 12 days postinfection and leptospires are spread to various organs. Lipid products of leptospiral metabolism can injure tissue and capillary endothelium (Arean, 1962). Reduced blood flow, intravascular coagulation, and thrombosis are sequelae to leptospiral infection, resulting in tissue hyposia and cell death.

The occurrence of naturally acquired leptospirosis in nonhuman primates is uncommon, even though experimental infection has been studied in a variety of monkeys (Perolat *et al.,* 1992). Naturally acquired infections have been reported in a tamarin, *Saguinus labiatus,* a chimpanzee, squirrel monkeys, baboons, *Papio* spp., and Barbary apes (*Macaca sylvana*) (Wilbert and Delorme, 1927; Fear *et al.,* 1968; Shive *et al.,* 1969; Perolat *et al.,* 1992; Reid *et al.,* 1993). Clinical disease in the tamarin was characterized by lethargy and icterus, rapidly progressing to dyspnea, epistaxis, hemorrhage from the mouth, and death (Reid *et al.,* 1993). Affected squirrel monkeys were found dead without previous clinical signs or presented with pyrexia, marked dehydration, and icterus (Perolat *et al.,* 1992). In addition, an unusually high rate of abortion was seen during the leptospiral epizootic in the squirrel monkey colony. Abortion was also the most common clinical finding in the outbreak among baboons (Fear *et al.,* 1968). In Barbary apes, clinical signs included convulsions, inactivity, and recumbency followed shortly by death (Shive *et al.,* 1969).

Presumptive diagnosis of leptospirosis was based on clinical signs and gross lesions, particularly icterus (Shive *et al.,* 1969; Perolat *et al.,* 1992; Reid *et al.,* 1993). Diagnosis of leptospirosis was confirmed by isolation of *Leptospira interrogans* serovar *copenhageni* from blood from clinically ill squirrel monkeys and urine of a feral rat (Perolat *et al.,* 1992) and of *L.* serovar *icterohemorrhagiae* from liver and kidney from affected macaques (Shive *et al.,* 1969). Leptospirosis was diagnosed in the tamarin from clinical signs and from gross and microscopic lesions, including the presence of filamentous spiral bacteria within kidney tubule epithelium in Warthin–Starry-stained sections (Reid *et al.*, 1993). Rising titers to leptospiral antigens have been a valuable means of diagnosis in other animal species.

Gross necropsy lesions in the tamarin included jaundice of all mucous membranes, subcutaneous tissues, and viscera (Reid *et al.*, 1993). Jaundice was also observed in squirrel monkeys and macaques at necropsy (Shive *et al.*, 1969; Perolat *et al.*, 1992). Hemorrhagic pneumonia was the primary lesion in the New World monkeys, with renal necrosis and hemorrhage, diffuse visceral hemorrhages, and hepatomegaly also occurring in the squirrel monkeys (Perolat *et al.*, 1992; Reid *et al.*, 1993). Isolated to extensive petechiation of viscera and marked hepatomegaly with increased friability were reported for Barbary apes (Shive *et al.*, 1969).

Microscopically, pulmonary hemorrhage and edema with inflammation were observed in New World monkeys (Perolat *et al.*, 1992; Reid *et al.*, 1993). Moderate, multifocal hepatocellular dissociation and mild, multifocal bile stasis were found in the tamarin (Reid *et al.*, 1993). Hepatocellular disassociation and focal hepatic necrosis were also found in Barbary apes (Shive *et al.*, 1969). Inflammatory infiltrates within the portal areas were observed in squirrel monkey livers, but there was no evidence of bile stasis and tissue architecture appeared normal (Perolat *et al.*, 1992). All monkeys had microscopic renal lesions of varying severity. Mild, multifocal interstitial nephritis and necrosis of tubular epithelial cells were reported in the tamarin (Reid *et al.*, 1993). Exudative glomerulopathy and interstitial nephritis were observed in squirrel monkeys (Perolat *et al.*, 1992). Congestion, vacuolar degeneration, and necrosis of renal tubular epithelium with and without marked mononuclear cell exudation and cast formation with hemorrhage in tubular lumens were reported for Barbary apes (Shive *et al.*, 1969). Spirochetes were revealed by silver stain of kidney tissues (Shive *et al.*, 1969; Reid *et al.*, 1993).

Treatment with benzylpenicillin (50,00 IU/kg/day for 10 days) and symptomatic treatment with intravenous fluids and phenobarbital (5 mg/kg/day) was used in squirrel monkeys with clinical leptospirosis with limited success (Perolat *et al.*, 1992). Prophylactic oral doxycycline was administered to the remaining asymptomatic squirrel monkeys at 200 mg/week for 4 weeks. Elimination of leptospiral infection from the squirrel monkey population was accomplished by immunization with an inactivated vaccine containing 2×10^8 cells/ml of *L. interrogans* serovar *copenhageni*. Monkeys were vaccinated subcutaneously with two 1-ml doeses given 3 weeks apart (Perolat *et al.*, 1992).

W. *Chromobacterium*

Chromobacterium violaceum is a facultative anaerobic, gram-negative, motile bacillus that produces a violet pigment, violacein, that is soluble in alcohol. *Chromobacterium violaceum* is an opportunistic pathogen found in soil or water and is geographically restricted to tropical and semitropical climates. Disease in humans and animals is rare, but mortality is high. Chromobacteriosis has been reported in a guenon, an Assam macaque (*Macaca assamensis*), colobus monkeys, and gibbons (Audebaud *et al.*, 1954; Groves *et al.*, 1969; Johnsen *et al.*, 1970; McClure and Chang, 1976; Kornegay *et al.*, 1991). The guenon and gibbons were infected in Africa and Asia (Audebaud *et al.*, 1954; Groves *et al.*, 1969; Johnsen *et al.*, 1970), respectively; the other cases occurred in the United States (McClure and Chang, 1976; Kornegay *et al.*, 1991).

The clinical histories were brief and nonspecific; most animals were found dead without previous clinical signs (McClure and Chang, 1976) or exhibited vague signs such as weakness or inappetence hours prior to death (Kornegay *et al.*, 1991). Abrasions and lacerations to the skin in 4 of 10 affected gibbons were determined to be the source of infection (Groves *et al.*, 1969); in other cases the source of infection was not determined.

Diagnosis of chromobacteriosis was based on culture of the organism from lesioned organs or blood and characteristic lesions at necropsy. *Chromobacterium violaceum* grows on a variety of standard laboratory media, including blood, chocolate, MacConkey, and EMB agars and thioglycollate broth at a temperature range of 10–40°C. The bacterium will grow under either aerobic or anaerobic conditions. Production of the characteristic water-insoluble, alcohol-soluble violet pigment provided presumptive diagnosis. The bacterium was further identified by a panel of biochemical tests. Gross lesions had a similar appearance to those described for yersiniosis and included hepatomegaly with multifocal necrosis and abscess formation, splenomegaly, and pneumonia or pulmonary edema and congestion (Audebaud *et al.*, 1954; Groves *et al.*, 1969; McClure and Chang, 1976; Kornegay *et al.*, 1991). Impression smears from the liver revealed necrotic debris, few polymorphonuclear cells, and many gram-negative, nonacid-fast bacteria (McClure and Chang, 1976; Kornegay *et al.*, 1991).

Gross lesions of chromobacteriosis were characteristic of septicemia and usually involved multiple organ systems, including lung, liver, spleen, bone marrow, kidney, and adrenal glands (Audebaud *et al.*, 1954; Groves *et al.*, 1969; McClure and Chang, 1976; Kornegay *et al.*, 1991). Pneumonia and multifocal pulmonary abscesses were reported for gibbons (Groves *et al.*, 1969); pulmonary congestion and edema (Kornegay *et al.*, 1991) with pinpoint white foci throughout the lobes were noted in other species (McClure and Chang, 1976). Severity and character of hepatic lesions also varied. In the Assam macaque, large, multifocal parenchymal and subcapsular, nodular lesions from 5 to 30 mm in diameter were found throughout the liver (McClure and Chang, 1976). The liver was enlarged and friable. Nodular lesions contained yellow-white, semifluid exudate; many appeared cavitary and encapsulated (Audebaud *et al.*, 1954; Groves *et al.*, 1969; McClure and Chang, 1976). In addition, there were pinpoint white foci of hepatic necrosis randomly distributed throughout the parenchyma (McClure and Chang, 1976). Sharply demarcated, random, off-white multifocal to patchy areas of necrosis <1 cm in diameter were observed in the livers of the colobus monkeys (Kornegay et al., 1991). Fibrinous peritonitis, splenomegaly, hyperemic congestion of the spleen, kidneys, and adrenal glands, and multifocal necrosis of the bone marrow were reported (McClure and Chang, 1976; Kornegay et al., 1991).

The primary microscopic lesion of chromobacteriosis consisted of severe multifocal to extensive hepatic necrosis with minimum inflammatory cell infiltrate and no encapsulation (Audebaud et al., 1954; Groves et al., 1969; McClure and Chang, 1976; Kornegay et al., 1991). Numerous, gram-negative, rod-shaped bacteria were found within areas of hepatic necrosis. In the colobus monkeys, necrotic hepatic foci with a central homogeneous core of basophilic debris and liquefaction bordered by a dense band of gram-negative bacteria and necrotic hepatocytes with pyknotic nuclei were seen (Kornegay et al., 1991). Hepatic vessels often were occluded by fibrinocellular thrombi with and without bacteria (Kornegay et al., 1991). Pulmonary lesions included moderate to severe edema with multifocal thickening, congestion, edema, and necrosis of interstitial septae and multifocal necrosis with inflammatory cell infiltrates and many gram-negative bacilli (Groves et al., 1969; McClure and Chang, 1976; Kornegay et al., 1991). Multifocal hemorrhages and congestion in the spleen and adrenal glands were noted. Multifocal necrosis with many bacteria and frequently without inflammation was observed in the hilar lymph nodes (McClure and Chang, 1976) and in the bone marrow (Kornegay et al., 1991).

X. *Mycobacterium*

Tuberculosis and mycobacteriosis are insidious diseases of New and Old World monkeys and apes capable of causing high morbidity and mortality within a group of primates and subsequent substantial financial loss. Tuberculosis is caused by *Mycobacterium tuberculosis* and *M. bovis* and is a disease acquired through human contact. There is no apparent difference in tuberculous disease in nonhuman primates caused by *M. tuberculosis* or *M. bovis* (McLaughlin, 1978); distribution and character of the lesions are identical. Kaufmann et al. (1975) estimated that up to 10% of tuberculosis outbreaks in nonhuman primates were caused by *M. bovis*.

Mycobacteriosis is a class of diseases caused by atypical mycobacteria. Included in this class are *M. avium-intracellulare*, *M. scrofulaceum*, *M. kansasii*, *M. africans*, and *M. gordanae*. Atypical bacteria were classified by Runyon groups based on pigment production and rate of growth *in vitro*. Most of these bacteria are saprophytic and opportunistic pathogens. Mycobacteriosis is usually acquired through contact with contaminated soil or water; affected monkeys may be immunosuppressed. In recent years, both Johne's disease due to *M. paratuberculosis* and leprosy due to *M. leprae* have been described in nonhuman primates.

1. Tuberculosis

Mycobacterium tuberculosis and *M. bovis* are acid-fast, faculative intracellular bacilli. They both grow on artificial media at 37°C but *M. tuberculosis* prefers media with glycerol, whereas glycerol inhibits the growth of *M. bovis*. *Mycobacterium tuberculosis* is niacin positive, and *M. bovis* is niacin negative.

The pathogenesis of tuberculosis via the respiratory tract begins with inhalation of fine particles containing one to three bacilli (Dannenberg, 1978). The bacilli are ingested by an alveolar macrophage upon reaching the alveolus. A macrophage lacking in microbicidal activity and enzyme content allows subsequent intracellular multiplication, resulting in macrophage death. The bacillary load is released and ingested by other macrophages recruited from alveoli and later from the blood. If these macrophages are unsuccessful in destroying the bacilli, a central core of necrotic cells, caseous necrosis, will develop at the center of the tubercle. New blood-borne macrophages are recruited to the site and must become activated locally in order to be effective in eliminating the bacilli. Following development of delayed hypersensitivity in the host, the turnover of macrophages and lymphocytes in the lesions becomes more rapid. Failure of macrophages to become activated prior to ingestion of bacilli continues the cycle of cellular death and bacilli release in the extracellular space. In the host with delayed hypersensitivity, bacillary products in high concentrations kill macrophages directly and indirectly, resulting in capillary thrombosis and subsequent caseation. Liquefaction of caseous foci is also mediated by delayed hypersensitivity, resulting in marked extracellular multiplication of bacilli, cavity formation, and spread of the bacilli through the respiratory tree (Dannenberg, 1978).

Tuberculosis is a disease acquired from humans. In the 1950s, when large numbers of macaques were imported from India, tuberculosis was common. Prior to shipping, monkeys were held in primitive cages, with inadequate sanitation and nutrition. With the adoption of rapid movement of the monkeys after capture into more sanitary housing conditions, improved nutrition, and expedited shipping, the incidence of tuberculosis declined. A survey of imported monkeys from June 1990 through May 1993 revealed tuberculosis infection in 0.4% of 22,913 nonhuman primates. All of the cases occurred in rhesus and cynomolgus monkeys with an incidence per shipment ranging from 0.8 to 80% (Centers for Disease Control, 1993). Recent increases in cases of tuberculosis in the human population in the 1990s may presage a rise in nonhuman primate tuberculosis. Routine yearly tuberculin testing of personnel in contact with nonhuman primates is an important measure in preventing the spread of disease from humans to animals.

Epizootic tuberculosis in nonhuman primates usually occurs by aerosol transmission, but transmission has occurred by ingestion, direct contact, and contact with fomites, including contaminated thermometers (Riordan, 1943) and a tatooing needle (Allen and Kinard, 1958).

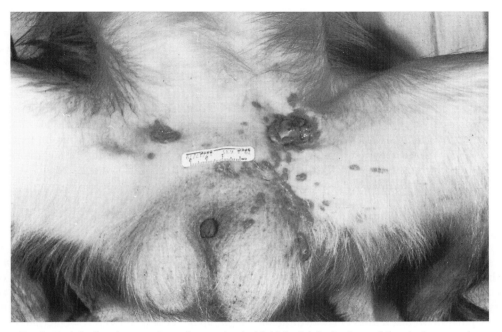

Fig. 4. Draining lymph note and pustules associated with *M. bovis* infection in an adult male rhesus monkey.

Tuberculosis has occurred in prosimians and in New and Old World monkeys and apes. Although particular species may be more or less susceptible to disease, all nonhuman primates can develop tuberculosis. Clinical signs of tuberculosis in nonhuman primates varied, depending on the location and severity of infection. Frequently monkeys were found dead with no previous clinical history (Renquist and Whitney, 1978). Clinical signs, when present, were nonspecific. A persistent cough indicated respiratory infection, but could also be attributed to lung mite infestation (Fourie and Odendaal, 1983). As tuberculosis progressed, monkeys may become fatigued, anorectic, and experience chronic weight loss or exertional dyspnea. Peripheral lymphadenopathy with or without draining tracts and cutaneous abscesses have been reported (Fig. 4) (Lindsey and Melby, 1966; Renquist and Whitney, 1978). Hepatomegaly and splenomegaly were discernable by palpation in some cases. Mild normocytic, normochromic anemia and leukocytosis with neutrophilia and lymphopenia were detected in rhesus monkeys with tuberculosis (Wolf *et al.*, 1988). The monkeys also had elevated serum globulin levels and an increased erythrocyte sedimentation rate, which has also been reported for baboons with tuberculosis (Tribe and Wellburn, 1976). A monkey with tuberculous spondylitis developed paraplegia and had severe kyphosis (Fox *et al.*, 1974).

Gross lesions included caseous nodules in the hilar lymph nodes and lung, large cavitary and coalescing lesions within the lung, and tubercles extending into the thoracic pleura. In animals with advanced disease there was secondary spread to the spleen, kidney, liver, and various lymph nodes with multifocal pinpoint, miliary disease, or larger nodular foci of caseation. Tuberculous nodules were found less frequently in the cerebrum (Machotka *et al.*, 1975), spinal column, omentum, uterus, ovary (McLaughlin, 1978), peripheral lymph nodes, skin (Lindsey and Melby, 1966), and mammary gland. A large, 2 × 6-cm paravertebral abscess and destruction of the second lumbar vertebra were seen in an individual monkey with kyphosis and spondylitis (Fox *et al.*, 1974).

Typical microscopic lesions consisted of granulomas of varying size. The granulomas were unencapsulated with a necrotic core. Surrounding the core were a layer of epithelioid macrophages and lesser numbers of neutrophils, with multinucleate Langhans giant cells at the periphery. Mineralization was uncommon. Acid-fast bacilli could be demonstrated within the lesions both intra- and extracellularly.

Diagnosis of tuberculosis antemortem is based on the intradermal tuberculin test. The tuberculin test consists of administration of 0.10-ml old tuberculin intradermally in either the eyelid or abdominal skin. The test site is observed at 24, 48, and 72 hr postinoculation and the reaction, if any, is graded. Swelling, erythema, edema, and ptosis are indicative of a suspect or positive reaction. McLaughlin and Marrs (1978) reported no advantage in using *M. bovis* PPD over mammalian tuberculin in the detection of monkeys infected with *M. bovis*; in fact, mammalian tuberculin was the superior diagnostic reagent.

The tuberculin test is limited in its efficacy in that animals with early or advanced disease may give false-negative reactions. Concomitant disease such as measles may also result in a false-negative reaction due to immunosuppression. Therapy with isoniazid will also negate the value of the tuberculin test. False positives may result from exposure to Freund's complete adjuvant (Pierce and Dukelow, 1988), trauma due to improper administration of the test, or nonspecific reactivity to the vehicle. Recent difficulties in obtaining old tuberculin further limit the efficacy of this test. For further discussion of tuberculin testing, please see Chapter 13: Medical Management, in *Nonhuman Primates in Biomedical Research: Biology and Management.*

Alternative tests have been used to detect specific antibodies to mycobacteria. The problem has been the lack of clear-cut differences in titer between uninfected and infected monkeys and in choosing a universal antigen for the test reagent (Corcoran and Thoen, 1991). However, repeated ELISA tests have been useful in categorizing monkeys into infected, suspect, and uninfected groups when tuberculin testing was ineffective (Corcoran and Thoen, 1991). Thoracic radiography may provide confirmation of pulmonary disease, but cannot distinguish between tuberculosis and other cavitary diseases of the lung such as nocardiosis or cryptococcosis.

Culture of either *M. bovis* or *M. tuberculosis* may be difficult especially early in disease when there are low numbers of mycobacteria present. In order to detect mycobacteria in sputum, lesions must have progressed into a bronchiole so that bacilli are coughed up into the mouth. Optimal conditions for culture of these two organisms are contradictory; *M. tuberculosis* needs glycerol for growth and glycerol is inhibitory for *M. bovis.* Laboratories must be advised to set up cultures under both conditions to increase the likelihood of recovery. Cultures must be held for 8 weeks before they can be considered negative. Detection of infection by screening feces or sputum by polymerase chain reaction (PCR) for mycobacterial DNA may provide a more rapid diagnosis of tuberculosis. Use of specific mycobacterial DNA primers in PCR amplification of DNA from tissues collected at necropsy can lead to an earlier diagnosis (Brammer *et al.*, 1995) than culture.

Treatment of monkeys and apes with tuberculosis has been undertaken and in some cases has been successful. Single drug therapy with isoniazid as a preventative or as sole therapeutic agent has proved to be ineffective (Burkholder *et al.*, 1967; Clarke and Schmidt, 1969). Use of isoniazid has the potential drawbacks of rendering tuberculin testing inaccurate, causing behavioral changes (Kraemer *et al.*, 1976), and causing pyridoxine deficiency (Wolf *et al.*, 1988). Multidrug chemotherapy of tuberculosis using two or more drugs has been effective in macaques and apes (Fremming *et al.*, 1957; Indzhila *et al.*, 1977; Brown *et al.*, 1980; McClure, 1980; Ward *et al.*, 1985; Wolf *et al.*, 1988). Use of multiple agents decreases the possibility of developing antibiotic resistance and allows for grouping agents that attack the mycobacterium at different stages in its life cycle (Wolf *et al.*, 1988). Effective drug combinations included isoniazid and streptomycin (Fremming *et al.*, 1957; Indzhila *et al.*, 1977; Ward *et al.*, 1985), isoniazid and *p*-aminosalicyclic acid (McClure, 1980), and isoniazid, etham-

butol, and rifampin (Brown *et al.*, 1980; Wolf *et al.*, 1988). In all cases of successful treatment, the organism had been isolated and antibiotic sensitivity determined. Failure to identify the organism and determine antibiotic sensitivity lead to treatment failure (Haberle, 1970; Dillehay and Huerkamp, 1990).

Treatment should only be undertaken if the infected animals can be isolated during therapy and if therapy can be provided over a prolonged period of time, usually 1 year. Failure to take drugs regularly is the primary cause of treatment failure in humans; this can be controlled in the laboratory situation. Animals will need to be reevaluated once treatment has been withdrawn to determine if there is recrudesence of disease.

2. Mycobacteriosis

a. *Mycobacterium avium-intracellulare.* *M. avium–M. intracellulare* complex, also known as *M. avium* complex, is composed of more than 30 serotypes. The first two serotypes are usually isolated from birds; serotypes 4–30 are usually recovered from humans or animals. These organisms are pathogenic saprophytic nontuberculous mycobacteria and can be contracted through exposure to soil, water, and tissues from infected animals. Entry into the body can be through respiratory, oral, and cutaneous routes. These organisms belonged to Runyon group III, characterized by slow growth, filamentous forms in culture, and formation of buff to yellow colonies regardless of light exposure.

Nonhuman primates are resistant to experimental infection with *M. avium-intracellulare,* although there are several reports of naturally acquired disease in macaques. Disease usually primarily involved the gastrointestinal tract and reticuloendothelial system (Sesline *et al.*, 1975; Sesline, 1978; Holmberg *et al.*, 1982, 1985), with rare thoracic disease (Sedgwick *et al.*, 1970), and two reports of cutaneous manifestations (Latt, 1975; Bellinger and Bullock, 1988). Clinical signs of infection ranged from none (Sedgwick *et al.*, 1970) to intermittent or continuous diarrhea refractory to treatment, accompanied by dramatic weight loss and generalized lymphadenopathy (Sesline, 1978). Infected macaques usually survived for 1 year after the onset of clinical signs (Sesline, 1978). One of the cutaneous cases presented as bilateral draining fistulas from the cheek pouches (Latt, 1975); the other case presented as an ulcerated cutaneous lesion on the posterior aspect of the left tarsus (Bellinger and Bullock, 1988). The lesion was soft, slightly raised, pale yellow, and friable (Bellinger and Bullock, 1988).

Clinical pathology associated with *M. avium-intracellulare* infection included normocytic, normochromic anemia, lymphopenia in conjunction with neutrophilic leukocytosis, hypoalbuminemia, and hypergammaglobulinemia (Sesline *et al.*, 1975; Sesline, 1978). Mild elevations in SGOT and SGPT were also reported. Thrombocytopenia was reported for one animal by Sesline *et al.* (1975). Abnormalities in lymphocyte rosette formation and phytomitogen responses were reported by Holmberg *et al.* (1985) and Sesline (1978). In retrospect, these abnormalities in immune function and the development of disease from *M. avium-interacellulare* infection were probably due to simian immunodeficiency virus (SIV) infection within the affected colonies of macaques.

In some macaques, no gross lesions were associated with infection (Sedgwick *et al.,* 1970). Those with intestinal illness had mild to severe thickening of the intestinal wall from the distal small intestine through the cecum and colon (Sesline, 1978; Holmberg *et al.,* 1982). Thickening of the intestinal mucosa was segmental to diffuse, and the mucosal surface had a granular or corrugated appearance (Holmberg *et al.,* 1985). The thickened mucosa was described as yellow-white with thick folds by Sesline *et al.* (1975). Lymphocytic channels in the mesentery were prominent, and small firm nodules were found along the channels (Sesline *et al.,* 1975; Holmberg *et al.,* 1985). Mesenteric lymph nodes were enlarged and edematous; the ileocecal nodes were most prominent. The spleen was enlarged to twice the normal size (Sesline, 1978) and firm. Small gray foci were observed rarely in the liver, kidney, and spleen (Sesline, 1978; Holmberg *et al.,* 1985). Malignant lymphoma or lymphosarcoma occurred concomitantly in some animals (Sesline *et al.,* 1975; Holmberg *et al.,* 1982).

The characteristic microscopic lesion was diffuse granulomatous inflammation due to infiltration of large, foamy macrophages with eosinophilic cytoplasm into the mucosa and submucosa of the intestine. The terminal ileum and proximal colon were most severely affected. In less severely affected areas, the infiltration of macrophages was confined to the lamina propria of the villous tips (Holmberg *et al.,* 1982). Numerous acid-fast bacilli were seen in the cytoplasm of macrophages in Ziehl–Niehlson-stained intestinal sections. In some cases there was a marked accumulation of amyloid within the mucosal lamina propria (Sesline, 1978). Involvement of the lymph nodes ranged from mild infiltrates of foamy macrophages into the subcapsular and cortical sinusoids to total effacement of the normal architecture (Holmberg *et al.,* 1982). Germinal centers were rare (Sesline, 1978). There were small, multifocal accumulations of macrophages within other organs, including the spleen, liver, lung, and brain. Acid-fast bacteria were less common in nonintestinal lesions. In the lung, acid-fast bacilli were found in foci of macrophages around lung mite lesions (Holmberg *et al.,* 1982). Granuloma formation was rare as were multinucleate giant cells (Sesline, 1978; Holmberg *et al.,* 1985). Only within brain lesions were moderate numbers of giant cells observed (Holmberg *et al.,* 1982). The macaque with focal cutaneous mycobacteriosis had numerous macrophages, epithelioid cells, and Langhans giant cells and granulation tissue within the lesion (Bellinger and Bullock, 1988). Acid-fast bacilli were found within the macrophages.

Diagnosis of *M. avium-intracellulare* infection can be difficult. Responses to tuberculin testing, even when using avium tuberculin, vary (Sedgwick *et al.,* 1970; Holmberg *et al.,* 1982). A positive test using old tuberculin may be only transitory erythema at 24 hr postinoculation (Sedgwick *et al.,* 1970). A clin-

ical history of chronic diarrhea and marked weight loss would indicate further diagnostic testing for *M. avium-intracellulare* as well as Johne's disease. Biopsy of colonic tissue or a suspect cutaneous site is a helpful diagnostic tool in that it can provide tissue for both histopathology and PCR analysis for mycobacterial DNA. Diffuse infiltration of foamy macrophages into the intestinal mucosa and the presence of numerous acid-fast bacilli within the macrophages can provide a presumptive diagnosis of mycobacteriosis. Culture of the organism from feces or lesions can be time-consuming as this is a slow-growing organism. Raised buff or yellow colonies may appear in 2–3 weeks when incubated at 37°C. The organism grows on standard mycobacterial media such as Lowenstein–Jensen. Specific serotypes may be identified from isolates. Serotypes 1, 2, 4, 8, and 18 have been recovered from macaques (Holmberg *et al.,* 1982).

Group-housed macaques in outdoor settings may be at risk, especially if they are immunocompromised due to SIV infection (Lowenstine *et al.,* 1992). Treatment should not be undertaken due to the multiple drug resistance characteristic of this organism. Several of the macaques reported to have mycobacteriosis due to *M. avium-intracellulare* had been on isoniazid preventive therapy prior to development of disease (Latt, 1975; Sesline *et al.,* 1975). It should be noted that the individual with a focal cutaneous lesion had spontaneous remission following biopsy of the site (Bellinger and Bullock, 1988).

b. *Mycobacterium paratuberculosis* (JOHNE'S DISEASE).
M. paratuberculosis requires mycobactin for *in vitro* growth. This organism causes chronic granulomatous intestinal disease in ruminants known as paratuberculosis or Johne's disease. The organism can survive for long periods of time in the environment. Infection of ruminant animal hosts usually occurs at a young age (<30 days); however, disease does not develop until 3–5 years of age. Johne's disease is characterized by chronic nonresponsive diarrhea that persists for months. Animals become unthrifty, experience chronic weight loss, and eventually die.

Mycobacterium paratuberculosis infection was reported in a colony of stump-tailed macaques (McClure *et al.,* 1987). Seventy-six percent of the 38 monkeys were infected and shed organisms in feces, even in the absence of overt disease. Clinical signs included recurrent chronic diarrhea and progressive weight loss. Average clinical course from the development of diarrhea to death was 5 months. Affected monkeys were juveniles and adults. Monkeys treated with Rifabutine, an experimental antimycobacterial drug, had a prolonged clinical course of 12–21 months (McClure *et al.,* 1987).

Thirteen macaques died over a 5-year period. At necropsy all monkeys were emaciated. Gross lesions were limited to thickening of the intestinal and colonic mucosa and mesenteric lymphadenopathy. Granulomatous inflammation of the entire intestinal tract was observed microscopically, with the most severe inflammation occurring in the jejunum and ileum. A histiocytic inflammatory cell infiltrate with numerous plasma cells was seen segmentally to diffusely throughout the intestine. In severe cases, the lamina propria of the intestinal villi was totally effaced. Acid-fast organisms were found throughout the small intestine and colon, with fewer organisms seen in the lower colon. Six monkeys had syncytial giant cells in the small intestine, and Langhans giant cells were seen occasionally. Histiocytic infiltrates in the lymph nodes ranged from mild to severe, with Langhans giant cells found frequently. Acid-fast bacilli were less apparent than in the intestine. Focal hepatic granulomas occurred in 9 monkeys. Acid-fast bacilli were identified in microgranulomas, spleen, and bone marrow (McClure *et al.*, 1987).

Mycobacterium paratuberculosis was isolated from feces and tissues cultured on medium containing mycobactin J. Nonchromogenic, rough colonies developed in 6–8 weeks. Growth was optimal at 37°C. Serologic testing of monkeys in the colony revealed specific antibodies in 84% of the monkeys. Six of the monkeys with clinical disease did not have serum antibodies to the organism (McClure *et al.*, 1987).

c. *Mycobacterium leprae* (LEPROSY). *M. leprae* is the etiologic agent of leprosy or Hansen' disease. The organism cannot be grown on artificial media. Leprosy is a chronic granulomatous disease affecting the skin and peripheral nerves and with lesions preferentially occurring in the cooler areas, i.e., the extremities, of the host.

Naturally acquired infections with *M. leprae* have been reported in a sooty mangabey, *Cercocebus atys* (Meyers *et al.*, 1985), and chimpanzees (Leininger *et al.*, 1978; Hubbard *et al.*, 1991b; Alford *et al.*, 1996). The mangabey presented multiple firm infiltrations in the skin of the forehead, periorbital region, muzzle, and lower lip. The ears were nodular and thickened, and there was slight thickening of the skin of the extensor surface of the forearms. Biopsy of affected areas revealed numerous acid-fast bacilli within the tissues. Over the next year, the lesions progressed to other areas, including the limbs and tail. Extensive ulceration of the skin, weight loss, and anemia developed. Deformities of the hands and feet developed with progressive paralysis of the intrinsic muscles of the hands and feet and some of the musculature of the legs. Initiation of antileprosy chemotherapy consisting of rifampin (10 mg/kg body weight/day orally for 1 month) and diacetyldiaminodiphenyl sulfone (20 mg intramuscularly every 77 days) resulted in gradual resolution of lesions over 16 months (Meyers *et al.*, 1985).

Multiple, eroded, nodular skin lesions of the face and ears occurred in chimpanzees with leprosy (Leininger *et al.*, 1978; Hubbard *et al.*, 1991b; Alford *et al.*, 1996). One chimpanzee had a 10-year history of self-mutilation of the hands and feet (Alford *et al.*, 1996). In this animal and another chimpanzee at the same facility, nodular and papular lesions were also found on the lateral surfaces of the arms and legs, scrotum, perineum, and penis. The face and extremities appeared edematous and swollen. Many of the nodular lesions became ulcerated. Multidrug therapy consisting of rifampin (600 mg daily), dapsone (100 mg daily), and clofazimine (100 mg daily) was utilized for 6 months in combination with topical therapy of sugar and saline

irrigating solution applied to deep ulcerated areas in one chimpanzee (Alford *et al.*, 1996). The chimpanzee showed improvement with resolution of some lesions, but developed a drug reaction characterized by pain and impairment of locomotion. Prednisone (60 mg daily) and aspirin (650 mg three times a day) were given to control these symptoms. The prednisone was stopped after 5 months and the aspirin therapy was continued with antibiotic therapy for 5 years. After 4 years of treatment, biopsy of previously lesioned skin sites revealed no acid-fast bacilli and no remarkable lesions. Rifampin and clofazimine were discontinued. Dapsone will be administered for the rest of the chimpanzee's life. The second chimpanzee received similar therapy but died suddenly after 1.5 years of therapy. Death occurred following routine ketamine immobilization and appeared to be due to heart failure resulting from acute myocardial necrosis and hemorrhage.

Microscopic lesions observed in biopsy and necropsy specimens revealed epidermal thinning and subepidermal clear zones (Meyers *et al.*, 1985; Leininger *et al.*, 1978; Hubbard *et al.*, 1991b). Dermal inflammation was primarily histiocytic, with lesser numbers of lymphocytes, plasma cells, and neutrophils. Inflammatory cells localized around neurovascular channels. Large numbers of acid-fast bacilli were observed in histiocytes and lesser numbers within nerves. Both the mangabey and a chimpanzee had negative tuberculin skin tests, positive lepromin skin tests, and specific antibodies to *M. leprae* (Meyers *et al.*, 1985; Hubbard *et al.*, 1991b). Repeated attempts to culture the organism on Lowenstein–Jensen media were unsuccessful.

d. *Mycobacterium kansasii*. *M. kansasii* is primarily a saprophytic, nonpathogenic mycobacterium; however, this organism has caused mycobacteriosis in humans and nonhuman primates (Valerio *et al.*, 1979; Jackson *et al.*, 1989; Wayne and Sramek, 1992; Brammer *et al.*, 1995). Photochromic, high catalase-producing strains are most frequently associated with clinical disease (Sommers and Good, 1985). Infections are believed to be acquired from the environment (Wayne and Sramek, 1992); the organism has been isolated from water samples (Wolinsky, 1979). In no case of mycobacteriosis due to *M. kansasii* infection in nonhuman primates has the source of the infection been identified (Valerio *et al.*, 1979; Jackson *et al.*, 1989; Brammer *et al.*, 1995).

Mycobacteriosis due to *M. kansasii* infection has been reported in rhesus monkeys and squirrel monkeys. One case occurred in a breeding colony of rhesus monkeys in which 71 monkeys developed positive tuberculin reactions and 60 monkeys were culture positive for *M. kansasii* (Valerio *et al.*, 1979). These monkeys developed mycobacteriosis after being placed in a new breeding facility following a long and uneventful quarantine. Infection was initially detected by conversion to a positive tuberculin test using mammalian tuberculin intradermally in both the eyelid and the abdomen. Positive tuberculin tests differed from those seen typically in monkeys infected with

M. tuberculosis; minimal ptosis, with mild thickening of the eyelid, and often no hyperemia were observed. A 1- to 2-cm area of blanched, thickened skin was found at the abdominal test site. Reactions in infants were more severe than in adults. The severity of tuberculin reactions became more pronounced in adults with questionable tests that were retested. Tuberculin testing with specific *M. kansasii* antigen or PPD was not diagnostically superior to testing with mammalian tuberculin (Valerio *et al.,* 1979).

Mycobacterium kansasii infection was diagnosed in a rhesus monkey that had developed a positive tuberculin reaction on semiannual testing and was subsequently euthanized (Jackson *et al.,* 1989). The monkey was 5 years old, originally from an outdoor, corncrib harem group, and had been singly housed for 7 months. The monkey was in a study to determine the effects of recombinant human granulocyte–macrophage stimulating factor and had been irradiated. The tuberculin reaction was characterized by mild erythema and moderate, diffuse swelling of the eyelid. Thoracic radiographs revealed multiple, 2- to 6-mm, radiodense foci throughout the right lung lobes (Jackson *et al.,* 1989).

Mycobacterium kansasii infection in squirrel monkeys was also detected by routine tuberculin testing of asymptomatic animals (Brammer *et al.,* 1995). A 1:10 dilution of mammalian tuberculin was used for testing. Diagnosis of *M. kansasii* infection was preliminarily confirmed by use of genus-specific probes for mycobacterial DNA in PCR testing of bronchial lymph nodes. The organism was isolated from three of five tuberculin reactors. The monkeys had been in the facility from 2 to 8 years.

Gross lesions of *M. kansasii* infection in rhesus monkeys included one to two pulmonary nodules, some of which contained yellow-green caseous matter and tuberculous-type lesions in the mediastinal lymph nodes (Valerio *et al.,* 1979). Some monkeys had miliary lesions in the liver and/or spleen. Those monkeys that had been held for prolonged periods after development of a positive tuberculin reaction had advanced lesions in multiple organ systems. An 8-mm cavitary lung lesion, a focal 2-mm nonexudative lung lesion, and enlargement of the right bronchial lymph node were noted in the irradiated monkey. (Jackson *et al.,* 1989). In the squirrel monkeys, gross lesions were confined to the lymph nodes (Brammer *et al.,* 1995). Four of five monkeys had enlarged bronchial lymph nodes; three monkeys had grossly enlarged cervical and mediastinal nodes. Microscopic lesions in all cases were indistinguishable from those of tuberculosis. Therapy was not attempted.

Unlike tuberculosis, in these three cases there was no evidence of animal-to-animal transmission. In the initial outbreak, there was no transmission from infected animals to other monkeys housed in adjacent enclosures separated by only a chain-link fence (Valerio *et al.,* 1979). The source of infection was believed to be the water supply. Similarly, disease was not transmitted from the singly infected rhesus monkey to the other 15 monkeys in the room, even though the monkeys were immu-

nosuppressed and the infected animal had a cavitary pulmonary lesion (Jackson *et al.,* 1989). Cagemates of infected squirrel monkeys did not develop disease (Brammer *et al.,* 1995).

e. *Mycobacterium gordonae.* Tuberculin testing of a colony of squirrel monkeys resulted in identification of three tuberculin reactors (Soave *et al.,* 1981). Subsequent tuberculin testing was also positive. Two monkeys were euthanized and necropsied. There were no gross or microscopic lesions. *Mycobacterium gordonae* was isolated from the mediastinal lymph nodes, spleen, and/or liver.

f. *Mycobacterium scrofulaceum.* Atypical tuberculin reactions were noted in some animals within a quarantine group of asymptomatic patas monkeys (Renquist and Rotkay, 1979). Mild edema, erythema, and, in some cases, induration of the test site in the eyelid were noted. Reactions were noticed at 24 hr posttest and frequently subsided after that. One patas monkey developed anorexia and weight loss. Radiographs revealed extensive opacity in the lungs. Necropsy lesions included numerous 0.5- to 2.0-cm white nodules in the liver, lungs, omentum, spleen, and mediastinal and mesenteric lymph nodes. In other patas, lesions were limited to enlargement of the mediastinal lymph nodes. Histopathologic findings included granulomas with giant cell formation in the lungs, liver, and spleen. *Mycobacterium scrofulaceum* was isolated from the lungs and liver.

Y. *Nocardia*

Nocardia spp. are aerobic actinomycetes found in richly fertilized soil existing as saprophytes on decaying vegetation. The organism is gram-positive, varies from being strongly to partially acid-fast, and is filamentous and branching. *Nocardia asteroides* is the most common isolate in nonhuman primates. Infection occurs following contact with skin wounds, inhalation, or ingestion. Secondary lesions occur in the brain or liver following dissemination through the blood or lymphatic system. Clinical signs include dyspnea and epistaxis (McClure *et al.,* 1976b), chronic weight loss, abdominal distension and discomfort (Liebenberg and Giddens, 1985), chronic intermittent diarrhea, lethargy or depression (Jonas and Wyand, 1966), and coma (Al-Doory *et al.,* 1969).

Gross pulmonary lesions characteristically include multinodular to diffuse, red to gray areas of consolidation in affected lobes (Jonas and Wayand, 1966; Al-Doory *et al.,* 1969; McClure *et al.,* 1976b; Sakakibara *et al.,* 1984). Pulmonary hemorrhage and edema; pleural adhesions; small to large focal abscesses; and cavitary lesions also occur (Jonas and Wayand, 1966; McClure *et al.,* 1976b; Liebenberg and Giddens, 1985). Pulmonary lesions without dissemination have been reported in macaques (Jonas and Wyand, 1966), a vervet (Al-Doory, 1972), and an orangutan (McClure *et al.,* 1976b). Disseminated nocardiosis with multifocal abscesses in the omentum, mesentery, liver, kidney, and stomach has been reported in macaques (Liebenberg and Giddens, 1985) as well as hemorrhage and multi-focal abscesses in the brain (Sakakibara *et al.,* 1984). A draining multinodular lesion on the hand of a baboon was infected with *N. caviae* (Boncyk *et al.,* 1975), and subcutaneous lesions in a squirrel monkey were diagnosed as nocardiosis based on histologic appearance (Kessler and Brown, 1981).

Multifocal to coalescing pyogranulomas are the characteristic microscopic lesion. Both acute and chronic lesions can be found within the same tissue section. Sulfur granules consisting of large colonies of filamentous bacteria may be found in a center of liquefactive necrosis, bordered by histiocytes, connective tissue, and mild lymphocytic infiltrates. Multinucleate giant cells are commonly found at the periphery. The branching filamentous organisms may be missed with standard hematoxylin and eosin stain and are demonstrated within lesions with gram, silver, or modified acid-fast stains. Differential diagnoses include any bacterial or fungal disease that produces a necrotizing or pyogranulomatous host response.

A tentative diagnosis of nocardiosis may be made based on the characteristic lesion morphology and identification of the organism within tissues. For definitive diagnosis by culture, samples should be collected anaerobically and transported immediately to the laboratory. Large tissue samples and large quantities of exudate give the best culture result (Attleberger, 1984). Samples cultured for *Nocardia* should be placed on blood agar and Sabouraud's dextrose agar and incubated aerobically at 25 and 37°C. Cultures should be held for 2 weeks. Nocardia is catalase positive and grows as yellow-white to orange colonies on Sabouraud's agar. Biochemical testing is necessary to differentiate among *Nocardia* spp.

There are no reports of successful treatment of nocardiosis in nonhuman primates.

Z. *Dermatophilus*

Dermatophilus congolensis, a gram-positive, nonacid-fast bacterium, is the causative agent of dermatophilosis or streptothricosis. The organism is an obligate pathogen of animals and humans. The zoospore or dormant phase is resistant to heat and dessication and can survive in infected scabs for months (Hyslop, 1980). Under favorable environmental conditions the zoospore germinates and produces filaments.

Dermatophilosis occurred in newly imported monkeys probably as a naturally acquired infection in the wild. It can be spread by direct contact between infected animals. Insect bites, skin trauma, and prolonged wetness of the skin may predispose an animal to infection (Migaki, 1986).

Dermatophilosis has been reported in owl monkeys (King *et al.,* 1971; McClure *et al.,* 1971a; Fox *et al.,* 1973) and titi monkeys (Migaki and Seibold, 1976). Affected monkeys were thin and in poor condition. The lesions were well-circumscribed areas of alopecia and exudative dermatitis that progressed into hairless papillomatous masses on the skin in some monkeys

(King *et al.,* 1971; McClure *et al.,* 1971a; Fox *et al.,* 1973). Lesions were usually discrete and circular, ranging from 0.2 to 3.0 cm in diameter. The face, head, distal extremities, and tail were involved most frequently, although lesions also occurred on the torso (Migaki and Seibold, 1976). Tail lesions tended to be more confluent (King *et al.,* 1971).

The affected epidermis was 10–15 times normal thickness with severe hyperkeratosis, parakeratosis, and acanthosis (Migaki and Seibold, 1976). A superficial crust composed of a dense layer of sebum, degenerating neutrophils, and keratin overlay the affected epidermis. In hematoxylin and eosin stained sections, numerous branching, filamentous basophilic organisms with septate and coccoid forms were visualized within the superficial keratin layers of the crusts (Migaki and Seibold, 1976). Proliferation of squamous cells with elongation of rete pegs, foci of ballooning degeneration and spongiosis, vesicle and pustule formation were found within the stratum spongiosum (King *et al.,* 1971). Dilated apocrine glands atrophied hair follicles and sebaceous glands, and occasional folliculitis also occurred (Migaki and Seibold, 1976).

Diagnosis can be made from demonstration of the organism in the lesion. Hair, crusts, and scabs submitted to the laboratory for isolation of *Dermatophilus* should be kept dry and submitted in paper envelopes to prevent growth of saprophytic organisms (Attleberger, 1984). In smears from moistened skin crusts, short lengths of narrow branching and divided hyphae, as well as numerous cocci, are seen with Gram or Giemsa stain. The organism can be isolated on blood agar, brain heart infusion media, or Sabouraud's media. The blood agar colonies are pinpoint with small zones of β hemolysis after 24 hr of growth; enlarging in 3–4 days of incubation and gray-white to orange in color. In culture the organism may appear only as cocci or as cocci and gram-positive branched filamentous organisms. Motile zoospores can be seen after growth in tryptose broth.

Penicillin alone or in combination with streptomycin has been effective in treating dermatophilosis in owl monkeys (Fox *et al.,* 1973; Weller, 1994). In some cases, lesions have regressed spontaneously as the overall condition of the monkey improved.

AA. *Actinomyces*

Organisms of the genus *Actinomyces* are gram-positive, nonacid-fast, pleomorphic coccobacilli that become filamentous within lesions. *Actinomyces* spp. grow in anaerobic to microaerophilic conditions of 10–15% CO_2. The colonies are nonhemolytic, serophilic, and visible in 3–5 days.

Actinomyces are obligate commensals of the gastrointestinal tract of a variety of animals and are opportunistic pathogens invading previously damaged tissue as contaminants or following penetration of the gastrointestinal mucosa. Granulomatous lesions on the face have been reported in a capuchin and a spider monkey in a zoological park (Weidman, 1935). *Actino-*

myces spp. was isolated from the abdominal wall of a moor macaque, *Macaca maura,* that died with acute hemorrhagic enteritis (Fiennes, 1967). *Actinomyces israeli* was recovered from a drill with multiple pyogranulomatous abscesses and adhesions in the peritoneum (Altman and Small, 1973) and from caseous lesions in the pancreas and liver of a gibbon, *Hylobates moloch* (Fiennes, 1967). Pyogranulomas with necrotic centers containing sulfur granules are the typical microscopic lesion. Sulfur granules are not diagnostic for actinomycosis as they may also occur in *Nocardia* infections.

III. MYCOTIC DISEASES

A. *Pneumocystis*

Pneumocystis carinii was originally described as an extracellular protozoa infecting the lungs of mammals and humans. Currently, *Pneumocystis* is recognized as a fungus; family Pneumocystidaceae, order Pneumocystidales (Ascomycota) based on DNA homology with other fungi (Wakefield *et al.,* 1992; Eriksson, 1994). *Pneumocystis* in different hosts are considered genetically distinct taxa (Eriksson, 1994).

The life cycle of the organism consists of a trophic and generative phase and is poorly understood as cultivation requires host cells. The trophic cells, previously termed trophozoites, are 1–5 μm, irregular in shape, and have a single nucleus. These cells undergo binary fission. Trophic cells develop tubular projections that enter invaginations in feeder cells in the lungs (Dei-Cas *et al.,* 1991). The generative phase consists of asci or cysts that are 5–8 μm in diameter and ovoid to rounded in shape. The asci produce eight unicellular ascospores, previously termed sporozoites. Asci turn over every 4 days (Schmatz *et al.,* 1991).

Pneumocystosis has been reported in nonhuman primates with debilitation due to recent importation, concomitant experimental or naturally acquired bacterial infection, and neoplasia or to immunodeficiency associated with experimental or naturally acquired retroviral infection (Poelma, 1975; Chandler *et al.,* 1976; Letvin *et al.,* 1983; Kestler *et al.,* 1990; Lowenstien *et al.,* 1992). *Pneumocystis* has also been reported as an endemic infection within a colony of tamarins, *Saguinus fusicollis* and *S. oedipus* (Richter *et al.,* 1978). Reports of clinical signs specifically due to *Pneumocystis* infection in nonhuman primates are few; progressive weight loss, anorexia, and failure to thrive, leading to death, were reported for an owl monkey with no other concomitant disease (Chandler *et al.,* 1976). Chimpanzees with pneumocystosis and erythroleukemia developed anorexia, pyrexia, dyspnea, cyanosis, and pneumonia (Chandler *et al.,* 1976). The chimpanzees were anemic with a marked leukocytosis, which was probably attributable to the erythroleukemia. Thoracic radiographs revealed extensive infiltrates in the lung lobes. Initial treatment with broad-spectrum antibiotics, supple-

mental oxygen, and corticosteroids resulted in short-lived clinical improvement before the chimpanzees relapsed. One chimpanzee was treated with pentamidine isethionate (4 mg/kg body weight intravenously for 14 days), resulting in mild clinical improvement (Chandler *et al.,* 1976).

Gross lesions attributable to pneumocystosis vary. In the owl monkeys, the lungs were partially collapsed, firm, rubbery, and pale pink in color (Chandler *et al.,* 1976). Gray-white foci, 0.5–1.5 mm in diameter, were found throughout the lung lobes. Irregular areas of hyperemia in the hilar region were noted in one owl monkey (Chandler *et al.,* 1976). Multifocal or diffuse consolidation with subpleural purpuric hemorrhages was noted in affected chimpanzees (Chandler *et al.,* 1976). Pulmonary edema, emphysema, and pneumonia were found in galagos, a woolly monkey, chimpanzee, and marmoset with pneumocystosis (Poelma, 1975). One affected tamarin had multiple 1- to 2-mm pale gray nodules throughout the lungs (Richter *et al.,* 1978).

Microscopic examination of hematoxylin and eosin stained lung sections from owl monkeys revealed multifocal areas in which alveoli were filled with a granular, eosinophilic foamy material (Fig. 5) (Chandler *et al.,* 1976). Alveoli also contained cell debris, foamy macrophages, desquamated alveolar cells, erythrocytes, and proteinaceous fluid; there was little to no inflammation in the interstitium. In chimpanzees, extensive interstitial pneumonia with a predominately mononuclear cell infiltrate was observed. *Pneumocystis* organisms were poorly defined in hematoxylin and eosin stained sections (Chandler *et al.,* 1976). Staining with Gomori methenamine silver or periodic acid–Schiff stains revealed cystic *Pneumocystis* organisms within a honeycomb matrix. Organisms were dark brown to black, round, ovoid, or cup-shaped cysts, 4–6 μm in diameter, in silver-stained tissues (Chandler *et al.,* 1976). In tamarins, inflammatory response to *Pneumocystis* consisted of mononuclear infiltration into the septal wall, varying numbers of foamy macrophages with an occasional giant cell, and occasional polymorphonuclear cells in the septae or alveoli (Richter *et al.,* 1978).

Diagnosis of *Pneumocystis* infection in nonhuman primates has usually been postmortem, based on characteristic histologic lesions. Certainly pneumocystosis should be considered as a diagnosis in an immunocompromised animal with dyspnea or other indications of pulmonary disease. Trimethoprim–sulfamethoxazole, dapsone, and aerosolized pentamidine have been effective in prophylaxis and treatment of *Pneumocystis* infections in humans. Dosages could be extrapolated from human data based on known safe dosages of these agents in nonhuman primates.

B. Superficial Infections

Dermatophytosis or ringworm in nonhuman primates is caused by organisms of the genera *Microsporum* and *Trichophyton.* This condition occurs rarely in nonhuman primates.

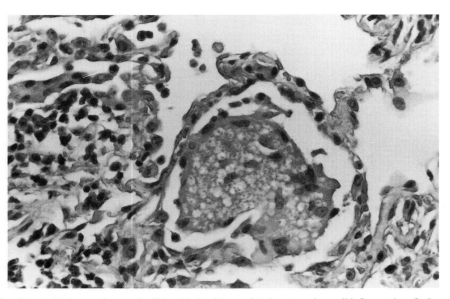

Fig. 5. Alveolus containing *Pneumocystis* organisms and cellular debris with associated mononuclear cell inflammation. Owl monkey lung. Hematoxylin and eosin stain. Magnification: ×200. (Photo by Jim Artwohl.) Courtesy of the Biologic Resources Laboratory, University of Illinois at Chicago.

Dermatophytes invade the horny layer of the skin and hair and produce a mild inflammatory response and hyperkeratosis. *Microsporum canis, M. gypseum,* and *T. mentagrophytes* produce arthrospores arranged on the outside of the hair shaft. Dermatophytes invade the anagen hairs and grow down the follicle to the layer of mitotic activity. The hair becomes brittle and breaks off, usually near the surface. Infection results from direct contact with infected animals or contaminated fomites.

Gross appearance of lesions in nonhuman primates varies, including baldness, typical circular or ring-shaped lesions, generalized scaliness, and patchy hair loss to generalized alopecia (Al-Doory, 1972). *Microsporum canis* has been isolated from affected New World monkeys (Kaplan *et al.,* 1957), a capuchin (Scully and Kligman, 1951), a rhesus monkey (Baker *et al.,* 1971) gibbons (Seeliger *et al.,* 1963; Taylor *et al.,* 1973), and a chimpanzee (Klokke and deVries, 1963). Other species of *Microsporum* isolated from skin lesions include *M. cookei, M. gypseum,* and *M. distortum* (Migaki, 1986). *Trichophyton mentagrophytes* was isolated from capuchins, rhesus monkeys, a gibbon, and a vervet (Bagnall and Grunberg, 1972; Gugnani, 1971; Hauck and Klehr, 1977). An epizootic of ringworm, in which the etiologic agent was *T. violaceum,* occurred in 60 baboons housed in the same cage in Sukhumi (Voronin *et al.,* 1948). The source of infection was believed to be dogs previously held in the cage. Chimpanzees were infected with an organism resembling *T. rubrum* (Otcenasek *et al.,* 1967), and *T. gallinae* was isolated from a cynomolgus monkey (Gordon and Little, 1967).

Diagnosis of dermatophytoses is based on the characteristic gross appearance of the lesions, cytologic examination of hairs or skin scrapings treated with potassium hydroxide, histologic examination of skin biopsy (Table I), and culture. Hair and scale samples are cultured for dermatophyte isolation and may be inoculated directly onto Sabouraud's agar or dermatophyte test medium (DTM). Dermatophyte test medium contains bacterial, yeast, and saprophytic fungi inhibitors and a color-based pH indicator. Growth of a dermatophyte utilizes the protein in the DTM, creating an alkaline pH and turning the media red in 5–8 days.

Marmosets and tamarins with varying degrees of alopecia were infected with an unidentified fungus that responded to therapy with griseofulvin (J. B. Deinhardt *et al.,* 1967).

C. Systemic Yeast Infections

Most systemic yeast infections have been diagnosed in nonhuman primates postmorten. Table II presents the characteristics of these yeasts in tissue.

1. Hypomycetes

a. *Coccidioides.* *C. immitis* is a soil saprophyte that inhabits semiarid areas in parts of the southwestern United States, Mexico, and Central and South America. A dimorphic fungus, the mycelial phase requires sandy alkaline soil, high environmental temperature, low rainfall, and low elevation (Walch, 1981). Transmission usually occurs by inhalation of arthrospores; dust storms in endemic areas may be the cause of epizootics (Flynn *et al.,* 1978).

Coccidiodes immitis grows on a wide range of fungal media and blood agar, and its growth is enhanced by supplementation with yeast extract. The mycelial phase grows best at 25 to 30°C,

TABLE I

HISTOLOGIC APPEARANCE OF DERMATOPHYTOSES

Agent	Appearance	Location	Inflammatory response
Microsporum spp.	Polygonal arthrospores	External surface of hair (ectothrix)	Orthokeratosis, parakeratosis with
Trichophyton spp.	Chains of round arthrospores	Within hair (endothrix) and on surface (ectothrix)	neutrophilic microabscesses

appearing in 3–4 days with varying pigment and texture. Microscopically the organism in culture is septate with racquet hyphae and barrel-shaped arthrospores. Because of the highly infectious nature of this organism, great care should be taken in handling cultures.

Several infections with *C. immitis* have been reported in nonhuman primates with baboons, macaques, and gorillas appearing to be most susceptible (McKenney *et al.,* 1944; Pappagianis *et al.,* 1973; Rapley and Long, 1974; Migaki, 1986). Clinical signs associated with respiratory disease included nasal discharge, cough, and dyspnea. *Coccidioides immitis* infection in the vertebrae caused lameness and reluctance to move in a baboon (Rosenberg *et al.,* 1984) and altered gait, leading to paralysis in a rhesus monkey (Castleman *et al.,* 1980). In all reports, affected monkeys and apes had a history of outdoor housing in California or Texas.

Coccidioides immitis infections usually result in disseminated disease involving multiple organ systems. Lesions in nonhuman primates are reported most frequently in the lung and vertebrae but have also occurred in the spleen, liver, kidneys, lymph nodes, and esophagus (Migaki, 1986). The lesion induced by *C. immitis* can be granulomatous, suppurative, or pyogranulomatous and range in size from miliary to massive. Pulmonary

lesions include multifocal firm white nodules, partial or complete collapse of a lung lobe, pleural adhesions, and cavitations (Bellini *et al.,* 1991; Breznock *et al.,* 1975; Castleman *et al.,* 1980). The hilar lymph nodes may be enlarged (Castleman *et al.,* 1980). Paravertebral masses or abscesses with invasion into the vertebrae and spinal cord were reported for those monkeys with lameness or paralysis (Rosenberg *et al.,* 1984; Castleman *et al.,* 1980).

Microscopic lesions are typically pyogranulomas bordered by multinucleate giant cells (Migaki, 1986), although primarily neutrophilic response has also been described (Breznock *et al.,* 1975). Lesions contain thick-walled spherules 10–60 μm in diameter filled with 2- to 4-μm round endospores (Fig. 6). Extensive destruction of airway walls and large bronchiectatic lesions may be observed in lungs with cavitary lesions (Breznock *et al.,* 1975). Vertebral lesions include lysis of bone, irregular trabeculae, necrosis, and osteomyelitis (Rosenberg *et al.,* 1984; Castleman *et al.,* 1980).

Radiography may be valuable in antemortem diagnosis of coccidioidomycosis. Radiographs can reveal severe pulmonary disease with multiple cavitary lesions or lysis of vertebral bone. Tuberculosis, neoplasia, and other disseminated mycotic dis-

TABLE II

HISTOLOGIC APPEARANCE OF SYSTEMIC YEAST INFECTION

Agent	Size (μm)	Appearance	Bud	Capsule	Inflammatory response
Hypomycetes					
Coccidiodes immitus	10–60	Thick-walled, spherule containing 2- to 4-μm endospores	None	No	Pyogranulomatous with multinucleate giant cells; neutrophilic
Histoplasma capsulatum var. *capsulatum*	2–4	Thin-walled yeast	Single, narrow-based attachment	No	Microgranulomas with multinucleate giant cells; histiocytic
H. capsulatum var. *duboisii*	8–15	Thick-walled yeast	Single, narrow-based attachment	No	Pyogranulomatous with multinucleate giant cells
Sporothrix schenkii	2–6	Pleomorphic, round, oval to cigar shaped	1–2	No	Granulomatous with multinucleate giant cells
Paracoccoidiodes braziliensis	8–20	Spherical yeast	Multiple peripheral buds	No	Granulomatous
Blastomycetes					
Candida albicans	3–5	Yeast, pseudohyphae, and blastospores	One or more	No	Neutrophilic
Cryptococcus neoformans	2–10	Thin-walled, varying size, spherical	Single, narrow-based attachment	Yes	None, neutrophilic, or histiocytic with giant cells
Owl monkey agent	7–8	Thin-walled yeast	Single, narrow-based attachment	Yes	Histiocytic

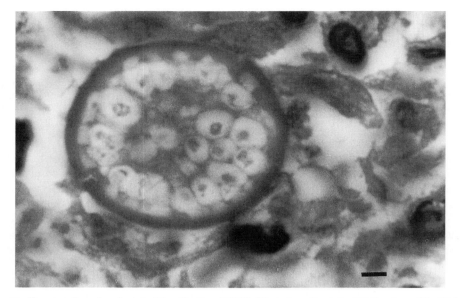

Fig. 6. Coccidiodes immitis. Hematoxylin and eosin stain. Magnification: ×1000. (Photo from Jim Artwohl.) Courtesy of the Biologic Resources Laboratory, University of Illinois at Chicago.

eases should be considered as diagnostic alternatives. Serologic testing for specific antibody by complement fixation or tube precipitin test or skin testing with coccidioidin may be helpful in reaching a diagnosis of coccidioidomycosis. Serologic testing requires changes in titer in paired serum samples over time, and a negative result does not preclude the possibility of disease. Skin testing is not very specific as cross-reactions with blastomycin and histoplasmin may occur. Definitive diagnosis can be made from the characteristic appearance of the organism in cytologic or histologic preparations and by culture.

b. *Histoplasma.* i. *H. capsulatum* var. *capsulatum:* This organism grows as a mycelium in soil, especially in areas enriched by feces of birds and bats, and as a yeast in cells of the reticuloendothelial system of infected hosts. Infection is spread by inhalation of spores. Only the yeast phase is pathogenic in mice; experimental infections with mycelia are cleared (Medoff *et al.,* 1987). Clinical disease in humans requires exposure to a heavy inoculum, preexisting pulmonary disease, or immunodeficiency (Medoff *et al.,* 1987).

There are few reports of spontaneous histoplasmosis due to *H. capsulatum* var. *capsulatum* in nonhuman primates. An epidemiologic survey of wild mammals in a zoological park in Brazil using delayed hypersensitivity skin tests revealed positive responses in 15% of capuchins, *Cebus apella,* and 6.25% of common marmosets, *Callithrix jacchus* (Costa *et al.,* 1994). No animal had overt disease. Systemic disease has been reported in a squirrel monkey with granulomatous pneumonia, hepatitis, and splenitis (Bergeland *et al.,* 1970), an owl monkey (Weller *et al.,* 1990), a de Brazza's monkey with granulomatous lesions in the kidneys, liver, and lungs (Frank, 1968), and a

rhesus monkey infected with SIV (Baskin, 1991). The owl monkey, *Aotus nancymai,* presented with weight loss and splenomegaly. Clinical pathological evaluation revealed neutropenia, eosinophilia, hypercalcemia, hypercholesterolemia, and hypophosphatemia (Weller *et al.,* 1990). The rhesus monkey experienced diarrhea, weight loss, anorexia, and dyspnea. Marked splenomegaly and enlargement of the mesenteric lymph nodes were found at necropsy (Baskin, 1991).

Microscopic lesions consisted of disseminated microgranulomas with multinucleated giant cells in the spleen, liver, kidneys, adrenal, and lymph nodes of the owl monkey (Weller *et al.,* 1990). In most granulomas there was a solid mass of histiocytes and multinucleate Langhans-type giant cells (Frank, 1968; Bergeland *et al.,* 1970; Weller *et al.,* 1990). In the rhesus, diffuse histiocytosis of many organs, including the lamina propria, submucosa and serosa of the intestines, sinuses of the mesenteric lymph nodes, and spleen, liver, adrenal peripheral lymph nodes, and bone marrow, was the prominent microscopic finding (Baskin, 1991). In all reports, small yeasts, 2–4 μm in diameter, with a thin cell wall and a central basophilic structure (Fig. 7), were found in the cytoplasm of macrophages or giant cells. The organisms are easily visible in hematoxylin and eosin stained sections, but will also stain with periodic acid–Schiff and methenamine silver stains.

Diagnosis can be made from the typical appearance of the organism and the resulting inflammatory response in tissue or in cytologic preparations. Serologic or skin testing using histoplasmin antigen is not sufficiently reliable for definitive diagnosis. Culture may be attempted, but samples must be plated rapidly to avoid overgrowth of contaminants. The yeast phase of *H. capsulatum* var. *capsulatum* grows on blood agar at 37°C

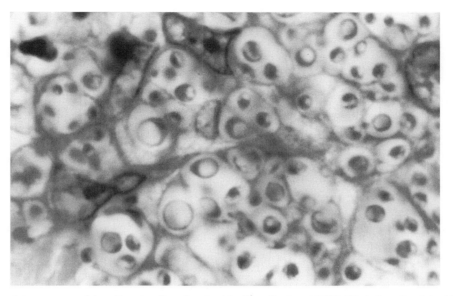

Fig. 7. Histoplasma capsulatum var. *capsulatum.* Hematoxylin and eosin stain. Magnification: ×1000. (Photo from Jim Artwohl.) Courtesy of the Biologic Resources Laboratory, University of Illinois at Chicago.

and the mycelial phase grows on Sabouraud's agar at room temperature. Care must be taken in the culture of the mycelial phase as the microconidia are infectious for personnel.

ii. *Histoplasma capsulatum* var. *duboissi:* This organism causes African or large-form histoplasmosis. Soil is believed to be the natural reservoir of *H. capsulatum* var. *duboisii* with direct dermal contact, inhalation, and ingestion as methods of transmission. The agent is indigenous to Africa, but infection has been spread among feral and laboratory-born baboons in Texas (Butler and Hubbard, 1991). Direct contact with infected baboons through grooming or licking of skin lesions appeared to be the most likely mode of transmission in this epizootic.

All reports of African histoplasmosis have occurred in baboons, both *Papio* and *Cynocephalus* (Courtois *et al.,* 1955; Mariat and Segretain, 1956; Walker and Spooner, 1960; Butler *et al.,* 1988; Butler and Hubbard, 1991). Lesions are usually confined to the skin, especially surfaces that contact the ground such as hands, buttocks, and tail but also occur on the face, ears, and scrotum. Lesions may appear as papules, pustules 5–10 mm in diameter, or ulcerative granulomas 1–2 cm in diameter (Butler *et al.,* 1988; Butler and Hubbard, 1991). Radiography may reveal osteolytic lesions in the skull, digits, and vertebrae underlying affected areas of skin (Butler *et al.,* 1988; Butler and Hubbard, 1991).

Numerous discrete elevated and ulcerated skin lesions on the face, ears, hands, feet, tail, and/or perineum and rarely the torso were found at necropsy (Butler and Hubbard, 1991). Superficial and retroperitoneal lymph nodes may be enlarged, particularly those lymph nodes draining areas with skin lesions (Butler *et al.,* 1988; Butler and Hubbard, 1991). Extension of cutaneous lesions to underlying bone resulted in osteolysis (Walker and

Spooner, 1960; Butler *et al.,* 1988; Butler and Hubbard, 1991). Discrete nodular lesions have been reported in liver and testis (Butler *et al.,* 1988; Butler and Hubbard, 1991).

Histopathologic examination of skin lesions revealed pyogranulomatous inflammation of the dermis and subcutaneous tissues characterized by marked histiocytic infiltrates, large numbers of both Langhans and foreign body type multinucleated giant cells, and neutrophils (Butler and Hubbard, 1991). Skin lesions are frequently ulcerative. Numerous intracellular and extracellular 8- to 15-μm uninucleate yeast cells occur throughout the lesions. The organisms have narrow-based budding and occur singly or in clusters (Fig. 8). Multinucleate giant cells contain numerous yeast. The microscopic appearance of lesions in other organs was similar to that in skin with the exception of lymph nodes in which there was little associated inflammation (Butler and Hubbard, 1991). *Histoplasma capsulatum* var. *duboisii* has similar staining characteristics to *H. capsulatum* var. *capsulatum.*

Diagnosis of *H. capsulatum* var. *duboisii* infection can be made based on the characteristic appearance of the organism and the resultant inflammation in tissue (Butler and Hubbard, 1991). Immunodiffusion and complement fixation tests cannot differentiate between the different varieties of histoplasmosis. *Histoplasma capsulatum* var. *duboisii* may be morphologically difficult to differentiate from *H. capsulatum* var. *capsulatum* in culture.

Treatment with ketaconazole administered orally at 10–40 mg/kg per day for 6 months was ineffective in treating African histoplasmosis (Butler *et al.,* 1988). Treatment with a daily oral dose of 160 mg trimethoprim and 800 mg sulfamethoxazole for 16 weeks was also ineffective (Butler and Hubbard, 1991). Sur-

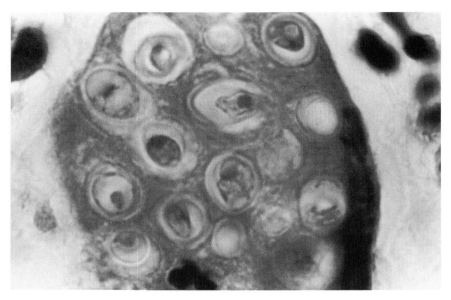

Fig. 8. Histoplasma capsulatum var. *duboisii.* Hematoxylin and eosin stain. Magnification: ×1000. (Photo from Jim Artwohl.) Courtesy of the Biologic Resources Laboratory, University of Illinois at Chicago.

gical excision of the lesion was effective in eliminating the infection from 13 baboons.

c. *Sporothrix.* *S. schenkii,* a saprophytic dimorphic fungus, is the etiologic agent of sporotrichosis. Distribution is worldwide throughout tropical and temporal climates. *Sporothrix schenkii* grows primarily in soil but also on tree bark, plants, and sphagnum moss. Sporotrichosis in humans and animals is associated with a puncture wound or other trauma to the skin. Lesions are usually confined to the skin, subcutaneous tissues, and lymphatics; there are rare reports of disseminated disease involving bone, lungs, and other viscera.

Sporotrichosis has been reported in a chimpanzee (Saliba *et al.,* 1968) that developed multiple nodules and pustules on the face and enlargement of the sublingual and submaxillary lymph nodes. Distinct granulomas composed of four well-defined zones were observed. A central core of necrosis and suppuration was bordered by a zone composed primarily of neutrophils with occasional macrophages, eosinophils, and erythrocytes. Peripheral to this zone was a border of epithelioid macrophages and Langhans giant cells with a final exterior border of connective tissue and mononuclear inflammation (Al-Doory, 1972). In tissue the organisms are large, 3 to 10 μm, spherical to oval yeasts that may have buds (Fig. 9). A survey of mammals in a zoological park in Brazil revealed 6% of *C. apella* and no *C. jacchus* had a positive response to a sporotrichin skin test (Costa *et al.,* 1994). Experimental sporotrichosis has been induced in a rhesus monkey by implanting an infected thorn in the finger (Benham and Kesten, 1932).

d. *Paracoccidioides.* *P. brasiliensis* is a dimorphic fungus endemic to South America. It is one of the most prevalent sys-

temic mycoses in humans and although disease in animals is rare, a survey of animals in Brazil revealed a 52% incidence of positive reactions to delayed hypersensitivity skin testing (Costa *et al.,* 1991). There is one report of granulomatous disease involving the liver and colon of a squirrel monkey imported from Bolivia to the United States (Johnson and Lang, 1977). *Paracoccidioides brasiliensis* is easily recognized in tissue sections as a large yeast form (8–50 μm) with multiple buds occurring around the periphery.

2. Owl Monkey Agent

A disseminated yeast infection was described in feral owl monkeys with a history of weight loss (Gibson *et al.,* 1993). All monkeys had splenomegaly at necropsy. Oval yeast cells, approximately 8 μm in diameter, with a distinct refractile capsule were found in many tissues with a minimal inflammatory response (Fig. 10). Organisms were located intracellularly in macrophages and were single budding. The yeast stained poorly with hematoxylin and eosin and was more distinct with either periodic acid–Schiff or Gomori methenamine silver stain.

3. Blastomycetes

a. *Candida.* Candidiasis, also known as moniliasis or thrush, is caused by yeast of the genus *Candida,* usually *C. albicans. Candida* organisms are acquired by neonatal animals in the birth canal and colonize the gastrointestinal and genital mucosa for life, usually with no deleterious effects. *Candida albicans* is a normal saprophytic inhabitant of the mucous membranes of the alimentary and genital tracts and skin of nonhu-

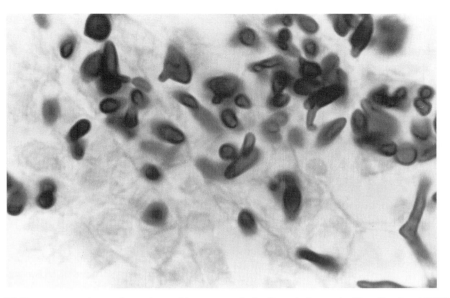

Fig. 9. *Sporothrix schenckii.* Numerous round to oval organisms with one to two buds. Gomori silver stain. Magnification: ×1000. (Photo from Jim Artwohl.) Courtesy of the Biologic Resources Laboratory, University of Illinois at Chicago.

man primates (Al-Doory, 1972; Hunt *et al.,* 1978; Wikse *et al.,* 1970; Migaki *et al.,* 1982b). Candidiasis is the most frequently reported and probably the most frequently occurring mycotic disease in nonhuman primates.

Candida is a dimorphic fungus that grows on Sabouraud agar at 25°C and blood agar at 37°C. Colonies are cream-colored and smooth with a yeasty odor. *Candida* form chlamydospores on cornmeal agar and are positive for the rapid germ tube test.

Candida spp. produce pseudohyphae and do not possess ascospores.

Spread of *Candida* is normally inhibited by normal microflora. The first step in dissemination of infection is localized proliferation of the yeast. Cell-mediated immunity may be an important determinant of infection. Antibiotic therapy, prolonged immunosuppression, neoplastic or infectious disease, or prolonged use of steroids has resulted in localized and dissemi-

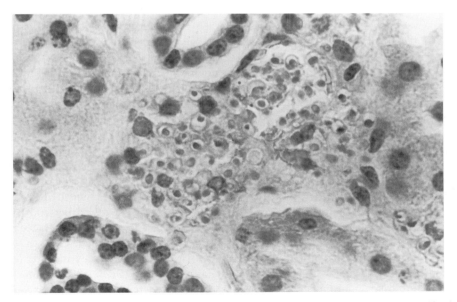

Fig. 10. Owl monkey agent. Note clusters of haloed organisms within renal tissue. Hematoxylin and eosin stain. Magnification: ×400. (Photo from Jim Artwohl.) Courtesy of the Biologic Resources Laboratory, University of Illinois at Chicago.

nated candidiasis (Seelig, 1966a,b). Circulating neutrophils may be a major defense to the development of candidiasis; neutropenic people are susceptible to disseminated candidiasis, as are dogs (Barsanti, 1984). Predisposing factors for the development of candidiasis in nonhuman primates include antibiotic therapy, recent importation, age, concomitant mycobacterial infection, retroviral infection, or parasitism (Migaki *et al.,* 1982b; Lowenstine *et al.,* 1992). Candidiasis has also occurred in monkeys during experimentation, including routine oral gavage in marmosets (Tucker, 1984), experimental schistosomiasis in a capuchin (McCullough *et al.,* 1977), and *T. cruzi* infection in a patas monkey (Thiry, 1913).

Clinical signs vary depending on the severity of infection and location of the lesions. Anorexia and dysphagia have been reported in rhesus monkeys with oral or esophageal lesions (Kaufmann and Quist, 1969b; Wikse *et al.,* 1970). Open mouth breathing (Wikse *et al.,* 1970) was associated with ulcers on the hard palate. Diarrhea may occur with intestinal involvement; however, many nonhuman primates that developed candidiasis had prior treatment with antibiotics for preexisting diarrhea (Migaki *et al.,* 1982b). Anorexia, dehydration, and diarrhea have been reported for owl monkeys with candidiasis (Weller, 1994). Infection of the nails, onychomycosis, with shortening, erosion, and deformation of the nails occurred in two rhesus monkeys (Kerber and Reese, 1968; Wikse *et al.,* 1970) that also had balanitis. One monkey became blind as the result of *C. curvata* infection of the brain (Herceg *et al.,* 1977).

Pseudomembrane formation results from candidal overgrowth. White or creamy plaques are found on the tongue, oral cavity, esophagus, and intestine. There are reports of localized lesions on the tongue in a patas monkey (Thiry, 1913), woolly monkey and a gorilla (Fiennes, 1967), in the buccal cavity of baboons (Saëz, 1970), and in the stomach in an infant gibbon (Saëz, 1975). Pseudomembranous or ulcerative esophagitis occurred in marmosets (Tucker, 1984), a rhesus monkey (Kaufmann and Quist, 1969b), and a chimpanzee (Schmidt and Butler, 1970). Candidiasis involving the tongue, mouth, esophagus, and intestines has been reported in newly imported tamarins, *Saguinus* spp. (Hunt *et al.,* 1978; Nelson *et al.,* 1966), and rhesus monkeys treated with antibiotics for diarrhea (Wikse *et al.,* 1970). Disseminated candidiasis in capuchins involved the oral cavity, lungs, liver, and intestine (Fiennes, 1967); nasal, pharyngeal, and intestinal mucosa (McCullogh *et al.,* 1977); and tongue and esophagus (Wikse *et al.,* 1970). Spider monkeys, *Ateles* spp., developed enterocolitis following antibiotic treatment for diarrhea (Patterson *et al.,* 1974).

The microscopic appearance of *Candida* infection in tissues is characterized by large clusters of pseudohyphae and blastospores (3–5 μm in diameter) in the superficial portion of the epithelium of the mucous membrane (Migaki *et al.,* 1982b). Pseudomembranes are composed of degenerate and sloughed epithelial cells, neutrophilic infiltrates, and numerous yeasts. Necrosis and ulceration result from deep invasion of the epithelium and lamina propria. Although *Candida* are readily appar-

ent with hematoxylin and eosin stain, morphology is best revealed by periodic acid–Schiff or Gomori methenamine silver stains (Migaki *et al.,* 1978).

Because *Candida* are normal flora of the gastrointestinal and genital tract, culture alone is not sufficient for diagnosis. Wet mounts of scrapings from lesions in 10% NaOH, 20% KOH, or lactophenol cotton blue can be used to demonstrate yeasts and hyphae. Gram-stained smears from lesions reveal gram-positive oval and budding yeast cells. Examination of tissue sections is most valuable for diagnosis in that tissue invasion can be demonstrated.

Oral nystatin suspension is an effective treatment for lesions of the oral cavity or digestive system.

b. *Geotrichum.* Geotrichosis is a rare mycotic disease of humans and animals caused by *Geotrichum candidum,* a common fungus found on fruits and vegetables, in soil and decaying matter, and in dairy products (Dolensek *et al.,* 1977). Geotrichosis occurred in six lowland gorillas that were fed hydroponically grown grasses infected with *G. candidum* (Dolensek *et al.,* 1977). The gorillas developed watery diarrhea over a 4-day period. Fungal elements were observed in fecal wet mounts, and *G. candidum* was cultured from the feces of all six gorillas. Treatment with oral nystatin for 10 days eliminated the infection, with diarrhea subsiding in five gorillas in 3–4 days. Disinfection of the hydroponic unit eliminated the source of the infection.

c. *Cryptococcus.* Cryptococcosis is a systemic infection of humans and animals caused by a yeast-like fungus, *Cryptococcus neoformans.* A saprophytic soil organism, *C. neoformans* has worldwide distribution. The most common source is pigeon droppings and old nests. Transmission usually occurs by inhalation of spores, but may occur as the result of direct contact (Migaki, 1986).

Cryptococcus neoformans is a thin-walled, oval to spherical budding cell 3.5 to 7 μm that forms a wide heteropolysaccharide capsule (1 to 30 μm) that is always present in the tissue form of the organism. The fungus forms white creamy colonies on Sabouraud's agar that yellow with age. It is distinguished from nonpathogenic cryptococci by its ability to grow at 37°C. *Cryptococcus neoformans* reproduces by budding one to two daughter cells connected to the mother cell by a narrow isthmus (Fig. 11).

Several cases of cryptococcosis have been described in nonhuman primates, including tamarins (Takos and Elton, 1953), a squirrel monkey (Roussilhon *et al.,* 1987), macaques (Garner *et al.,* 1969; Griner, 1983; Miller and Boever, 1983; Pal *et al.,* 1989), a black lemur, a purple-faced langur (Migaki, 1986), proboscis monkeys (Griner, 1983), a sooty mangabey (Migaki *et al.,* 1978) a de Brazza's monkey (Al-Doory, 1972), and a patas monkey (Sly *et al.,* 1977). Clinical signs vary as infection is usually disseminated. Central nervous system signs included seizures (Migaki, 1986; Sly *et al.,* 1977), depression (Miller and Boever, 1983), and blindness (Sly *et al.,* 1977). The affected

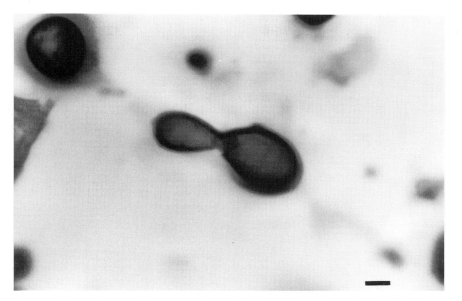

Fig. 11. Cryptococcus neoformans. Note single bud with a narrow isthmus. Periodic acid–Schiff stain. Magnification: ×1000. (Photo from Jim Artwohl.) Courtesy of the Biologic Resources Laboratory, University of Illinois at Chicago.

squirrel monkey had a deforming mass of the lower jaw, significant weight loss, and leukopenia with lymphopenia and anemia (Roussilhon *et al.,* 1987). Cutaneous lesions occurred in a patas monkey (Sly *et al.,* 1977) and a de Brazza's monkey (Al-Doory, 1972).

Gross lesions in primates are usually disseminated widely, involving lung, brain, spinal cord, spleen, lymph nodes, thyroid, pancreas, adrenal glands, tonsils, skin, and/or muscle. There has been one case of primary cryptococcal endometriosis (Griner, 1983). There are two general forms of gross lesions: a gelatinous mass loosely organized with no defined capsule or a solid granulomatous mass. Emaciation, splenomegaly, granulomatous pneumonia, and lymphadenopathy involving the hilar or peripheral lymph nodes were common features (Takos and Elton, 1953; Garner *et al.,* 1969; Al-Doory, 1972; Sly *et al.,* 1977; Roussilhon *et al.,* 1987).

Histologically, large, irregularly sized yeast cells with abundant capsular polysaccharide were observed. Organisms occurred singly, in small aggregates, or in large masses. The degree and type of inflammation ranged from none, to acute inflammation, or granulomatous inflammation. The granulomatous cellular response contained primarily macrophages and giant cells with few plasma cells and lymphocytes.

Cytologic evaluation of cutaneous masses or spinal fluid can provide rapid diagnosis of cryptococcal infection. In gram-stained impression smears, the organism is gram positive and the capsule light yellow. India ink preparations allow visualization of the organism against a black background but are not diagnostic unless budding is observed. The latex agglutination test for capsular antigen in CSF, serum, or urine is an effective method of diagnosis in cases of disseminated disease. Commer-

cial kits are available. Serologic and CSF testing of an affected monkey for antibody to *C. neoformans* did show a marked rise in titer prior to development of clinical signs and immediately prior to death (Sly *et al.,* 1977). The organism can be cultured from exudate, CSF, or tissues on Sabouraud agar without cyclohexamide incubated at both 25 and 37°C. Morphology, growth at 37°C, hydrolysis of urea, and mouse virulence tests can be used for confirmation.

D. Systemic Hyphal Infections

The histologic appearance of hyphal infections in nonhuman primates is described in Table III.

1. Hyphomycetes

a. *Aspergillus.* *A. fumigatus* is the most common causative agent of aspergillosis. *Aspergillus* spp. are very common ubiquitous saprophytic organisms growing in soil, decaying vegetation, and organic debris. Spores are common in dust, hay, and straw. Reports of infection in nonhuman primates are limited to an outbreak at the London zoo involving dual infection with tuberculosis (Fiennes, 1967). The infection was limited to Old World monkeys, including macaques, a roloway monkey, and a black mangabey. The lesions were disseminated in the lungs, liver, kidneys, and spleen. The microscopic lesion consisted of a caseous necrotic core bordered by a wide zone of fibroblasts, epithelioid cells, multinucleate giant cells, and lymphocytes (Migaki *et al.,* 1978). Uniform diameter, septate hyphae 3–6

TABLE III

HISTOLOGIC APPEARANCE OF SYSTEMIC HYPHAL INFECTIONS

Agent	Size	Appearance	Inflammatory response
Hyphomycetes			
Aspergillus spp.	3–6 μm uniform diameter	Septate hyphae, branching at 45° angle	Granulomatous with giant cells
Paecilomyces spp.	Short	Septate hyphae with pleomorphic vesicles and pleomorphic conidia	Granulomatous with giant cells
Zygomycetes			
Mucorales	4–24 μm diameter, 10–60 μm long	Irregularly branched, bulbous, rare septae	Granulomatous with giant cells
Entomophthorales	6–12 μm diameter	Irregularly branched, thin-walled hyphae with dense eosinophilic precipitate (Splendore–Hoeppli phenomenon)	Pyogranulomatous with eosinophils and multinucleate giant cells

μm in width, branching at 45° angles, were observed in the lesions (Fig. 12).

b. *Paecilomyces.*   Organisms of the genus *Paecilomyces* are saprophytic molds related to *Penicillium* and *Aspergillus,* ubiquitous in soil and decaying matter. *Paecilomyces* have septate, branching hyphae bearing long chains of conidia from the tips of conidiaphores. Paecilomycosis in humans and animals is rare; there is a single case report in a rhesus macaque (Fleischman and McCracken, 1977). Chronic slight wheezing progressed over 8 months to labored breathing when stressed and stridor immediately prior to death. Multifocal subcutaneous nodules and a large occlusive laryngeal mass were noted at necropsy. Microscopic examination of the laryngeal and subcutaneous masses revealed granulomatous inflammation with many Langhans and foreign body giant cells. Fungal elements, including short septate hyphae with pleomorphic vesicles and swellings, and pleomorphic conidia were observed within the cytoplasm of epithelioid and giant cells. Fungal morphology was most clearly demonstrated with periodic acid–Schiff and Gomori methenamine silver stains.

2. Zygomycetes

Mycotic disease caused by fungi in the class Zygomycetes (formerly Phycomycetes) is termed zygomycosis. Zygomycosis has replaced all previous designations for mycotic infections from organisms of the orders Mucorales and Entomophthorales. Zygomycetes are characterized by nonseptate hyphae and for-

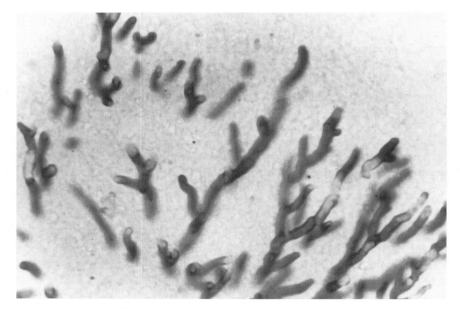

Fig. 12. Aspergillus. Note hyphae branching at 45° angles. Gomori silver stain. Magnification ×400. (Photo from Jim Artwohl.) Courtesy of the Biologic Resources Laboratory, University of Illinois at Chicago.

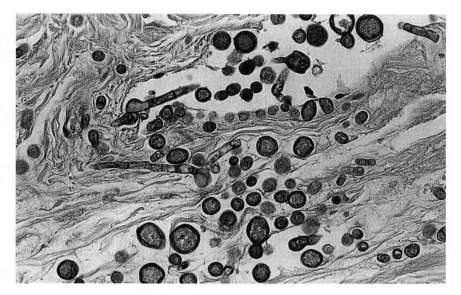

Fig. 13. Cutaneous zygomycosis with angioinvasion. Hematoxylin and eosin stain. Magnification: ×400.

mation of spores by cleavage within a sporangium. All grow rapidly at 25 and 37°C on blood and Sabouraud agar. Growth is inhibited by cycloheximide.

a. MUCORALES. Fungi of the order Mucorales are opportunistic pathogens ubiquitous in the soil that occur worldwide. Genera implicated in animal infections include *Absidia, Rhizopus, Rhizomucor, Mucor,* and *Mortierella.*

Human patients are predisposed to zygomycosis by chronic debilitating diseases, including lymphatic cancer, by immunosuppression, by antibiotic and or corticosteroid use, and by acidosis (Lehrer *et al.,* 1980). Nonhuman primates that have developed zygomycosis were subject to the stresses of recent capture and quarantine (Hessler *et al.,* 1967; Martin *et al.,* 1969), fungus-contaminated feed (Lucke and Linton, 1965), diabetes mellitus (Martin *et al.,* 1969), and fight trauma with probable metabolic acidosis (Baskin *et al.,* 1984).

Zygomycosis or mucormycosis caused by fungi of the order Mucorales has three primary clinical forms in humans: cutaneous, rhinocerebral, and systemic (Chandler *et al.,* 1980). Cases similar to these three forms have been described in nonhuman primates. Zygomycosis with primary gastric or intestinal lesions is the most frequently reported form in nonhuman primates. Gastrointestinal disease with no systemic involvement occurred in an adult female rhesus monkey with gastric ulcers (Hessler *et al.,* 1967) and in two spider monkeys, *Ateles hybridus,* with ulcerative colitis (Fiennes, 1967). Severe ulcerative colitis with liver involvement was reported in two rhesus monkeys (Gisler and Pitcock, 1962). Mycotic ulcerative gastroenteritis in a mandrill, *Mandrillus sphinx* (Lucke and Linton,

1965), and in a golden-bellied mangabey, *Cercocebus galeritus chrysogaster* (Kageruka *et al.,* 1972), also involved the heart, kidneys, liver, lung, and spleen.

Cutaneous zygomycosis has been reported in two adult female rhesus monkeys following extensive fight wound trauma (Baskin *et al.,* 1984). In both monkeys there was extensive bruising, lacerations, and puncture wounds to the skin. Severe necrosis occurred in affected areas that were blackened, edematous, friable, and covered with a fibrinopurulent exudate. Rhinoorbital lesions occurred during quarantine in a rhesus monkey believed to have diabetes mellitus (Martin *et al.,* 1969). The facial lesions began as severe pustular dermatitis that progressed to extensive ulcerative and excoriated skin lesions with erosion of the orbit and sinuses. The monkey also had a large draining submandibular mass.

The hallmark microscopic lesion of zygomycosis due to Mucorales, regardless of site, is angioinvasion and thrombosis, which was found in all cases in nonhuman primates. Histologic lesions in the gastrointestinal tract were characterized by ulcerative and necrotizing granulomatous inflammation containing fungal hyphae (Migaki *et al.,* 1982b). Large hyphae, 7–15 μm in diameter, irregularly branched, bulbous, with rare septae were observed. Cutaneous zygomycosis was characterized microscopically by full thickness necrosis with a loss of normal architecture in the skin, subcutaneous tissue, and underlying muscle from affected areas (Baskin *et al.,* 1984). Adjacent areas contained diffuse edema, hemorrhage, and mixed inflammatory cell infiltrates. Broad, 10–20 μm, irregularly branched, thin-walled hyphae, 10–60 μm long with infrequent septae, were found in skin (Fig. 13), subcutaneous tissue, and muscle. Microscopic lesions in the case of rhinoorbital zygomycosis consisted of ulceration and suppuration of the epidermis and confluent granulomatous inflammation with giant cells within the dermis (Martin *et al.*, 1969). Amphophilic, aseptate, irregularly branching fungal hyphae, 4–24 μm wide, were found in the granulomas. The bone of the orbit, the frontal and paranasal sinuses, and the turbinates were diffusely infiltrated with granulumatous inflammation containing numerous hyphae. The submandibular mass consisted of granulomatous inflammation infiltrating the contiguous lymph nodes and salivary gland.

Presumptive diagnosis of zygomycosis caused by fungi of the order Mucorales can be made from the microscopic appearance of fungal hyphae in the lesions and the presence of hyphal invasion of blood vessels and thrombosis (Migaki *et al.*, 1982b). Fungal elements usually stain well with hematoxylin and eosin and may stain poorly with Gomori methenamine silver. Immunofluoresence techniques may be used to aid in identifying fungi in formalin-fixed tissues (Baskin *et al.*, 1984). Because these organisms are ubiquitous in the environment, isolation of the agent is not sufficient for diagnosis.

b. ENTOMOPHTHORALES. Fungi of the order Entomophthorales, including genera *Basidiobolus* and *Conidiobolus*, are found in Africa, Asia, and South America. These fungi differ from Mucorales in culture in that hyphae are septate and either conidia or sporangia are produced. In humans, *Basiobolus haptosporus* infection is associated with subcutaneous nodules. *Conidiobolus* (*Entomophthora*) *coronatus* causes rhinophycomycosis. These forms of zygomycosis are referred to as entomophthoromycosis.

In nonhuman primates there are two reports of entomophthoromycosis. A feral chimpanzee developed lesions on the nose and eyebrows due to infection with *Entomophthora coronata* (Roy and Cameron, 1972) and a mandrill died from disseminated systemic entomophthoromycosis (Migaki *et al.*, 1982a). The mandrill had been treated symptomatically for a nonspecific disease that presented as depression, weakness, excessive salivation, and respiratory distress. Necropsy findings included pleural adhesion and consolidation of the left lung lobes with firm masses within the lobes; a large solid multiloculated mediastinal mass; thickening of the pericardium and epicardium with pericardial effusion; and mesenteric lymphadenopathy. Thickening of the gastric wall, hepatomegaly, and lesions in the kidneys were also noted. Cut sections of masses in affected tissues revealed large yellow-white caseonecrotic lesions. Microscopically these lesions were chronic pyogranulomas with a large central core of neutrophils and eosinophils bordered by a wide zone of macrophages, multinucleate giant cells, and fibrocytes. Irregularly branching thin-walled hyphae, 6–12 μm in diameter, were found in the necrotic centers. The Splendore–Hoeppli phenomenon, a wide collar of eosinophilic material around the hyphae characteristic of Entomophthorales, was observed. Diagnosis was based on the histologic appearance of the hyphae and the accompanying eosinophilic precipitate (Migaki *et al.*, 1982a).

ACKNOWLEDGMENTS

The author thanks Jim Artwohl and Mary Lang of the Biologic Resources Laboratory, University of Illinois at Chicago, for assistance with the figures in this chapter. The author also recognizes G. Baskin, T. Butler, M. Kessler, and the University of Missouri Research Animal Diagnostic and Investigative Laboratory for providing specimens.

REFERENCES

Agarwal, K. C., and Chakravarti, R. N. (1969). Preliminary observations on the intestinal bacterial flora of wild rhesus monkeys with special reference to shigellosis, salmonellosis, and vibriosis. *J. Assoc. Phys. India* **17**, 409–412.

Al-Doory, Y. (1972). Fungal and bacterial diseases. *In* "Pathology of Simian Primates" (R. N. T.-W. Fiennes, ed.), pp. 206–241. Karger, Basel.

Al-Doory, Y., Pinkerton, M. E., and Vice, T. E. (1969). Pulmonary nocardiosis in a vervet monkey. *J. Am. Vet. Med. Assoc.* **155**(7), 1179–1180.

Alford, P. L., Lee, D. R., Binhazim, A. A., Hubbard, G. B., and Matherne, C. M. (1996). Naturally acquired leprosy in two wild-born chimpanzees. *Lab. Anim. Sci.* **46**(3), 341–346.

Allen, A. M., and Kinard, R. F. (1958). Primary cutaneous inoculation of tuberculosis in *Macaca mulatta* monkeys. *Am. J. Pathol.* **34**, 337–345.

Altman, N. H., and Small, J. D. (1973). Actinomycosis in a primate confirmed by fluorescent antibody technics in formalin fixed tissue. *Lab. Anim. Sci.* **23**, 696–700.

Altwegg, M., and Geiss, H. K. (1989). *Aeromonas* as a human pathogen. *Crit. Rev. Microbiol.* **16**, 253–286.

Anderson, K. F., Kiehlbauch, J. A., and Anderson, D. C. (1993). *Arcobacter (Campylobacter) butzleri*-associated diarrheal illness in a nonhuman primate population. *Infect. Immun.* **61**, 2220–2223.

Arean, V. M. (1962). Studies on the pathogenesis of leptospires. II. A clinicopathologic evaluation of hepatic and renal function in experimental leptospiral infections. *Lab. Invest.* **11**, 273–288.

Arya, S. C., Verghese, A., and Agarwal, D. S. (1973). Shigellosis in rhesus monkeys in quarantine. *Lab. Anim.* **7**, 101–109.

Attleberger, M. H. (1984). Laboratory diagnosis of fungal and achloric algal infections. *In* "Clinical Microbiology and Infectious Diseases of the Dog and Cat" (C. E. Greene, ed.), pp. 129–136. Saunders, Philadelphia.

Audebad, G., Ganzin, M., Ceccaldi, J., and Merville, P. (1954). Isolement d'un *Chromobacterium violaceum* à partir de lésions hépatiques observées chez un singe *Cercopithecus cephus* étude et pouvoir pathogène. *Ann. Inst. Pasteur* **87**, 413–417.

Baggs, R. B., Hunt, R. D., Garcia, F. G., Hajema, E. M., Blake, B. J., and Fraser, C. E. O. (1976). Pseudotuberculosis (*Yersinia enterocolitica*) in the owl monkey (*Aotus trivirgatus*). *Lab. Anim. Sci.* **26**(6), 1079–1083.

Bagnall, B. G., and Grunberg, W. (1972). Generalized *Trichophyton mentagrophytes* ringworm in capuchin monkeys (*Cebus nigrivitatus*) *Br. J. Dermatol.* **87**, 655–570.

Baker, H. J., Bradford, L. G., and Montes, L. F. (1971). Dermatophytosis due to *Microsporum canis* in a rhesus monkey. *J. Am. Vet. Med. Assoc.* **159**, 1607–1611.

Banish, L. D., Sims, R., Sack, D., Montali, R. J., Phillips, L., Jr., and Bush, M. (1993a). Prevalence of shigellosis and other enteric pathogens in a zoologic collection. *J. Am. Vet. Med. Assoc.* **203**(1), 126–132.

Banish, L. D., Sims, R., Bush, M., Sack, D., and Montali, R. J. (1993b). Clearance of *Shigella flexneri* carriers in a zoologic collection of primates. *J. Am. Vet. Med. Assoc.* **203**(1), 133–136.

Barsanti, J. A. (1984). Miscellaneous fungal infections. *In* "Clinical Microbiology and Infectious Diseases of the Dog and Cat" (C. E. Greene, ed.), pp. 738–746. Saunders, Philadelphia.

Baskerville, A., and Newell, D. G. (1988). Naturally occurring chronic gastritis and *C. pylori* infection in the rhesus monkey: A potential model for gastritis in man. *Gut* **29**, 465–472.

Baskerville, M., Wood, M., and Baskerville, A. (1983). An outbreak of *Bordetella bronchiseptica* in a colony of common marmosets (*Callithrix jacchus*). *Lab. Anim.* **17**, 350–355.

Baskin, G. B. (1991). Disseminated histoplasmosis in a SIV-infected rhesus monkey. *J. Med. Primatol.* **20**, 251–253.

Baskin, G. B., Chandler, F. W., and Watson, E. A. (1984). Cutaneous zygomycosis in rhesus monkeys (*Macaca mulatta*). *Vet. Pathol.* **21**, 125–128.

Bellinger, D. A., and Bullock, B. C. (1988). Cutaneous *Mycobacterium avium* infection in a cynomologus monkey. *Lab. Anim. Sci.* **38**(1), 85–86.

Bellini, S., Hubbard, G. B., and Kaufman, L. (1991). Spontaneous fatal coccidioidomycosis in a native-born hybrid baboon (*Papio cynocephalus anubis/Papio cynocephalus cynocephalus*). *Lab. Anim. Sci.* **41**(5), 509–511.

Bemis, D. A., Griesen, H. A., and Appel, M. J. G. (1977). Pathogenesis of canine bordetellosis. *J. Infect. Dis.* **135**, 735–762.

Benham, R. W. and Keston, B. (1932). Sporothricosis: Its transmission to plants and animals. *J. Infec. Dis.* **50**, 437–458.

Benjamin, S. A., and Lang, C. M. (1971). Acute pasteurellosis in owl monkeys (*Aotus trivirgatus*). *Lab. Anim. Sci.* **21**(2), 258–262.

Bennett, B. T., Causay, L., Welsh, T. J., Belhun, F. Z., and Schofield, L. (1980). Acute gastric dilatation in monkeys: A microbiologic study of gastric contents, blood and feed. *Lab. Anim. Sci.* **30**(2), 241–244.

Bergeland, M. E., Barnes, D. M., and Kaplan, W. (1970). "Spontaneous Histoplasmosis in a Squirrel Monkey," Primate Surveillance Zoonosis Rep. No. 1, pp. 10–11. CDC, Atlanta, GA.

Bernadini, M. L., Fontaine, A., and Sansonetti, P. J. (1990). The two-component regulatory system OmpR-EnvZ controls the virulence of *Shigella flexneri*. *J. Bacteriol.* **172**, 6274–6281.

Blaser, M. J. (1990). *Helicobacter pylori* and the pathogenesis of gastroduodenal inflammation. *J. Infect. Dis.* **161**, 626–633.

Blaser, M. J. (1993). *Helicobacter pylori:* Microbiology of a 'slow' bacterial infection. *Trends Microbiol.* **1**(7), 255–259.

Boncyk, L. H., Brack, M., and Kalter, S. S. (1972). Hemorrhagic enteritis in a baboon (*Papio cynocephalus*) due to *Vibrio fetus*. *Lab. Anim. Sci.* **22**(5), 734–738.

Boncyk, L. H., McCullough, B., Grotts, D. D., and Kalter, S. S. (1975). Localized nocardiosis due to *Nocardia caviae* in a baboon (*Papio cynocephalus*). *Lab. Anim. Sci.* **25**(1), 88–91.

Brack, M., and Hosefelder, F. (1992). In vitro characteristics of *Yersinia pseudotuberculosis* of nonhuman primate origin. *Zentralbl. Bakteriol.* **277**, 280–287.

Brack, M., Bonyck, L. H., Moore, G. T., and Kalter, S. S. (1975). Bacterial meningo-encephalitis in newborn baboons (*Papio cynocephalus*). *Contemp. Primatol., Proc. Int. Congr. Primatol., 5th, 1974*, pp. 493–501.

Brammer, D. W., O'Rourke, C. M., Heath, L. A., Chrisp, C. E., Peter, G. K., and Hofing, G. L. (1995). *Mycobacterium kansasii* infection in squirrel monkeys (*Saimiri sciureus sciureus*). *J. Med. Primatol.* **24**, 231–235.

Brendt, R. F., McDonough, W. E., and Walker, J. S. (1974). Persistence of *Diplococcus pneumoniae* after influenza virus infection in *Macaca mulatta*. *Infect. Immun.* **10**, 369–374.

Bresnahan, J. F., Whitworth, U. G., Hayes, Y., Summers, E., and Pollock, J. (1984). *Yersinia enterocolitica* infection in breeding colonies of ruffed lemurs. *J. Am. Vet. Med. Assoc.* **185**(11), 1354–1356.

Breznock, A. W., Henrickson, R. V., Silverman, S., and Schwartz, L. W. (1975). Coccidioidomycosis in a rhesus monkey. *J. Am. Vet. Med. Assoc.* **167**(7), 657–661.

Bronsdon, M. A., and DiGiacomo, R. F. (1993). *Pasteurella multocida* infections in baboons (*Papio cynocephalus*). *Primates* **34**(2), 205–209.

Bronsdon, M. A., and Schoenknecht, F. D. (1988). *Campylobacter pylori* isolated from the stomach of the monkey, *Macaca nemestrina*. *J. Clin. Microbiol.* **26**(9), 1725–1728.

Bronsdon, M. A., Goodwin, C. S., Sly, L. I., Chilvers, T., and Schoenknecht, F. D. (1991). *Helicobacter nemestrinae* sp. nov., a spiral bacterium found in the stomach of a pigtailed macaque (*Macaca nemestrina*). *Int. J. Syst. Bacteriol.* **41**(1), 148–153.

Bronson, R. T., May, B. D., and Ruebner, B. H. (1972). An outbreak of infection by *Yersinia pseudotuberculosis*. *Am. J. Pathol.* **69**, 289–303.

Brown, T. M., Clark, H. W., and Bailey, J. S. (1980). Rheumatoid arthritis in the gorilla: A study of mycoplasma-host interaction into the pathogenesis and treatment. *In* "The Comparative Pathology of Zoo Animals" (R. J. Montali and G. Migaki, eds.), pp. 259–266. Smithsonian Institution Press, Washington, DC.

Bryant, J. L., Stills, H. F., Jr., Lentsch, R. H., and Middleton, C. C. (1983). *Campylobacter jejuni* isolated from patas monkeys with diarrhea. *Lab. Anim. Sci.* **33**(3), 303–305.

Buhles, W. C., Jr., Vanderlip, J. E., Russell, S. W., and Alexander, N. L. (1981). *Yersinia pseudotuberculosis* infection: Study of an epizootic in squirrel monkeys. *J. Clin. Microbiol.* **13**, 519–525.

Burkholder, C. R., Hirsh, D. W., Hickman, R. L., and Soave, O. A. (1967). Influence of isoniazid therapy on the course of tuberculosis in a rhesus monkey. *J. Am. Vet. Med. Assoc.* **151**(7), 918–919.

Butler, T. M., and Hubbard, G. B. (1991). An epizootic of *Histoplasmosis duboisii* (African histoplasmosis) in an American baboon colony. *Lab. Anim. Sci.* **41**(5), 407–410.

Butler, T. M., Schmidt, R. E., and Wiley, G. L. (1971). Melioidosis in a chimpanzee. *Am. J. Vet. Res.* **32**(7), 1109–1117.

Butler, T. M., Gleiser, C. A., Bernal, J. C., and Ajello, L. (1988). Case of disseminated African histoplasmosis in a baboon. *J. Med. Primatol.* **17**, 153–161.

Cambre, R. C., Wilson, H. L., Spraker, T. R., and Favara, B. E. (1980). Fatal airsacculitis and pneumonia, with abortion, in an orangutan. *J. Am. Vet. Med. Assoc.* **177**(9), 822–824.

Campos, M. F., Alvares, J. N., Arruda, M. F., and do Vale, N. B. (1981). Surto epizoótico por *Klebsiella* sp num núcleo de reprodução de sagüis (*Callithrix jacchus*), em cativiero. *Rev. Biotérios* **1**, 95–99.

Carpenter, K. P., and Cooke, E. F. N. (1965). An attempt to find shigellae in wild primates. *J. Comp. Pathol.* **75**, 201–208.

Carvalho, A. C. T., Queiroz, D. M. M., Mendes, E. N., Rocha, G. A., Cisalpino, E. O., Pereira, L. H., and Melo, A. L. (1987). *Campylobacter jejuni* intestinal infection in an outdoor colony-born *Callithrix penicillata*. *Int. J. Primatol.* **8**, 502.

Castleman, W. L., Anderson, J., and Holmberg, C. A. (1980). Posterior paralysis and spinal osteomyelitis in a rhesus monkey with coccidioidomycosis. *J. Am. Vet. Med. Assoc.* **177**(9), 933–934.

Centers for Disease Control. (1993). Tuberculosis in imported nonhuman primates—United States, June 1990–May 1993. *Morbid. Mortal. Wkly. Rep.* **42**(29), 572–576.

Chalifoux, L. V., and Hajema, E. M. (1981). Septicemia and meningoencephalitis caused by *Listeria monocytogenes* in a neonatal *Macaca fasicularis*. *J. Med. Primatol* **10**, 336–339.

Chalifoux, L. V., Hajema, E. M., and Lee-Parritz, D. (1993). *Aeromonas hydrophilia* peritonitis in a cotton-top tamarin (*Saguinus oedipus*), and retrospective study of infections in seven primate species. *Lab. Anim. Sci.* **43**(4), 355–358.

Chalmers, D. T., Murgatroyd, L. B., and Wadsworth, P. F. (1983). A survey of the pathology of marmosets (*Callithrix jacchus*) derived from a marmoset breeding unit. *Lab. Anim.* **17**, 270–279.

Chandler, F. W., McClure, H. M., Campbell, W. G., Jr., and Watts, J. C. (1976). Pulmonary pneumocystosis in nonhuman primates. *Arch. Pathol. Lab. Med.* **100**, 163–167.

Chandler, F. W., Kaplan, W., and Aiello, L. (1980). "Color Atlas and Text of the Histopathology of Mycotic Diseases," pp. 122–127. Year Book Med. Publ., Chicago.

Chang, J., Wagner, J. L., and Kornegay, R. W. (1980). Fatal *Yersinia pseudotuberculosis* infection in captive bushbabies. *J. Am. Vet. Med. Assoc.* **177**(9), 820–821.

Chapman, W. L., Jr. (1967). Acute gastric dilatation in *Macaca mulatta* and *Macaca speciosa* monkeys. *Lab. Anim. Care* **17**, 130–136.

Chapman, W. L., and Crowell, W. A. (1977). Amyloidosis in rhesus monkeys with rheumatoid arthritis and enterocolitis. *J. Am. Vet. Med. Assoc.* **177**(9), 855–858.

Cicmanec, J. L. (1977). Medical problems encountered in a callitrichid colony. *In* "The Biology and Conservation of the Callitrichidae" (D. G. Kleinman, ed.), pp. 331–336. Smithsonian Institution Press, Washington, DC.

Clarke, G. C., and Schmidt, J. P. (1969). Effects of prophylactic isoniazid on early developing tuberculosis in *Macaca mulatta. Am. Rev. Respir. Dis.* **100,** 224–227.

Cole, R. J., Jr. (1990). *Streptococcus* and related cocci. *In* "Diagnostic Procedures in Veterinary Microbiology" (G. R. Carter and J. R. Cole, Jr., eds.), pp. 211–220. Academic Press, San Diego, CA.

Cooper, J. E., and Needham, J. R. (1976). An outbreak of shigellosis in laboratory marmosets and tamarins. *J. Hyg.* **76**(3), 415–424.

Corcoran, K. D., and Thoen, C. O. (1991). Application of an enzyme immunoassay for detecting antibodies in sera of *Macaca fascicularis* naturally exposed to *Mycobacterium tuberculosis. J. Med. Primatol.* **20,** 404–408.

Cornelius, G., Laroche, Y., Ballingand, G., Sory, M.-P., and Wauters, G. (1987). *Yersinia enterocolitica,* a primary model of bacterial invasiveness. *Rev. Infect. Dis.* **9**(1), 64–87.

Costa, E. O., Diniz, L. S. M., Dagli, M. L. Z., and Arruda, C. (1991). Delayed hypersensitivity test: Paracocciodioidin in Latin American wild mammals considering 'habitats' terrestrial X tree-dwellings. *In* "Congresso Mundial de Medicina Veterinária," p. 320. Anais, Rio de Janeiro.

Costa, E. O., Diniz, L. S. M., Netto, C. F., Arruda, C., and Dagli, M. L. Z. (1994). Epidemiological study of sporotrichosis and histoplasmosis in captive Latin American wild mammals, Sao Paulo, Brazil. *Mycopathologia* **125,** 19–22.

Courtois, G., Segretain, G., Mariat, F., and Levaditi, J. C. (1955). Mycose cutanée à corps levuriformes observée chez des singes africains en captivité. *Ann. Inst. Pasteur, Paris* **89,** 124–127.

Curry, A., Jones, D. M., and Eldridge, J. (1987). Spiral organisms in the baboon stomach. *Lancet* **2,** 634–635.

Dance, D. A. B. (1990). Melioidosis. *Rev. Med. Microbiol.* **1,** 143–150.

Dance, D. A. B. (1991). Melioidosis: The tip of the iceberg? *Clin. Microbiol. Rev.* **4**(1), 52–60.

Dannenberg, A. M., Jr. (1978). Pathogenesis of pulmonary tuberculosis in man and animals: Protection of personnel against tuberculosis. *In* "Mycobacterial Infections in Zoo Animals" (R. J. Montali, ed.), pp. 65–75. Smithsonian Press, Washington, DC.

Dei-Cas, E., Jackson, H., Palluault, F., Aiouat, E. M., Hancock, V., Soulez, B., and Camus, D. (1991). Ultrastructural observations on the attachment of *Pneumocystis carinii in vitro. J. Protozol.* **38,** 205S–207S.

Deinhardt, F., Holmes, A. W., Devine, J., and Deinhardt, J. (1967). Marmosets as laboratory animals. IV. The microbiology of laboratory-kept marmosets. *Lab. Anim. Care* **17,** 48–70.

Deinhardt, J. B., Devine, J., Passavoy, M., Pohlman, R., and Deinhardt, F. (1967). Marmosets as laboratory animals. I. Care of marmosets in the laboratory, pathology and outline of the statistical evaluation of data. *Lab. Anim. Care* **17,** 11–29.

DiGiacomo, R. F., and Missakian, E. A. (1972). Tetanus in a free-ranging colony of *Macaca mulatta:* A clinical and epizootiologic study. *Lab. Anim. Sci.* **22**(3), 378–383.

Dillehay, D. L., and Huerkamp, M. J. (1990). Tuberculosis in a tuberculin-negative rhesus monkey (*Macaca mulatta*) on chemoprophylaxis. *J. Zoo Wildl. Med.* **21**(4), 480–484.

Dolensek, E. P., Napolitano, R. L., and Kazimiroff, J. (1977). Gastrointestinal geotrichosis in six adult gorillas. *J. Am. Vet. Med. Assoc.* **171,** 975–976.

Dow, S. W., Jones, R. L., and Rosychuk, R. A. (1989). Bacteriologic specimens, selection, collection and transport for optimum results. *Compend. Contin. Educ. Pract. Vet.* **11,** 686–702.

Doyle, L., Young, C. L., Jang, S. S., and Hillier, S. L. (1991). Normal vaginal aerobic and anaerobic bacterial flora of the rhesus macaque (*Macaca mulatta*). *J. Med. Primatol.* **20,** 409–413.

Drazek, E. S., Dubois, A., and Holmes, R. K. (1994). Characterization and presumptive identification of *Helicobacter pylori* isolates from rhesus monkeys. *J. Clin. Microbiol.* **32**(7), 1799–1804.

Dubois, A., Tarnawski, A., Newell, D. G., Fiala, N., Dabros, W., Stachura, J., Krivan, H., and Heman-Ackah, L. M. (1991). Gastric injury and invasion of parietal cells by spiral bacteria in rhesus monkeys. *Gastroenterology* **100,** 884–891.

Dubois, A., Fiala, N., Heman-Ackah, L. M., Drazek, E. S., Tarnawski, A., Fishbein, W. N., Perez-Perez, G. I., and Blaser, M. J. (1994). Natural gastric infection with *Helicobacter pylori* in monkeys: A model for spiral bacteria infection in humans. *Gastroenterology* **106,** 1405–1417.

Duncan, A. J., Carman, R. J., and Olson, G. J. (1993). Assignment of the agent of Tyzzer's disease to *Clostridium piliforme* comb. nov. On the basis of 16S rRNA sequence analysis. *Int. J. Syst. Bacteriol.* **43,** 314–318.

Duncan, M., Nichols, D. K., Montali, R. J., and Thomas, L. A. (1994). An epizootic of *Salmonella enteritidis* at the National Zoological Park. *Proc. Am. Assoc. Zoo Vet.,* pp. 256–248.

Emmons, R. W., Woodie, J. D., Taylor, M. S., and Nygaard, G. S. (1970). Tularemia in a pet squirrel monkey (*Saimiri sciureus*). *Lab. Anim. Care* **20**(6), 1149–1153.

Eriksson, O. E. (1994). *Pneumocystis carinii,* a parasite in lungs of mammals, referred to a new family and order (*Pneumocystidaceae, Pneumocystidales, Ascomycota*). *Syst. Ascomycetum* **13**(2), 164–180.

Euler, A. R., Zurenko, G. E., Moe, J. B., Ulrich, R. G., and Yagi, Y. (1990). Evaluation of two monkey species (*Macaca mulatta* and *Macaca fascicularis*) as possible models for human *Helicobacter pylori* disease. *J. Clin. Microbiol.* **28**(10), 2285–2290.

Fear, F. A., Pinkerton, M. E., Cline, J. A., Kriewaldt, F., and Kalter, S. S. (1968). A leptospirosis outbreak in a baboon (*Papio* sp.) Colony. *Lab. Anim. Care* **18,** 22–28.

Fiennes, R. (1967). "Zoonoses of Primates: The Epidemiology and Ecology of Diseases in Relation to Man." Cornell University Press, Ithaca, NY.

Fitzgeorge, R. B., Baskerville, A., and Lander, K. P. (1981). Experimental infection of rhesus monkeys with a human strain of *Campylobacter jejuni. J. Hyg.* **86,** 343–351.

Fleischman, R. W., and McCracken, D. (1977). Paecilomycosis in a nonhuman primate (*Macaca mulatta*). *Vet. Pathol.* **14,** 387–391.

Flynn, N. M., Hoeprich, P. D., and Kawachi, M. M. (1979). An unusual outbreak of windborne coccidioidomycosis. *N. Engl. J. Med.* **301,** 358–361.

Fourie, P. B., and Odendaal, M. W. (1983). *Mycobacterium tuberculosis* in a closed colony of baboons (*Papio ursinus*). *Lab. Anim.* **17,** 125–128.

Fox, J. G. (1975). Transmissible drug resistance in *Shigella* and *Salmonella* isolated from pet monkeys and their owners. *J. Med. Primatol.* **4**(3), 165–171.

Fox, J. G., and Frost, W. W. (1974). *Corynebacterium ulcerans* mastitis in a bonnet macaque (*Macaca radiata*). *Lab. Anim. Sci.* **24**(5), 820–822.

Fox, J. G., and Rohovsky, M. W. (1975). Meningitis caused by *Klebsiella* spp in two rhesus monkeys. *J. Am. Vet. Med. Assoc.* **167**(7), 634–636.

Fox, J. G., and Wikse, S. E. (1971). Bacterial meningoencephalitis in rhesus monkeys: Clinical and pathological features. *Lab. Anim. Sci.* **21**(4), 558–563.

Fox, J. G., Campbell, L. H., Reed, C., Snyder, S. B., and Soave, O. A. (1973). *Dermatophilus* (cutaneous streptothricosis) in owl monkeys. *J. Am. Vet. Med. Assoc.* **163,** 642–644.

Fox, J. G., Campbell, L. H., Snyder, S. B., Reed, C., and Soave, O. A. (1974). Tuberculous spondylitis and Pott's paraplegia in a rhesus monkey. *Lab. Anim. Sci.* **24**(2), 335–339.

Frank, H. (1968). Systemiche Histoplasmose bei einem afrikanischen Affen. *Dtsch. Tierërztl. Wochenschr.* **75,** 371–374.

Fremming, B., D., Benson, R. E., Young, R. J., and Harris, M. D., Jr. (1957). Antituberculous therapy in *Macaca mulatta* monkeys. *Am. Rev. Tuberc. Pulm. Dis.* **76,** 225–231.

Fritz, P. E., Miller, J. G., Slayter, M., and Smith, T. J. (1986). Naturally occurring melioidosis in a colonized rhesus monkey (*Macaca mulatta*). *Lab. Anim.* **20,** 281–285.

Fuchs, G., Mobassaleh, M., Donahue-Rolfe, A., Montgomery, R. K., Grand, R. J., and Keusch, G. T. (1986). Pathogenesis of *Shigella* diarrhea: Rabbit intestinal cell microvillus membrane binding site for *Shigella* toxin. *Infect. Immun.* **53**(2), 372–377.

Galton, M. M., Mitchell, R. B., Clark, G., and Riessen, A. H. (1948). Enteric infections in chimpanzees and spider monkeys with special reference to a sulfadiazine resistant *Shigella. J. Infect. Dis.* **83**, 147–154.

Garner, F. M., Ford, D. F., and Ross, M. A. (1969). Systemic cryptococcosis in 2 monkeys. *J. Am. Vet. Med. Assoc.* **155**, 1163–1168.

Garvey, W., Fathi, A., and Bigelow, F. B. (1985). Modified Steiner for the demonstration of spirochetes. *J. Histotechnol.* **8**(1), 15–17.

George, J. W., and Lerche, N. W. (1990). Electrolyte abnormalities associated with diarrhea in rhesus monkeys: 100 cases (1986–1987). *J. Am. Vet. Med. Assoc.* **196**(10), 1654–1658.

Gianella, R. A., Gots, R. E., Charney, A. N., Greenough, W. B., and Formal, S. B. (1975). Pathogenesis of *Salmonella*-mediated intestinal fluid secretion: Activation of adenylate cyclase and inhibition by indomethacin. *Gastroenterology* **69**, 1238–1245.

Gibson, S., Matherne, C., Brady, A., and Abee, C. (1993). Disseminated yeast infection in wild-caught owl monkeys (*Aotus vociferans* and *Aotus nancymai*). *Lab. Anim. Sci.* **43**(4), 391.

Gilbert, S. G., Reuhl, K. R., Wong, J. H., and Rice, D. C. (1987). Fatal pneumococcal meningitis in a colony-born monkey (*Macaca fasicularis*). *J. Med. Primatol.* **16**, 333–338.

Giles, R. C., Jr., Hildebrandt, P. K., and Tate, C. (1974). *Klebsiella* air sacculitis in the owl monkey (*Aotus trivirgatus*). *Lab. Anim. Sci.* **24**(4), 610–616.

Giorgi, W., Matera, A., Mollaret, H. H., and Pestana de Castro, A. F. (1969). Isolamento de *Yersinia enterocolitica* de abscessos hepaticos de sagüis (*Callithrix penicillata* e *Callithrix jacchus*). *Arq. Inst. Biol., Sao Paulo* **36**, 123–127.

Gisler, D. B., and Pitcock, J. A. (1962). Intestinal mucormycosis in the monkey (*Macaca mulatta*). *Am. J. Vet. Res.* **23**, 365–367.

Good, R. C., and May, B. D. (1971). Respiratory pathogens in monkeys. *Infect. Immun.* **3**, 87–99.

Good, R. C., May, B. D., and Kawatomari, T. (1969). Enteric pathogens in monkeys. *J. Bacteriol.* **97**(3), 1048–1055.

Goodwin, B. T., Jerome, C. P., and Bullock, B. C. (1988). Unusual lesion morphology and skin test reaction for *Mycobacterium avium* complex in macaques. *Lab. Anim. Sci.* **38**(1), 20–24.

Goodwin, W. J., Haines, R. J., and Bernal, J. C. (1987). Tetanus in baboons of a corral breeding colony. *Lab. Anim. Sci.* **37**(2), 231–232.

Gordon, M. A., and Little, G. N. (1967). *Trichophyton (microsporum) gallinae* ringworm in a monkey. *Sabaraudia* **6**, 207–212.

Gormus, B. J., Xu, K., Alford, P. A., Lee, D. R., Hubbard, G. B., Eichberg, J. W., and Meyers, W. M. (1991). A serologic study of naturally acquired leprosy in chimpanzees. *Int. J. Lepr.* **59**(3), 450–457.

Gozalo, A., and Montoya, E. (1991a). *Klebsiella pneumoniae* infection in a New World nonhuman primate center. *Lab. Primate Newsl.* **30**(2), 13–15.

Gozalo, A., and Montoya, E. (1991b). Mortality causes in the moustached tamarin (*Saguinus mystax*) in captivity. *J. Med. Primatol.* **21**, 35–38.

Gozalo, A., Block, K., Montoya, E., Moro, J., and Escamilla, J. (1991). A survey for *Campylobacter* in feral and captive tamarins. *Primatol. Today,* pp. 675–676.

Gozalo, A., Montoya, E., and Revolledo, L. (1992). *Pasteurella hemolytica* infection in a Goeldie's monkey. *J. Med. Primatol.* **21**, 387–388.

Graczyk, T. K., Cranfield, M. R., Kempske, S. E., and Eckhaus, M. A. (1995). Fulminant *Streptococcus pneumoniae* meningitis in a lion-tailed macaque (*Macaca silenus*) without detected signs. *J. Wildl. Dis.* **31**(1), 75–77.

Graham, D. Y., Lew, G. M., Klein, P. D., Evans, D. G., Evans, D. J., Jr., Saeed, Z. A., and Malaty, H. M. (1992). Effect of treatment of *Helicobacter pylori* infection on the long-term recurrence of gastric or duodenal ulcer. *Ann. Intern. Med.* **116**(9), 705–708.

Graves, J. L. (1968). *Bordetella bronchiseptica* isolated from a fatal case of bronchopneumonia in an African green monkey. *Lab. Anim. Care* **18**, 405–406.

Greenberg, B., and Sanati, M. (1970). Enteropathogenic types of *Escherichia coli* from primates and cockroaches in a zoo. *J. Med. Entomol.* **7**(6), 744.

Greene, C. E. (1984). Tetanus. *In* "Clinical Microbiology and Infectious Diseases of the Dog and Cat" (C. E. Greene, ed.), pp. 608–616. Saunders, Philadelphia.

Greenstein, E. T., Doty, R. W., and Lowy, K. (1965). An outbreak of a fulminating infectious disease in the squirrel monkey (*Saimiri sciureus*). *Lab. Anim. Care* **15**(1), 74–80.

Griner, L. A. (1983). "Pathology of Zoo Animals." Zoological Society of San Diego, San Diego, CA.

Groves, M. G., Strauss, J. M., Abbas, J., and Davis, C. E. (1969). Natural infection of gibbons with a bacterium producing violet pigment (*Chromobacterium violaceum*). *J. Infect. Dis.* **120**, 605–610.

Gugnani, H. C. (1971). *Trichophyton mentagrophytes* infection in monkeys and its transmission to man. *Hind. Antibiot. Bull.* **14**, 11–13.

Haberle, A. J. (1970). Tuberculosis in an orangutan. *J. Zoo Anim. Med.* **1**, 10–15.

Haider, K., Albert, M. J., Hossain, A., and Nahir, S. (1991). Contact-haemolysin production by entero-invasive *Escherichia coli* and shigellae. *J. Med. Microbiol.* **35**, 330–336.

Harkness, J. E., and Wagner, J. E. (1988). "The Biology and Medicine of Rabbits and Rodents." Lea & Febiger, Philadelphia.

Hartley, E. G. (1975). The incidence and antibiotic sensitivity of *Shigella* bacteria isolated from newly imported macaque monkeys. *Br. Vet. J.* **131**, 205–212.

Hauck, H., and Klehr, N. (1977). Meerkatzenfavus als ursache für die pilzinfektion eines menschen. *Z. Allg. Med.* **53**, 331–332.

Hazell, S. L., Lee, A., Brady, L., and Hennessy, W. (1986). *Campylobacter pyloridis* and gastritis: Association with intracellular spaces and adaptation to an environment of mucus as important factors in colonization of the gastric epithelium. *J. Infect. Dis.* **153**(4), 658–663.

Hazell, S. T., Eichberg, J. W., Lee, D. R., Alpert, L., Evans, D. G., Evans, D. J., Jr., and Graham, D. Y. (1992). Selection of the chimpanzee over the baboon as a model for *Helicobacter pylori* infection. *Gastroenterology* **103**, 848–854.

Herceg, M., Marzan, B., Hajsig, M., Naglic, T., and Huber, I. (1977). Pathomorphological observations of spontaneous candidal encephalitis in a monkey. *Vet. Arh.* **47**, 183–187.

Herman, P. H., and Fox, J. G. (1971). Panophthalmitis associated with diplococcic septicemia in a rhesus monkey. *J. Am. Vet. Med. Assoc.* **159**(5), 560–562.

Hessler, J. R., Woodard, J. C., Beattie, R. J., and Moreland, A. F. (1967). Mucormycosis in a rhesus monkey. *J. Am. Vet. Med. Assoc.* **151**, 909–913.

Hirai, K., Suzuki, Y., Kato, N., Yagami, K., Miyoshi, A., Mabuchi, Y., Nigi, H., Inagaki, H., Otsuki, K., and Tsubokura, M. (1974). *Yersinia pseudotuberculosis* infection occurred spontaneously in a group of patas monkeys (*Erythrocebus patas*). *Jpn. J. Vet. Sci.* **36**, 351–355.

Hird, D. W., Anderson, J. H., and Bielitski, J. T. (1984). Diarrhea in nonhuman primates: A survey of primate colonies for incidence rates and clinical opinion. *Lab. Anim. Sci.* **34**(5), 465–470.

Hirsh, D. C., Boorman, G. A., and Jang, S. S. (1975). Erysipelas in a black and red tamarin. *J. Am. Vet. Med. Assoc.* **167**, 646–647.

Holmberg, C. A., Henrickson, R. V., Malaga, C., Schneider, R., and Gribble, D. (1982). Nontuberculous mycobacterial disease in rhesus monkeys. *Vet. Pathol.* **19**, Suppl., 9–16.

Holmberg, C. A., Henrickson, R., Lenninger, R., Anderson, J., Hayashi, L., and Ellingsworth, L. (1985). Immunologic abnormality in a group of *Macaca arctoides* with high mortality due to atypical mycobacterial and other disease processes. *Am. J. Vet. Res.* **46**(5), 1192–1196.

Hoopes, P. J., McKay, D. W., Daisley, G. W., Kennedy, S., and Bush, M. (1978). Suppurative arthritis in an infant orangutan. *J. Am. Vet. Med. Assoc.* **173**(9), 1145–1147.

Hu, P. J., Mitchell, H. M., Li, Y. Y., Zhou, M. H., and Hazell, S. L. (1994). Association of *Helicobacter pylori* with gastric cancer and observations on the detection of this bacterium in gastric cancer cases. *Am. J. Gastroenterol.* **89**(10), 1806–1810.

Hubbard, G. B., Lee, D. R., and Eichberg, J. W. (1991a). Diseases and pathology of chimpanzees at the Southwest Foundation for Biomedical Research. *Am. J. Primatol.* **24**, 273–282.

Hubbard, G. B., Lee, D. R., Eichberg, J. W., Gormus, B. J., Xu, K., and Meyers, W. M. (1991b). Spontaneous leprosy in a chimpanzee. *Vet. Pathol.* **28**, 546–548.

Hunt, D. E., Pitillo, R. F., Deneau, G. A., Schaebel, F. M., Jr., and Mellet, L. B. (1968). Control of an acute *Klebsiella pneumoniae* infection in a rhesus monkey colony. *Lab. Anim. Care* **18**, 182–185.

Hunt, R. D., Anderson, M. P., and Chalifoux, L. V. (1978). Spontaneous infectious diseases of marmosets. *Primates Med.* **10**, 239–253.

Hyslop, N., St.G. (1980). Dermatophilosis (streptothricosis) in animals and man. *Comp. Immunol. Microbiol. Infect. Dis.* **2**, 389–404.

Indzhila, L. V., Yakovleva, L. A., Simovonjan, V. G., Dshikidze, E. K., Kovaljova, I., and Popova, V. N. (1977). The character and results of comparative experimental therapy of tuberculosis in *Macaca arctoides* monkeys. *Z. Versuchstierkd.* **19**, Suppl., 13–25.

Issacson, P. G., and Spencer, J. (1993). Is gastric lymphoma an infectious disease? *Hum. Pathol.* **24**, 569–570.

Jackson, R. K., Juras, R. A., Stiefal, S. M., and Hall, J. E. (1989). *Mycobacterium kansasii* in a rhesus monkey. *Lab. Anim. Sci.* **39**(5), 415–428.

Johnson, W. D., and Lang, C. W. (1977). Paracoccidioidomycosis (South American blastomycosis) in a squirrel monkey (*Saimiri sciureus*). *Vet. Pathol.* **14**, 368–371.

Johnsen, W. M., Pulliam, J. D., and Tanticharoenyos, P. (1970). *Chromobacterium* septicemia in the gibbon. *J. Inf. Dis.* **122**, 563.

Jonas, A. M., and Wyand, D. S. (1966). Pulmonary nocardiosis in the rhesus monkey: Importance of differentiation from tuberculosis. *Pathol. Vet.* **3**, 588–600.

Jones, E. E., Alford, P. L., Reingold, A. L., Russell, H., Keeling, M. E., and Broome, C. V. (1984). Predisposition to invasive pneumococcal illness following parainfluenza type 3 virus infection in chimpanzees. *J. Am. Vet. Med. Assoc.* **185**(11), 1351–1353.

Kageruka, P., and De Vroey, C. (1972). Generalized mucormycosis in the golden-bellied mangabey (*Cercocebus galeitus chrysogaster*, Lydekker). *Acta Zool. Pathol. Antverp.* **55**, 19–28.

Kaplan, W., Georg, L. K., Hendricks, S. L., and Leeper, R. A. (1957). Isolation of *Microsporum distortum* from animals in the United States. *J. Invest. Dermatol.* **28**, 449–453.

Karasek, E. (1969). Streptokokkeninfektionen bei zootieren. *Int. Symp. Dis. Zoo Anim., 11th,* Zagreb, pp. 81–84.

Kaufmann, A. F., and Quist, K. D. (1969a). Pneumococcal meningitis and peritonitis in rhesus monkeys. *J. Am. Vet. Med. Assoc.* **155**(7), 1158–1162.

Kaufmann, A. F., and Quist, K. D. (1969b). Thrush in a rhesus monkey: Report of a case. *Lab. Anim. Care* **19**, 526–527.

Kaufmann, A. F., Alexander, A. D., Allen, A. M., Cronin, R. J., Dillingham, L. A., Douglas, J. D., and Moore, T. D. (1970). Melioidosis in imported nonhuman primates. *J. Wildl. Dis.* **6**, 211–219.

Kaufmann, A. F., Moulthrop, J. I., and Moore, R. M., Jr. (1975). A perspective of simian tuberculosis in the United States–1972. *J. Med. Primatol.* **4**, 278–286.

Keeling, M. E., and McClure, H. M. (1974). Pneumococcal meningitis and fatal enterobiasis in a chimpanzee. *Lab. Anim. Sci.* **24**(1), 92–95.

Kennedy, F. M., Astbury, J., and Cheasty, T. (1993). Shigellosis due to occupational contact with nonhuman primates. *Epidemiol. Infect.* **110**(2), 247–251.

Kent, T. H., Formal, S. B., and LaBrec, E. H. (1966). *Salmonella* gastroenteritis in rhesus monkeys. *Arch. Pathol.* **82**, 272–279.

Kent, T. H., Formal, S. B., LaBrec, E. H., Spronz, H., and Maenza, R. M. (1967). Gastric shigellosis in rhesus monkeys. *Am. J. Pathol.* **51**, 259–267.

Kerber, W. T., and Reese, W. H. (1968). Balanitis, paronychia, and onychia in a rhesus monkey. *Lab. Anim. Care* **18**, 506–507.

Kessler, M. J., and Brown, R. J. (1979). Clinical description of tetanus in squirrel monkeys (*Saimiri sciureus*). *Lab. Anim. Sci.* **29**(2), 240–242.

Kessler, M. J., and Brown, R. J. (1981). Mycetomas in a squirrel monkey (*Saimiri sciureus*). *J. Zoo Anim. Med.* **12**, 91–93.

Kessler, M. J., Berard, J. D., and Rawlins, R. G. (1988). Effect of tetanus toxoid inoculation on mortality in the Cayo Santiago macaque population. *Am. J. Primatol.* **15**, 93–101.

Kestler, H., Kodama, T., Ringler, D., Marthas, M., Pederson, N., Lackner, A., Regier, D., Sehgal, P., Daniel, M., King, N., and Desrosiers, R. (1990). Induction of AIDS in rhesus monkeys by molecularly cloned simian immunodeficiency virus. *Science* **248**, 1109–1112.

Kiehlbauch, J. A., Brenner, D. J., and Nicholson, M. A. (1991). *Campylobacter butzleri* sp. nov. isolated from humans and animals with diarrheal illness. *J. Clin. Microbiol.* **29**, 365–376.

Kim, J. C. S. (1976). *Corynebacterium pseudotuberculosis* as a cause of nephritis in a chimpanzee. *VM/SAC, Vet. Med. Small Anim. Clin.* **71**, 1093–1095.

King, N. W., Frazier, C. E. O., Garcia, F. G., Wolf, L. A., and Williamson, M. E. (1971). Cutaneous streptothricosis (dermatophiliasis) in owl monkeys. *Lab. Anim. Sci.* **21**, 67–74.

Kinsey, M. D., Dammin, G. J., Formal, S. B., and Giannella, R. A. (1976). The role of altered intestinal permeability in the pathogenesis of *Salmonella* diarrhea in the rhesus monkey. *Gastroenterology* **71**, 429–434.

Klipstein, F. A., Engert, R. F., Short, H., and Schenk, E. A. (1985). Pathogenic properties of *Campylobacter jejuni:* Assay and correlation with clinical manifestations. *Infect. Immun.* **50**(1), 43–49.

Klokke, A. H., and deVries, G. A. (1963). *Tinea capitis* in a chimpanzee caused by *Microsporum canis* Bodin 1902 resembling *M. obesum* Conant 1937. *Sabaraudia* **2**, 268–270.

Klumpp, S. A., and McClure, H. M. (1993a). Dermatophilosis, skin. *In* "Nonhuman primates" (T. C. Jones, U. Mohr, and R. D. Hunt, eds.), Vol. 2, pp. 14–18. Springer-Verlag, Berlin and Heidelberg.

Klumpp, S. A., and McClure, H. M. (1993b). Nocardiosis, lung. *In* "Nonhuman Primates" (T. C. Jones, U. Mohr, and R. D. Hunt, eds.), Vol. 2, pp. 99–104. Springer-Verlag, Berlin and Heidelberg.

Klumpp, S. A., Weaver, D. S., Jerome, C. P., and Jokinen, M. P. (1986). *Salmonella* osteomyelitis in a rhesus monkey. *Vet. Pathol.* **23**, 190–197.

Kohn, D. F., and Haines, D. E. (1977). *Bordetella bronchiseptica* infection in the lesser bushbaby (*Galago senegalensis*). *Lab. Anim. Sci.* **27**(2), 279–280.

Kornegay, R. W., Piric, G., Brown, C. C., and Newton, J. C. (1991). Chromobacteriosis (*Chromobacterium violaceum*) in three colobus monkeys (*Colobus polykomos*). *J. Zoo Wildl. Med.* **22**(4), 476–484.

Kraemer, G. W., McKinney, W. T., Jr., Prange, A. J., Jr., Breese, G. R., McMurray, T. M., and Kemnitz, J. (1976). Isoniazid: Behavioral and biochemical effects in rhesus monkeys. *Life Sci.* **19**, 49–60.

Lang, C. M., and Benjamin, S. A. (1969). Acute pyometra in a rhesus monkey (*Macaca mulatta*). *J. Am. Vet. Med. Assoc.* **155**(7), 1156–1157.

Langner, P. H., Brightman, A. H., and Tranquilli, W. J. (1986). Maxillofacial abscesses in captive squirrel monkeys. *J. Am. Vet. Med. Assoc.* **189**(9), 1218.

Latt, R. H. (1975). Runyon group III atypical mycobacteria as a cause of tuberculosis in a rhesus monkey. *Lab. Anim. Sci.* **25**(2), 206–209.

Lausen, N. C. G., Richter, A. G., and Lage, A. L. (1986). *Pseudomonas aeruginosa* infection in squirrel monkeys. *J. Am. Vet. Med. Assoc.* **189**(9), 1216–1218.

Leelarasamee, A., and Bovornkitti, S. (1989). Melioidosis: Review and update. *Rev. Infect. Dis.* **11**(3), 413–425.

Lehrer, R. J., Howard, D. H., Sypherd, P. S., Edwards, J. E., Segal, G. P., and Winston, D. J. (1980). Mucormycosis. *Ann. Intern. Med.* **93**, 93–108.

Leininger, J. R., Donham, K. J., and Rubino, M. J. (1978). Leprosy in a chimpanzee: Morphology of the skin lesions and characterization of the organism. *Vet. Pathol.* **15**, 339–346.

Letcher, J. (1992). Survey of *Saguinus* mortality in a zoo colony. *J. Med. Primatol.* **21**, 24–29.

Letvin, N. L., Eaton, K. A., Aldrich, W. R., Sehgal, P. K., Blake, B. J., Schlossman, S. F., King, N. W., and Hunt, R. D. (1983). Acquired immunodeficiency syndrome in a colony of macaque monkeys. *Proc. Natl. Acad. Sci. U.S.A.* **80**, 2718–2722.

Liebenberg, S. P., and Giddens, W. E. (1985). Disseminated nocardiosis in three macaque monkeys. *Lab. Anim. Sci.* 35(2), 162–166.

Lindsey, J. R., and Melby, E. C. (1966). Naturally occurring primary cutaneous tuberculosis in the rhesus monkey. *Lab. Anim. Care* 16, 369–385.

Lindsey, J. R., Hardy, P. H., Baker, H. J., and Melby, E. C. (1971). Observations on shigellosis and development of multiply resistant *Shigellas* in *Macaca mulatta*. *Lab. Anim. Sci.* 21(6), 832–844.

Line, A. S., Paul-Murphy, J., Aucoin, D. P., and Hirsh, D. C. (1992). Enrofloxacin treatment of long-tailed macaques with acute bacillary dysentery due to multiresistant *Shigella flexneri* IV. *Lab. Anim. Sci.* 42(3), 240–244.

Line, S., Dorr, T., Roberts, J., and Ihrke, P. (1984). Necrotizing cellulitis in a squirrel monkey. *J. Am. Vet. Med. Assoc.* 185(11), 1378–1379.

Lowenstine, L. J., Lerche, N. W., Yee, J. L., Jennings, M. B., Munn, R. J., McClure, H. M., Anderson, D. C., Fulz, P. N., and Gardner, M. B. (1992). Evidence for a lentiviral etiology in an epizootic of immune deficiency and lymphoma in stump-tailed macaques (*Macaca arctoides*). *J. Med. Primatol.* 21, 1–14.

Lucke, V. M., and Linton, A. H. (1965). Phycomycosis in a mandrill (*Mandrillus sphinx*). *Vet. Rec.* 77, 1306–1309.

Luechtefeld, N. W., Cambre, R. C., and Wang, W.-L. L. (1981). Isolation of *Campylobacter fetus* subspecies *jejuni* from zoo animals. *J. Am. Vet. Med. Assoc.* 179(11), 1119–1122.

Lund, E., and Petersen, K. B. (1959). Pneumococci in monkeys. *Acta Pathol. Microbiol. Scand.* 45, 309–313.

MacArthur, J. A., and Wood, M. (1983). Yersiniosis in a breeding unit of *Macaca fasicularis* (cynomolgus monkeys). *Lab. Anim.* 17, 151–155.

Machotka, S. V., Chapple, F. E., and Stookey, J. L. (1975). Cerebral tuberculosis in a rhesus monkey. *J. Am. Vet. Med. Assoc.* 167, 648–650.

Mair, N. S., White, G. D., Schubert, F. K., and Harbourne, J. F. (1970). *Yersinia enterocolitica* infection in the bush-baby (*Galago*). *Vet. Rec.* 86, 69–71.

Mannheimer, H. S., and Rubin, L. D. (1969). An epizootic of shigellosis in a monkey colony. *J. Am. Vet. Med. Assoc.* 155(7), 1181–1185.

Mariat, F., and Segretain, G. (1956). Etude mycologique d'une histoplasmose spontanée du singe african cynocephalus babuin. *Ann. Inst. Pasteur, Paris* 91, 874–891.

Marshall, B. J. (1994). *Helicobacter pylori. Am. J. Gastroenterol.* 89(8), S116–S128.

Martin, J. E., Kroe, D. J., Bostrum, R. E., Johnson, D. J., and Whitney, R. A. (1969). Rhino-orbital phycomycosis in a rhesus monkey (*Macaca mulatta*). *J. Am. Vet. Med. Assoc.* 155, 1253–1257.

Maurelli, A. T., and Sansonetti, P. J. (1988). Identification of a chromosomal gene controlling temperature-regulated expression of *Shigella* virulence. *Proc. Natl. Acad. Sci. U.S.A.* 85, 2820–2824.

May, B. D. (1972). *Corynebacterium ulcerans* infections in monkeys. *Lab. Anim. Sci.* 22(4), 509–513.

McClure, H. M. (1980). Bacterial diseases of nonhuman primates. *In* "The Comparative Pathology of Zoo Animals" (R. J. Montali and G. Migaki, eds.), pp. 197–217. Smithsonian Institution Press, Washington, DC.

McClure, H. M., and Chang, J. (1976). *Chromobacterium violaceum* infection in a nonhuman primate (*Macaca assamensis*). *Lab. Anim. Sci.* 26(5), 807–810.

McClure, H. M., and Strozier, L. M. (1975). Perinatal listeric septicemia in a Celebese black ape. *J. Am. Vet. Med. Assoc.* 167, 637–638.

McClure, H. M., Kaplan, W., Bonner, W. B., and Keeling, M. E. (1971a). Dermatophilosis in owl monkeys. *Sabauraudia* 9, 185–190.

McClure, H. M., Weaver, R. E., and Kaufmann, A. F. (1971b). Pseudotuberculosis in nonhuman primates: Infection with organisms of the *Yersinia enterocolitica* group. *Lab. Anim. Sci.* 21(3), 376–382.

McClure, H. M., Strozier, L. M., and Keeling, M. F. (1972). Enteropathogenic *Escherichia coli* infection in anthropoid apes. *J. Am. Vet. Med. Assoc.* 161(6), 687–689.

McClure, H. M., Alford, P., and Swenson, B. (1976a). Nonenteric *Shigella* infections in nonhuman primates. *J. Am. Vet. Med. Assoc.* 169(9), 938–939.

McClure, H. M., Chang, J., Kaplan, W., and Brown, J. M. (1976b). Pulmonary nocardiosis in an orangutan. *J. Am. Vet. Med. Assoc.* 169(9), 943–945.

McClure, H. M., Brodie, A. R., Anderson, D. C., and Swenson, R. B. (1986). *In* "Primates: The Road to Self-sustaining Populations" (K. Benirschke, ed.), pp. 531–556. Springer-Verlag, New York.

McClure, H. M., Chiodini, R. J., Anderson, D. C., Swenson, R. B., Thayer, W. R., and Coutu, J. A. (1987). *Mycobacterium paratuberculosis* infection in a colony of stumptail macaques (*Macaca arctoides*). *J. Infect. Dis.* 155(5), 1011–1019.

McCullough, B., Moore, J., and Kuntz, R. E. (1977). Multifocal candidiasis in a capuchin monkey (*Cebus apella*). *J. Med. Primatol.* 6, 186–191.

McKenney, F. D., Traum, J., and Bonestall, A. E. (1944). Acute coccidioidomycosis in a mountain gorilla (*Gorilla beringeri*) with anatomical notes. *J. Am. Vet. Med. Assoc.* 104, 136–140.

McLaughlin, R. M. (1978). *Mycobacterium bovis* in nonhuman primates. *In* "Mycobacterial Infections in Zoo Animals" (R. J. Montali, ed.), pp. 151–155. Smithsonian Press, Washington, DC.

McLaughlin, R. M., and Marrs, G. E. (1978). Tuberculin testing in nonhuman primates: OT vs. PPD. *In* "Mycobacterial Infections in Zoo Animals" (R. J. Montali, ed.), pp. 123–127. Smithsonian Press, Washington, DC.

Medoff, G., Kobayashi, G. S., Painter, A., and Travis, S. (1987). Morphogenesis and pathogenicity of *Histoplasma capsulatum. Infect. Immun.* 55(6), 1355–1358.

Mellins, R. B., Levine, O. R., Wigger, H. J., Leidy, G., and Curnen, E. C. (1972). Experimental meningococcemia: Model of overwhelming infection in unanesthetized monkeys. *J. Appl. Phys.* 32(3), 309–314.

Meyers, W. M., Walsh, G. P., Brown, H. L., Binford, C. H., Imes, G. D., Jr., Hadfield, T. L., Schlagel, C. J., Fukunishi, Y., Gerone, P. J., Wolf, R. H., Gormus, B. J., Martin, L. T., Harboe, M., and Imaeda, T. (1985). Leprosy in a mangabey monkey-naturally acquired infection. *Int. J. Lepr.* 53(1), 1–14.

Middlebrook, J. L., and Dorland, R. B. (1984). Bacterial toxins: Cellular mechanisms of action. *Microbiol. Rev.* 48(3), 199–221.

Migaki, G. (1980). Mycotic diseases in captive animals—a mycopathologic overview. *In* "The Comparative Pathology of Zoo Animals" (R. J. Montali and G. Migaki, eds.), pp. 267–275. Smithsonian Institution Press, Washington, DC.

Migaki, G. (1986). Mycotic infections in nonhuman primates. *In* "Primates: The Road to Self-Sustaining Populations" (K. Benirschke, ed.), pp. 557–570. Springer-Verlag, New York.

Migaki, G., and Seibold, H. R. (1976). Dermatophilosis in a titi monkey (*Callicebus moloch*). *Am. J. Vet. Res.* 37, 1225–1226.

Migaki, G., Voelker, F. A., and Sagartz, J. W. (1978). Fungal diseases. *In* "Pathology of Laboratory Animals" (K. Benirschke, F. M. Garner, and T. C. Jones, eds.), Vol. 2, pp. 1552–1586. Springer-Verlag, New York.

Migaki, G., Asher, D. M., Casey, H. W., Locke, L. N., Gibbs, C. J., Jr., and Gajdusek, C. (1979). Fatal suppurative nephritis caused by *Pseudomonas* in a chimpanzee. *J. Am. Vet. Med. Assoc.* 175(9), 957–959.

Migaki, G., Toft, J. D., and Schmidt, R. E. (1982a). Disseminated entomophthoromycosis in a mandrill (*Mandrillus sphinx*). *Vet. Pathol.* 19, 551–554.

Migaki, G., Schmidt, R. E., Toft, J. D., and Kaufmann, A. F. (1982b). Mycotic infections of the alimentary tract of nonhuman primates: A review. *Vet. Pathol., Suppl.* 7, 93–103.

Migaki, G., Hubbard, G. B., and Butler, T. M. (1993). *Histoplasma capsulatum* var. *duboisii* infection, baboon. *In* "Nonhuman Primates" (T. C. Jones, U. Mohr, and R. D. Hunt, eds.), Vol. 2, pp. 19–22. Springer-Verlag, Berlin.

Miller, R. E., and Boever, W. J. (1983). Cryptococcosis in a lion-tailed macaque (*Macaca silenus*). *J. Zoo Anim. Med.* 14, 110–114.

Mobley, H. L., Hu, L.-T., and Foxall, P. A. (1991). *Helicobacter pylori* urease: Properties and role in pathogenesis. *Scand. J. Gastroenterol., Suppl.* 187, 39–46.

Moisson, P., and Gysin, J. (1994). Reproductive performances and pathological findings in a breeding colony of squirrel monkeys (*Saimiri sciureus*). *In* "Current Primatology: Behavioral Neuroscience, Physiology and Reproduction" (J. R. Anderson, J. J. Roeder, B. Thierry, and N. Herrenschmidt, eds.), Vol. 3, pp. 263–272. University Louis Pasteur, Strasbourg.

Morton, W. R., Bronsdon, M., Mickelsen, G., Knitter, G., Rosenkranz, S., Kuller, L., and Sajuthi, D. (1983). Identification of *Campylobacter jejuni* in *Macaca fascicularis* imported from Indonesia. *Lab. Anim. Sci.* **33**(2), 187–188.

Mulder, J. B. (1971). Shigellosis in nonhuman primates: A review. *Lab. Anim. Sci.* **21**(5), 734–738.

Murphy, B. L., Maynard, J. E., Krushak, D. H., and Berquist, K. R. (1972). Microbial flora of imported marmosets: Viruses and enteric bacteria. *Lab. Anim. Sci.* **22**, 339–343.

Mutalib, A. R., Sheikh-Omar, A. R., and Zamari, M. (1984). Melioidosis in a banded leaf-monkey (*Presbytis melalophos*). *Vet. Rec.* **115**, 438–439.

Nayar, G. P. S., Crawshaw, G. J., and Neufeld, J. L. (1979). Tularemia in a group of nonhuman primates. *J. Am. Vet. Med. Assoc.* **175**(9), 962–963.

Nelson, B., Cosgrove, G. E., and Gengozian, N. (1966). Diseases of an imported primate *Tamarinus nigricollis*. *Lab. Anim. Care* **16**, 255–275.

Newton, W. M., Beamer, P. D., and Rhoades, H. E. (1971). Acute bloat syndrome in stumptailed macaques (*Macaca arctoides*): A report of four cases. *Lab. Anim. Sci.* **21**(2), 193–196.

Niven, J. S. F. (1968). Tyzzer's disease in laboratory animals. *Z. Versuchstierkd.* **10**, 168–174.

Noach, L. A., Rolf, T. M., and Tytgat, G. N. (1994). Electron microscopic study of association between *Helicobacter pylori* and gastric and duodenal mucosa. *J. Clin. Pathol.* **47**, 699–704.

Obaldia, N., III. (1991). Detection of *Klebsiella pneumoniae* antibodies in *Aotus lemurinus* (Panamanian owl monkey) using a enzyme linked immunosorbent assay (ELISA) test. *Lab. Anim.* **25**, 133–141.

O'Brien, A. D., and Holmes, R. K. (1987). Shiga and shiga-like toxins. *Microbiol. Rev.* **51**, 206–220.

Ogawa, H., Takahashi, R., Honjo, S., Takasaka, M., Fujiwara, T., Ando, K., Nakagawa, M., and Muto, T. (1964). Shigellosis in cynomolgus monkeys (*Macaca irus*) III. Histopathological studies on natural and experimental shigellosis. *Jpn. J. Med. Sci. Biol.* **17**, 321–332.

Ogawa, H., Honjo, S., Takaska, M., Fujiwara, T., and Imaizumi, K. (1966). Shigellosis in cynomolgus monkeys (*Macaca irus*) IV. Bacteriological and histopathological observations on the earlier stage of experimental infection with *Shigella flexneri* 2A. *Jpn. J. Med. Biol. Sci.* **19**, 23–32.

Olsen, L. C., Bergquist, D. Y., and Fitzgerald, D. L. (1986). Control of *Shigella flexneri* in Celebese black macaques (*Macaca nigra*). *Lab. Anim. Sci.* **36**(3), 240–242.

Otcenasek, M., Dvorak, J., and Ladzianska, K. (1967). *Trichophyton rubrum*-like dermatophytosis in chimpanzees. *Mycopathol. Mycol. Appl.* **31**, 33–37.

Padovan, D., and Cantrell, C. (1983). Causes of death of infant rhesus and squirrel monkeys. *J. Am. Vet. Med. Assoc.* **183**(11), 1182–1184.

Pal, T., Newland, J. W., Tall, B. D., and Hale, T. L. (1989). Intracellular spread of *Shigella flexneri* associated with the kcpA locus and a 140-kilodalton protein. *Infect. Immun.* **57**, 477–486.

Pappagianis, D., Vanderlip, J., and May, B. (1973). Coccidioidomycosis naturally acquired by a monkey, *Cercocebus atys*, in Davis California. *Sabouraudia* **11**, 52–55.

Parsons, R. (1991). Pseudotuberculosis at the zoological society of London (1981 to 1987). *Vet. Rec.* **128**, 130–132.

Patterson, D. R., Wagner, J. E., Owens, D. R., Ronald, N. C., and Frisk, C. S. (1974). *Candida albicans* infections associated with antibiotic and corticosteroid therapy in spider monkeys. *J. Am. Vet. Med. Assoc.* **164**, 721–722.

Paul-Murphy, J. (1993). Bacterial enterocolitis in nonhuman primates. *In* "Zoo and Wildlife Medicine: Current Therapy 3" (M. Fowler, ed.), pp. 334–351. Saunders, Philadelphia.

Paul-Murphy, J., Markovits, J. E., Wesby, I., and Roberts, J. A. (1990). Listeriosis causing stillbirths and neonatal septicemia in outdoor housed macaques. *Lab. Anim. Sci.* **40**, 547.

Pazzaglia, G., Widja, S., Soebecki, D., Tjaniadi, P., Simanjuntak, L., Lesmana, M., and Jennings, G. (1994). Persistent, recurring diarrhea in a colony of orangutans (*Pongo pygmaeus*) caused by multiple strains of *Campylobacter* spp. *Acta Trop.* **57**, 1–10.

Pernikoff, D. S., and Orkin, J. (1991). Bacterial meningitis syndrome: An overall review of the disease complex and considerations of cross infectivity between great apes and man. *Proc. Am. Assoc. Zoo Vet.*, pp. 235–241.

Perolat, P., Poingt, J., Vie, J., Jouaneau, C., Baranton, G., and Gysin, J. (1992). Occurrence of severe leptospirosis in a breeding colony of squirrel monkeys. *Am. J. Trop. Med. Hyg.* **46**(5), 538–545.

Peterson, P. K. (1980). Host defense against *Pseudomonas aeruginosa*. *In* "*Pseudomonas aeruginosa*, the Organism, the Diseases it Causes, and Their Treatment" (L. H. Sabath, ed.), pp. 103–108.

Phadnis, S. H., Ilver, D., Janzoni, L., Normark, S., and Westblom, T. U. (1994). Pathological significance and molecular characterization of the vacuolating toxin gene of *Helicobacter pylori*. *Infect. Immun.* **62**(5), 1557–1565.

Pierce, D. L., and Dukelow, W. R. (1988). Misleading positive tuberculin reactions in a squirrel monkey colony. *Lab. Anim. Sci.* **38**(6), 729–730.

Pinheiro, E. S., Simon, F., Cassaro, K., and Soares, M. E. G. (1993). Outbreak of diarrhea due to *Campylobacter jejuni* in lion-tamarins (*Leontopithecus* spp.) in captivity. *Verh. Ber. Zootiere* **35**, 159–161.

Pinkerton, M. E. (1968). Shigellosis in the baboon (*Papio* sp.). *Lab. Anim. Care* **18**(1), 11–21.

Pinkerton, M. (1972). Miscellaneous organisms. *In* "Pathology of Simian Primates" (R. N. T.-W.-Fiennes, ed.), Part II, pp. 283–313. Karger, Basel.

Plesker, R., and Claros, M. (1992). A spontaneous *Yersinia pseudotuberculosis*-infection in a monkey colony. *J. Vet. Med. B* **39**, 201–208.

Poelma, F. G. (1975). *Pneumocystis carinii* infections in zoo animals. *Z. Parasitenkd.* **46**, 61–68.

Poelma, F. G., Borst, G. H. A., and Zwart, P. (1977). *Yersinia enterocolitica* infections in nonhuman primates. *Acta Zool. Soc. London* **46**, 61–68.

Postal, J. M., Gysin, J., and Crenn, Y. (1988). Protection against fatal *Klebsiella pneumoniae* sepsis in the squirrel monkey *Saimiri sciureus* after immunization with a capsular polysaccharide vaccine. *Ann. Inst. Pasteur/Immunol.* **139**, 401–407.

Potkay, S. (1992). Diseases of the Callitrichidae: A review. *J. Med. Primatol.* **21**, 189–236.

Pucak, G., Orcutt, R. P., Judge, R. J., and Rendon, F. (1977). Elimination of the *Shigella* carrier state in rhesus monkeys (*Macaca mulatta*) by trimethoprim-sulfamethoxazole. *J. Med. Primatol.* **6**(2), 127–132.

Rapley, W. A., and Long, J. R. (1974). Coccidioidomycosis in a baboon recently imported from California. *Can. Vet. J.* **15**, 39–41.

Rawlins, R. G., and Kessler, M. T. (1982). A five-year study of tetanus in the Cayo Santiago rhesus monkey colony: Behavioral description and epizootiology. *Am. J. Primatol.* **3**, 23–39.

Reid, A. C., Herron, A. J., Hines, M. E., Orchard, E. A., and Altman, N. H. (1993). Leptospirosis in a white-lipped tamarin (*Saguinus labiatus*). *Lab. Anim. Sci.* **43**(3), 258–259.

Renquist, D. M., and Potkay, S. (1979). *Mycobacterium scrofulaceum* infection in *Erythrocebus* patas monkeys. *Lab. Anim. Sci.* **29**(1), 97–101.

Renquist, D. M., and Whitney, R. A. (1978). Tuberculosis in nonhuman primates—an overview. *In* "Mycobacterial Infections in Zoo Animals" (R. J. Montali, ed.), pp. 9–16. Smithsonian Press, Washington, DC.

Retnasabapathy, A., and Joseph, P. G. (1966). A case of melioidosis in a macaque monkey. *Vet. Rec.* **79**(3), 72–73.

Richter, C. B., Humason, G. L., and Godbold, J. H., Jr. (1978). Endemic *Pneumocystis carinii* in a marmoset colony. *J. Comp. Pathol.* **88**, 221–223.

Riordan, J. T. (1943). Rectal tuberculosis in monkeys from the use of contaminated thermometers. *J. Infect. Dis.* **73**, 93–94.

Rosenberg, D. P., and Blouin, P. (1979). Retrobulbar abscess in an infant rhesus monkey. *J. Am. Vet. Med. Assoc.* **175**(9), 994–996.

Rosenberg, D. P., Lerche, N. W., and Henrickson, R. V. (1980). *Yersinia pseudotuberculosis* infection in a group of *Macaca fasicularis*. *J. Am. Vet. Med. Assoc.* **177**(9), 818–819.

Rosenberg, D. P., Gleiser, C. A., and Carey, K. D. (1984). Spinal coccidioidomycosis in a baboon. *J. Am. Vet. Med. Assoc.* **185**(11), 1379–1381.

Roussilhon, C., Postal, J. M., and Ravisse, P. (1987). Spontaneous cryptococcosis of a squirrel monkey (*Saimiri sciureus*) in French Guyana. *J. Med. Primatol.* **16**, 39–47.

Rout, W. R., Formal, S. B., Dammin, G. J., and Gianella, R. A. (1974). Pathophysiology of *Salmonella* diarrhea in the rhesus monkey: Intestinal transport, morphological, and bacteriological studies. *Gastroenterology* **67**, 59–70.

Rout, W. R., Formal, S. B., Giannella, R. A., and Dammin, G. J. (1975). Pathophysiology of *Shigella* diarrhea in the rhesus monkey: Intestinal transport, morphological, and bacteriological studies. *Gastroenterology* **68**, 270–278.

Roy, A. D., and Cameron, H. M. (1972). Rhinophycomycosis entomophthorae occurring in a chimpanzee in the wild in East Africa. *Am. J. Trop. Med. Hyg.* **21**, 234–237.

Russell, R. G. (1992). *Campylobacter jejuni* colitis and immunity in primates: epidemiology of natural infection. *In* "*Campylobacter jejuni*: Current Status and Future Trends" (I. Nachamkin, ed.), pp. 148–157. *Am. Soc. Microbiol.*, Washington, DC.

Russell, R. G., and DeTolla, L. J. (1993). Shigellosis. *In* "Nonhuman Primates" (T. C. Jones, U. Mohr, and R. D. Hunt, eds.), Vol. 1, pp. 46–53. Springer-Verlag, Berlin.

Russell, R. G., Rosenkranz, S. L., Lee, L. A., Howard, H., DiGiacomo, R. F., Bronsdon, M. A., Blakley, G. A., Tsia, C.-C., and Morton, W. R. (1987). Epidemiology and etiology of diarrhea in colony-born *Macaca nemestrina*. *Lab. Anim. Sci.* **37**(3), 309–316.

Russell, R. G., Krugner, L., Tsai, C.-C., and Ekstrom, R. (1988). Prevalence of *Campylobacter* in infant, juvenile and adult laboratory primates. *Lab. Anim. Sci.* **38**(6), 711–714.

Russell, R. G., Blaser, M. J., Sarmiento, J. I., and Fox, J. (1989). Experimental *Campylobacter jejuni* infection in *Macaca nemestrina*. *Infect. Immun.* **57**, 1438–1444.

Russell, R. G., O'Donnoghue, M., Blake, D. C., Jr., Zulty, J., and DeTolla, L. J. (1993). Early colonic damage and invasion of *Campylobacter jejuni* in experimentally challenged infant *Macaca mulatta. J. Infect. Dis.* **168**, 210–215.

Saëz, H. (1970). Levures del a cavité buccale du baboun, *Papio papio* (Desm). *Zentralbl. Veterinaermed.* **17**, 381–388.

Saëz, H. (1975). Candidose de l'estomac chez un gibbon a'facoris blancs-*Hylobates concolor leucogenys. Mykosen* **18**, 519–525.

Sakakibara, I., Sugimoto, Y., Takasaka, M., and Honjo, S. (1984). Spontaneous nocardiosis with brain abscess caused by *Nocardia asteroides* in a cynomolgus monkey. *J. Med. Primatol.* **13**, 89–95.

Saliba, A. M., Matera, E. A., and Moreno, G. (1968). Sporotrichosis in a chimpanzee. *Mod. Vet. Pract.* **49**, 74.

Sato, T., and Takeuchi, A. (1982). Infection by spirilla in the stomach of the rhesus monkey. *Vet. Pathol.* **19**, Suppl., 17–25.

Schiff, L. J., Barbera, P. W., Port, C. D., Yamashiroya, H. M., Shefner, A. M., and Poiley, S. M. (1972). Enteropathogenic *Escherichia coli* infections: Increasing awareness of a problem in laboratory animals. *Lab. Anim. Sci.* **22**(5), 705–708.

Schiller, C. A., Wolff, M. J., Munson, L., and Montali, R. J. (1989). *Streptococcus zooepidemicus* infections of possible horsemeat source in red-bellied tamarins and Goeldi's monkeys. *J. Zoo Wildl. Med.* **20**(3), 322–327.

Schmatz, D. M., Powles, M., McFadden, D. C., Pittarelli, L. A., Liberator, P. A., and Anderson, J. W. (1991). Treatment and prevention of *Pneumocystis carinii* pneumonia and further elucidation of *P. carinii* life cycle with 1,3-B-glucan synthesis inhibitor L-671, 329. *J. Protozol.* **38**, 151S–153S.

Schmidt, R. E., and Butler, T. M. (1970). Esophageal candidiasis in a chimpanzee. *J. Am. Vet. Med. Assoc.* **157**(5), 722–723.

Schmidt, R. E., and Butler, T. M. (1971). *Klebsiella-Enterobacter* infections in chimpanzees. *Lab. Anim. Sci.* **21**(6), 946–949.

Scimeca, J. M., and Brady, A. G. (1990). Neonatal mortality in the captive breeding squirrel monkey colony associated with an invasive *Escherichia coli. Lab. Anim. Sci.* **40**(5), 546–547.

Scully, J. P., and Kligman, A. M. (1951). Coincident infection of a human and an anthropoid with *Microsporum audouini. Arch. Dermatol. Syphilol.* **64**, 495–498.

Sedgwick, C., Parcher, J., and Durham, R. (1970). Atypical mycobacterial infection in the pig-tailed macaque (*Macaca nemestrina*). *J. Am. Vet. Med. Assoc.* **157**(5), 724–725.

Seelig, M. S. (1966a). Mechanisms by which antibiotics increase the incidence and severity of candidiasis and alter the immunologic defenses. *Bacteriol. Rev.* **30**, 422–459.

Seelig, M. S. (1966b). The role of antibiotics in the pathogenesis of Candida infections. *Am. J. Med.* **40**, 887–917.

Seeliger, H. P. R., Bisping, W., and Brandt, H. P. (1963). Über eine Microsporum Enzootie bie Kappen-Gibbons (*Hylobates lar*) verursacht durch eine variante von *Microsporum canis. Mykosen.* **6**, 61–68.

Seibold, H. R., Perrin, E. A., Jr., and Garner, A. C. (1970). Pneumonia associated with *Bordetella bronchiseptica* in *Callicebus* species primates. *Lab. Anim. Care* **20**(3), 456–461.

Sesline, D. H. (1978). *Mycobacterium avium* enteritis in nonhuman primates. *In* "Mycobacterial Infections in Zoo Animals" (R. J. Montali, ed.), pp. 157–159. Smithsonian Press, Washington, DC.

Sesline, D. H., Schwartz, L. W., Osburn, B. I., Thoen, C. O., Terrell, T., Holmberg, C., Anderson, J. H., and Henrickson, R. V. (1975). *Mycobacterium avium* infection in three rhesus monkeys. *J. Am. Vet. Med. Assoc.* **167**(7), 639–645.

Sharma, R. D., Kwatra, M. S., Dhillon, S. S., and Dua, K. (1990). Tetanus in a domestic monkey. *J. Res. (Punjab Agric. Univ.)* **27**(4), 661–662.

Shive, R. J., Green, S. S., Evans, L. B., and Garner, F. M. (1969). Leptospirosis in Barbary apes (*Macaca sylvana*). *J. Am. Vet. Med. Assoc.* **155**(7), 1176–1178.

Skavlen, P. A., Stills, H. F., Jr., Steffen, E. K., and Middleton, C. C. (1985). Naturally occurring *Yersinia enterocolitica* septicemia in patas monkeys (*Erythrocebus patas*). *Lab. Anim. Sci.* **35**(5), 488–490.

Sly, D. W., London, W. T., Palmer, A. E., and Rice, J. M. (1977). Disseminated cryptococcosis in a patas monkey (*Erythrocebus patas*). *Lab. Anim. Sci.* **27**, 694–699.

Smart, J. L., Roberts, T. A., McCullagh, K. G., and Pearson, H. (1980). An outbreak of type C botulism in captive monkeys. *Vet. Rec.* **107**, 445–446.

Smith, N. R., and Damit, M. (1982). Fatal bronchopneumonia in a young orangutan caused by *Pseudomonas pseudomallei. Vet. Rec.* **110**, 251.

Snook, S., Reimann, K., and King, N. (1992). Neonatal mortality in cottontop tamarins: Failure of passive immunoglobin transfer. *Vet. Pathol.* **29**(5), 444.

Snyder, S. B., Lund, J. E., Bone, J., Soave, O. A., and Hirsch, D. C. (1970). A study of *Klebsiella* infection in owl monkeys (*Aotus trivirgatus*). *J. Am. Vet. Med. Assoc.* **157**(11), 1935–1939.

Soave, O. (1978). Observations on acute gastric dilatation in nonhuman primates. *Lab. Anim. Sci.* **28**(3), 331–334.

Soave, O., Jackson, S., and Ghumman, J. S. (1981). Atypical mycobacteria as the probable cause of positive tuberculin reactions in squirrel monkeys (*Saimiri sciureus*). *Lab. Anim. Sci.* **31**(3), 295–296.

Solleveld, H. A., van Zweitten, M. J., Heidt, P. J., and van Eerd, P. M. C. A. (1984). Clinicopathologic study of six cases of meningitis and meningoencephalitis in chimpanzees (*Pan troglodytes*). *lab. Anim. Sci.* **34**(1), 86–90.

Stein, F. J., and Stott, G. (1979). *Corynebacterium equi* in the cottontop marmoset (*Saguinus oedipus*): A case report. *Lab. Anim. Sci.* **29**(4), 519–520.

Stein, F. J., Lewis, D. H., Stott, G. G., and Sis, R. F. (1981). Acute gastric dilatation in common marmosets (*Callithrix jacchus*). *Lab. Anim. Sci.* **31**(5), 522–523.

Stills, H. F., Jr., Bond, M. G., and Bullock, B. C. (1979). Bacterial myocarditis in African green monkeys (*Cercopithecus aethiops*). *Vet. Pathol.* **16**, 376–380.

Strauss, J. M., Jason, S., Lee, H., and Gan, E. (1969). Meliodosis with spontaneous remission of osteomyelitis in a macaque (*Macaca nemestrina*). *J. Am. Vet. Med. Assoc.* **155**(7), 1169–1175.

Swindle, M. M., Craft, C. F., Marriott, B. M., Strandberg, J. D., and Luzarraga, M. (1982). Ascending uterine infections in rhesus monkeys. *J. Am. Vet. Med. Assoc.* **181**(11), 1367–1370.

Takasaka, M., Honjo, S., Fujiwara, T., Hagiwara, T., Ogawa, H., and Imaizumi, K. (1964). Shigellosis in cynomolgus monkeys (*Macaca irus*) I. Epidemiological surveys of *Shigella* infection rate. *Jpn. J. Med. Sci. Biol.* **17**, 259–265.

Takasaka, M., Kohono, A., and Sakakibara, I. (1988). An outbreak of salmonellosis in newly imported cynomolgus monkeys. *Jpn. J. Med. Sci. Biol.* **41**, 1–8.

Takos, M. J., and Elton, N. W. (1953). Spontaneous cryptococcosis of marmoset monkeys in Panama. *Arch. Pathol.* **55**, 403–407.

Taylor, N. S., Ellenberger, M. A., Wu, P. Y., and Fox, J. G. (1989). Diversity of serotypes of *Campylobacter jejuni* and *Campylobacter coli* isolated in laboratory animals. *Lab. Anim. Sci.* **39**(3), 219–221.

Taylor, R. L., Cadigan, F. C., and Chaicumpa, V. (1973). Infections among Thai gibbons and humans caused by atypical *Microsporum canis. Lab. Anim. Sci.* **23**, 226–231.

Telford, J. L., Ghiara, P., Dell-Orco, M., Comanducci, M., Burroni, D., Bugnoli, M., Teece, M. F., Censini, S., Covacci, A., Xiang, Z., Papini, E., Montecucco, C., Parente, L., and Rappuoli, R. (1994). Gene structure of the *Helicobacter pylori* cytotoxin and evidence of its key role in gastric disease. *J. Exp. Med.* **179**, 1653–1658.

Thiry, G. (1913). Muguet spontanéchez le singe. *Arch. Parasitol.* **16**, 168–176.

Thurman, J. D., Morton, R. J., and Stair, E. L. (1983). Septic abortion caused by *Salmonella heidelberg* in a white-handed gibbon. *J. Am. Vet. Med. Assoc.* **183**(11), 1325–1326.

Tribe, G. W., and Fleming, M. P. (1983). Biphasic enteritis in imported cynomolgus (*Macaca fascicularis*) monkeys infected with *Shigella, Salmonella,* and *Campylobacter* species. *Lab. Anim.* **17**, 65–69.

Tribe, G. W., and Wellburn, A. E. (1976). Value of combining the erythrocyte sedimentation rate test with tuberculin testing in the control of tuberculosis in baboons. *Lab. Anim.* **10**, 39–43.

Tribe, G. W., MacKensie, P. S., and Fleming, M. P. (1979). Incidence of thermophilic *Campylobacter* species in newly imported simian primates with enteritis. *Vet. Rec.* **105**, 333–337.

Tucker, M. J. (1984). A survey of the pathology of marmosets (*Callithrix jacchus*). *Lab. Anim.* **18**, 351–358.

Valerio, D. A., Dalgard, D. W., Voelker, R. W., McCarrol, N. E., and Good, R. C. (1979). *Mycobacterium kansasii* infection in rhesus monkeys. *In* "Mycobacterial Infections in Zoo Animals" (R. J. Montali, ed.), pp. 65–75. Smithsonian Press, Washington, DC.

VandeWoude, S. J., and Luzarraga, M. B. (1991). The role of *Branhamella catarrhalis* in the "bloody-nose syndrome" of cynomolgus macaques. *Lab. Anim. Sci.* **41**(5), 401–406.

Vetési, F., Balsai, A., and Kemenes, F. (1972). Abortion in Gray's monkey (*Cercopihecus mona*) associated with *Listeria monocytogenes. Acta Microbiol. Acad. Sci. Hung.* **19**, 441–443.

Voronin, L. G., Kanfor, I. S., Lakin, G. F., and Tikh, N. N. (1948). Spontaneous diseases of lower monkeys, their prophylaxis, diagnosis, and treatment. *In* "Experimentation on the Keeping and Raising of Monkeys at Sukhami." *Acad. Med. Sci.,* Moscow.

Wagner, J. D., Jayo, M. J., Bullock, B. C., and Washburn, S. A. (1992). Gestational diabetes mellitus in a cynomolgus monkey with group A streptococcal metritis and hemolytic uremic syndrome. *J. Med. Primatol.* **21**, 371–374.

Wakefield, A. E., Peters, S. E., Banerji, S., Bridge, P. D., Hall, G. S., Hawksworth, D. L., Guiver, L. A., Allen, A. G., and Hopkin, J. M. (1992). *Pneumocystis carinii* shows DNA homology with the ustomycetous red yeast fungus. *Mol. Microbiol.* **6**(14), 1903–1911.

Walch, H. A. (1981). *Coccidioides immitis. In* "Medical Microbiology and Infectious Diseases" (A. I. Braude, ed.), pp. 658–664. Saunders, Philadelphia.

Wallach, J. D. (1977). Erisipelas in two captive Diana monkeys. *J. Am. Vet. Med. Assoc.* **171**(9), 979–980.

Walker, J., and Spooner, E. T. C. (1960). Natural infection of the African baboon *Papio papio* with the large-cell form of *Histoplasma. J. Pathol. Bacteriol.* **80**, 436–438.

Ward, G. S., Elwell, M. R., Tingpalapong, M., and Pomsdhit, J. (1985). Use of streptomycin and isoniazid during a tuberculosis epizootic in a rhesus and cynomolgus breeding colony. *Lab. Anim. Sci.* **35**(4), 395–399.

Wayne, L. G., and Sramek, H. A. (1992). Agents of newly recognized or infrequently encountered Mycobacterial diseases. *Clin. Microbiol. Rev.* **5**, 1–25.

Weidman, F. D. (1935). Dermatoses of monkeys and apes. *9th Int. Congr. Dermatol.* **1**, 600–606.

Weller, R. E. (1994). Infectious and noninfectious diseases of owl monkeys. *In* "Aotus: The Owl Monkey" (J. F. Baer, R. E. Weller, and I Kakoma, eds.), pp. 178–215. Academic Press, San Diego, CA.

Weller, R. E., Dagle, G. E., Malaga, C. A., and Baer, J. F. (1990). Hypercalcemia and disseminated histoplasmosis in an owl monkey. *J. Med. Primatol.* **19**, 675–670.

Wikse, S. E., Fox, J. G., and Kovatch, R. M. (1970). Candidiasis in simian primates. *Lab. Anim. Care* **20**, 957–963.

Wilbert, R., and Delorme, M. (1927). Note sur la spirochetose icterohémorrhagique du chimpanzee. *C. R. Soc. Bull.* **98**, 343–345.

Wolf, R. H., Gibson, S. V., Watson, E. A., and Baskin, G. B. (1988). Multidrug chemotherapy of tuberculosis in rhesus monkeys. *Lab. Anim. Sci.* **38**(1), 25–33.

Wolinsky, E. (1979). Nontuberculsus mycobacteria and associated diseases. *Am. Rev. Respir. Dis.* **199**, 107–159.

Xiang, Z., Censini, S., Bayell, P. F., Telford, J. L., Figura, N., Rappuoli, R., and Covacci, A. (1995). Analysis of expression of CagA and VacA virulence factors in 43 strains of *Helicobacter pylori* reveals that clinical isolates can be divided into two major types and that CagA is not necessary for expression of the vacuolating cytotoxin. *Infect. Immun.* **63**(1), 94–98.

Chapter 3

Parasitic Diseases

John D. Toft, II and Mark L. Eberhard

I. INTRODUCTION

Those who have had more than cursory experience in the husbandry of nonhuman primate colonies will agree that parasitism is one of the most common disease entities that affects these animals. Numerous protozoan and metazoan genera have been described as infecting the members of all major nonhuman primate groups. Some of these are considered to be nonpathogenic, or at least their detrimental effects on the host have yet to be elucidated. A large number, however, can result in physiologic disturbances, nutritional loss, or produce lesions that re-

sult in serious debilitation, and can create opportunities for secondary infections that may be fatal. This process appears to be exacerbated by the stress of capture and confinement.

This chapter discusses the histomorphologic features of protozoan and metazoan parasitic infections of nonhuman primates. Since the chapter is essentially a review of the literature, an extensive bibliography is included for those readers who wish to pursue the subject in greater detail. All tables in the text follow a published system (373). Major nonhuman primate groups are classified according to a published taxonomy system (815). Prosimians include the species in the families Tupaiidae; New World monkeys include the species in the families Calli-

TABLE I

PARASITIC FLAGELLATES DESCRIBED FROM NONHUMAN PRIMATES

Parasite Genus species	Location in host	Prosimians	New World monkeys	Old World monkeys	Great apes	Reference
Phylum Sarcomastigophora, order Trichomonadida, family Trichomonadidae						
Trichomitus wenyoni	Cecum, colon			X		124, 373, 1162
Trichomonas buccalis	Mouth			X		491, 967
T. tenax	Mouth			X	X	124, 373, 491, 519, 699
T. foetus	Intestine	X				89
T. hominis	Intestine				X	656, 659
Tritrichomonas mobilensis	Intestine		X			94, 203, 1010
Tetratrichomonas macacovaginae	Vagina			X		203, 487
Trichomonas sp.	Intestine	X	X			224, 514, 564, 1110, 1157
Pentatrichomonas hominis	Cecum, colon		X	X	X	373, 489, 491, 699, 891
Phylum Sarcomastigophora, order Trichomonadida, family Monocercomonadidae						
Dientamoeba fragilis	Cecum, colon			X		124, 373, 491, 624, 651, 652, 699, 700
Phylum Sarcomastigophora, order Diplomonadida, family Enteromonadidae						
Enteromonas hominis	Cecum			X	X	124, 373, 656, 700, 929
Phylum Sarcomastigophora, order Retortamonadida, family Retortamonadidae						
Retortamonas intestinalis	Cecum			X	X	124, 373, 699, 700
Chilomastix mesnili	Cecum, colon		X	X	X	21, 124, 373, 489, 491, 650, 656, 700, 804, 855, 891, 929
C. tarsii	Intestine	X				89, 514, 896
Chilomastix sp.	Intestine		X			804
Phylum Sarcomastigophora, order Diplomonadida, family Hexamitidae						
Hexamita pitheci	Cecum, colon			X	X	209, 373, 699
Hexamita sp.	Cecum			X	X	124, 373, 489, 1160
Giardia intestinalis (syn. *G. lamblia*)	Anterior small intestine		X	X	X	124, 373, 507, 640, 699, 700, 873, 967
G. wenyoni	Anterior small intestine	X				640
Giardia sp.	Intestine		X	X		224, 564, 1110, 1157

trichidae and Cebidae; Old World monkeys include the species in the family Cercopithedidae; and the great apes include the species in the families Hylobatidae and Pongidae.

The numerous articles published previously that discuss the subject of nonhuman primate parasitology as a specific entity or as a part of an overall discussion of general parasitology, systemic pathology, or the broad topic of nonhuman primate diseases are outlined as follows: enteric and somatic protozoans (40, 103, 124, 131, 247, 393, 445, 446, 489, 490, 536, 581, 593, 640, 699, 798, 818, 1106); hemoprotozoans (3, 29, 162, 175, 181–183, 312, 376, 415, 416, 418–421, 444, 492, 735, 740, 1030, 1075, 1131, 1139, 1196); nematodes (37, 851); trematodes (192, 647); cestodes (803); acanthocephalans (996); arthropods (126, 268, 361, 364, 373, 523, 544, 554, 555, 608, 1209); pentastomids (1019); general parasitology (52, 449, 558, 570, 649, 652, 662, 664, 698, 700, 701, 1023, 1044); systemic pathology (30, 134, 486, 572, 712, 756, 784, 1001, 1055, 1092, 1093); nonhuman primate diseases (2, 16, 55, 56, 151, 173, 408, 436, 493, 500, 510, 546, 567, 579, 588, 590, 617, 627, 673, 694, 754, 771, 772, 939, 967, 972, 1121, 1126); and diseases/pathology of zoo animals (436, 451–453).

In addition, there are many papers in the literature concerning parasitological surveys and parasite checklists for specific species of nonhuman primates. These are referenced as follows: rhesus monkey (*Macaca mulatta* (1, 285, 364, 582, 583, 597, 881, 891, 933, 965, 1109, 1178); cynomolgus monkey (*Macaca fascicularis*) (1, 69, 479, 521, 989, 1178); pig-tail monkey (*Macaca nemestrina*) (1178); bonnet monkey (*Macaca radiata*) (1178); stump-tail monkey (*Macaca arctoides*) (1178); Japanese monkey (*Macaca fuscata*) (1113); Barbary ape (*Macaca sylvanus*) (125); Formosan rock macaque (*Macaca cyclopis*) (655, 659); African green monkey (*Cercopithecus* sp.) (685, 1064); patas monkey (*Erythrocebus patas*) (1064); silvered leaf monkey (*Presbytis cristatus*) (4, 859–861); chacma baboon (*Papio ursinus*) (21, 441, 763, 879); yellow baboon (*Papio cynocephalus*) (650, 662, 811); olive baboon (*Papio anubis,* syn. *P. doguera*) (651, 653, 806); baboons (*Papio* sp.) (1, 385, 757, 765, 804, 805, 872, 1058); gelada baboon (*Theropithecus gelada*) (658); tamarin (*Saquinus fuscicollis*) (194); owl monkey (*Aotus trivirgatus*) (160, 1157); squirrel monkey (*Saimiri sciureus*) (771); New World monkeys (29, 585, 657); slender loris (*Loris tradigradus*)

TABLE I—*Continued*

PARASITIC FLAGELLATES DESCRIBED FROM NONHUMAN PRIMATES

Parasite Genus species	Location in host	Prosimians	New World monkeys	Old World monkeys	Great apes	Reference
Phylum Sarcomastigophora, order Kinetoplasida, family Trypanosomatidae (hemoflagellates)						
Trypanosoma cruzi	Blood, RE cells, muscle, heart, other tissues		X	X	X	10, 28, 40, 42, 52, 121, 148, 149, 212, 215–217, 273, 282, 373, 435, 676, 694, 738–741, 1013, 1020, 1046
T. cruzi-like	Blood			X		740
T. sanmartini	Blood		X			40, 273, 373, 425
T. minasense	Blood		X			40, 148, 216, 218, 273, 373, 738–740, 954
T. rangeli	Blood		X			40, 212, 273, 373, 456, 457, 694, 698, 740
T. saimirii	Blood		X			40, 219 273, 373, 740, 954
T. diasi	Blood		X			40, 219, 220, 273, 373, 740
T. lambrechti	Blood		X			40, 223, 273, 738–740
T. primatum	Blood				X	40, 103, 281, 373, 740, 930, 1008, 1009, 1207
T. brucei	Blood			X		40
T. perodictici	Blood	X				40, 58, 62, 63, 103, 516, 740, 930, 1009
T. irangiense	Blood	X				40, 61, 63, 516, 740
T. cyclops	Blood			X		740, 1154–1156
T. conorhini	Blood			X		740
T. devei	Blood		X			740
T. advieri	Blood		X			740
T. mycetae	Blood		X			740
Trypanosoma sp.	Blood	X				174, 264, 274, 469, 472, 661, 816, 1203

(636); tarsiers (*Tarsius bancanus*) (89,514); chimpanzee (*Pan* sp.) (365,656,808,812,1115); orangutan (179); and laboratory primates (881,929,990,1066,1177,1178).

References for additional reading on nonhuman primate parasitology, associated lesions, and related subjects outside the scope of this chapter are as follows: pathology (59,373,545,570, 571,967,1023); necropsy techniques (1176); recognition of parasites (802); comparative parasitology (166,267); experimental parasitology (648,843); identification of parasitic eggs (563); identification of parasites in tissue sections (167,400,848,1094); parasitic zoonoses (182,515,569,580,699,934,1139,1200); and parasite control (208).

II. PROTOZOAN PARASITES

A. Flagellates

1. Enteric Flagellates

The enteric flagellates described from nonhuman primates are listed in Table I. Many of the enteric flagellates are consid-

ered to be nonpathogenic with the exception of *Giardia* sp. and *Tritrichomonas mobilensis*. These will be discussed in detail below.

a. GIARDIASIS. *Giardia,* once considered a harmless parasite of humans and animals, is now recognized as a pathogen (22). *Giardia intestinalis* (synonym *G. lamblia, duodenalis*) is found throughout the world and is a common inhabitant of the small intestine of humans, rhesus monkey, cynomolgus monkey, chimpanzee, and other nonhuman primates (373,698,929, 967).

Giardia intestinalis trophozoites are bilaterally symmetrical and measure 9 to 21 μm long, 5 to 15 μm wide, and 2 to 4 μm thick (373,698). The body of the parasite is pear-shaped with a broadly rounded anterior end, an extended posterior end, and a large sucking disc on the anterior ventral side. In addition, there are two anterior nuclei, two slender axostyles, eight flagella which emerge at different locations, and a pair of darkly staining median bodies that are curved bars shaped like the claws of a claw hammer. The two nuclei and the rod-like median bodies resemble a face with eyes and mouth (373,698,934). The cysts are ovoid, measure 8 to 12 μm by 7 to 10 μm, and contain four nuclei when mature (373). Reproduction is by binary longitudinal fission (373).

Giardia intestinalis has been reported to cause diarrhea in monkeys (373,967). Also, *Giardia* cysts were observed in the feces of two gibbons, two chimpanzees, a gorilla, an orangutan, and three of the animal's attendants during an outbreak of giardiasis at the Kansas City Zoo in 1978 (22). Clinical signs in this outbreak consisted of diarrhea and vomiting in both nonhuman and human primate patients.

Giardia sp. cysts, morphologically consistent with those of *G. intestinalis,* also have been reported in a chimpanzee (*Pan troglodytes*) and four marmosets (*Callithrix argentata*) housed at the Poznan Zoo, Poznan, Poland (873). These infections were essentially asymptomatic and responded to treatment with metronidazole (Flagyl) for the chimpanzee and furazolidone for the marmosets (873).

The ability of *Giardia* to cause disease in humans and other primates is variable, however, and the factors that govern its pathogenicity are not completely understood (22,640,699). Although clinical illness associated with *Giardia* infection is documented in both medical and veterinary medical literature, the fact remains that *Giardia* infection does not always result in overt clinical illness. Many persons infected with *Giardia* are asymptomatic and animals frequently show no signs indicative of infection (22,640).

Diagnosis of giardiasis can be made by finding the characteristic *Giardia* trophozoites and/or cysts in the feces or intestine of the affected nonhuman primate with diarrhea. Both a fluorescent antibody and a fecal antigen detection assay have been developed and used for the detection of *Giardia lamblia* cysts in fecal smears (1048).

However, because of the unpredictable pathogenicity of *Giardia,* the finding of *Giardia* cysts in the stool of an animal with diarrhea cannot be considered as incontrovertible proof that this parasite is the cause of the illness (22). Critical assessment of the clinical signs, in addition to appropriate cultures to exclude bacterial and viral infections, is required to establish a definitive causation (22). Appropriate treatment with resolution of symptoms would also be highly suggestive that *Giardia* was the causative agent. Strict sanitary practices are necessary for control. The cysts are relatively resistant in the environment, but 2–5% phenol or cresol will destroy the cysts (373), as will heat and desiccation.

Nonhuman primates can be asymptomatic carriers and hence be a source of infection to humans, with infection via direct contact (934): the report from the Kansas City Zoo provides evidence that fecal–oral transmission of *Giardia* between apes and their attendants is possible (22).

Although most parasitology textbooks indicate that *Giardia* is host specific, studies have shown that at least some species of *Giardia* are transmissible from animals to humans and vice versa, thus making it potentially both a zoonotic and an anthropozoonotic infection (22,215,574).

Therefore, personnel working with or caring for nonhuman primates should always follow accepted personal hygiene practices, wear protective clothing, gloves, etc. Nonhuman primates and their excrement should be handled with caution at all times to prevent contamination and the possibility of fecal–oral transmission.

Treatment with quinacrine at 10 mg/kg per day, three times a day, for 5 days is 70–95% effective but is not tolerated well by squirrel monkeys, often causing some gastrointestinal disturbances (934). Treatment with metronidazole (Flagyl), via stomach tube, at a dose of 30–50 mg/kg for 5 to 10 days, is usually effective in both New and Old World primates and apes (694, 873). Furazolidone at a dose level of 1.5 mg/kg for 7 days is reported to be effective treatment for marmosets (873).

b. TRICHOMONIASIS. *Tritrichomonas mobilensis* is a newly isolated trichomonad flagellate from the lower intestinal tract of squirrel monkeys.

This trichomonad has been characterized morphologically and taxonomically (203). The trophozoites are lanceolate shaped, 7–10.5 μm in length and 1.5–3 μm in width. The organism has three anterior flagella of about body length and a well-developed undulating membrane that continues in a free acroneme-type posterior flagellum as long as the body. The nucleus is ovoid and situated in the anterior portion of the body (203). This parasite is common in squirrel monkeys, and trophozoites were reported in 100% of animals by 8 weeks of age in a large breeding colony (94,887,1010).

The clinical significance of this enteric trichomonad in squirrel monkeys is uncertain (94,887). However, this particular organism has been shown to cause cytopathic effects in tissue culture (94,204,887,1010), and supernatants from cultures contained a potent hemagglutinin that has been identified as a sialic acid-specific lectin that binds sialoglycoproteins (887, 888, 1010, 1158). Virulence and invasiveness have been demonstrated using the standardized "subcutaneous mouse inoculation assay," a standard measure of protozoan pathogenicity (94,205,1010).

A retrospective study of cecal and colonic tissues, stained with hematoxylin and eosin (HE), from a group of squirrel monkeys demonstrated *T. mobilensis* within luminal crypts (1010). These organisms were also seen to invade the mucosal epithelium, beneath the superficial luminal mucosal epithelium, and between the basement membrane and crypt epithelial cells. Immunoperoxidase staining also identified organisms within the lamina propria and submucosa. Histologically, mucosal ulceration, multifocal cryptitis, and focal epithelial necrosis also were observed, but most areas containing trichomonads did not have an associated inflammatory response (1010). Although trichomonads were not identified in mucosal ulcers, their occasional association with these lesions suggests the possibility that *T. mobilensis* may be pathogenic in the squirrel monkey (1010).

Invasive trichomoniasis has been previously reported involving the colonic mucosa in a New World Monkey (Titi monkey)

(122) and the stomach and pelvic cavity in Old World Monkeys (Rhesus monkeys) (79,773).

The diagnosis of trichomonads can be made using a combination of immediate microscopic examination and culture of fecal samples. The use of both techniques provides greater sensitivity than microscopic examination alone (94).

Some of the enteric trichomonads that infect nonhuman primates also are known to infect humans but are probably nonpathogenic to humans (373). Nevertheless, personnel working with/or caring for nonhuman primates should follow the same control measures outlined earlier for *Giardia*. As with *Giardia*, strict sanitary practices are vital for control.

An effective treatment regimen for adult monkeys is reported to be 25 mg/kg body weight of metronidazole (Flagyl) given orally, twice daily for 5 days. This treatment schedule appears to clear squirrel monkeys of *T. mobilensis* permanently, provided that animals are not reexposed (94).

2. Hemoflagellates

The hemoflagellates described in nonhuman primates are listed in Table I. The majority of the hemoflagellates reported from nonhuman primates are also considered to be nonpathogenic. An exception is *Trypanosoma cruzi*, which is an important pathogen and is the cause of Chagas disease in humans. Many species of wild and domestic animals have been found to be infected with this parasite, including nonhuman primates, and it is speculated that most mammals are susceptible. In addition, because it is an important pathogen of humans, it has potentially serious public health implications and will be discussed in detail below.

a. SOUTH AMERICAN TRYPANOSOMIASIS OR CHAGAS DISEASE. The cause of this disease, the hemoflagellate *T. cruzi,* is distributed throughout South and Central America with extension into the southern and southwestern regions of the United States.

Dr. Chagas made the original description of this parasite in *Callithrix penicillata* from Brazil (40,148). He also reported the first case of natural infection in the squirrel monkey (149).

Natural *T. cruzi* infection has been reported from numerous New World primate species (squirrel monkeys, owl monkeys, marmosets, tamarins, spider monkeys, woolly monkeys, cebus monkeys, and uakaris) (10,28,42,52,121,216,217,273,282,373, 453,676,694,738,741,1046,1066). It has also been reported as a congenital infection in a colony-born squirrel monkey (*Saimiri sciureus*) (289). *Trypanosoma cruzi* also has been reported from Old World Monkeys that originated in Asia (*Macaca* sp.) (40, 373,1020,1023), a colony-born baboon (*Papio cynocephalus*) (435), and great apes (gibbon) (1013).

Despite the reports in nonhuman primates other than New World monkeys, the question as to whether *T. cruzi* exists outside the Western Hemisphere remains unanswered. A review of some of the earlier reports of this parasite in Asian monkeys concluded that infection was most probably acquired after the animals were in captivity (40). Two additional cases have been reported involving rhesus monkeys that were members of colonies that were part of long-term research projects. Infection in these monkeys was considered also to have occurred during captivity, especially since they were housed outdoors in an endemic area of the United States (171,584).

Two forms of *T. cruzi* are found in susceptible animals. The trypomastigote (trypanosomal) form occurs in the blood; the amastigote (leishmanial) form is found in pseudocysts in the cells of skeletal and cardiac muscle, the reticuloendothelial system, and other tissues.

The life cycle is indirect with species of several genera of triatomid bugs belonging to the family Reduviidae (cone-nose bugs, assassin bugs, or kissing bugs) as biological vectors for New World monkeys. For a detailed description of the morphology and life cycle of this parasite, the reader is referred to the following references (373,698,700,1023).

Infection with *T. cruzi* causes rather nonspecific clinical signs (373). Generalized edema without necrosis or hemorrhage is said to be common. Anemia, hepatosplenomegaly, and lymphadenitis also can occur (373,1023). Depression, anorexia, weight loss, and dehydration were seen in the case involving the gibbon (1013). Electrocardiographic patterns consistent with that of right bundle branch block are reported from cebus monkeys and squirrel monkeys (121,694,1175). Also, a case of intrauterine death from congenital trypanosomiasis in marmosets has been reported (726).

The lesion mentioned most frequently in all of the naturally occurring cases of *T. cruzi* infection in nonhuman primates is myocarditis, which results in the destruction of myocardial fibers (121,373,435,676,1013). Histopathologically, the infected myocardium contains numerous, randomly scattered, cystic structures of varying sizes, occupying individual myocardial fibers. These structures are pseudocysts that contain many individual circular to oval-shaped organisms from 1.5 to 4 μm in diameter, with a central nucleus and a prominent bar-shaped structure (kinetoplast). These organisms can also be seen filling the cytoplasm of large mononuclear reticuloendothelial (RE) cells, some of which can be multinucleated and have the characteristics of giant cells. Degenerating pseudocysts elicit a focal mononuclear cell inflammatory response, and there may be mild dystrophic mineralization of individual myocardial fibers in some of these areas (584).

The diagnosis of *T. cruzi* can be made by demonstrating and identifying the parasites in blood or other body fluids, or in histological sections. Thin and thick blood smears should be stained with Giemsa preparations and examined for the presence of trypanosomes. The size and morphology of *T. cruzi* make it relatively easy to distinguish from the other trypanosomes commonly seen in neotropical primates (Fig. 1). It measures about 20 μm in length, but because it very often is curved in a c-shaped attitude, it appears smaller. The nucleus is located near midbody and a large kinetoplast is situated near the posterior end of the body. The flagellum runs along a narrow undu-

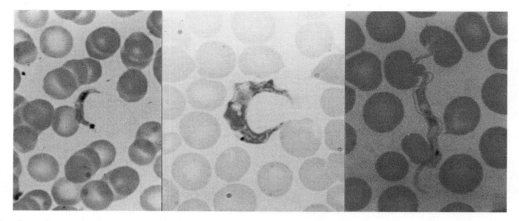

Fig. 1. Composite photomicrograph of trypanosomes in thin blood smears from infected neotropical primates. (Left) *Trypanosoma cruzi*-like organism from squirrel monkey (*Saimiri sciureus*) illustrating the small size. C-shaped attitude, and large, prominent kinetoplast near the end of the organism. (Middle) *Trypanosoma* species (possibly *T. lambrechti*) from a squirrel monkey (*S. sciureus*) illustrating the large, broad trypanosome with a very small kinetoplast not located terminally. (Right) *Trypanosoma rangeli*-like organism (= *T. minasense*) from a moustached marmoset (*Saguinus mystax mystax*) showing the long, slender body, again with a small kinetoplast not located terminally. Giemsa stain. (Reprinted from Toft, II, J. D. (1982). *Veterinary Pathology.* With permission.)

lating membrane and projects as a free flagellum from the anterior end. Animal inoculation and xenodiagnosis also can be used to allow the organism to complete its life cycle, or blood from suspected nonhuman primates can be cultured on NNN medium. Xenodiagnosis involves the examination of known vectors for trypanosomes after they have been allowed to feed on suspected hosts (40,373,694). Serologic testing, including complement fixation or ELISA-based assays, is used to test for infection in people and also may be helpful in screening for infections in monkeys.

Control is based on elimination of the insect vector. There is no reported effective treatment for *T. cruzi* in nonhuman primates (373,354,694).

Because *T. cruzi* can cause serious disease in humans, all people involved with the care and use of nonhuman primates should exercise extreme care to avoid exposure either by accidental inoculation with trypanosomes or by contamination of mucous membranes or skin with infected material. This should be especially true for those persons working with New World monkeys or with any nonhuman primate maintained in an endemic area in the United States (40,373).

B. Sarcodines: Ameba

The parasitic amebae described in nonhuman primates are listed in Table II. All are considered nonpathogenic except *Dientamoeba*, which sometimes can be pathogenic, and *Entamoeba histolytica* and *Balamuthia mandrillus,* which can cause severe enteric disease in humans and nonhuman primates. *Entamoeba histolytica* and *Balamuthia mandrillus* will be discussed in detail.

1. Amebiasis: *Entamoeba histolytica*

The cause of this disease, *E. histolytica,* has a worldwide distribution and has been reported in New World monkeys (spider monkeys, cebus monkeys, woolly monkeys, howler monkeys, squirrel monkeys, and marmosets), Old World monkeys (rhesus monkeys, pig-tailed macaques, bonnet macaques, cynomolgus monkeys, Barbary ape, colobus monkeys, proboscis monkeys, African green monkeys, baboons, guenons, and langurs), and the great apes (gibbons, orangutans, and chimpanzees) (14,60,75,126,228,268,293,294,367,373,387,430,431, 451,453,489,497,566,585,595,651,656–659,716,718,776,791, 794,862,929,967,972,973,995,1023,1115,1197).

Infection is said to be common in Old World monkeys but uncommon or rare in New World monkeys obtained from their natural habitat (258,967,1023,1121). Young monkeys and New World monkeys are reported to sustain more severe lesions from infection with this parasite (70,124,268,294,921,967,1121).

The morphology of this parasite has been reviewed (124,238, 373,517,694,699,700,974,1023). Two distinct but related species occur in humans and other primates. *Entamoeba histolytica* is considered pathogenic whereas *E. dispar* is not. The pathogenic *E. histolytica* is slightly larger; the trophozoites measure 20–30 μm in diameter. The smaller nonpathogenic *E. dispar* has trophozoites that measure 12–15 μm in diameter. Only the pathogenic organisms ingest red blood cells; the presence of erythrocytes within trophozoites is helpful in distinguishing pathogenic from nonpathogenic amoebae. Nuclear morphology also can be used to distinguish pathogenic *E. histolytica* from nonpathogenic species (191,694). Cysts are formed in the large intestine and may be uninucleate or binucleate. Mature cyst forms are 10–20 μm in diameter and contain four nuclei and

TABLE II

PARASITIC AMEBAE DESCRIBED FROM NONHUMAN PRIMATES

Parasite Genus species	Location in host	Prosimians	New World monkeys	Old World monkeys	Great apes	Reference
Phylum Sarcomastigophora, order Amoebida, family Entamoebidae (ameba)						
Entamoeba histolytica	Cecum, colon		X	X	X	4, 14, 60, 124, 224, 228, 268, 293, 367, 373, 390, 430, 431, 449, 451, 453, 480, 489, 564, 650–652, 656, 658, 659, 699, 700, 776, 791, 794, 805, 806, 811, 855, 862, 866, 895, 897, 898, 929, 967, 995, 1023, 1065, 1115, 1120, 1121, 1168
E. hartmanii	Cecum, colon			X	X	84, 124, 373, 564, 650, 656, 659, 699, 700, 806, 811
E. coli	Cecum, colon			X	X	21, 124, 224, 373, 564, 650–652, 656, 658, 659, 699, 700, 763, 765, 811, 855, 891, 929, 966, 1115
E. chattoni	Cecum, colon			X		124, 373, 594, 595, 650, 656, 699, 700, 811
E. gingivalis	Mouth			X	X	124, 373, 491, 699, 700, 967
E. polecki	Cecum, colon				X	656, 659, 806
Entamoeba sp.	Cecum, colon		X	X	X	651, 652, 656, 659, 757, 763, 1157
Iodamoeba buetschlii	Cecum, colon		X	X	X	21, 124, 268, 373, 489, 491, 564, 650–652, 658, 659, 699, 700, 730, 765, 806, 811, 929, 1161
I. wallacei	Intestine			X		937
Iodamoeba sp.	Cecum, colon		X	X		658, 659, 757, 763, 1157
Endolimax nana	Cecum, colon		X	X	X	21, 124, 268, 373, 489, 491, 564, 650–652, 658, 659, 699, 700, 730, 806, 811, 855, 929, 966
Endolimax sp.	Cecum, colon		X			1157
Phylum Sarcomastigophora, order Amoebida, family Acanthamoebidae						
Acanthamoeba-like	Brain, lung			X		18
Phylum Sarcomastigophora, Order Amoebida, family Hartmanellidae						
Hartmanella sp.	Brain			X		454
Phylum Sarcomastigophora, order Schizopyrenida, family Vahlkampfiidae						
Naegleri sp.	Brain			X		451
Phylum Sarcomastigophora, order Leptomyxida, family Leptomyxidae						
Balamuthia mandrillaris	Brain, lung, liver, kidney, mammary gland			X	X	942, 1123, 1124

rod-like chromatin bodies when mature. Maturation may occur in the intestine or outside the body.

These organisms reproduce by binary fission (124,373,700). Prior to producing the cyst form, the amebae become round and small. A cyst wall is formed; the nucleus divides twice, resulting in four small nuclei. The nuclei and cytoplasm divide on rupture of the cyst wall; thus each original cyst typically separates into four trophozoites.

Infection with *E. histolytica* may be asymptomatic or produce mild to severe clinical signs. There is a great variability in virulence among strains of organisms (124, 373, 699, 1023).

Pathogenicity is affected by the host species infected, the nutritional status of the host, environmental factors, and the bacterial flora present in the gastrointestinal tract (124,373,699,751,1023). *Entamoeba histolytica* usually lives in the intestinal lumen where it is nonpathogenic (699). Only when it invades the mucosa does it become pathogenic and lead to amebic dysentery (699).

Clinically, affected animals may show the following signs: apathy, lethargy, weakness, dehydration, gradual weight loss, anorexia, vomiting, and severe diarrhea, which may be hemorrhagic or catarrhal (124, 294, 373, 503, 512, 617, 694, 700, 776, 866,921,1065,1120,1121,1149).

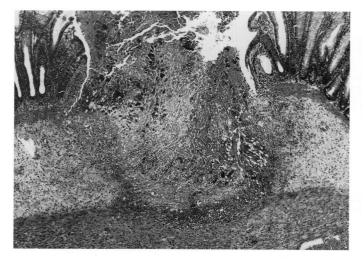

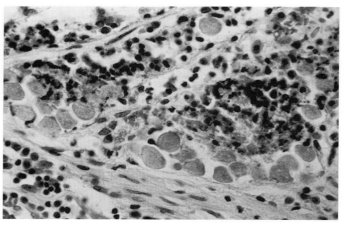

Fig. 3. Photomicrograph of spider monkey (*Ateles* sp.) showing *Entamoeba histolytica* trophozoites aggregating along advancing margin of ulcer between necrotic and normal tissue. HE stain.

Fig. 2. Photomicrograph of flash-shaped ulcer in colon of callicebus monkey (*Callicebus* sp.) with *Entamoeba histolytica* infection. Hematoxyline–eosine (HE) stain.

The gross and microscopic lesions associated with amebiasis in nonhuman primates have been described (84, 88, 124, 373, 390, 617, 694, 776, 866, 921, 967, 1023, 1065, 1121).

At necropsy, a mild to severe necroulcerative colitis can be seen. *Entamoeba histolytica* trophozoites can be found in wet smears from material from the colon of clinically ill animals or from the colonic contents overlying the lesions seen at necropsy (494).

Histologically, the colonic mucosa is necrotic and ulcerated down to the level of the muscularis mucosae; typical flask-shaped ulcers may be seen (Fig. 2). These ulcers can be as small as a few millimeters or may become large and confluent and involve extensive areas of the colon. Ulcerative extension through the muscular coats of the large intestine is possible, resulting in peritonitis. Trophozoites may be seen in or adjacent to the ulcers (Fig. 3). Amebae do not stain well with HE, but stain bright red with the periodic acid–Schiff stain. Trichrome, Giemsa, or iron hematoxylin stains may be used to demonstrate nuclear structure (694). Often, the host response is minimal unless secondary bacterial invasion has occurred (373, 617, 694, 921, 1023). Extensive hemorrhage with neutrophilic and mononuclear inflammatory cell infiltrates has been described in lesions from New World monkeys (617).

Some trophozoites may enter lymphatic channels or even the venules of the mesenteric vasculature. Most are filtered by the regional lymph nodes; a few, however, may be carried to distant parts of the body where they can produce the so-called amebic abscesses, particularly in the liver, lungs, or central nervous system (CNS) (373, 390, 694, 776, 866, 1023).

Fatal amebiasis with abscess formation has been reported in a baboon (390), a chimpanzee (776), an orangutan (866), a group of spider monkeys (14), douc langurs (387), and several colobus monkeys (387, 716, 718).

Gastric amebiasis and death due to infection with *E. histolytica* has been reported in the silver leaf monkey, douc langurs, proboscis monkey, and colobus monkey (387, 431, 716, 718, 794, 862).

The diagnosis of amebiasis depends on the microscopic recognition of the causative organisms in the feces or in intimate association with typical lesions. These organisms are also common as nonpathogenic commensals in the digestive tract of nonhuman primates. Their presence in the feces of animals with clinical signs is not definitive evidence that protozoa are the cause of the gastrointestinal disease (373, 700, 1023). Wet-mount preparations may be used to examine the feces for trophozoites. This requires a fresh sample, which must be placed immediately in a saline or buffer solution and examined while the preparation is still warm. The movement of the organisms can be seen. *Entamoeba histolytica* makes the most obvious kinds of progressive movement of all the intestinal amoebae. Staining for *E. histolytica* can be accomplished easily and rapidly with trichrome or Giemsa stains. Smears may be stained with Lugol's iodine solution, which identifies the nuclei and stains glycogen. Smears also may be fixed in Schaudinn's fluid and stained with Heidenhain's iron hematoxylin (124, 1023).

Strict sanitation is paramount in the prevention of amebiasis. The trophozoites are killed with common disinfectants; however, the cysts are more resistant, and hot water or steam is necessary to destroy them (373). Infected humans are a potential source of infection for monkeys, particularly if they are involved in the preparation or handling of feed. Also, insects such as flies and cockroaches may serve as mechanical carriers of the amebic cysts (694). Routine screening of laboratory animal technicians and an active program of vermin control and prevention should be part of any nonhuman primate colony management program.

Entamoeba histolytica causes amebic dysentery in humans; therefore, this organism in nonhuman primates poses a serious potential public health problem. The disease has been transmitted from laboratory primates to humans (72,430). These primates should be considered potential sources of infection for both humans and other monkeys, and proper care and hygiene should be exercised in all phases of their handling to prevent direct oral contact with their feces. The high incidence of asymptomatic carriers complicates this problem (934).

The treatment of choice for both intestinal and extraintestinal amebiasis is metronidazole (Flagyl) at a dose of 30–50 mg/kg/day given orally in three divided doses for 5–10 days. Combination with diiodohydroxyquin (Diodoquin, Yodoxin) at a dose of 30–40 mg/kg/day in three individual doses may be required in severe cases. Tetracycline, at a dose of 25–50 mg/kg for 5 to 10 days, and/or chloroquin, at a dose of 5 mg/kg for 14 days, or chloramphenicol, at a dose of 50–100 mg/kg twice daily, also may be used. Three negative stools obtained on three successive days are usually indicative of cure. Reexamination of the stools at 1, 3, and 6 months after treatment is recommended (213, 694,934).

2. Balamuthiasis

This free-living, soil-dwelling ameba (family Leptomyxidae, order Leptomyxida) has been isolated and described from brain tissue of a mandrill (*Papio sphinx*) that died of acute suppurative meningoencephalitis at the San Diego Wild Animal Park (1123,1124). The parasite was named *Balamuthia mandrillaris*. Since then, infections in a white-cheeked gibbon (*Hylobates concolor leucogenys*), two western lowland gorillas (*Gorilla gorilla gorilla*), and a kibuya colobus monkey (*Colobus guereza kikuyuensis*) have been identified (942). There have also

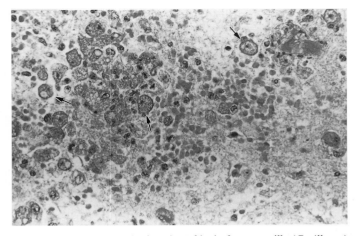

Fig. 5. Photomicrograph of section of brain from a gorilla (*Gorilla* sp.) infected with *Balamuthia mandrillarus*. At greater magnification, trophozoites (arrows) are more readily seen. HE stain. (Courtesy of Dr. G. Visvesvara.)

been at least 60 reported cases of human infection with this same ameba, all resulting in amoebic meningoencephalitis (743).

Not a great deal is known about the life cycle, but it is presumably direct through contact with soil or other environmental surfaces. Identification is through detection of organisms in brain (Figs. 4 and 5) or other tissues in either routine-stained sections or through immunofluorescent staining (942). *Balamuthia* probably cannot be distinguished readily from *Acanthamoeba* in tissue sections, based on morphologic features. Immunofluorescent staining, electron microscopic study, or *in vitro* isolation are required to separate these two causes of amebic meningoencephalitis (942).

Clinically, animals experienced either an acute to subacute course that was as short as 2 days in some cases. Animals generally exhibited prominent CNS signs, including limb paresis or paralysis, depression, and weakness. Because of the rapid progression of the disease, supportive care was unrewarding. Animals with chronic disease, in one instance of over a year, typically exhibited variable lethargy, depression, and weight loss. In addition, disseminated lesions or tissue masses were noted in the mammary glands, lung, liver, and kidney (942).

No effective treatment for *Balamuthia* infections are recognized currently, although pentamidine isethionate has shown promise in *in vitro* studies (1007).

The likelihood of animal to humans transmission of *Balamuthia* would seem to be small, although exposure during necropsy could pose increased risk.

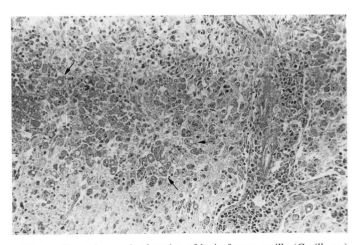

Fig. 4. Photomicrograph of section of brain from a gorilla (*Gorilla* sp.) infected with *Balamuthia mandrillarus* infection. Numerous trophozoites (arrows) are discernable in the granulomatous inflammatory lesion. HE stain. (Courtesy of Dr. G. Visvesvara.)

C. Apicomplexa: Coccidians

The coccidian parasites described from nonhuman primates are listed in Table III. Infection with most of the common en-

TABLE III

PARASITIC COCCIDIANS DESCRIBED FROM NONHUMAN PRIMATES

Parasite Genus species	Location in host	Prosimians	New World monkeys	Old World monkeys	Great apes	Reference
Phylum Apicomplexa, order Eucoccidiorida, family Eimeriidae						
Eimeria galago	Intestine	X				124, 373, 889
E. lemuris	Intestine	X				124, 373, 889
E. otolicni	Intestine	X				124, 373, 889
E. pachylepyron	Intestine	X				180
E. tupaiae	Intestine	X				798
E. modesta	Intestine	X				798
E. ferruginea	Intestine	X				798
Eimeria sp.	Intestine	X				224, 514
Isospora arctopitheci	Intestine		X			124, 373, 498, 499, 952
I. callimico	Intestine		X			280, 532
I. papionis	Intestine			X		759, 760, 763
Isospora sp.	Intestine	X			X	124, 373, 650, 889, 943
Cyclospora	Intestine			X	X	25, 1038
Phylum Apicomplexa, order Eucoccidiorida, family Cryptosporidiidae						
Cryptosporidium sp.	Intestine	X	X	X		116, 178, 507, 578, 631, 777, 1023, 1171
Phylum Apicomplexa, order Eucoccidiorida, family Klossiellidae						
Klossiella sp.	Kidney	X				125, 1003
Phylum Apicomplexa, order Eucoccidiorida, family Haemogregerinidae						
Haemogregarina cynomolgi	Blood			X		81, 373, 670, 693, 1163
Phylum Apicomplexa, order Piroplasmorida, family Babesiidae						
Babesia pitheci	Erythrocytes			X		40, 373, 411, 512, 513, 599, 963, 1079
Babesia sp.	Erythrocytes	X				103
Entopolypoides macaci	Erythrocytes			X		40, 346, 373, 434, 481, 650, 748, 749, 786
Phylum Apicomplexa, order Eucoccidiorida, family Theileriidae						
Theileria cellii	Erythrocytes			X		135, 136, 373
Phylum Apicomplexa, order Eucoccidiorida, family Plasmodiidae						
Plasmodium cynomolgi	Erythrocytes			X		101, 183, 187, 236, 312, 315, 319, 373, 412, 415, 420, 557, 747, 795, 919, 998, 999
P. knowlesi	Erythrocytes			X		112, 165, 183, 319, 373, 414, 415, 420, 623, 667, 999, 1030, 1193
P. inui (syn. *P. shortti*)	Erythrocytes			X		101, 102, 183, 242, 312, 313, 373, 415, 420, 467, 557, 667, 1027, 1029, 1051
P. coatneyi	Erythrocytes			X		183, 312, 316, 317, 320, 373, 415, 420, 744, 859, 860, 863, 1140
P. fieldi	Erythrocytes			X		183, 312, 318, 373, 415, 494, 1140
P. gonderi	Erythrocytes			X		183, 315, 373, 415, 423, 958

TABLE III—*Continued*

PARASITIC COCCIDIANS DESCRIBED FROM NONHUMAN PRIMATES

Parasite Genus species	Location in host	Prosimians	New World monkeys	Old World monkeys	Great apes	Reference
P. fragile	Erythrocytes			X		183, 236, 373, 415, 920
P. siminovale	Erythrocytes			X		183, 236, 237, 373, 415
Plasmodium sp.	Erythrocytes			X		312, 373
P. brasilianum	Erythrocytes		X			183, 222, 266, 272, 373, 415, 420, 442, 742, 901, 1076
P. simium	Erythrocytes		X			183, 221, 222, 373, 375, 413, 415, 420
P. pitheci	Erythrocytes				X	183, 373, 415, 420, 430, 467
P. malariae (syn. *P. rodhaini*)	Erythrocytes				X	99, 100, 373, 420, 422, 955, 956
P. reichenowi	Erythrocytes				X	96, 97, 102, 183, 373, 415, 420, 422, 430, 931, 1034
P. schwetzi	Erythrocytes				X	98, 101, 113, 183, 373, 415, 420, 957
P. hylobati	Erythrocytes				X	102, 183, 184, 373, 415, 420, 430, 953
P. eylesi	Erythrocytes				X	183, 373, 415, 420, 1141
P. jefferyi	Erythrocytes				X	183, 373, 415, 420, 1142, 1143
P. youngi	Erythrocytes				X	183, 320, 373, 415, 420
P. silvaticum	Erythrocytes				X	183, 420, 426, 712
P. girardi	Erythrocytes	X				59, 117, 183, 197, 373, 417, 421
P. lemuris	Erythrocytes	X				183, 373, 538
P. foleyi	Erythrocytes	X				59, 197, 417, 421
Hepatocystis kochi (syn. *H. simiae*)	Erythrocytes			X		3, 99, 348, 373, 385, 409, 410, 416, 424, 602, 652, 653, 685, 692, 763, 775, 805, 853, 882, 883, 1058, 1105, 1119
H. semnopitheci	Erythrocytes			X		313, 314, 348, 373, 416, 484, 622, 892, 931, 969
H. taiwanensis	Erythrocytes			X		101, 348, 373, 416, 969
H. bouillezi	Erythrocytes			X		348, 416
H. cercopitheci	Erythrocytes			X		348, 416
H. foleyi	Erythrocytes	X				101, 117, 373
Hepatocystis sp.	Erythrocytes				X	230, 231, 757, 1026
Sergentella anthropopitheci	Blood				X	229, 373
Phylum Apicomplexa, order Eucoccidiorida, family Sarcocystidae						
Sarcocystis kortei	Striated muscle, oral cavity, heart, tongue, esophagus			X		40, 250, 373, 463, 476, 491, 733, 836
S. nesbitti	Striated muscle, oral cavity, heart, tongue, esophagus			X		40, 373, 733
Sarcocystis sp.	Striated muscle, oral cavity, heart, tongue, esophagus	X	X	X		44, 224, 373, 489, 497, 616, 757, 763, 819, 909, 1070, 1074, 1202
Toxoplasma gondii	Brain, lungs, liver, heart, kidney, lymph nodes, blood, other tissues	X	X	X	X	17, 40, 57–59, 86, 113, 114, 158, 197, 210, 234, 238, 249, 373, 421, 505, 560, 628, 696, 762, 763, 766, 824, 829, 923–926, 949, 1014, 1052, 1068, 1088, 1108, 1110, 1179, 1181, 1204, 1205

teric coccidian parasites is considered essentially innocuous; there are no known lesions or diseases associated with their presence in the nonhuman primate gastrointestinal tract. An exception is *Cryptosporidium* sp., which has been described from the gastrointestinal tract of monkeys and *Cyclospora* sp.; they will be discussed in greater detail. In addition, the malarial parasites, toxoplasmasids (*Sarcocystis* and *Toxoplasma*), piroplasmids (*Babesia* and *Entopolypoides*), and microsporidains (*Encephalitozoon*), will be discussed in detail.

1. Cryptosporidiosis

This disease, caused by coccidian parasites of the genus *Cryptosporidium,* has been shown to cause gastroenteritis and diarrhea in many species of animals, including humans, domestic and exotic mammals, reptiles, and fish (507,818,1106).

The life cycle of this parasite is monoxenous and generally follows that of other enteric coccidia (808,1106). Mature sporulated oocysts passed in the feces of infected animals are immediately infective for other susceptible animals, are relatively resistant to drying, highly resistant to chemical disinfection, and remain viable for months in water (777,818). After ingestion, sporozoites are released from the oocyst in the gastrointestinal tract of the new host and develop into trophozoites, which are the earliest developmental stage of this parasite to be observed so far. This and all other developmental stages are found just under the surface of various epithelial membranes, never within the cytoplasm of the epithelial cells or beneath the epithelial layer (818).

Trophozoites undergo three nuclear divisions to form eight daughter merozoites resulting in a structure termed a first-generation schizont. These eight first-generation merozoites are released from the schizont and reinfect other epithelial cells. After attachment, the elongated merozoite becomes round and undergoes two nuclear divisions resulting in the second-generation schizont, which contains four second-generation merozoites (818).

As with other apicomplexans, both macrogametocytes and microgametocytes occur. Macrogametocytes undergo little change as they become macrogametes, but microgametocytes undergo nuclear division and form several microgametes. When a microgamete joins with a macrogamete, a zygote is formed. The zygote then develops into a oocyst and the life cycle is complete (818). *Cryptosporidium* sp. organisms have been reported in the digestive tract of rhesus monkeys (*Macaca mulatta*) (Fig. 6), including those with acquired immune deficiency syndrome (178,501,631,951), cynomolgus monkey (*Macaca fascicularis*) and bonnet monkey (*Macaca radiata*) (1171), pigtailed macaques (*Macaca nemestrina*) (641,777), red-ruffed lemur (*Varecia variegata*), and a cotton-topped tamarin (*Saguinus oedipus*) (507).

In one study, the organisms were seen in the epithelium of the common bile duct, the intrahepatic and pancreatic ducts, and the gallbladder of one monkey (631). Histologic changes

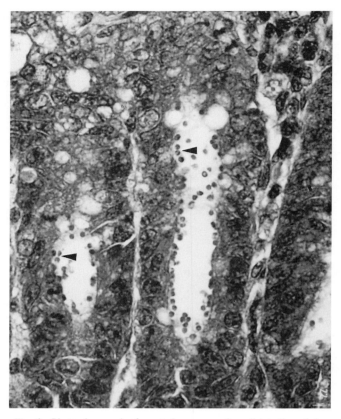

Fig. 6.   Photomicrograph of crypts in mucosa of small intestine of rhesus monkey (*Macaca mulatta*). Many *Cryptosporidium* organisms are attached to the luminal surface of crypt epithelial cells (arrowheads). HE stain. (Reprinted from Toft, II, J. D. (1982). *Veterinary Pathology.* With permission.)

consisted of epithelial hyperplasia and mucosal inflammation.

In another study, cryptosporidial organisms were found on the small intestinal epithelium of seven rhesus monkeys and on both the small and the large intestinal epithelium of one infant monkey. No lesions were associated with the organisms in any of the monkeys except the infant. In this infant, the changes were characterized by atrophy of villi associated with many parasites in the brush border of the epithelium lining the villi and intestinal crypts (178).

Severe intestinal disease in four juvenile macaques due to infection with *Cryptosporidium* sp. has been documented (1171). Two of the animals died naturally and the other two were humanely killed due to the illness, despite extensive therapy.

Clinical signs in these young monkeys consisted of depression, dehydration, weight loss, and intractable diarrhea (1171).

At necropsy, the animals were considered to be underweight for their age and dehydrated. The intestines were distended with gas and liquid, and the mesenteric lymph nodes were enlarged in three of the four monkeys (1171).

Histopathologically, the lesions in the small intestine consisted of blunting and fusion of villi, variation in height of the intestinal epithelium, necrosis of individual epithelial cells, and an increased mitotic index in the crypts. Variable numbers of organisms with both light microscopic and ultrastructural morphologic features consistent with *Cryptosporidium* sp. were seen adherent to enterocytes along the tips and side of villi, as well as within the crypts (1171).

These cases indicate that cryptosporidial infection in young macaques can be a severe and potentially fatal disease. The cryptosporidia were associated with ultrastructural changes in the enterocytes, which can result in malabsorption, as well as fluid loss in the infected host (1171).

In another report (777), 81 cases of acute cryptosporidiosis were diagnosed among a group of 157 infant primates, mainly *Macaca nemestrina,* housed in a nursery unit.

Clinical signs in this outbreak consisted of profuse, watery diarrhea, and dehydration. Fever was not a common finding, but hypothermia was seen as a secondary complication in dehydrated animals. The younger infants also exhibited anorexia (777). Infected animals excreted oocysts for a mean of 36 days. No reinfections occurred and no deaths were reported (777).

The disease just described in infant macaques is considered to be clinically, histologically, and microbiologically indistinguishable from that seen in young children. This has led to the development of a reproducible experimental model of cryptosporidiosis in pig-tailed macaques (*Macaca nemestrina*) that has been used to study the infectious dose of oocysts and the effect of inoculum size on the severity of the disease (778).

Diagnosis is based on histological demonstration of the endogenous stages of the parasite attached to the brush border of epithelial cells either by light or electron microscopic examination or by the identification of *Cryptosporidium* oocysts in stool samples of infected patients (818,1106). Techniques used to identify oocysts include acid-fast staining of fecal smears or concentrates with carbolfuchsin [cold Kinyoun stain, dimethyl sulfoxide (DMSO)–carbolfuchsin, or Ziehl–Neelsen stain] (107, 502,507,818,1048,1106), fluorescence staining with auramine O (507,1048), or a modification of the traditional Sheather's sucrose coverslip flotation followed by phase microscopy (507, 818,1048). Other effective methods of oocyst detection include a modified zinc sulfate centrifugal flotation method (1106), the fecal flotation technique (1106), Giemsa staining (507,1106, 1048), iodine staining (507,1048), safranin–methylene blue staining (507,1048), Hemacolor staining (1048), methylene blue–eosine staining (1048), and negative staining by periodic acid–Schiff reagent (1048). The use of combinations of some of these methods of oocyst detection have been commonly reported (1048). Direct and indirect fluorescent antibody procedures have been developed that provide potentially more specific and sensitive ways of visualizing *Cryptosporidium* oocysts in fecal smears or concentrates (1048), and the use of a stool antigen detection assay is even more sensitive, in that whole organisms need not be present for a positive test.

Fecal specimens suspected of containing oocysts can be preserved in 5 or 10% formalin for future examination. Some workers prefer 2.5% potassium dichromate as a preservative;

the sporozoites within oocysts become easier to recognize after 1 week in potassium dichromate because much of the oocyst residuum disappears during this time (818). Because oocysts may remain viable when preserved in potassium dichromate, extra care should be taken while handling specimens preserved in this medium (818).

Control should be aimed at isolation of infected animals in conjunction with proper sanitation and management. Control and/or elimination of the disease is hampered by the fact that cryptosporidial occysts are extremely resistant to the action of common laboratory disinfectants (1106), including full-strength Clorox.

Because *Cryptosporidium* lacks host specificity, a characteristic uncommon among other enteric coccidia, these organisms should be considered to have a high potential for zoonotic transmission (1106). Cases of crytosporidiosis among animal handlers caring for infected infant nonhuman primates in a nursery have been reported (777). The occurrence of these cases during the nursery outbreak strongly suggests transmission from the infected primates to humans (777). All primate handlers should be considered at risk for occupational exposure to *Cryptosporidium* (777). Care in handling these animals, in addition to the wearing of approved protective clothing and proper personal hygiene practices, should be standard operating procedures for all personnel who work with and care for nonhuman primates.

A large number of antimicrobial agents have been tested against *Cryptosporidium;* none have been found to be effective (507,777,818,1106). Therapy for affected animals should be mainly supportive, consisting of fluid and electrolyte replacement, antidiarrheal compounds, antibiotics, and other supportive measures (507).

2. Cyclosporiasis

Cyclospora cayetenensis has been recognized and described as an important cause of diarrheal illness in humans. A similar if not identical parasite has been reported from nonhuman primates. First reported from chimpanzees in Uganda (26), *Cyclospora* has since been found to be common in baboons (*Papio* sp.) in Tanzania (1038). The full range of potential primate hosts for this parasite may be extensive.

Cyclospora is diagnosed by finding the characteristic oocysts in feces. The oocysts are unsporulated when passed and can be identified readily using fluorescence microscopy; they stain variably with acid fast and uniformly with safranin if heated during the staining process (291,1125). The oocysts measure 8–10 μm in diameter, thus they are about twice the size of *Cryptosporidium* oocysts. If held under appropriate conditions, oocysts sporulate in about 10 days and contain two sporocysts, each with two sporozoites. Infection is through oral ingestion of sporulated, infective oocysts. Because of the time required for sporulation, it is not likely that transmission between nonhuman primates and humans occurs in institutional settings, but in nature, it may well be a shared parasite.

In humans, *Cyclospora* infection frequently results in severe, watery diarrhea, weight loss, and fatigue. Treatment with trimethoprim–sulfamethoxazole (Septra) results in rapid clinical improvement in humans and should be equally effective in treating nonhuman primates. A clinical course of infection has not been established for infections in chimpanzees or baboons, and it may be that a less severe clinical course is experienced by these animals.

The intestinal stages of the parasite have not been well documented, but there appear to be similarities to other coccidian infections.

3. Malaria

This disease, caused by parasites in the family Plasmodiidae, genus *Plasmodium,* affects both humans and animals (52,102, 182,188,373,415,420,694,967,985,1023,1131). Malaria is one of the most important hemoprotozoal parasitic diseases of primates in the tropical and semitropical regions of the world. The species reported to occur in nonhuman primates are listed in Table III.

Natural infection is universal among nonhuman primates, with the exception of a few species: rhesus monkey (*Macaca mulatta*), tamarins and marmosets (*Callithrix* sp. and *Saquinus* sp.), and owl monkeys (*Aotus* sp.). *Aotus* and members of the Callithrichidae, however, are susceptible to experimental infection (694,742).

Malaria parasites that infect the anthropoid apes are a different group of *Plasmodium* than those that afflict monkey species. They are virtually homologous to the malaria parasites of humans and they are considered to be indistinguishable morphologically. Cross-infection to humans has been documented.

In the natural host these organisms do not produce a very severe disease, as there are no outward signs of illness seen and usually no fever. There may be a slight anemia associated with a low-grade parasitemia in some animals, but they appear outwardly normal. In the aberrant host, infection with malarial parasites produces severe disease and debilitation which can, and often does, lead to death.

Malaria parasites can be classified on the basis of the host infected, human, monkey, or anthropoid ape; on the morphology of the parasite; or on the basis of the type of cyclic fever produced. Thus, quotidian malaria has a 24-hr cycle, tertian malaria has a 48-hr cycle, and quartan malaria has a 72-hr cycle. The periodicity of the cyclic fever is determined by the length of time the organisms parasitize the host erythrocytes.

The life cycle of malaria parasites has been reviewed in detail (175,181–183,312,373,415,700,735,1023,1131). It is indirect with numerous mosquitoes in the genus *Anopheles* serving as biological vectors.

Basically, the life cycle consists of two major phases: the sexual or sporogonic phase in the mosquito vector and the asexual or schizogonic/gametogonic phase in the vertebrate host. The schizogonic phase is further divided into the exoerythrocytic or liver phase and the erythrocytic or blood phase.

Clinical signs reported in nonhuman primates infected with malaria consist of irritability, cyclic fever, depression, listlessness, anorexia, and weight loss. Thrombocytopenia, leukopenia, progressive anemia, and reticulocytosis also have been reported. Diarrhea may be an accompanying symptom (182, 373, 694, 1023, 1051, 1076, 1131). Hematocrit, hemoglobin, mean corpuscular volume, and erythrocyte values are reported to be lower in infected nonhuman primates (242,496). In general, young animals exhibit more severe symptoms than older animals (1131).

Fever in infected nonhuman primates is less severe than in their human counterparts. The onset of fever coincides with the rupture of the parasitized erythrocytes and the release of toxic metabolic products into the bloodstream. Depending on the species of *Plasmodium* involved, this event can occur at 24-, 48-, or 72-hr intervals. Usually the natural nonhuman primate host of a species of plasmodia is asymptomatic.

Histopathology consists of hepatosplenomegaly, hyperplasia of lymphoid elements, and macrophages in the spleen, liver, and bone marrow. Myeloid hyperplasia of the bone marrow may be seen in conjunction with erythropoiesis. Malarial pigment (hemazoin) deposition occurs in the Kupffer cells of the liver, in macrophages in the bone marrow, and in red pulp of the spleen. Hemorrhages in the brain, splenic rupture, and lower nephron (tubular) necrosis of the kidney also have been reported (373,694,712,962,1023,1075,1131).

The diagnosis of malaria depends on the demonstration and identification of the organisms in erythrocytes in thin or thick blood smears stained with Giemsa or Wright–Giemsa stains (182,183,373,1023). A negative blood smear from a feral nonhuman primate does not necessarily mean that the animal is in a malaria-free state.

Serologic tests (fluorescent antibody) have been developed for the examination of nonhuman primates to determine the presence of past or present malaria infection. Many of these infections persist at patent or subpatent levels for many years and will rise to higher levels if the animal is splenectomized (182).

Effective mosquito control is essential to prevent transmission of malaria in laboratory animal colonies or other facilities in which possibly infected nonhuman primates are housed.

Malaria in most nonhuman primates is generally not fatal. However, it may cause debilitation and overt disease can be precipitated by stress, concurrent disease, splenectomy or immunosuppression. Handlers of malarious nonhuman primates are at a great risk from acquiring infection through the blood-borne route. Infected nonhuman primates may also serve as sources of infection for man provided the required mosquito vectors are present (165,188,374,1139). However, many more laboratory accidents are through the blood-borne route than through mosquito transmission. All people actively working with or caring for nonhuman primates should be alert to the possible existence and potential liabilities of malarial infection.

Treatment of malaria in nonhuman primates consists of intramuscular administration of chloroquine, 2.5–5 mg/kg of body weight for 4–7 days, followed by oral administration of primaquine, 0.75 mg/kg of body weight for 14 days (2, 373, 694). Because of increased toxicity when given together, these two drugs should be given separately (694).

a. MALARIA OF OLD WORLD MONKEYS. i. *Plasmodium knowlesi:* This is the only known quotidian (24-hr) malarial parasite. It is distributed geographically throughout southeast Asia and the natural hosts include the cynomolgus monkey (*Macaca fascicularis*), leaf monkey (*Presbytis malalophus*), and the pig-tailed macaque (*Macaca nemestrina*).

Plasmodium knowlesi produces a virulent infection in the rhesus monkey (*Macaca mulatta*), which is almost always fatal, and resembles acute *P. falciparum* infection of humans (101, 112, 165, 312, 319, 373, 414, 415, 420, 623, 667, 712, 999, 1030, 1131, 1193). Naturally acquired cases of *P. knowlesi* infection have been reported in humans (165, 374, 420).

ii. *Plasmodium cynomolgi:* This is a tertian malarial parasite with a geographic distribution including the East Indies, southeast Asia, and the Philippine Islands. Natural hosts include a wide variety of *Macaca* species, including the cynomolgus monkey (*M. fascicularis*), Toque monkey (*Macaca sinica*), pig-tailed macaque (*M. nemestrina*), bonnet macaque (*Macaca radiata*), Formosan rock macaque (*Macaca cyclopis*), and several species of leaf monkeys (*Presbytis cristatus* and *P. entellus*). Infection in the rhesus monkey (*M. mulatta*) with this organism is not as severe as with *P. knowlesi* and usually consists of low-grade parasitemia of long duration. This organism is similar to *P. vivax* of humans and is also transmissible to humans (101, 187, 236, 312, 319, 373, 412, 415, 420, 712, 747, 795, 919, 999, 1131).

iii. *Plasmodium gonderi:* This tertian malarial parasite is distributed throughout west Africa and tropical central Africa, and is the only simian *Plasmodium* found in Africa. Natural hosts include mangabeys (*Cercocebus* sp.), and drills (*Mandrillus* sp.). This parasite produces a high, chronic parasitemia in the rhesus monkey (*M. mulatta*). Baboons (*Papio* sp.) and guenons (*Cercopithecus* sp.) are also susceptible. Humans have proven to be susceptible in experimental studies (99, 175, 373, 415, 423, 442, 712, 958, 1030, 1131).

iv. *Plasmodium fieldi:* *P. fieldi* is a tertian malarial parasite found on the Malay Peninsula. Natural hosts include the Asian species of *Macaca*, including the cynomolgus monkey (*M. fascicularis*), and the pig-tailed macaque (*M. nemestrina*). Infection with *P. fieldi* produces a severe disease in the rhesus monkey (*M. mulatta*), which is often fatal. Humans seem to be resistant to infection with this organism (318, 373, 415, 494, 712, 1131, 1140).

v. *Plasmodium fragile* This is also a tertian malarial parasite with a geographic range throughout southern India and on the island of Sri Lanka. Natural hosts include the Toque monkey (*Macaca sinica*) and the bonnet macaque (*Macaca radiata*). Infection in the rhesus monkey (*M. mulatta*) produces severe

disease, which often kills the host (175, 236, 373, 415, 712, 920, 1131).

vi. *Plasmodium siminovale:* This tertian malarial parasite is found on the island of Sri Lanka. The natural host is the Toque monkey (*M. sinica*). Even though the parasitemia is not particularly severe, a pronounced anemia has been reported to accompany this infection. This parasite is considered to be similar to *P. ovale* of humans (237, 373, 415, 712, 1131).

vii. *Plasmodium coatneyi:* This species of malarial parasite causes a mild tertian malaria in susceptible hosts. Its geographic distribution includes the Malay Peninsula and the Philippine Islands. The natural nonhuman primate host is the cynomolgus monkey (*M. fascicularis*). It is quite closely related morphologically to *P. knowlesi,* and the infection in the rhesus monkey (*M. mulatta*) is similar to *P. knowlesi,* producing a severe and often fatal disease accompanied by severe anemia (316, 317, 320, 340, 373, 415, 420, 712, 1131, 1140).

viii. *Plasmodium inui:* *P. inui* is a mildly pathogenic species that produces a quartan malaria in susceptible hosts. It is very widespread throughout southeast Asia and extends from India to the Philippine Islands. The natural hosts include the Asian species of *Macaca;* cynomolgus monkey (*M. fascicularis*) and pig-tailed macaque (*M. nemestrina*). It has also been reported from members of the genus *Presbytis* and the Celebes black ape (*Cynopithecus niger*). This infection is frequently encountered in asian monkeys and can persist for at least several years even in animals removed from endemic areas. Infection in rhesus monkeys (*M. mulatta*) produces a mild to moderate, usually nonfatal illness. The presence of clinical signs has been reported in as many of 16–22% of infected animals (1000, 1004).

The parasite is considered to be homologous to *P. malariae* of humans, and humans are susceptible to infection with this organism (101, 102, 312, 313, 373, 415, 420, 467, 531, 667, 712, 999, 1027, 1029, 1131).

ix. *Plasmodium shortti:* This quartan malarial parasite is found in India and on the island of Sri Lanka. Natural nonhuman primate hosts include the Toque monkey (*M. sinica*) and the bonnet macaque (*M. radiata*). This organism has been transmitted experimentally to humans (101, 312, 373, 415, 420, 1027).

b. MALARIAL PARASITES OF NEW WORLD MONKEYS. i. *Plasmodium simium:* This is a tertian malarial parasite with a geographic distribution in the region of southern Brazil. The natural nonhuman primate hosts are howler monkeys (*Alouatta* sp.) and woolly spider monkeys (*Brachyteles arachnoides*). The organism is similar to *P. vivax* of humans, and infection with this parasite has been reported in humans (175, 221, 373, 375, 413, 415, 420, 712, 1131).

ii. *Plasmodium brazilianum:* *P. brazilianum* is sometimes a markedly pathogenic species and is the most common malarial parasite of New World monkeys. The natural nonhuman primate hosts include howler monkeys (*Alouatta* sp.), spider monkeys (*Ateles* sp.), woolly spider monkeys (*Brachyteles* sp.), Uakaris (*Cacajao* sp.), titis (*Callicebus* sp.), bearded sakis (*Chiroptes* sp.), capuchin monkeys (*Cebus* sp.), woolly monkeys (*Lagothrix* sp.), and squirrel monkeys (*Saimiri* sp.) (3,175,272, 373,415,442,712,742,901,1076,1131). The geographic distribution ranges from Mexico throughout Central America and into South America down to Peru. *Plasmodium brazilanum* causes quartan malaria, which can produce severe symptoms due to extensive destruction of erythrocytes, and even adult monkeys have been known to die from this infection (415,694, 712, 1076). Usually it is seen as an infection at equilibrium, having a low parasitemia that may persist for several years (1131). This organism is considered to be the same as *P. malariae* of humans, and humans are susceptible to experimental infection (420). This species may actually be *P. malariae* introduced into the New World by early explorers and modified through numerous passages in wild monkeys (266,373).

c. MALARIA OF ANTHROPOID APES. i. *Plasmodium pitheci* and *Plasmodium silvaticum:* These two species of malaria parasites are found in orangutans, often as double infections (420). These are tertian malarial parasites; the former was originally described in 1907 from Borneo in an orangutan (*Pongo* sp.) (415,418,467,712). Orangutans are the only nonhuman primates in which this parasite has been reported and there are few details about the organism and the disease it produces (420). It has proved to be noninfectious for gibbons and monkeys in limited experimental studies.

ii. *Plasmodium rodhaini:* P. rodhaini is found in west to central tropical Africa where it causes quartan malaria in its natural nonhuman primate hosts: chimpanzees (*Pan* sp.) and gorillas (*Gorilla* sp.). There is no morphological difference between this organism and *Plasmodium malariae* of humans; these two parasites are considered to be synonymous. This is the only malarial parasite that occurs as a natural infection in humans and nonhuman primates to any great extent. Infection is easily transmitted from humans to chimpanzees and vice versa (99,100,373,420,422,712,955,956,1131).

iii. *Plasmodium reichenowi:* This mildly pathogenic species occurs in west, central, and east tropical Africa. The natural nonhuman primate hosts include chimpanzees (*Pan* sp.) and gorillas (*Gorilla* sp.). *Plasmodium reichenowi* causes a mild quartan malaria in these species. This organism is very similar to *P. falciparum* of humans. There is only a slight morphological difference between the two organisms, but attempts to transmit *P. reichenowi* to humans have been unsuccessful (96,97,99, 101,102,373,415,422,712,931,1034,1131).

iv. *Plasmodium schwetzi:* P. schwetzi is a mildly pathogenic plasmodium species that is found in west Africa. The natural nonhuman primate hosts are chimpanzees (*Pan* sp.) and gorillas (*Gorilla* sp.), and this parasite causes a mild tertian malaria in these species (420). The disease is often subclinical and not obvious unless the animal is splenectomized. *Plasmodium schwetzi* is very similar to *P. vivax* of humans. This organism can infect humans and has been transmitted from chimpanzees to humans via mosquitoes (420). The disease in humans consists of a mild febrile period followed by a spontaneous cure (98,101,102,113,373,415,712,957,1131).

v. *Plasmodium hylobati, Plasmodium eylesi, Plasmodium jefferyi,* and *Plasmodium youngi:* These four closely related parasites are found in the East Indies. They produce a quartan malaria in gibbons (*Hylobates* sp.), which are the natural nonhuman primate hosts for these parasites. *Plasmodium hylobati, P. youngi,* and *P. eylesi* are reported to be pathogenic. A febrile response associated with the parasitemia has been seen in gibbons infected with *P. hylobati* and *P. youngi.* Details of the clinical disease and pathology have not been reported (184,320, 373,415,420,712,953,1131,1141–1143).

4. Hepatocystosis

This disease is caused by parasites classified in the genus *Hepatocystis* in the family Plasmodiidae. The species reported to occur in nonhuman primates are listed in Table III. This parasite does not infect humans.

These sporozoan parasites are distributed in India to the East Indies subcontinent and throughout the African continent south of the Sahara Desert. Nonhuman primates reported to be affected with *Hepatocystis kochi* [synonyms including *H. joyeuxi, H. cercopitheci, H. bovilliezi* and *H. simiae,* and *Plasmodium kochi* (373)] or *Hepatocystis* sp. include Old World monkeys (African green monkeys, other guenons, mangabeys, baboons, patas monkeys, colobus monkeys, Formosan rock macaques, other *Macaca* sp., and leaf monkeys) and great apes (gibbons) (3,230,231,373,385,409,416,424,652,712,736,882,1026,1119, 1131, 1143). *Hepatocystis semnopitheci* has been reported in numerous Old World monkeys (Rhesus monkeys, other *Macaca* sp., and langurs) (419,484,969).

The incidence of *Hepatocystis* can exceed that of malaria (712) and has been reported from 42 to 56% in nonhuman primates obtained from west central Africa (99,373,692), from 40 to 75% in species from east central Africa (373,385,775,882, 883, 1058, 1105, 1119), and 48% for chacma baboons from southern Africa (768). The reported incidence of *H. semnopitheci* in Asian monkeys ranges from 24 to 43% and is 13% in macaques imported into England (419,484).

The life cycle of *Hepatocystis* is indirect with midges (*Culicoides* sp.) serving as the biological vector for the gamont stage (348,373,416,424,712,1023). *Hepatocystis kochi* is the only species in which the life cycle is completely known (409,410, 416,700,775).

The life cycle resembles that of *Plasmodium* sp. with the major exception that asexual schizogony does not take place in the erythrocytes of the hosts. Schizogony in the liver produces grossly visible cysts called merocysts (348,373,416,712,1131).

Because schizogony occurs in the liver, *Hepatocystis* infection in the nonhuman primate produces no cyclic fever or waves

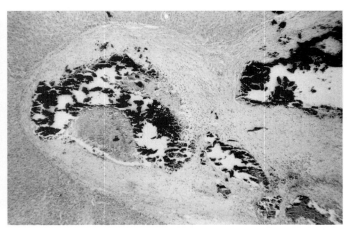

Fig. 7. Gross photograph of a liver from a rhesus monkey (*Macaca mulatta*) with *Hepatocystis*. Large, developing merocyst (large arrowhead) and multiple scars (small arrows) representative of healed merocysts can be seen scattered randomly over the hepatic lobes.

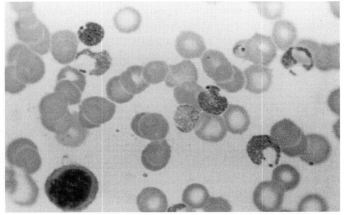

Fig. 9. Photomicrograph of liver from a baboon (*Papio cynocephalus*) infected with *Hepatocystis*. This illustrates an old, chronic lesion in which the merocyst has undergone calcification. HE stain.

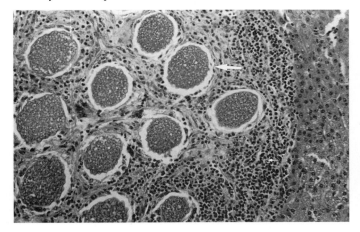

Fig. 8. Photomicrograph of a liver from a cynomolgus monkey (*Macaca fascicularis*) with *Hepatocystis*. Developing merocyst containing numerous schizonts filled with merozoites (large arrow). Note early granulomatous inflammatory reaction (small arrow). HE stain. (Courtesy of Dr. Michael Ryan.)

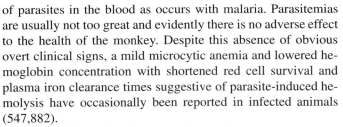

Fig. 10. Photomicrograph of a thin blood smear from a green monkey (*Cercopithecus aethiops*) infected with *Hepatocystis*. At least six trophozoites with heavy pigment and stippling are evident. Giemsa stain.

of parasites in the blood as occurs with malaria. Parasitemias are usually not too great and evidently there is no adverse effect to the health of the monkey. Despite this absence of obvious overt clinical signs, a mild microcytic anemia and lowered hemoglobin concentration with shortened red cell survival and plasma iron clearance times suggestive of parasite-induced hemolysis have occasionally been reported in infected animals (547,882).

Grossly, infected nonhuman primates have numerous, randomly scattered, grayish white, translucent foci on the surface of the liver that correspond to the mature merocysts (Fig. 7) (373,416,712,969,1119). Histopathologically, there is no tissue reaction in the liver until the merocysts are formed. After the cyst develops there is usually a neutrophilic exudate surrounding it (Fig. 8). Following rupture of the cyst and release of the merozoites, a chronic eosinophilic granulomatous inflammatory

reaction ensues with the infiltration of lymphocytes and macrophages (Fig. 9). Healing results in fibrosis in and around the area where the cyst was located. These appear as white foci grossly (Fig. 7) (373,416,712,969,1119).

Diagnosis is based on demonstration and identification of the parasite in thick or thin blood smears (Fig. 10) or finding the typical hepatic lesions at necropsy and/or on histologic sections (373,416,883,1119).

An effective vector control program prevents spread within nonhuman primate colonies as transmission (with the exception of blood transfusion associated spread) of these parasites is impossible in the absence of the insect vector. Treatment with antimalarial drugs is reported not to be effective (373,775,967).

There are no public health considerations with this parasite as *Hepatocystis* sp. are not known to infect humans (373).

5. Toxoplasmosis

The cause of this disease, *Toxoplasma gondii,* is a cosmopolitan protozoan parasite in the family Sarcocystidae. Naturally occurring infection with *T. gondii* has been reported in New World monkeys (squirrel monkeys, spider monkeys, sakis, owl monkeys, uakaris, marmosets, tamarins, woolly monkeys, titi monkeys, howler monkeys, woolly monkeys, and cebus monkeys), Old World monkeys (rhesus monkeys, stump-tailed macaques, cynomolgus monkeys, and baboons), great apes (chimpanzees), and prosimians (Malayan tree shrew, ring-tailed lemur, ruffed lemur, and slow loris) (17,40,57,58,69,158,234, 239,249,373,505,560,628,694,696,762,766,824,829,923–926, 949,1014,1052,1068,1088,1108,1179,1181,1204,1205).

New World monkeys are reported to be more susceptible to this disease (40,505,572,766,967,1023,1179); marmosets are very susceptible and may die within 5–6 days after contracting the disease (58). Also, marmosets and owl monkeys have proven to be very susceptible to experimental infection with *T. gondii.* They uniformly develop acute fatal infections after inoculation by a wide variety of routes (950). The fulminant character of this disease in naturally occurring and experimental infections and the occurrence of the disease in many New World primates attest to the marked susceptibility and lack of resistance of these animals to toxoplasmosis (694).

There is some question as to whether the infection in the baboon (*Papio cynocephalus*) and the chimpanzee (*Pan* sp.) was acquired naturally, as both animals had been inoculated intracerebrally with material from guinea pigs and rabbits shortly before death (40,967).

Also, there is some doubt about the validity of the diagnosis regarding two fatal cases of toxoplasmosis in lemurs (*Lemur catta*) from Japan (40). The diagnosis was based on the microscopic demonstration of the parasites, and the published photomicrographs are reported not to be entirely convincing (40).

The morphology of *T. gondii* has been reviewed previously (247,373,393,394,569,700). *Toxoplasma* tachyzoites (formerly called trophozoites) are crescent or banana-shaped structures that measure 4–8 μm by 2–4 μm. One end is pointed and the other is rounded and contains a centrally located nucleus. Tachyzoites can be found in various cells throughout the host and also in blood and peritoneal fluid. Initially they occupy vacuoles in the host cells (current preferred terminology, group stage or colony) (393,394,1023). As they multiply, a cyst forms around them. The encysted forms are known as bradyzoites (formerly called merozoites). Oocysts seen in the intestinal epithelial cells and feces of the cat measure 10 by 12 μm and are the smallest of the three common cat coccidia.

For an in-depth discussion of the life cycle of this interesting parasite, the reader is referred to the following references (247, 373,392–394,569).

Briefly, the life cycle consists of an enteroepithelial phase, which occurs only in the definitive host, and a extraintestinal or tissue phase, which occurs in all susceptible species (intermediate hosts). Asexual reproduction (endodyogeny, endopolygeny, and schizogony) and sexual reproduction (gametogony), which leads to the production of oocysts, occur in the intestinal epithelium of various domestic and feral members of the family Felidae. Unsporulated oocysts are shed by these animals, the only known definitive hosts, and sporogony occurs in the feces. In the extraintestinal cycle, multiplication of tachyzoites occurs by endodyogeny in all other tissues of the intermediate hosts, which include a wide variety of domestic and wild animals (including cats), birds, and some nonmammalian species (247, 373,392,394,1023).

Infection with *Toxoplasma* can occur via transplacental transmission, consumption of tissue cysts, or consumption of oocysts. The organisms also can be spread mechanically and by insect vectors, such as cockroaches (280, 373, 393, 394, 1023, 1137). Many of the cases reported in the literature document the association between feeding raw meat to New World monkeys and fatal toxoplasmosis (86,694). Human infection acquired through ingestion of oocyst-contaminated water has been reported (53).

Nonspecific clinical signs reported in nonhuman primates infected with *T. gondii* include listlessness, lethargy, depression, somnolence, anorexia, emesis, diarrhea, fever, cough, weakness, ocular and nasal discharges, pale mucous membranes, leukopenia, dyspnea, tachypnea, premature birth, abortion, recumbency, and death without any signs or evidence of illness (86, 294, 373, 572, 694, 1023, 1181). The peripheral blood may contain organisms terminally (694).

Neurologic signs include circling, grasping and holding of the head, leaning head against or hitting head on cage, incoordination, paresis, and terminal convulsions (373,572,694).

At necropsy, the most frequently observed abnormalities reported are dehydration; cardiomegaly; myocardial necrosis; hemorrhagic lymphadenopathy; pulmonary edema with frothy fluid in the bronchi; hepatic and pulmonary congestion; petechial to ecchymotic pulmonary hemorrhages; generalized, acute pneumonia; hepatocellular necrosis; splenomegaly; splenic hyperplasia; hepatomegaly; enlarged kidneys; and mottled spleen, liver, and kidneys (57,86,249,694,1181).

Histopathologically, focal hepatic necrosis; focal to diffuse necrotic lymphadenitis, splenitis, and nephritis; segmental intestinal necrosis; interstitial and fibrinous pneumonia; and focal myocarditis and myositis have been reported. Necrotic foci and extracellular and/or intercellular tachyzoites are frequently found in conjunction with inflammatory lesions. Lesions seen in the central nervous system include gliosis, focal hemorrhage, microscopic infarcts, and cellular degeneration (necrosis) (86, 249,393,572,694,1023,1181). *Toxoplasma gondii* cysts and free organisms have been noted in capillary endothelial cells and in the brain tissue, frequently with associated perivascular cuffing and cellular necrosis (572,628,766).

Diagnosis of toxoplasmosis depends on the demonstration and identification of the causative organism in smear preparations or in histopathologic sections or by animal inoculation (40,247,373,572,694,700). Laboratory serological tests include the complement fixation test, indirect fluorescent antibody test, the Sabin–Feldman dye test, and the hemagglutination test. Isolation of *T. gondii* itself by mouse inoculation of biopsy specimens is most reliable, but is time-consuming and expensive (694). Toxoplasmosis should be considered in the differential diagnosis of nonspecific acute illnesses in New World primates. A history of feeding raw animal tissues, exposure to cats, lymphadenopathy, or evidence of encephalitis are reasons to consider a decision to initiate anti-*Toxoplasma* therapy (694).

Recognition of oocysts in fecal samples of cats is important for the prevention and control of both animal and human toxoplasmosis (373,572,1023). The following references should be consulted for information about preparing fecal samples and the morphological differences between common feline coccidial oocysts (245,247,248).

To prevent toxoplasmosis in susceptible animals, all meat used for feed should be frozen to −20°C for 2 days and/or be cooked to 60°C for 30 min (694). This is especially important for meat being fed to felines because a single cat can excrete millions of *T. gondii* oocysts and because oocysts can survive in soil for several months (249). Strict sanitation practices should be employed at all times, and under no circumstances should cats be allowed to contaminate the monkeys' environment (694).

Because toxoplasmosis can occur in humans, reasonable care should be taken to prevent infection in those personnel responsible for the care and use of nonhuman primates. Feces from Felidae should be removed frequently (within 24 hr) and preferably incinerated or disposed of in some other way that will prevent contact of vectors and fomites with sporulated oocysts (373). Also, it is probably a good idea to maintain a reasonable distance between the cages of primates and cats and to train all caretakers on techniques that will minimize cage-to-cage contamination (249).

The effectiveness of chemotherapy for toxoplasmosis in monkeys is unknown (694). Lehner (694) suggests that the combined treatment used for humans—pyrimethamine and a sulfonamide such as sulfadiazine or trisulfapyrimidine—be used for monkeys. Pyrimethamine is a folic acid antagonist and acts synergistically with the sulfa drug. These drugs act on the trophozoites and are suppressive rather than toxoplasmocidal. Because the dose of pyrimethamine for New World monkeys has not been established, it is recommended that pediatric human doses may be a good starting point for treatment of sick monkeys (694). Clinicians should be aware that pyrimethamine may depress the bone marrow, so hematologic examinations should be performed to monitor for these effects (694). Folic acid (1 mg per day) may be administered to alleviate the depressive effects on bone marrow and will not interfere with the therapeutic action of the drugs (694).

6. Sarcocystosis

This disease is caused by coccidian parasites in the genus *Sarcocystis,* family Sarcocystidae. The cystic phase of this parasite (Miescher's tubes) has been described in skeletal muscle

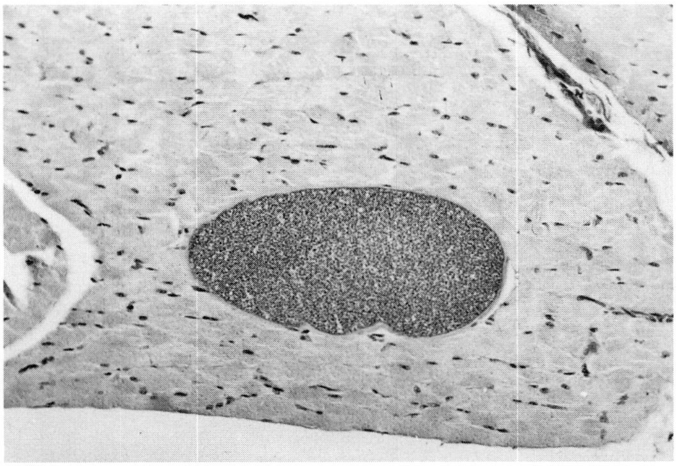

Fig. 11.   Photomicrograph of large cyst containing *Sarcocystis* organisms in the skeletal muscle of tongue of rhesus monkey (*Macaca mulatta*). HE stain. (Reprinted from Toft, II, J. D. (1982). *Veterinary Pathology.* With permission.)

fibers and occasionally in cardiac or smooth muscle fibers in a wide variety of animals throughout the world (40,296,373,617, 700,702). They are cylindrical, spindle shaped, ellipsoidal, or irregular in structure and lie lengthwise in the muscle cells (373). Mature trophozoites (Rainey's corpuscles) are banana shaped; the anterior end is slightly pointed and the posterior end is rounded. Their size varies with the species (373).

These cysts are observed commonly in the skeletal muscle of the tongue or the esophageal muscle of many nonhuman primates (Fig. 11). *Sarcocystis kortei* and *S. nesbitti* have been described in the rhesus monkey, and other unnamed species have been reported in both Old and New World monkeys (40, 250,347,373,476,497,602,630,704,727,733,819,836,909,1023, 1058).

It is now known that *Sarcocystis* has an obligatory two-host life cycle. The reader is referred to the definitive works published outlining the intricacies of the life cycle of this unique and interesting parasite (246,247,392,394,968).

Lesions associated with naturally occurring infections in nonhuman primates are rare (296,373,617,1023). Inflammation characterized by infiltrates of lymphocytes, plasma cells, and eosinophils is associated with degeneration of the cysts within the muscle fibers. With time, there is a proliferation of fibrous connective tissue and resulting scar formation (1023,1086).

Sarcocystosis is usually an incidental finding, and its diagnosis depends on identification of the characteristic intramuscular cysts during histopathologic examination. There is no effective treatment (373).

7. Babesiosis

Two organisms are associated with this disease in nonhuman primates; both are in the order Piroplasmorida, family Babesiidae. *Babesia pitheci* has been reported from Old World monkeys (mangabeys, guenons, macaques, and baboons) (40,373,

TABLE IV

MICROSPORIDIAN PARASITES DESCRIBED FROM NONHUMAN PRIMATES

Parasite Genus species	Location in host	Prosimians	New World monkeys	Old World monkeys	Great apes	Reference
Phylum Microsporida, order Pleistophoridida, family Pleistophoridae (microsporidia)						
Encephalitozoon cuniculi	Brain, kidneys, heart, lungs, adrenals, other tissues		X			20, 111, 857, 1022, 1206
Microsporidian sp.	Intestine		X			1012
Enterocytozoon bienusi	Intestine, liver, gallbladder		X			734

411,512,513,599,962,1079) and New World monkeys (marmosets) (512).

Its distribution and incidence in nature are unknown (373, 712). Also, the complete life cycle is unknown, but ticks are thought to be the biological vectors (40,373,712). Natural infections are restricted to Africa.

This babesial parasite is considered to be only slightly pathogenic in normal intact monkeys but can result in severe anemia and death after splenectomy. Marked poikilocytosis and anisocytosis are associated with the anemia (40,373,411,599,712, 1079).

Babesia pitheci organisms are pyriform in shape and measure 2–6 μm long. Round, elliptical, oval, lanceolate, and ameboid stages have also been observed in peripheral blood smears (40, 373,712).

The second babesia-like organism, *Entopolypoides macaci*, is a mildly pathogenic hemosporozoal parasite that has been described in Old World monkeys (cynomolgus monkeys, rhesus monkeys, baboons, and guenons) and great apes (chimpanzees) (52,346,373,434,481,748,749,786,1023).

This organism does not have true pyriform stages, but early ring-shaped stages and ameboid stages with polypoid projections of cytoplasm similar to the true *Babesia* species have been seen. *Entopolypoides macaci* is smaller than *Babesia* and *Plasmodium* species parasites and is morphologically distinct (434, 712). Parasitized erythrocytes are not enlarged and pigment is not formed (712).

Fever, monocytosis, and anemia have been reported in parasitized nonhuman primates; generally, however, infection with *E. macaci* appears to have little effect on the host (373,712, 749). Chronic, latent infections are known to occur, and splenectomy or immunosuppression will result in recurrence of the parasitemia and a marked increase in the intensity of hemolytic anemia and icterus.

In one report, *E. macaci* parasitemias developed in two cynomolgus monkeys secondary to stress (type D retrovirus/severe trauma) (294). Under these conditions, the disease may be fatal (1023). There are indications that this organism is common in nonhuman primates (712).

Diagnosis of these two organisms depends on the demonstration and identification of the parasites within the erythrocytes

of the host in stained blood smears (294,373,1023). In the case of the two cynomolgus monkeys, antibodies against *Babesia* sp. were detected by immunofluorescence assay (IFA) in one of the infected macaques (294).

Proper vermin control with elimination of any possible arthropod vectors will prevent the spread of these two organisms within a nonhuman primate colony (373). However, the potential for transmission through the blood-borne route exists for both *Babesia* and *Entopolypoides*.

Treatment for *B. pitheci* with 1% Trypan blue solution intravenously at a dose rate of 1 mg/kg of body weight per day for 2 days in combination with a single injection of 0.5% acriflavine solution at a dose rate of 0.2 ml/kg of body weight is reported to be helpful, but will not completely eliminate the parasite (373,1079). Treatment for *E. macaci* has not been reported.

There is no public health significance associated with either *B. pitheci* or *E. macaci* infections as neither parasite has been reported in humans (373).

D. Microsporidia

The causes of this disease, *Encephalitozoon cuniculi*, *Enterocytozoon bienusi,* and other microsporidia, are obligate intracellular protozoan parasites in the family Pleistophoridae, phylum Microsporida. Table IV lists those reported from nonhuman primates. They have been reported in a wide variety of vertebrate and invertebrate species (1023).

Naturally occurring cases have been reported in nonhuman primates, all in New World monkeys. All of these cases involved squirrel monkeys, except one that involved an unidentified microsporidian parasite in a dusky titi monkey (*Callicebus moloch*) (20,111,133,1012,1206).

Shadduck and Baskin (1022) reported on the high prevalence of seropositivity to *E. cuniculi* in a colony of squirrel monkeys that has proved to be relatively stable, occurs at a 60–70% frequency rate, and is especially prevalent in older animals (1022).

Encephalitozoon cuniculi is a small, oval parasite that measures approximately 2.5 by 1.5 μm. Division occurs by binary fission and produces two spores per sporont. The organisms can

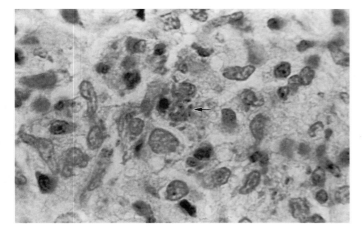

Fig. 12. Photomicrograph of *Encephalitozoon* sp. cyst (arrow) in brain of squirrel monkey (*Saimiri sciureus*). Gram stain.

be distinguished from *Toxoplasma* and other parasites by their location, size, PAS(+) filament attachment site, and positive staining characteristics with the Gram stain (Fig. 12) and various silver impregnation methods. A coiled polar filament, with four to five coils, is a distinctive ultrastructural feature of *E. cuniculi* (1023).

The life cycle of this parasite is monoxenous. Transmission normally occurs when spores contaminating the environment or the diet are ingested by a new host. Spores extrude thin polar filaments, invade gut epithelium, and spread hematogenously to several organs (1206). A variety of cell types are invaded in different tissues of the body, but there is a predilection for peritoneal macrophages and for unidentified cells of the central nervous system and renal tubular epithelium in chronically infected animals. The hatching of spores and the migration from the intestine to the viscera, as occurs in some other microsporida, have not been observed for *E. cuniculi*. Asexual division by binary fission or schizogony occurs in peritoneal macrophages, resulting in the development of a parasitophorous vacuole. Sporonts with thickened walls transform into pairs of sporoblasts that ultimately develop into spores. Repeated sporogony results in macrophages that are engorged with spores. In chronic infections, development localizes in cells of the viscera, especially the kidney and the brain. Spores are passed out with the urine (133).

Clinical signs in infected monkeys are usually absent or the animals exhibit nonspecific clinical disorders prior to death (1206).

Those clinical signs that have been described in nonhuman primates infected with *E. cuniculi* consist of nervous symptoms (intermittent petit mal seizures) displayed by a 2-month-old squirrel monkey for approximately 1 month prior to death (111). Lesions in this animal were focal granulomatous meningoencephalitis, hepatitis, and nephritis. Characteristic *E. cuniculi* organisms were seen by both light and electron microscopy.

Also, a granulomatous encephalitis due to *E. cuniculi* infection has been reported in a newborn squirrel monkey (20).

In the case involving the dusky titi (*Callicebus moloch*) (1012), gram-positive, acid-fast-positive microsproidial organisms having a polar filament with as many as seven coils were found in the jejunal epithelium. It was felt that this organism was one that normally infects arthropods rather than *E. cuniculi* and that the monkey became infected through ingestion of the arthropods that it was able to capture in its outdoor environment. No host response to the presence of the organisms in the intestinal epithelium was reported (1012). *Encephalitozoon cuniculi* infection also has been reported as the cause of death in two infant squirrel monkeys (857).

Zeman (1206) reported on the finding of 22 naturally occurring cases of encephalitozoonosis in squirrel monkeys. At least 7 of these cases were considered to be congenital, whereas 10 of the others occurred in monkeys less than 9 months of age. Characteristic foci of granulomatous inflammation and *E. cuniculi* organisms were observed in the brains, kidneys, lungs, adrenals, and livers of infected animals. Vasculitis and perivasculitis also were seen commonly in these organs, in addition to the heart, skeletal muscle, and pancreas. A granulomatous placentitis was present in one of the infected monkeys (1206).

Diagnosis of *E. cuniculi* can be made by finding the parasites associated with the typical lesions during histopathological examination of the tissues or by demonstration of the organisms in the urine. *Encephalitozoon cuniculi* stains poorly with HE, but stains well with Giemsa and Goodpasture stains and are gram positive (694). The use of a modified Gram–chromotrope staining procedure greatly improves detection of microsporidia parasites in urine, stool, and tissue. Currently, indirect immunofluorescence and dot–enzyme-linked immunosorbent assay (ELISA) tests, which detect antibodies against the organisms, and an intradermal test have proved reliable (512,1022,1023).

Encephalitozoon cuniculi must be differentiated from *T. gondii* in tissue sections. *Toxoplasma* cysts are usually small (up to 60 μm in diameter), whereas the pseudocysts of *E. cuniculi* are larger (between 60 and 120 μm in diameter). Mature organisms of *Toxoplasma* are larger and crescent shaped (2×6 μm), whereas those of *E. cuniculi* are somewhat oval rods (1.5×2.5 μm). *Encephalitozoon cuniculi* spores are variably acid fast and gram positive and iron–hematoxylin positive whereas *T. gondii* is not (1206).

The public health importance of this organism is unclear at this time, but there are recognized infections in humans. For this reason, personnel working or caring for nonhuman primates should follow accepted personal hygiene practices, and because urinary excretion is now known as the mode of transmission, excrement from nonhuman primates should be handled with caution. Also, care should be taken to ensure that captive nonhuman primates are protected from exposure to species known to be carriers of this organism (373).

There is no chemotherapeutic agent known that is effective against *Encephalitozoon* in vertebrates (694).

TABLE V

PARASITIC CILIATES DESCRIBED FROM NONHUMAN PRIMATES

Parasite Genus species	Location in host	Prosimians	New World monkeys	Old World monkeys	Great apes	Reference
Phylum Ciliophora, order Vestibuliferida, family Balantidiidae						
Balantidium coli	Cecum, colon		X	X	X	21, 60, 124, 364, 373, 433, 463, 480, 488, 564, 589, 612, 617, 650–652, 656, 659, 699, 765, 791, 793, 806, 811, 906, 929, 1023, 1085, 1115, 1170, 1197
Balantidium sp.	Cecum, colon			X		451, 757, 763
Phylum Ciliophorida, order Entodiniomorphida, family Cycloposthiidae						
Troglodytella abrassarti	Cecum, colon				X	114, 211, 365, 373, 404, 619, 656, 699, 765, 791, 820, 1103, 1115
T. gorillae	Cecum, colon				X	124, 373, 404

E. Ciliates

The parasitic ciliates in the phylum Ciliophora described from nonhuman primates are listed in Table V. *Balantidium coli* (family Balantiidae, order Vestibuliferida) is the only species that has been associated with lesions of the intestinal tract. It is discussed below.

1. Balantidiasis

The cause of this disease, *B. coli,* has a worldwide distribution and has been reported in a number of nonhuman primate species, including New World monkeys (howler monkeys, spider monkeys, and cebus monkeys), Old World monkeys (rhesus monkeys, cynomolgus monkeys, and baboons), and great apes (orangutans, chimpanzees, and gorillas) (60,124,126,367,373, 381,433,451,463,488–491,585,593,612,617,652,754,791,891, 898,906,945,1023,1085,1115,1170,1178).

The organism is usually nonpathogenic and is a common inhabitant of the cecum of nonhuman primates (124,126,373, 476,617,659,806,906,929,1115). Some nonhuman primates have been reported to be symptomless carriers (177,1135).

Balantidium coli trophozoites are large, ovoid structures with a heavily ciliated outer surface (26,123,373,465,632,700,1021, 1023,1163). This form measures 30 to 150 μm by 25 to 120 μm. Internal structures consist of a macronucleus and micronucleus, two contractile vacuoles, and numerous food vacuoles. Cyst forms are spherical to ovoid and measure 40 to 60 μm in diameter. Reproduction occurs by conjugation or by transverse binary fission. Infection occurs through ingestion of trophozoites or cysts (124,373,700,1023).

Infection with *B. coli* can cause severe ulcerative enterocolitis, which can be fatal in great apes (77,169,367,612,967).

Signs of clinically ill animals are weight loss, anorexia, muscle weakness, lethargy, watery diarrhea, tenesmus, and rectal prolapse (124,489,788,1085).

At necropsy, lesions may resemble those seen in amebiasis and may consist primarily of an ulcerative colitis (124,617, 1023).

Histologically the ulcers may be large and may extend down to the muscularis mucosae (373,1023). There may be an accompanying lymphocytic infiltrate and, at times, coagulation necrosis and hemorrhage (373,1023). Typical large *B. coli* organisms can be seen in masses associated with lesions in the tissues or in capillaries, lymphatics, or regional lymph nodes (124,373, 1023,1135). (Fig. 13).

Diagnosis depends on identification of the characteristic *B. coli* organisms associated with the typical colonic lesions (373, 617,1023). Their presence as secondary invaders to a primary

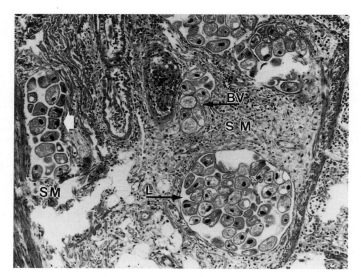

Fig. 13. Photomicrograph of submucosa of colon from chimpanzee (*Pan* sp.) with severe *Balantidium coli* infection. Many large organisms (thick white arrow) with typical morphologic features in submucosal tissue (SM), blood vessels (BV), and lymphatics (L) are seen. HE stain. (Reprinted from Toft, II, J. D. (1982). *Veterinary Pathology.* With permission.)

TABLE VI

Parasite of Uncertain Taxonomic Position Reported from Nonhuman Primates

Parasite Genus species	Location in host	Prosimians	New World monkeys	Old World monkeys	Great apes	Reference
Pneumocystis carinii	Lungs		X	X	X	156, 714, 890, 941, 1055, 1130

disease caused by other microorganisms should always be considered and must be ruled out (373).

Control is based on consistently maintaining strict sanitation practices within the nonhuman primate colony (373). Good nutrition and the routine treatment of newly procured, asymptomatic carriers also are recommended (72,373,967). *Balantidium coli* may cause diarrhea in humans; therefore, care should be taken in handling captive nonhuman primates to avoid infection (373).

Treatment for balantidiasis in nonhuman primates is similar to that used for lumenal amebiasis. Effective drugs are metronidazole (Flagyl) at a dose of 35–50 mg/kg/day per os divided into three daily doses for 10 days; tetracycline at a dose of 40 mg/kg/day per os divided into three daily doses for 10–14 days; and diiodohydroxyquin (Yodoxin) at a dose of 40 mg/kg/day per os divided into three daily doses for 14–21 days (694,1072).

F. Pneumocystis

Pneumocystis carinii is now recognized to have closer affinity with certain fungal groups than to the parasitic agents. However, because reports of this organism from primates were originally included under the heading of parasitic diseases, Table VI is included for the readers use. It is likely that in subsequent considerations, *Pneumocystis* will not be included.

III. METAZOAN PARASITES

A. Nematodes

The parasitic nematode genera described from nonhuman primates are listed in Table VII. Because nematodiasis is such a common occurrence in nonhuman primates, the majority of the genera listed will be discussed in detail.

1. Rhabditoids

a. STRONGYLOIDIASIS. This disease results from infection by the parasitic members of the genus *Strongyloides*. These small nematodes are prevalent in most tropical and subtropical areas, but their occurrence in the temperate zones is sporadic.

Several species have been reported to affect nonhuman primates: *Strongyloides cebus* has been found in New World monkeys (cebus monkeys, woolly monkeys, spider monkeys, squirrel monkeys, and marmosets) (268,373,585,617,626,657, 830,851,978,1023), *Strongyloides fulleborni* (threadworm) in Old World monkeys and great apes (rhesus monkeys, cynomolgus monkeys, Japanese monkeys, guenons, baboons, and chimpanzees) (373, 459, 463, 830, 851, 855, 929, 966, 967, 978, 990,1023,1113,1115,1189,1197), and *Strongyloides stercoralis* and *Strongyloides* sp. in Old World monkeys (patas monkeys) and great apes (gibbons, chimpanzees, gorillas, and orangutans) (60,227,233,293,366,373,475,669,690,754,851,874,898,1002, 1023,1107,1112,1189).

Only adult (parthenogenic) females and larvae are found in the gastrointestinal tract of the host animal. Migrating larvae can be found in the lungs and other parenchymatous organs. There are no parasitic males (373).

The life cycle of *Strongyloides* sp. is complex and consists of both parasitic and free-living generations (155,373). The reader is referred to the recognized parasitology texts and referenced papers for a detailed discussion of this unique life cycle (49, 159,350,373,410,1023,1045).

A variation in this life cycle seen only in *S. stercoralis,* known as autoinfection, is a direct reinvasion of the host animal by filariform larvae that have developed during passage through the lower intestinal tract (227,624). This phenomenon results in hyperinfection of the infected host and is most responsible for sustained infections that result in clinical disease, severe damage to affected organs, and death (109,129,227,373).

There also is evidence of intrauterine or transcolostral transmission (373,746,779,1054).

Fatal cases of strongyloidiasis have been reported in the chimpanzee, gibbon, orangutan, patas monkey, and woolly monkey (74,75,227,232,300,475,565,669,695,755,833,851, 886,1107,1112).

The disease in gibbons has been reported in detail (227). Diarrhea, which may be hemorrhagic or mucoid, is the most common clinical sign described in infected animals (227). Other common clinical signs are dermatitis, urticaria, anorexia, depression, listlessness, debilitation, vomiting, emaciation, reduced growth rate, dehydration, constipation, dyspnea, cough, prostration, and death (227,352,373,617,967,1023,1044). Paralytic ileus is described in infected gibbons (227).

TABLE VII
Parasitic Nematodes Described from Nonhuman Primates

Parasite Genus species	Location in host	Prosimians	New World monkeys	Old World monkeys	Great apes	Reference
Subclass Secernentea (phasmidia), order Rhabditida, superfamily Rhabditoidea						
Strongyloides fulleborni	Intestines			X	X	4, 364, 365, 373, 459, 463, 475, 765, 793, 851, 879, 966, 967, 990, 1023, 1113, 1115, 1136, 1188, 1189, 1197
S. cebus	Intestines		X			194, 373, 617, 693, 711, 1023
S. stercoralis	Intestines				X	232, 373, 690, 701, 711, 851, 1023, 1044, 1110, 1189
S. simiae	Intestines			X		564
S. papillosus	Intestines			X	X	373, 711
Strongyloides sp.	Intestines		X	X	X	200, 598, 754, 763, 765, 855, 859, 1170, 1189
Pelodera strongyloides	Skin lesions			X		700, 967
Subclass Secernentea, order Strongylida, superfamily Ancylostomatoidea						
Ancylostoma duodenale	Small intestine				X	60, 155, 200, 373, 822, 851, 1023, 1197
Ancylostoma sp.	Small intestine		X			1081
Necator americanus	Small intestine		X	X	X	60, 106, 241, 360, 373, 651, 652, 656, 804, 851, 945, 967, 1023, 1087, 1197
Globocephalus simiae	Small intestine			X		373, 1183
Characostomum asimilium	Small intestine	X		X		373, 1186
Necator sp.	Small intestine	X	X	X	X	514, 765, 1081
Uncinaria sp.	Small intestine	X				143
Subclass Secernentea, order Strongylida, superfamily Strongyloidea						
Oesophagostomum apiostomum	Colon, mesentery			X		4, 200, 354, 364, 373, 463, 464, 700, 851, 859, 967, 1023, 1188
O. bifurcum	Colon			X	X	68, 71, 354, 373, 449, 459, 650–653, 658, 659, 700, 763, 804, 851, 879, 967, 1023, 1115
O. aculeatum	Colon			X		354, 357, 373, 479, 700, 851, 929, 967, 1023, 1077, 1113
O. stephanostomum	Colon			X	X	354, 360, 373, 656, 700, 804, 851, 929, 967, 1023, 1115
O. blanchardi	Colon				X	373, 851, 1023, 1186
Oesophagostomum sp.	Colon, abdominal viscera			X	X	1, 21, 440, 653, 656, 725, 757, 813, 855, 859, 860, 863, 1189
Ternidens deminutus	Cecum, colon			X	X	13, 68, 200, 373, 440, 449, 463, 700, 763, 804, 822, 851, 929, 967, 990, 1023, 1077
Ternidens sp.	Cecum, colon			X		21, 659
Subclass Secernentea; order Strongylida, superfamily Trichostrongyloidea						
Molineus torulosus	Small intestine		X			260, 268, 373, 617, 674, 1023, 1194
M. vexillarius	Small intestine, stomach		X			194, 224, 260, 268, 373, 617, 900, 1023
M. elegans	Small intestine		X			260, 268, 373, 528, 617, 1023
M. teocchii	Small intestine	X				448
M. vogelianus	Small intestine	X				260, 373, 448
Pithecostrongylus alatus	Intestine			X	X	373, 1031, 1098, 1186
Trichostrongylus colubriformis	Small intestine			X	X	354, 373, 658, 674, 700, 763, 929, 1044, 1114
T. falculatus	Small intestine			X		879
Graphidioides berlai	Intestine		X			373, 617, 1186
Nematodirus weinbergi	Small intestine				X	373, 916, 1186
Longistriata dubia	Small intestine		X			194, 268, 373, 617, 900
L. cristata	Small intestine	X				801
Nochtia nochti	Stomach			X		1, 85, 262, 449, 479, 673, 851, 967, 1015, 1023, 1036, 1098, 1189

TABLE VII—*Continued*

PARASITIC NEMATODES DESCRIBED FROM NONHUMAN PRIMATES

Parasite Genus species	Location in host	Prosimians	New World monkeys	Old World monkeys	Great apes	Reference
Tupaiostrongylus liei	Small intestine	X				262, 277, 278
T. major	Small intestine	X				279
T. minor	Small intestine	X				279
Anoplostrongylus liei	Intestine	X				278
Hepatojarakus malayae	Intestine	X				278
Nycteridosytrongylus petersi	Intestine, lungs	X				278
Trichostrongylus sp.	Small intestine			X		650–652, 656, 659, 811, 859
Mammanidula siamensis	Mammary gland	X				840
Subclass Secernentea, order Strongylida, superfamily Metastrongyloidea						
Filaroides barretoi	Lungs		X			268, 373, 449, 771, 967
F. gordius	Lungs		X			268, 373, 449, 967
F. cebus	Lungs		X			92
Filaroides sp.	Lungs		X			194, 373
Filariopsis arator	Lungs		X			373, 1186
F. asper	Lungs		X			268, 617, 1117
Angiostrongylus costaricensis	Mesenteric arteries		X			841, 1035, 1092
A. malaysiensis	Brain, spinal cord, heart, lung, pulmonary arteries	X				705
A. cantonensis	Heart		X			625
Stefanskostrongylus pottoi	Various viscera, liver	X				448
Subclass Secernentea, order Oxyurida, superfamily Oxyuridea						
Enterobius vermicularis	Large intestine				X	21, 130, 170, 373, 479, 549, 564, 813, 851, 879, 936, 945, 967, 1110
E. (Trypanoxyuris) bipapillata	Large intestine			X	X	68, 373, 549, 851, 945, 1186
E. brevicauda	Large intestine			X		373, 549, 577, 650, 851, 985, 1186
E. anthropopitheci	Large intestine				X	270, 429, 549, 656, 765, 851, 929, 945, 967
E. buckleyi	Large intestine				X	373, 549, 851, 985, 1186
E. lerouxi	Large intestine				X	373, 549, 851, 985, 1186
E. pitheci	Large intestine			X		549
E. parallela	Large intestine			X		549
E. zakiri	Large intestine			X		549
E. microon	Large intestine		X			373, 851, 1186
E. chabaudi	Large intestine			X		577
E. lemuris	Large intestine	X				31, 577
E. inglisi	Large intestine			X		577, 1133
E. pesteri	Large intestine			X		1133
E. macaci	Large intestine			X		577, 1192
E. presbytis	Large intestine			X		577, 1192
Enterobius sp.	Large intestine	X	X	X	X	89, 453, 514, 519, 598, 650, 859, 860, 863, 929, 1110, 1189
Buckleyenterobius dentata	Large intestine			X		549
Trypanoxyuris (Trypanoxyuris) trypanuris	Large intestine		X			132, 540, 541, 549
T. (Trypanoxyuris) atelis	Large intestine		X			118, 130, 373, 540, 541, 549, 985, 1186
T. (Trypanoxyuris) duplicideus	Large intestine		X			118, 373, 540, 541, 549, 1186
T. (Trypanoxyuris) lagothricis	Large intestine		X			118, 373, 540, 541, 549, 551, 1081, 1186
T. (Trypanoxyuris) clementinae	Large intestine		X			540, 541
T. (Trypanoxyuris) minutus	Large intestine		X			373, 540, 541, 549, 550, 617, 851, 894, 1087, 1189
T. (Trypanoxyuris) microon (syn. *Trypanoxyruis interlabiata*)	Large intestine		X			373, 540, 541, 549, 851, 985, 1186
T. (Trypanoxyuris) satanas	Large intestine		X			540, 541

TABLE VII—*Continued*

PARASITIC NEMATODES DESCRIBED FROM NONHUMAN PRIMATES

Parasite Genus species	Location in host	Prosimians	New World monkeys	Old World monkeys	Great apes	Reference
T. (Trypanoxyuris) sceleratus	Large intestine		X			268, 373, 528, 540, 541, 549, 553, 617, 851
T. (Trypanoxyuris) brachytelesi	Large intestine		X			540, 541, 549
T. callithricis	Large intestine		X			539, 549
T. callicebi	Large intestine		X			542
T. tamarini	Large intestine		X			194, 224, 373, 539, 550, 553, 600, 617, 900
T. oedipi	Large intestine		X			539, 550
T. goeldii	Large intestine		X			539, 550
Enterobius lemuris	Large intestine	X				549
Lemuricola nycticebi	Large intestine	X				552
L. malaysensis	Large intestine	X				47, 269, 552
L. contagiosus	Large intestine	X				552
Labatorobius scleratus	Large intestine		X			373, 1186
Oxyuronema atelophorum	Large intestine		X			373, 449, 633, 1186
Primasubulura jacchi	Large intestine		X			224, 528, 1081
P. otolicini	Large intestine	X				307
Trypanoxyuris sp.	Large intestine		X			789, 804, 900
Probstmayria nainitalensis	Rectum			X		24
P. gombensis	Intestine				X	363, 365, 765
P. gorillae	Intestine				X	365, 635
P. simiae	Intestine				X	365, 737
Subclass Secernentea, order Ascaridida, superfamily Ascaridoidea						
Ascaris lumbricoides	Small intestine		X	X	X	132, 270, 373, 674, 700, 851, 885, 929, 945, 967, 1023, 1189
Ascaris sp.	Intestine			X		200, 656
Polydelphis sp.	Larvae: mesentery				X	288
Baylasascaris sp.	Larvae: brain, viscera		X			405
Subclass Secernentea, order Ascaridida, superfamily Subuluroidea						
Subulura distans	Stomach, small intestine	X		X		132, 373, 460, 804, 822, 967, 1189
S. malayensis	Colon			X		373, 1189
S. jacchi	Small intestine		X			132, 194, 224, 373, 731, 900, 967, 1087, 1189
Subulura sp.	Intestine		X			453
S. otolicni	Cecum	X				448
S. perarmata	Cecum, colon	X				89
S. indica	Large intestine, cecum	X				636
S. prosimiae	Large intestine	X				31
S. pigmentata	Large intestine	X				801
Subclass Secernentea, order Spirurida, superfamily Habronematoidea						
Chitwoodspirura serrata	Stomach, small intestine				X	146, 373, 1186
Subclass Secernentea, order Spirurida, superfamily Spiruroidea						
Spirura guianensis	Esophagus		X			80, 194, 373, 528, 819, 913
S. tamarini	Esophagus		X			193
S. talpae	Esophagus	X				801
S. malayensis	Esophagus	X				914
Protospirura (Mastophorus) muricola	Stomach		X	X		138, 373, 377, 653
Streptopharagus armatus	Stomach			X	X	373, 463, 763, 804, 1077
S. pigmentatus	Stomach			X	X	68, 373, 449, 479, 650, 653, 659, 804, 879, 929, 990, 1113
S. baylisi	Stomach			X		650–652
S. guptai	Rectum			X		1043
Streptopharagus sp.	Stomach			X	X	650, 765, 811
Gongylonema macrogubernaculum	Esophagus, stomach		X	X		373, 449, 617, 703, 722, 723, 804, 851, 1023

TABLE VII—*Continued*

PARASITIC NEMATODES DESCRIBED FROM NONHUMAN PRIMATES

Parasite Genus species	Location in host	Prosimians	New World monkeys	Old World monkeys	Great apes	Reference
G. pulchrum	Tongue, oral cavity, esophagus, stomach		X	X		259, 373, 617, 701, 722, 723, 851, 1023
Physocephalus sp.	Stomach			X		563, 855, 1177
Spirocerca lupi	Wall of aorta	X				59, 197
Subclass Secernentea, order Spirurida, superfamily Thelazioidea						
Trichospirura leptostoma	Pancreas		X			44, 194, 195, 373, 617, 657, 850, 851, 1040, 1041
Oxyspirura youngi	Conjunctival sac	X				8
O. conjunctivalis	Conjunctival sac	X				8, 31
Metathelazia ascaroides	Lungs			X		243, 244, 373, 1186
Thelazia callipaeda	Eyes			X		349, 373, 701, 1044
Subclass Secernentea, order Spirurida, superfamily Rictularioidea						
Pterygodermatites nycticebi	Small intestine	X	X			706, 783, 911, 912, 1104, 1198
P. (Rictularia) alphi	Small intestine		X			78, 373, 787, 911, 912, 1186, 1189
P. lemuri	Small intestine	X				911
Rictularia sp.	Small intestine	X	X			5, 453, 781, 782, 801, 1199
Pseudophysaloptera vincenti	Stomach	X				448
Subclass Secernentea, order Spirurida, superfamily Physalopteroidea						
Physaloptera tumefaciens	Stomach			X		357, 373, 479, 659, 701, 851, 990, 1077, 1172, 1188, 1189, 1201
P. dilatata	Stomach		X			224, 373, 851, 1186
P. masoodi	Stomach	X				636
P. multiuteri	Stomach, esophagus		X			132, 645
P. cebi	Stomach			X		1201
Physaloptera sp.	Stomach	X	X	X		132, 380, 697, 765, 807, 812, 855, 1087, 1172, 1177
Physaloptera (Abbreviata) caucasica	Stomach			X	X	21, 104, 132, 200, 364, 365, 373, 561, 650, 652, 701, 763, 765, 804, 822, 879, 967, 1186, 1201
P. turgida	Stomach			X		132
Abbreviata poicilometra	Stomach			X		373, 982, 1032, 1186
Abbreviata sp.	Stomach			X		811
Subclass Secernentea, order Spirurida, superfamily Dracunculoidea						
Dracunculus medinensis	Skin, subcutis, viscera			X		354, 373, 701, 804, 967
Subclass Secernentea, order Spirurida, superfamily Filarioidea						
Dirofilaria magnilarvatum	Subcutis, peritoneal membranes			X		19, 139, 373, 665, 764, 799, 905, 988, 1084, 1166
D. corynodes (syn. *D. aethiops, D. schoutedeni*)	Subcutis			X		19, 139, 360, 373, 482, 672, 707, 764, 1132, 1144–1147
D. immitis (syn. *D. pongoi*)	Subcutis, muscle, right ventricle			X	X	19, 43, 139, 373, 764, 967, 1129, 1144
D. repens (syn. *D. macacae*)	Subcutis			X		799, 980, 1144
Dirofilaria sp.	Blood			X		744, 1006
Edesonfilaria malayensis	Peritoneal cavity			X		373, 402, 701, 796, 799, 831, 929, 1187, 1191
Loa loa	Subcutis, mesentery, eyes			X	X	252, 254, 257, 360, 373, 680, 701, 804, 822, 846, 959, 981, 1099, 1128, 1145
Macacanema formosana	Peritracheal connective tissue			X		65, 373, 701, 994
Meningonema peruzzii	Subdural space, medulla oblongata			X		849
Brugia pahangi	Lymphatic system	X		X		19, 139, 292, 373, 701, 860, 863, 992, 993, 1044

Parasite Genus species	Location in host	Prosimians	New World monkeys	Old World monkeys	Great apes	Reference
B. malayi	Lymphatic system	X		X		19, 120, 139, 360, 373, 672, 701, 744, 799, 860, 863, 1044, 1165
B. tupaiae	Lymphatic system	X				842
Wuchereria kalimantani	Inguinal lymph nodes, testicles			X		744, 860, 861, 863
Dipetalonema gracile	Peritoneal cavity		X			44, 76, 128, 132, 194, 224, 225, 240, 271, 373, 406, 528, 634, 673, 701, 707, 750, 752, 753, 764, 852, 967, 1081, 1082, 1117, 1144, 1148
D. caudispina	Peritoneal cavity		X			271, 373, 407, 764
D. graciliformis	Peritoneal cavity		X			389
D. robini	Peritoneal cavity		X			878
D. freitasi	Peritoneal cavity		X			33
D. tenue	Subcutis, body cavity		X			139, 140, 373, 1186
D. petteri	Subcutis, pleura, peritoneum	X				59, 142, 197
Protofilaria furcata	Thoracic cavity	X				153, 1145
Mansonella barbascalensis	Peritoneal cavity		X			306
M. zakii	Peritoneal cavity		X			271, 306, 617, 814, 1145
M. obtusa	Periesophagal connective tissue		X			302, 373, 701, 764, 1190
M. marmosetae	Subcutis		X			271, 351, 373, 764, 967, 1091, 1144, 1190
M. mariae	Subcutis		X			878
M. tamarinae	Subcutis		X			225, 271, 302, 373
M. atelenis	Subcutis		X			373, 764, 967, 1144, 1186, 1190
M. parvum	Subcutis		X			268, 373, 764, 967, 1144, 1189, 1190
M. nicollei	Peritoneal cavity		X			271, 1144
M. dunni	Subcutis	X				797
M. mystaxi	Subscapular connective tissue		X			283
M. panamensis	Subcutis		X			287, 303, 621, 1081
M. saimiri	Subcutis		X			304
M. colombiensis	Subcutis		X			305
Mansonella sp.	Peritoneal cavity		X			1081
M. perstans	Subcutis, body cavity				X	139, 162, 255, 354, 373, 450, 462, 544
M. vanhoofi	Peritoneal cavity				X	64, 137, 138, 373, 701, 804, 846, 870–872, 964, 967, 1144, 1190
M. rodhaini	Subcutis				X	373, 846, 872, 967, 1144, 1186, 1190
M. streptocerca	Subcutis				X	161, 253, 255, 354, 373, 701, 846, 872, 967, 1144, 1190
M. digitatum	Peritoneal cavity			X	X	139, 140, 153, 373, 799, 967, 984, 1144, 1148, 1186, 1190
M. leopoldi	Subcutis				X	64
M. gorillae	Subcutis				X	64
M. lopeensis	Subcutis				X	34
Dipetalonema sp.	Subcutis	X				452
Cercopithifilaria papionis	Subcutis			X		763
C. kenyensis	Subcutis			X		284
C. degraffi	Subcutis			X		32
C. verveti	Subcutis			X		36
C. narokensis	Subcutis			X		35
C. eberhardi	Subcutis			X		35
Onchocerca volvulus	Connective tissue				X	64, 846

TABLE VII—*Continued*

Parasitic Nematodes Described from Nonhuman Primates

Parasite Genus species	Location in host	Prosimians	New World monkeys	Old World monkeys	Great apes	Reference
Subclass Adenophorea (Aphasmidia), order Enoplida, superfamily Trichuroidea						
Trichuris trichiura	Cecum, colon		X	X	X	4, 68, 106, 108, 132, 200, 354, 364, 373, 449, 464, 617, 651, 652, 659, 793, 851, 855, 879, 899, 929, 967, 1023, 1077, 1113, 1188, 1189
Trichuris sp.	Cecum, colon, stomach	X		X		68, 89, 514, 519, 564, 653, 656, 658, 659, 765, 811, 859, 860, 863, 1110, 1189
Capillaria hepatica	Liver		X	X	X	354, 373, 378, 463, 464, 562, 646, 672, 701, 967, 1044, 1101, 1103
Capillaria sp.	Liver		X	X	X	1189
Anatrichosoma cutaneum	Nasal mucosa, skin			X		12, 105, 354, 373, 477, 851, 929, 967, 1023, 1073
A. cynomolgi (syn: *Anatrichosoma nacepobi, Anatrichosoma rhina*)	Nasal mucosa			X		12, 168, 186, 364, 373, 715, 851, 1039
A. ocularis	Eye	X				362
Anatrichosoma sp.	Eye			X		286

Gross lesions consist of catarrhal to hemorrhagic or necrotizing enterocolitis (227,373,617,1023). There may be a secondary peritonitis associated with the enterocolitis (373, 571). Pulmonary hemorrhage is the most common lesion outside the digestive tract (227,373,617,1023). Histologic examination of the small intestine of the infected animal shows a multifocal erosive and ulcerative enteritis caused by adults, eggs, and rhabditiform larvae (227). The mucosa contains numerous parasites, most of which are in interepithelial tunnels or lumina of intestinal glands (Fig. 14). These lesions may be infiltrated by neutrophils. Mononuclear cells and an occasional eosinophil can be seen in the lamina propria. Intestinal villi are short and blunt, and in severe infections bridging and loss of villi are seen (183). In cases where autoinfection has occurred, changes in the small and large intestines in response to invasion by the filariform larvae range from a mild inflammatory cell response to severe, acute, or granulomatous or necrotizing enterocolitis. Larval invasion of the submucosal and serosal lymphatics results in a severe granulomatous endolymphangitis (227) (Fig. 15). These changes are associated with various degrees of lymphatic obstruction and submucosal and serosal edema, fibrosis, or both. In the lungs, acute multifocal or diffuse hemorrhage is most common. Larval granulomas may be seen over the surface of the pleura. Filariform larvae also are seen in many tissues throughout the body, most commonly in the lymph nodes and liver (227). Fatal strongyloidiasis has been described in lowland gorillas and chimpanzees (874).

This condition may be diagnosed by identification of typical larvae in the stool, by clinical signs, or by demonstration of parasitic adult females, eggs, and larvae at necropsy or at histologic examination (373).

The primary methods of control consist of strict sanitary practices and proper management due to the short life cycle of this nematode. Because first-stage larvae in the feces can develop into third-stage infective larvae within 48 hr, it is imperative that feces be removed daily and that food and water be kept free of contamination (373,464,1115). Special care needs to be taken to prevent the free-living stages of this parasite from breeding in cages, runs, enclosures, or any other areas where

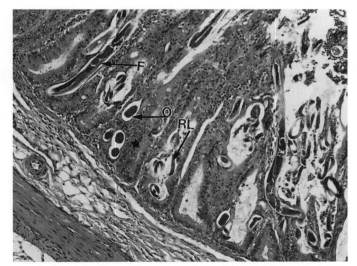

Fig. 14. Photomicrograph of mucosa of small intestine of gibbon (*Hylobates* sp.) with severe strongyloidiasis. Many adult female parasites (F), rhabditiform larvae (RL), and ova (O) in interepithelial tunnels are seen throughout mucosa. HE stain. (Reprinted from Toft, II, J. D. (1982). *Veterinary Pathology.* With permission.)

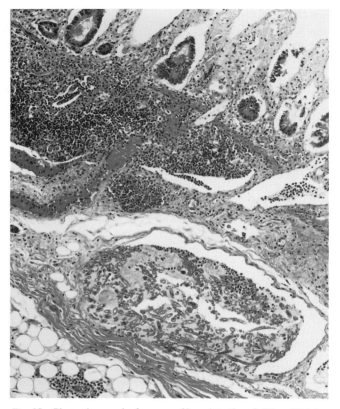

Fig. 15. Photomicrograph of mucosa of large intestine of gibbon (*Hylobates* sp.) with severe strongyloidiasis and autoinfection. Masses of filariform larvae in subserosal lymphatic and associated granulomatous endolymphangitis are seen. HE stain. (Reprinted from Toft, II, J. D. (1982). *Veterinary Pathology.* With permission.

nonhuman primates are housed. Keeping surfaces dry will aid greatly in controlling this parasite as moisture is necessary for the survival of the larvae (373). Use of dry bedding may facilitate the control of strongyloidiasis greatly. Newly acquired nonhuman primates should be examined on arrival and, if infected, should be either treated or eliminated (373).

Strongyloidiasis in nonhuman primate colonies is considered a potential public health problem. Infections by *S. fulleborni* that have been transmitted naturally from monkeys or apes to humans have been reported (95, 373, 851, 967, 1136). Experimental infections in humans by *Strongyloides* sp. isolated from nonhuman primates also have been reported (73, 232, 350, 373, 851, 978). All personnel handling, caring, or otherwise working with nonhuman primates should be instructed in proper personal hygiene practices and safe methods of handling infected animals and excrement (373). All animal care personnel should be required to wear the proper protective clothing, gloves, masks, etc. at all times to avoid potential skin penetration of the infective larvae (934).

Ivermectin (Ivomec), administered at a dose level of 200 mcg/kg intramuscularly, repeated after 3 weeks if needed, is reported to be an effective anthelminthic against strongyloid-

iasis in nonhuman primates (46,90,213). Other effective drugs are thiabendazole (Omnizole) administered at a dose level of 50–100 mg/kg orally for 1, 2, or 5 days, depending on the dosage used (2,71,206,373,459,694,934,1072,1115); Telmin (18% mebendazole) at a dose of 22 mg/kg/day per os for 3 days; levamisole phosphate (Levisole, Ripercol) at a dose of 10 mg/kg per os or subcutaneously for 2–3 days; or pyrantel pamoate (Strongid-T, Nemex) in a single dose of 11 mg/kg per os (213, 1072). Thiabendazole (Omnizole), particularly in high doses, may produce vomiting, resulting in loss of the drug (1072). Treatment with drugs listed other than ivermectin should be repeated in 10 days to 2 weeks (373,934,1072,1115). Sanitation is essential in preventing reinfection (934,1072).

Leeflang (690) has published a 6-week treatment regimen for the elimination of *S. stercoralis* in orangutans. This schedule includes treatments with mebendazole (Telmin: 18% mebendazole) biweekly, 50 mg/kg body weight/day (2 equal doses) for 7 days during weeks 1 and 5; 100 mg/kg body weight/day (two equal doses) for 7 days during week 3. During weeks 2 and 4 the animals are rested from therapy and their enclosure steam cleaned. At week 6 the enclosure is again steam cleaned and a fecal sample from each animal is examined for evidence of *Strongyloides* infection. If this sample is negative for *Strongyloides,* the animals are released into their outdoor daytime enclosure (690,746).

Note: The death of a cynomolgus monkey (*Macaca fascicularis*) was attributed to the side effects of filarial nematodes (*Edesonfilaria malayensis*) located in the pulmonary blood vessels that died following a single dose of ivermectin. The resulting parasitic emboli caused pulmonary infarction and a severe inflammatory reaction. This condition compromised pulmonary function and contributed to the death of the monkey after anesthesia for experimental purposes (629). These authors suggested that it might be prudent to give ivermectin earlier during the quarantine period so that lesions associated with parasite death can resolve prior to the subsequent stresses of experimental procedures. However, this drug has been used extensively in the treatment of nematode infections, including filariasis, in humans, monkeys, and various other animals without adverse reactions. It seems likely that this may well have been an isolated instance, although clinicians should be alert to the possibility.

2. Oxyurids

a. OXYURIASIS. Commonly known as pinworms (family: Oxyuridae), these small nematode parasites inhabit the colon and cecum of nonhuman primate hosts.

Genera described in nonhuman primates are *Trypanoxyuris* and *Oxyuronema* species found in New World monkeys (268, 550, 553, 617), *Enterobius vermicularis* and other *Enterobius* species found in Old World monkeys and great apes, *Enterobius anthropopitheci* in the chimpanzee (126,130,170,293,373,479, 549,754,813,851,897,929,936,944,967,983,985,1001,1186,

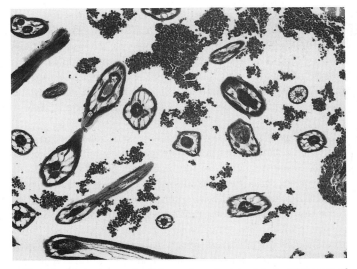

Fig. 16. Photomicrograph of focus of purulent exudate in submucosa of colon of chimpanzee. Many nematode parasites, probably *Enterobius* sp., with morphologic features of oxyurid parasites are seen. Movat stain. (Reprinted from Toft, II, J. D. (1982). *Veterinary Pathology.* With permission.)

1189), and several species in prosimian primates (47,63,144, 145,147).

These parasites are considered cosmopolitan in geographic distribution. The life cycle is direct.

Most reports of oxyuriasis in nonhuman primates state that these infections are essentially innocuous (373,617,851,1023). Clinical signs usually are limited to anal pruritus and irritation, which may lead to self-multilation, restlessness, and increased aggressiveness (170,214,258,373,617,754,851,967,1001,1023). Heavy pinworm infections are reported to be common in chimpanzees, and their coprophagic habits make constant reinfection inevitable (936).

Fatal cases of enterobiasis have been reported in chimpanzees (518,589,1001,1002,1100), characterized by extensive ulcerative enterocolitis, peritonitis, and necrogranulomatous lymphadenitis involving the mesenteric lymph nodes. Numerous parasites with the morphologic characteristics of *E. vermicularis* were associated with these lesions (Fig. 16). There is also an early report of the death of a red spider monkey caused by an overwhelming pinworm infection (633).

Multiple intestinal polyps associated with immature male oxyurid parasites have been described in a male chimpanzee (1095). The gross and histologic characteristics of these lesions were identical to those produced by *Nochtia nochti* in the stomach and esophagus of Old World primates. It was thought that the lesion resulted from hypersensitivity to oxyurid infection in an aberrant host.

Pinworm infection can be diagnosed by observing adult oxyurids emerging from the anus. Perianal swabs or cellophane tape also can be used to recover the typical ellipsoid, asymmetrical pinworm eggs (354,373).

Control is based on maintaining rigid sanitary practices, isolation and treatment of infected animals, and quarantine of newly arrived nonhuman primates coupled with fecal examinations to identify infected animals. Positive animals should be treated prior to introduction into the colony.

Naturally infected nonhuman primates may be sources of infection in humans. Also, captive primates can acquire *E. vermicularis* infection from humans and then can act as reservoirs to reinfect humans (72,373). The same procedures outlined for animal care personnel to guard against the possible transmission of *Strongyloides* from nonhuman primates also apply here.

Effective drugs for the treatment of oxyuriasis are thiabendazole (Omnizole) at a dose of 50–100 mg/kg per os (694); mebendazole (Telmin: 18% mebendazole) at a dose of 100 mg (active drug) per os as a single dose for adult apes and 10 mg/ kg for infants and small species; and pyrantel pamoate (Strongid-T, Nemex) in a single dose of 11 mg/kg per os. Total maximum dose should not exceed 1 g (1072). All drugs should be repeated in 10 days (213,1072).

3. Strongylids

a. OESOPHAGOSTOMIASIS.   This disease is caused by infection of nematodes in the genus *Oesophagostomum,* the nodular worm. These parasites are considered to be the most common nematode parasite found in Old World monkeys and great apes (64,373,592,754,845,851,929,967,1023). They have been described in baboons, mangabeys, guenons, macaques, chimpanzees, and gorillas (60,71,126,367,373,449,459,464,479,486, 520,588,602,651,659,763,805,813,855,929,965,1001,1023, 1077,1113,1115,1153). They are rare in New World monkeys (268,851,1189).

Their geographic distribution is widespread, almost universal. At least 11 different species have been proposed but not clearly defined (845,1189). The species mentioned most frequently are *O. apiostomum, O. bifurcum, O. aculeatum,* and *O. stephanostomum* (354,373,701,967,990). The life cycle is direct, but requires about a week for infective larvae to develop.

Infected monkeys usually are asymptomatic, and light infections usually go unrecognized (373,967,1023). Monkeys with severe infections may show general unthriftiness and debilitation characterized by increased weight loss and diarrhea; the mortality rate increases for this group (373,967,1023).

Lesions seen at necropsy consist of typical *Oesophagostomum* nodules, which are elevated, smooth, 2–4 mm in diameter, and firm (Fig. 17). They are seen most frequently on the serosal surface of the large intestine and cecum and in the mesentery supporting these organs (126,373,813,845,967,1023,1121), but also in ectopic sites, such as the peritoneal wall, mesentery of the small intestine, omentum, kidney, liver, lungs, or diaphragm (157,845,851,1023). The nodules may be black or brown if there is associated hemorrhage; older nodules usually are white because of caseation of the contents. Viable worms may be seen in relatively young nodules; usually, however, the parasite is

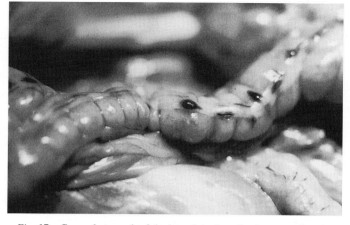

Fig. 17. Gross photograph of the large intestine of a rhesus monkey (*Macaca mulatta*) showing numerous small black nodules on the serosal surface consistent with a diagnosis of oesophagostomiasis.

dead and surrounded by a mass of caseous debris. Older nodules may contain foci of mineralization (373,463,1023). Sometimes ulcers form in the colonic mucosa at the point where the larval penetration occurred, and a migratory tract filled with inflammatory exudate connects the nodule in the wall with the intestinal lumen (373,463,464,1023).

Histopathologically, the parasite and cell detritus are surrounded by a mantle of inflammatory cells, mainly neutrophils and macrophages with scattered eosinophils, lymphocytes, and plasma cells (Fig. 18). Foreign-body giant cells may be present in the cellular exudate. A fibrous capsule of various degrees of thickness and maturity, depending on the age of the nodule, surrounds the centrally located necroinflammatory mass (126, 373,813,1023).

Research with *O. aculeatum* in Japanese macaques has resulted in the detection of a low molecular weight product released from the larvae of this parasite, which is chemotactic for neutrophils. It is postulated that this compound may be responsible for the formation of the pyogranulomatous nodules found in *Oesophagostomum* infections in monkeys (527). Granulomatous lesions, without caseation, involving the submucosa and subserosa of the colon, the kidney, the adventitial tissue of the prostate, the pancreas, and the heart have been reported in rhesus monkeys infected with *Oesophagostomum* sp. nematodes (584,725).

Death of a chimpanzee from septicemia due to bacterial invasion of *Oesophagostomum* nodules in the colon has been reported (1151–1153). Rupture of the nodules may result in acute or chronic peritonitis with fibrous peritoneal adhesions (845, 1023). Adhesions may restrict intestinal motility and result in obstruction or rarely in ascites (373,967,1023).

Oesophagostomum infection can be diagnosed by identifying the eggs in the feces. A problem arises, however, because the eggs of the different *Oesophagostomum* species cannot be dif-

ferentiated from one another and also are indistinguishable from those of *Ternidens* and other hookworm species. The diagnosis of oesophagostomiasis based solely on typical eggs in the feces always should be questioned. Positive identification of larvae can be made following stool culture. Occasionally, adults are passed and can be identified. The postmortem diagnosis is based on typical nodular lesions, identification of adults, or both (373,1023).

The primary methods of control consist of adherence to strict sanitation practices and good management, which together result in a rapid reduction of the incidence of this infection in a colony (373,464). Fecal examination of newly acquired nonhuman primates should be accomplished during quarantine. Infected animals should be either treated or eliminated.

This parasite has been reported to infect humans and therefore should be considered to have zoonotic potential (373,461, 719). Appropriate care in handling nonhuman primates should be exercised.

Effective drugs for the treatment of oesophagostomiasis are thiabendazole (Omnizole) as a single dose of 100 mg/kg per os, 50 mg/kg once daily per os for 2 days, or 25 mg/kg twice daily per os for 2 days; levamisole phosphate (Levisole, Ripercol) at a single dose of 10 mg/kg subcutaneously or per os; and Telmin (18% mebendazole) at a dose of 40 mg/kg per os, divided three times daily for 3–5 days (1072). All treatments should be repeated in 10 to 14 days (1072).

b. TERNIDENIASIS.   The cause of this disease, *Ternidens deminutus,* is a strongyle that is related to the oesophagostomes and hookworms (373,851). These parasites inhabit the cecum and colon and have been reported in Old World monkeys (macaques, especially *Macaca arctoides,* guenons, and baboons)

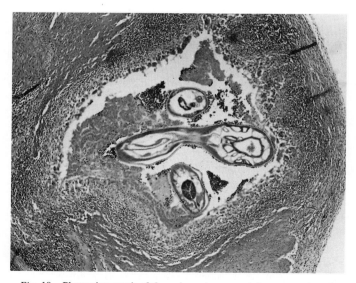

Fig. 18. Photomicrograph of *Oesophagostomum* nodule on serosal surface of colon of rhesus monkey (*Macaca mulatta*). Larvae in center and typical host response comprise the inflammatory nodule. HE stain. (Reprinted from Toft, II, J. D. (1982). *Veterinary Pathology.* With permission.)

and in the great apes (gorilla and chimpanzee) (13,373,449,463, 701,804,822,929,967,990,1077,1114,1186).

The morphologic features of the adult worms and their eggs are similar to those of *Oesophagostomum* (373,967,1077). The life cycle is direct and also is similar to *Oesophagostomum* (373).

There is little macroscopic evidence of any lesions associated with this parasite; however, as the worms move about within the intestinal lumen there can be extensive mucosal damage and blood loss, which can cause anemia and the formation of cystic nodules in the colonic wall (373,701,851).

This parasite can infect humans; it causes intestinal nodules. Infected captive animals should be handled with caution (373).

Control and treatment for this parasite are the same as that outlined for the treatment of *Oesophagostomum* sp.

4. Ancylostomatids

a. ANCYLOSTOMIASIS AND NECATORIASIS. The cause of these diseases, the hookworms usually found in humans, *Ancylostoma duodenale* and *Necator americanus,* are recorded occasionally in nonhuman primates, including monkeys, mandrills, baboons, gibbons, chimpanzees, and gorillas (60,241, 293,360,373,470,473,708,754,804,847,898,936,1197). Reports of their presence in South American monkeys are rare (851). These parasites have a direct life cycle, but require about a week for infective larvae to develop.

Clinical signs associated with heavy hookworm infection in nonhuman primates are similar to those produced by these parasites in humans and other animals and include anemia, eosinophilia, "pot-belly" appearance, dyspnea on exertion, and a general debilitation (373,470,473,967).

Necropsy findings have included a general pallor of all tissues. The mucosa of the small intestine was thickened by a chronic inflammatory reaction. Small hemorrhages were seen throughout the intestinal mucosa, and large numbers of hookworms were attached to the mucosa (473).

The diagnosis of hookworm disease is based on finding eggs in the feces or mature worms in the bowel at necropsy (373). Because hookworm eggs are morphologically identical to those of several species of strongyles that also infect nonhuman primates, diagnosis based on the eggs alone should be viewed with caution (851). Again, identification of larvae can be performed following culture of stool.

Control of this parasite is best achieved by following strict sanitation practices within the colony, by the removal of all conditions that present a favorable environment for the development of eggs and larvae, and by the elimination or regular treatment of all infected animals (373,1044).

Because humans are the normal definitive host for these parasites, infected captive primates should be handled with caution (373).

Effective drugs for the treatment of ancylostomiasis are ivermectin (Ivomec) at a dose level of 200 mcg/kg intramuscularly,

repeated after 3 weeks if needed; tetramisol (Concurat) as a single oral dose of 12–16 mg/kg (active ingredients); mebendazole (Telmin: 18% mebendazole) at a dose of 15 mg/kg (active ingredients) per os for 2 days or at a dose of 3 mg/kg per os for 10 days (436); and levamisole (Nemicide) at a dose of 7.5 mg/kg subcutaneously, equivalent to 0.1 mg/kg. Two doses are given, 2 weeks apart (213,1159).

5. Trichostrongylids

a. MOLINEIASIS. This disease is caused by trichostrongyles in the genus *Molineus.* These are small, slender, pale red worms that inhabit the upper digestive tract, duodenum, and sometimes the pyloric region of the stomach of nonhuman primates. Occasionally they may involve the pancreas and mesentery (91, 194,224,260,268,373,617,674,694,1023,1186). They always are found lying on the mucosa, never attached.

Geographically they are distributed throughout Central and South America, with one species occurring in Africa (260,268, 373). Species described in nonhuman primates include *M. vexillarius* in marmosets; *M. elegans* in squirrel monkeys, cebus monkeys, and howler monkeys; *M. vogelianus* in pottos; and *M. torulosus* in cebus monkeys, squirrel monkeys, and owl monkeys (194,260,268,373,617,694,1023,1194). *Molineus torulosus* is the only species reported to be a specific pathogen (91,373,617,674,694,1023).

The life cycle and method of transmission of these parasites are unknown. Infection with *M. torulosus* has been reported to cause hemorrhagic or ulcerative enteritis, sometimes associated with diverticula of the intestinal wall (91,373,617,674,694, 1023). Serosal nodules that involved the upper portion of the small intestine have been seen in capuchin monkeys (91) (Fig. 19). These nodules communicated with the intestinal lumen through 1-mm reddish brown ulcers.

Histologically, the nodules were composed of an intense granulomatous inflammatory response surrounded by a rim of proliferating fibrous connective tissue (Fig. 20). The central portion contained a mass of nematode parasites and their eggs surrounded by eosinophilic debris. Neutrophils, histiocytes, and other chronic inflammatory cells were present adjacent to the worms (Fig. 21). Chronic pancreatitis also was seen, with worms and eggs in inflamed pancreatic ducts (91,694,1023).

Diagnosis rests on the identification of typical eggs in the feces or the presence of adult worms associated with typical lesions in the digestive tract (373,701,850).

Procedures for control of this parasite have not been described. Sanitation and good management appear to be sufficient. Reports from laboratories that have experienced heavy infections in newly arrived susceptible nonhuman primates indicate a decline in incidence with time and an absence of this parasite in laboratory-reared primates (194,224,373,674).

Nothing is known of the public health significance of this parasite (373), and no treatment has been described.

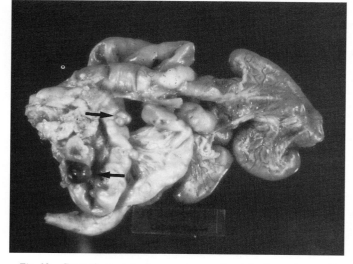

Fig. 19. Gross photograph of numerous serosal nodules (arrows) caused by *Molineus torulosus* in upper small intestine of cebus monkey (*Cebus* sp.). (Courtesy of Dr. R. E. Schmidt.) (Reprinted from Toft, II, J. D. (1982). *Veterinary Pathology.* With permission.)

b. NOCHTIASIS. This disease results from infection by trichostrongyles in the genus *Nochtia*. *Nochtia nochti* is a small, slender, bright red worm that has been described in prepyloric region of the stomach of Asian macaques (85,373,673,851,972, 1023,1036,1098).

Eggs are thin-shelled and ellipsoid, typical of members of the strongyles. *Nochtia* eggs can be differentiated from those of other members of the order Strongylida as they are larger and more pointed and are embryonated when passed in the feces. Free parasites are not found in the feces or the gastrointestinal tract. The life cycle is direct (85,373).

At necropsy, hyperemic, cauliflower-like masses are seen protruding from the gastric mucosa at the junction of the fundus and prepyloric regions. These lesions must be differentiated from the gastric hyperplasia caused by polychlorinated biphenols present in concrete sealers.

Histologically, these masses are benign inflammatory polyps composed of hyperplastic fronds of gastric mucosa and inflammatory tissue. Adult worms and their eggs can be found deep at the base of the lesion (85,373,817,851,972,1023,1036,1098) (Fig. 22).

Diagnosis depends on identification of typical eggs in the feces of affected animals or on the finding at necropsy of characteristic gastric polyps containing the parasite (373,1023).

Nothing is known about control of this parasite. As with any parasite, effective control can probably be obtained through proper sanitation procedures and good management practices (373).

Also, nothing is known of the public health aspects of this nematode (373), and no treatment has been described.

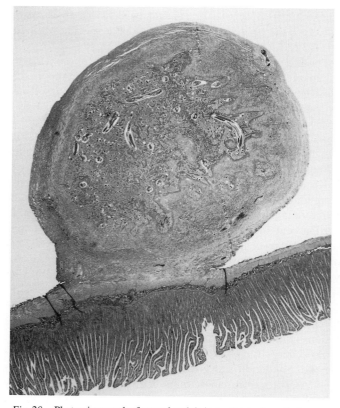

Fig. 20. Photomicrograph of serosal nodule in small intestine of cebus monkey (*Cebus* sp.) showing granulomatous inflammatory reaction associated with *Molineus torulosus* parasites in center and surrounding capsule of fibrous connective tissue. HE stain. (Reprinted from Toft, II, J. D. (1982). *Veterinary Pathology.* With permission.)

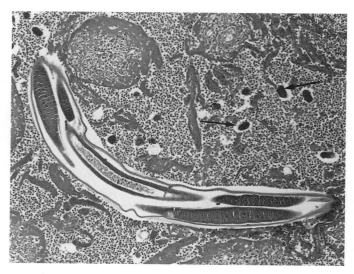

Fig. 21. Higher magnification of nodule in Fig. 18: *Molineus torulosus* parasite, many ova (arrows) and associated eosinophilic debris, and mixed inflammatory cell population. HE stain. (Reprinted from Toft, II, J. D. (1982). *Veterinary Pathology.* With permission.)

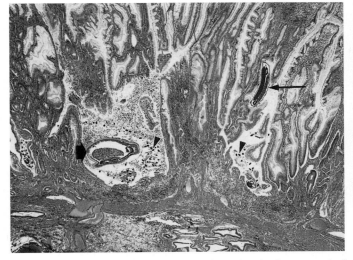

Fig. 22. Photomicrograph of section through gastric polyp from stomach of rhesus monkey (*Macaca mulatta*) infected with *Nochtia nochti*. Hyperplastic gastric epithelium, female worm (thick arrow), male worm (thin arrow), many ova (arrowheads). HE stain. (Reprinted from Toft, II, J. D. (1982). *Veterinary Pathology*. With permission.)

6. Metastrongylids

a. ANGIOSTRONGYLIASIS. The cause of this disease, the metastrongyle *Angiostrongylus costaricensis,* normally is found in rats in South and Central America (395). It also causes a clinical syndrome in humans, particularly in children who reside in this geographic region. This syndrome is characterized by an inflammatory granulomatous mass that usually is located in the wall of the appendix, but which can extend to the ileum, the cecum and ascending colon, and regional lymph nodes (395). Histologically, the granulomatous mass is composed of chronic inflammatory cells and nematode eggs. Adult parasites reside in arteries of the intestinal wall and mesentery (395).

Similar parasitic granulomas in the wall of the small intestine have been reported from two mustached marmosets (*Saguinus mystax*) (1035, 1092). The histomorphologic features of these lesions were identical to those described previously for *A. costaricensis* infection in humans. In addition to the chronic inflammatory cells, the granulomas contained numerous nematode eggs and many larvae. The eggs of this particular parasite are reported to hatch within the rat or monkey host, then migrate to the gut and pass out in the feces to complete the life cycle (395). Adult parasites with morphologic features consistent with a diagnosis of *Angiostrongylus* sp. were found in the mesenteric arteries associated with the granuloma.

On the basis of the nonhuman primate species involved, the fact that this species originated in the geographical region where this parasite has been reported to occur, the gross and histological appearance of the lesions, and the finding of adult *Angiostrongylus* sp. in the mesenteric arteries intimately involved with the granulomas, these parasites were identified as *A. costaricensis.*

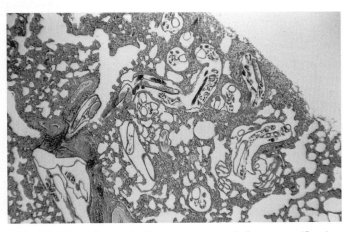

Fig. 23. Photomicrograph of lung of a moustached marmoset (*Saguinus mystax mystax*) infected with *Filariopsis* sp. At this power, the nature of the worm embedded in the lung parenchyma is illustrated. HE stain.

People who work with marmosets should be aware of the presence of this parasite and look for additional cases to document further its occurrence in South American monkeys.

b. PULMONARY METASTRONGYLIASIS. This condition is the result of infection with the metastrongylid lungworms in the genera *Filaroides* and *Filariopsis.* These parasites are most commonly seen in New World monkeys (marmosets, squirrel monkeys, cebus monkeys, and howler monkeys) (92, 194, 268, 373, 449, 617, 694, 819, 851, 967, 1023, 1024, 1117, 1186).

In the live state, these parasites are very slender and fragile (850). Adults are found in the terminal bronchioles, respiratory bronchioles, and pulmonary alveoli (Figs. 23 and 24) (373, 617, 694, 851, 1023, 1024). The adult female is viviparous. They produce larvae that are coughed up, swallowed by the host, and passed in the feces. The remainder of the life cycle, and whether

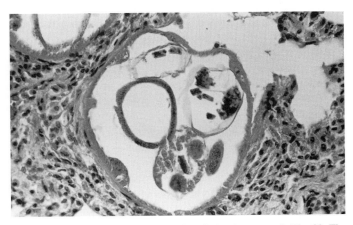

Fig. 24. Photomicrograph of a female *Filariopsis* sp. seen in Fig. 22. The features of this metastrongyle worm, including the thin cuticle and low muscle cells, reproductive tubes, and gut (to right), are evident. HE stain.

any intermediate hosts are required, is not known (617,851, 1024).

Gross lesions in the pulmonary parenchyma are subtle. The lung appears normal except for the presence of varying numbers of randomly located, small, elevated, subpleural nodules, which may be hyperpigmented, and cause the pleura to bulge.

Histopathologically, there are varying degrees of atelectasis and foci of chronic inflammatory cells infiltrating the affected alveolar spaces and intraalveolar septae.

Most infections are considered to be subclinical in nature, and although the parasite is common in certain species of New World monkeys, there is no evidence to suggest that the presence of lungworms has been a cause of death (617,851,1024).

Diagnosis can be made by finding and identifying the typical lungworm larvae in fresh feces. In dead animals, the presence of characteristic gross and histopathologic pulmonary lesions associated with metastrongylid parasites is also diagnostic.

Methods of control have not been described for these parasites. However, strict sanitation within the colony and good management practices are probably effective in preventing the dissemination of this parasite.

The public health significance of these parasites in unknown (373), and no treatment has been described.

7. Ascarids

a. ASCARIASIS. This disease results from infection with members of the genus *Ascaris,* commonly known as roundworms. They are a common finding in the intestinal tract of nonhuman primates (851). The specimens that have been recovered are reported to be indistinguishable from *Ascaris lumbricoides* in humans (27, 270, 1090, 1189). Both Old World monkeys and great apes have been reported to be infected (60, 270,293,359,463,470,626,885,929,967,1047,1049,1189).

The life cycle of this parasite is direct.

Although roundworm infection in nonhuman primates is thought to be relatively innocuous and of little clinical significance (754,851), fatal cases of ascariasis have been reported in both monkeys and great apes (463,885,1047). Death in the great apes was thought to be due to the presence of many worms, blockage of the bowel, and migration of the worms into the bile duct and liver.

Diagnosis of ascariasis is based on the presence of typical eggs in the feces or adults in the digestive tract at necropsy.

Because the ascarids reported in nonhuman primates are morphologically identical to *A. lumbricoides* in humans, cross-infection from infected animals to humans is possible; however, no reports were found that documented such an occurrence. Nevertheless, infected nonhuman primates should be considered a potential zoonotic threat and should be handled accordingly.

Piperazine compounds (Uvilon) at a dose rate of 0.5 ml/kg body weight orally for 2 days is reported to safely eliminate this parasite (436). Mebendazole (Telmin) at a dose rate of 22 mg/kg per os for 3 days and pyrantel pamoate (Strongid T) at a dose

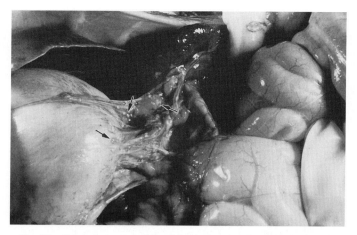

Fig. 25. Gross photograph of the abdominal cavity of a green monkey (*Cercopithecus aethiops*) showing numerous encysted ascarid larvae (arrows) in the genus *Polydelphis.*

rate of 11 mg/kg per os, repeated in 10–14 days, also are reported to be effective therapeutic agents (213).

Occasionally, nematode larvae consistent with larval ascarids are identified in various primate hosts from a wide range of tissues (Figs. 25–28). These larvae are frequently encased in a marked granulomatous nodule, but not always. Typically there is little clinical indication of infection.

8. Spirurids

a. TRICHOSPIRURIASIS. The cause of this disease, *Trichospirura leptostoma,* is a spirurid nematode that parasitizes the pancreatic ducts of several species of New World monkeys,

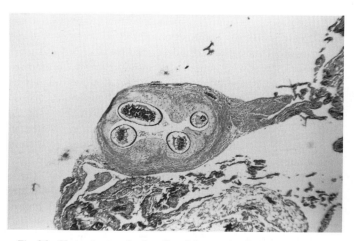

Fig. 26. Photomicrograph of small nodule, seen in Fig. 24, on the serosa of a green monkey (*Cercopithecus aethiops*) containing a coiled larval ascarid in the genus *Polydelphis.* At this level, the marked lateral alae are not evident. Trichrome stain.

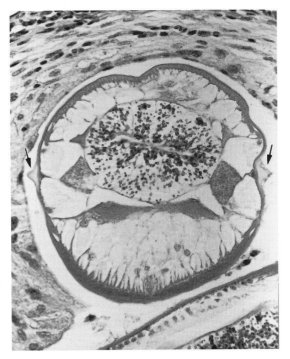

Fig. 27. Photomicrograph of section through *Polydelphis* larva from the case illustrated in Fig. 24 and 25 showing the typical ascarid morphology, especially the prominent lateral alae (arrows). HE stain.

including marmosets, tamarins, squirrel monkeys, and owl monkeys.

Geographic distribution is confined to Central and South America (194,195,373,510,617,850,851,1040,1041).

Male and female adult parasites measure up to 15 and 120 mm, respectively. The eggs are medium sized and are typically spirurid in that they are thick shelled and contain a larva (704). The complete life cycle is unknown (373,617).

The parasite usually is found incidentally on histological examination. Infection usually causes little tissue destruction or inflammatory reaction (Fig. 29). Tissue response apparently varies in proportion to the number of parasites present (617, 851). Chronic pancreatitis in association with the worms has been described in marmosets (*Callithrix* sp.) (851,1041). Acute pancreatitis in owl monkeys (*Aotus* sp.) consisting of a patchy granulocytic interstitial infiltrate adjacent to intralobular ducts was thought to be associated with leakage of retained pancreatic secretions. Larger ducts containing gross sections of worms also contained granulocytes (850,851). Occasional obstructive jaundice, due to blocking of the bile ducts by this parasite, has been reported in marmosets and tamarins (510).

Diagnosis is made postmortem by finding sections of the parasite in slides made of pancreatic tissue or by flotation of the pancreas in normal saline at necropsy; the parasites leave the tissue and can be seen in the fluid (510).

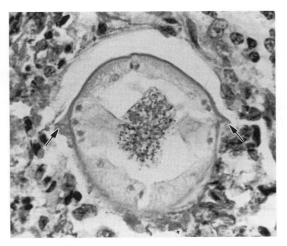

Fig. 28. Photomicrograph of a larval ascarid in the brain of a mangabey monkey (*Cercocebus atys*). The sharply pointed lateral alae (arrows) are clearly evident. HE stain.

Nothing is known about the public health significance of this parasite, and there is no known treatment.

b. PTERYGODERMATITIASIS. The cause of this disease, *Pterygodermatites nycticebi* and/or *Pterygodermatites alphi,* is spirurid nematodes that have been reported from prosimians (slow loris), New World monkeys (tamarins and marmosets), and the great apes (gibbons) (78,706,783,1104). Several reports in members of the family Callitrichidae refer to this parasite by a synonym, *Rictularia nycticebi* (5,781,782,1199).

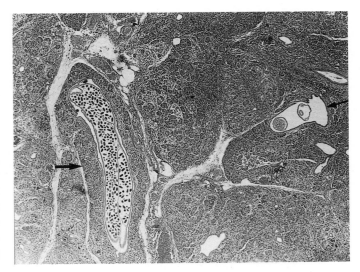

Fig. 29. Photomicrograph of several *Trichospirura leptostoma* parasites in pancreatic ducts of marmoset (*Callithrix* sp.). A female worm with many ova in uterus in the duct is shown on the left (thick arrow), and a smaller male worm in the duct is shown on the right (thin arrow). No host response. HE stain. (Reprinted from Toft, II, J. D. (1982). *Veterinary Pathology.* With permission.)

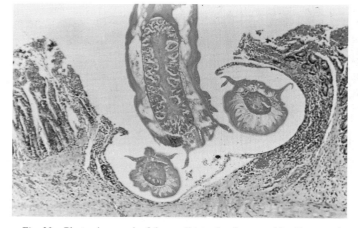

Fig. 30. Photomicrograph of the small intestine from a golden lion tamarin (*Leontopithecus rosalia*) showing an adult *Pterygodermatites nycticebi* parasite embedded in the mucosa. HE stain.

The life cycle of *P. nycticebi* is indirect. Several species of insects in the orthopterans, coleopterans, and dermapterans groups have been incriminated as suitable intermediate hosts for several species of *Pterygodermatites* that parasitize rodents (912,915,1198). Cockroaches have proven to be viable intermediate hosts for infections involving nonhuman primates (783,1198).

Morbidity and mortality associated with infection of *P. nycticebi* have been reported in golden lion tamarins (*Leontopithecus rosalia* (783).

Clinical signs in heavily infected animals included extreme weakness, passage of watery diarrhea containing adult parasites, anemia, leukopenia, and hypoproteinemia (783).

At necropsy, masses of *P. nycticebi* parasites were found throughout the gastrointestinal tract. Histopathologically, the anterior end of the adult worms was embedded in the mucosa of the small intestine (Fig. 30). Larvae were seen deeper in the submucosa. In a few cases, worms were seen in the tunica muscularis and the pancreatic ducts. There was severe clubbing of the small intestinal villi and randomly located foci composed of a necrotic pseudomembrane containing spirurid eggs, numerous yeasts, and pseudohyphae consistent with *Candida* sp. (783).

Diagnosis depends on demonstrating and identifying the characteristic spirurid eggs, adult worms, or larvae in the feces, in the gastrointestinal tract at necropsy, or in histopathological slide preparations.

Methods of control should be directed against the cockroach intermediate host through reducing populations and preventing consumption by susceptible hosts.

Nothing is known about the public health significance of this parasite.

Successful treatment, which resulted in elimination of this parasite from infected animals, has been obtained with the injectable anthelminthic, ivermectin (Ivomec). Infected marmosets were injected subcutaneously, on 3 consecutive days, with ivermectin at a dose rate of 0.5 mcg/kg body weight [Ivomec: 1%(w/v), 10mg/ml]. This is equivalent to 0.005 ml per 100 g body weight. Dilution of the dose with sterile water is recommended, especially when administering to smaller nonhuman primates (78). The only disadvantage of this treatment is the stress caused to the animals in having to catch and restrain them on 3 consecutive days (78).

Also, the use of mebendazole (Telmin: 18% mebendazole) at a dose rate of 40 mg/kg body weight for 3 consecutive days, repeated three to four times yearly, keeps this infection under control (78).

c. STREPTOPHARAGIASIS. This disease is caused by parasitic members of the genus *Streptopharagus*. These are thelaziid nematodes that have been described in the stomach of Old World monkeys and great apes (373). *Streptopharagus armatus* has been reported in the rhesus monkey, cynomolgus monkey, Japanese macaque, other macaques, guenons, patas monkey, baboon, and gibbon (373,463,1077). *Streptopharagus pigmentatus* has been reported in the rhesus monkey, cynomolgus monkey, Japanese monkey, guenon, baboon, and gibbon (373,449, 479,929,1113).

The life cycle of *S. pigmentatus* has been reviewed (728).

Little is known about the anatomic effects of these parasites (373); however, there is one report of the death of a baby chimpanzee (*Pan* sp.) that died as a result of a perforated esophagus secondary to the migration of *Streptopharagus* sp. larvae (166).

Nothing is known about the public health significance of this parasite (373), and no treatment has been reported.

d. GONGYLONEMIASIS. The cause of this disease, parasites in the genus *Gongylonema*, are small filiform nematodes that have been reported in many nonhuman primates, including both Old and New World monkeys (23,373,617,703,851,1177,1186, 1189).

These parasites have a cosmopolitan geographic distribution, and the species most commonly mentioned as infecting nonhuman primates are *G. macrogubernaculum* and *G. pulchrum*.

A characteristic feature of the adults is several rows of conspicuous oval to round cuticular bosses located at the anterior extremity (693).

The life cycle is indirect, with cockroaches or dung beetles serving as intermediate hosts (270,851).

Infection with this parasite is asymptomatic. Its presence usually is recognized only histologically and is considered to be an incidental finding. Adults are found in tunnels in the stratum malpighii of the squamous epithelium of the esophagus, lip, tongue, and other parts of the buccal cavity (Fig. 31). They also have been recovered from bronchi and the stomach. There is little or no tissue reaction (373,617,851).

Gongylonema pulchrum has been reported to occur in humans (373).

There is no treatment for this parasite in nonhuman primates.

e. PHYSALOPTERIASIS. This disease is caused by infection by members of the genus *Physaloptera*. Nine species of phys-

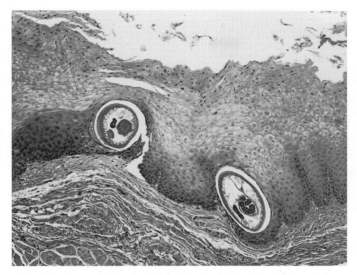

Fig. 31. Photomicrograph of several cross sections through *Gongylonema* sp. parasite in deep layers of squamous epithelium of esophagus of rhesus monkey (*Macaca mulatta*) showing a complete lack of host response. HE stain. (Reprinted from Toft, II, J. D. (1982). *Veterinary Pathology.* With permission.)

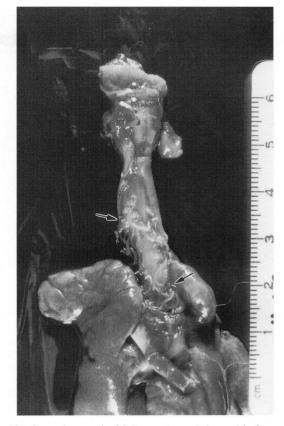

Fig. 32. Gross photograph of *Spirura quianensis* (arrows) in the esophagus of a squirrel monkey (*Saimiri sciureus*).

alopterids have been reported to occur in the upper gastrointestinal tract of nonhuman primates (1201). *Physaloptera tumefaciens* is common in the stomach of Asian macaques (373, 479). *Physaloptera dilatata* is found in the stomach of New World monkeys (titi monkeys, bearded sakis, and marmosets) (224,268,373,657,1186). *Physaloptera (Abbreviata) caucasica* has been found in the esophagus, stomach, and small intestine of the rhesus monkey, baboon, and orangutan (373,561,701, 872,967,1186). *Abbreviata poicilometra* has been found in the stomach of mangabeys and guenons (373,632,982,1186).

The life cycle of the physalopterids is indirect; an arthropod intermediate host is required. The entire life cycle is not completely understood, and a second intermediate or paratenic host may also be necessary (373,1044). Lesions result from the attachment of the worms to the wall of the affected organ. Gastritis, esophagitis, enteritis, erosion, and ulceration of the mucosa at the point of attachment are seen at necropsy (373). Hyperplastic gastric lesions and perforation of the stomach wall associated with *Physaloptera* sp. infection in cynomolgus monkeys (*Macaca fascicularis*) have been described (370,972).

Diagnosis depends on identification of the eggs in the feces or on the presence of adult worms attached to the mucosa of the upper digestive tract (373). A formol–ether sedimentation method of fecal concentration has been found to be quite reliable for qualitative detection of *Physaloptera* infection (645, 946).

Control measures should include sanitation and extermination of the possible arthropod or paratenic hosts from the nonhuman primate colony, coupled with diagnosis and treatment of the infection (373,645).

The public health aspects of these parasites are unknown.

Effective treatments for the elimination of *Physaloptera* sp. parasites from nonhuman primates include thiabendazole (Om-

nizole) at a dose rate of 300 mg/day for 6 consecutive days in cynomolgus monkeys (*M. fascicularis*) (989); levamisole hydrochloride (L-Spartakon) at a dose rate of 10 mg/kg body weight for 3 days produced complete cure in spider monkeys (*Ateles* sp.) as could be determined from the observed worm elimination and fecal examination records (645); and a mixture of *n*-butyl chloride and toluene (Nemacide) at a dose level of 0.1 ml/kg of body weight, given orally in a single dose, is effective in eliminating the adult worms (373). Carbon bisulfide and dichlorvos (Task) also have been reported to be effective for the treatment of physalopterid infections (645).

f. Other Spirurids. A wide range of other spirurid nematodes have been reported from nonhuman primates, including those such as *Spirura guianensis,* which, as adults, live attached to the epithelium of the esophagus (Fig. 32) and produce severe clinical manifestations or death (88).

g. Filariasis. This condition is caused by a variety of filarial nematodes, all in the superfamily Filarioidea, that are commonly encountered parasites of nonhuman primates. The adult filarids are long, slender worms that inhabit various tissue sites in the host animal outside the gastrointestinal tract (373, 617,701,851,967,1023,1148).

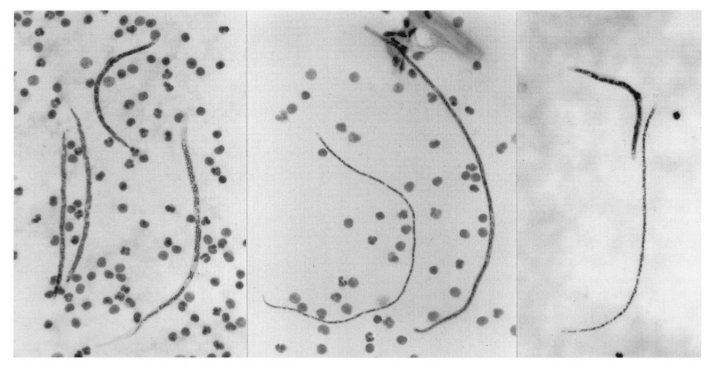

Fig. 33. Composite photomicrograph of microfilariae (all at the same relative magnification) from neotropical primates. (Left) Three *Dipetalonema gracile* and one *Dipetalonema caudispina* (to right) microfilariae in the blood of a squirrel monkey (*Saimiri sciureus*); Knott's preparation stained with hematoxylin. (Middle) *Mansonella marmosetae* microfilaria (left) and *Mansonella panamensis* (right) in the blood of a squirrel monkey (*Saimiri sciureus*); Knott's preparation stained with hematoxylin. (Right) One *Dipetalonema graciliformis* microfilaria (top) and one *Mansonella mystaxi* microfilaria (bottom) recovered in the blood of a marmoset (*Saguinus* sp.); thick blood film stained with hematoxylin.

The length of the adult worm varies, depending on the species, from a few centimeters to as much as 30 cm. Female filariae are typically much larger than the males. The female worms produce small, primitive larvae called microfilariae that circulate throughout the peripheral blood or live in the skin of the definitive host (224,225,373,617,851,967,1148).

The life cycle for these parasites is indirect. Obligatory intermediate hosts include an extensive variety of biting and blood or lymph-sucking insects (617,1023).

The filarial worms reported from nonhuman primates are listed in Table VII.

i. Filariasis in New World Monkeys: At least 13 different species of filariid nematodes have been described from New World monkeys (marmosets, squirrel monkeys, cebus monkeys, spider monkeys, and owl monkeys). These include 5 species of *Dipetalonema* and 9 species of *Mansonella* (*Tetrapetalonema*) (76,194,224,240,268,271,290,302,306,373,406,407,617,673, 764, 967, 1023, 1066, 1091, 1148, 1190). Mixed infections (Fig. 33) in the same animal are reported to be very common, with some animals containing as many as 4 different species at the same time (617).

These species live in the abdominal (Fig. 34) or thoracic cavities or in the subcutaneous tissues (Fig. 35) of the definitive host. Worms that locate in the subcutaneous tissues cause very little, if any, inflammatory response (617,851). Those species that are found in the serous cavities (*D. gracile, D. graciliformis, D. caudispina, D. robini,* and *D. freitasi*) can cause a fibrinopurulent peritonitis or pleuritis with associated fibrinous adhesions that frequently results in entrapment of the worms (617,851).

ii. Filariasis in Old World Monkeys: *Dirofilaria corynodes* is reported to be the most prevalent filarial parasite of African Old World monkeys (vervets, mangabeys, colobus monkeys, and patas monkeys). These are large parasites that are found in the subcutaneous tissues of the trunk and lower extremities where their presence causes very little tissue reaction (851). Two closely related species, *D. magnilarvatum* and *D. macacae,* have been reported from Asian Old World monkeys (cynomolgus monkeys) (851).

Macacanema formosana has been reported from Asian Old World monkeys (Taiwan macaque and cynomolgus monkey). This parasite commonly inhabits the peritracheal connective tissue and the diaphragm of the infected host (65,373,701,851, 994).

Edesonfilaria malayensis has been described in Old World monkeys (cynomolgus and rhesus monkeys) (373,402,701,831,

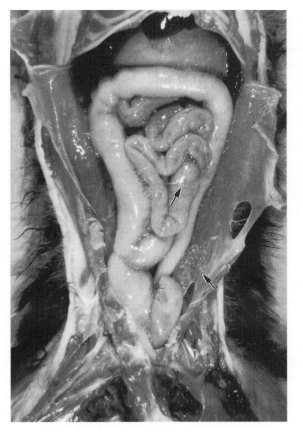

Fig. 34. Gross photograph of the opened abdominal cavity of a moustached marmoset (*Saguinus mystax mystax*) showing a natural infection with *Dipetalonema* sp. The worms (arrows) are long but slender and lie entwined in the mesenteries or viscera.

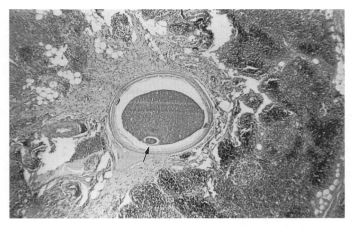

Fig. 36. Photomicrograph of the thymus of a cynomolgus monkey (*Macaca fascicularis*) containing a section through the filarial worm *Edesonfilaria malayensis*. This section, through the esophageal region of the worm, illustrates the peculiar nature of the esophagus (arrow) in this genus, which is embedded in a column of glandular material. HE stain.

929, 1187, 1191). The adult worms (Fig. 36) usually are found free in the peritoneal cavity, but have been reported from the subserosal connective tissue of the abdominal and thoracic cavities. In one report they were associated with retroperitoneal masses composed of fibrous connective tissue and multiple foci of lymphoplasmocytic infiltrates. Numerous migratory tracts containing amorphous eosinophilic debris or adult *E. malayensis* worms were scattered throughout the masses (402). In another report (831), six female adult cynomolgus (*Macaca fascicularis*) monkeys were found to be infected with *E. malayensis*.

Clinical pathological findings in the infected monkeys included reduced values of hemoglobin and hematocrit, eosino-

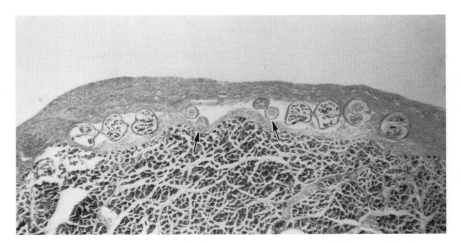

Fig. 35. Photomicrograph of subcutaneous connective tissues overlying muscles of the chest wall of a moustached marmoset (*Saguinus mystax mystax*) containing numerous sections of male (arrows) and female *Mansonella mystaxi*. Trichrome stain.

philia, an elevated level of total protein, and a decreased A/G ratio (831).

Gross lesions consisted of thickening of the connective tissues, hemorrhage, and adhesions of the serosa involving the site occupied by the worms. Mechanical damage was seen occasionally in tissues adjacent to the location of the parasites such as the pancreas and iliopsoas muscle. Splenic nodules were seen in five of the six infected monkeys (831).

Histopathologically, there was hemorrhage, fibroplasia of connective tissue, and proliferation of granulation tissue with infiltration of eosinophils, lymphocytes, and other inflammatory cells associated with the presence of worms in the tissues. Nodular lesions in the spleen consisted of a highly vascular network of large reticuloendothelial cells, reticulum fibers, eosinophils, and erythrocytes. Microfilariae were present in some of these lesions, and it was felt that the splenic nodules were most likely associated with their existence in the spleen (831).

Loa papionis, very similar to *L. loa* of humans, has been reported from a variety of Old World monkeys (drills, baboons, mangabeys, and vervets) (257, 851, 981, 1099). Except for size, the worms described from both humans and nonhuman primates are nearly identical morphologically.

Another variation is the different circadian rhythm displayed by the microfilariae produced by the worms that infect nonhuman primates. These larvae circulate in the peripheral blood with a nocturnal periodicity (851). Infection is usually asymptomatic, and significant lesions related to the presence of the adult *L. papionis* in the subcutaneous tissues of nonhuman primate hosts have not been reported (851). However, there has been a report of splenic lesions in drills experimentally infected with *L. loa.* Grossly, there were multiple nodules over the surface of the spleen due to the presence of granulomas that arose in the red pulp. Microscopically, the nodules were composed of fibrous connective tissue and numerous multinucleated giant cells, many of which contain disintegrating microfilariae within their cytoplasm. These lesions were attributed to the destruction of microfilariae within the spleen (256).

Brugia malayi and *B. pahangi* have been reported from a wide variety of Asian monkeys, particularly *Macaca* species (120,665,851). *Brugia malayi* is also a parasite of humans. The adult parasites are found in the lymphatic and perilymphatic tissues of their nonhuman primate hosts. Another species, *B. tupaiae,* has been described from the lymphatic system of prosimians (tree shrews) (851).

Symptoms and histopathology in the lymphatic system similar to that seen in human malayan filariasis have not been reported in infected nonhuman primates (851).

Meningonema peruzzii is a filariid parasite that has been reported from African Old World monkeys (vervets and talapoin monkeys) (849). These worms were found only in the subarachnoid space along the dorsum of the brain stem at the level of the medulla oblongata.

Female *M. peruzzii,* unlike most other filariae, are quadridelphic. Symptoms and lesions associated with infection by this parasite were not reported (849). Human infection with this parasite has been reported on several occasions and included marked symptoms of central nervous system involvement. However, because transmission is by insect intermediate host, there is virtually no risk of transmission under laboratory settings.

iii. Filariasis in Great Apes: *Onchocerca volvulus,* a parasite of humans, has been reported from the gorilla (64,851). The parasite was located in a subcutaneous fibrous nodule morphologically similar to that formed by the parasite in the human host (64,851).

Mansonella streptocerca and *M. rodhaini* are two filariid parasites reported from the chimpanzee. These two parasites, along with *O. volvulus* from the gorilla, are different from other filarids in that the microfilariae produced by the female remain in the dermis rather than circulating in the peripheral blood (846, 851).

Several other filarids have been reported from the great apes, including *Dirofilaria pongoi* (=*D. immitis*) from the heart of an orangutan (851,1129) and *Dirofilaria immitis* in the abdominal cavity of another orangutan (851,986). *Loa loa* also has been reported from the chimpanzee and gorilla (64,959).

Mansonella vanhoofi, a filariid parasite of the chimpanzee, inhabits the mesenteries and the connective tissue adjacent to the gallbladder, bile duct, liver, pancreas, and kidney and the loose connective tissues and lymphatics surrounding the hepatic blood vessels (851,872). They also have been described from the periadrenal connective tissue (846, 851). This parasite is very similar, if not identical, to *M. perstans* found in humans.

Diagnosis is based on demonstration and identification of the adult worms in the body cavities or subcutaneous connective tissues or on the characteristic microfilariae in the blood (150, 373,1023).

Transmission of these filarial parasites within a nonhuman primate colony is unlikely, and no special control measures are required other than extermination of possible arthropod vectors (373).

Several filarial nematodes affect humans (*Dirofilaria, Onchocerca, Loa*), but the public health significance for the majority of these species is unknown (354,373).

Recommended treatment for filariid parasites (adults and microfilaria) in nonhuman primates is diethylcarbamazine (Hetrazan, Carizid, Banozide) given orally at a dose level of 20–40 mg/kg body weight for 7–21 days (287,436). A regimen of thiacetarsamide sodium (0.22 ml/kg twice daily for 2 days) plus levamisole phosphate (11 mg/kg/day for 10 days) has been reported to be effective in clearing microfilariae from the blood of tamarins (1080).

9. Trichurids

a. TRICHURIASIS.   This disease is caused by parasites, commonly known as whipworms, in the genus *Trichuris.* Trichurid

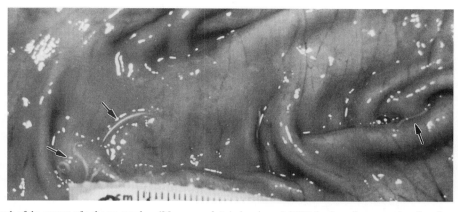

Fig. 37. Gross photograph of the cecum of a rhesus monkey (*Macaca mulatta*) showing adult *Trichuris* on the mucosal surface (arrows). The enlarged posterior end of the worms is visible while the thin anterior end is embedded in the mucosa.

parasites are frequent inhabitants of the cecum (Figs. 37 and 38) and large intestine of nonhuman primates (354, 373, 701, 754, 851, 967).

These nematodes have a worldwide distribution but are more prevalent in the tropics and subtropics (373).

Nonhuman primates reported to be affected include New World species (howler monkeys, woolly monkeys, and squirrel monkeys) (108, 269, 483, 657, 851, 1049), Old World species (rhesus monkeys, cynomolgus monkeys, Japanese macaques, Formosan macaques, African green monkeys, and baboons) (106, 373, 449, 479, 652, 659, 804, 929, 966, 990, 1077, 1113, 1189), and great apes (gibbons and chimpanzees) (293, 373, 474, 754, 897, 900, 929, 1089, 1115, 1152).

These parasites are morphologically identical to and indistinguishable from *T. trichiura* in humans (373, 754, 851, 967). The life cycle of this parasite is direct.

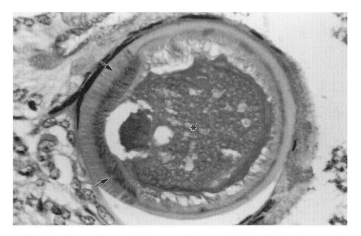

Fig. 38. Photomicrograph from case illustrated in Fig. 37 showing the thin anterior end of *Trichuris* embedded in the mucosal epithelium. The single bacillary band (arrows) and stichocyte (asterisk) are clearly evident. HE stain.

Trichuriasis in nonhuman primates usually does not cause any significant clinical problems (754). Light infections are reported to cause no apparent lesions; heavy infections, however, have been reported to result in anorexia, a gray mucoid diarrhea, and sometimes death (373, 449, 967, 1089).

Fatal whipworm infections have been reported in two chimpanzees and a gibbon. Death of one chimpanzee was attributed to a severe parasitic enteritis; the second death was thought to be the result of a secondary bacterial infection resulting from the *Trichuris* infection (1089, 1152). The death of a gibbon with chronic colitis caused by an overwhelming infection with *Trichuris* and oxyurid parasites also has been reported (474).

Diagnosis depends on the identification of the eggs, with characteristic polar plugs, in the feces, or adults in the cecum (373). Because the trichurid species that affects nonhuman primates is morphologically similar to the whipworm found in humans, cross-infection from animals to humans is possible (373, 754, 967), and experimental transmission of *Trichuris* eggs from monkeys to humans has been reported (526). Because of the direct life cycle, appropriate care in the handling of infected captive nonhuman primates and their excreta is recommended. All laboratory animal care personnel should be trained in proper personal hygiene (373).

The following drugs are reported to be effective against *T. trichiura* in nonhuman primates: butamisole (Styquin: 1.1%), at a dose rate of 0.2 ml/kg subcutaneously (213); mebendazole (Telmin: 18% mebendazole), given at a dose level of 40 mg/kg/ day by mouth twice daily for 5 days; dichlorvos (Task), given at a dose level of 10 mg/kg by mouth once daily for 1–2 days (1072); and levamisole (Nemicide), given at a dose rate of 7.5 mg/kg body weight subcutaneously, equivalent to 0.1 mg/kg, in two doses, 2 weeks apart (1159).

Flubendazole 5% administered orally at a dose rate of 27–50 mg of the active ingredient per kg body weight twice daily for 5 days has been reported to be efficient in eliminating *Trichuris trichiura* infection in baboons (*Papio hamadryas*). The drug

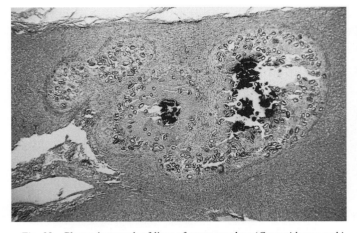

Fig. 39. Photomicrograph of liver of green monkey (*Cercopithecus aethiops*) infected with *Capillaria hepatica.* This low power view shows a large lesion containing many eggs but no adult worms. Some calcification is evident in the central area of the lesion. HE stain.

was found to be safe, without toxic side effects, and its palatability was excellent (643).

b. CAPILLARIASIS.   This disease results from infection with the cosmopolitan trichurid parasite *Capillaria hepatica.* It has been reported in the liver of a wide variety of mammalian hosts throughout the world (176), including New World monkeys (squirrel monkeys, cebus monkeys, and spider monkeys), Old World monkeys (rhesus monkeys), and great apes (chimpanzee) (354, 373, 378, 463, 464, 562, 672, 701, 967, 1023, 1044, 1101, 1102).

The anterior portion of these parasites is more slender than the posterior, but it is not as pronounced as in the whipworms. The eggs have bipolar plugs and the shell contains many small perforations, giving it a striated or pitted appearance (176,373, 851,1023).

The life cycle is direct and unique. Adult worms are found only in the hepatic parenchyma, and eggs are retained within the liver until the host dies or is killed. The eggs must be liberated from the liver either by decomposition of the original host or by passage through a predator or scavenger. Ingestion of infected liver tissue produces only spurious passage of the eggs in the feces. To become infective, the eggs must undergo embryonation under aerobic conditions. Infection occurs when embryonated eggs are ingested (176,373,378,464,851,1023).

Grossly, the liver of infected animals reveals randomly placed white or yellow patches or nodules over the surface.

Histopathologically, these foci are composed of adult *C. hepatica* and masses of eggs (Figs. 39 and 40) that are surrounded and infiltrated by proliferating fibrous connective tissue, chronic inflammatory cells, and foreign body giant cells. These lesions are ultimately converted to scar tissue, and the liver

becomes cirrhotic. Fatal hepatitis has been reported in infected nonhuman primates (360,373,851,967,1023).

Neither eggs nor adult parasites are found in the feces; therefore, diagnosis depends on demonstration and identification of the typical eggs and/or worms through liver biopsy or at necropsy (373,1023).

This parasite is pathogenic for humans (176), but because of the unusual life cycle of *C. hepatica,* infective nonhuman primates do not constitute a public health menace for persons caring for or working with them (354,373).

No special control procedures are required, and there is no treatment for this parasite in nonhuman primates (373).

c. ANATRICHOSOMIASIS.   This condition is the result of infection with the anatrichosomatid parasite *Anatrichosoma cynomolgi* (synonyms *Anatrichosoma cutaneum, A. rhina,* or *A. nacepobi*).

This species (by one name or another) has been described from both Asian and African Old World nonhuman primates (rhesus monkeys, cynomolgus monkeys, Assamese macaque, celebes crested macaque, moor macaque, pig-tailed macaque, patas monkeys, vervets, talapoin monkeys, mangabeys, spectacled langur, and baboons) (12,168,185,186,354,373,477,596, 772,844,929,967,1039,1073), New World primates (common marmoset) (477), and great apes (orangutan, siamang, and gibbon) (105,477).

The adult worms are small and slender. The eggs are large, barrel shaped, have bipolar opercula, and, unlike *Trichuris* and *Capillaria,* contain a larva (393, 851).

The life cycle and method of transmission are not known, but the cycle is thought to probably be direct. The female worms migrate through the stratified layers of squamous epithelium,

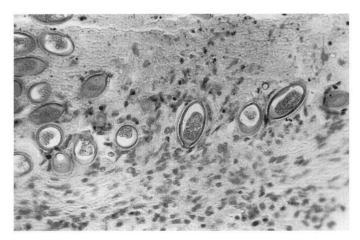

Fig. 40. Photomicrograph at higher magnification of lesion illustrated in Fig. 39 showing the typical bipolar eggs. HE stain.

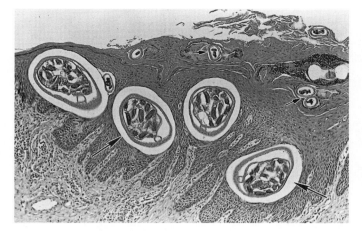

Fig. 41. Photomicrograph of the hyperplastic nasal mucosa of a rhesus monkey (*Macaca mulatta*) showing cross sections through female *Anatrichosoma cynomolgi* nematodes within intraepithelial tunnels (large arrows). There is a minimal host inflammatory response. Eggs can be seen admixed with the keratin debris on the surface (small arrows). HE stain.

forming tunnels in which the embryonated eggs are deposited (Fig. 41) (12,373,844,851). These tunnels are composed of epithelial cells and maintain their integrity. They are sloughed with the superficial keratin layers of the squamous epithelium and accumulate on the mucosal surface of the nares or skin of the extremities (Fig. 41). Eggs are excreted from the host in the nasal secretions and less often in the feces or during the normal exfoliation of the skin of the soles and palms of the extremities (12,373,844,851).

The original report of this parasite in nonhuman primates concerns its ability to cause cutaneous creeping eruption (CE) in the soles and palms of the extremities (1073). Since then there has been only one additional report of CE that involved primates in a zoological collection and in the primate colony of a contract research laboratory (477).

Grossly, these lesions had the appearance of white, serpentine tracks on the palms and/or soles of the hands and feet. These are caused by the adult parasites migrating through the epithelial and subepithelial dermal layers of the skin (477,851,1073). These tracts may contain seropurulent to purulent exudate in early stages of the infection (477).

Tissue reaction to the parasite involving the hands and feet can be severe and result in marked irritation (pruritus) of the soles and palms and concurrent regional lymphadenopathy (477). Vesicle–bulla–pustule formation within the dermis and epidermis and rupture of affected lymph nodes also have been reported (477).

All other reports concern the presence of this parasite in the stratified squamous epithelium of the external nares. Infection of the nares does not produce serious disease and is usually subclinical, but is considered to be common in susceptible animals. A mild serous nasal discharge may occasionally be seen clinically (477).

Histopathologically, the affected epithelium is diffusely hyperplastic and parakeratotic, and there is a mild inflammatory infiltrate composed of leukocytes and plasma cells in the underlying lamina propria (12,373,477,844,851,1023).

Diagnosis in the living animal can be made through the use of nasal, mucosal, or peripheral epidermal scrapings or swabs, which reveal the characteristic eggs. In the dead animal finding of the parasite in microscopic slides of the nasal mucosa or epidermis is considered to be diagnostic (12,373,851,1023).

Control procedures have not been reported (373).

This parasite has been reported in humans where it causes a type of creeping eruption. Even though infection in humans is considered to be uncommon, those personnel who work with and care for nonhuman primates should handle those species known to be infected or susceptible to infection with proper caution (354,373,851).

Treatment of the cutaneous creeping eruption with fenbendazole (Panacur) at 10–25 mg/kg per os once daily for 3–10 days, depending on the patient, is reported to initiate clinical remission of lesions in 10–14 days (477). Also, thiabendazole (Omnizole), at a dose rate of 100 mg/kg, repeated in 2 weeks, has been reported to be effective in reducing infection; however, it may not completely eliminate it (500,1114).

A new species, *Anatrichosoma ocularis,* has been reported from the eye of a tree shrew (*Tupaia glis*) (362).

B. Trematodes

The parasitic trematodes described from nonhuman primates are listed in Table VIII. The species most frequently mentioned in the literature are discussed below.

1. Trematodiasis

This disease in nonhuman primates can be caused by infection with a number of species of trematodes. Several of the more commonly encountered species are discussed in detail.

a. GASTRODISCOIDIASIS. *Gastrodiscoides hominis* is a small, orange-red fluke that attaches to the mucosa of the cecum and colon (373,449,504,1023) (Fig. 42). The parasite is distributed throughout the tropical orient and has been described in various *Macaca* species that range throughout this geographic area (354,373,449,479,504,535,754,907,929,990,1023,1168, 1121). It is the most common fluke of Old World monkeys.

The life cycle is indirect with a snail serving as the intermediate host (354,373,965).

Infection usually is asymptomatic when the parasites are present in small numbers. Heavy infections produce a mucoid diarrhea and mild chronic colitis.

TABLE VIII

PARASITIC TREMATODES DESCRIBED FROM NONHUMAN PRIMATES

Parasite Genus species	Location in host	Prosimians	New World monkeys	Old World monkeys	Great apes	Reference
Subclass Digenea, order Protostomata, family Brachylaimidae						
Brachylaima sp.	Intestine	X				67
Subclass Digenea, order Protostomata, family Plagiorchiidae						
Plagiorchis multiglandularis	Intestine			X		647
Subclass Digenea, order Protostomata, family Lecithodendriidae						
Novetrema nycticebi	Intestine	X				647
Odeningotrema apidion	Intestine	X				67, 265, 647
O. bivesicularis	Intestine	X				647, 961
Odeningotrema sp.	Intestine	X				67
Phaneropsolus bonnei	Intestine	X		X		647
P. lakdivensis	Intestine	X				192, 443, 647, 904
P. longipenis	Intestine	X			X	192, 647, 904
P. perodictici	Intestine	X				443
P. orbicularis	Intestine		X			192, 194, 373, 617, 647, 900, 904, 1087, 1184
P. oviforme	Intestine	X		X		192, 373, 647, 904
P. simiae	Intestine			X		647
P. aspinosus	Intestine			X		858
Primatotrema macacae	Intestine			X		192, 373, 647, 904
Pithecotrema kelloggi	Intestine			X		1078
Subclass Digenea, order Protostomata, family Dicrocoelidae						
Athesmia foxi	Bile ducts		X			44, 87, 192, 311, 353, 360, 373, 407, 438, 617, 647, 900, 967
A. heterolecithodes	Bile ducts		X			388, 647, 1081, 1087
Brodenia laciniata	Bile ducts, pancreas			X		192, 373, 647, 651, 652
B. serrata	Pancreas			X		192, 373, 647
Concinnum brumpti (syn. Eurytrema brumpti)	Bile duct, pancreas				X	192, 360, 373, 647, 906, 918, 1023, 1063, 1189
Controrchis biliophilus	Gallbladder, bile ducts		X			192, 617, 647
Dicrocoelium colobusicola	Bile ducts			X		192, 647
D. lanceatum	Bile ducts			X	X	192, 486, 647, 1189
D. macaci	Bile ducts			X	X	192, 360, 373, 471
Euparadistomum cercopitheci	Gallbladder			X		647
Euparadistomum sp.	Gallbladder	X				67
Eurytrema pancreaticum	Pancreatic ducts			X		647
E. satoi	Bile ducts, pancreas			X	X	192, 360, 373, 647
Leipertrema rewelli	Pancreas				X	192, 373, 647, 986
Leipertrema sp.	Small intestine	X				67, 508
Platynosomum amazonensis (syn. Conspicuum conspicuum)	Gallbladder, bile ducts		X			192, 194, 373, 617, 618, 647, 1081
P. marmoseti (syn. Conspicuum conspicuum)	Gallbladder, bile ducts		X			192, 194, 373, 617, 618, 647, 1081
P. fastosum	Gallblader, bile ducts		X			1081
P. minutum	Gallbladder, bile ducts		X			1081
Skrjabinus sp.	Gallbladder, bile ducts	X				67
Zonorchis goliath	Bile ducts		X			617, 647
Z. microcebi	Bile ducts		X			647
Zonorchis sp.	Gallbladder, bile ducts	X				67
Subclass Digenea, order Protostomata, family Fasciolidae						
Fasciola hepatica	Liver			X		68, 192, 373, 449, 479, 647
Fasciolopsis buski	Duodenum, stomach			X		192, 354, 373, 476, 647
Subclass Digenea, order Protostomata, family Opisthorchiidae						
Chonorchis sinensis	Bile ducts			X		647, 655
Opisthorchis felineus	Bile and pancreatic ducts			X		647

TABLE VIII—*Continued*

PARASITIC TREMATODES DESCRIBED FROM NONHUMAN PRIMATES

Parasite Genus species	Location in host	Prosimians	New World monkeys	Old World monkeys	Great apes	Reference
Subclass Digenea, order Protostomata, family Heterophyidae						
Haplorchis pumilio	Intestine			X		647
H. yokogawai	Intestine			X		192, 647
Metagonimus yokogawai	Intestine			X		192, 647
Pygidiopsis summa	Intestine			X		647
Subclass Digenea, order Protostomata, family Microphallidae						
Spelotrema brevicaeca	Intestine			X		647
Subclass Digenea, order Protostomata, family Echinostomatidae						
Artyfechinostomum sp.	Intestine			X		192, 373, 647
Echinostoma aphylactum	Small intestine		X			192, 617, 647, 1087
E. ilocanum	Intestine			X		72, 192, 354, 373, 647
Reptiliotrema primata	Intestine			X		192, 373, 647
Subclass Digenea, order Protostomata, family Notocotylidae						
Ogmocotyle ailuri	Small intestine			X		647
O. indica	Small intestine, stomach			X		68, 192, 373, 449, 647, 655, 1195
Subclass Digenea, order Protostomata, family Paragonimidae						
Paragonimus westermani	Lungs, pleural cavity, diaphragm, body cavity, brain			X		192, 354, 371, 373, 479, 800, 967, 987, 1044
P. africanus	Lungs			X		970
Subclass Digenea, order Protostomata, family Achillurbainiidae						
Achillurbania sp.	Parotid gld.	X				67, 856
Subclass Digenea, order Protostomata, family Trogletrematidae						
Beaveria sp.	Intestine/liver	X				67
Subclass Digenea, order Protostomata, family Schistosomatidae						
Schistosoma bovis	Mesenteric and abdominal veins			X		647
S. haematobium	Mesenteric, visceral, and abdominal veins			X	X	192, 226, 298, 354, 373, 647, 821, 823, 910
S. japonicum	Mesenteric and portal veins			X	X	192, 533, 647
S. mansoni	Mesenteric and abdominal veins		X	X	X	163, 192, 298, 354, 356, 360, 373, 397, 447, 486, 534, 576, 647, 651, 652, 663, 672, 765, 774, 910, 935, 1057, 1071
S. mattheei	Mesenteric and abdominal veins			X		73, 354, 647, 763, 804, 1058
Schistosoma sp.	Mesenteric and abdominal veins	X		X	X	59, 647
Subclass Digenea, order Protostomata, family Diplostomidae						
Diplostomid mesocercariae	Visceral and pulmonary cysts		X	X		647
Neodiplostomum tamarini	Intestine			X		192, 194, 251, 373, 617, 647
Subclass Digenea, order Protostomata, family Paramphistomatidae						
Chiorchis noci	Intestine			X		192, 373, 647
Gastrodiscoides hominis	Cecum, colon			X		192, 354, 373, 449, 479, 504, 535, 647, 859, 863, 871, 907, 929, 990, 1023, 1169
Watsonius deschiensi	Intestine			X		192, 354, 373, 647, 804, 967, 1023
W. watsoni	Intestine			X		192, 354, 360, 373, 449, 479, 647, 804, 967, 1023
W. macaci	Intestine			X		192, 354, 373, 479, 647, 1023

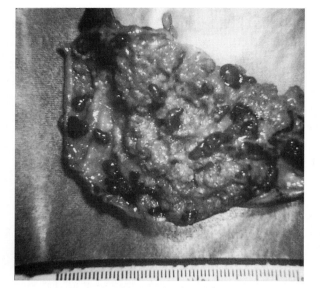

Fig. 42. Gross photograph of numerous trematode parasites. *Gastrodiscoides hominis,* attached to colonic mucosa of rhesus monkey (*Macaca mulatta*).

Attachment of the flukes to the intestinal mucosa results in focal lesions characterized by hyperemia, loss of surface epithelium, and necrosis. Neutrophilic infiltrates may be associated with these lesions. The submucosa may be sclerotic because of proliferation of fibrous connective tissue and a lymphoplasmacytic cell infiltrate (354,373,383,504,535,1023).

Diagnosis can be made by identifying the characteristic eggs in the feces or by finding the typical adult flukes in the lumen of the cecum or colon at necropsy (373,1023).

Because natural transmission cannot occur in the laboratory, no special control measures are necessary. No treatment has been reported (373).

This parasite has been reported to cause a mild diarrhea in humans, but because of the obligatory snail intermediate host in the life cycle, infected captive monkeys are not a direct health hazard for humans (354,373).

b. WATSONIASIS. *Watsonius watsoni, W. deschieni,* and *W. macaci* have been reported to inhabit the intestinal tract of several Old World primate species (guenons, baboons, and cynomolgus monkeys) (354, 360, 373, 449, 479, 804, 967). Adult trematodes of this genus are translucent, orange, and pear shaped. The complete life cycle is not known, but probably involves a snail intermediate host and is thought to be similar to that of *Fasciola hepatica* (354,373,967).

Watsonius watsoni and *W. deschieni* have been reported to be associated with diarrhea, severe enteritis, and death in monkeys (373,449,967). Little else is known about the anatomic effects of these species (373).

Diagnosis can be made from the characteristic eggs in the feces or adults in the intestine at necropsy (373).

The control and public health considerations for these flukes are the same as described for *G. hominis.* No treatment has been reported for these parasites.

c. PARAGONIMIASIS. This disease, caused by the oriental lung fluke, *Paragonimus westermanii,* has been reported in the cynomolgus monkey (*Macaca fascicularis*). Infection in this animal is directly associated with the ingestion of infected raw crabs or crayfish as part of its dietary regimen (354,371,373, 479,800,967,987,1044).

Adult flukes have a brown, plump, ovoid body with scale-like spines. The eggs are oval shaped, golden brown in color, and have a partly flattened operculum at one end.

The life cycle is indirect with snails and crabs or crayfish serving as intermediate hosts (354,373,1023).

Adult flukes are found primarily in the lung but sometimes occur in ectopic sites such as the brain, liver, and other organs.

Clinical signs reported in infected animals include coughing, wheezing, bloody or rusty tinged sputum, moist rales, and progressive emaciation (373,1023).

At necropsy, lesions consist of focal areas of emphysema and soft, dark red-to-brown cysts that measure 2–3 cm in diameter, and are randomly located throughout the pulmonary parenchyma. These cysts may be elevated above the lung surface and pleural adhesions can sometimes be present. Two or more flukes occupy each cyst (373,647,1023).

Histopathologically, the presence of the flukes provokes a leukocytic infiltration and there is usually a mature fibrous capsule around the parasites which in turn are surrounded by a purulent exudate containing blood and groups of typically appearing fluke eggs. Hemorrhage into the cyst often occurs, which may lead to hemoptysis. Additional lesions described include hyperplasia of bronchial epithelium and submucosal glands and focal areas of inflammation in the lung parenchyma associated with groups of fluke eggs (373,647,1023).

The diagnosis depends on the demonstration and identification of the typical eggs in the feces or the adult flukes in the pulmonary tissue at necropsy (373,506,1023).

Paragonimus westermanii can affect humans; however, because of the obligatory molluscan and crustacean intermediate hosts in the life cycle, infected captive nonhuman primates are not a direct health hazard for humans (373,647), and no special control procedures are required (373).

Treatment for this parasite in nonhuman primates has not been reported.

d. SCHISTOSOMIASIS. Several species of schistosomatid flukes have been reported to infect nonhuman primates naturally. These include *Schistosoma mansoni* in New World monkeys (squirrel monkeys) (647, 1071), Old World monkeys (mangabeys, patas monkeys, guenons, and baboons) (163,298, 354,356,360,373,647,652,663,774,910,1023,1057), and the great apes (chimpanzees) (486,534,647,935,1023); *S. haematobium* in Old World monkeys (mangabeys, guenons, and baboons) (298,354,373,647,821,823,910,1023) and the great apes (chimpanzees) (226, 373, 647); and *S. mattheei* in Old World monkeys (baboons) (73, 354, 647, 763, 804, 1023, 1058).

Although schistosomatids are considered to be extremely serious pathogens for humans, they are of little consequence in captive nonhuman primates and are usually found incidentally at necropsy (373, 652).

In the schistosomatids, both male and female forms are present and differ in appearance. They are usually found together in constant copulation with the long, slender female in the sex canal of the short, muscular male.

The egg of *S. mansoni* is elongated ovoid in shape, rounded at both ends, and bears a lateral spine. The egg of *S. haematobium* is also elongated ovoid in shape, rounded at the anterior end, and bears a posterior terminal spine.

Adult *S. mansoni* and *S. mattheei* inhabit the mesenteric veins, whereas *S. haematobium* adults are found in the pelvic or portal veins of susceptible hosts (373, 1023).

The life cycle is indirect with snails serving as intermediate hosts (373, 1023).

The reported clinical signs include pyrexia, hemorrhagic diarrhea or hematuria, and ascites (354, 373, 1023).

The principal pathologic effects are caused by the presence of eggs in the tissues (354, 373, 571, 647). The eggs may be found almost anywhere in the abdominal or pleural cavities. The most frequently encountered lesion is thickening of the intestinal or urinary bladder walls due to chronic inflammation. Microgranulomas surrounding typical schistosome eggs are also very common in the liver (Fig. 43), brain, spleen, wall of the gastrointestinal tract and urinary bladder, and other organs. Continued insult can lead to stenosis of portions of the gastrointestinal tract, urinary bladder and other parts of the urogenital system, and cirrhosis of the liver (227, 354, 373, 571, 647, 910).

Diagnosis is made based on the finding and identification of the characteristic eggs in the feces or urine, the presence of adult schistosomes in the blood vessels at necropsy, or the finding of the typical lesions during histopathological examination of appropriate tissues (373, 647, 1023).

Natural transmission cannot occur in the laboratory; therefore, no special control measures are required (373).

Infected captive nonhuman primates are not of direct public health significance to humans because of the requirement for an obligatory molluscan intermediate host. However, because schistosomiasis is such an important and serious disease in humans, excreta from nonhuman primates should be decontaminated before disposal (373).

Treatment with 56.8 mg/ml praziquantel (Droncit), at an empirical dose of 0.2 cm³ for primates less than 1 kg and 0.1 cm³/kg for primates greater than 2 kg, is said to be effective (213).

e. ATHESMIASIS. The cause of this disease, a trematode parasite cited in the primate literature as *Athesmia foxi,* is considered to be a moderately pathogenic fluke that inhabits the bile ducts of susceptible nonhuman primate species. Some parasitologists feel that the proper terminology for this parasite is

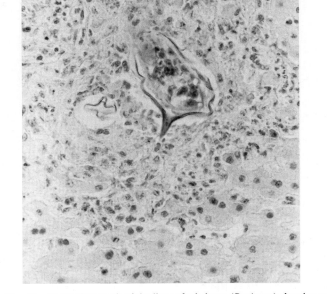

Fig. 43. Photomicrograph of the liver of a baboon (*Papio* sp.) showing an egg of the trematode parasite *Schistosoma mansoni* and associated microgranuloma. The lateral spine is clearly evident. HE stain.

Athesmia heterolecithoides. They feel that because this is a species that is very variable in its characteristics and shows a high range of intraspecific variation, this name is the only valid name for the genus (388, 1081, 1087). Regardless of what it is called, it is a common finding in nonhuman primates obtained from South America and has been reported in a variety of New World monkeys (cebus monkeys, squirrel monkeys, tamarins, and titi monkeys) (87, 192, 311, 353, 360, 373, 407, 438, 617, 900, 967, 1059).

The adult flukes are long and slender and measure 8.5 by 0.7 mm. Eggs are ovoid and golden brown in color; they have a thick shell and are operculated (373, 1023, 1059).

The life cycle is indirect with a mollusk serving as a required intermediate host. However, because the method of infection of the vertebrate host is unknown, our knowledge about the life cycle of this particular fluke is incomplete (373, 1023).

Infections in nonhuman primates are usually asymptomatic and most often considered an incidental finding. Aside from causing a moderate to marked distension of affected ducts, these parasites cause very little damage or invoke much of a host inflammatory response (Figs. 44 and 45). Heavy infections can result in hyperplasia of the biliary epithelium and fibroplasia around eggs and the ducts. Extremely severe infections can re-

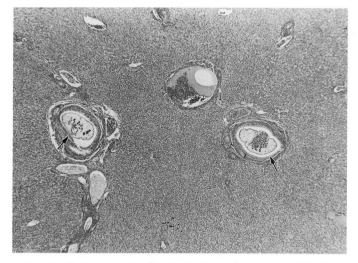

Fig. 44. Photomicrograph of the liver of a squirrel monkey (*Saimiri sciureus*) showing cross sections of the trematode parasite *Athesmia heterolecithoides* (syn. *foxi*) within bile duct lumens (arrows). Note the paucity of host response. HE stain.

and identification of the characteristic eggs in the feces (373, 1023).

Transmission in the laboratory cannot occur because of the obligate need for an intermediate host; therefore, no special control measures are required (373).

Nonhuman primates infected with *A. heterolecithoides* (*foxi*) do not pose any public health problems for humans. This parasite has not been reported in humans. Infected nonhuman primates are not a direct hazard to humans because of the need of a required molluscan intermediate host to complete the life cycle (360,373).

No treatment has been reported for this parasite (2,373).

f. OTHER TREMATODES.   Many other trematodes have been described from primates. Most incite little host response (Fig. 46) and there is little in the way of clinical manifestations, unless overwhelming infections are present.

C. Cestodes

1. Cestodiasis

This condition results from infection by one of any number of numerous tapeworm genera that have been described in the intestinal tract of nonhuman primates, including prosimians, New and Old World monkeys, and great apes (198,261,263, 293,360,373,479,483,617,651,652,763,803,855,898,929,997, 1001,1060,1061,1071,1077,1114,1173,1185).

Cestode genera and the primate group they parasitize are listed in Table IX.

sult in pronounced thickening of the bile ducts with resultant pressure and trauma to adjacent hepatic parenchyma, leading to fatty degeneration of affected hepatocytes (87, 311, 373, 407, 617,644,967,1023,1059).

Diagnosis depends on the demonstration and identification of the adult flukes in the bile duct either at necropsy or on histopathological examination of liver sections or by demonstration

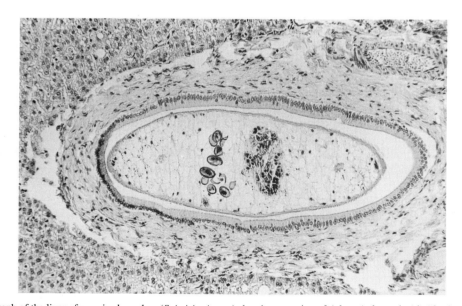

Fig. 45. Photomicrograph of the liver of a squirrel monkey (*Saimiri sciureus*) showing a section of *Athesmia heterolecithoides* (syn. *foxi*) within the lumen of a bile duct. Again, note the absence of inflammatory response. The eggs contained within the worm are evident. HE stain.

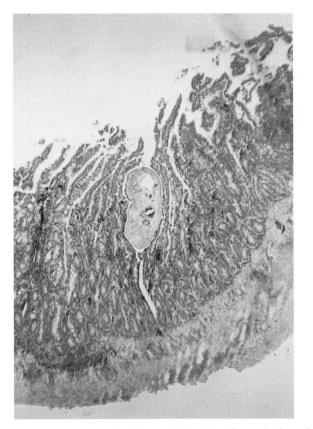

Fig. 46. Photomicrograph of the small intestine of a squirrel monkey (*Saimiri sciureus*) with the small trematode, *Phaneropsolus* sp., lying deep in mucosal folds of the epithelium.

Life cycles for all the genera listed, except one, are indirect and require an arthropod intermediate host for completion of the cycle. *Hymenolepis nana* can complete its life cycle through either direct or indirect means (373,617).

Although these parasites may be present in large numbers, clinical disease or enteric lesions are seldom associated with tapeworm infection (Fig. 47). *Hymenolepis* can cause a catarrhal enteritis with abscessation of the mesenteric lymph nodes.

The principal clinical signs reported in affected nonhuman primates are diarrhea and abdominal pain, evidenced in the patient by crouching and tucking of the abdomen (934).

Diagnosis depends on the identification of characteristic eggs in the feces, passing of proglottids of adult worms, or the recovery of adult worms at necropsy (373).

Control of *H. nana* is difficult because infection with this tapeworm can be transmitted in many ways (373). Strict sanitation practices and effective rodent and insect control are necessary to prevent spread or establishment of this infection within a nonhuman primate colony (373,464). All newly arrived nonhuman primates should be examined during the quar-

antine period and, if infected, either treated or eliminated. All caging should be cleaned and sterilized frequently and contamination of food and water prevented (373). Other tapeworm species can best be controlled through elimination of the intermediate insect vectors (373).

Some tapeworm genera (*Hymenolepis, Raillietina, Bertiella*) rarely affect humans. Proper precautions in handling captive nonhuman primates, good personal hygiene by the caretakers, and care in disposing of bedding and feces of infected animals should be stressed in order to rule out accidental transfer of infection to humans (373).

Drugs reported to be effective in the treatment of cestodes in nonhuman primates are niclosamide (Yomesan) at a dosage of 100 mg/kg orally as a single dose (1072); bunamidine (Scolaban) at a dosage of 25–100 mg/kg orally as a single dose (1072); and praziquantel (Droncit) at a dosage level of 1.25 mg praziquantel per animal mixed in food (tree shrews) (93) or injected intramuscularly at a dose rate of 0.1 ml/kg body weight in other nonhuman primates (1159).

2. Larval Cestodiasis

Nonhuman primates may serve as intermediate hosts for several species of tapeworm parasites and thus develop various larval forms of these parasites in their somatic tissues. The larval cestode species and the primate group they parasitize are listed in Table IX.

Cestode larvae are classified as solid and bladder forms. Solid larvae are represented by the sparganum. Bladder larvae consist of cysticercus, coenurus, hydatid, and tetrathyridium. Each will be discussed in detail below.

a. SPARGANOSIS. This term denotes infection with the elongate, nonspecific plerocercoid larvae of cestodes in the order Pseudophylloidea (617,1023). The adult tapeworms belong to genera *Diphyllobothrium* and *Spirometra*, which are intestinal parasites of various carnivores, birds, and reptiles (803).

Spargana have been described in New World monkeys (squirrel monkeys and marmosets) (194,263,268,373,401,617, 803), Old World monkeys (rhesus monkeys, cynomolgus monkeys, vervets, baboons, and talapoin monkeys (373,660,792, 804,805), and prosimians (tree shrew) (997).

These larvae are solid with a scolex that contains a pseudosucker. Larvae are white, ribbon-like, and of variable size and motility. They resemble the adult except they lack proglottids and mature genitalia. Spargana can vary from a few millimeters to several centimeters in length (803,1023,1094).

In nonhuman primates spargana may be found in any part of the body: retroperitoneal tissues, in abdominal or pleural cavities, or in subcutaneous (Fig. 48) and muscular tissues. They are commonly encased by a connective tissue capsule and they do not incite much of an inflammatory response unless they die. These degenerating larvae may cause local inflammation and edema. Most infections in nonhuman primates are usually

TABLE IX
PARASITIC CESTODES DESCRIBED FROM NONHUMAN PRIMATES

Parasite Genus species	Location in host	Prosimians	New World monkeys	Old World monkeys	Great apes	Reference
Subclass Cestoda, order Cyclophyllidea, family Anoplocephalida						
Bertiella studeri	Small intestine			X	X	52, 68, 199, 354, 373, 432, 447, 448, 479, 617, 637, 650–652, 659, 763, 803, 879, 929, 1023, 1060, 1077, 1114, 1173, 1189
B. mucronata	Small intestine		X		X	52, 198, 263, 360, 373, 803, 893, 900
B. fallax	Small intestine		X			263, 360, 373, 803
B. satyri	Small intestine		X	X		152
B. okabei	Small intestine			X		991
Bertiella sp.	Small intestine			X	X	198, 642, 656, 754, 811, 855, 860, 990
Anaplocephala sp.	Small intestine				X	803, 979
Parabertiella sp.	Small intestine			X		4, 859, 860, 863
Moniezia rugosa	Small intestine		X			263, 360, 373, 617, 803
Thysanotaenia sp.	Small intestine	X				803, 1185
Tupaiataenia guentini	Small intestine	X				93, 997
Intermicapsifer sp.	Small intestine			X		709, 803
Atriotaenia megastoma	Small intestine	X	X			194, 224, 263, 373, 407, 528, 617, 803, 819
Matheovataenia brasiliensis	Small intestine		X			638
M. cruzsilvai	Small intestine			X		769
Matheovataenia sp.	Small intestine		X			42, 617, 803
Paratriotaenia oedipomidatus	Small intestine		X			268, 373, 617, 803, 900, 1061
Subclass Cestoda, order Cyclophyllidea, family Davaineidae						
Raillietina alouattae	Small intestine		X			263, 373, 803, 967
R. demerariensis	Small intestine		X			52, 263, 373, 647, 1087
R. rothlisbergeri	Small intestine	X				31
Raillietina sp.	Small intestine	X	X			224, 373, 617, 803, 819
Subclass Cestoda, order Cyclophyllidea, family Dilepididae						
Dilepis sp.	Small intestine			X		803
Choanotaenia infundibulum	Small intestine			X		568
Subclass Cestoda, order Cyclophyllidea, family Hymenolepidae						
Hymenolepis nana	Small intestine		X	X	X	60, 354, 373, 463, 617, 771, 803, 967, 990, 1023, 1042, 1138
H. diminuta	Small intestine	X		X		354, 357, 373, 463, 617, 803, 967, 990, 997, 1023, 1138

asymptomatic and their presence is considered to be an incidental finding at necropsy (Fig. 49) (803,1023).

Diagnosis can be made in the live animal by radiography, which may reveal calcified nodules. Also, one may palpate mobile nodules in the subcutaneous tissue in association with localized edema. In the dead animal diagnosis is made through demonstration and identification of the characteristic spargana larvae either grossly at necropsy or microscopically in histopathologic specimens (803,1023).

b. CYSTICERCOSIS. This condition is the result of infection with the larval form of various members of the family Taeniidae. Adult tapeworms of this family commonly parasitize birds and mammals (617,803).

Cysticerci have been described in New World monkeys (squirrel monkeys and marmosets) (617), Old World monkeys (rhesus monkeys, baboons, mangabeys, patas monkeys, langurs, and vervets) (360,373,449,803,804,967,1122,1134), great apes (gibbons and chimpanzees) (803,970,1189), and prosimians (lemur) (119,511,803).

Cysticerci are oval, translucent cysts (Fig. 50) that contain a single invaginated scolex with four suckers. In those species that have them, a circle of hooks is present (617,803,1094).

These cysts may be found in the abdominal or thoracic cavities, muscle, subcutaneous tissue (Fig. 51), and central nervous system. Usually there is very little host inflammatory reaction to the presence of viable cysts. As the cysts enlarge, there may be compression of adjacent tissues. Dead cysts will provoke an intense, chronic inflammatory reaction (617,803,1122).

TABLE IX—*Continued*

PARASITIC CESTODES DESCRIBED FROM NONHUMAN PRIMATES

Parasite Genus species	Location in host	Prosimians	New World monkeys	Old World monkeys	Great apes	Reference
H. cebidarum	Small intestine		X			263, 373, 819
Hymenolepis sp.	Small intestine	X			X	89, 514, 754, 990, 1189
Vampirolepis sp.	Small intestine		X			617, 803
Subclass Cestoda, order Cyclophyllidea, family Mesocestoididae						
Mesocestoides sp. (*Tetrathyridium*)	Larva: peritoneal cavity			X	X	321, 369, 373, 449, 537, 803, 804, 929, 932, 977, 1177
Subclass Cestoda, order Cyclophyllidea, family Cyclophyllidae						
Taenia crocutae (*Cysticercus*)	Larva: skeletal muscle			X		763
T. hydatigena (*Cysticercus tenuicollis*)	Larva: liver, peritoneal cavity			X		52, 68, 360, 373, 449, 653, 671, 672, 803, 804, 1044, 1064
T. solium (*Cysticercus cellulosae*)	Larva: brain, heart, muscle, subcutis			X	X	52, 360, 373, 672, 803, 804, 967, 971, 1122, 1134
Multiceps (*Taenia*) *serialis* (*Coenurus serialis*)	Larva: subcutis, skeletal muscle			X		52, 297, 373, 447, 451, 586, 721, 967
M. multiceps (*Coenurus cerebralis*)	Larva: thorax			X		1005
M. brauni (*Coenurus*)	Larva: subcutis, pleural and abdominal cavities, brain			X		52, 324, 373
Coenurus sp.	Retrobulbar				X	677
Echinococcus granulosus (Hydatid cyst)	Larva: liver, lungs, peritoneal cavity, intraocular	X	X	X	X	11, 52, 66, 82, 201, 235, 295, 354, 373, 403, 437, 485, 529, 530, 548, 617, 666, 809, 810, 838, 864, 865, 902, 1011, 1044, 1067, 1083
Cysticercus	Larva: liver, lungs, peritoneal cavity	X				59
Subclass Cestoda, order Pseudophylloidea, family Diphyllobothriidae						
Diphyllobothrium erinacei (Sparganum)	Larva: subcutis, muscle		X	X		52, 194, 263, 360, 373, 674, 804, 967, 1044
Spirometra (= *Lueheelia*) *reptans* (Sparganum)	Larva: subcutis		X			263, 268, 373
Spirometra (= *Lueheelia*) sp. (Sparganum)	Larva: abdominal cavity, subcutis, muscle	X		X		89, 373, 660, 763, 792, 805, 997, 1177
Sparganum sp.	Larva: abdominal cavity, subcutis, muscle		X	X		401, 448

Symptoms in nonhuman primates are directly related to the tissue in which the cysticercus develops and the number present (803). Involvement of the central nervous system can produce neurological disorders, but this appears to be less of a problem in infected nonhuman primates than in cerebral cysticercosis in the human patient (803,1122,1134).

Diagnosis depends on the finding of the characteristic bladder-shaped structure in the tissues. Identification of the specific species involved is based on the characteristic hook size and structure (803).

c. COENUROSIS. This condition is the result of infection with the larval form of the tapeworms *Multiceps multiceps* or *M. serialis,* which are intestinal cestodes of dogs and related carnivores (373,617).

Coenurosis has been reported in Old World monkeys (macaques, vervets, gelada baboon, and baboons) (172, 297, 324, 373, 451, 654, 666, 803, 917, 960, 967, 983, 1111) and prosimians (lemur) (803).

The coenurus is a polycephalid larval form that produces both internal and external daughter cysts. The inner layer of the cyst wall is composed of germinal epithelium from which numerous scolices develop (373, 803, 1094).

Coenuri have been described in the subcutaneous tissues, peritoneal cavity, liver, brain, and other organs of affected nonhuman primates (373, 617, 803, 983).

Clinical signs and histopathology depend on the number of coenuri present and their location. In general, infection in nonhuman primates has produced minimal symptoms and lesions (297, 666, 803, 917, 960, 1111). However, in those cases where

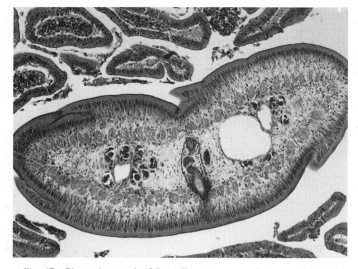

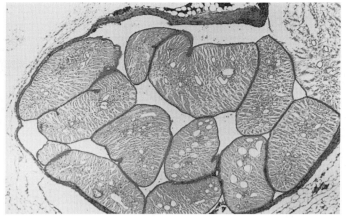

Fig. 49. Photomicrograph of a sparganum. An incidental finding in the axillary connective tissue of a cynomolgus monkey (*Macaca fascicularis*) is shown. Note capsule and the lack of host response. HE stain.

Fig. 47. Photomicrograph of *Bertiella* sp. tapeworm in lumen of small intestine of cebus monkey (*Cebus* sp.). No tissue destruction or host response is seen. HE stain. (Reprinted from Toft, II, J. D. (1982) *Veterinary Pathology.* With permission.)

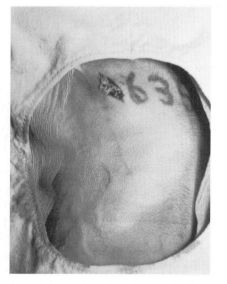

Fig. 48. Gross photograph of a sparganum emerging from a surgical incision in the chest wall of a marmoset (*Saguinus* sp.).

found in the intestinal tract of dogs, wolves, bush dogs, other members of the canine family, and related carnivores (373,617, 803).

Hydatid cysts caused by *E. granulosus* have been described from a number of Old World monkeys (guenons, colobus monkey, mangabeys, mandrills, rhesus monkeys, other macaques, Celebes ape, and baboons) (11,82,201,235,258,295,373,485, 529, 548, 666, 803, 809, 810, 864, 865, 902, 1067, 1083), New World monkeys (marmoset) (617), great apes (chimpanzee, gorilla, and orangutan) (66,403,838), and prosimians (galago and lemurs) (373, 864, 1011). In addition, hydatid cysts from the tapeworm *E. vogeli* have been reported from a group of young great apes (gorillas, orangutans, and chimpanzees) (530).

Hydatid cysts are large, unilocular cysts. The inner layer of the cyst wall is composed of germinal epithelium from which

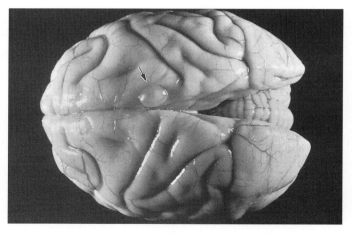

Fig. 50. Gross photograph of a brain from a rhesus monkey (*Macaca mulatta*) showing a solitary *Taenia solium* cysticercus (arrow) involving the cerebrum. (Courtesy of Dr. Marion Valario.)

there is involvement of the central nervous system, typical neurological symptoms are observed (803,1111).

Diagnosis can be made by radiography or the finding of a tumor-like mass in the subcutaneous tissues. Identification of the species of cestode is based on the hook structure of the scolex (373,803).

d. HYDATIDOSIS. This disease, also known as echinococcosis, is the result of infection by the larval stage of cestode parasites in the genus *Echinococcus*. Adult tapeworms are

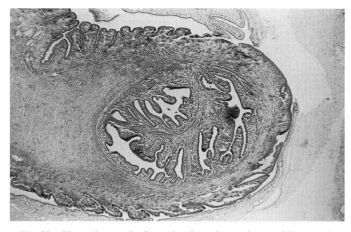

Fig. 51. Photomicrograph of a section through a cysticerus of *Taenia solium* in the subcutaneous tissue of a rhesus monkey (*Macaca mulatta*). This section is through the highly coiled neck region, although the scolex and hooklets are not evident at this level. HE stain.

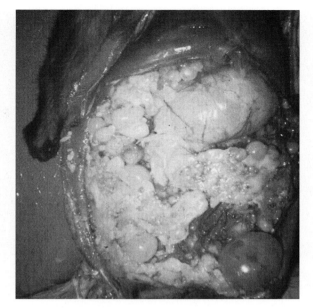

Fig. 52. Gross photograph of the abdominal cavity of a male rhesus monkey (*Macaca mulatta*). Normal abdominal architecture has been replaced by a mass of varying sized cysts of *Echinococcus granulosus* (hydatid disease). (Courtesy of Dr. Marion Valario.)

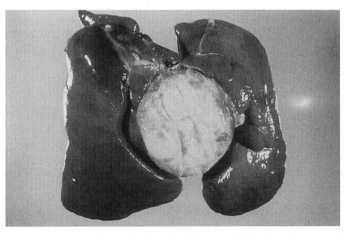

Fig. 53. Gross photograph of a sterile hydatid cyst in the thoracic cavity of a rhesus monkey (*Macaca mulatta*).

numerous brood capsules develop. Multiple scolices then develop from the wall of the brood capsule. The cyst wall of *E. granulosa* is characteristically laminated and composed of a thick hyaline material (373,617,1023,1094).

Hydatid cysts may be located in the abdominal or thoracic cavity, liver, lungs, retrobulbar area, subcutis, or throughout the body (201, 235, 258, 373, 548, 617, 803, 810, 902, 1023, 1083) (Figs. 52 and 53).

The size of the cyst and the amount of involvement and host reaction depend on its age and the location within the host. Abdominal distention, exophthalmia, or localized subcutaneous swellings are sometimes seen, but usually the presence of cysts causes no clinical signs or ill effects and is found incidently at necropsy (201,373,485,672,803,1023,1067).

The gross appearance of the cyst is that of a variably sized, spherical mass, usually in the liver, but may sometimes be embedded in the lungs, subcutis, retrobulbar area, or be free in the abdominal cavity. Rupture of pulmonary hydatid cysts and resulting anaphylactic shock have been suggested as the cause of death in several cases of echinococcosis in nonhuman primates (11,803,922). Free scolices from ruptured cysts can implant in other tissues and produce additional cysts (803).

The diagnosis of hydatidosis is usually not made until after the cyst reaches considerable size. Symptoms may mimic a neoplasm. Radiographs can be helpful in detecting the presence of pulmonary or calcified hepatic cysts. However, pulmonary changes can be mistaken for tuberculosis or neoplasia. Serological tests such as the Casoni intradermal skin test or tanned cell hemagglutination test are of value in the diagnosis of hydatid disease in nonhuman primates. Abdominal ultrasonic scanning has been used successfully in diagnosing echinococcosis in gorillas (838).

Specific identification is based on the finding of detached scolices, or daughter cysts, in the cyst fluid. The hook is consid-

ered characteristic for the genus. If scolices are not present, the histomorphology of the cyst wall can be used as identifying criteria (201,373,575,803,1023).

e. TETRATHYRIDIOSIS. This condition results from infection with the larval stage of cestode parasites in the genus *Mesocestoides*. The adult tapeworms of this genus parasitize various birds and mammals (373,803,1023). This larval cestode has been described in Old World monkeys (rhesus monkeys, guenons, cynomolgus monkeys, and baboons) (321,373,449,

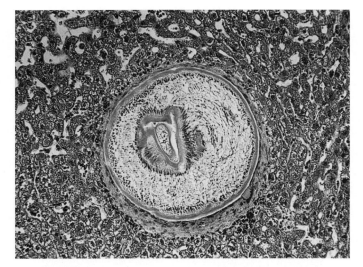

Fig. 54. Photomicrograph of a tetrathyridia in the liver of a squirrel monkey (*Saimiri sciureus*). The solid body with invaginated protoscolex of this cysticercoid type larval cestode is typical of tetrathyridia. HE stain.

Diagnosis depends on demonstration and identification of the characteristic larval form in the body cavities or encysted in the host tissues (373,803,1023).

Larval cestodes in nonhuman primates are of little public health importance to humans because infection can occur only by ingestion of the larval form. Of more importance to both humans and captive nonhuman primates is the possible ingestion of eggs passed by the infected definitive host. For this reason, feces from domestic and feral canids should be handled and disposed of with extreme care. Control of these parasites can only be accomplished through programs aimed at eliminating them from the definitive host (373).

No effective therapeutic agent for the treatment of larval cestodes has been reported. Small cysts and spargana can be removed surgically if they are diagnosed in time. If surgery is attempted, care must be taken so as not to result in seeding of the host through rupture of the original cysts. Usually, however, these cysts are of such a size when diagnosed that surgical removal is impossible and impractical.

803,804,929,932) and great apes (gibbon) (977), but its occurrence in nonhuman primates is considered to be uncommon, or even rare (373).

The tetrathyridial larva is flat and has an extremely contractile body. They may be confused with spargana. The anterior end is knot-like and contains an invaginated holdfast apparatus with four suckers but no rostellum. Length can vary from 2 to 70 mm, depending on the species of cestode and species of host. The tetrathyridium is proglottid shaped in the monkey (373, 449,803,1023).

These larvae usually are found free in the serous cavities of the body or are found encysted in various tissues (Fig. 54). Tetrathyridium evokes little host response and are usually considered to be an incidental finding in nonhuman primates (321, 373,449,803,1023).

D. Acanthocephalans

The parasitic acanthocephalans (common name thornyheaded worms) described in the alimentary tract of nonhuman primates are listed in Table X. Those species most frequently encountered in nonhuman primates are discussed below.

1. Acanthocephaliasis

This disease in nonhuman primates is most frequently the result of infection with acanthocephalan parasites in the genus *Prosthenorchis.*

These parasites are distributed throughout Central and South America and have been reported in a variety of New World monkeys. Prosimians, Old World primates, and great apes can become infected under laboratory or captive conditions (154, 263,373,967,996). The species involved are *P. elegans,* which

TABLE X

PARASITIC ACANTHOCEPHALANS DESCRIBED FROM NONHUMAN PRIMATES

Parasite Genus species	Location in host	Prosimians	New World monkeys	Old World monkeys	Great apes	Reference
Phylum Acanthocephala						
Moniliformis moniliformis	Small intestine				X	48, 373, 617, 967, 996, 1023, 1174, 1189
Prosthenorchis elegans	Ileum, cecum, colon		X			36, 54, 154, 224, 225, 263, 282, 373, 407, 528, 617, 729, 819, 900, 938, 967, 996, 1023, 1074, 1081, 1082, 1087, 1182
P. spirula	Ileum, cecum, colon	X	X			115, 154, 263, 373, 819, 900, 967, 996, 1023, 1087

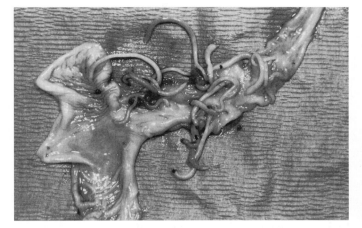

Fig. 55. Gross photograph of the ileocecal junction from a moustached marmoset (*Saguinus mystax mystax*). Numerous thorny-headed worms (*Prosthenorchis elegans*) attached to the intestinal mucosa are shown.

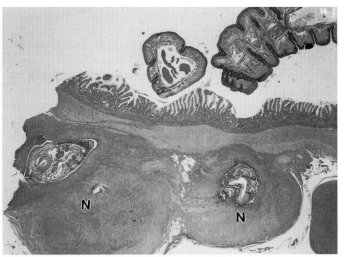

Fig. 56. Photomicrograph of many *Prosthenorchis elegans* embedded in mucosa of terminal ileum of squirrel monkey (*Saimiri sciureus*). Inflammatory nodules (N) on the serosal surface contain embedded proboscis of worm, nodules can be seen grossly. HE stain. (Reprinted from Toft, II, J. D. (1982). *Veterinary Pathology.* With permission.)

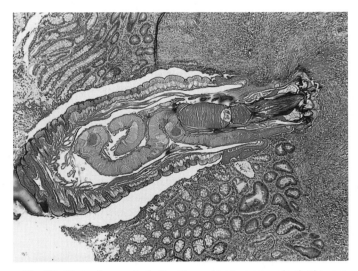

Fig. 57. Photomicrograph of a *Prosthenorchis elegans* parasite that has penetrated through the mucosal surface and embedded proboscis into submucosa, invoking a severe granulomatous inflammatory response. HE stain. (Reprinted from Toft, II, J. D. (1982). *Veterinary Pathology.* With permission.)

inhabits the cecum or colon, and *P. spirula,* which favors the terminal ileum (Fig. 55) (154,224,263,268,373,407,453,617, 729,770,819,878,938,940,967,996,1023,1062,1074,1118).

The life cycle is indirect, with cockroaches and beetles acting as the intermediate hosts (301,373,449,617,827,996,1023).

No distinctive symptoms accompany infection with acanthocephalans. Suspected cases must be confirmed by diagnostic methods. Clinical signs vary, depending on the severity of the infection. Diarrhea, anorexia, debilitation, abdominal distention, dehydration, and death all have been associated with acanthocephaliasis in New World monkeys. In cases of massive infection, there is often cachexia caused by secondary complications, and perhaps pain, sometimes of sudden onset; death follows rapidly. Squirrel monkeys have been observed eating large amounts of feed followed by diarrhea and steady weight loss. This syndrome was considered to be the result of hyperperistalsis and malabsorption. Most often the parasite does not contribute directly to the death of the animal, but rather produces lesions that allow secondary pathogens to become established, resulting in debilitation and the ultimate demise of the host (2,154,224,373,617,787,936,996,1023,1074).

Attachment of the proboscis of these parasites to the intestinal mucosa causes a pronounced, usually severe, granulomatous inflammatory response, and the nodules formed usually can be seen from the serosal surface (Fig. 56). The proboscis often penetrates the mucosa and invades the muscular layers of the intestinal wall. If complete penetration of the intestinal wall occurs, a fatal peritonitis results. Adult parasites sometimes are found in the abdominal cavity. Severe infections can cause mechanical blockage of the intestinal tract, intussusception, or rectal prolapse. Under these circumstances, infected animals will be depressed and pass bright red blood and scanty feces (2,224, 225,263,373,407,617,770,819,938,966,1023,1074).

Histologically, a chronic, active inflammatory response is seen, with ulcers of the mucosa and granuloma and abscess formation in the intestinal wall associated with penetration of the proboscis and the resulting destruction of existing tissues (Fig. 57). A focal suppurative to fibrinopurulent serositis also may be present in areas where the parasites approach penetration or actually rupture the intestinal wall (115,373,617,996, 1023). A hepatic abscess and granulomatous myositis (diaphragm) associated with migration of an unidentified acanthocephalan have been reported from an adult bushbaby (*Galago crassicaudatus*) (110).

Diagnosis depends on a combination of clinical signs, identification of the characteristic thick-walled eggs, or, more rarely, the worm itself in the feces. Conventional fecal flotation methods are ineffective as a means of demonstrating the eggs of these worms; fecal smears or formalin–ether sedimentation techniques must be used. Infection with these parasites is often detected at necropsy, when few to many typical "thorny-headed worms" are found attached to the intestinal mucosa (2,224,373, 617,996,1023).

The diagnostic accuracy of flexible fiber-optic proctoscopy, formalin–ether fecal sedimentation, and sodium nitrate fecal flotation has been compared, and proctoscopy proved to be the best of the three methods evaluated for the diagnosis of *Prosthenorchis* infections (2,790).

Management of acanthocephalid infections should be directed at providing supportive treatment for newly imported parasitized primates and development of a strong sanitation program aimed at preventing reinfection. Because a cockroach intermediate host is required to complete the life cycle, an effective vermin control program is necessary to eliminate the possibility of reinfection and spread within the primate colony. Richter (940) reported on a devastating epidemic of acanthocephaliasis in a marmoset colony mediated by *Blattella germanica*. At least 20 deaths were attributed to infection by this parasite, and larval *P. elegans* were readily found in cockroaches (939,993). Many New World monkeys consider cockroaches a culinary delicacy, and the observation of insect parts in the fecal collection pans should alert laboratory care personnel to the potential hazard (2).

Anthelminthics used for treatment of other helminth parasites are not effective for *Prosthenorchis* (2). The oral administration of carbon tetrachloride at a dosage of 0.5 ml/kg of body weight has been reported to be an effective treatment with minimal side effects (2, 510, 729). However, the efficiency and long-term safety of this treatment have not been established (2).

Infection with these parasites has not been reported in humans. Human infection is theoretically possible because of the broad host spectrum of this parasite; however, is unlikely because it would require the ingestion of an infected cockroach (373).

E. Annelida

The species of annelids that parasitize nonhuman primates are listed in Table XI.

1. Dinobdellaiasis

The cause of this condition is the leech, *Dinobdella ferox*, which is distributed geographically throughout southern Asia (354,373,1055). It is a frequent parasite of the nasal cavities of macaques that range throughout this region of the world. *Dinobdella ferox* has been reported from several Old World monkey species (rhesus monkeys and Formosan macaques) (127, 373,382,659,908,1055).

The life cycle of this parasite is direct. Adults are hermaphroditic and eggs are laid in cocoons that are attached to objects at the surface of a pond. After hatching, the immature leeches stay at the surface of the water. Infection of the host occurs during drinking; the leech enters the body through the oral or nasal cavities, attaches to the mucosa of the upper respiratory tract, sucks blood for periods that may last a few days or many weeks, grows and matures, detaches, and drops out through the nostrils. The adult leeches are not parasitic (123,373,908).

Infection with a few parasites is usually asymptomatic, but heavy infection is reported to cause restlessness, epistaxis, anemia, weakness, asphyxiation, and sometimes death (373,908, 1055).

Histopathologically, lesions are composed of a mild, focal, chronic inflammatory infiltrate and increased mucous production involving the nasopharyngeal mucosa (373,908,1055).

Diagnosis is based on recognizing and identifying the parasite in its typical anatomical location within the host (373,908).

All newly arrived nonhuman primates from endemic areas should be examined during their quarantine period and treated, if infected (373). Gentle traction with a forceps is usually sufficient to remove the leech (373,908).

This leech does present some public health significance because it does infect humans; however, infection under laboratory conditions is improbable. Nevertheless, precautions should be taken when removing leeches from affected monkeys (373).

F. Arthropods: Insecta

The parasitic genera of *Siphonaptera* (fleas), *Diptera* (flies), and *Mallophaga* and *Anoplura* (lice) described from nonhuman primates are listed in Tables XII, XIII, and XIV, respectively. The most important members of these Orders are discussed in detail below.

For detailed information regarding the morphology and life cycle of these parasites, the reader is referred to any one of a number of recognized standard pathology or parasitology texts (52,373,571,1023,1045).

1. Flea Infestation

There is a relative paucity of information regarding the extent of flea infestation in nonhuman primates. The available reports concern fleas that, for the most part, are natural parasites of animals other than nonhuman primates (dogs, cats, and chickens). There is no suggestion about the importance of siphonapterids in nonhuman primates or of any potential role they may play in transmission of disease to humans (361).

TABLE XI
LEECHES DESCRIBED FROM NONHUMAN PRIMATES

TABLE XI

LEECHES DESCRIBED FROM NONHUMAN PRIMATES

Parasite Genus species	Location in host	Prosimians	New World monkeys	Old World monkeys	Great apes	Reference
Phylum Annelida, order Gnathobdellida						
Limnatus africana	Nasal cavities			X		164, 373, 671
Dinobdella ferox	Nasal cavities, pharynx			X		127, 354, 373, 382, 659, 908

Tunga penetrans (stick-tight, jigger, or chigoe flea) has been reported from Old World monkeys (guenons and baboons) (360,361,373,1023) and great apes (gorilla) (361,1049).

These parasites frequently invade the hard skin covering the ischial callosities where the female *T. penetrans* becomes firmly attached and penetrates into the epidermis that proliferates around the parasite. The implanted female fleas elicit severe irritation and pruritus, and secondary bacterial infections can occur, particularly after removal of the parasite from the site of attachment (360,361,373,466,1023).

Tunga penetrans is only a problem in nonhuman primates obtained directly from their natural habitat (373). If infected, treatment consists of surgical removal of the parasite and sterilization of the wound (360,373).

Humans are often infected in endemic areas, but infection under laboratory conditions is probably remote, provided that all newly arrived nonhuman primates are quarantined, examined, and treated, as appropriate, for any parasites they may be harboring.

Infestation with these parasites produces dermal cysts or swellings, containing a central pore, primarily in the cervical region. A chronic inflammatory reaction occurs around these sites, and a seropurulent exudate containing the dark feces of the larvae may exude through the pore. Healing of these lesions is usually rapid after emergence of the larvae. Secondary bacterial infections can occur, which may be more severe than the primary infection (373).

Diagnosis depends on demonstrating and identifying the typical larvae from the characteristic dermal cysts (373).

Control can best be achieved through the insect proofing of animal housing areas (373).

Although these flies do affect humans in the geographical locations where they normally occur, captive nonhuman primates are not considered a direct human public health hazard (373).

Treatment consists of surgical removal of the encysted fly larvae, flushing the cyst cavity with saline or and antiseptic solution, and applying an antibiotic powder or ointment (373).

2. Dermal Myiasis

The larvae (bots) of several species of flies in the families Cuterebridae and Calliphoridae are reported to infect nonhuman primates (361,373).

New World monkeys (howler monkeys) are reported to be a natural host for *Cuterebra* sp. larvae (361,373,1024).

3. Pediculosis

a. MALLOPHAGA. The mallophagans, or biting lice, are reported to be relatively rare on nonhuman primates, and apparently are unimportant in regard to zoonoses (361). Species of biting lice have been reported from prosimians (loris, indri, and mongoose lemur), New World monkeys (woolly spider mon-

TABLE XII

FLEAS DESCRIBED FROM NONHUMAN PRIMATES

Parasite Genus species	Location in host	Prosimians	New World monkeys	Old World monkeys	Great apes	Reference
Phylum Arthropoda, class Insecta, order Siphonoptera, family Pulicidae						
Ctenocephalides felis	Hair, skin	X		X		361, 373, 804, 1049
Pulex irritans	Hair, skin			X		373, 1200
Ctenocephalides canis	Hair, skin			X		361, 1049
Phylum Arthropoda, class Insecta, order Siphonoptera, family Tungidae						
Tunga penetrans	Skin			X	X	360, 361, 373, 1049
Echidnophaga gallinacea	Skin	X				361, 1049

TABLE XIII

FLIES DESCRIBED FROM NONHUMAN PRIMATES

Parasite Genus species	Location in host	Prosimians	New World monkeys	Old World monkeys	Great apes	Reference
Phylum Arthropoda, class Insecta, order Diptera, family Cuterebridae						
Cuterebra sp.	Skin, subcutis		X	X		361, 373, 1024
Dermatobia hominis	Skin, subcutis		X			373, 771
Alouattamyia sp.	Skin		X			268
Phylum Arthropoda, class Insecta, order Diptera, family Calliphoridae						
Cordylobia anthropophaga	Skin			X		360, 361, 373
Cochliomyia hominivorax	Skin			X		785

TABLE XIV

LICE DESCRIBED FROM NONHUMAN PRIMATES

Parasite Genus species	Location in host	Prosimians	New World monkeys	Old World monkeys	Great apes	Reference
Phylum Arthropoda, class Insecta, order Anoplura						
Pedicinus eurigaster	Hair			X		373, 639, 656, 1126
P. obtusus	Hair			X		373, 639, 656, 804
P. patas	Hair			X		373, 639
P. hamadryas	Hair			X		373, 804
P. mjobergi	Hair			X		373, 893
P. schaeffi	Hair			X	X	361, 373, 524, 613, 1049
Docophthirus acionetus	Hair	X				275, 361, 524, 1049
Phthiropediculus propitheci	Hair	X				361, 524, 1049
Lemurphthirus galagus	Hair	X	X			51, 276, 361, 524, 615, 1049
L. stigmosus	Hair	X				276, 354, 614
Pediculus lobatus pseudohumanus	Hair		X			361, 524, 1049
P. lobatus atelophilus	Hair		X			361, 524, 1049
Harrisonia uncinata	Hair		X			361, 524, 1049
Gliricola pintoi	Hair		X			361, 524, 1049
Pediculus humanus friedenthali	Hair				X	361, 524, 1049
Phthirus pubis	Hair				X	361, 524, 1049
P. gorillae	Hair				X	361, 524, 1049
Pediculus humanus capitis	Hair		X		X	207, 361, 524, 1049
Pediculus sp.	Hair		X			268, 832
Sathrax durus	Hair	X				275
Pedicinus longiceps	Hair			X		655
Phylum Arthropoda, class Insecta, order Mallophaga						
Trichodectes armatus	Hair		X			361, 1049
T. colobi	Hair			X		361, 1049
T. mjoebergi	Hair	X				361, 1049
T. semiarmatus	Hair		X			361, 1049
Trichodectes sp.	Hair		X			361, 1049
Trichophilopterus babakotophilus	Hair	X				361, 1049
Tetragynopus aotophilus	Hair		X			361, 1049
Trichophilopterus ferrisi	Hair	X				361, 524
Eutrichophilus setosus	Hair			X		355, 361
Aotiella aotophilus	Skin		X			268, 524
Cebidicola armatus	Skin		X			268, 524
C. semiarmatus	Skin		X			268, 524

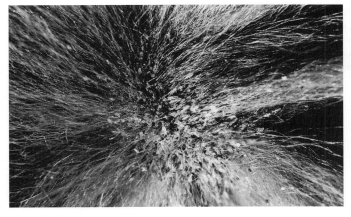

Fig. 58. Gross photograph of the hair of a rhesus monkey (*Macaca mulatta*) infested with *Pediculus* lice.

keys, howler monkeys, and owl monkey), and Old World monkeys (colobus monkeys) (361, 1049). There is also a single report of infestation of rhesus monkeys with *Eutrichophilus setosus,* the porcupine-biting louse. These monkeys were housed in close proximity to a cage of porcupines, resulting in cross-infestation (355,361). There are no reports of Mallophaga infestations involving great apes or humans.

b. ANOPLURA. Numerous species of anoplurans, or sucking lice, have been reported from a wide variety of nonhuman primates, including prosimians (tree shrew, lemurs, and galagos), Old World monkeys (macaques, langurs, green monkeys, guenons, baboons, colobus monkeys) (Fig. 58), New World monkeys (sakis, uakaris, howler monkeys, spider monkeys, marmosets, and tamarins), and great apes (gibbons, siamangs, chimpanzees, and gorilla) (309,310,361,524,891,1049,1169). There has been at least one report of a black spider monkey (*Ateles paniscus*) infestation with the human head louse. This infestation was thought to have been the result of contact with an infested person, indicating that the Anoplura can be shared by humans and the New World monkeys, but not the Old World monkeys (207,361).

Fiennes (361) regards sucking lice as interchangeable among humans, great apes, and New World monkeys, with the possible exception of marmosets and tamarins. Old World monkeys are not affected by the species of Anoplura that infest humans, great apes, and New World monkeys.

Quarantine and inspection of all newly arrived nonhuman primates with isolation and treatment of infested animals are essential to prevent infestation from becoming established within a primate colony (373).

There are no reports of transmission of rickettsial diseases by lice from great apes or New World monkeys to humans, or vice versa, although in theory such transmission would seem possible (361).

Treatment for lice in nonhuman primates consists of spraying with dichlorvos (Nuvan top) and, in severe cases, bathing with gamma benzene hydrochloride (Quellada shampoo) (1159). Alugan powder has also been recommended for the treatment of ectoparasites infesting nonhuman primates (436). Treatment should be repeated at weekly intervals for 2–3 weeks. Ivermectin (Ivomec), at a dose rate of 200 mg/kg subcutaneously, has also proved to be effective. This can be repeated in 3 weeks if necessary (213). Cages, bedding, and equipment should be cleaned and disinfected at the same time the animals are treated (373).

G. Arachnida

The parasitic genera of ticks and mites described from nonhuman primates are listed in Tables XV and XVI, respectively. The most important members are discussed in detail below.

As for the parasitic insecta, the reader is referred to any one of a number of recognized standard pathology or parasitology texts for detailed information regarding the morphology and life cycle of these parasites (52,373,455,571,1045).

1. Tick Infestation

According to Fiennes (361), the problem of ticks on captive monkeys is not important because when engorged, the ticks drop off the host, and under the conditions of captivity, reinfestion does not occur (361).

Species of ixodid ticks have been reported from numerous nonhuman primates, including prosimians (bushbabies), New World monkeys (spider monkeys), and Old World monkeys (rhesus monkeys, cynomolgus monkeys, baboons, colobus monkeys, bonnet macaques, langurs, and green monkeys) (361, 373, 522, 804, 1049, 1096, 1097). Argasid ticks have been reported infrequently from Old World monkeys (cynomolgus monkeys). In addition, the argasid tick, *Argas reflexus,* normally parasitic on pigeons and other avians, has been reported from an otherwise unidentified monkey (361,1049).

It appears that feral, nonhuman primates are parasitized by ticks in most of the geographical areas in which they live and that they are infested by a variety of different species. The importance of ticks as parasites is their worldwide geographic distribution and their role as vectors of a wide variety of diseases, many of which are zoonotic. Because they can infect other animals and contaminate the premises, producing long-term difficulties in parasite control, procedures aimed at eliminating them from newly acquired animals are of primary importance (361, 1023).

Most cases of tick infestation are asymptomatic; however, heavy parasite loads can result in irritation, restlessness, weight loss, and anemia. Tick bites cause a local inflammatory reaction characterized by hyperemia, edema, and focal hemorrhage. Bite

TABLE XV

Ticks Described from Nonhuman Primates

Parasite Genus species	Location in host	Prosimians	New World monkeys	Old World monkeys	Great apes	Reference
Phylum Arthropoda, subclass Acari, suborder Ixodida, family Ixodidae						
Rhipicephalus sanguineus	Skin	X		X		361, 373, 522, 523, 804, 1114
R. appendiculatus	Skin	X		X		373, 522, 523, 651, 804
R. pulchellus	Skin			X		480, 653
R. haemaphysaloides	Skin			X		1097
R. evertsi	Skin			X		523
R. pravus	Skin			X		523
R. simus	Skin	X		X		523
Dermacentor auratus	Skin			X		1097
Ixodes ceylonensis	Skin			X		1097
I. petauristae	Skin			X		1097
I. calvipalpus	Skin			X		361, 523, 1049
I. loricatus	Skin		X			189, 268, 361, 1049
I. schillingeri	Skin			X		361, 373, 522, 523, 1049
I. rasus	Skin			X		523, 653
I. lemuris	Skin	X				523
Ixodes sp.	Skin	X				523
Amblyomma hebraeum	Skin	X		X		373, 522, 523, 763, 804
A. variegatum	Skin	X				523
Amblyomma sp.	Skin			X		523, 653, 1097
Boophilus annulatus	Skin			X		361, 1049

wounds may be involved with secondary bacterial infections (1023).

Diagnosis is based on the signs and on the demonstration and identification of the specific species of tick on the host (373).

Control is based primarily on prevention of infestation of buildings within the primate colony and on prompt elimination of infestation should it occur (373). All buildings used to house nonhuman primates should be constructed in such a manner to minimize cracks and crevices, and all cages should be of a material that can be readily cleaned and disinfected (373). All newly acquired nonhuman primates should be quarantined and examined on arrival and treated, if infested (373).

Because ticks can be the vectors of zoonotic diseases, nonhuman primates infested with ticks should be handled with caution. Care should be taken when removing ticks manually to prevent the contamination of open wounds or mucous membranes with any blood from crushed ticks (373).

If treatment for ticks is required for nonhuman primates, Alugan powder is recommended (436). Ticks also can be removed manually with a forceps. Care should be taken when removing ticks from the skin so as not to leave the parasites' mouthparts in the host. Firmly grasping the tick near the skin will usually result in removal of the entire parasite (373).

2. Cutaneous Acariasis

a. Scabies (Mange).   The cause of this disease, *Sarcoptes scabiei,* the human itch mite, has been reported from Old World monkeys (cynomolgus monkeys and drills) (38, 373, 379, 396, 691, 1150) and the great apes (gorillas, chimpanzees, orangutans, gibbons, and siamangs) (361, 373, 439, 923, 936, 967, 1116, 1149, 1150).

A closely related species, *Prosarcoptes pitheci,* has been reported in Old World monkeys (African green monkeys and baboons) and New World monkeys in captivity (cebus monkeys) (334, 337, 342, 373, 880).

Two sarcoptiform species, *Dunnalges lambrechti* and *Rosalialges cruciformis,* have been reported from New World monkeys (marmosets and owl monkeys) (617, 681). There appears to be no reports of *S. scabiei* infestion in prosimians (361).

Signs associated with *S. scabiei* infestion in nonhuman primates include intense pruritus, anorexia, weakness, weight loss, tremors, and emaciation. Gross lesions include thickening and scaling of the skin and severe alopecia. The severe itching can result in self-mutilation, with secondary hemorrhage and suppurative bacterial dermatitis (373, 439, 691, 1023, 1116, 1150). Death of a chimpanzee has been ascribed to a severe *S. scabiei* infestion (884).

TABLE XV—*Continued*

TICKS DESCRIBED FROM NONHUMAN PRIMATES

Parasite Genus species	Location in host	Prosimians	New World monkeys	Old World monkeys	Great apes	Reference
Hyalomma truncatum	Skin			X		523
Hyalomma sp.	Skin			X		523
Haemaphysalis wellingtoni	Skin			X		1097
H. aculeata	Skin			X		1097
H. cuspidata	Skin			X		1097
H. kyasanurensis	Skin			X		1097
H. minuta	Skin			X		1097
H. leachii	Skin	X				523
H. lemuris	Skin	X				523
H. palmata	Skin			X		361, 523, 1049
H. spinigera	Skin			X		373, 1096, 1097, 1114
H. koningsbergi	Skin	X				15
H. hylobatis	Skin				X	15
H. bispinosa	Skin			X		834, 1097
H. turturis	Skin			X		1097
H. papuanakinneari	Skin			X		1097
Haemaphysalis sp.	Skin			X		1095
Phylum Arthropoda, subclass Acari, suborder Ixodida, family Argasidae						
Ornithodorus talaje	Skin			X		189, 361, 373, 1049
Argas reflexus	Skin			X		361, 1049

Histopathologically, the infested skin is characterized by hyperkeratosis, parakeratosis, and crusting. The epidermis contains burrows in which many parasites and eggs are seen (373, 396,439,967,1023).

The tentative diagnosis of scabies is based on the signs and lesions and is confirmed by demonstrating and identifying the parasites and/or eggs in deep skin scrapings (373,1023).

Sarcoptes scabiei infestions in nonhuman primates are transmissible to humans by direct contact (373,439,967,1150,1200). Thus infested nonhuman primates, or those suspected of being infested, should be handled with caution by those responsible for their care and management (373).

Successful treatment for *S. scabiei* infestation in nonhuman primates has been accomplished with the application of a 4% solution of Alugan at 4-day intervals (436) and/or by the subcutaneous injection of ivermectin (Ivomec) at a dose level of 200 mg/kg, repeated in 3 weeks if necessary (213).

Control of the various lice, mites, fleas, flies, and ticks that can infest nonhuman primates is basically through environmental sanitation and direct treatment of the primate. Therapy is difficult because of the grooming, licking nature of primates; however, dusts and ointments suitable for cats and humans can be used with discretion on the primate (934).

b. OTHER MANGE MITES. Various other mites, such as *Psorergates cercopitheci* (Figs. 59 and 60), can cause skin lesions similar to sarcoptic mange. Control and treatment would be the same as for *Sarcoptes*.

3. Pulmonary Acariasis

The cause of this condition is any one of at least 10 species of lung mites in the genus *Pneumonyssus* that have been reported from the lower respiratory tract of Old World monkeys (rhesus monkeys, cynomolgus monkeys, pigtail macaques, patas monkeys, Celebes black apes, mangabeys, baboons, numerous members of the genus *Cercopithecus*, colobus monkeys, langurs, and proboscis monkeys) and the great apes (chimpanzees, gorillas, and orangutans) (41,83,308,322,323,325,328, 330,347,373,427,451,463,545,555,605,607,608,767,772,825, 826,867,948,967,1209). Also, there has been one species of lung mite in the genus *Pneumonyssoides* that has been reported from the lungs, larynx, nasal cavities, and sinuses in New World monkeys (woolly monkeys and howler monkeys) (331, 373, 545,555,967,1127).

The most commonly encountered member of this genus, *Pneumonyssus simicola,* is found in the lungs of essentially

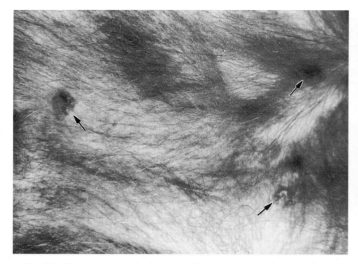

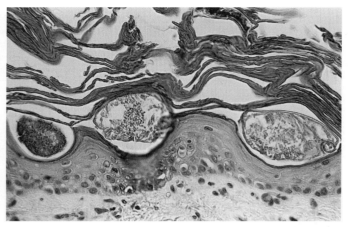

Fig. 60. Photomicrograph of section through several *Psorergates cercopitheci* mites in dermal lesions seen in Fig. 59. HE stain.

Fig. 59. Gross photograph of crusted skin lesions (arrows) on the chest of a mangabey monkey (*Cercocebus atys*) infested with *Psorergates cercopitheci* mange mites.

100% of imported rhesus monkeys (*Macaca mulatta*) (368,373, 391,427,554–556,603,604,607,947). Also, this mite has been seen in the lungs of infant rhesus monkeys allowed to remain with their wild-caught parents after birth (684). Reports of *P. simicola* infestation in other macaque species are less frequent (41,328,331,373,521,554,1056). Despite the common occurrence in feral *M. mulatta*, *P. simicola* has not been seen in laboratory-born monkeys taken from their mothers at birth (373,554,621). A high incidence of lung mite infestation with species other than *P. simicola* has been reported from baboons (601,602,1058).

The complete life cycle of this parasite is unknown (373,391, 604,607). Hull (544) first demonstrated the existence of the protonymph and deutonymph in the life cycle, thus correcting the widely held misconception that these mites transformed directly from larvae to adults.

The infestation in the rhesus monkey is usually nonsymptomatic and clinical signs are uncommon (373,388,554–556,605, 608,1023). There have been reports of paroxysms of sneezing and coughing, but these may be the result of associated pulmonary disease (373,495,554,555).

Gross lesions are located randomly throughout the pulmonary parenchyma and consist of varying sized pale spots or yellowish gray foci that are usually flat or slightly umbilicated on the surface and contain translucent areas. Those located near the surface of the lungs elevate the visceral pleura (Fig. 61). The lesions can resemble tubercles but are soft to the touch rather than firm. Adjacent lesions may become confluent. Bullous emphysematous lesions and hemorrhagic lesions may be seen in some cases. Many animals have fine, violin string-like fibrous adhesions between visceral and parietal pleural surfaces and between all of the lung lobes.

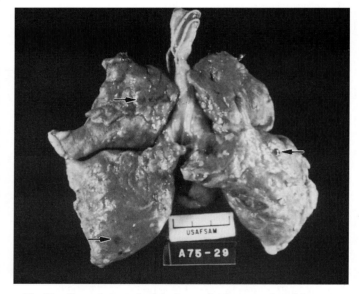

Fig. 61. Gross photograph of the lungs of a rhesus monkey (*Macaca mulatta*) showing numerous, randomly scattered nodules ("mite houses") (arrows) associated with infestation by the lung mite *Pneumonyssus semicola*.

Under the dissecting microscope, the lesions present as pale, white, jelly-like masses that have a small opening or slit in the center. These so-called "mite houses" can contain from 1 to 20 mites. The majority of these are females, but sometimes eggs, larvae, and male mites are also present. A characteristic golden brown to black pigment permeates the lesions and surrounding pulmonary parenchyma (373,427,455,463,554–556,605,607, 609,668,1023).

Histopathologically, lung mite lesions are characterized by a localized bronchiolitis, peribronchiolitis, focal lobular pneumonitis, alveolar collapse or consolidation, and sometimes bronchiolectasis. There is thickening of the bronchiolar wall, loss of the lining epithelium, hyperplasia of the bronchiolar smooth muscle, and formation of peribronchiolar lymphoid aggregations. A pleocellular inflammatory cell exudate consisting of neutrophils, eosinophils, lymphoplasmocytes, and macrophages infiltrates the affected bronchiolar wall. There is little or no tissue necrosis or giant cell formation (Fig. 62) (373,427, 455,463,554–556,605,607,609,668,1023).

Macrophages, whose cytoplasm is laden with a golden brown to blackish pigment and refractile crystals, are always present in and around the lesions and throughout the lung tissues. This pigment, which is not seen in the lungs of mite-free monkeys, does not contain carbon or melanin, but is iron positive and birefringent under polarized light. The exact source of the pigment is not known, but it is felt that it probably results from the breakdown and excretion of the hosts' blood proteins by the mites (373,427,455,463,554–556,605,607,609,668,837,1023).

The immunological response to pulmonary acariasis has been reviewed by Kim (606–608).

Lung mite infestation has been reported to be associated with pneumothorax (925) and pulmonary arteritis (675,688,1180) in the rhesus monkey. There is also a report that describes extensive pleuritis and pericarditis associated with ruptured lung mite lesions (610). The disease also hinders the interpretation of cardiopulmonary experiments done with affected animals (554, 573,575,925).

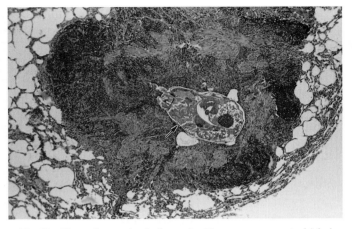

Fig. 62. Photomicrograph of a lung mite (*Pneumonyssus semicola*) lesion involving the bronchiole of a rhesus monkey (*Macaca mulatta*). Mite (arrow) located centrally surrounded by a mantle of chronic inflammatory cells. Note destruction of normal pulmonary architecture and large amount of dark pigment within macrophages located around the periphery of the lesion. HE stain.

Even though several earlier reports ascribe fatalities to *P. simicola* infestation, death probably results only under conditions of massive infestations. Such cases of massive infestations and resultant death have been reported in the rhesus monkey,

TABLE XVI

Mites Described from Nonhuman Primates

Parasite Genus species	Location in host	Prosimians	New World monkeys	Old World monkeys	Great apes	Reference
Phylum Arthropoda, subclass Acari, order Parasitiformes, suborder Gamasida (= Mesotigmata), family Halarachnidae						
Pneumonyssus simicola	Lungs		X		X	1, 38, 41, 328, 331, 347, 368, 373, 391, 398, 427, 451, 463, 521, 544, 555, 556, 601, 602, 605, 607, 608, 688, 745, 754, 767, 772, 825, 947, 948, 1056, 1114, 1127, 1209
P. duttoni	Bronchi, trachea			X		190, 328, 330, 344, 373, 544, 555, 607, 826
P. santos-diasi	Lungs			X		328, 373, 544, 555, 607, 650, 653, 804, 1209
P. longus	Lungs, bronchi, trachea			X	X	328, 330, 373, 544, 555, 607
P. oudemansi	Lungs, bronchi, trachea			X	X	83, 325, 328, 330, 373, 544, 555, 607
P. africanus	Bronchi			X		328, 373, 544, 555, 607
P. mossambicencis	Lungs			X		328, 373, 544, 555, 607, 650, 653, 763, 804, 1209
P. congoensis	Trachea, lungs			X		308, 328, 373, 544, 555, 607, 653, 804
P. rodhaini	Lungs, nasal fossae			X		322, 544, 555, 607
P. vitzthumi	Lung bronchi, maxillary sinuses, nasal fossae			X		83, 544, 555, 607

TABLE XVI—*Continued*

MITES DESCRIBED FROM NONHUMAN PRIMATES

Parasite Genus species	Location in host	Prosimians	New World monkeys	Old World monkeys	Great apes	Reference
P. vocalis	Laryngeal ventricles, vocal pouch			X		757, 761, 763
Pneumonyssus sp.	Lungs			X		544, 555
Rhinophaga dinolti	Nasal cavities, lungs			X		323, 373, 398, 544, 555, 607, 854
R. cercopitheci	Lungs, frontal sinuses			X		323, 345, 373, 544, 555, 607, 1056
R. papionis	Lungs, nasal fossae			X		323, 345, 373, 544, 555, 607, 653, 757, 758, 763, 804, 1056
R. pongicola	Maxillary sinuses, nasal fossal				X	327, 544, 555
R. elongata	Nasal mucosa			X		653, 757, 758, 763
Pneumonyssoides stammeri	Large bronchiole, larynx, nasal cavities, sinuses		X			331, 373, 428, 544, 555, 607, 1127

Phylum Arthropoda, subclass Acari, order Parasitiformes, suborder Trombidiformes (= Actinedida)

Psorergates cercopitheci	Skin			X		37, 373, 683, 927, 1025, 1209, 1210
Psorergates sp.	Skin			X		679, 683, 687
Demodex canis	Skin		X		X	361, 880
D. saimiri	Skin		X			686
D. intermedius	Skin	X				724
Demodex sp.	Skin		X			509, 617, 869
Trombicula sp.	Skin			X		361, 1095

Phylum Arthropoda, subclass Acari, order Parasitiformes, suborder Sarcoptiformes (= Acaridida)

Sarcoptes scabiei	Skin			X	X	38, 361, 373, 379, 396, 439, 691, 884, 923, 936, 967, 1116, 1149, 1150, 1200
S. pitheci	Skin			X		361, 880, 967
Prosarcoptes pitheci	Skin		X	X		334, 337, 342, 373, 880
Pithesaroptes talapoini	Skin			X		337, 342, 373
Cosarcoptes scanloni	Skin			X		342, 373, 1037
Notoedres galagoensis	Skin	X				334, 336, 342, 373
Alouattalges corbeti	Skin		X			340, 373
Fonsecalges saimirii	Skin		X			194, 268, 340, 372, 373
Galagalges congolonsis	Skin	X				276, 334
Paracoroptes gordoni	Skin			X		334, 373, 678
Pangorillages pani	Skin				X	333, 373
Listrocarpus cosgrovei	Skin		X			194, 341, 373
L. hapalei	Skin		X			341, 373
L. saimirii	Skin		X			341, 373
L. lagothrix	Skin		X			341, 373
Rhyncoptes anastosi	Skin		X			338, 373
R. cebi	Skin		X			338, 373
R. cercopitheci	Skin			X		338, 373
Saimirioptes paradoxus	Skin		X			343, 373
Audycoptes greeri	Hair follicles		X			268, 343, 373, 681
A. lawrenci	Hair follicles		X			268, 343, 373, 681
Lemurnyssus galagoensis	Nasal cavities	X				276, 326, 335, 373
Mortelmansia brevis	Nasal cavities		X			194, 268, 329, 335, 373
M. longis	Nasal cavities		X			194, 268, 329, 335, 373
M. duboisi	Nasal cavities		X			194, 268, 335, 373, 657
Dunnalges lambrechti	Skin		X			268, 617, 681, 682
Rosalialges cruciformis	Skin		X			268, 617, 681, 682
Prosarcoptes sp.	Skin			X		1037
Pithesarcoptes sp.	Skin			X		1037
Kutzerocoptes sp.	Skin			X		683, 1037

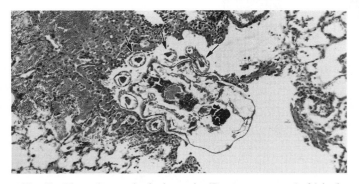

Fig. 63. Photomicrograph of a lung mite (*Pneumonyssus semicola*) in the lung of a rhesus monkey (*Macaca mulatta*). Three pair of legs (arrows) are clearly visible in this section. This may be an immature mite as four pair of legs are present on adults. HE stain.

proboscis monkey, "lion macaque," pig-tailed macaque, douc langurs, and chimpanzee (16,55,386,458,472,844,608,767,948, 1053).

The gross lesions and histopathology of lung mite infestation in baboons and chimpanzees are similar to that described for rhesus monkeys (609,754).

Diagnosis of lung mite infestation in live monkeys is difficult. Thoracic X-rays or hematologic studies are of little value (373,556,1023). There has been some success in demonstrating lung mite larvae in tracheobronchial washings, but a negative finding is not conclusive proof that infestation does not exist (399). Gross lesions are rather characteristic but must be differentiated from tuberculosis. Tissue sections containing the mites (Figs 62 and 63) and/or the characteristic pigment and crystals are diagnostic of lung mite infestation (373,556,1023). Lung mites can be found in the feces of infested nonhuman primates (868).

Complete control can only be achieved through the development of infestation-free colonies that are initiated by rearing newborn monkeys in isolation from their mothers (373,1114).

There is no evidence that *P. simicola* infests humans. Therefore, there is no public health significance associated with lung mite infestations in nonhuman primates (373).

Therapy for pulmonary acariasis has been attempted, but with little success (573). The organic arsenical tryparsamide failed to reduce the number of mites present in infected monkeys (368,573). The organophosphate ronnel reduced but did not eliminate mite infestation and resulted in organophosphate toxicity in some animals (368,573). Joseph (573) has reported that a single injection of ivermectin (200 μg/kg) in rhesus monkeys appeared to be effective in the elimination of *Pneumonyssus* sp. infestation in nonhuman primates.

4. Nasal Acariasis

Five species of nasal mites of the genus *Rhinophaga* have been described from the upper skull and olfactory mucosa of

Old World monkeys (rhesus monkeys, baboons, *Cercopithecus* sp.) and great apes (orangutan) (325,345,544,555,600,608,757, 758,854).

Rhinophaga papinois is found in the maxillary sinuses of the chacma baboon (*Papio ursinus*) where it causes mucosal polyps (608,722,757). In the lungs it causes pneumonitis and excessive mucous production.

Rhinophaga elongata, also reported from the chacma baboon, is an extremely long mite that has been described in the apex of small mucosal nodules distributed randomly throughout the nasal cavity. The anterior third of the mite was embedded deeply in the nasal mucosa and, in some cases, in the adjacent bone. An inflammatory reaction and obstruction of the mucosal glands, which became greatly dilated, were associated with the presence of this mite (608,757,758).

Rhinophaga dinolti has been reported from the lungs and nasal cavities of the rhesus monkey (*Macaca mulatta*). Lesions associated with the presence of this parasite in tissues have not been reported (323,373,388,555,854). *Rhinophaga cercopitheci* has been reported from the lungs and frontal sinuses of several species of guenons (*Cercopithecus ascanius, C. mitis*). Lesions include pneumonitis and excessive mucous production (345, 373,555,1056).

Rhinophaga pongicola has been reported from the maxillary sinuses and nasal fossae of an orangutan (*Pongo pygmaeus*) (327,555).

5. Laryngeal Acariasis

A newly recognized mite, *Pneumonyssus vocalis,* has been reported from the mucosa of the laryngeal ventricles and vocal pouch of the chacma baboon where it elicits a mild local inflammatory response (608,757,761).

There is no known control or treatment for the various respiratory mites that infest nonhuman primates other than that outlined earlier. The public health significance of these parasites has not been reported.

H. Pentastomids

The parasitic pentastomid nymphs described from nonhuman primates are listed in Table XVII. They are discussed in detail below.

1. Pentastomiasis

The parasites that cause this disease are considered to be highly aberrant arthropods (332,373,617,1016,1019).

Four genera have been described: *Linguatula,* which has a worldwide distribution; *Porocephalus,* found in both South America and Africa; *Armillifer,* which occurs in Africa, Asia, and Australia; and *Gigliolella,* found on the Island of Madagascar.

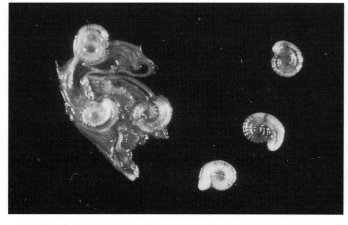

Fig. 64. Gross photograph of mesentery of cynomolgus monkey (*Macaca fascicularis*) containing several encysted pentastome larvae. *Armillifer* sp. The C-shaped coiling and pseudosegmentation are evident.

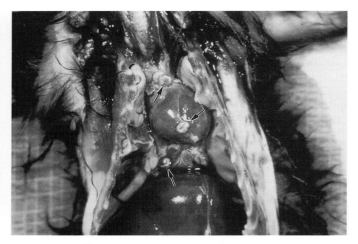

Fig. 65. Gross photograph of chest cavity of moustached marmoset (*Saguinus mystax mystax*) showing several encysted pentastome larvae (arrows), *Porocephalus* sp., lying on the heart and diaphragm.

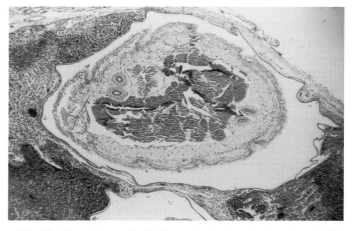

Fig. 66. Photomicrograph of a *Porocephalus* larva in a lymph node of a moustached marmoset (*Saguinus mystax mystax*) from the case illustrated in Fig. 65. HE stain.

The nymph form occurs in nonhuman primates, which serve as intermediate hosts in the pentastome life cycle (202,233,301, 373,617,1019,1023,1208). The adult forms of *Linguatula* are found in the nasal passages of dogs, other canids, domestic animals, and humans. Adults of the other three genera are found in the lungs and air sacs of various snakes (373,617,1019,1023). Pentastomid nymphs have been reported in a wide variety of nonhuman primates, including prosimians, New and Old World monkeys, and great apes (194,196,332,339,360,373,384,470, 506,521,617,658,804,819,1018,1019,1033,1208).

Infection with this parasite is usually asymptomatic. Dead nymphs act as foreign bodies and invoke an intense inflammatory response in the host. Fatal peritonitis has been reported in overwhelming infections with penetration of the intestinal wall by nymphs. When one infection follows another of considerable duration, there may be a lymphocytic response due to presensitization by the initial infection (33,196,373,384,617,1017,1018, 1033,1167).

Diagnosis is usually based on an incidental finding at necropsy and hinges on the identification of the characteristic "C"-shaped nymph in the tissues (373) (Fig. 64). Nymphs have been described in the lungs, liver, omentum, and serosa of the intestinal tract of nonhuman primates (373, 617, 819, 1019, 1023) (Fig. 65), but may be found in almost any tissue (Fig. 66), including the brain (373,1019).

Pentastomids have been reported in humans in tropical Africa and Asia, but the parasite in captive animals is of no public health significance (373,903,975). Infections in humans can occur only through the ingestion of eggs passed in the feces or in the saliva of the definitive host (373).

There is no reported treatment for this parasite in nonhuman primates.

ACKNOWLEDGMENTS

Portions of this chapter are reprinted from Toft (1092,1093), which are used by permission of Veterinary Pathology and the American College of Veterinary Pathologists and Springer-Verlag, respectively. Figures 1, 6, 11, 13–16, 18–22, 29, 31, 47, 56, and 57 were reprinted by permission of Veterinary Pathology and the American College of Veterinary Pathologists. We acknowledge the following people for their assistance and support during the preparation of this manuscript: Ms. Anne L. Killman-Inabnitt for assistance in formating and typing the manuscript; Mr. David L. Blum, Battelle librarian, for assistance in obtaining copies of many of the references cited in the bibliography; Mr. Anthony J. Stuart and Ms. Dana Hall, Battelle, and Mr. James Gathany, CDC, for assistance with the photography; and Dr. Stanley D. Dannemiller for review of the manuscript and helpful editorial comments.

TABLE XVII

PENTASTOMIDS DESCRIBED FROM NONHUMAN PRIMATES

Parasite Genus species	Location in host	Prosimians	New World monkeys	Old World monkeys	Great apes	Reference
Phylum Arthropoda, class Pentastomida						
Linguatula serrata	Mesenteric lymph nodes, viscera		X	X		373, 658, 1019
Porocephalus clavatus	Peritoneum, viscera, brain		X			194, 373, 468, 617, 819, 900, 976, 1016, 1018, 1023, 1033, 1050
P. subulifer	Viscera	X		X		332, 373, 1019, 1023
Porocephalus sp.	Omentum/mesentery			X		713
Gigliolella brumpti	Mesentery	X				141, 373
Armillifer armillatus	Thoracic and abdominal cavities	X	X	X	X	202, 233, 268, 276, 332, 360, 373, 449, 479, 506, 521, 617, 651, 839, 976, 1019, 1023, 1050, 1167
A. moniliformis	Viscera, peritoneal cavity			X		69, 339, 373, 1019, 1023
Armillifer sp.	Omentum		X			713
Porocephalus crotali	Peritoneal cavity		X			233, 268, 1050
Nephridiacanthus sp. (juvenile)	Rectal wall			X		651, 652

REFERENCES

1. Abbott, D. P., and Majeed, S. K. (1984). A survey of parasitic lesions in wild-caught laboratory-maintained primates: (rhesus, cynomolgus, and baboon). *Vet. Pathol.* **21,** 198–207.

2. Abee, C. R. (1985). Medical care and management of the squirrel monkey. *In* "Handbook of Squirrel Monkey Research" (L. A. Rosenblum and C. L. Cole, eds.), pp. 447–488. Plenum, New York.

3. Aberle, S. D. (1945). "Primate Malaria." Natl. Acad. Sci.—Natl. Res. Counc. Publ., Washington, DC.

4. Abrambulo, P. V., III, Abass, J. B., and Walker, J. S. (1974). Silvered leaf monkey (*Presbytis cristatus*) II Gastrointestinal parasites and their treatment. *Lab. Anim. Sci.* **24,** 299–306.

5. Adams, L. (1980). Research scores breakthrough in answer to marmoset disease. *Zoo Sounds* **16,** 11.

6. Adams, M. R., Lewis, J. C., and Bullock, B. C. (1983). Hemobartonellosis in a squirrel monkey breeding colony. *34th Annu. Sessi. Am. Assoc. Lab. Anim. Sci.,* Abstr. No. 5.

7. Adams, M. R., Lewis, J. C., and Bullock, B. C. (1984). Hemobartonellosis in squirrel monkeys (*Saimiri sciureus*) in a domestic breeding colony. *Lab. Anim. Sci.* **34,** 82–85.

8. Addison, E. M., Forrester, D. J., Whitley, R. D., and Curtis, M. M. (1986). *Oxyspirura youngi* sp. in (Nematoda): Thelaziidae) from the patas monkey, *Erythrocebus patas. Proc. Helminthol. Soc. Wash.* **53,** 89–93.

9. Aikawa, M., and Nassenzweig, R. (1972). Fine structure of *Haemobartonella* sp. in the Squirrel monkey. *J. Parasitol.* **58,** 628–630.

10. Albuquerque, R. D. R., and Barretto, M. P. (1969). Estudos sobre reservatorios e vectores silvestres de *Trypanosoma cruzi,* XXXII-Infecção natural do simio *Callicebus nigrifons* (Spix, 1823) pelo *T. cruzi. Rev. Inst. Med. Trop. Sao Paulo* **11,** 115–122.

11. Allen, A. M. (1957). Pulmonary hydatid in a rhesus monkey. *Arch. Pathol.* **64,** 148–151.

12. Allen, A. M. (1960). Occurrence of the nematode, *Anatrichosoma cutaneum,* in the nasal mucosae of *Macaca mulatta* monkeys. *Am. J. Vet. Res.* **21,** 389–392.

13. Amberson, J. M., and Schwarz, E. (1952). *Ternidens deminatus* Railliet and Henry, a nematode parasite of man and primates. *Ann. Trop. Med. Parasitol.* **46,** 227–237.

14. Amyx, H. L., Asher, D. M., Nash, T. E., Gibbs, C. J., Jr., and Gajdusek, D. C. (1978). Hepatic amebiasis in spider monkeys. *Am. J. Trop. Med. Hyg.* **27,** 888–891.

15. Anastos, G. (1950). The scutate ticks of Ixodidae of Indonesia. *Entomol. Am.* [N. S.] **30,** 1–144.

16. Andersen, S., Christensen, N. O., and Eriksen, E. (1972). Disease in freshly imported proboscis monkeys (*Nasalis larvatus*). *Verh. Int. Symp. Erk. Zootiere, 14th,* Berlin, pp. 307–312 (in German).

17. Anderson, D. C., and McClure, H. M. (1982). Acute disseminated fatal toxoplasmosis in a squirrel monkey. *J. Am. Vet. Med. Assoc.* **181,** 1363–1366.

18. Anderson, M. P., Oosterhuis, J. E., Kennedy, S., and Benirschke, K. (1986). Pneumonia and meningoencephalitis due to amoeba in a lowland gorilla. *J. Zoo Anim. Med.* **17,** 87–91.

19. Anderson, R. C. (1957). The life cycles of dipetalonematid nematodes (Filaroidea: Dipetalonematidae): The problem of their evolution. *J. Helminthol.* **31,** 203–224.

20. Anver, M. R., King, N. W., and Hunt, R. D. (1972). Congenital encephalitozoonosis in a squirrel monkey (*Saimiri sciureus*). *Vet. Pathol.* **9,** 475–480.

21. Appleton, C. C., Henzi, S. P., Whiten, A., and Byrne, R. (1986). The gastrointestinal parasites of *Papio ursinus* from the Drakensberg Mountains, Republic of South Africa. *Int. J. Primatol.* **7,** 449–456.

22. Armstrong, J., Hertzog, R. E., Hall, R. T., and Hoff, G. L. (1979). Giardiasis in apes and zoo attendants, Kansas City, Missouri. *CDC Vet. Publ. Health Notes,* Jan., Page 7.

23. Artigas, P. de T. (1933). Sobre o parasitismo do *Saimiris sciureus* por um *Gongylonema* (*G. saimirsi, N. sp.*) e as possibilidades de infestação humana. *Rev. Soc. Paulista Med. Vet.* **3,** 83–91; cited by Dunn (268).

24. Arya, S. N. (1981). A new species of the genus *Probstmayria* Ransom, 1907 (Nematoda:Atractidae) from the rhesus macaque, *Macaca mulatta. Primates* **22,** 261–265.

25. Ashford, R. W., Warhurst, D. C., and Reid, G. D. (1993). Human infection with cyanobacterium-like bodies. *Lancet* **341**, 1034.

26. Auerbach, E. (1953). A study of *Balantidium coli* Stein, 1863 in relation to cytology and behavior in culture. *J. Morphol.* **93**, 404–445.

27. Augustine, D. L. (1939). Some observations on some ascarids from a chimpanzee (*Pan troglodytes*) with experimental studies on the susceptibility of monkeys (*Macaca mulatta*) to infection with human and pig ascaris. *Am. J. Hyg.* **30**, 29–33.

28. Ayala, F. M. (1961). Hallazgo de *Trypanosoma cruzi* Chagas, 1909 en el mono *Saimiri boliviensis* de la Amazonia Peruana. *Rev. Bras. Malaiol. Doencas Trop.* **13**, 99–105.

29. Ayala, S. C., D'Alessandro, A., MacKenzie, R., and Angel, D. (1973). Hemoparasite infection in 830 wild animals from the eastern llanos of Colombia. *J. Parasitol.* **59**, 52–59.

30. Ayers, K. M., and Jones, S. R. (1978). The cardiovascular system. *In* "Pathology of Laboratory Animals" (K. Benirschke, F. M. Garner, and T. C. Jones, (eds.), Vol. I, Chapter 1, pp. 2–69. Springer-Verlag, New York.

31. Baer, J. G. (1935). Etudes de quelques helminthes de Lémuriens. *Rev. Suisse Zool.* **42**, 275–292.

32. Bain, O., Baker, M., and Chabaud, A. G. (1982). Nouvelles données sur la lignée *Dipetalonema* (Filarioidea, Nematoda). *Ann. Parasitol. Hum. Comp.* **57**, 593–620.

33. Bain, O., Diagne, M., and Muller, R. (1987). Une cinquieme filaire du genre *Dipetalonema*, parasite de singes Sud-Americains. *Ann. Parasitol. Hum. Comp.* **62**, 262–270.

34. Bain, O., Moisson, P., Huerre, M., Landsoud-Soukate, J., and Tutin, C. (1995). Filariae from a wild gorilla in Gabon with description of a new species of *Mansonella. Parasite* **2**, 315–322.

35. Bain, O. I., Wamae, C. N., and Reid, G. D. (1988). Diversity of filariae of the genus *Cecopithifilaria* in baboons in Kenya. *Ann. Parasitol. Hum. Comp.* **63**, 224–239.

36. Bain, O. I., Wamae, C. N., and Reid, G. D. (1989). Description de *Cercopithifilaria verveti* n. sp., filaire sous-cutanée d'un cercopitheque au Kenya. *Ann. Parasitol. Hum. Comp.* **64**, 42–45.

37. Bakarr, M. I., Gbakima, A. A., and Bah, Z. (1991). Intestinal helminth parasites in free-living monkeys from a West African rainforest. *Afr. J. Ecol.* **29**, 170–172.

38. Baker, E. W., Evans, T. M., Gould, D. J., Hull, W. B., and Keegan, H. L. (1956). "A Manual of Parasitic Mites of Medical or Economic Importance," Tech. Publ. Natl. Pest Control Assoc., New York.

39. Baker, H. J., Cassell, G. H., and Lindsey, J. R. (1971). Research complications due to *Haemobartonella* and *Eperythrozoon* infections in experimental animals. *Am. J. Pathol.* **64**, 625–652.

40. Baker, J. R. (1972). Protozoa of tissues and blood (other than the Haemosporina). *In* "Pathology of Simian Primates" (R. N. T.-W. Fiennes, ed.), Part 2, pp. 29–56. Karger, Basel.

41. Banks, N. (1901). A new genus of endoparasitic acarians. *Geneeskd. Tidschr. Ned.-Indie* **41**, 334–336.

42. Barretto, M. P., Siqueira, A. F., Ferriolli, F., and Carvalheiro, J. R. (1966). Estudos sôbre reservatorios e vectores silvestres do *Trypanosoma cruzi. Rev. Inst. Med. Trop. Sao Paulo* **8**, 103–112.

43. Baskin, G., and Eberhard, M. L. (1982). *Dirofilaria immitis* infection in a rhesus monkey *Macaca mulatta. Lab. Anim. Sci.* **32**, 401–402.

44. Baskin, G. B., Wolf, R. H., Worth, C. L., Soike, K., Gibson, S. V., and Bieri J. G. (1983). Anemia, steatitis, and muscle necrosis in marmosets (*Saguinus labiatus*). *Lab. Anim. Sci.* **33**, 74–80.

45. Baskin, G. B., Eberhard, M. L., Watson, E., and Fish, R. (1984). Diagnostic exercise: Skin lesions in sooty mangabeys. *Lab. Anim. Sci.* **34**, 602–603.

46. Battles, A. H., Greiner, E. C., and Collins, B. R. (1988). Efficacy of ivermectin against natural infection of *Strongyloides* spp. in squirrel monkeys (*Saimiri sciureus*). *Lab. Anim. Sci.* **38**, 474–476.

47. Baylis, H. A. (1928). Some further parasitic worms from Sarawak. *Ann. Mag. Nat. Hist.* [10] **1**, 606–608; cited by Inglis and Dunn (552).

48. Baylis, H. A. (1929). "A Manual of Helminthology, Medical and Veterinary." Wm. Wood; cited by Ruch (967).

49. Beach, T. D. (1936). Experimental studies on human and primate species of *Strongyloides*. V. The free-living phase of the life cycle. *Am. J. Hyg.* **23**, 243–277.

50. Beddard, F. E. (1916). On two new species of cestodes belonging to the genera *Linstowia* and *Cotugnia. Proc. Zool. Soc. London* **87**, 695–706.

51. Bedford, G. A. H. (1927). Description of a new genus and species of Anoplura (*Lemurphthirus galagus*) from a lemur. *Parasitology* **19**, 263–264.

52. Belding, D. L. (1965). "Textbook of Parasitology," 3rd ed. Appleton-Century-Crofts, New York.

53. Benenson, M. W., Takafuji, E. T., Lemon, S. M., Greenup, R. L., and Sulzar, A. J. (1982). Oocyst-transmitted toxoplasmosis associated with ingestion of contaminated water. *N. Engl. J. Med.* **307**, 666–669.

54. Benirschke, K. (1979). Diagnostic exercise. *Lab. Anim. Sci.* **29**, 33–34.

55. Benirschke, K. (1983). Occurrence of spontaneous diseases. *In* "Viral and Immunological Diseases in Nonhuman Primates" (S. S. Kalter, ed.), pp. 17–30. Liss, New York.

56. Benirschke, K., and Adams, F. D. (1980). Gorilla diseases and causes of death. *J. Reprod. Fertil. Suppl.* **28**, 139–148.

57. Benirschke, K., and Low, R. J. (1970). Acute toxoplasmosis in woolly monkey (*Lagothrix* spp). *Comp. Pathol. Bull* **2**, 3–4.

58. Benirschke, K., and Richart, R. (1960). Spontaneous acute toxoplasmosis in a marmoset monkey. *Am. J. Trop. Med. Hyg.* **9**, 269–273.

59. Benirschke, K., Miller, C., Ippen, R., and Heldstab, A. (1985). The pathology of prosimians, especially lemurs. *Adv. Vet. Sci. Comp. Med.* **30**, 167–208.

60. Benson, R. E., Fremming, B. D., and Young, R. J. (1955). "Care and Management of Chimpanzees at the Radiobiological Laboratory of the University of Texas and the United States Air Force, School of Aviation Medicine," U. S. Air Force Rep. No. 55-48.

61. Berghe van den, L., Peel, E., and Chardome, M. (1956). *Trypanosoma irangiense*, n. sp. parasite du singe de nuit *Protodicticus* [sic] *potto ibeanus* an Congo belge. *Folia Sci. Afr. Cent.* **2**, 17.

62. Berghe van den, L., Chardome, M., and Peel, E. (1956). Etude d'an trypanosome du potto. *Folia Sci. Afr. Cent.* **2**, 20.

63. Berghe van den, L., Chardome, M., and Peel, E. (1963). Trypanosomes of the African lemurs, *Perodicticus potto ibeanus* and *Galago demidovi thomasi. J. Protozool.* **10**, 133–135.

64. Berghe van den, L., Chardome, M., and Peel, E. (1964). The filarial parasites of the eastern gorilla in the Congo. *J. Helminthol.* **38**, 349–368.

65. Bergner, J. F., Jr., and Jachowski, L. A., Jr. (1968). The filarial parasite *Macacanema formosana*, from the Taiwan monkey and its development in various arthropods. *Formosan Sci.* **22**, 1–68.

66. Bernstein, J. J. (1972). An epizootic of hydatid disease in captive apes. *J. Zoo Anim. Med.* **3**, 16–20.

67. Betterton, C., and Lim, B. L. (1975). Digenetic trematodes from rats, squirrels and tree shrews in Malaysia. *Southeast Asian J. Trop. Med. Public Health* **6**, 343–358.

68. Bezubik, B., and Furmaga, S. (1959). The helminth parasites in *Macacus rhesus* Audeb., from China. *Acta Parsitol. Pol.* **7**, 591–598.

69. Bezubik, B., and Fermaga, S. (1960). The parasites in *Macacus cynomolgus* L. from Indonesia. *Acta Parasitol. Pol.* **8**, 334–344.

70. Biagi, F. F., and Beltran, F. H. (1969). The challenge of amoebiasis: Understanding pathogenic mechanisms. *Int. Rev. Trop. Med.* **3**, 219–239.

71. Bingham, G. A., and Rabstein, M. M. (1964). A study of the effectiveness of thiabendazole in the rhesus monkey. *Lab. Anim. Care* **14**, 357–365.

72. Bisseru, B. (1967). "Diseases of Man Acquired from his Pets." Heinemann, London.

73. Blackie, W. K. (1932). A helminthological survey of southern Rhodesia. *Mem. London Sch. Hyg. Trop. Med.* **9**, 91.

74. Blacklock, B., and Adler, S. (1922). A parasite resembling *Plasmodium falciparum* in a chimpanzee. *Ann. Trop. Med. Parasitol.* **16**, 99–106.

75. Blacklock, B., and Adler, J. (1922). The pathological effects produced by *Strongyloides* in a chimpanzee. *Ann. Trop. Med. Parasitol.* **16**, 283–290.

76. Blair, W. R. (1904). Internal parasites in wild animals. *Rep. N.Y. Zool. Soc.* **8**, 129.

77. Blair, W. R. (1912). Some common affections of the respiratory tract and digestive organs among primates. *Zoologica (N.Y.)* **1**, 175–186; cited by Ruch (967).

78. Blampied, N. Le Q., Allchurch, A. F., and Tagg, J. (1983). Diagnosis, treatment and control of *Pterygodermatites* (*Mesopectines*) *alphi* (Nematoda: Spirurida) in the collection of Callitrichidae and Callimiconidae at the Jersey Wildlife Preservation Trust. *J. Jersey Wildl. Trust* **20**, 90–91.

79. Blanchard, J. L., and Baskin, G. B. (1988). Trichomonas gastritis in rhesus monkeys infected with the simian immunodeficiency virus. *J. Infect. Dis.* **157**, 1092–1093.

80. Blanchard, J. L., and Eberhard, M. L. (1986). Clinical note—Case Report: Esophageal *Spirura* infection in a squirrel monkey (*Saimiri sciureus*). *Am. J. Primatol.* **10**, 279–282.

81. Blanchard, R., and Langeron, M. (1913). Le paludisme des macaques (*Plasmodium cynomolgi* Mayer, 1907). *Arch. Parasitol.* **15**, 529–542.

82. Boever, W. J., and Britt, J. (1975). Hydatid disease in a mandrill baboon. *J. Am. Vet. Med. Assoc.* **167**, 619–621.

83. Böhm, L. K., and Supperer, R. (1955). Zwei neue lungenmilben aus menschenaffen: *Pneumonyssus oudemansi* and *Pneumonyssus vitzthumi* (Ascarina, Halarachnidae). *Oesterr. Zool. Z.* **6**, 11–29.

84. Bond, V. P., Bostic, W., Hansen, E. L., and Anderson, A. H. (1946). Pathologic study of natural amebic infection in macaques. *Am. J. Trop. Med.* **26**, 625–629.

85. Bonne, C., and Sandground, J. H. (1939). On the production of gastric tumors, bordering on malignancy in Javanese monkeys through the agency of *Nochtia nochti*, A parasitic nematode. *Am. J. Cancer* **37**, 173–185.

86. Borst, G. H. A., and van Knapen, F. (1984). Acute acquired toxoplasmosis in primates in a zoo. *J. Zoo Anim. Med.* **15**, 60–62.

87. Bostrom, R. C., and Slaughter, L. J. (1968). Trematode (*Athesmia foxi*) infection in two squirrel monkeys (*Saimiri sciureus*). *Lab. Anim. Care* **18**, 493–495.

88. Bostrom, R. E., Ferrell, J. F., and Martin, J. E. (1968). Simian amebiasis with lesions simulating human amebic dysentery. *19th Annu. Sess. Am. Assoc. Lab. Anim. Sci.,* Las Vegas, Abstr. No. 51.

89. Brack, M., and Niemitz, C. (1984). The parasites of wild-caught tarsiers (*Tarsiurs bancanus*). *In* "Biology of Tarsius" (C. Niemitz, ed.), pp. 77–84. Fischer, New York.

90. Brack, M., and Rietschel, W. (1986). Ivermectin for the control of *Strongyloides fuelleborni* in rhesus monkeys. *Kleintier-Prax.* (Short commun.) **31**, 29 (in German); cited by Battles *et al.* (46).

91. Brack, M., Myers, B. J., and Kuntz, R. E. (1973). Pathogenic properties of *Molineus torulosus* in capuchin monkeys, *Cebus apella. Lab. Anim. Sci.* **23**, 360–365.

92. Brack, M., Boncyk, L. H., and Kalter, S. S. (1974). *Filaroides cebus* (Gebauer, 1933)—Parasitism and respiratory infections in *Cebus apella. J. Med. Primatol.* **3**, 164–173.

93. Brack, M., Naberhaus, F., and Heymann, E. (1987). *Tupaiataenia quentini* (Schmidt & File, 1977) in *Tupaia belangeri* (Wagner, 1841): Transmission experiments and praziqantel treatment. *Lab. Anim.* **21**, 18–19.

94. Brady, A. G., Pindak, F. F., Abee, C. R., and Gardner, W. A., Jr. (1988). Enteric trichomonads of squirrel monkeys (*Saimiri* sp.): Natural infestation and treatment. *Am. J. Primatol.* **14**, 65–71.

95. Brannon, M. J. C., and Faust, E. C. (1949). Preparation and testing of a specific antigen for diagnosis of human strongyloidiasis. *Am. J. Trop. Med. Hyg.* **29**, 229–239.

96. Bray, R. S. (1956). Studies on malaria in chimpanzees: I. The erythrocytic forms of *Plasmodium reichenowi. J. Parasitol.* **42**, 588–592.

97. Bray, R. S. (1957). Studies on malaria in chimpanzees: III. Gametogony of *Plasmodium reichenowi. Ann. Soc. Belge Med. Trop.* **37**, 169–174.

98. Bray, R. S. (1958). Studies on malaria in chimpanzees: V. The sporogonous cycle and mosquito transmission of *Plasmodium vivax schwetzi. J. Parasitol.* **44**, 46–51.

99. Bray, R. S. (1959). Pre-erythrocytic stages of human malaria parasites: *Plasmodium malariae. Br. Med. J.* **2**, 679–680.

100. Bray, R. S. (1960). Studies on malaria in chimpanzees: VIII. The experimental transmission and pre-erythrocytic phase of *Plasmodium malariae*, with a note on the host-range of the parasite. *Am. J. Trop. Med. Hyg.* **9**, 455–465.

101. Bray, R. S. (1963). Malaria infections in primates and their importance to man. *Ergeb. Mikrobiol., Immunitaetsforsch. Exp. Ther.* **36**, 168–213.

102. Bray, R. S. (1963). The malaria parasites of anthropoid apes. *J. Parasitol.* **49**, 888–898.

103. Bray, R. S. (1964). A check-list of the parasitic protozoa of west Africa with some notes on their classification. *Bull. Inst. Fr. Afr. Noire, Ser. A* **26**, 238–315.

104. Brede, H. D., and Burger, P. J. (1977). *Physaloptera caucasica* (= *abbreviata caucasica*) in the South African baboon (*Papio ursinus*). *Arb. Paul-Ehrlich-Inst. Georg-Speyer-Haus Ferdinand-Blum-Inst. Frankfurt am Main* **71**, 119–122.

105. Breznock, A. W., and Pulley, T. L. (1975). *Anatrichosoma* infection in two white-handed gibbons. *J. Am. Vet. Med. Assoc.* **167**, 631.

106. Britz, W. E., Jr., Fineg, J., Cook, J. E., and Miksche, E. D. (1961). Restraint and treatment of young chimpanzees. *J. Am. Vet. Med. Assoc.* **138**, 653–658.

107. Bronsdon, M. A. (1984). Rapid dimethyl sulfoxide-modified acid-fast stain of *Cryptosporidium* oocysts in stool specimens. *J. Clin. Microbiol.* **19**, 952–953.

108. Brooks, B. A. (1963). More notes on *Saimiri sciureus. Lab. Primate Newsl.* **2**, 3–4.

109. Brown, H. W., and Perna, V. P. (1958). An overwhelming *Strongyloides* infection. *J. Am. Vet. Med. Assoc.* **138**, 653–658.

110. Brown, R. J. (1969). Acanthocephalan myositis in a bushbaby. *J. Am. Vet. Med. Assoc.* **155**, 1141–1143.

111. Brown, R. J., Hinkle, D. K., Trevethan, S. P., Kupper, J. L., and McKee, A. E. (1972). Nosematosis in a squirrel monkey (*Saimiri sciureus*). *J. Med. Primatol.* **2**, 114–123.

112. Brug, S. L. (1934). Observations on monkey malaria. *Riv. Malariol.* **13**, 121–142.

113. Brumpt, E. (1939). Les parasites du paludisme des chimpanzés. *C. R. Seances Soc. Biol. Ses Fil.* **130**, 837–840.

114. Brumpt, E., and Joyeux, E. (1912). Sur un infusoire nouveau parasite du chimpanzé *Troglodytella abrassarti*, n. g, n. sp. *Bull. Soc. Pathol. Exot.* **5**, 499–503.

115. Brumpt, E., and Urbain, A. (1938). Épizootie vermineuse por canthocéphales (*Prosthenorchis*) ayant sévi ala singerie due Muséum de Paris. *Ann. Parasitol. Hum. Comp.* **16**, 289–300.

116. Bryant, J. L., Stills, H. F., and Middleton, C. C. (1983). *Cryptosporidia* in squirrel monkeys (*Saimiri sciureus*). *34th Annu./Sess., Am. Assoc. Lab. Anim. Sci.,* Abstr. No. 6.

117. Buck, G., Coudurier, J., and Quesnel, J. J. (1952). Sur deux nouveaux *Plasmodium* observés chez un lémurien de Madagascar splénectomise. *Arch. Inst. Pasteur Algé.* **30**, 240–243.

118. Buckley, J. J. C. (1931). On two new species of *Enterobius* from the monkey *Lagothrix humboldti. J. Helminthol.* **9**, 133–140.

119. Buckley, J. J. C. (1949). Cysticerci in liver and lung of ring-tailed lemur. *Trans. R. Soc. Trop. Med. Hyg.* **43**, 2.

120. Buckley, J. J. C. (1960). On *Brugia* gen. nov. for *Wuchereria* sp. of the "*malayi*" group, i.e. *W. malayi* (Brug, 1927), *W. pahangi* Buckley and Edeson, 1956, and *W. pateri* Buckley, Nelson and Heisch, 1958. *Ann. Trop. Med. Parasitol.* **54**, 75–77.

121. Bullock, B. C., Wolf, R. H., and Clarkson, T. B. (1967). Myocarditis associated with trypanosomiasis in a cebus monkey (*Cebus albifrons*). *J. Am. Vet. Med. Assoc.* **151**, 920–922.

122. Bunton, T. E., Lowenstine, L. V., and Leininger, R. (1983). Invasive trichomoniasis in a *Callicebus moloch. Vet. Pathol.* **20**, 491–494.

123. Burrows, R. B. (1965). "Microscopic Diagnosis of the Parasites of Man VI." Yale University Press, New Haven, CT.

124. Burrows, R. B. (1972). Protozoa of the intestinal tract. *In* "Pathology of Simian Primates" (R. N. T.-W. Fiennes, ed.), Part 2, pp. 2–28. Karger, Basel.

125. Burton, F. D., and Underwood, C. (1976). Intestinal helminths in *Macaca sylvanus* of Gibraltar. *Can. J. Zool.* **54**, 1406–1407.

126. Butler, T. M. (1973). The chimpanzee. *In* Selected Topics in Laboratory Animal Medicine," Aeromed. Rev. 1–73, Vol. 16, U.S.A.F. Sch. Aerosp. Med., Aerosp. Med. Div. (AFSC), Brooks Air Force Base, Texas.

127. Bywater, J. E. C., and Mann, K. H. (1960). Infestation of a monkey with the leech *Dinobdella ferox. Vet. Rec.* **72**, 955.

128. Caballero, C. E., and Peregrina, D. I. (1938). Nemátodes de los mamiferos de México, I. *An. Inst. Biol., Univ. Nac. Auton. Méx.* **18**, 169.

129. Cahill, K. M. (1967). Thiabendazole in massive strongyloidiasis. *Am. J. Trop. Med. Hyg.* **16**, 451–453.

130. Cameron, T. W. M. (1929). The species of *Enterobius* Leach, in primates. *J. Helminthol.* **7**, 161–182.

131. Caminiti, B. (1970–1984). "Parasites of the Digestive System of Nonhuman Primates and Tupaiidae: A Bibliography." Primate Information Center, University of Washington, Seattle.

132. Canavan, W. P. N. (1929). Nematode parasites of vertebrates in the Philadelphia Zoological Garden and vicinity. *Parasitology* **21**, 63–102.

133. Canning, E. U. (1977). Microsporidea. *In* "Parasitic Protozoa" (J. P. Kreier, ed.), Vol. 4, pp. 155–196. Academic Press, New York.

134. Casey, H. W., Ayers, K. M., and Robinson, F. R. (1978). The urinary system. *In* "Pathology of Laboratory Animals" (K. Benirschke, F. M. Garner, and T. C. Jones, eds.), Vol. I, Chapter 3, pp. 116–173. Springer-Verlag, New York.

135. Castellani, A., and Chalmers, A. J. (1910). "Manual of Tropical Medicine." Baillière, Tindall and Cox, London.

136. Castellani, A., and Chalmers, A. J. (1913). "Manual of Tropical Medicine," 2nd ed. Baillière, Tindall and Cox, London.

137. Chabaud, A. G. (1952). Le genre *Dipetalonema* Diesing 1861: Essai de classification. *Ann. Parasitol. Hum. Comp.* **27**, 250–285.

138. Chabaud, A. G. (1955). Essai d'interprétation phylétique des cycles évolutifs chez les nématodes parasites de vértébres. Conclusions taxomoniques. *Ann. Parasitol. Hum. Comp.* **30**, 83–126.

139. Chabaud, A. G., and Anderson, R. C. (1959). Nouvel essai de classification des filaires (superfamille des Filarioidea) II. *Ann. Parasitol. Hum. Comp.* **34**, 64–87.

140. Chabaud, A. G., and Choquet, M. T. (1953). Nouvel essai de classification des filaires superfamille des Filarioidea. *Ann. Parasitol. Hum. Comp.* **28**, 172–192.

141. Chabaud, A. G., and Choquet, M. T. (1954). Nymphes du pentastome *Gigliolella* (n. gen.) *brumpti* (Giglioli, 1922) chez un Lémurien. *Riv. Parassitol.* **15**, 331–336.

142. Chabaud, A. G., and Choquet, M. T. (1955). Deux nématodes parasites de lémurien. *Ann. Parasitol. Hum. Comp.* **30**, 329.

143. Chabaud, A. G., and Durette-Desset, M. C. (1975). *Uncinaria* (*Megadeirides*) *olseni* n.sp., nematode a caracteres archaiques parasite d'un *Tupaia* a Borneo. *Ann. Parasitol. Hum. Comp.* **50**, 789–793.

144. Chabaud, A. G., and Petter, A. J. (1958). Les nématodes parasites de lémuriens Malgaches. I. *Mém. Inst. Sci. Madagascar, Ser. A* **12**, 139–158; cited by Inglis and Dunn (552).

145. Chabaud, A. G., and Petter, A. J. (1959). Les nématodes parasites de lémuriens Malgaches. II. Un nouvel oxyure: *Lemuricola contagiosus. Mém. Inst. Sci. Madagascar, Ser. A* **13**, 127–132; cited by Inglis and Dunn (552).

146. Chabaud, A. G., and Rousselot, R. (1956). Un nouveau spiruridae parasite du gorille *Chitwoodspirura wehri* n.g., n.sp. *Bull. Soc. Pathol. Exot.* **49**, 467–472.

147. Chabaud, A. G., Petter, A. J., and Golvan, Y. J. (1961). Les nématodes parasites de lémuriens Malgaches. III. Collection recolteé par M et Mme Francis Petter. *Ann. Parasitol. Hum. Comp.* **36**, 113–126; cited by Inglis and Dunn (552).

148. Chagas, C. (1909). Neue Trypanosomen. *Vorläufige Mitt. Arch. Schiffs Trop.-Hyg.* **13**, 120–122.

149. Chagas, C. (1924). Infection naturelle des singes du para (*Chrysothrix sciureus* L.) par *Trypanosoma cruzi. C. R. Seances Soc. Biol. Ses Fil.* **90**, 873–876.

150. Chalifoux, L. V., Hunt, R. D., Garcia, F. G., Sehgal, P. K., and Comiskey, J. R. (1973). Filariasis in New World monkeys: Histochemical differentiation of circulating microfilariae. *Lab. Anim. Sci.* **23**, 211–220.

151. Chalmers, D. T., Murgatroyd, L. B., and Wadsworth, P. F. (1983). A survey of the pathology of marmosets (*Callithrix jacchus*) derived from a marmoset breeding unit. *Lab. Anim.* **17**, 270–279.

152. Chandler, A. C. (1925). New records of *Bertiella satyri* (cestoda) in man and apes. *Parasitology* **17**, 421–425.

153. Chandler, A. C. (1929). Some new genera and species of nematode worms, Filarioidea, from animals dying in the Calcutta Zoological Garden. *Proc. U.S. Natl. Mus.* **75**, 1.

154. Chandler, A. C. (1953). An outbreak of *Prosthenorchis* (Acanthocephala) infection in primates in the Houston Zoological Garden, and a report of this parasite in *Nasua narica* in Mexico. *J. Parasitol.* **39**, 226.

155. Chandler, A. C., and Read, C. P. (1961). "Introduction to Parasitology, with Special Reference to the Parasites of Man," 10th ed. Wiley, New York.

156. Chandler, F. W., McClure, H. M., Campbell, W. G., Jr., and Watts, J. C. (1976). Pulmonary pneumocystosis in nonhuman primates. *Arch. Pathol. Lab. Med.* **100**, 163–167.

157. Chang, J., and McClure, H. M. (1975). Disseminated oesophagostomiasis in the rhesus monkey. *J. Am. Vet. Med. Assoc.* **167**, 628–630.

158. Chang, J., Kornegay, R. W., Wagner, J. L., Mikat, E. M., and Hackel, D. B. (1980). Toxoplasmosis in a sifaka. *In* "The Comparative Pathology of Zoo Animals" (R. J. Montali and G. Migaki, eds.), pp. 347–352. Smithsonian Institution Press, Washington, DC.

159. Chang, P. C. H., and Graham, G. L. (1957). Parasitism, parthenogenesis and polyploidy: The life cycle of *Strongyloides papillosus. J. Parasitol. Suppl.* **43**, 13.

160. Chapman, W. L., Crowell, W. A., and Isaac, W. (1973). Spontaneous lesions seen at necropsy in 7 owl monkeys (*Aotus trivirgatus*). *Lab. Anim. Sci.* **23**, 434–442.

161. Chardome, M., and Peel, E. (1949). La répartition des filaires dans la région de Coquilhatville et la transmission de *Dipetalonema streptocerca* par *Culicoides grahami. Ann. Soc. Belge Med. Trop.* **29**, 99–119.

162. Chase, R. E., and Degaris, C. F. (1938). Anomalies of venae cavae superiores in an orang. *Am. J. Phys. Anthropol.* **24**, 61–65.

163. Cheever, A. W., Kirschstein, R. L., and Reardon, L. V. (1970). *Schistosoma mansoni* infection of presumed natural origin in *Cercopithecus* monkeys from Tanzania and Ethiopa. *Bull. W. H. O.* **42**, 486–490.

164. Cheng, T. C. (1964). "The Biology of Animal Parasites." Saunders, Philadelphia.

165. Chin, W., Contacos, P. G., Coatney, G. R., and Kimball, H. R. (1965). A naturally acquired quotidian-type malaria in man transferable to monkeys. *Science* **149**, 865.

166. Chitwood, M. (1970). Comparative relationships of some parasites of man and Old and New World subhuman primates. *Lab. Anim. Care* **20**, 389–394.

167. Chitwood, M., and Lichtenfels, J. R. (1972). Identification of parasitic metazoa in tissue sections. *Exp. Parasitol.* **32**, 407–519.

168. Chitwood, M. B., and Smith, W. N. (1958). A redescription of *Anatrichosoma cynomolgi* Smith and Chitwood 1954. *Proc. Helminthol. Soc., Wash.* **25**, 112–117.

169. Christeller, E. (1922). Über die balantidienruhr bei den schimpansen des Berliner Zoologischen Gartens. *Virchows Arch. A: Pathol. Anat.* **238**, 396–422; cited by Ruch (967).

170. Christensen, L. T. (1964). Chimp and owners share worm infestation. *Vet. Med.* **59**, 801–803.

171. Cicmanec, J. L., Neva, F. A., McClure, H. M., and Loeb, W. F. (1974). Accidental infection of laboratory-reared *Macaca mulatta* with *Trypanosma cruzi. Lab. Anim. Sci.* **24**, 783–787.

172. Clark, J. D. (1969). Coenurosis in a Gelada baboon (*Theropithecus gelada*). *J. Am. Vet. Med. Assoc.* **155**, 1258–1263.

173. Clarkson, T. B., Bullock, B. C., Lehner, N. D. M., and Manning, P. J. (1970). Diseases affecting the usefulness of nonhuman primates for nutrition research. *In* "Feeding and Nutrition of Nonhuman Primates" (R. S. Harris, ed.), pp. 233–250. Academic Press, New York.

174. Coatney, G. R., Elbel, R. E., and Kocharatana, P. (1960). Some blood parasites found in birds and mammals from Loei Province, Thailand. *J. Parasitol.* **46**, 701–702.

175. Coatney, G. R., Collins, W. E., Warren, McW., and Contacos, P. G. (1971). "The Primate Malarias." U.S. Govt. Printing Office, Washington, DC.

176. Cochrane, J. C., Sagorin, L., and Wilcocks, M. G. (1957). *Capillaria hepatica* infection in man. A syndrome of extreme eosinophilia, hepatomegaly and hyperglobulinemia. *S. Afr. Med. J.* **31**, 751–755.

177. Cockburn, T. A. (1948). *Balantidium* infection associated with diarrhoea in primates. *Trans. R. Soc. Trop. Med. Hyg.* **42**, 291–293.

178. Cockrell, B. Y., Valerio, M. G., and Garner, F. M. (1974). Cryptosporidiosis in the intestines of rhesus monkeys (*Macaca mulatta*). *Lab. Anim. Sci.* **24**, 881–887.

179. Collet, J.-Y., Galdikas, B. M. F., Sugarjito, J., and Jojosudharmo, S. (1986). A coprological study of parasitism in orangutans (*Pongo pygmaeus*) in Indonesia. *J. Med. Primatol.* **15**, 121–129.

180. Colley, F. C., and Mullin, S. W. (1972). *Eimeria pachylepyron* sp. n. (Protozoa: Eimeriidae) from the slow loris in Malaysia. *J. Parasitol.* **58**, 110–111.

181. Collins, W. E. (1974). Primate malarias. *Adv. Vet. Sci. Comp. Med.* **18**, 1–23.

182. Collins, W. E. (1982). Simian malaria. *In* "Parasitic Zoonoses" (L. Jacobs and P. Arambulo, eds.), CRC Handb. Ser. Zoonoses, Sect. C, Vol. I, pp. 141–150. CRC Press, Boca Raton, FL.

183. Collins, W. E., and Aikawa, M. (1977). Plasmodia of nonhuman primates. *In* "Parasitic Protozoa" (J. P. Kreier, ed.), Vol. 3, pp. 467–492. Academic Press, New York.

184. Collins, W. E., Contacos, P. G., Garnham, P. C. C., Warren, McW., and Skinner, J. C. (1972). *Plasmodium hylobati:* A malaria parasite of the gibbon. *J. Parasitol.* **58**, 123–128.

185. Conrad, H. D., and Wong, M. M. (1969). *Anatrichosoma* sp in Old World non-human primates. *Program Abstr., 44th Annu. Meet. Am. Soc. Parasitol.* No. 52, p. 41; cited by Orihel (844).

186. Conrad, H. D., and Wong, M. M. (1973). Studies of *Anatrichosoma* (Nematoda: Trichinellida) with descriptions of *Anatrichosoma rhina* sp. n. and *Anatrichosoma nacepobi* sp. n. from the nasal mucosa of *Macaca mulatta. J. Helminthol.* **57**, 289–302.

187. Conran, P. B. (1967). Monkey malaria. *18th Annu. Meet., Am. Assoc. Lab. Anim. Sci.,* Washington, DC, Abstr. No. 38.

188. Contacos, P. G., Lunn, J. S., Coatney, G. R., Kilpatrick, J. W., and Jones, F. E. (1963). Quartan-type malaria parasite of new world monkeys transmissible to man. *Science* **142**, 676.

189. Cooley, R. A., and Kohls, G. M. (1944). The Argasidae of North America, Central America and Cuba. *Am. Midl. Nat. Monogr.* **1**.

190. Cooreman, J. (1946). Observations sur *Pneumonyssus duttoni* Newstead et Todd. Acarien parasite de la trachée de *Cercopithecus ascanius* Audebert au Congo belge. *Rev. Zool. Bot. Afr.* **39**, 331–335.

191. Copeland, B. E., and Kimber, J. (1968). Nuclear size in diagnosis of *Entamoeba histolytica* on stained smears. *Am. J. Clin. Pathol.* **38**, 664–668.

192. Cosgrove, G. E. (1966). The trematodes of laboratory primates. *Lab. Animal Care* **16**, 23–29.

193. Cosgrove, G. E., Nelson, B. M., and Jones, A. W. (1963). *Spirura tamarini* sp. n. (Nematoda: Spiruridae) from an Amazon primate, *Tamarinus nigricolis* (Spix, 1823). *J. Parasitol.* **49**, 1010–1013.

194. Cosgrove, G. E., Nelson, B., and Gengozian, N. (1968). Helminth parasites of the tamarin, *Saguinus fusciollis. Lab. Anim. Care* **18**, 654–656.

195. Cosgrove, G. E., Humason, G., and Lusbaugh, C. C. (1970). *Trichospirura leptostoma,* a nematode of the pancreatic ducts of marmosets (*Saguinus* spp.) *J. Am. Vet. Med. Assoc.* **157**, 696–698.

196. Cosgrove, G. E., Nelson, B. M., and Self, J. T. (1970). The pathology of pentastomid infection in primates. *Lab. Anim. Care* **20**, 354–360.

197. Coulanges, P., Zeller, H., Clark, Y., Rodhain, F., and Albignac, R. (1979). La pathologie des lémuriens malgaches et ses relations avec la pathologie humaine. *Bull. Soc. Pathol. Exot.* **72**, 272–278.

198. Cram, E. B. (1928). A species of the genus *Bertiella* in man and chimpanzees in Cuba. *Am. J. Trop. Med. Hyg.* **8**, 339–344.

199. Crockett, E. C. (1985). *Bertiella studeri* in a mona monkey (*Cercopithecus mona mona*) in Nigeria. *Vet. Rec.* **116**, 268.

200. Crockett, E. C., and Dipeolu, O. O. (1984). A survey of helminth parasites of game animals in Kainji Lake National Park of Nigeria. *Int. J. Zoonoses* **11**, 204–215.

201. Crosby, W. M., Ivey, M. H., Shaffer, W. L., and Holmes, D. D. (1968). *Echinococcus* cysts in the savannah baboon. *Lab. Anim. Care* **18**, 395–397.

202. Cruz, A. A. da, and De Sousa, L. (1959). *Armillifer armillatus* in chimpanzee (*Pan satyrus verus*). *Rev. Cienc. Vet. (Lisbon)* **54**, 21–24.

203. Culberson, D. E., Pindak, F. F., Gardner, W. A., and Honigberg, B. M. (1986). *Tritrichomonas mobilensis* n. sp. (Zoomastigophorea: Trichomonadida) from the Bolivian squirrel monkey *Saimiri boliviensis boliviensis. J. Protozool.* **33**, 301–304.

204. Culberson, D. E., Scimeca, J. M., Jr., Pindak, F. F., and Gardner, W. A., Jr. (1987). *Tritrichomonas mobilensis* pathogenicity: A microscopic perspective. *Trans. Am. Microsc. Soc.* **106**, 94.

205. Culberson, D. E., Scimeca, J. M., Jr., Gardner, W. A., and Abee, C. R. (1988). Pathogenicity of *Tritrichomonas mobilensis:* Subcutaneous inoculation in mice. *J. Parasitol.* **74**, 774–780.

206. Cullum, L. E., and Hamilton, B. R. (1965). Thiabendazole as an anthelmintic in research monkeys. *Am. J. Vet. Res.* **26**, 779–780.

207. Cummings, B. F. (1916). Studies on the Anoplura and Mallophaga being a report upon a collection from the mammals and birds in the Society's gardens. *Proc. Zool. Soc. London* **1**, 253–295.

208. Cummins, L. B., Keeling, M. E., and McClure, H. M. (1973). Preventive medicine in anthropoids: Parasite control. *Lab. Anim. Sci.* **23**, 819–822.

209. Cunha A. da, and Muniz, J. (1929). Nota sobre os parasitas intestinaes do *Macacus rhesus* com a descripção de una nova especie de *Octomitus. Mem. Inst. Oswaldo Cruz, Suppl.* **5**, 34–35.

210. Cunningham, A. A., Buxton, D., and Thomson, K. M. (1992). An epidemic of toxoplasmosis in a captive colony of squirrel monkeys (*Saimiri sciureus*). *J. Comp. Pathol.* **107**, 207–219.

211. Curasson, G. C. M. (1929). *Troglodytella abrassarti* infusoire pathogène du chimpanzé. *Ann. Parasitol. Hum. Comp.* **7**, 465–468.

212. D'Allessandro, A., Eberhard, M., de Hincopie, O., and Holstead, S. (1986). *Trypanosoma cruzi* and *Trypanosoma rangeli* in *Saimiri sciurius* from Bolivia and *Saguinus mystax* from Brazil. *Am. J. Trop. Med. Hyg.* **35**, 285–289.

213. Dannemiller, S. D. (1991). Personal communication.

214. Das, K. M. (1965). Discussion. *In* "Pathology of Laboratory Animals" (W. E. Ribelin and J. R. McCoy, eds.), pp. 363–364. Thomas, Springfield, IL.

215. Davies, R. B., and Hibler, C. P. (1979). Animal reservoirs and cross-species transmission of *Giardia. In* "Waterborne Transmission of Giardiasis" (W. Jakubowski and J. C. Hoff, eds.), pp. 104–126, U. S. Environmental Protection Agency, Office of Research & Development, Environmental Research Center, Springfield, VA.

216. Deane, L. M. (1962). Infecção natural sagüi *Callithrix jacchus* por tripanosoma do tipo *cruzi. Rev. Inst. Med. Trop. Sao Paulo* **4,** 255–229.

217. Deane, L. M. (1964). Animal reservoirs of *Trypanosoma cruzi* in Brazil. *Rev. Bras. Malariol. Doencas Trop.* **16,** 27–48.

218. Deane, L. M. (1967). Tripanosomídeos de mamiferos de regiao Amazônico. *Rev. Inst. Med. Trop. Sao Paulo* **9,** 143–148.

219. Deane, L. M., and Damasceno, R. G. (1961). Tripanosomídeos de mamiferos de regiano Amazô-nico: II. Tripanosomas de macacos de zona de Salgado, estado do Para. *Rev. Inst. Med. Trop. Sao Paulo* **3,** 61–70.

220. Deane, L. M., and Martins, R. (1952). Sobre um tripansoma encontrado em macaco da Amazô-nica e que evolui em triatomineos. *Rev. Bras. Malariol. Doencas Trop.* **4,** 47–61.

221. Deane, L. M., Deane, M. P., and Neto, J. F. (1966). Studies on transmission of simian maliaria and on a natural infection of man with *Plasmodium simium* in Brazil. *Bull. W. H. O.* **35,** 805–808.

222. Deane, L. M., Ferreira, N., and Sitonio, J. G. (1968). Novo hospedeiro natural do *Plasmodium simium* e do *Plasmodium brasilianum:* O mono, *Brachyteles arachnoides. Rev. Inst. Med. Trop. Sao Paulo,* **10,** 287–288.

223. Deane, L. M., Batista, D., Ferreria Neto, J. A., and DeSouza, H. (1970). Tripanosomídeos de maniferos da Regiã Amazô-nico V-*Trypanosoma lambrechti* Marinkelle, 1968, em macacos de Estado do Amazonas, Brasil. *Rev. Inst. Med. Trop. Sao Paulo.* **12,** 1–7.

224. Deinhardt, F., Holmes, A. W., Devine, J., and Deinhardt, J. (1967). Marmosets as laboratory animals. IV. The microbiology of laboratory kept marmosets. *Lab. Anim. Care* **17,** 48–70.

225. Deinhardt, J. B., Devine, J., Passovoy, M., Pohlman, R., and Deinhardt, F. (1967). Marmosets as laboratory animals. I. Care of marmosets in the laboratory. Pathology and outline of statistical evaluation of data. *Lab. Anim. Care* **17,** 11–29.

226. DePaoli, A. (1965). *Schistosoma haematobium* in the chimpanzee—A natural infection. *Am. J. Trop. Med. Hyg.* **14,** 561–565.

227. De Paoli, A., and Johnsen, D. O. (1978). Fatal strongyloidiasis in gibbons (*Hylobates lar*). *Vet. Pathol.* **15,** 31–39.

228. Deschiens, R. E. A. (1927). Sur les protozoaires intestinaux des singes. *Bull. Soc. Pathol. Exot.* **20,** 19–23; cited by Miller and Bray (776).

229. Deschiens, R. E. A., Limousin, H., and Troisic, J. (1927). Eléments présentant les caractères d'un protozoaire sanguicole observés chez le chimpanzé. *Bull. Soc. Pathol. Exot.* **20,** 597–600.

230. Desowitz, R. S. (1968). *Hepatocystis* sp. from a gibbon. *Trans. R. Soc. Trop. Med. Hyg.* **62,** 4.

231. Desowitz, R. S. (1970). Observations on *Hepatoystis* of white-cheeked gibbon (*Hylobates concolor*) *J. Parasitol.* **56,** 444–446.

232. Desportes, C. (1945). Sur *Strongyloides stercoralis* (Bavay 1876) et sur les *Strongyloides* des primates. *Ann. Parasitol. Hum. Comp.* **20,** 160–190.

233. Desportes, C., and Roth, P. (1943). Helminthes rècoltées au cours d'autopsies pratiquées sur différents mammifères morts à la ménagerie due Muséum de Paris. *Bull. Mus. Hist. Nat. (Paris)* **15,** 108–114; cited by Dunn (268).

234. Dickson, J., Fry, J., Fairfax, R., and Spence, T. (1983). Epidemic toxoplasmosis in captive squirrel monkeys (*Saimiri sciureus*). *Vet. Rec.* **12,** 302.

235. Dissanaike, A. S. (1958). On hydatid infection in a Ceylon toque monkey *Macaca sinica. Ceylon Vet.* **7,** 33–35.

236. Dissanaike, A. S., Nelson, P., and Garnham, P. C. C. (1965). Two new malaria parasites, *Plasmodium cynomolgi ceylonensis* subsp. nov. and *Plasmodium fragile* sp. nov., from monkeys in Ceylon. *Ceylon J. Med. Sci.* **14,** 1–9.

237. Dissanaike, A. S., Nelson, P., and Garnham, P. C. C. (1965). *Plasmodium simiovale* sp. nov. a new simian malaria parasite from Ceylon. *Ceylon J. Med. Sci.* **14,** 27–32.

238. Dobell, C. (1931). Researches on the intestinal protozoa of monkeys and man. IV. An experimental study of the *histolytica*-like species of *Entamoeba* living naturally in macaques. *Parasitology* **23,** 1–72.

239. Döbereiner, J. (1955). Toxoplasmose espontânea em macaco. *Veterinaria* **9,** 44–55.

240. Dodd, K., and Murphy, E. (1970). *Dipetalonema gracile* in a capuchin monkey (*Cebus capucinus*). *Vet. Rec.* **87,** 538–539.

241. Dollifus, R. P., and Chabaud, A. G. (1955). Cinq espèces de nématodes chez un atèle mort à la ménagerie du muséum. *Arch. Mus. Natl. Hist. Nat.* **3,** 27–40; cited by Dunn (268).

242. Donovan, J. C., Stokes, W. S., Montrey, R. D., and Rozmiarek, H. (1983). Hematologic characterization of naturally occurring malaria (*Plasmodium inui*) in cynomolgus monkeys (*Macaca fascicularis*). *Lab. Anim. Sci.* **33,** 86–89.

243. Dougherty, E. C. (1943). The genus *Filaroides* van Beneden, 1858, and its relatives. Preliminary note. *Proc. Helminthol. Soc. Wash.* **10,** 69–74.

244. Dougherty, E. C. (1952). A note on the genus *Metathelazia* Skinker, 1931 (Nematoda:Metastrongylidae). *Proc. Helminthol. Soc. Wash.* **19,** 55–63.

245. Dubey, J. P. (1973). Feline toxoplasmosis and coccidiosis: A survey of domiciled and stray cats. *J. Am. Med. Assoc.* **162,** 873–877.

246. Dubey, J. P. (1976). A review of sarcocystis of domestic animals and of other coccidia of cats and dogs. *J. Am. Vet. Med. Assoc.* **169,** 1061–1078.

247. Dubey, J. P. (1977). *Toxoplasma, Hammondia, Besnoitia, Sarcocystis,* and other tissue cyst-forming coccidia of man and animals. *In* "Parasitic Protozoa" (J. P. Kreier, ed.), Vol. 3, pp. 101–239. Academic Press, New York.

248. Dubey, J. P., Swan, G. V., and Frenkel, J. K. (1972). A simplified method for isolation of *Toxoplasma gondii* from the feces of cats. *J. Parasitol.* **58,** 1005–1006.

249. Dubey, J. P., Kramer, L. W., and Weisbrode, S. E. (1985). Acute death associated with *Toxoplasma gondii* in ring-tailed lemurs. *J. Am. Vet. Med. Assoc.* **187,** 1272–1273.

250. Dubin, I. N., and Wilcox, A. (1947). *Sarcocystis* in *Macaca mulatta. J. Parasitol.* **33,** 151–153.

251. Dubois, G. (1966). Un néodiplostome (Trematoda: Diplostomatidae) chez le tamarin *Leontocebus nigricollis* (Spix). *Rev. Suisse Zool.* **73,** 37–42.

252. Duke, B. O. L. (1954). The transmission of loiasis in the forest-fringe area of the British Cameroons. *Ann. Trop. Med. Parasitol.* **48,** 349–355.

253. Duke, B. O. L. (1954). The uptake of the microfilariae of *Acanthocheilonema streptoerca* by *Culicoides grahamii,* and their subsequent development. *Ann. Trop. Med. Parasitol.* **48,** 416–420.

254. Duke, B. O. L. (1955). The development of *Loa* in flies of the genus *Chrysops* and the probable significance of the different species in the transmission of loiasis. *Trans. R. Soc. Trop. Med. Hyg.* **49,** 115–121.

255. Duke, B. O. L. (1956). The intake of the microfilariae of *Acanthocheilonema perstans* by *Culicoides grahamii* and *C. inornatipennis,* and their subsequent development. *Ann. Trop. Med. Parasitol.* **50,** 32–38.

256. Duke, B. O. L. (1960). Studies on loiasis in monkeys. III. The pathology of the spleen in drills (*Mandrillus leucophaeus*) infected with *Loa. Ann. Trop. Med. Parasitol.* **54,** 141–146.

257. Duke, B. O. L., and Wijers, D. J. B. (1958). Studies on loiasis in monkeys: I. The relationship between humans and simian *Loa* in the rainforest zone of the British Cameroons. *Ann. Trop. Med. Parasitol.* **52,** 158–175.

258. Dumas, J. (1953). "Les animaux de laboratoire Paris." Médicales Flammarion, Paris; cited by Ruch (967).

259. Duncan, M., Tell, L., Gardiner, C. H., and Montali, R. J. (1995). Lingual gongylonemiasis and pasteurellosis in Goeldi's monkeys (*Callimico goeldii*). *J. Zoo Wildl./Med.* **26,** 102–108.

260. Dunn, F. L. (1961). *Molineus vexillarius* sp. n. (Nematoda: Trichostrongylidae) from a Peruvian primate *Tamarinus nigricollis* (Spix, 1823). *J. Parasitol.* **47**, 953–956.

261. Dunn, F. L. (1962). *Raillietina (R.) trinitatae* (Cameron and Reesal, 1951), Baer and Sandars, 1956 (Cestoda) from a Peruvian primate. *Proc. Helminthol. Soc. Wash.* **29**, 148–152.

262. Dunn, F. L. (1963). A new trichostrongylid nematode from an oriental primate. *Proc. Helminthol. Soc. Wash.* **30**, 161–165.

263. Dunn, F. L. (1963). Acanthocephalans and cestodes of South American monkeys and marmosets. *J. Parasitol.* **49**, 717–722.

264. Dunn, F. L. (1964). Blood parasites of Southeast Asian primitive primates. *J. Parasitol.* **50**, 214–216.

265. Dunn, F. L. (1964). *Odeningotrema apidion* n. sp. (Trematoda: Lecithodendriidae) from a Malayan primitive primate. *Proc. Helminthol. Soc., Wash.* **31**, 21.

266. Dunn, F. L. (1965). On the antiquity of malaria in the Western Hemisphere. *Hum. Biol.* **37**, 385–393.

267. Dunn, F. L. (1966). Patterns of parasitism in primates: Phylogenetic and ecological interpretations, with particular reference to the Hominoidea. *Folia Primatol.* **4**, 329.

268. Dunn, F. L. (1968). The parasites of *Saimiri* in the context of Platyrrhine parasitism. *In* "The Squirrel Monkey" (L. A. Rosenblum and R. W. Cooper, eds.), pp. 31–68. Academic Press, New York.

269. Dunn, F. L. (1970). Natural infection in primates: Helminths and problems in primate phylogeny, ecology, and behavior. *Lab. Anim. Care* **20**, 383–388.

270. Dunn, F. L., and Greer, W. E. (1962). Nematodes resembling *Ascaris lumbricoides* L., 1758, from a Malayan gibbon, *Hylobates agilis* F. Cuvier, 1821. *J. Parasitol.* **48**, 150.

271. Dunn, F. L., and Lambrecht, F. L. (1963). On some filarial parasites of South American primates with a description of *Tetrapetalonema tamarinae* n. sp. from the Peruvian tamarin marmoset, *Tamarinus nigricollis* (Spix, 1823). *J. Helminthol.* **37**, 261–286.

272. Dunn, F. L., and Lambrecht, F. L. (1963). The hosts of *Plasmodium brasilianum* Gonder and von Berenberg-Gossler, 1908. *J. Parasitol.* **49**, 316–319.

273. Dunn, F. L., Lambrecht, F. L., and du Plessis, R. (1963). Trypanosomes of South American monkeys and marmosets. *Am. J. Trop. Med. Hyg.* **12**, 524–534.

274. Dunn, F. L., Lim, B. L., and Yap, L. F. (1968). Endoparasite patterns in mammals of the Malayan rain forest. *Ecology* **49**, 1179–1184.

275. Durden, L. A., and DeBruyn, E. J. (1984). Louse infestations of tree shrews (*Tupaiaglis*). *Lab. Anim. Sci.* **34**, 188–190.

276. Durden, L. A., Sly, D. L., and Buck, A. T. (1985). Parasitic arthrodods of bushbabies (*Galago senegalensis* and *G. crassicaudatus*) recently imported to the U.S.A. *Lab. Primate Newsl.* **24**, 5–6.

277. Durette-Desset M. C. (1968). Nematodes heligmosomes d'Amerique du Sud. III. Nuvelles données morphologiques sur cinq espècies parasites de rongeurs ou de primates. *Bull. Mus. Natl. Hist. Nat.* [2] **40**, 1215–1221.

278. Durette-Desset, M. C., and Chabaud, A. G. (1975). Sur trois nematodes trichostrongylides parasites de Tupaiidae. *Ann. Parasitol.* **50**, 173–185.

279. Durette-Desset, M. C., Palmieri, J. R., Puronomo, and Cassone, J. (1981). Two new species of *Tupaiostongylus* Dunn, 1963 (Nematoda: Molineidae) from a tree shrew (*Tupaia tana*) of Indonesia. *Syst. Parasitol.* **3**, 237–242.

280. Duszynski, D. W., and File, S. K. (1974). Structure of oocyst and excystation of sporozoites of *Isospora endocallimici* n. sp. from marmoset *Callimico goeldii.* *Trans. Am. Microsc. Soc.* **93**, 403–408.

281. Dutton, J. E., Todd, J. L., and Tobey, E. N. (1906). Concerning certain parasitic protozoa observed in Africa. *Mem. Liverpool Sch. Trop. Med.* **21**, 87–97.

282. Eastin, C. E., and Roeckel, I. (1968). *Trypanosoma cruzi* complicating *Prosthenorchis* infestation in the squirrel monkey (*Saimiri sciureus*). *19th Annu. Meet., Am. Assoc. Lab. Anim. Sci.,* Las Vegas, Abstr. No. 52.

283. Eberhard, M. L. (1978). *Tetrapetalonema (T.) mystaxi* sp. n. (Nematoda: Filariodea) from Brazilian moustached marmosets, *Saguinus m. mystax.* *J. Parasitol.* **64**, 204–207.

284. Eberhard, M. L. (1980). *Dipetalonema (Cercopithifilaria) kenyensis* from African baboons. *J. Parasitol.* **66**, 551–554.

285. Eberhard, M. L. (1981). Intestinal parasitism in an outdoor breeding colony of *Macaca mulatta.* *Lab. Anim. Sci.* **31**, 282–285.

286. Eberhard, M. L. (1982). *Anatrichosoma* from the eye of a cynomolgus monkey. *Proc. Helminthol. Soc. Wash.* **49**, 154–155.

287. Eberhard, M. L. (1982). Chemotherapy of filariasis in squirrel monkey, *Saimiri sciureus.* *Lab. Anim. Sci.* **32**, 397–400.

288. Eberhard, M. L., and Baskin, G. B. (1982). *Polydelphis* (Nematoda: Ascarididae) larvae encysted in a feral African green monkey (*Cercopithecus aethiops*). *Proc. Helminthol. Soc. Wash.* **49**, 157–159.

289. Eberhard, M. L. and D'Alessandro A. (1982). Congenital *T. cruzi* infection in a laboratory born squirrel monkey *Saimiri Sciurius.* *Am. J. Trop. Med. Hyg.* **31**, 931–933.

290. Eberhard, M. L., and Orihel, T. C. (1984). The genus *Mansonella* (syn. *Tetrapetalonema*): A new classification. *Ann. Parasitol. Hum. Comp.* **59**, 483–496.

291. Eberhard, M. L., Pieniazek, N. J., and Arrowood, M. J. (1997). Laboratory diagnosis of *Cyclospora* infections. *Arch. Pathol.* **121**, 792–797.

292. Edeson, J. F. B., Wharton, R. H., and Laing, A. B. G. (1960). A preliminary account of the transmission, maintenance and laboratory vectors of *Brugia pahangi.* *Trans. R. Soc. Trop. Med. Hyg.* **54**, 439–449.

293. Edsall, G., Gaines, S., Landy, M., Tigertt, W. D., Sprinz, H., Trapani, R. J., Mandel, A. D., and Benenson, A. S. (1960). Studies on infection and immunity in experimental typhoid fever. I. Typhoid fever in chimpanzees orally infected with *Salmonella typhosa.* *J. Exp. Med.* **112**, 143–166.

294. Eichhorn, A., and Gallagher, B. (1916). Spontaneous amoebic dysentery in monkeys. *J. Infect. Dis.* **19**, 395–407.

295. Eisenbrandt, D. L., Floering, D. A., David, T. D., and McKee, A. E. (1978). Scanning electron microscopy of a cryofractured hydatid cyst. *Scanning Electron Microsc.* **2**, 229–233.

296. Eisenstein, R., and Innes, J. R. M. (1956). Sarcosporidiosis in man and animals. *Vet. Rev. Annot.* **2**, 61–78.

297. Elek, S. R., and Finkelstein, L. E. (1939). *Multiceps serialis* infestation in a baboon. Report of a case exhibiting multiple connective tissue masses. *Zoologica (N.Y.)* **24**, 323–328.

298. Else, J. G., Satzger, M., and Sturrock, R. F. (1982). Natural infections of *Schistosoma mansoni* and *S. haematobium* in *Cercopithecus* monkeys in Kenya. *Ann. Trop. Med. Parasitol.* **76**, 111–112.

299. Emerson, C. L., Tsai, C.-C., Holland, C. J., Ralston, P., and Diluzio, M. E. (1990). Recrudescence of *Entopolypoides macaci* Mayer, 1933 (Babesiidae) infection secondary to stress in long-tailed macaques (*Macaca fascicularis*). *Lab. Anim. Sci.* **40**, 169–171,

300. Essbach, H. (1949). Strongyloidose beim schimpansen. *Beitr. Pathol. Anat.* **110**, 319–345; cited by Ruch (967).

301. Esslinger, J. H. (1962). Hepatic lesions in rats experimentaliy infected with *Porocephalus crotali* (Pentastomida). *J. Parasitol.* **48**, 631–638.

302. Esslinger, J. H. (1966). *Dipetalonema obtusa* (McCoy, 1936) comb. n. (Filarioidea: Onchocercidae) in Colombian primates, with a description of the adult. *J. Parasitol.* **52**, 498–502.

303. Esslinger, J. H. (1979). *Tetrapetalonema (T.) panamensis* (McCoy 1936) comb. n. (Filarioidea: Onchocercidae) in Colombia primates, with a description of the adults. *J. Parasitol.* **65**, 924–927.

304. Esslinger, J. H. (1981). *Tetrapetalonema (T.) saimiri* sp. n. (Nematoda: Filarioidea) from Colombian squirrel monkeys, *Saimiri sciureus.* *J. Parasitol.* **67**, 268–271.

305. Esslinger, J. H. (1981). *Tetrapetalonema (T.) colombiensis* sp. n. (Nematoda:Filarioidea) from Colombian primates. *J. Parasitol.* **68**, 1138–1141.

306. Esslinger, J. H., and Gardiner, C. H. (1974). *Dipetalonema barbascalensis* sp. n. (Nematoda: Filarioidea) from the owl monkey, *Aotus trivirga-*

tus, with a consideration of the status of *Parlitomosa zakii* Nagaty, 1935. *J. Parasitol.* **60**, 1001–1005.

307. Evans, L. B. (1978). Fatal parasitism among free living bushbabies. *J. S. Afr. Vet. Assoc.* **49**, 67–69.

308. Ewing, H. E. (1929). Notes on the lung mites of primates (Acarina, Dermanyssidae), including the description of a new species. *Proc. Entomal. Soc. Wash.* **31**, 126–130.

309. Ewing, H. E. (1932). A new sucking louse from the chimpanzee. *Proc. Biol. Soc. Wash.* **45**, 117–118.

310. Ewing, H. E. (1938). The sucking lice of American monkeys. *J. Parasitol.* **24**, 13–33.

311. Ewing, S. A., Helland, D. R., Anthony, H. D., and Leipold, H. W. (1968). Occurrence of *Athesmia* sp. in the cinnamon ringtail monkey *Cebus albifrons. Lab. Anim. Care* **18**, 488–492.

312. Eyles, D. E. (1963). The species of simian malaria: Taxonomy, morphology, life cycle, and geographical distribution of the monkey species. *J. Parasitol.* **49**, 866–887.

313. Eyles, D. E., and Warren, McW. (1962). *Plasmodium inui* in Sulawesi. *J. Parasitol.* **48**, 739.

314. Eyles, D. E., and Warren, McW. (1963). *Hepatocystis* from *Macaca irus* in Java. *J. Parasitol.* **49**, 891.

315. Eyles, D. E., Coatney, G. R., and Getz, M. E. (1960). *Vivax*-type malaria parasite of macaques transmissible to man. *Science* **131**, 1812–1813.

316. Eyles, D. E., Fong, Y. L., Warren, McW., Guinn, E., Sandosham, A. A., and Wharton, R. H. (1962). *Plasmodium coatneyi*, a new species of primate malaria from Malaya. *Am. J. Trop. Med. Hyg.* **11**, 597–604.

317. Eyles, D. E., Laing, A. B. G., and Dobrovolny, C. G. (1962). The malaria parasites of the pig-tailed macaque *Macaca nemestrina nemestrina* (Linnaeus), in Malaya. *Indian J. Malariol.* **16**, 285–298.

318. Eyles, D. E., Laing, A. B. G., and Fong, Y. L. (1962). *Plasmodium fieldi* sp. nov., a new species of malaria parasite from the pig-tailed macaque in Malaya. *Ann. Trop. Med. Parasitol.* **56**, 242–247.

319. Eyles, D. E., Warren, McW., Fong, Y. L., Sandosham, A. A., and Dunn, F. L. (1962). A malaria parasite of Malayan gibbons. *Med. J. Malaya* **17**, 86.

320. Eyles, D. E., Fong, Y. L., Dunn, F. L., Guinn, E., Warren, McW., and Sandosham, A. A. (1964). *Plasmodium youngi* n. sp., A malaria parasite of the Malayan gibbon, *Hylobates lar lar. Am. J. Trop. Med. Hyg.* **13**, 248–255.

321. Ezzat, M. A. E., and Gaafar, S. M. (1951). *Tetrathyridium* sp. in a Syke's monkey (*Cerccopithecus alboqulars*) from Giza Zoological Gardens, Egypt. *J. Parasitol.* **37**, 392–394.

322. Fain, A. (1952). Sur les acariens parasites du genre *Pneumonyssus* au Congo belge. Description de deux espèces nouvelles chez le daman et le colobe. *Rev. Zool. Bot. Afr.* **45**, 358–382.

323. Fain, A. (1955). Deux nouveaux acariens de la famille Halarachnidae Oudemans, parasites des fosses nasales des singes au Congo Belge et au Ruanda-Urandi. *Rev. Zool. Bot. Afr.* **51**, 307–324.

324. Fain, A. (1956). *Coenurus* of *Taenia brauni* setti parasitic in man and animals from the Belgian Congo and Ruanda-Ufundi. *Nature (London)* **178**, 1353.

325. Fain, A. (1957). L'acariase pulmonaire chez le chimpanzé et le gorille par des acariens du genre *Pneumonyssus* Banks. *Rev. Zool. Bot. Afr.* **56**, 234–242.

326. Fain, A. (1957). Notes sur l'acariase des voies respiratoires chez l'homme et les animaux. Description de deux nouveaux acariens chez un lemurien et des rongeurs. *Ann. Soc. Belge Med. Trop.* **37**, 469–482.

327. Fain, A. (1958). Un nouveau parasite de l'orang-outan *Rhinophaga pongoicola* n. sp. (Acarina-Halarachnidae). *Rev. Zool. Bot. Afr.* **58**, 323–327.

328. Fain, A. (1959). Les acariens du genre *Pneumonyssus* Banks, parasites endopulmonaires des singes au Congo Belge (Halarchnidae: Mesotigmata). *Ann. Parasitol. Hum. Comp.* **34**, 126–148.

329. Fain, A. (1959). Deux nouveaux acariens nasicoles chez un singe platyrrhinien *Saimiri sciurea* (L). *Bull. Soc. Zool. Anvers* **12**, 3–12.

330. Fain, A. (1961). *Pneumonyssus duttoni* Newstead et Todd (1906) est une espèce composite. Description des deux espèces du complex duttoni (Mesostigmata: Halarachnidae). *Rev. Zool. Bot. Afr.* **63**, 213–226.

331. Fain, A. (1961). Sur le statut de deux espèces d'arïens du genre *Pneumonyssus* Banks décrites par H. Vitzthum. Designation d'un néotype pour *Pneumonyssus simicola* Banks, 1901 (Mesostigmata: Halarchnidae). *Z. Parasitenkd.* **21**, 141–150.

332. Fain, A. (1961). Le pentastomidés de l'Afrique Centrale. *Ann. Mus. R. Afr. Centr., Tervuren, Belg., Ser 8, Sci. Zool.* **92**, 1–115.

333. Fain, A. (1962). *Pangorillages pani* g. n., sp. n. Acarien psorique du chimpanzé (Psoralqidae: Sarcoptiformes). *Rev. Zool. Bot. Afr.* **66**, 283–290.

334. Fain, A. (1963). Les acariens producteurs de gale chez les lémuriens et les singes avec une étude des Psoroptidae (Sarcoptiformes). *Bull. Inst. R. Sci. Nat. Belg.* **39**, 1–125.

335. Fain, A. (1964). Les Lemurnyssidae parasites nasicoles des Lorisidae africains et des Cebidae sud-américains. Description d'une espèce nouvelle (Acarina: Sarcoptiformes). *Ann. Soc. Belge Med. Trop.* **44**, 453–458.

336. Fain, A. (1965). Notes sur le genre *Notoedres* Railliet, 1893 (Sarcoptidae: Sarcoptiformes). *Acarologia* **7**, 321–342.

337. Fain, A. (1965). Nouveaux genres et espèces d'Acariens Sarcoptiformes parasites (Note Préliminaire). *Rev. Zool. Bot. Afr.* **72**, 252–256.

338. Fain, A. (1965). A review of the family Rhyncptidae: Lawrence, parasitic on porcupines and monkeys (Acarina: Sarcoptiformes). *Adv. Acarol.* **2**, 135–159.

359. Fain, A. (1966). Pentastomida of snakes—their parasitological role in man and animals. *Mem. Inst. Butantan, São Paulo* **33**, 167–174.

340. Fain, A. (1966). Les acariens producteurs de gale chez les lémuriens et les singes. II. Nouvelles observations avec description d'une espèce nouvelle. *Acarologia* **8**, 94–114.

341. Fain, A. (1967). Diagnoses d'Acariens Sarcoptiformes nouveaux. *Rev. Zool. Bot. Afr.* **65**, 378–382.

342. Fain, A. (1968). Étude de la variabilité de *Sarcoptes scabei* avec une revision des Sarcoptidae. *Acta Zool. Pathol. Antverp.* **47**, 3–196.

343. Fain, A. (1968). Notes sur trois acariens remarquables (Sarcoptiformes). *Acarologia* **10**, 276–291.

344. Fain, A., and Schobbens, S. (1947). Lesions histopathologiques produites per l'acarïen parasite *Pneumonyssus duttoni*. Newst. et Todd. *Rev. Zool. Bot. Afr.* **40**, 12–16.

345. Fain, A., Mignolet G., and Bereznay, Y. (1958). L'acariase des voies respiratoires chez les singes due Zoo d'Anvers. *Bull. Soc. Zool. Anvers* **9**, 15–19.

346. Fairbairn, H. (1948). The occurrence of a piroplasm *Entopolypoides macaci*, in East African monkeys. *Ann. Trop. Med. Parasitol.* **42**, 118.

347. Fairbrother, R. W., and Hurst, E. W. (1932). Spontaneous diseases observed in 600 monkeys. *J. Pathol. Bacteriol.* **35**, 867–873.

348. Fallis, M., and Desser, S. S. (1977). On species of *Leucocytozoon, Haemoproteus*, and *Hepatocystis*. *In* "Parasitic Protozoa" (J. P. Kreier, ed.), Vol. 3, pp. 239–266. Academic Press, New York.

349. Faust, E. C. (1928). Studies on *Thelazia callipaeda*, Railliet and Henry, 1910. *J. Parasitol.* **15**, 75–86.

350. Faust, E. C. (1933). Experimental studies on human and primate species of *Strongyloides*. II. The development of *Strongyloides* in the experimental host. *Am. J. Hyg.* **18**, 114–132.

351. Faust, E. C. (1935). Notes on helminths from Panama. III: Filarial infection in the marmosets, *Leontocebus geoffroyi* (Pucheron) and *Saimiri orstedii* (Reinhardt) in Panama. *Trans. R. Soc. Trop. Med. Hyg.* **28**, 627.

352. Faust, E. C. (1936). *Strongyloides* and strongyloidiasis. *Rev. Parasitol. (Habana)* **2**, 315–341.

353. Faust, E. C. (1967). *Athesmia* (Trematoda: Dicrocoeliidae) Odhner, 1911 liver fluke of monkeys from Colombia, South America, and other mammalian hosts. *Trans. Am. Microsc. Soc.* **86**, 113–119.

354. Faust, E. C., Beaver, P. C., and Jung, R. C. (1968). "Animal Agents and Vectors of Human Disease," 3rd. ed. Lea & Febiger, Philadelphia.

355. Fenstermacher, R., and Jellison, W. L. (1932). Porcupine louse infesting the monkey. *J. Parasitol.* **18**, 294.

356. Fenwick, A. (1969). Baboons as reservoir hosts of *Schistosoma mansoni. Trans. R. Soc. Trop. Med. Hyg.* **63**, 557–567.

357. Fernando, C. H., and Jothy, A. A. (1981). Helminth parasites from miscellaneous hosts in Malaysia with a note on some Malaysian type material. *Indian J. Zool.* **9**, 61–70.

358. Ferris, G. F. (1954). A new species of Anoplura. *Ann. Natal. Mus.* **13**, 91–94.

359. Fiennes, R. N. T.-W. (1959). Report of the Society's pathologist for the year 1957. *Proc. Zool. Soc. London* **132**, 129–146.

360. Fiennes, R. N. T.-W. (1967). Zoonoses of Primates. "The Epidemiology and Ecology of Simian Diseases in Relation to Man." Weidenfeld & Nicolson, London.

361. Fiennes, R. N. T.-W. (1972). Ectoparasites and vectors. *In* "Pathology of Simian Primates" (R. N. T.-W. Fiennes, ed.), Part 2, pp. 158–176. Karger, New York.

362. File, S. K. (1974). *Anatrichosoma ocularis* sp. n. (Nematoda: Trichosomodidae) from the eye of the common tree shrew, *Tupaia glis. J. Parasitol.* **60**, 985–988.

363. File, S. K. (1976). *Probstmayria gombensis* sp. n. (Nematoda: Atractidae) from the chimpanzee. *J. Parasitol.* **62**, 256–258.

364. File, S. K., and Kessler, M. J. (1989). Parasites of free-ranging Cayo Santiago macaques after 46 years of isolation. *Am. J. Primatol.* **18**, 231–236.

365. File, S. K., McGrew, W. C., and Tutin, C. E. G. (1976). The intestinal parasites of a community of feral chimpanzees, *Pan troglodytes schweinfurthii. J. Parasitol.* **62**, 259–261.

366. Deleted in proof.

367. Fineg, J., Britz, W. E., Jr., Cook, J. E., and Edwards, R. H. (1961). "Clinical Observations and Methods Used in the Treatment of Young Chimpanzees," Rep. No. AFMCD-TR-61-12. Air Force Missile Development Center, Holloman Air Force Base, New Mexico.

368. Finegold, M. J., Seaquist, M. E., and Doherty, M. J. (1968). Treatment of pulmonary acariasis in rhesus monkeys with an organic phosphate. *Lab. Anim. Care* **18**, 127–130.

369. Fincham, J. E., Seier, J. V., Verster, A., Rose, A. G., Taljaard, J. J. F., Woodroof, C. W., and Rutherfoord, G. S. (1995). Pleural *Mesocestoides* and cardiac shock in an obese vervet monkey (*Cercopithecus aethiops*). *Vet. Pathol.* **32**, 330–333.

370. Finkeldey, W. (1931). Pathologisch-anatomischo Befunde bei der Oesophagostomiasis des *Javeneraffen. Z. Infekionskr., Parasit. Kr. Hyg. Haustiere* **40**, 146–164; cited by Ruch (987).

371. Fischthal, J. H., and Kuntz, R. E. (1965). Six digenetic trematodes of mammals from North Borneo (Malaysia). *Proc. Helminthol. Soc. Wash. D.C.* **32**, 154–159.

372. Flatt, R. E., and Patton, N. M. (1969). A mite infestation in squirrel monkeys (*Saimiri sciureus*). *J. Am. Vet. Med. Assoc.* **155**, 1233–1235.

373. Flynn, R. J. (1973). "Parasites of Laboratory Animals." Iowa State University Press, Ames.

374. Fong, Y. L., Codigan, F. C., and Coatney, J. R. (1971). A presumptive case of naturally occurring *Plasmodium knowlesi* malaria in man in Malaysia. *Trans. R. Soc. Trop. Med. Hyg.* **65**, 839–840.

375. Fonseca, F. da (1951). Plasmódio de primata do Brasil. *Mem. Inst. Oswaldo Cruz* **49**, 543–553.

376. Fooden, J. (1994). Malaria in macaques. *In. J. Primatol.* **15**, 573–596.

377. Foster, A. O., and Johnson, C. M. (1939). A preliminary note on the identity, life cycle, and pathogenicity of an important nematode parasite of captive monkeys. *Am. J. Trop. Med.* **19**, 265–277.

378. Foster, A. O., and Johnson, C. M. (1939). An explanation for the occurrence of *Capillaria hepatica* ova in human faeces suggested by the finding of three new hosts used as food. *Trans. R. Soc. Trop. Med. Hyg.* **32**, 639–644.

379. Fox, H. (1926). Scabies in a male drill. *Rep. Lab. Comp. Pathol. Philadelphia*, pp. 27–28.

380. Fox, H. (1927). Notes on special animals. *Rep. Lab. Comp. Pathol. Philadelphia*, pp. 11–18; cited by Kumar *et al.* (645).

381. Fox, H. (1928). *Balantidium* in the red howler (*Alouatta seniculus*). *Rep. Lab. Comp. Pathol. Philadelphia*, p. 27.

382. Fox, J. G., and Ediger, R. D. (1970). Nasal leach infestation in the rhesus monkey. *Lab. Anim. Care* **20**, 1137–1138.

383. Fox, J. G., and Hall, W. C. (1970). Fluke (*Gastrodiscoides hominis*) infection in a rhesus monkey with related intussusception of the colon. *J. Am. Vet. Med. Assoc.* **157**, 714–716.

384. Fox, J. G., Diaz, J. R., and Barth, R. A. (1972). Nymphal *Porocephalus clavatus* in the brain of a squirrel monkey, *Saimiri sciureus. Lab. Anim. Sci.* **22**, 908–910.

385. Foy, H., Kondi, A., and Mbaya, V. (1965). Hematologic and biochemical indices in the East African baboon. *Blood* **26**, 682–686.

386. Frank, H. (1962). Durch milben verursachte tödliche lungenerkrankung bei einem affen. *Berl. Muench. Tieraerztl. Wochenschr.* **76**, 135–137.

387. Frank, H. (1982). Pathology of amebiasis in leaf monkeys (*Colobidae*). *Proc. Int. Symp. Dis. Zoo Anim., 24th*, pp. 321–326.

388. Freitas, J. F. T. (1962). Notas sobre o gênero *Athesmia* Loos, 1899 Trematoda, Dicrocoeliidae). *Arq. Mu. Nac. (Rio de Janeiro)* **52**, 85–104.

389. Freitas, J. F. T. (1964). Achegas helmintologicas. *Rev. Cienc./Biol. (Belem)* **2**, 3–40.

390. Fremming, B. D., Vogel, F. S., Benson, R. E., and Young, R. J. (1955). A fatal case of amebiasis with liver abscesses and ulcerative colitis in a chimpanzee. *J. Am. Vet. Med. Assoc.* **126**, 406–407.

391. Fremming, B. D., Harris, M. D., Jr., Young, R. J., and Benson, R. E. (1957). Preliminary investigation into the life cycle of the monkey lung mite (*Pneumonyssus foxi*). *Am. J. Vet. Res.* **18**, 427–428.

392. Frenkel, J. K. (1971). Protozoal diseases of laboratory animals. *In* "Pathology of Protozoal and Helminthic Diseases" (R. A. Marcial-Rojas, ed.), pp. 318–369. Williams & Wilkins, Baltimore.

393. Frenkel, J. K. (1973). Toxoplasmosis: Parasite life cycle, pathology and immunology. *In* "The Coccidia: *Eimeria, Toxoplasma, Isospora,* and Related Genera" (D. M. Hammond and P. Long, eds.), pp. 343–410. University Park Press, Baltimore.

394. Frenkel, J. K. (1974). Advances in the biology of sporozoa. *Z. Parasitenkd.* **45**, 125–162.

395. Frenkel, J. K. (1976). *Angiostrongylus costaricensis* infections. *In* "Pathology of Tropical and Extraordinary Diseases, An Atlas" (C. H. Binford and D. H. Connor, eds.), Vol. 2, Sec. 9, Chapter 10, pp. 452–454. Armed Forces Institute of Pathology, Washington, DC.

396. Fuerstenberg, M. H. F. (1861). "Die Kraetzmilben der Menschen und Tiere." Engelmann, Leipzig.

397. Fuller, G. K., Lemma, A., and Haile, T. (1989). Schistosomiasis in Omo National Park of southwest Ethiopia. *Am. J. Trop. Med. Hyg.* **28**, 526–530.

398. Furman, D. P. (1954). A revision of the genus *Pneumonyssus* (Acarina: Halarachnidae). *J. Parasitol.* **40**, 31–42.

399. Furman, D. P., Bonasch, H., Springsteen, D., and Rahlmann, D. F. (1974). Studies on the biology of the lung mite, *Pneumonyssus simicola,* Bank (Acarina: Halaracnidae) and diagnosis of infestation in macaques. *Lab. Anim. Sci.* **24**, 622–629.

400. Gardiner, C. H. (1982). "Syllabus: Identification of Animal Parasites in Histologic Section." Reg. Vet. Pathol., A.F.I.P., Washington, DC.

401. Gardiner, C. H., and Imes, G. D., Jr. (1986). Sparganosis in a saddleback tamarin: Another case of viral-induced proliferation? *J. Wildl. Dis.* **22**, 437–439.

402. Gardiner, C. H., Nold, J. B., and Sanders, J. E. (1982). Diagnostic exercise. *Lab. Anim. Sci.* **32**, 601–602.

403. Gardner, M. B., Esra, G., Cain, M. J., Rossman, S., and Johnson, C. (1978). Myelomonocytic leukemia in an organgutan. *Vet. Pathol.* **15**, 667–770.

404. Garin, Y., Tutin, C. E. G., Fernandez, M., and Goussard, B. (1982). A new intestinal parasitic entodiniomorph ciliate from wild lowland gorillas (*Gorilla gorilla gorilla*) in Gabon. *J. Med. Primatol.* **11**, 186–190.

405. Garlick, D. S., Marcus, L. C., Pokras, M., and Schelling, S. H. (1996). *Baylisacaris* larva migrans in a spider monkey (*Ateles* sp.). *J. Med. Primatol.* **25**, 133–136.

406. Garner, E. (1967). *Dipetalonema gracile* infection in squirrel monkeys (*Saimiri sciureus*). *Lab. Anim. Dig.* **3**, 16–17.

407. Garner, E., Hemrick, R., and Rudiger, H. (1967). Multiple helminth infections in cinnamon-ringtailed monkeys (*Cebus albifrons*). *Lab. Anim. Care* **17**, 310–315.

408. Garner, F. M., and Stookey, J. L. (1968). "Syllabus: Diseases of Nonhuman Primates," pp. 22–28, 36–53. Am. Reg. Pathol., A.F.I.P., Washington, DC.

409. Garnham, P. C. C. (1947). Exoerythrocytic schizogony in *Plasmodium kochi* Laveran: A preliminary note. *Trans. R. Soc. Trop. Med. Hyg.* **40**, 719–722.

410. Garnham, P. C. C. (1948). The development cycle of *Hepatocystis* (*Plasmodium*) *kochi* in the monkey host. *Trans. R. Soc. Trop. Med. Hyg.* **41**, 601–616.

411. Garnham, P. C. C. (1950). Blood parasites of East African vertebrates with a brief description of exoerythrocytic schizogony in *Plasmodium pitmani*. *Parasitology* **40**, 328–337.

412. Garnham, P. C. C. (1959). A new sub-species of *Plasmodium cynomolgi*. *Riv. Parassitol.* **20**, 273–278.

413. Garnham, P. C. C. (1963). Distribution of simian malaria parasites in various hosts. *J. Parasitol.* **49**, 905–911.

414. Garnham, P. C. C. (1963). A new sub-species of *Plasmodium knowlesi* in the long-tailed macaque. *J. Trop. Med. Hyg.* **66**, 156–158.

415. Garnham, P. C. C. (1966). "Malaria Parasites and Other Haemosporidia." Blackwell, Oxford.

416. Garnham, P. C. C. (1966). *Hepatocystis* of African monkeys. *In* "Malaria Parasites and other Haemosporidia" (P. C. C. Garnham, ed.), pp. 829–861. Blackwell, Oxford.

417. Garnham, P. C. C. (1973). Distribution of malaria parasites in primates, insectivores and bats. *Symp. Zool. Soc. London* **33**, 377–404.

418. Garnham, P. C. C. (1973). Recent research on malaria in mammals excluding man. *Adv. Parasitol.* **11**, 603–630.

419. Garnham, P. C. C. (1977). A malaria parasite and a trypanosome of the talapoin monkey, with a discussion on the genus *Hepatocystis*. *Protozoology* **30**, 135–142.

420. Garnham, P. C. C. (1980). Malaria in its various vertebrate hosts. *In* "Malaria, Epidemiology, Chemotherapy, Morphology, and Metabolism" (J. P. Kreier, ed.), Vol. 1. pp. 95–144. Academic Press, New York.

421. Garnham, P. C. C., and Gonzales-Mugaburu, L. (1962). A new trypanosome in *Saimiri* monkeys from Colombia. *Rev. Inst. Med. Trop. Sao Paulo* **4**, 79–84.

422. Garnham, P. C. C., and Uilenberg, G. (1975). Malaria parasites of lemurs. *Ann. Parasitol.* **50**, 409–418.

423. Garnham, P. C. C., Lainson, R., and Gunders, A. E. (1956). Some observations on malaria parasites in a chimpanzee, with particular reference to the persistence of *Plasmodium reichenowi* and *Plasmodium vivax*. *Ann. Soc. Belge Med. Trop.* **36**, 811–822.

424. Garnham, P. C. C., Lainson, R., and Cooper, W. (1958). The complete life cycle of a new strain of *Plasmodium gonderi* from the drill (*Mandrillus leucophaeus*), including its sporogony in *Anopheles aztecus* and its pre-erythrocytic schizogony in the rhesus monkey. *Trans. R. Soc. Trop. Med. Hyg.* **2**, 509–517.

425. Garnham, P. C. C., Heisch, R. B., and Minter, D. M. (1961). The vector of *Hepatocystis* (*Plasmodium*) *kochi;* the successful conclusion of observations in many parts of tropical Africa. *Trans. R. Soc. Trop. Med. Hyg.* **55**, 497–502.

426. Garnham, P. C. C., Rajapaksa, N., Peters, W., and Killick-Kendrick, R. (1972). Malaria parasites of the orang-utan (*Pongo pygmaeus*). *Ann. Trop. Med. Parasitol.* **66**, 287–294.

427. Gay, D. M., and Branch, A. (1927). Pulmonary acariasis in monkeys. *Am. J. Trop. Med.* **7**, 49–55.

428. Gebauer, O. (1933). Beitrag zur kenntnis von nematoden aus affenlungen. *Z. Parasitenkd.* **5**, 724–734.

429. Gedoelst, L. (1916). Notes sur la faune parasitaire du Congo Belge. *Rev. Zool. Afr.* **5**, 1–90.

430. Geiman, Q. M. (1964). Shigellosis, amebiasis, and simian malaria. *Lab. Anim. Care* **14**, 441–454.

431. Geisel, O., Krampitz, H. E., and Willaert, E. (1975). Invasive amoebiasis caused by *Entamoeba histolytica* in a douc langur (*Pyrathrix nemaeus* L. 1771). *Berlin. Muench. Tieraerztl. Wochenschr.* **88**, 52–55.

432. Ghosh, R. K. (1982). On *Bertiella studeri* (Blanchard 1891) Stiles and Hassal, 1902 (Cestoda, Anaplocephalidae) from crab-eating macaque of Great Nicobar Islands. *J. Zool. Soc. India* **34**, 32–36.

433. Gisler, D. B., Benson, R. E., and Young, R. J. (1960). Colony husbandry of research monkeys. *Ann. N.Y. Acad. Sci.* **85**, 758–768.

434. Gleason, N. N., and Wolfe, R. E. (1974). *Entopolypoides macaci* (Babesiidae) in *Macaca mulatta*. *J. Parasitol.* **60**, 844–847.

435. Gleiser, C. A., Yaeger, R. G., and Ghidoni, J. J. (1986). *Trypanosoma cruzi* infection in a colony-born baboon. *J. Am. Vet. Med. Assoc.* **189**, 1225–1226.

436. Goeltenboth, R. (1982). Special section: Diseases of zoo animals. Nonhuman primates (apes, monkeys, prosimians). *In* "Handbook of Zoo Medicine" (H-G. Kloes and E. M. Lang, eds.), pp. 46–85. Van Nostrand-Reinhold, New York.

437. Goldberg, G. P., Fortman, J. D., Beluhan, F. Z., and Bennett, B. T. (1991). Pulmonary *Echinococcus granulosus* in a baboon (*Papio anubis*) *Lab. Anim. Sci.* **41**, 177–180.

438. Goldberger, J., and Crane, C. (1911). A new species of *Athesmia* (*A. foxi*) from a monkey. *Bull. Hyg. Lab. (Tokyo)* **71**, 48–55.

439. Goldman, L., and Feldman, M. D. (1949). Human infestation with scabies of monkeys. *Arch. Dermatol. Syphilol.* **59**, 175–178.

440. Goldsmid, J. M. (1974). The intestinal helminthzoonoses of primates in Rhodesia. *Ann. Soc. Belge Med. Trop.* **54**, 87.

441. Goldsmid, J. M., and Rogers, S. (1978). A parasitological study on the chacma baboon (*Papio ursinus*) from the Nothern Transvaal. *J. S. Afr. Vet. Assoc.* **49**, 109–111.

442. Gonder, R., and von-Berenberg-Gossler, H. (1908). Untersuchungen über malaria-plasmodien der affen. *Malaria (Leipzig)* **1**, 47–56.

443. Goodman, J. D., and Panesar, T. S. (1986). *Phaneropsolus* (*Phaneropsolus*) n. sp. (Trematoda: Lecithodendriidae) from the potto *Perodicticus potto* in Uganda. *Trans. Am. Microsc. Soc.* **105**, 76–78.

444. Gothe, R., and Kreier, J. P. (1977). *Aegyptianella, Eperythrozoon,* and *Haemobartonella*. *In* "Parasitic Protozoa" (J. P. Kreier, ed.), Vol. 4, pp. 251–294. Academic Press, New York.

445. Goussard, B., Collet, J.-Y., Garin, Y., Tutin, C. E. G., and Fernandez, M. (1983). The intestinal entodiniomorph ciliates of wild lowland gorillas (*Gorilla gorilla gorilla*) in Gabon, West Africa. *J. Med. Primatol.* **12**, 239–249.

446. Gozalo, A., and Tantalean, M. (1996). Parasitic protozoa in neotropical primates. *Lab. Primate Newsl.* **35**, 1–7.

447. Graber, M. (1975). Helminths and helminthiasis of different domestic and wild animals of Ethiopia. *Bull. Anim. Health Prod. Afr.* **23**, 57.

448. Graber, M. (1981). Endoparasites in domestic and wild animals of the Central African Republic (CAR). *Bull. Anim. Health Prod. Afr.* **29**, 25–47.

449. Graham, G. L. (1960). Parasitism in monkeys. *Ann. N.Y. Acad. Sci.* **85**, 842–860.

450. Grigorova, O., and Nesturch, M. (1934). Filariosis in a young chimpanzee. *Trans. Lab. Exp. Biol. Zoo Park Moscow* **6**, 210–211.

451. Griner, L. A. (1983). "Pathology of Zoo Animals." Zoological Society of San Diego, San Diego, CA.

452. Griner, L. A. (1983). "Pathology of Zoo Animals," pp. 319–325. Zoological Society of San Diego, San Diego, CA.

453. Griner, L. A. (1983). "Pathology of Zoo Animals," pp. 326–345. Zoological Society of San Diego, San Diego, CA.

454. Griner, L. A., and Monroe, L. S. (1974). "Amoebiasis of Mammals at San Diego Zoo." Proc. Cent. Symp. Sci. Res., Philadelphia, pp. 99–105.

455. Grinker, J. A., Karlin, D. A., and Estrella, P. M. (1962). Lung mites: Pulmonary acariasis in the primate. *Aerosp. Med.* **33,** 841–844.

456. Groot, H. (1951). Nuevo foco de trypanosomiasis humana en Colombia. *An. Soc. Biol. Bogota* **4,** 220–221.

457. Groot, H., Renjifo, S., and Uribe, C. (1951). *Trypanosoma ariarii,* n. sp., from man, found in Colombia. *Am. J. Trop. Med.* **31,** 673–691.

458. Grizimek, B. (1951). Tod durch lungenmilben bei einem schimpansen. *Zool. Garten (Leipzig)* **18,** 249.

459. Guilloud, N. B., King, A. A., and Lock, A. (1965). A study of the efficacy of thiabendazole and dithiazanine iodide-piperazine citrate suspension against intestinal parasites in the *Macaca mulatta. Lab. Anim. Care* **15,** 354–358.

460. Gupta, N. K., and Dutt, K. (1975). On three nematode parasites of the genus *Subulura* Molin, 1860 from India. *Riv. Parassitol.* **36,** 185–188.

461. Haaf, E., and Soest van, A. H. (1964). Oesophagostomiasis in man in North Ghana. *Trop. Geogr. Med.* **16,** 49–53.

462. Habermann, R. T., and Menges, R. W. (1968). Filariasis (*Acanthocheilonema perstans*) in a gorilla (a case history). *VM/SAC, Vet. Med. Small Anim. Clin.* **63,** 1040–1043.

463. Habermann, R. T., and Williams, F. P., Jr. (1957). Diseases seen at necropsy of 708 *Macaca mulatta* (rhesus monkey) and *Macaca philippinensis* (cynomolgus monkey). *Am. J. Vet. Res.* **18,** 419–426.

464. Habermann, R. T., and Williams, F. P., Jr. (1958). The identification and control of helminths in laboratory animals. *J. Natl. Cancer Inst. (U.S.)* **20,** 979–1009.

465. Habermann, R. T., Williams, F. P., Jr., and Thorp, W. T. S. (1954). "Identification of Some Internal Parasites of Laboratory Animals," Public Health Serv. Publ. No. 343. U.S. Dept. of Health, Education, and Welfare, Washington, DC.

466. Haddow, A. J., Williams, M. C., Woodall, J. P., Simpson, D. I. H., and Goma, L. K. H. (1964). 12 Isolations of Zika virus from *Aedes stegomyia africanas* (Theobald) taken in and above a Uganda forest. *Bull. W. H. O.* **31,** 57–69.

467. Halberstadter, L., and von Prowazek, S. (1907). Untersuchungen über die malariaparisiten der affen. *Arb. Gesundheits. amte (Berlin)* **26,** 37–43.

468. Hall, J. E., Haines, D. E., and Frederickson, R. G. (1985). Pentastomid nymph from the brain of a squirrel monkey (*Saimiri sciureus*). I. Morphology of the nymph. *J. Med. Primatol.* **14,** 195–208.

469. Hamerton, A. E. (1932). Report on the deaths occurring in the Society's gardens during the year 1931. *Proc. Zool. Soc. London* **1,** 613–638.

470. Hamerton, A. E. (1933). Report on deaths occurring in the Society's gardens during the year 1932. *Proc. Zool. Soc. London* **2,** 451–482.

471. Hamerton, A. E. (1937). Report on the deaths occurring in the Society's gardens during 1936. *Proc. Zool. Soc. London* **107,** 443–474.

472. Hamerton, A. E. (1938). Report on the deaths occurring in the Society's gardens during the year 1937. *Proc. Zool. Soc. London* **108,** 489–526.

473. Hamerton, A. E. (1941–1942). Report on the deaths occurring in the Society's gardens during 1939–1940. *Proc. Zool. Soc. London* **111,** 151–184.

474. Hamerton, A. E. (1943). Report on the deaths occurring in the Society's gardens during 1942. *Proc. Zool. Soc. London* **113,** 149.

475. Harper, J. S., III, Rice, J. M., London, W. T., Sly, D. L., and Middleton, C. (1982). Disseminated strongyloidiasis in *Erythrocebus patas. Am. J. Primatol.* **3,** 89–98.

476. Hartman, H. A. (1961). The intestinal fluke (*Fasciolopsis buski*) in a monkey. *Am. J. Vet. Res.* **22,** 1123–1126.

477. Harwell, G., and Dalgard, D. (1979). Clinical *Anatrichosoma cutaneum* dermatitis in non-human primates. *Annu. Proc., Am. Assoc. Zoo Vet.,* pp. 83–86a.

478. Hasegawa, H., Kano, T., and Mulavwa, M. (1983). A parasitological survey on the feces of pygmy chimpanzees, *Pan paniscus,* as Wamba, Zaire. *Primates* **24,** 419–423.

479. Hashimoto, I., and Honjo, S. (1966). Survey of helminth parasites in cynomologus monkeys (*Macaca irus*). *Jpn. J. Med. Sci. Biol.* **19,** 218.

480. Hausfater, G., and Sutherland, R. (1984). Little things that tick off baboons. *Nat. Hist. (N.Y.)* **93,** 54–62.

481. Hawking, F. (1972). *Entopolypoides macaci,* a *Babesia*-like parasite in *Cercopithecus* monkeys. *Parasitology* **65,** 89–109.

482. Hawking, F., and Webber, W. A. F. (1955). *Dirofilaria aethiops* Webber, 1955, a filerial parasite of monkeys: II. Maintenance in the laboratory. *Parasitology* **45,** 378–387.

483. Hayama, S., and Nigi, H. (1963). Investigation on the helminth parasites in the Japan Monkey Centre during 1959–61. *Primates* **4,** 97–112.

484. Hayes, C. G., Garnham, P. C. C., and Bagar, S. (1981). *Hepatocystis semopitheci* in rhesus monkey populations from northern Pakistan. *Indian J. Malariol.* **18,** 57–59.

485. Healy, G. R., and Hayes, N. R. (1963). Hydatid disease in rhesus monkeys. *J. Parasitol.* **49,** 837.

486. Healy, G. R., and Myers, B. J. (1973). Intestinal helminths. *In* "The Chimpanzee" (G. H. Bourne, ed.), Vol. 6, pp. 265–296. University Park Press, Baltimore.

487. Hegner, R., and Ratcliffe, H. (1927). Trichomonads from the vagina of the monkey; from the mouth of the cat and man, and from the intestine of the monkey, opossum and prairie-dog. *J. Parasitol.* **14,** 27–35.

488. Hegner, R. W. (1934). Specificity in the genus *Balantidium* based on size and shape of body and macronucleus with descriptions of six new species. *Am. J. Hyg.* **19,** 38–67.

489. Hegner, R. W. (1934). Intestinal protozoa of chimpanzees. *Am. J. Hyg.* **19,** 480–501.

490. Hegner, R. W. (1935). Intestinal protozoa from Panama monkeys. *J. Parasitol.* **21,** 60–61.

491. Hegner, R. W., and Chu, H. J. (1930). A survey of protozoa parasitic in plants and animals of the Philippine Islands. *Philipp. J. Sci.* **43,** 451–482.

492. Held, J. R. (1969). Primate malaria. *Ann. N.Y. Acad. Sci.* **162,** 587–593.

493. Held, J. R., and Whitney, R. A., Jr. (1978). Epidemic diseases of primate colonies. *Recent Adv. Primatol.* **4,** 23–41.

494. Held, J. R., Contacos, P. G., and Coatney, G. R. (1967). Studies of the exoerythrocytic stages of simian malaria. I. *Plasmodium fieldi. J. Parasitol.* **53,** 225–232.

495. Helwig, F. C. (1925). Arachnid infection in monkeys (*Pneumonyssus foxi* of Weidman). *Am. J. Pathol.* **1,** 389.

496. Henderson, J. D., Jr. (1992). Diagnostic exercise: Anemia in a baboon. *Lab. Anim. Sci.* **42,** 514–515.

497. Henderson, J. D., Jr., Webster, W. S., Bullock, B. C., Lehner, N. D. M., and Clarkson, T. B. (1970). Naturally occurring lesions seen at necropsy in eight woolly monkeys (*Lagothrix* sp.). *Lab. Anim. Care* **20,** 1087–1097.

498. Hendricks, L. D. (1974). A redescription of *Isospora arctopitheci* Rodhain, 1933 (Protozoa: Eimeriidae) from primates of Panama. *Proc. Helminthol. Soc. Wash.* **41,** 229–233.

499. Hendricks, L. D. (1977). Host range characteristics of the primate coccidian *Isospora arctopitheci* Rodhain 1933 (Protozoa: Eimeriidae). *J. Parasitol.* **63,** 32–35.

500. Henrickson, R. V. (1984). Biology and diseases of old world primates. *In* "Laboratory Animal Medicine" (B. G. Fox, B. J. Cohen, and F. M. Loew, eds.), Chapter 11, pp. 297–321. Academic Press, Orlando, FL.

501. Henrickson, R. V., Maul, D. H., Osborn, K. G., Sever, J. L., Madden, D. L., Ellingsworth, L. R., Anderson, J. A., Lowenstone, L. J., and Gardner,

M. B. (1983). Epidemic of acquired immunodeficiency in rhesus monkeys. *Lancet* **1**, 388–390.

502. Henriksen, Sv. Aa., and Pohlenz, J. F. L. (1981). Staining of cryptosporidiosis by a modified Ziehl-Neelsen technique. *Acta Vet. Scand.* **22**, 594–596.

503. Herman, C. M., and Schroeder, C. R. (1939). Treatment of ameobic dysentery in an orang-utan. *Zoologica (N.Y.)* **24**, 339.

504. Herman, L. H. (1967). *Gastrodiscoides hominis* infestation in two monkeys. *Vet. Med.* **62**, 355–356.

505. Hessler, J., Woodard, J., and Tucek, P. (1971). Lethal toxoplasmosis in a woolly monkey. *J. Am. Vet. Med. Assoc.* **159**, 1588–1594.

506. Heuschele, W. P. (1961). Internal parasitism of monkeys with the pentastomid, *Armillifer armillatus*. *J. Am. Vet. Med. Assoc.* **139**, 911–912.

507. Heuschele, W. P., Oosterhuis, J., Janssen, D., Robinson, P. T., Ensley, P. K., Meier, J. E., Olson, T., Anderson, M. P., and Benirschke, K. (1986). Cryptosporidial infections in captive wild animals. *J. Wild. Dis.* **22**, 493–496.

508. Heyneman, D., and Lim, B.-L. (1965). *Leipertrema* from squirrels, bats and tree shrews: A species complex. *Med. J. Malaya* **20**, 154.

509. Hickey, T. E., Kelly, W. A., and Sitzman, J. E. (1983). Demodectic mange in a tamarin (*Saguinus geoffroyi*). *Lab Anim. Sci.* **33**, 192–193.

510. Hiddleston, W. A. (1984). Veterinary care of marmosets and tamarins. *Proc. Symp. Assoc. Br. Wild Anim. Keepers B*, pp. 68–71.

511. Hill, W. C. O. (1951). Report of the Society's prosector for the year 1950. *Proc. Zool. Soc. London* **121**, 641–650.

512. Hill, W. C. O. (1953). Report of the Society's prosector for the year 1952. *Proc. Zool. Soc. London* **123**, 227–251.

513. Hill, W. C. O. (1954). Report of the Society's prosector for the year 1953. *Proc. Zool. Soc. London* **124**, 303–311.

514. Hill, W. C. O., Porter, A., and Southwich, M. D. (1952). The natural history, endoparasites, and pseudoparasites of the tarsiers (*Tarsius carbonarius*) recently living in the Society's menagerie, *Proc. Zool. Soc. London* **122**, 79–119.

515. Hira, P. R. (1978). Some helminthozoonotic infections in Zambia. *Afr. J. Med. Sci.* **7**, 1–7.

516. Hoare, C. A. (1932). On protozoal blood parasites collected in Uganda. *Parasitology* **24**, 210–224.

517. Hoare, C. A. (1958). The enigma of host-parasite relations in amebiasis. *Rice Inst. Pam.* **45**, 23–35.

518. Holmes, D. D., Kosanke, S. D., and White, G. L. (1980). Fatal enterobiasis in a chimpanzee. *J. Am. Vet. Med. Assoc.* **177**, 911–913.

519. Honigberg, B. M., and Lee, J. J. (1959). Structure and division of *Trichomonas tenax* (O. F. Muller). *Am. J. Hyg.* **69**, 177–201.

520. Honjo, R., and Imaizumi, K. (1965). Diseases observed in monkeys. *Bull. Exp. Anim.* **14**, 162–163.

521. Honjo, S., Muto, K., Fujiwara, T., Suzuki, Y., and Imaizumi, K. (1963). Statistical survey of internal parasites in cynomolgus monkeys (*Macaca irus*). *Jpn. J. Exp. Med.* **16**, 217–224.

522. Hoogstraal, H. (1956). "African Ixodoidea: I. ticks of the Sudan (with special reference to Equatoria province and with preliminary reviews of the genera *Boophilus, Margaropus*, and *Hyalomma*)," Res. Rep. NM 005 050.29.07. U.S. Navy Dept., Washington, DC.

523. Hoogstrall, H., and Theiler, G. (1959). Ticks (Ixodoidea, Ixodidae) parasitizing lower primates in Africa, Zanzibar, and Madagascar. *J. Parasitol.* **45**, 217–222.

524. Hopkins, G. H. E. (1949). The host associations of the lice of mammals. *Proc. Zool. Soc. London* **119**, 387–604.

525. Hori, Y., Imada, I., Yanuqida, T., Usui, M., and Mori, A. (1982). Parasite changes on the influence of body weight of Japanese monkeys in the Hoshimi troop. *Primates* **23**, 416–431.

526. Horii, Y., and Usui, M. (1985). Experimental transmission of *Trichuris* ova from monkeys to man. *Trans. R. Soc. Trop. Med. Hyg.* **79**, 423.

527. Horii, Y., Ishii, A., Owhashi, M., Miyoshi, M., and Usui, M. (1985). Neutrophilic nodules in the intestinal walls of Japanese monkeys associated with the neutrophil chemotactic activity of larval extracts and secretions of *Oesophagostomum aculeatum*. *Res. Vet. Sci.* **38**, 115–119.

528. Horna, M., and Tantalean, V. M. (1983). Parasitos de primates peruanos: Helmintos del "mono fraile" y del "pichico barba blanca." *Bol. Lima* **5**, 54–58 (in Spanish with English summary).

529. Houser, W. D., and Paik, S. K. (1971). Hydatid disease in a macaque. *J. Am. Vet. Med. Assoc.* **159**, 1574–1577.

530. Howard, E. B., and Gendron, A. P. (1980). *Echinococcus vogeli* infection in higher primates at the Los Angeles zoo. *In* "The Comparative Pathology of Zoo Animals" (R. J. Montali and G. Migaki eds.), pp. 379–382. Smithsonian Institution Press, Washington, DC.

531. Howard, L. M., and Cabrera, B. D. (1961). Simian malaria in the Philippines. *Science* **134**, 555–556.

532. Hsu, C.-K., and Melby, E. C., Jr. (1974). *Isospora callimico*, n. sp. (Coccidia Eimeriidae) from Goldi's marmoset (*Callimico goeldii*). *Lab. Anim. Sci.* **24**, 476–479.

533. Hsu, H. F., Davis, J. R., and Hsu, S. Y. L. (1969). Histopathological lesions of rhesus monkeys and chimpanzees infected with *Schistosoma japonicum*. *Z. Tropenmed. Parasitol.* **20**, 184–205.

534. Hsu, S. Y. L., and Hsu, H. F. (1968). A chimpanzee naturally infected with *Schistosoma mansoni:* Its resistance against a challenge infection of *S. japonicum*. *Trans. R. Soc. Trop. Med. Hyg.* **62**, 901–902.

535. Hubbard, G. B., and Butcher, W. I. (1983). What's your diagnosis? Passengers. Trematodiasis and typhlitis caused by *Gastrodiscoides hominis*. *Lab. Anim.* **12**, 12, 14.

536. Hubbard, G. B. (1995). Protozal diseases of nonhuman primates. *Semin. Avian Exotic Pet Med.* **4**, 145–149.

537. Hubbard, G. B., Gardiner, C. H., Bellini, S., Ehler, W. J., Conn, D. B., and King, M. M. (1993). *Mesocestoides* infection in captive olive baboons (*Papio cynocephalus anubis*). *Lab. Anim. Sci.* **53**, 625–627.

538. Huff, C. G., and Hoogstraal, H. (1963). *Plasmodium lemuris* n. sp. from *Lemur collaris*. *J. Infect. Dis.* **112**, 233–236.

539. Hugot, J.-P. (1984). The genus *Trypanoxyuris* (Oxyuridae, Nematoda): II. Subgenus *Hapaloxyuris* parasite of primates Callitrichidae. *Bull. Mus. Natl. Hist. Nat., Ser. A* **6**(4), 1007–1019.

540. Hugot, J.-P. (1985). The genus *Trypanoxyuris* (Oxyuridae. Nematoda): III. Subgenus *Trypanoxyuris* parasite of Cebidae and Atelidae primates. *Bull. Mus. Natl. Hist. Nat., Ser. A* **7**(1), 131–155 (in French w/English summary).

541. Hugot, J.-P. (1985). Sur le genre *Trypanoxyuris* (Oxyuridae, Nematoda). III. Sous genre *Trypanoxyuris* parasite de primates Cebidae et Atelidae. *Bull. Mus. Natl. Hist. Nat., Ser. A* **7**, 131–155.

542. Hugot, J.-P., and Vaucher, C. (1985). The genus *Trypanoxyuris* (Oxyuridae, Nematoda): IV. Subgenus *Trypanoxyuris* parasite of Cebidae and Atelidae primates (continuation). Morphological study of *Trypanoxyuria callicebi* n. sp. *Bull. Mus. Natl. Hist. Nat., Ser. A* **7**(3), 633–636.

543. Hull, W. B. (1956). The nymphal stages of *Pneumonyssus simicola* Banks, 1901 (Acarina: Halarachnidae). *J. Parasitol.* **42**, 653–565.

544. Hull, W. B. (1970). Respiratory mite parasites in non-human primates. *Lab. Anim. Care* **20**, 402.

545. Hunt, R. D., Jones, T. C., and Williamson, M. (1970). Mechanisms of parasitic damage and the host response. *Lab. Anim. Care* **20**, 345–353.

546. Hunt, R. D., Anderson, M. P., and Chalifoux, L. V. (1978). Spontaneous infectious diseases of marmosets. *Primate Med.* **10**, 239–253.

547. Huser, H. J., Rieber, E. E., Sheehy, T. W., and Berman, A. R. (1967). Erythrokinetic studies in the baboon under normal and experimental conditions. *In* "The Baboon in Medical Research" (H. Vagtborg, ed.), pp. 390–406. University of Texas Press, Austin.

548. Ilievski, V., and Esber, H. (1969). Hydatid disease in a rhesus monkey. *Lab. Anim. Care* **19**, 199–204.

549. Inglis, W. G. (1961). The oxyurid parasites (nematoda) of primates. *Proc. Zool. Soc. London* **136**, 103–122.

550. Inglis, W. G., and Cosgrove, G. E. (1965). The pinworm parasites (Nematoda: Oxyuridae) of the Hapalidae (Mammalia: Primates). *Parasitology* **55**, 731–737.

551. Inglis, W. G., and Diaz-Ungria, C. (1960). Nematodes parasitos de vertebrados venezolanos. I. Una revision del género *Trypanoxyuris* (Ascardiata: Oxyuridae). *Mem.—Soc. Cienc. Nat. La Salle* **19**, 176–212.

552. Inglis, W. G., and Dunn, F. L. (1963). The occurrence of *Lemuricola* (Nematoda Oxyurinae) in Malaya: with description of a new species. *Z. Parasitenkd.* **23**, 354–359.

553. Inglis, W. G., and Dunn, F. L. (1964). Some Oxyurids (Nematoda) from neotropical primates. *Z. parasitenkd.* **24**, 83–87.

554. Innes, J. R. M. (1969). Pulmonary acariasis: An enzootic disease caused by *Pneumonyssus simicola* particularly in *Macaca mulatta*. *Lab. Anim. Handb.* **4**, 101–105.

555. Innes, J. R. M., and Hull, W. B. (1972). Endoparasites—lung mites. *In* "Pathology of Simian Primates" (R. N. T.-W. Fiennes, ed.), Part 2, pp. 177–193. Karger, New York.

556. Innes, J. R. M., Colton, M. W., Yevich, P. P., and Smith, C. L. (1954). Pulmonary acariasis as an enzootic disease caused by *Pneumonyssus simicola* in imported monkeys. *Am. J. Pathol.* **30**, 813–835.

557. Inoki, S., Takemura, S., Makiura, Y., and Hotta, F. (1942). Studies on *Plasmodium inui var. Cyclopis* n. sp., new malaria parasite found in Formosan macaques (*Macaca cyclopis*). *Osaka Igakkai Zassi* **41**, 1327–1343.

558. Irving, G. W., III (1972). Parasitology. *In* "Selected Topics in Laboratory Animal Medicine," Aeromed. Rev. 2-72, Vol 8, pp. 1–44. U.S.A.F. Sch. Aerosp. Med. Aerosp. Med. Div. (AFSC), Brooks Air Force Base, Texas.

559. Irving, G. W., III (1972). Zoonoses of primates. *In* "Selected Topics in Laboratory Animal Medicine," Aeromed. Rev. 13-72, Vol. 16. U.S.A.F. Sch. of Aerosp. Med. Aerosp. Med. Div. (AFSC), pp. 1–74. Brooks Air Force Base, Texas.

560. Itakura, C., and Nigi, H. (1968). Histopathological observations on two spontaneous cases of toxoplasmosis in the monkey (*Lemur catta*). *Jpn. J. Vet. Sci.* **30**, 341–346.

561. Jaskoski, B. J. (1960). Physalopteran infection in an orangutan. *J. Am. Vet. Med. Assoc.* **137**, 307.

562. Jensen, J. M., and Huntress, S. L. (1982). *Capillaria hepatica* infestation in a gelada baboon (*Theropithecus gelada*) troop. *Annu. Proc., Am. Assoc. Zoo. Vet.*, pp. 48–49.

563. Jessee, M. T., Schilling, P. W., and Stunkard, J. A. (1970). Identification of intestinal helminth eggs in Old World primates. *Lab. Anim. Care* **20**, 83–87.

564. Jindal, B. R., Vinayak, V. K., and Chhuttani, P. N. (1977). Intestinal parasitosis of rhesus monkeys (*Macaca mulatta*) in health and disease. *Bull. Postgrad. Inst. Med. Educ. Res., Chandigarh* **11**, 110–113.

565. Johnsen, D. O., Gould, D. J., Tanticharoenyos, P., Diggs, C. L., and Wooding, W. L. (1970). Experimental infection of gibbons with *Dirofilaria immitis*. *Trans. R. Soc. Trop. Med. Hyg.* **64**, 937–938.

566. Johnson, C. M. (1941). Observations on natural infections of *Endamoeba histolytica* in *Ateles* and rhesus monkeys. *Am. J. Trop. Med.* **21**, 49–61.

567. Jones, D. M. (1982). Veterinary aspects of the maintenance of orangutans in captivity. *In* "The Orang-utan: Its Biology and Conservation" (L. E. M. de Boer, ed.), pp. 171–199. Dr. W. Junk Publishers, The Hague.

568. Jones, N. D., Brooks, D. R., and Harris, R. L. (1980). *Macaca mulatta*—A new host for *Choanotaenia* Cestodes. *Lab. Anim. Sci.* **30**, 575–577.

569. Jones, S. R. (1973). Toxoplasmosis: A review. *J. Am. Vet. Med. Assoc.* **163**, 1038–1042.

570. Jones, T. C., and Hunt, R. D. (1983). Diseases due to protozoa. *In* "Veterinary Pathology," 5th ed., pp. 719–777. Lea & Febiger, Philadelphia.

571. Jones, T. C., and Hunt, R. D. (1983). Diseases caused by parasitic helminths and arthropods. *In* "Veterinary Pathology," 5th ed., pp. 778–879. Lea & Febiger, Philadelphia.

572. Jortner, B. S., and Percy, D. H. (1978). The nervous system. *In* "Pathology of Laboratory Animals" (K. Benirschke, F. M. Garner, and T. C. Jones, eds.), Vol. I, Chapter 5, pp. 320–421. Springer-Verlag, New York.

573. Joseph, B. E., Wilson, D. W., and Henrickson, R. V. (1984). Treatment of pulmonary acariasis in rhesus macaques with ivermectin. *Lab. Anim. Sci.* **34**, 360–364.

574. Juranek, D. (1979). Waterborne giardiasis. *In* "Waterborne Transmission of Giardiasis" (W. Jakubowski and J. C. Hoff, eds.), pp. 150–163.

575. Kagan, I. G., Allain, D. S., and Norman, L. (1959). An evaluation of the hemagglutination and flocculation tests in the diagnosis of *Echinococcus* disease. *Am. J. Trop. Med. Hyg.* **8**, 51–55.

576. Kagei, N., and Yoshida, M. (1976). *Schistosoma mansoni* infection in a green monkey, *Cercopithecus aethiops* (Linneaus) imported from Africa. *Bull. Inst. Public Health (Tokyo)* **25**, 82–85.

577. Kalia, D. C., and Gupta, N. K. (1982). On an oxyurid nematode, *Enterobius chabaudi* n. sp., from langur, *Presbytis entellus*. *Indian J. Parasitol.* **6**, 141–143.

578. Kalishman, J., Paul-Murphy, J., Scheffler, J., and Thompson, J. A. (1996). Survey of *Cryptosporidium* and *Giardia* spp in a captive population of common marmosets. *Lab. Anim. Sci.* **46**, 116–119.

579. Kalter, S. S. (1980). Infectious diseases of the great apes of Africa. *J. Reprod. Fertil., Suppl.* **28**, 149–159.

580. Kalter, S. S., and Heberling, R. L. (1978). Health hazards associated with newly imported primates and how to avoid them. *Recent Adv. Primatol.* **4**, 5–21.

581. Karr, S. L., Jr., and Wong, M. M. (1975). A survey of *Sarcocystis* in nonhuman primates. *Lab. Anim. Sci.* **25**, 641–645.

582. Karr, S. L., Jr., Henrickson, R. V., and Else, J. G. (1979). A survey for *Anatrichosoma* (Nematoda: Trichinellida) in wild-caught *Macaca mulatta*. *Lab. Anim. Sci.* **29**, 789–790.

583. Karr, S. L., Jr., Henrickson, R. V., and Else, J. G. (1980). A survey for intestinal hemlinths in recently wild-caught *Macaca mulatta* and results of treatment with mebendazole and thiabendazole. *J. Med. Primatol.* **9**, 200–204.

584. Kasa, T. J., Lathrop, G. D., Dupuy, H. J., Bonney, C. H., and Toft, J. D., II (1977). An endemic focus of *Trypanosoma cruzi* infection in a subhuman primate research colony. *J. Am. Vet. Med. Assoc.* **171**, 850–854.

585. Kaufmann, A. F., Morris, G., Richardson, J. H., Healy, G., and Kaplan, W. (1970). A survey of newly arrived South American monkeys for potential human pathogens. *In* "Primate Zoonoses Surveillance," Rep. No. 1. Center for Disease Control, Atlanta, GA.

586. Kaufmann, P. H., and Whittaker, F. H. (1972). Coenurosis in a zoo collection of Gelada baboons (*Theropithecus gelada*). *VM/SAC, Vet. Med. Small Anim. Clin.* **67**, 1100–1104.

587. Kaur, J., Chakravarti, R. N., Chugh, K. S., and Chhuttani, P. N. (1968). Spontaneously occurring renal disease in wild rhesus monkeys. *J. Pathol.* **95**, 31–36.

588. Keeling, M. E., and McClure, H. M. (1972). Clinical management, diseases and pathology of the gibbon and siamang. *In* "Gibbon and Siamang" (D. M. Rumbaugh, ed.), Vol. 1, pp. 207–249. Karger, Basel.

589. Keeling, M. E., and McClure, H. M. (1974). Pneumoncoccal meningitis and fatal enterobiasis in a chimpanzee. *Lab. Anim. Sci.* **24**, 92–95.

590. Keeling, M. E., and Wolf, R. H. (1975). Medical management of the rhesus monkey. *In* "The Rhesus Monkey" (G. H. Bourne, ed.), Vol. 2, pp. 11–96. Academic Press, New York.

591. Kellogg, V. L. (1913). Ectoparasites of the monkeys, apes and man. *Science* **38**, 601.

592. Kennard, M. A. (1981). Abnormal findings in 246 consecutive autopsies on monkeys. *Yale J. Biol. Med.* **13**, 701–712.

593. Kessel, J. F. (1928). Intestinal protozoa of monkeys. *Univ. Calif., Berkeley, Publ. Zool.* **31**, 275–306.

594. Kessel, J. F., and Johnstone, H. G. (1949). The occurrence of *Endamoeba polecki* Prowazek, 1912, in *Macaca mulatta* and in man. *Am. J. Trop. Med.* **29**, 311–317.

595. Kessel, J. F., and Kaplan, F. (1949). The effect of certain arsenicals on natural infections of *Endamoeba histolytica* and of *Endamoeba polecki* in *Macaca mulatta*. *Am. J. Trop. Med.* **29**, 319–322.

596. Kessler, M. J. (1982). Nasal and cutaneous anatrichosomiasis in the free-ranging rhesus monkeys (*Macaca mulatta*) of Cayo Santiago. *Am. J. Primatol.* **3**, 55–60.

597. Kessler, M. J., Yarbrough, B., Rawlins, R. G., and Bérard, J. (1984). Intestinal parasites of the free-ranging Cayo Santiago rhesus monkeys (*Macaca mulatta*). *J. Med. Primatol.* **13**, 57–66.

598. Keymer, I. F. (1976). Report of the pathologist, 1973 and 1974. *J. Zool.* **178**, 456–493.

599. Kikuth, W. (1927). Piroplasmose bei affen. *Arch. Schiffs-Trop.-Hyg.* **31**, 37–40.

600. Kim, C. S., and Bang, B. G. (1970). Nasal mites parasitic in nasal and upper skull tissues in the baboon (*Paplo* sp). *Science* **169**, 372–373.

601. Kim, C. S., and Kalter, S. S. (1972). Unilateral renal aplasia in an African baboon (*Papio* sp). *Folia Primatol.* **2**, 352.

602. Kim, C. S., Eugster, A. K., and Kalter, S. S. (1968). Pathologic study of the African baboon (*Papio* sp.) in his native habitat. *Primates* **9**, 93–104.

603. Kim, C. S., Bank, F. B., and DiGiacomo, R. F. (1972). Hemagglutination assay of antibodies associated with pulmonary acariasis in rhesus monkeys. *Infect. Immun.* **5**, 138–140.

604. Kim, J. C. S. (1974). Distribution and life cycle stages of lung mites (*Pneumonyssus* sp). *J. Med. Primatol.* **3**, 105–119.

605. Kim, J. C. S. (1977). Pulmonary acariases in Old World monkeys. *Vet. Bull.* **47**, 249–255.

606. Kim, J. C. S. (1977). Lung mite infection in old world monkeys. *Lab. Anim.* **6**(5), 44–50.

607. Kim, J. C. S. (1977). Pathobiology of pulmonary acariasis in old world monkeys. *Acarologia* **19**, 371–383.

608. Kim, J. C. S. (1980). Pulmonary acariasis in Old World monkeys: A review. *In* "The Comparative Pathology of Zoo Animals" (R. J. Montali and G. Migaki, eds.), pp. 383–394. Smithsonian Institution Press, Washington, DC.

609. Kim, J. C. S., and Kalter, S. S. (1975). Pathology of pulmonary acariasis in baboons (*Papio* sp.). *J. Med. Primatol.* **4**, 70.

610. Kim, J. C. S., and Kalter, S. S. (1976). Scanning electron microscopic studies of simian lung mites (*Pneumonyssus santos-diasi,* Zumpt and Till, 1954). *J. Med. Primatol.* **5**, 3–12.

611. Kim, J. C. S., and Wolf, R. J. (1980). Diseases of moustached marmosets. *In* "The Comparative Pathology of Zoo Animals" (R. J. Montali and G. Migaki, eds.), pp. 431–435. Smithsonian Institution Press, Washington, DC.

612. Kim, J. C. S., Abee, C. R., and Wolf, R. H. (1978). Balantidiosis in a chimpanzee (*Pan troglodytes*). *Lab. Anim.* **12**, 231–233.

613. Kim, K. C., and Emerson, K. C. (1968). Descriptions of two species of Pediculidae (Anoplura) from great apes (Primates, Pongidae). *J. Parasitol.* **54**, 690–695.

614. Kim, K. C., and Emerson, K. C. (1970). Anoplura from Mozambique with descriptions of a new species and nymphal stages. *Rev. Zool. Bot. Afr.* **81**, 383–416.

615. Kim, K. C., and Emerson, K. C. (1973). Anoplura of tropical West Africa with descriptions of new species and nymphal stages. *Rev. Zool. Bot. Afr.* **87**, 425–455.

616. Kimura, T., Ito, J., Suzuki, M., and Inokuchi, S. (1987). *Sarcocystis* found in the skeletal muscle of common squirrel monkeys. *Primates* **28**, 247–255.

617. King, N. W., Jr. (1976). Synopsis of the pathology of new world monkeys. *Sci. Publ. Pan. Am. Health Org.* **317**, 169–198.

618. Kingston, N., and Cosgrove, G. E. (1967). Two new species of *Platynosomum* (Trematode: Dicrocoeliidae) from South American monkeys. *Proc. Helminthol. Soc. Wash.* **34**, 147–151.

619. Kirby, H., Jr. (1928). Notes on some parasites from chimpanzees. *Proc. Soc. Exp. Biol. Med.* **25**, 698–700.

620. Klumpp, S. A., Anderson, D. C., McClure, H. M., and Dubey, J. P. (1994). Encephalomyelitis due to a *Sarcocystis neurona*-like protozoan in a rhesus monkey (*Maacaca mulatta*) infected with simian immunodeficiency virus. *Am. J. Trop. Med. Hyg.* **51**, 332–338.

621. Knezevich, A. L., and McNulty, W. P., Jr. (1970). Pulmonary acariasis (*Pneumonyssus simicola*) in colony bred *Macaca mulatta*. *Lab. Anim. Care* **20**, 693–696.

622. Knowles, R. (1919). Notes on the monkey *Plasmodium* and on some experiments in malaria. *Indian J. Med. Res.* **7**, 195–202.

623. Knowles, R., and Das Gupta, B. M. (1932). A study of monkey malaria and its experimental transmission to man. *Indian Med. Gaz.* **67**, 213–268.

624. Knowles, R., and Das Gupta, B. M. (1936). Some observations on the intestinal protozoa of macaques. *Indian J. Med. Res.* **24**, 547–556.

625. Ko, R. C. (1978). Occurrence of *Angiostrongylus cantonensis* in the heart of a spider monkey. *J. Helminthol.* **52**, 229.

626. Kobayashi, H. (1925). On the animal parasites in Korea. *Jpn. Med. World* **5**, 9–16.

627. Kohn, D. F., and Haines, D. E. (1982). Diseases of the Prosimii: A review. *In* "The Lesser Bushbaby (*Galago*) as an Animal Model: Selected Topics" (D. E. Haines, ed.), pp. 285–301. CRC Press, Boca Raton, FL.

628. Kopciowska, L., and Nicolau, S. (1938). Toxoplasmose spontanée du chimpanzé. *C. R. Seances Soc. Biol. Ses. Fil.* **129**, 179–181.

629. Kornegay, R. W., Giddens, W. E., Jr., Morton, W. R., and Knitter, G. H. (1986). Verminous vasculitis, pneumonia and pulmonary infarction in a cynomolgus monkey after treatment with ivermectin. *Lab. Anim. Sci.* **36**, 45–47.

630. Korte, W. F. de (1905). On the presence of a sarcosporidium in the thigh muscles of *Macaca rhesus*. *J. Hyg.* **5**, 451–452.

631. Kovatch, R. M., and White, J. D. (1972). Cryptosporidiosis in two juvenile rhesus monkeys. *Vet. Pathol.* **9**, 426–440.

632. Krascheninnikow, S., and Wenrich, D. H. (1958). Some observations on the morphology and division of *Balantidium coli* and *Balantidium caviae* (?). *J. Protozool.* **5**, 196–202.

633. Kreis, H. A. (1932). A new pathogenic nematode of the family Oxyuroidea, *Oxyuronema atelophora* n. g., n. sp in the red-spider monkey, *Ateles geoffroyi*. *J. Parasitol.* **18**, 295–302.

634. Kreis, H. A. (1945). Beiträge zur Kenntnis parasitischer Nematoden. XII: Parasitische Nematoden aus den Tropen. *Rev. Suisse Zool.* **52**, 551.

635. Kreis, H. A. (1955). Beiträge zur Kenntnis parasitischer Nematoden XVIII. Das genus *Probstmayria* Ransom, 1907. *Schweiz. Arch. Tierheilkd.* **97**, 422–433.

636. Krishnamoorthy, R. V., Srihari, K., Rahaman, H., and Rajasekharaiah, G. L. (1978). Nematode parasites of the slender loris. *Loris tardigradus*. *Proc.–Indian Acad. Sci., Sect. B* **87B**, 17–22.

637. Krishnasamy, M., Jeffery, J., and Sirimanne, R. A. (1988). A new record of *Bertiella studeri* (Blanchard 1891) Stiles and Hassal, 1902 from the crab-eating macaque *Macaca fascicularis* in peninsular Malaysia. *Trop. Biomed.* **5**, 89–90.

638. Kugi, G., and Sawada, I. (1970). *Mathevotaenia brasiliensis* n. sp., a tapeworm from the squirrel monkey, *Saimiri sciureus*. *Jpn. J. Parasitol.* **19**, 467–470.

639. Kuhn, H.-J., and Ludwig, H. W. (1967). Die affenläuse der gattung *Pedicinus*. *Z. Zool. Syst. Evol.* **5**, 144–256.

640 Kulda, J., and Nohynkova, E. (1978). *Giardia* and Giardiasis. *In* "Parasitic Protozoa" (J. P. Kreier, ed.), Vol. 2, pp. 69–104. Academic Press, New York.

641. Kuller, L., Morton, W. R., and Bronsdon, M. A. (1984). Occurrence of *Cryptosporidium* in a nonhuman primate nursery. *Am. J. Primatol.* **6**, 411 (abstr.).

642. Kumar, V., and de Meurichy, W. (1982). Efficacy of Yomesan against *Bertiella* sp (Anoplochephalidae/Cestoda) of a chimpanzee, *Pan schweinfurthii*. *Riv. Parassitol.* **43**, 161–163.

643. Kumar, V., Ceulemans, F., and de Meurichy, W. (1978). Chemotherapy of helminthiasis among wild animals. IV. Efficacy of flubendazole against *Trichuris trichiura* infections of baboons, *Papio hamadryas* L. *Acta Zool. Pathol. Antverp.* **73**, 3–9.

644. Kumar, V., de Meurichy, W., and Van Peer, L. (1980). Microscopic pathology of liver of capucchin monkey (*Cebus albifrons*) infected with *Athesmia foxi* (Dicroelidae: Trematoda): A pictorial illustration. *Acta Zool. Pathol. Antverp.* **75**, 71–77.

645. Kumar, V., de Meurichy, W., Delahaye, A.-M., and Mortelmans, J. (1981). Chemotherapy of helminthiasis among wild mammals. V. Gastric involvement of spider monkeys with *Physaloptera* sp. and chemotherapy of the infection. *Acta Zool. Pathol. Antverp.* **76**, 191–199.

646. Kumar, V., de Meurichy, W., Delahaye, A.-M., and Mortelmans, J. (1983). Tissue dwelling capillarid nematode infections in the fauna of Zoological Garden, Antwerp. *Acta Zool. Pathol. Antverp.* **77**, 87–95.

647. Kuntz, R. E. (1972). Trematodes of the intestinal tract and biliary passages. *In* "Pathology of Simian Primates" (R. N. T.-W. Fiennes, ed.), Part 2, pp. 104–123. Karger, Basel.

648. Kuntz, R. E. (1973). Models for investigation in parasitology. *In* "Nonhuman Primates in Biomedical Research" (G. H. Bourne, ed.), pp. 167–201. Academic Press, New York.

649. Kuntz, R. E. (1982). Significant infections in primate parasitology. *J. Hum. Evol.* **11**, 185–194.

650. Kuntz, R. E., and Moore, J. A. (1973). Commensals and parasites of African baboons (*Papio cynocephalus* L. 1766) captured in rift valley province of central Kenya. *J. Med. Primatol.* **2**, 236–241.

651. Kuntz, R. E., and Myers, B. J. (1966). Parasites of baboons (*Papio doguera* Pucheran, 1856) captured in Kenya and Tanzania, East Africa. *Primates* **7**, 27–32.

652. Kuntz, R. E., and Myers, B. J. (1967). Microbiological parameters of the baboon (*Papio* sp): Parasitology. *In* "The Baboon in Medical Research (H. Vagtborg, ed.), Vol. 2, pp. 741–755. University of Texas Press, Austin.

653. Kuntz, R. E., and Myers, B. J. (1967). Parasites of the Kenya baboon: Arthropods, blood protozoa and helminths. *Primates* **8**, 75–82.

654. Kuntz, R. E., and Myers, B. J. (1967). Primate cysticercosis: *Taenia hydatigena* in Kenya vervets (*Cercopithecus aethiops* Linnaeus, 1758) and Taiwan macaques (*Macaca cyclopis* Swinhoe, 1864). *Primates* **8**, 83–88.

655. Kuntz, R. E., and Meyers, B. J. (1969). A checklist of parasites and commensals reported for the Taiwan macaque (*Macaca cyclopis* Swinhoe, 1862). *Primates* **10**, 71–80.

656. Kuntz, R. E., and Myers, B. J. (1969). Parasitic protozoa, commensals and helminths of chimpanzees imported from the Republic of the Congo. *Proc. Int. Congr. Primatol., 2nd,* Atlanta, *1968,* Vol. 3, pp. 184–190.

657. Kuntz, R. E., and Myers, B. J. (1972). Parasites of South American primates. *Int. Zoo Yearb.* **12**, 61–68.

658. Kuntz, R. E., Myers, B. J., and Vice, T. C. (1967). Intestinal protozoans and parasites of the gelada baboon (*Theropithecus gelada* Ruppel, 1835). *Proc. Helminthol. Soc. Wash.* **34**, 65–66.

659. Kuntz, R. E., Myers, B. J., Bergner, J. F., Jr., and Armstrong, D. E. (1968). Parasites and commensals of the Taiwan macaque (*Macaca cyclopis* Swinhoe, 1862). *Formosan Sci.* **22**, 120–136.

660. Kuntz, R. E., Myers, B. J., and Katzberg, A. (1970). Sparganosis and "proliferative-like" spargana in vervets and baboons from East Africa. *J. Parasitol.* **56**, 196–197.

661. Kuntz, R. E., Myers, B. J., and McMurray, T. S. (1970). *Trypanosoma cruzi*-like parasites in the slow loris (*Nycticebus coucang*) from Malaysia. *Trans. Am. Microsc. Soc.* **89**, 304–307.

662. Kuntz, R. E., Myers, B. J., and Moore, J. A. (1973). Parasitology. *In* "Primates in Medicine" (S. S. Kalter, ed.), Vol. 8, pp. 79–104. Karger, Basel.

663. Kuntz, R. E., Huang, T., and Moore, J. A. (1977). Patas monkey (*Erythrocebus patas*) naturally infected with *Schistosoma mansoni*. *J. Parasitol.* **63**, 166–167.

664. Kupper, J. L., and Britz, W. E. (1972). The squirrel monkey. *In* "Selected Topics in Laboratory Animal Medicine," Aeromed. Rev. 5-72. Vol 18, pp. 1–16. USAF Sch. Aerosp. Med., Aerosp. Med. Div. (AFSC), Brooks Air Force Base, Texas.

665. Laing, A. B. G., Edeson, J. F. B., and Wharton, R. H. (1960). Studies on filariasis in Malaya; the vertebrate hosts of *Brugia malayi* and *B. pahangi*. *Ann. Trop. Med. Parasitol.* **54**, 92–99.

666. Lambert, R. A. (1918). *Echinococcus* cysts in a monkey. *Proc. N.Y. Pathol. Soc.* **18**, 29–30.

667. Lambrecht, F. L., Dunn, F. L., and Eyles, D. E. (1961). Isolation of *Plasmodium knowlesi* from Philippine macaques. *Nature (London)* **191**, 1117–1118.

668. Landois, F., and Hoepke, H. (1914). Ein endoparasitäre milbe in der lunge von Macacus rhesus. *Zentralbl. Bakteriol., Parasitenkd., Infektionstr. Hyg., Abt. 1: Orig.* **73**, 384.

669. Lang, E. M. (1966). The care and breeding of anthropoids. *Symp. Zool. Soc. London* **17**, 113–125.

670. Langeron, M. (1920). Note additionhelle sur une hémogrégarine d'um macaque. *Bull. Soc. Pathol. Exot.* **13**, 394.

671. Lapage, G. (1962). "Monnig's Veterinary Helminthology and Entomology," 5th ed. Williams & Wilkins, Baltimore.

672. Lapage, G. (1968). "Veterinary Parasitology." Oliver & Boyd, Edinburgh and London.

673. Lapin, B. A. (1962). Disease in monkeys within the period of acclimatization and during long-term stay in animal houses. *In* "The Problems of Laboratory Animal Disease" (R. J. C. Harris, ed.), pp. 143–149. Academic Press, New York.

674. Lapin, B. A., and Yakovleva, L. A. (1960). "Comparative Pathology in Monkeys." Thomas, Springfield, IL.

675. Lapin, B. A., and Yakovleva, L. A. (1963). Diseases of the cardiovascular system. *In* "Comparative Pathology in Monkeys," pp. 132–177. Thomas, Springfield, IL.

676. Lasry, J. E., and Sheridan, B. W. (1965). Chagas myocarditis and heart failure in the red uakari. *Int. Zoo Yearb.* **5**, 182–187.

677. Lau, D. T., Casey, W. J., and Jones, M. D. (1973). Coenurosis in a whitehanded gibbon. *J. Am. Vet. Med. Assoc.* **163**, 633–635.

678. Lavoipierre, M. M. J. (1955). A description of a new genus of sarcopiform mites and of three new species of Acarina parasitic on primates in the British Cameroons. *Ann. Trop. Med. Parasitol.* **49**, 299–307.

679. Lavoipierre, M. M. J. (1955). The occurrence of a mange mite, *Psoregates* sp. (*Acarina*), in a West African monkey. *Ann. Trop. Med. Parasitol.* **49**, 351.

680. Lavoipierre, M. M. J. (1958). Studies on the host-parasite relationships of filarial-nematodes and their arthropod hosts: I. The sites of development and the migration of *Loa loa* in *Chrysops silacea*, the escape of the infective forms from the head of the fly, and the effect of the worm on its insect host. *Ann. Trop. Med. Parasitol.* **52**, 103–121.

681. Lavoipierre, M. M. J. (1964). A new family of acarines belonging to the suborder Sarcoptiformes parasitic in the hair follicles of primates. *Ann. Natal. Mus.* **16**, 1–18.

682. Lavoipierre, M. M. J. (1964). A note on the family Psoralgidae (Acari: Sarcoptiformes) together with a description of two new genera and two new species parasitic on primates. *Acarologia* **6**, 342–352.

683. Lavoipierre, M. M. J. (1970). A note on the scarcoptic mites of primates. *J. Med. Entomol.* **7**, 376–380.

684. Leathers, C. W. (1978). Pulmonary acariasis in a infant, colony-born rhesus monkey (*Macaca mulatta*). *Lab. Anim. Sci.* **28**, 102–103.

685. Leathers, C. W. (1978). The prevalence of *Hepatocystis kochi* in African green monkeys. *Lab. Anim. Sci.* **28**, 186–189.

686. Lebel, R. R., and Nutting, W. B. (1973). Demodectic mites of subhuman primates I: *Demodex saimiri* sp. n. (Acari: Demodicidae) from the squirrel monkey, *Saimiri sciureus*. *J. Parasitol.* **59**, 719–722.

687. Lee, K. J., Lang, C. M., Hughes, H. C., and Hartshorn, R. D. (1981). Psorergatic mange (Acari: Psorergatidae) of the stumptail macaque (*Macaca arctoides*). *Lab. Anim. Sci.* **31**, 77–79.

688. Lee, R. E., Williams, R. B., Jr., Hull, W. B., and Stein, S. N. (1954). Significance of pulmonary acariasis in rhesus monkeys (*Macaca mulatta*). *Fed. Proc., Fed. Am. Soc. Exp. Biol.* **13**, 85–86.

689. Lee, R. V., Prowten, A. W., Anthone, S., Satchidanand, S. K., Fisher, J. E., and Anthone, R. (1990). Typhlitis due to *Balantidium coli* in captive lowland gorillas. *Rev. Infect. Dis.* **12**, 1052–1059.

690. Leeflang, P. D., and Markham, R. J. (1986). Strongyloidiasis in orangutans *Pongo pygmaeus* at Perth zoo. *Int. Zoo Yearb.* **24/25**, 256–260.

691. Leerhoy, J., and Jensen, H. S. (1967). Sarcoptic mange in a shipment of cynomolgus monkeys. *Nord. Veterinaermed.* **19**, 128–130.

692. Lefrou, G., and Martignoles, J. (1955). Contribution à l'étude de *Plasmodium kochi*. *Plasmodium* des singes africans. *Bull. Soc. Pathol. Exot.* **48**, 227–234.

693. Leger, M., and Bedier, E. (1922). Hémogrégarine du cynocéphale, *Papio sphinx* E. Geoffrey. *C. R. Seances Soc. Biol. Ses. Fil.* **87**, 933–934.

694. Lehner, N. D. M. (1984). Biology and diseases of Cebidae. *In* "Laboratory Animal Medicine" (B. G. Fox, B. J. Cohen, and F. M. Loew, eds.), Chapter 11, pp. 321–353. Academic Press, Orlando, FL.

695. Leibegott, G. (1962). Pericarditis verminosa (*Strongyloides*) beim schimpansen. *Virchows Arch. A: Pathol. Anat.* **335**, 211–225.

696. Levaditi, C., and Schoen, R. (1933). Présence d'um toxoplasme dans l'encéphale du cynocephalus babuin. *Bull. Soc. Pathol. Exot.* **26**, 402–405.

697. Le-Van-Hoa. (1965). Redescription de *Physaloptera tumefaciens*, Henry et Blanc, 1912 parasite des primates *Macaca cynomolgus* L. *Bull. Soc. Pathol. Exot.* **58**, 518–519.

698. Levine, N. D. (1961). "Protozoan Parasites of Domestic Animals and of Man." Burgess, Minneapolis, MN.

699. Levine, N. D. (1970). Protozoan parasites of nonhuman primates as zoonotic agents. *Lab. Anim. Care* **20**, 377–382.

700. Levine, N. D. (1973). "Protozoan Parasites of Domestic Animals and of Man," 2nd ed. Burgess, Minneapolis, MN.

701. Levine, N. D. (1976). "Nematode Parasites of Domestic Animals and of Man." Burgess, Minneapolis, MN.

702. Levine, N. D. (1977). Nomenclature of *Sarcocystis* in the ox and sheep and of fecal coccidia of the dog and cat. *J. Parasitol.* **63**, 36–51.

703. Lichtenfels, J. R. (1971). Morphological variation in the gullet nematode. *Gongylonema pulchrum* Molin, 1857, from eight species of definitive hosts with a consideration of *Gongylonema* from *Macacca* spp. *J. Parasitol.* **57**, 348–355.

704. Lillie, R. D. (1947). Reactions of various parasitic organisms in tissues to the Bauer Feulgen Gram and Gram-Weigert methods. *J. Lab. Clin. Med.* **32**, 76–88.

705. Lim-Boo-Liat (1974). New hosts of *Angiostrongylus malaysiensis* Bhaibulaya and Cross 1971, in Malaysia. *Southeast Asian J. Trop. Med. Public Health* **5**, 379–384.

706. Lindquist, W. D., Bieletzki, J., and Allison, S. (1980). *Pterygodermatites* sp. (Nematode: Rictulariidae) from primates in Topeka, Kansas Zoo. *Proc. Helminthol. Soc. Wash.* **47**, 224–227.

707. Linstow, von O. F. B. (1899). Nematoden aus der berliner zoologischen Sammlung. *Mitt. Zool. Mus. Berlin* **1**(2), 1.

708. Linstow, von O. F. B. (1903). The American hookworm in chimpanzees. *Am. Med.* **6**, 611.

709. Linstow, von O. F. B. (1912). Cestoda and cestodaria. *In* "Stiles and Hassall Index-Catalogue of Medical and Veterinary Zoology," Bull. 85, Hyg. Lab, U. S. Public Health and Marine Hospital Service, Washington, DC.

710. Little, M. D. (1962). Experimental studies on the life cycle of *Strongyloides*. *J. Parasitol.* **48**, Suppl., 41.

711. Little, M. D. (1966). Comparative morphology of six species of *Strongyloides* (Nematoda) and redefinition of the genus. *J. Parasitol.* **52**, 69–84.

712. Loeb, W. F., Bannerman, R. M., Rininger, B. F., and Johnson, A. J. (1978). Hematologic disorders. *In* "Pathology of Laboratory Animals" (K. Benirschke, F. M. Garner, and T. C. Jones, eds.), Vol. I, Chapter 11, pp. 1000–1021, 1032–1050. Springer-Verlag, New York.

713. Lok, J. B., and Kirkpatrick, C. E. (1987). Pentastomiasis in captive monkeys. *Lab. Anim. Sci.* **37**, 494–496.

714. Long, G. G., White, J. D., and Stookey, J. L. (1975). *Pneumocystis carinii* infection in splenectomized owl monkeys. *J. Am. Vet. Med. Assoc.* **167**, 651–654.

715. Long, G. G., Lichtenfels, J. R., and Stookey, J. L. (1976). *Anatrichosoma cynamolgi* (Nematoda: Trichinellida) in rhesus monkeys, *Macaca mulatta*. *J. Parasitol.* **62**, 111–115.

716. Loomis, M. R., and Britt, J. O. (1983). An epizootic of *Entamoeba histolytica* in colobus monkeys. *Annu. Proc., Am. Assoc. Zoo Vet.,* p. 10.

717. Loomis, M. R., and Wright, J. F. (1986). Gastric trichuriasis in a black and white colobus monkey. *J. Am. Vet. Med. Assoc.* **189**, 1214–1215.

718. Loomis, M. R., Britt, J. O., Gendron, A. P., Holshuh, H. J., and Howard, E. B. (1983). Hepatic and gastric amebiasis in black and white colobus monkeys. *J. Am. Vet. Med. Assoc.* **183**, 1188–1191.

719. Lothe, D. F. (1958). An immature *Oesophagostomum* sp. from an umbilical swelling in an African child. *Trans. R. Soc. Trop. Med. Hyg.* **52**, 12.

720. Lourenco-de-Oliveira, R., and Deane, L. M. (1995). Simian malaria at two sites in the Brazilian Amazon. I. The infection rates of *Plasmodium brasilianum* in non-human primates. *Mem. Inst. Oswaldo Cruz* **90**, 331–339.

721. Lozano-Alarcon, F., Stewart, T. B., and Pirie, G. J. (1985). Taeniasis in a purple-faced langur. *J. Am. Vet. Med. Assoc.* **187**, 1271.

722. Lucker, J. T. (1933). *Gongylonema macrogubernaculum* Lubimov, 1931: Two new hosts. *J. Parasitol.* **19**, 243.

723. Lucker, J. T. (1933). Two new hosts *Gongylonema pulchrum* Molin, 1857. *J. Parasitol.* **19**, 248.

724. Lukoschus, F. S., Mertens, L. J. A. M., Nutting, W. B., and Nadchatram, M. (1984). *Demodex intermedius* sp.nov. (Acarina: Prostigmata: Demodicidae) from the meibomian glands of the tree shrew *Tupaia glis* (Mammalia: Scandentia). *Malay. Nat. J.* **36**, 233–245.

725. Lumb, G. D., Beamer, P. R., and Rust, J. H. (1985). Oesphagostomiasis in feral monkeys (*Macaca mulatta*). *Toxicol. Pathol.* **13**, 209–214.

726. Lushbaugh, C. C., Humason, G., and Gengozian, N. (1969). Intrauterine death from congenital Chagas disease in laboratory marmosets (*Saguinus fusciocollis labonotus*). *Am. J. Trop. Med.* **18**, 662–665.

727. Lussier, G., and Marois, P. (1964). Animal sarcosporidiosis in the province of Quebec. *Can. J. Public Health* **55**, 243–246.

728. Machida, M., Araki, J., Koyama, T., Kumada, M., Horii, Y., Imada, I., Takasaka, M., Honjo, S., Matsubayashi, K., and Tibat, T. (1978). The life cycle of *Streptopharagus pigmentatus* (Nematoda, Spiruroidea) from the Japanese monkey. *Bull. Natl. Sci. Mus., Ser. A* **4**, 1–9.

729. MacKenzie, P. S. (1979). Pathogenicity, identification and treatment of *Prosthenorchis elegans* infestation in squirrel monkeys (*Saimiri sciureus*). *Primates, Suppl.* **4**, 5–7.

730. MacKinnon, D. L., and Dibb, M. J. (1938). Report on intestine protozoa of some mammals in the zoological gardens at Regent's Park. *Proc. Zool. Soc. London, Ser. B* **108**, 323–345.

731. Magalhaes, Pinto R. (1970). Occurrence of *Subulura jacchi* (Marcel, 1857) Railliet and Henry, 1913 (Nematoda, Subuluroidea) in a new host: *Callithrix aurita coelestis* (M. Ribeiro, 1924). *Atas Soc. Biol. Rio de Janeiro* **13**, 143–145.

732. Mak, J. W., Inder-Singh, Yen, P. K. F., and Yap, L. F. (1980). *Dipetalonema digitatum* (Chandler, 1929) infection in the leaf monkey, *Presbytis obscura* (Reid). *Southeast Asian J. Trop. Med. Public Health* **11**, 141.

733. Mandour, A. M. (1969). *Sarcocystis nesbitti* n. sp. from the rhesus monkey. *J. Protozool.* **16**, 353–354.

734. Mansfield, K. G., Carville, A., Shvetz, D., MacKey, J., Tzipori, S., and Lackner, A. A. (1997). Identification of an *Enterocytozoon bienusi*-like microsporidian parasite in simian-immunodeficiency-virus-innoculated macaques with hepatobiliary disease. *Am. J. Pathol.* **190**, 1396–1405.

735. Manwell, R. D. (1968). Simian malaria. *In* "Infectious Blood Diseases of Man and Animals" (D. Weinman and M. Ristic, eds.), Vol. 2, pp. 78–88. Academic Press, New York.

736. Manwell, R. D., and Kuntz, R. E. (1966). *Hepatocystis* in Formosan mammals with a description of a new species. *J. Protozool.* **13**, 670–672.

737. Maplestone, P. A. (1931). Parasitic nematodes obtained from animals dying in the Calcutta Zoological Gardens. Pt. 4-8. *Rec. Indian Mus.* **33**, 71–171.

738. Marinkelle, C. J. (1966). Observations on man, monkey, and bat trypanosomes and their vectors in Colombia. *Trans. R. Soc. Trop. Med. Hyg.* **60**, 109–116.

739. Marinkelle, C. J. (1968). *Trypanosoma lambrechti* n. sp. aislado de micos (*Cebus albifrons*) de Colombia. *Caldasia* **10**, 155–165.

740. Marinkelle, C. J. (1976). The biology of the trypanosomes of non-human primates. *In* "Biology of the Kinetoplastida" (W. H. R. Lumsden and D. A. Evans, eds.), Vol. 1, pp. 217–256. Academic Press, New York.

741. Marinkelle, C. J. (1982). The prevalence of *Trypanosoma* (*Schizotrypanum*) *cruzi* infection in Colombian monkeys and marmosets. *Ann. Trop. Med. Parasitol.* **76**, 121–124.

742. Marinkelle, C. J., and Grose, E. (1968). *Plasmodium brasilianum* in Colombian monkeys. *Trop. Geogr. Med.* **20**, 276–280.

743. Martinez, A. J., Guerra, A. E., Garcia-Tamayo, J., Cespedes, G., Gonzales-Alfano, J. E., and Visvesvara, G. S. (1994). Granulomatous amebic encephalitis: A review and report of a spontaneous case from Venezuela. *Acta Neuropathol.* **87**, 430–434.

744. Masbar, S., Palmieri, J. R., Marwoto, H. A., Purnomo, and Darwis, D. F. (1981). Blood parasites of wild and domestic animals from South Kalimantan (Borneo), Indonesia. *Southeast Asian J. Trop. Med. Public Health* **12**, 42–46.

745. Masse, R., Geneste, M., and Thiery, G. (1965). Acariose pulmonaire du singe traitement, prophylaxie. *Recl. Méd. Vét.* **141**, 1227–1234.

746. Matern, B. (1976). Zur strongyloidose der menschenaffen in Zoologischen Gärten. Doctoral Dissertation, University of Giessen; cited by Leeflang and Markham (690).

747. Mayer, M. (1907). Über malaria beim affens. *Med. Klin.* **3**, 579–580.

748. Mayer, M. (1933). Über einen neuen blutparasiten des affen (*Entopolypoides macaci* n. g. n. sp.). *Arch. Schiffs.- Trop.-Hyg.* **37**, 504–505.

749. Mayer, M. (1934). Ein neuer, eigenartiger blutparasit des affen (*Entopolypoides macaci* n. g. et n. sp.). *Zentralbl. Bakteriol., Parasitenkd., Abt. I: Infektionskr. Hyg., Orig.* **131**, 132–136.

750. Mazza, S. (1930). Doble parasitismo por filarias en monos *Cebus* del norte. *5a Reun. Soc. Argent. Patol. Reg. Norte* **2**, 1140.

751. McCarrison, R. (1920). The effects of deficient dietaries on monkeys. *Br. Med. J.* Feb. 21, pp. 249–253.

752. McClure, G. W. (1932). Nematode parasites of mammals with a description of a new species, *Wellcomia branickii* from specimens collected in the New York Zoological Park, 1930. *Zoologica (N.Y.)* **15**, 1.

753. McClure, G. W. (1934). Nematode parasites of mammals from specimens collected in the New York Zoological Park, 1932. *Zoologica (N.Y.)* **15**, 49.

754. McClure, H. M., and Guilloud, N. B. (1971). Comparative pathology of the chimpanzee. *In* "The Chimpanzee" (G. H. Bourne, ed.), Vol. 4, pp. 103–272. University Park Press, Baltimore.

755. McClure, H. M., Strozier, L. M., Keeling, M. E., and Healy, G. R. (1973). Strongyloidosis in two infant orangutans. *J. Am. Vet. Med. Assoc.* **163**, 629–632.

756. McClure, H. M., Chapman, W. L., Jr., Hooper, B. E., Smith, F. G., and Fletcher, O. J. (1978). The digestive system. *In* "Pathology of Laboratory Animals" (K. Benirschke, F. M. Garner, and T. C. Jones, eds.), Vol. I, Chapter 4, pp. 176–317. Springer-Verlag, New York.

757. McConnell, E. E. (1977). Parasitic diseases observed in free-ranging and captive baboons. *Comp. Pathol. Bull.* **9**, 2.

758. McConnell, E. E., Basson, P. A., and DeVos, V. (1971). Nasal acariasis in the chacma baboon. *Papio ursinus* Kerr 1792. *Onderstepoort J. Vet. Res.* **38**, 207.

759. McConnell, E. E., DeVos, A. J., Basson, P. A., and DeVos, V. (1971). *Isopora papionis* n. sp. (Eimeriidae) of the Chacma baboon *Papio ursinus* (Kess, 1792). *J. Protozool.* **18**, 28–32.

760. McConnell, E. E., Basson, P. A., Thomas, S. E., and DeVos, V. (1972). Oocysts of *Isopora papionis* in the skeletal muscle of Chacma baboons. *Onderstepoort J. Vet. Res.* **39**, 113–116.

761. McConnell, E. E., Basson, P. A., and DeVos, V. (1972). Laryngeal acariasis in the chacma baboon. *J. Am. Vet. Med. Assoc.* **161**, 678–682.

762. McConnell, E. E., Basson, P. A., Wolstenholme, B., DeVos, V., and Malherbe, H. (1973). Toxoplasmosis in "free-ranging" chacma baboons (*Papio ursinus*) from the Krueger National Park. *Trans. R. Soc. Trop. Med. Hyg.* **67**, 851–855.

763. McConnell, E. E., Basson, P. A., DeVos, V., Myers, B. J., and Kuntz, R. E. (1974). A survey of diseases among 100 free-ranging baboons (*Papio ursinus*) from Krueger National Park. *Onderstepoort J. Vet. Res.* **41**, 97–167.

764. McCoy, O. R. (1936). Filarial parasites of monkeys of Panama. *Am. J. Trop. Med.* **16**, 383–403.

765. McGrew, W. C., Tutin, C. E. G., Collins, D. A., and File, S. K. (1989). Intestinal parasites of sympatric *Pan troglodytes* and *Papio* spp. at two sites: Gombe (Tanzania) and Mt. Assirik (Senegal). *Am. J. Primatol.* **17**, 147–155.

766. McKissick, G. E., Ratcliffe, H. L., and Koestner, A. (1968). Enzootic toxoplasmosis in caged squirrel monkeys. *Saimiri sciureus. Pathol. Vet.* **5**, 538–560.

767. Meir, J. E. (1978). Lung mites in a douc langur (*Pygathrix nemaeus*). *Annu. Proc., Am. Assoc. Zoo Vet.*, pp. 139–142.

768. Melton, D. A., and Melton, C. L. (1981). Blood parameters of the wild chacma baboon, *Papio ursinus. Am. J. Zool.* **17**, 85–90.

769. Mendonca, de M. M. (1983). *Mathevotaenia cruzsilvai* n. sp. (cestoda Anoplocephalidae), parasite of *Macaca irus* F. Cuvier, 1818. *Bull. Mus. Natl. Hist. Nat., Ser. A* **3**, 1081–1086.

770. Middleton, C. C. (1966). Acanthocephala (*Prosthenorchis elegans*) infection in squirrel monkeys (*Saimiri sciureus*). *Lab. Anim. Dig.* **2**, 16–17.

771. Middleton, C. C., Clarkson, T. B., and Garner, F. M. (1964). Parasites of squirrel monkeys (*Saimiri sciureus*). *Lab. Anim. Care* **14**, 335.

772. Migaki, G., Seibold, H. R., Wolf, R. H., and Garner, F. M. (1971). Pathologic conditions in the patas monkey. *J. Am. Vet. Med. Assoc.* **159**, 549–556.

773. Migaki, G., Bernirschke, K., McKee, A. E., and Casey, H. W. (1978). Trichomonal granuloma of the pelvic cavity in a rhesus monkey. *Vet. Pathol.* **15**, 679–681.

774. Miller, J. H. (1959). The dog face baboon, *Papio doguera*, a primate reservoir host for *Schistosoma mansoni* in East Africa. *J. Parasitol.* **45**, 22–25.

775. Miller, J. H. (1959). *Hepatocystis* (= *Plasmodium*) *kochi* in the dog face baboon, *Papio doguera. J. Parasitol.* **45**, Suppl., 53.

776. Miller, M. J., and Bray, R. S. (1966). *Entamoeba histolytica* infections in the chimpanzee (*Pan satyrus*). *J. Parasitol.* **52**, 386–388.

777. Miller, R. A., Bronsdon, M. A., Kuller, L., and Morton, W. R. (1990). Clinical and parasitologic aspects of cryptosporidiosis in nonhuman primates. *Lab. Anim. Sci.* **40**, 42–46.

778. Miller, R. A., Bronsdon, M. A., and Morton, W. R. (1990). Experimental cryptosporidiosis in a primate model. *J. Infect. Dis.* **161**, 312–315.

779. Moncol, D. J., and Batte, E. G. (1966). Transcolostral infection of newborn pigs with *Strongyloides ransomi*. *VM/SAC, Vet. Med. Small Anim. Clin.* **61**, 583–586.

780. Monnig, H. O. (1920). *Filaria nycticebi* eine nene filaria aus dem *Nycticebus*. *Zentralbl. Bakteriol. Parasitenkd., Infektionskr. Hyg., Abt. I: Orig.* **85,** 216–221.

781. Montali, R. J., and Bush, M. (1980). Diagnostic exercise. *Lab. Anim. Sci.* **30,** 33–34.

782. Montali, R. J., and Bush, M. (1981). Rictulariasis in Callitrichidae at the National Zoological Park. *Int. Symp. Erkr. Zootiere Halle/Saale, 23rd,* pp. 197–202.

783. Montali, R. J., Gardiner, C. H., Evans, R. E., and Bush, M. (1983). *Pterygodermatites nycticebi* (Nematoda: Spirurida) in Golden Lion Tamarins. *Lab. Anim. Sci.* **33,** 194–197.

784. Montgomery, C. A. (1978). Muscle diseases. *In* "Pathology of Laboratory Animals" (K. Benirschke, F. M. Garner, and T. C. Jones, eds.), Vol. I, Chapter 10, pp. 841–853, 880–887. Springer-Verlag, New York.

785. Moore, G., and Myers, B. J. (1974). Parasites of non-human primates. *Annu. Proc., Am. Assoc. Zoo Vet.,* Washington, DC, pp. 79–86.

786. Moore, J. A., and Kuntz, R. E. (1975). *Entopolypoides macaci* Mayer 1934 in the African baboon (*Papio cynocephalus* L. 1776). *J. Med. Primatol.* **4,** 1–7.

787. Moore, J. G. (1970). Epizootic of acanthocephaliasis among primates. *J. Am. Vet. Med. Assoc.* **157,** 699–705.

788. Mooreman, A. E. (1941). *Balantidium coli* and pinworm in a chimpanzee. *J. Parasitol.* **27,** 366.

789. Moreina, R. A., Lombardero, O. J., and Coppo, J. A. (1979). Nuevos parasitos de primates para la Argentina. *Acta Zool. Lilloana* **35,** 13–19.

790. Morin, M. L., Renquist, D. M., Johnson, D. K., and Strumpf, I. J. (1980). Flexible fiberoptic protoscopy compared with fecal examination techniques for diagnosis of *Prosthenorchis* infection in squirrel monkeys (*Saimiri sciureus*). *Lab. Anim. Sci.* **30,** 1009–1011.

791. Mortelman, J., Vercruysse, J., and Kageruka, P. (1971). Three pathogenic intestinal protozoa of anthropoid apes: *Entamoeba histolytica, Balantidium coli* and *Troglodytella abrassarti. Proc. Int. Cong. Primatol., 3rd,* Zurich, *1970,* Vol. 2, pp. 187–191.

792. Morton, H. L. (1969). Sparganosis in African green monkeys (*Cercopithecus aethiops*). *Lab. Anim. Care* **19,** 253–255.

793. Movcan, A. T., and Tscherner, W. A. (1982). Parasitisation of hamadryas baboon (*Papio hamadryas*). *Erkr. Zootiere* **24,** 337–339 (in German w/ English, French and Russian summaries).

794. Muller, R., and Ruedi, D. (1981). Gastric amebiasis in a proboscis monkey (*Nasalis larvatus*). *Acta Zool. Pathol. Antverp.* **76,** 9–16.

795. Mulligan, H. W. (1935). Description of two species of monkey *Plasmodium* isolated from *Silenus irus. Arch. Protistenkd.* **84,** 285–314.

796. Mullin, S. W. (1971). A description of the microfilariae of *Edensonfilaria malayensis* Yeh, 1960. *Southeast Asian J. Trop. Med. Public Health* **2,** 256.

797. Mullin, S. W., and Orihel, T. C. (1972). *Tetrapetalonema dunni* sp. n. (Nematoda: Filaroidea) from Malaysian tree shrews. *J. Parasitol.* **58,** 1047–1051.

798. Mullin, S. W., Colley, F. C., and Stevens, G. S. (1972). Coccidia of Malaysian mammals: New host records and descriptions of three new species of *Eimeria. J. Protozool.* **19,** 260–263.

799. Mullin, S. W., Dondero, T. T., Jr., Sivanandam, S., and Dewey,, R. (1972). Filarial parasites of malaysian monkeys. *Southeast Asian J. Trop. Med. Public Health* **3,** 548–551.

800. Murphy, J. C., Fox, J. G., and Shalev, M. (1979). *Paragonimus westermani* infection in a cynomolgus monkey. *J. Am. Vet. Med. Assoc.* **175,** 981–984.

801. Myers, B. J. (1960). A note on some helminths from Malayan animals. *Can. J. Zool.* **38,** 440–441.

802. Myers, B. J. (1970). Techniques for recognition of parasites. *Lab. Anim. Care* **20,** 342–344.

803. Myers, B. J. (1972). Echinococcosis, coenurosis, cysticercosis, sparganosis, etc. *In* "Pathology of Simian Primates" (R. N. T.-W. Fiennes, ed.), Part 2, pp. 124–143. Karger, Basel.

804. Myers, B. J., and Kuntz, R. E. (1965). A checklist of parasites reported for the baboon. *Primates* **6,** 137–194.

805. Myers, B. J., and Kuntz, R. E. (1967). Parasites of baboons taken by the Cambridge Mwanza expedition (Tanzania 1965). *East Afr. Med. J.* **44,** 322–324.

806. Myers, B. J., and Kuntz, R. E. (1968). Intestinal protozoa of the baboon *Papio doguera* Pucheran 1856. *J. Protozool.* **15,** 363–365.

807. Myers, B. J., and Kuntz, R. E. (1969). Nematode parasites of mammals (Dermoptera, Primates, Pholidata, Rodentia, Carnivora, and Atiodactyla) from North Borneo (Malaysia). *Can. J. Zool.* **47,** 419–421.

808. Myers, B. J., and Kuntz, R. E. (1972). A checklist of parasites and commensals reported for the chimpanzee (*Pan*). *Primates* **13,** 433–471.

809. Myers, B. J., Kuntz, R. E., and Vice, T. E. (1965). Hydatid disease in captive primates (*Colobus* and *Papio*). *J. Parasitol., Suppl.* **51,** 22.

810. Myers, B. J., Kuntz, R. E., Vice, T. E., and Kim, C. S. (1970). Natural infection of *Echinococcus granulosus* (Batsch, 1786) Rudolph, 1805 in the Kenya baboon (*Papio* sp.). *Lab. Anim. Care* **20,** 283–286.

811. Myers, B. J., Kuntz, R. E., and Malherbe, H. (1971). Intestinal commensals and parasites of the South African baboon (*Papio cynocephalus*). *Trans. Am. Microsc. Soc.* **90,** 80–83.

812. Myers, B. J., Kuntz, R. E., and Kamara, J. A. (1973). Parasites and commensals of chimpanzees captured in Sierra Leone, West Africa. *Proc. Helminthol. Soc. Wash.* **40,** 298–299.

813. Mysorekar, N. R., Chakravarti, R. N., Chawla, L. S., and Chhuttani, P. N. (1966). Diseases of rhesus monkeys—III. Large intestine. *J. Assoc. Physicians India* **14,** 583–587.

814. Nagaty, H. F. (1935). *Parlitomosa zakii* (Filariinae). A new genus and species and its microfilaria from *Leontocebus rosalia. J. Egypt. Med. Assoc.* **18,** 483–496.

815. Napier, J. R., and Napier, P. H. (1967). "A Handbook of Living Primates." Academic Press, New York.

816. Naquira, C. (1963). Estudio preliminar sobre la infeccion celomica de *Triatoma infestans* por *Trypanosoma cruzi* y *Trypanosoma* sp. de mono. *Biologica, Santiago* **35,** 3–8.

817. Narama, I., Tsuchitani, M., Umemura, T., and Tsuruta, M. (1983). The morphogenesis of a papillomatous gastric polyp in the crab-eating monkey (*Macaca fascicularis*). *J. Comp. Pathol.* **93,** 195–203.

818. Navin, T. R., and Juranek, D. D. (1984). Cryptosporidiosis: Clinical, epidemiologic and parasitologic review. *Rev. Infect. Dis.* **6,** 313–327.

819. Nelson, B., Cosgrove, G. E., and Gengozian, N. (1966). Diseases of an imported primate *Tamarinus nigricollis. Lab. Anim. Care* **16,** 255–275.

820. Nelson, E. C. (1932). The cultivation of a species of *Troglodytella*, a large ciliate, from the chimpanzee. *Science* **75,** 317–318.

821. Nelson, G. S. (1960). Schistosome infections as zoonoses in Africa. *Trans. R. Soc. Trop. Med. Hyg.* **54,** 301–316.

822. Nelson, G. S. (1965). The parasitic helminths of baboons with particular reference to species transmissible to man. *In* "The Baboon in Medical Research" (H. Vagtborg, ed.), pp. 441–470. University of Texas Press, Austin.

823. Nelson, G. S., Teesdale, C., and Highton, R. B. (1962). The role of animals as reservoirs of bilharziasis in Africa. *Bilharziasis, Ciba Found. Symp.* pp. 127–149.

824. Nery-Guimaraes, F., Franken, A. J., and Chagas, W. A. (1971). Toxoplasmose em primates não humanos. I. Infeccões naturais em *Macaca mulatta* e *Cebus apella. Mem. Inst. Oswaldo Cruz* **69,** 77–96.

825. Newstead, R. (1906). On another new Dermanyssid Acarid parasitic in the lungs of the rhesus monkey (*Macaca rhesus*). *Mem. Liverpool Sch. Trop. Med.* **18,** 45.

826. Newstead, R., and Todd, J. L. (1906). On a new dermanyssid acarid found living in the lungs of monkeys (*Cercopithecus schmidti*) from the upper Congo. *Mem. Liverpool Sch. Trop. Med.* **18,** 41–44.

827. Nicholas, W. L. (1967). The biology of acanthocephala. *Adv. Parasitol.* **5,** 205–246.

828. Nielsen, D. H. (1980). *Prosthenorchis elegans* infection in a primate colony. *Annu. Proc., Am. Assoc. Zoo Vet.*, pp. 113–116.

829. Nigi, H., and Itakura, C. (1968). Spontaneous toxoplasmosis in *Lemur cata. Primates* 9, 155–160.

830. Noda, S. (1962). Comparative studies on morphology of free-living stages of *Strongyloides* parasitic in monkeys. *Jpn. J. Parasitol.* 11, 207–229.

831. Nonoyama, T., Sugitani, T., Orita, S., and Miyajima, H. (1984). A pathological study in cynomolgus monkeys infected with *Edesonfilaria malayensis. Lab. Anim. Sci.* 34, 604–609.

832. Norman, R. C., and Wagner, J. E. (1973). Pediculosis of spider monkeys: A case report with zoonotic implications. *Lab. Anim. Sci.* 23, 872–875.

833. Nouvell, J., and Prot-Lassele, J. (1963). Shigella dysenteriae 2 chez des chimpanzé en captivité. *Bull. Acad. Vet. Fr.* 36, 373–379.

834. Nuttall, G. H. F., and Warburton, C. (1915). The genus *Haemaphysalis. In* "Ticks, A Monograph of the *Ixodoidea*, Part III, pp. 349–550. Cambridge University Press, Cambridge, UK.

835. O'Farrell, L., and Griffith, J. W. (1995). What's your diagnosis? Esophageal parasite in a cynomolgus monkey. *Lab. Anim.* 24(7), 17–19.

836. Offutt, E. P., Jr., and Telford, I. R. (1945). *Sarcocystis* in the monkey. A report of two cases. *J. Parasitol., Suppl.* 21, 15.

837. Ogata, T., Imai, H., and Coulston, F. (1971). Pulmonary acariasis in rhesus monkeys: Electron microscopic study. *Exp. Mol. Pathol.* 15, 137.

838. O'Grady, J. P., Yeager, C. H., Esra, G. N., and Thomas, W. (1982). Ultrasonic evaluation of echinococcosis in four lowland gorillas. *J. Am. Vet. Med. Assoc.* 181, 1348–1350.

839. Ogunsusi, R. A., and Mohammed, A. N. (1978). The chimpanzee (*Pan troglodytes*), a new host for nymphal *Armillifer armillatus* (Pentastomida: Porocephalida) in West Africa. *Rev. Elev. Med. Vet. Pays Trop.* 1, 361–362.

840. Ohbayashi, M., and Vajrasthira, S. (1983). A new nematode, *Mammanidula siamensis* n. sp., from the mammary gland of *Tupaia glis* and *Rattus surifer* of Thailand. *Jpn. J. Vet. Res.* 31, 1–5.

841. Oku, Y., Kudo, N., Ohbayashi, M., Narama, I., and Umemura, T. (1983). A case of abdominal angiostrongyliasis in a monkey. *Jpn. J. Vet. Res.* 31, 71–75.

842. Orihel, T. C. (1966). *Brugia tupaiae* sp. n. (Nematoda: Filarioidea) in three shrews (*Tupaia glis*) from Malaysia. *J. Parasitol.* 52, 162–165.

843. Orihel, T. C. (1970). Primates as models for parasitological research. *In* "Medical Primatology" (E. I. Goldsmith and J. Moor-Jankowski, eds.), pp. 772–782. Karger, Basel.

844. Orihel, T. C. (1970). Anatrichosomiasis in African monkeys. *J. Parasitol.* 56, 982–985.

845. Orihel, T. C. (1970). The helminth parasites of nonhuman primates and man. *Lab. Anim. Care* 20, 395–401.

846. Orihel, T. C. (1970). Filariasis in chimpanzees. *In* "The Chimpanzee" (G. H. Bourne, ed.), Vol. 3, pp. 56–70. University Park Press, Baltimore.

847. Orihel, T. C. (1971). *Necator americanus* infection in primates. *J. Parasitol.* 57, 117–121.

848. Orihel, T. C., and Ash, L. R. (1995). "Parasites in Human Tissues." Am. Soc. Clin. Pathol. Press, Chicago.

849. Orihel, T. C., and Esslinger, J. H. (1973). *Meningonema peruzzii* gen. et sp. n. (Nematoda: Filarioidea) from the central nervous system of African monkeys. *J. Parasitol.* 59, 437–441.

850. Orihel, T. C., and Seibold, H. R. (1971). Trichospirurosis in South American monkeys. *J. Parasitol.* 57, 1366–1368.

851. Orihel, T. C., and Seibold, H. R. (1972). Nematodes of the bowel and tissues. *In* "Pathology of Simian Primates" (R. N. T.-W. Fiennes, ed.), Part 2, pp. 76–103. Karger, Basel.

852. Ortlepp, R. J. (1924). On a collection of helminths from Dutch Guiana. *J. Helminthol.* 2, 15.

853. Otsuru, M., and Sekikawa, H. (1968). A survey of simian malaria in Japan. *Trans. R. Soc. Trop. Med. Hyg.* 62, 558–561.

854. Oudemans, A. C. (1935). Kritische literaturubersicht zue gattung *Pneumonyssus* beschreibung dreier arten, darunter einer neuen. *Z. Parasitenkd.* 7, 466–512.

855. Owen, D., and Casillo, S. (1973). A preliminary survey of the nematode parasites of some imported Old-World monkeys. *Lab. Anim.* 7, 265–269.

856. Ow-Yang, C. K., and Wah, M. J. (1975). A remarkable trematode from the parotid gland of *Tupaia glis. Southeast Asian J. Trop. Med. Public Health* 6, 449.

857. Padovan, D., and Cantrell, C. (1983). Causes of death of infant rhesus and squirrel monkeys. *J. Am. Vet. Med. Assoc.* 183, 1182–1184.

858. Palmieri, J. R., and Krishnasamy, M. (1978). *Phaneropsolus aspinosus* sp. n. (Lecithodendriidae Phaneropsoline) from leaf monkey *Macaca fascicularis* (Raffles). *J. Helminthol.* 52, 155–158.

859. Palmieri, J. R., Krishasamy, M., and Sullivan, J. T. (1977). Helminth parasites of the Old World leaf monkey *Presbytis* sp. from west Malaysia. *Southeast Asian J. Trop. Med. Public Health* 8, 409.

860. Palmieri, J. R., Purnomo, Lee, V. H., Dennis, D. T., and Marwoto, H. A. (1980). Parasites of the silvered leaf monkey, *Presbytis cristatus* Eschscholtz 1921, with a note on a *Wuchereria*-like nematode. *J. Parasitol.* 66, 170–171.

861. Palmieri, J. R., Purnomo, Dennis, D. T., and Marwoto, H. A. (1980). Filarid parasites of South Kalimantan (Borneo) Indonesia. *Wuchereria kalimantani* sp. n. (Nematoda: Filarioidea) from the silvered leaf monkey, *Presbytis cristatus* Eschscholtz 1921. *J. Parasitol.* 66, 645–651.

862. Palmieri, J. R., Dalgard, D. W., and Conner, D. H. (1984). Gastric amebiasis in a silvered leaf monkey. *J. Am. Vet. Med. Assoc.* 185, 1374–1375.

863. Palmieri, J. R., Van Dellen, A. F., Tirtokusumo, S., Masbar, S., Rusch, J., and Connor, D. H. (1984). Trapping, care, and laboratory management of the silvered leaf monkey (*Presbytis cristatus*). *Lab. Anim. Sci.* 34, 194–197.

864. Palotay, J. L., and Uno, H. (1975). Hydatid disease in four nonhuman primates. *J. Am. Vet. Med. Assoc.* 167, 615–618.

865. Parker, G. A., Gilmore, C. J., and Roberts, C. R. (1979). Diagnostic exercise. *Lab. Anim. Sci.* 29, 457–458.

866. Patten, R. A. (1939). Amoebic dysentery in orang-utans (*Simia satyrus*). *Aust. Vet. J.* 15, 68–71.

867. Paulicki, A. (1872). Beiträge zur vergleichenden pathologischen anatomie aus dem Hamburger Zoologischen Garten II. *Grune Psorospermienheerde in der Affenlunge Magges Thierheilk* 38, 1.

868. Pavor, M. L. (1965). Lung mites (*Pneumonyssus simicola*) in the feces of *Macaca mulatta. Lab. Primate Newsl.* 4, 4.

869. Peddie, J. F., and Larson, E. J. (1971). Demodectic acariasis in a woolly monkey. *VM/SAC, Vet. Med. Small Anim. Clin.* 66, 485–488.

870. Peel, E., and Chardome, M. (1946). Note préliminaire sur des filaridés de chimpanzés, *Pan panicus* et *Pan satyrus* au Congo belge. *Recl. Trav. Sci. Méd. Congo Belge* 5, 244.

871. Peel, E., and Chardome, M. (1946). Sur des filaridés de chimpanzés "*Pan paniscus*" et "*Pan satyrus*" au Congo belge. *Ann. Soc. Belge Med. Trop.* 26, 117–156.

872. Peel, E., and Chardome, M. (1947). Note complémentaire sur des filaridés de chimpanzés, *Pan paniscus* et *Pan satyrus* Congo belge. *Ann. Soc. Belge Med. Trop.* 27, 241–250.

873. Peisert, W., Taborski, A., Pawlowski, Z., Karlewiczowa, R., and Zdun, M. (1983). *Giardia* infection in animals in Poznan Zoo. *Vet. Parasitol.* 13, 183–186.

874. Penner, L. R. (1981). Concerning threadworm (*Strongyloides stercoralis*) in great apes—lowland gorillas (*Gorilla gorilla*) and chimpanzees (*Pan troglodytes*). *J. Zoo Anim. Med.* 12, 128–131.

875. Pessoa, S. B., and Prado, A. (1927). Sobra uma nova *Bartonella* parasita do mocaco *Pseudocebus appela* (L.). *Rev. Biol. Hyg. Sao Paulo* 1, 116–117.

876. Peters, W., Howells, R. E., and Molyneux, D. H. (1973). *Eperythrozoon* and *Haemobartonella* in primates. *Trans. R. Soc. Trop. Med. Hyg.* 67, 21.

877. Peters, W., Molyneux, D. H., and Howells, R. E. (1974). *Eperythrozoon* and *Haemobartonella* in monkeys. *Ann. Trop. Med. Parasitol.* **68**, 47–50.

878. Petit, G., Bain, O., and Roussilhon, C. (1985). Deux nouvelles filaires chez un singe, *Saimiri sciureus,* au Guyana. *Ann. Parasitol. Hum. Comp.* **60**, 65–81.

879. Pettifer, H. L. (1984). The helminth fauna of the digestive tracts of chacma baboons, *Papio ursinus,* from different localities in the Transvaal. *Onderstepoort J. Vet. Res.* **51**, 161–170.

880. Phillipe, J. (1948). Note sur les gales du singe. *Bull. Soc. Pathol. Exot.* **41**, 597–600.

881. Phillippi, K. M., and Clarke, M. R. (1982). Survey of parasites of rhesus monkeys housed in small social groups. *Am. J. Primatol.* **27**, 293–302.

882. Phillips-Conroy, J. E., Lambrecht, F. L., and Jolly, C. J. (1988). *Hepatocystis* in populations of baboons (*Papio hamadryas* s. l.) of Tanzania and Ethiopia. *J. Med. Primatol.* **17**, 145–152.

883. Pietrzyk, J., and Uminski, J. (1967). Malaria u malp *Cercopithecus* wywolana prezez *Hepatocystis kochi. Zwierzeta Lab.* **2**, 72–79.

884. Pillers, A. W. N. (1921). Sarcoptic scabies (or itch) in the chimpanzee. *Br. Vet. J.* **77**, 329–333.

885. Pillers, A. W. N. (1924). *Ascaris lumbricoides* causing fatal lesions in a chimpanzee. *Ann. Trop. Med. Parasitol.* **18**, 101–102.

886. Pillers, A. W. N., and Southwell, T. (1929). Strongyloidosis of the woolly monkey (*Lagothrix humboldti*). *Ann. Trop. Med. Parasitol.* **23**, 129.

887. Pindak, F. F., Mora de Pindak, M., Abee, C. R., and Gardner, W. A., Jr. (1985). Detection and cultivation of intestinal trichomonads of squirrel monkeys (*Saimiri sciureus*). *Am. J. Primatol.* **9**, 197–205.

888. Pindak, F. F., Gardner, W. A., Jr., Mora de Pindak, M., and Abee, C. R. (1987). Detection of hemagglutinins in cultures of squirrel monkey intestinal trichomonads. *J. Clin. Microbiol.* **25**, 609–614.

889. Poelma, F. G. (1966). *Eimeria lemuris* n. sp., *E. galago* n. sp. and *E. otolicni* n. sp. from a galago *Galago senegalensis. J. Protozool.* **13**, 547–549.

890. Poelma, F. G. (1975). *Pneumocystis carinii* infections in zoo animals. *Z. Parasitenkd.* **46**, 61–68.

891. Poindexter, H. A. (1942). A study of the intestinal parasites of the monkeys of the Santiago Island primate colony. *P. R. J. Public Health Trop. Med.* **18**, 175–191.

892. Poisson, R. (1953). Sous-ordre des hémosporidies (Haemosporidiidea Danilewsky, 1889 emend.; Doflein, 1901). *In* "Traité de Zoologie Anatomie-Systématique Biologie" (P.-P. Grassé, ed.), Vol. I, Fasc. II, pp. 798–906. Masson, Paris.

893. Pope, B. L. (1966). Some parasites of the howler monkey of northern Argentina. *J. Parasitol.* **52**, 166–168.

894. Pope, B. L. (1968). XV. Parasites. *In* "Biology of the Howler Monkey (*Alouatta caraya*)" (M. R. Malinow, ed.), Bibl. Primatol. No. 7, pp. 204–208. Karger, Basel.

895. Porter, A. (1945). Report of the honorary parasitologist for 1944. *Proc. Zool. Soc. London* **115**, 384–386.

896. Porter, A. (1952). *Chilomastix tarsii* sp. n., a new flagellate from the gut of *Tarsius carbonarius. Proc. Zool. Soc. London* **121**, 915.

897. Porter, A. (1953–1954). Report of the honorary parasitologist for the year 1952. *Proc. Zool. Soc. London* **123**, 253–257.

898. Porter, A. (1954). Report of the honorary parasitologist for the year 1953. *Proc. Zool. Soc. London* **124**, 313–316.

899. Porter, A. (1955). Summary of the report of the honorary parasitologist for the year 1954. *Proc. Zool. Soc. London* **125**, 541.

900. Porter, J. A., Jr. (1972). Parasites of marmosets. *Lab. Anim. Sci.* **22**, 503–506.

901. Porter, J. A., Jr., Johnson, C. M., and DeSousa, L. (1966). Prevalence of malaria in Panamanian primates. *J. Parasitol.* **52**, 669–670.

902. Powers, R. D., Price, R. A., Houk, R. P., and Mattlin, R. H. (1966). Echinococcosis in a drill baboon. *J. Am. Vet. Med. Assoc.* **149**, 902–905.

903. Prathap, K., Law, K. S., and Bolton, J. M. (1969). Pentastomiasis. A common finding at autopsy among Malaysian Aborigines. *Am. J. Trop. Med. Hyg.* **18**, 20–27.

904. Premvati. (1959). *Primatotrema macacae* gen. nov. sp. nov. from macaque rhesus monkeys, and a redescription of *Phaneropsolus oviforme* (Poirier, 1886) Looss 1899 (Lecithodendriidae). *J. Parasitol.* **44**, 639–642.

905. Price, D. L. (1959). *Dirofilaria magnilarvatum* n. sp. (Nematoda: Filarioidea) from *Macaca irus* Cuvier: I. Description of the adult filarial worms. *J. Parasitol.* **45**, 499–504.

906. Prine, J. R. (1968). Pancreatic flukes and amoebic colitis in a gorilla. *19th Annu. Meet. Am. Assoc. Lab. Anim. Sci.,* Las Vegas, Abstr. No. 50.

907. Prosl, H., and Tamer, A. (1979). The parasite fauna of the rhesus monkey (*Macaca mulatta*) and the Java ape (*Macaca irus*). *Zentralbl. Veterinaermed., Reihe B* **26**, 696–709.

908. Pryor, W. H., Jr., Bergner, J. F., and Raulston, G. L. (1970). Leech (*Dinobdella ferox*) infection of a Taiwan monkey (*Macaca cyclopis*). *J. Am. Vet. Med. Assoc.* **157**, 1926–1927.

909. Pucak, G. J., and Johnson, D. K. (1972). *Sarcocystis* in a Patas monkey (*Erythrocebus patas*). *Lab. Anim. Dig.* **8**, 36–39.

910. Purvis, A. J., Ellison, I. R., and Husting, E. L. (1965). A short note on the findings of schistosomes in baboons (*Papio rhodesiae*). *Cent. Afr. J. Med.* **11**, 368.

911. Quentin, J.-C. (1969). Essai de classification des nématodes rictularies. *Mem. Mus. Natl. Hist. Nat., Ser. A (Paris)* **54**, 57–115.

912. Quentin, J.-C. (1969). Cycle biologique de *Pterygodermatites desportesi* (Chabaud et Rousselot, 1956) *Nematoda Rictulariidae. Ann. Parasitol. Hum. Comp.* **44**, 47–58.

913. Quentin, J.-C. (1973). Présence de *Spirura guianensis* (Ortlepp, 1924) chez des Marsupiaux néotropicaux. Cycle évolutif. *Ann. Parasitol. Hum. Comp.* **48**, 117–133.

914. Quentin, J.-C., and Krishnasamy, M. (1975). Nematodes *Spirura* parasites des *Tupaia* et du *Nycticebe* en Malaisie. *Ann. Parasitol. Hum. Comp.* **50**, 795–812.

915. Quentin, J.-C., and Seureau, C. (1974). Cycle biologique de *Pterygodermatites hispanica* Quentin, 1973 (*Nematoda Rictulariidae*). *Ann. Parasitol. Hum. Comp.* **49**, 701–719.

916. Railliet, A., and Henry, A. (1909). Sur la classification des Strongylidae. I. Metastrongylinae. *C. R. Seances Soc. Biol. Ses Fil.* **66**, 85–88.

917. Railliet, A., and Marullaz, M. (1919). Sur un cénure nouveau du bonnet chinois (*Macacus sinicus*). *Bull. Soc. Pathol. Exot.* **12**, 223–228.

918. Railliet, A., Henry, A., and Joyeux, C. (1912). Sur deux trématodes de primates. *Bull. Soc. Pathol. Exot.* **5**, 833–837.

919. Ramakrishnan, S. P., and Mohan, B. N. (1961). Simian malaria in the Nilgiris, Madras State, India. *Bull. Natl. Soc. Indian Malariol. Mosq. Dis.* **9**, 139–140.

920. Ramakrishnan, S. P., and Mohan, B. N. (1962). An enzootic focus of simian malaria in *Macaca radiata radiata.* Geoffrey of Nilgiris, Madras State, India. *Indian J. Malariol.* **16**, 87–94.

921. Ratcliffe, H. L. (1931). A comparative study of amoebiasis in man, monkeys and cats, with special reference to the formation of the early lesions. *Am. J. Hyg.* **14**, 337–352.

922. Ratcliffe, H. L. (1942). Deaths and important diseases. *Rep. Penrose Res. Lab.,* pp. 11–25.

923. Ratcliffe, H. L. (1955). Causes of death in the animal collection. *Rep. Penrose Res. Lab.,* pp. 6–16.

924. Ratcliffe, H. L. (1962). Causes of death in the animal collection. *Rep. Penrose Res. Lab.,* pp. 6–18.

925. Ratcliffe, H. L. (1963). Causes of death in the animal collection. *Rep. Penrose Res. Lab.,* pp. 13–24.

926. Ratcliffe, H. L., and Worth, C. B. (1951). Toxoplasmosis of captive wild birds and mammals. *Am. J. Pathol.* **27**, 655–667.

927. Raulston, G. L. (1972). Psorergatic mites in patas monkeys. *Lab. Anim. Sci.* **22**, 107–108.

928. Rawling, C. A., and Splitter, G. A. (1973). Pneumothorax associated with lung mite lesions in a rhesus monkey. *Lab. Anim. Sci.* **23**, 259–261.

929. Reardon, L. V., and Rininger, B. F. (1968). A survey of parasites in laboratory animals. *Lab. Anim. Care* **18**, 577–580.

930. Reichenow, E. (1917). Parásitos de la sangre y del intestino de los monos antropomorfos africanos. *Bol. R. Soc. Esp. Hist. Nat., Secc. Biol.* **17**, 312–332.

931. Reichenow, E. (1949–1953). "Lehrbuch der Protozoenkunde," 6th ed., 3 vols. Fischer, Jena.

932. Reid, W. A., and Reardon, M. J. (1976). *Mesocestoides* in the baboon and its development in laboratory animals. *J. Med. Primatol.* **5**, 345–352.

933. Remfry, J. (1982). The endoparasites of rhesus monkeys (*Macaca mulatta*) before and after capture. *Microbiologica (Bologna)* **5**, 143–147.

934. Renquist, D. M., and Whitney, R. A., Jr. (1987). Zoonoses acquired from pet primates. *Vet. Clin. North Am.: Small Anim. Pract.* **17**(1), 219–240.

935. Renquist, D. M., Johnson, A. J., Lewis, J. C., and Johnson, D. J. (1975). A natural case of *Schistosoma mansoni* in the chimpanzee (*Pan troglodytes*). *Lab. Anim. Sci.* **25**, 763–768.

936. Rewell, R. E. (1948). Diseases of tropical origin in captive wild animals. *Trans. R. Soc. Trop. Med. Hyg.* **42**, 17–36.

937. Reyes, E. (1970). *Iodamoeba wallacei* n. sp. of amoeba found in *Cercopithecus diana* L. (Mammalia-Primate) (Sarcodina-Endamoebidae). *Bol. Soc. Biol. Concepcion* **42**, 215–256.

938. Richart, R., and Benirschke, K. (1963). Causes of death in a colony of marmoset monkeys. *J. Pathol. Bacteriol.* **86**, 221–223.

939. Richter, C. B. (1984). Biology and diseases of Callitrichidae. *In* "Laboratory Animal Medicine" (B. G. Fox, B. J. Cohen, and F. M. Loew eds.), Chapter 11, pp. 353–383. Academic Press, Orlando, FL.

940. Richter, C. B., Humason, G. L., and Tankersley, B. (1976). Acanthocephaliasis in caged marmosets. *27th Annu. Sess., Am. Assoc. Lab. Anim. Sci.*, Abstr. 50.

941. Richter, C. B., Humason, G. L., and Godbold, J. H., Jr. (1978). Endemic *Pneumocystis carinii* in a marmoset colony. *J. Comp. Pathol.* **88**, 171–180.

942. Rideout, B. A., Gardiner, C. H., Stalis, I. H., Zuba, J. R., Hadfield, T., and Visvesvara, G. S. (1997). Fatal infections with *Balamuthia mandrillaris* (a free-living amoebae) in gorillas and other old world primates. *Vet. Pathol.* **34**, 15–22.

943. Rijpstra, A. C. (1967). Sporocysts of *Isospora* sp. in a chimpanzee (*Pan troglodytes*, L.). *Proc. K. Ned. Akad. Wet.* **70**, 395–401.

944. Riopelle, A. J. (1967). The Chimpanzee. *In* "UFAW Handbook on the Care and Management of Laboratory Animals" (UFAW Staff, ed.), 3rd ed., pp. 696–708. Livingstone and the Universities Federation for Animal Welfare, London.

945. Riopelle, A. J., and Daumy, O. J. (1962). Care of chimpanzees for radiation studies. *Proc. Int. Symp. Bone Marrow Ther. Chem. Prot. Irradiat. Primates, 1962*, pp. 205–223.

946. Ritchie, L. S. (1948). An ether sedimentation technique for routine stool examination. *Bull. U.S. Army Med. Dep.* **8**, 326.

947. Robertson, O. H., Loosli, C. G., Puck, T. T., Wise, H., Lemon, H. M., and Lester, W., Jr. (1947). Tests for the chronic toxicity of propylene glycol and triethylene glycol on monkeys and rats by vapor inhalation and oral administration. *J. Pharmacol. Exp. Ther.* **91**, 52–76.

948. Robinson, P. T., and Bush, M. (1981). Clinical and pathologic aspects of pulmonary acariasis in douc langur and proboscis monkeys. *Zool. Garten, Leipzig* **51**, 161–169.

949. Rodaniche, de E. D. (1954). Spontaneous toxoplasmosis in the white-face monkey, *Cebus capucinus*, in Panama. *Am. J. Trop. Med. Hyg.* **3**, 1023–1025.

950. Rodaniche, de E. D. (1955). Susceptibility of the marmoset *Marikina geoffroyi* and the night monkey, *Aotus zonalis*, to experimental infection with *Toxoplasma*. *Am. J. Trop. Med. Hyg.* **3**, 1026–1032.

951. Rodger, R. F., and Bronson, R. T. (1983). A rhesus monkey with acquired immune deficiency syndrome and cryptosporidiosis. *34th Annu. Sess. Am. Assoc. Lab. Anim. Sci.*, Abstr. No. 7.

952. Rodhain, J. (1933). Sur une coccidie de l'intestin de l'ouistiti: *Hapale jacchus penicillalus* (Geoffroy) *C. R. Seances Soc. Biol. Ses Fil.* **114**, 1357–1358.

953. Rodhain, J. (1941). Sur un *Plasmodium* du gibbon *Hylobates leusciscus* Geoff. *Acta Biol. Belg.* **1**, 118–123.

954. Rodhain, J. (1941). Notes sur *Trypanosoma minasense* Chagas: Identité spécifique du trypanosome du saimiri: *Chrysothrix sciureus*. *Acta Biol. Belg.* **1**, 187–193.

955. Rodhain, J. (1948). Contribution à l'étude des plasmodiums des anthropoides africains. Transmission du *Plasmodium malariae* de l'homme au chimpanzé. *Ann. Soc. Belge Med. Trop.* **28**, 39–49.

956. Rodhain, J., and Dellaert, R. (1943). L'infection a *Plasmodium malariae* du chimpanzé chez l'homme. Étude d'une première souche isolée de l'anthropoïde *Pan satyrus verus*. *Ann. Soc. Belge Med. Trop.* **23**, 19–46.

957. Rodhain, J., and Dellaert, R. (1955). Contribution a l'étude de *Plasmodium schwetzi* E. Brumpt: II. Transmission du *Plasmodium schwetzi* á l'homme. *Ann. Soc. Belge Med. Trop.* **35**, 73–76.

958. Rodhain, J., and van den Berghe, L. (1936). Contribution á l'étude des plasmodiums des singes africains. *Ann. Soc. Belge Med. Trop.* **16**, 521–531.

959. Rodhain, J., and van den Berghe, L. (1939). *Paraloa anthropopitheci* genre et espèce nouveaux de Filaroidea chez le chimpanzé du Congo Belge. *Ann. Soc. Belge Méd. Trop.* **19**, 445.

960. Rodhain, J., and Wanson, M. (1954). Un nouveau cas de coenurose chez le babouin (*Theropithecus gelada* Ruppell. *Riv. Parassitol.* **15**, 613–620.

961. Rohde, K. (1962). Zwei Trematoden-Arten, *Odenigotrema bivesicularis* n.g., n. sp. und *Novetrema nycticebi* n. g., n. sp. (Odeningotrematini n.subfam. Lecithodendriidae), aus dem darm von *Nycticebus coucang* in Malaya. *Z. Parasitenkd.* **21**, 465 (in German).

962. Rosen, S., Hono, J. E., and Barry, K. G. (1968). Malarial nephropathy in the rhesus monkey. *Arch. Pathol.* **85**, 36–44.

963. Ross, P. H. (1905). A note on the natural occurrence of piroplasmosis in the monkey (*Cercopithecus*). *J. Hyg.* **5**, 18–23.

964. Rousselot, R. (1956). Hepatite filariènne des anthropides. *Bull. Soc. Pathol. Exot.* **49**, 301–303.

965. Rousselot, R., and Pellissier, A. (1952). Pathologie du gorille. III. Oesophagostomose nodulaire a *Oesophagostomum stephanostomum* du gorille et du chimpanzé. *Bull. Soc. Pathol. Exot.* **45**, 568–574.

966. Rowland, E., and Vandenbergh, J. G. (1965). A survey of intestinal parasites in a new colony of rhesus monkeys. *J. Parasitol.* **51**, 294–295.

967. Ruch, T. C. (1959). "Diseases of Laboratory Primates." Saunders, Philadelphia.

968. Ruiz, A., and Frenkel, J. K. (1976). Recognition of cyclic transmission of *Sarcocystis muris* by cats. *J. Infect. Dis.* **133**, 409–418.

969. Ryan, M. J., Cousins, D. B., and Bhandari, J. C. (1986). Diagnostic excercise: Hepatic granulomas in a cynomolgus monkey. *Lab. Anim. Sci.* **36**, 56–58.

970. Sachs, R., and Voelker, J. (1975). A primate, *Mandrillus leucophaeus*, as natural host of the African lung fluke *Paragonimus africanus* in West Cameroon. *Tropenmed. Parasitol.* **26**, 205–206.

971. Sagartz, J. W., and Tingpalapong, M. (1974). Cerebral cysticercosis in a white-handed gibbon. *J. Am. Vet. Med. Assoc.* **165**, 844–845.

972. Sakakibara, I. (1981). Naturally occurring diseases in cynomolgus monkeys. *Jpn. J. Med. Sci. Biol.* **34**, 263–267.

973. Sakakibara, I., Sugimoto, Y., Koyama, T., and Honjo, S. (1982). Natural transmission of *Entamoeba histolytica* from mother cynomolgus monkeys (*Macaca fascicularis*) to their newborn infants under indoor rearing conditions. *Exp. Anim.* **31**, 135–138.

974. Salis, H. (1941). Studies on the morphology of the *E. histolytica*-like amoebae found in monkeys. *J. Parasitol.* **27**, 327–341.

975. Sambon, L. W. (1910). Porocephaliasis in man. *J. Trop. Med. Hyg.* **13**, 17–24, 212–217, 258–263.

976. Sambon, L. W. (1922). A synopsis of the family Linguatulidae. *J. Trop. Med. Hyg.* **25**, 188–206, 391–428.

977. Sambon, L. W. (1924). The elucidation of cancer. *J. Trop. Med. Hyg.* **27**, 124–174.

978. Sandground, J. H. (1925). Speciation and specificity in the nematode genus *Strongyloides*. *J. Parasitol.* **12**, 59–80.

979. Sandground, J. H. (1930). Notes and descriptions of some parasitic helminths collected by the expedition. *Contrib. Dep. Trop. Med. Inst. Trop. Biol. Med.* **5**, 462–486.

980. Sandground, J. H. (1933). Report on the nematode parasites collected by the Kelley-Roosevelts expedition to Indo-China with descriptions of several new species. I: Parasites of birds. 2: Parasites of mammals. *Z. Parasitenkd.* **5**, 542.

981. Sandground, J. H. (1936). On the occurrence of a species of *Loa* in monkeys in the Belgian Congo. *Ann. Soc. Belge Med. Trop.* **16**, 273.

982. Sandground, J. H. (1936). Scientific results of an expedition to rain forest regions in Eastern Africa. *Bull. Mus. Comp. Zool.* **79**, 343–366.

983. Sandground, J. H. (1937). On a coenurus from the brain of a monkey. *J. Parasitol.* **23**, 482–490.

984. Sandground, J. H. (1938). Some parasitic worms in the helminthological collection of the Museum of Comparative Zoology. 2: A redescription of *Tetrapetalonema digitata* (Chandler 1929) comb. nov., a filariid parasite of gibbon apes with an enumeration of its congeners. *Bull. Mus. Comp. Zool.* **85**, 49.

985. Sandosham, A. A. (1950). On *Enterobius vermicularis* (Linnaeus, 1758) and some related species from primates and rodents. *J. Helminthol.* **24**, 171–204.

986. Sandosham, A. A. (1951). On two helminths from the orang-utan, *Leipertrema rewelli*, n.g., n. sp. and *Dirofilaria immitis* (Leidy, 1856). *J. Helminthol.* **25**, 19–26.

987. Sandosham, A. A. (1954). Malaysian parasites. XV. Seven new worms from miscellaneous hosts. *Stud. Inst. Med. Res., Fed. Malay States* **26**, 213–226.

988. Sandosham, A. A., Wharton, R. H., Warren, McW., and Eyles, D. E. (1962). Microfilariae in the rhesus monkey (*Macaca mulatta*) from East Pakistan. *J. Parasitol.* **48**, 489.

989. Sano, M., Kino, H., deGuzman, T. S., Ishii, A. I., Kino, J., Tanaka, T., and Tsuruta, M. (1980). Studies on the examination of imported laboratory monkey *Macaca fascicularis* for *E. histolytica* and other intestinal parasites. *Int. J. Zoonoses* **7**, 34–39.

990. Sasa, M., Tanaka, H., Fukui, M., and Takata, A. (1962). Internal parasites of laboratory animals. *In* "The Problems of Laboratory Animal Disease" (R. J. C. Harris, ed.), pp. 195–214. Academic Press, New York.

991. Sawada, I., and Kifune, T. (1974). A new species anoplocephaline cestode from *Macaca irus*. *Jpn. J. Parasitol.* **23**, 366–368.

992. Schacher, J. F. (1962). Morphology of the microfilaria of *Brugia pahangi* and of the larval stages in the mosquito. *J. Parasitol.* **48**, 679–692.

993. Schacher, J. F. (1962). Developmental stages of *Brugia pahangi* in the final host. *J. Parasitol.* **48**, 693–706.

994. Schad, G. A., and Anderson, R. C. (1963). *Macacanema formosana* n. g., n. sp. (Onchocercidae:Dirofilariinae) from *Macaca cyclopis* of Formosa. *Can J. Zool.* **41**, 797–800.

995. Schiefer, B., and Loew, F. M. (1978). Amebiasis and salmonellosis in a woolly monkey (Lagothrix). *Vet. Pathol.* **15**, 428–431.

996. Schmidt, G. D. (1972). Acanthocephala of captive primates. *In* "Pathology of Simian Primates" (R. N. T.-W. Fiennes, ed.), Part 2, pp. 144–156. Karger, Basel.

997. Schmidt, G. D., and File, S. (1977). *Tupaiataenia quentini* gen. et sp. n. (Anoplocephalidae:Linstowiinae) and other tapeworms from the common tree shrew, *Tupaia glis*. *J. Parasitol.* **63**, 473–475.

998. Schmidt, L. H., Greenland, R., and Genther, C. S. (1961). The transmission of *Plasmodium cynomolgi* to man. *Am. J. Trop. Med. Hyg.* **10**, 679–688.

999. Schmidt, L. H., Greenland, R., Rossan, R., and Genther, C. (1961). Natural occurrence of malaria in rhesus monkeys. *Science* **133**, 753.

1000. Schmidt, L. H., Fradkin, R., Harrison, J., Rossan, R. N., and Squires, W. (1980). The course of untreated *Plasmodium inui* infections in the rhesus monkey (*Macaca mulatta*). *Am. J. Trop Med. Hyg.* **29**, 158–169.

1001. Schmidt, R. E. (1978). Systemic pathology of chimpanzees. *J. Med. Primatol.* **7**, 274–318.

1002. Schmidt, R. E., and Prine, J. R. (1970). Severe enterobiasis in a chimpanzee. *Pathol. Vet.* **7**, 56–59.

1003. Schoeb, T. R. (1984). *Klossiella* sp. infection in a galago. *J. Am. Vet. Med. Assoc.* **185**, 1381–1382.

1004. Schofield, L. D., Bennett, B. T., Collins, W. E., and Beluhan, F. Z. (1985). An outbreak of *Plasmodium inui* malaria in a colony of diabetic rhesus monkeys. *Lab. Anim. Sci.* **35**, 167–168.

1005. Schuerer, U. (1979). [A tapeworm (*Multiceps multiceps*) of a baboon (*Theropithecus gelada*)]. *Zool. Garten, Leipzig* **49**, 80–81 (in German).

1006. Schultz, A. H. (1939). Notes on diseases and healed fractures of wild apes, and their bearing on the antiquity of pathological conditions in man. *Bull. Hist. Med.* **7**, 571–582; cited by Ruch (967).

1007. Schuster, F. L., and Visvesvara, G. S. (1996). Axenic growth and drug sensitivity studies of *Balamuthia mandrillaris*, an agent of amebic meningoencephalitis in humans and other animals. *J. Clin. Microbiol.* **34**, 385–388.

1008. Schwetz, J. (1933). Trypanosomes rares de la région de Stanleyville (Congo belge). *Ann. Parasitol. Hum. Comp.* **11**, 287–296.

1009. Schwetz, J. (1934). Sur quelgues trypanosomes rares de la région de Stanleyville (deuxièine note). *Ann. Parasitol. Hum. Comp.* **12**, 278–282.

1010. Scimeca, J. M., Culberson, D. E., Abee, C. R., and Gardner, W. A., Jr. (1989). Intestinal trichomonads (*Tritrichomonas mobilensis*) in the natural host *Saimiri sciureus* and *Saimiri boliviensis*. *Vet. Pathol.* **26**, 144–147.

1011. Scott, H. H. (1926). Report on the deaths occurring in the Society's gardens during the year 1925. *Proc. Zool. Soc. London* **97**, 231–244.

1012. Seibold, H. R., and Fussell, E. N. (1973). Intestinal microsporidiosis in *Callicebus moloch*. *Lab. Anim. Sci.* **23**, 115–118.

1013. Seibold, H. R., and Wolf, R. H. (1970). American trypanosomiasis in *Hylobates pileatus*. *Lab. Anim. Sci.* **20**, 514–517.

1014. Seibold, H. R., and Wolf, R. H. (1971). Toxoplasmosis in *Aotus trivirgatus* and *Callicebus moloch*. *Lab. Anim. Sci.* **21**, 118–120.

1015. Seibold, H. R., and Wolf, R. H. (1973). Neoplasms and proliferative lesions in 1065 nonhuman primate necropsies. *Lab. Anim. Sci.* **23**, 533–539.

1016. Self, J. T. (1969). Biological relationships of the Pentastomida. A bibliography on the Pentastomida. *Exp. Parasitol.* **24**, 63–119.

1017. Self, J. T. (1972). Pentastomiasis host responses to larval and nymphal infections. *Trans. Am. Microsc. Soc.* **91**, 2–8.

1018. Self, J. T., and Cosgrove, G. E. (1968). Pentastome larvae in laboratory primates. *J. Parasitol.* **54**, 969.

1019. Self, J. T., and Cosgrove, G. E. (1972). Pentastomida. *In* "Pathology of Simian Primates" (R. N. T.-W. Fiennes, ed.), Part 2, pp. 194–204. Karger, Basel.

1020. Seneca, H., and Wolf, A. (1955). *Trypanosoma cruzi* infection in the Indian monkey. *Am. J. Trop. Med. Hyg.* **4**, 1009–1014.

1021. Sen Gupta, P. C., and Ray, H. N. (1955). A cytochemical study of *Balantidium coli* Malmsten, 1857. *Proc. Zool. Soc. India* **8**, 103–110.

1022. Shadduck, J. A., and Baskin, G. (1989). Serologic evidence of *Encephalitozoon cuniculi* infection in a colony of squirrel monkeys (*Saimiri sciureus*). *Lab. Anim. Sci.* **39**, 328–330.

1023. Shadduck, J. A., and Pakes, S. P. (1978). Protozoal and metazoal diseases. *In* "Pathology of Laboratory Animals" (K. Benirschke, F. M.

Garner, and T. C. Jones, eds.), Vol. 2, Chapter 17, pp. 1587–1696. Springer-Verlag, New York.

1024. Shannon, R. C., and Greene, C. T. (1926). A bottfly parasite in monkeys. *Zoopathologica* **1**, 285.

1025. Sheldon, W. G. (1966). Psoregatic mange in the sooty mangabey (*Cercocebus torquates atys*) monkey. *Lab. Anim. Care* **16**, 276–279.

1026. Shiroishi, T., Davis, J., and Warren, McW. (1968). *Hepatocystis* in white-cheeked gibbon *Hylobates concolor. J. Parasitol.* **54**, 168.

1027. Shortt, H. E., Rao, G., Qadri, S. S., and Abraham, R. (1961). *Plasmodium osmaniae*, a malaria parasite of an Indian *Macaca radiata. J. Trop. Med. Hyg.* **64**, 140–143.

1028. Shute, P. G., and Maryon, M. (1970). Specimen demonstrating a blood film of a splenectomized rhesus monkey showing *P. c. bastianellii* and *Bartonella* in erythrocyte. *Trans. R. Soc. Trop. Med. Hyg.* **64**, 5.

1029. Sinton, J. A. (1934). A quartan malaria parasite of the lower oriental monkey, *Silenus irus* (*Macaca cynomolgus*). *Rec. Malaria Surv. India* **4**, 379–410.

1030. Sinton, J. A., and Mulligan, H. W. (1932–1933). A critical review of the literature relating to the identification of the malaria parasites recorded from monkeys of the families Cercopithecidae and Colobidae. *Rec. Malaria Surv. India* **3**, 357–380, 381–444.

1031. Skrjabin, K. I., Shirhobalova, N. P., and Shults, R. S. (1954). Trichostrongylids of animals and man. *In* "Essentials of Nematodology" (K. I. Skrjabin, ed.), Vol. 3. Acad. Sci., Moscow. (English edition, Israel Program for Scientific Translations, Jerusalem, 1960).

1032. Slaughter, L. J., and Bostrom, R. E. (1969). Physalopterid (*Abbreviata poicilometra*) infection in a sooty mangabey monkey. *Lab. Anim. Care* **19**, 235–236.

1033. Slaughter, L. J., Dade, A. W., Chineme, C., and Andrews, E. J. (1974). Pentastoma larvae in a squirrel monkey. *J. Am. Vet. Med. Assoc.* **164**, 711.

1034. Sluiter, C., Wellengrebel, N., and Ihle, J. (1922). "De Dierlyke Parasieten Van Den Mensch en Van Onze Hursdieren." Scheltema & Holkema, Amsterdam.

1035. Sly, D. L., Toft, J. D., II, Gardiner, C. H., and London, W. T. (1982). Spontaneous occurrence of *Angiostrongylus costaricensis* in marmosets (*Saguinus mystax*). *Lab. Anim. Sci.* **32**, 286–288.

1036. Smetana, H. F., and Orihel, T. C. (1969). Gastric papillomata in *Macaca speciosa* induced by *Nochtia nochti* (Nematoda:Trichostrongyloidea). *J. Parasitol.* **55**, 349–351.

1037. Smiley, R. L., and O'Connor, B. M. (1980). Mange in *Macaca arctoides* (Primates:Cercopithecidae) caused by *Cosarcoptes scanloni* (Acari: Sarcoptidae) with possible human involvement and descriptions of the adult male and immature stages. *Int. J. Acarol.* **6**, 283–290.

1038. Smith, H. V., Paton, C. A., Girdwood, R. W. A., and Mtambo, M. M. A. (1996). *Cyclospora* in non-human primates in Gombe, Tanzania. *Vet. Rec.* **138**, 528.

1039. Smith, W. N., and Chitwood, M. B. (1954). *Anatrichosoma cynamolgi*, a new trichrid nematode from monkeys. *J. Parasitol., Suppl.* **40**, 12.

1040. Smith, W. N., and Chitwood, M. B. (1967). *Trichospirura leptostoma* gen et sp n (Nematoda:Thelazioidea) from the pancreatic ducts of the white-eared marmoset, *Callithrix jacchus. J. Parasitol.* **53**, 1270–1272.

1041. Smith, W. N., and Levy, B. M. (1969). The effects of *Trichospirura leptostoma* on the pancreas of *Callithrix jacchus. Program Abstr., 44th Annu. Meet., Am. Soc. Pathol.* Washington, DC, No. 7, pp. 45.

1042. Soave, O. A. (1963). Diagnosis and control of common diseases of hamsters, rabbits, and monkeys. *J. Am. Vet. Med. Assoc.* **142**, 285–290.

1043. Sood, M. L., and Toong, R. (1973). *Streptopharagus guptai* n. sp. (Nematoda: Spiruridae) from the rectum of a rhesus macaque *Macaca mulatta* from India. *Zool. Anz.* **190**, 132–136.

1044. Soulsby, E. J. L. (1965). "Textbook of Veterinary Clinical Parasitology," Vol. I. Davis, Philadelphia.

1045. Soulsby, E. J. L. (1968). "Helminths, Arthropods and Protozoa of Domesticated Animals (Monnig)," 6th ed. Williams & Wilkins, Baltimore.

1046. Sousa, O. E., Rossan, R. N., and Baerg, D. C. (1974). The prevalence of trypanosomes and microfilarae in Panamanian monkeys. *Am. J. Trop. Med. Hyg.* **23**, 862–868.

1047. Stam, A. B. (1960). Fatal ascaridosis in a dwarf chimpanzee. *Ann. Parasitol. Hum. Comp.* **35**, 675.

1048. Stibbs, H. H., and Ongerth, J. E. (1986). Immunofluorescence detection of *Cryptosporidium* oocysts in fecal smears. *J. Clin. Microbiol.* **24**, 517–521.

1049. Stiles, C. W., and Hassall, A. (1929). "Key-catalogue of Parasites Reported for Primates (Monkeys and Lemurs) with their Possible Public Health Importance," Hyg. Lab. Bull. No. 152, pp. 409–601. Public Health Serv., Washington, DC; cited by Dunn (268).

1050. Stiles, C. W., and Nolan, M. O. (1929). "Key-catalogue of Primates for Which Parasites are Reported," Hyg. Lab. Bull. No. 152, Public Health Serv., Washington, DC; cited by Dunn (268).

1051. Stokes, W. S., Donovan, J. C., Montrey, R. D., Thompson, W. L., Wannemacher, R. W., Jr., and Rosmiarek, H. (1983). Acute clinical malaria (*Plasmodium inui*) in a cynomolgus monkey (*Macaca fascicularis*). *Lab. Anim. Sci.* **33**, 81–85.

1052. Stolz, G. (1962). Spontaneous lethal toxoplasmosis in a woolly monkey. *Schweiz. Arch. Tierheilkd.* **104**, 162–166.

1053. Stone, W. B., and Hughes, J. A. (1969). Massive pulmonary acariasis in the pig-tail macaque. *Bull. Wildl. Dis. Assoc.* **5**, 20.

1054. Stone, W. M. (1964). *Strongyloides ransomi* prenatal infection in swine. *J. Parasitol.* **50**, 568.

1055. Stookey, J. L., and Moe, J. B. (1978). The respiratory system. *In* "Pathology of Laboratory Animals" (K. Benirschke, F. M. Garner, and T. C. Jones, eds.), Vol. 1, Chapter 2, pp. 72–113. Springer-Verlag, New York.

1056. Strandtmann, R. W., and Wharton, G. W. (1958). "A Manual of Mesostigmatid Mites Parasitic on Vertebrates," Contrib. No. 4. Institute of Acarology, University of Maryland, College Park.

1057. Strong, J. P., McGill, H. C., Jr., and Miller, J. H. (1961). *Schistosomiasis mansoni* in the Kenya baboon. *Am. J. Trop. Med. Hyg.* **10**, 25–31.

1058. Strong, J. P., Miller, J. H., and McGill, H. C., Jr. (1965). Naturally occurring parasitic lesions in baboons. *In* "The Baboon in Medical Research" (H. Vagtborg, ed.), pp. 503–512. University of Texas Press, Austin.

1059. Stunkard, H. W. (1923). On the structure, occurrence and significance of *Athesmia foxi*, a liver fluke of American monkeys. *J. Parasitol.* **10**, 71–79.

1060. Stunkard, H. W. (1940). The morphology and life history of the cestode, *Bertiella studeri. Am. J. Trop. Med.* **20**, 305–333.

1061. Stunkard, H. W. (1965). *Paratriotaenia oedipomidatis* gen. et sp. n. (Cestoda), from a marmoset. *J. Parasitol.* **51**, 545–551.

1062. Stunkard, H. W. (1965). New intermediate hosts in the life cycle of *Prosthenorchis elegans* (Diesing 1851), an acanthocephalan parasite of primates. *J. Parasitol.* **51**, 645–649.

1063. Stunkard, H. W., and Goss, L. J. (1950). *Eurytrema brumpti* Railliet, Henry and Joyeux, 1912 (Trematoda:Dicrocoeliidae), from the pancreas and liver of African anthropoid apes. *J. Parasitol.* **36**, 574–581.

1064. Sulaiman, S., Williams, J. F., and Wu, D. (1986). Natural infections of vervet monkeys (*Cercopithecus aethiops*) and African red monkeys (*Erythrocebus patas*) in Sudan with taeniid cysticerci. *J. Wildl. Dis.* **22**, 586–587.

1065. Suldey, E. W. (1924). Dysentérie amibienne spontanée chez le chimpanzé (*Troglodytes niger*). *Bull. Soc. Pathol. Exot.* **17**, 771–773.

1066. Sullivan, J. J., Steurer, F., Benavides, G., Tanleton, R. L., Eberhard, M. L., and Landry, S. (1993). Trypanosomes and microfilariae in feral owl and squirrel monkeys maintained in research colonies. *Am. J. Trop. Med. Hyg.* **49**, 254–259.

1067. Summers, W. A. (1960). A case of hydatid disease in the rhesus monkey (*Macaca mulatta*). *Allied Vet.* **31**, 141–143.

1068. Sureau, P., Raynaud, J. P., Lapeire, C., and Brygoo, E. R. (1962). Premier isolement de *Toxoplasma gondii* à Madagascar. Toxoplasmose spontanée et expérimentale du *Lemur catta. Bull. Soc. Pathol. Exot.* **55**, 357–362.

1069. Susseville, V. G., Pauley, D., Mackey, J. J., and Simon, M. A. (1995). Concurrent central nervous system toxoplasmosis and simian immunodeficiency virus-induced AIDS encephalomyelitis in a Barbary macaque (*Macaca sylvana*). *Vet. Pathol.* **32**, 81–83.

1070. Suzuki, T., Miura, H., Narita, K., Suzuki, H., Miki, H., and Sado, T. (1978). Quarantine and health control of the squirrel monkey (*Saimiri sciureus*). *Exp. Anim.* **27**, 161–166 (in Japanese w/ English summary).

1071. Swellengrebel, N. H., and Rijpstra, A. C. (1965). Lateral-spined schistosome ova in the intestine of a squirrel monkey from Surinam. *Trop. Geogr. Med.* **17**, 80–84.

1072. Swenson, B., Strobert, E., and Orkin, J. (1979). "AALAS Workshop on Nonhuman Primate Parasitology." Emory University, Atlanta, GA.

1073. Swift, H. F., Boots, R. H., and Miller, C. P. (1922). A cutaneous nematode infection in monkeys. *J. Exp. Med.* **35**, 599–620.

1074. Takos, M. J., and Thomas, L. J. (1958). The pathology and pathogenesis of fatal infections due to an acanthocephalid parasite of marmoset monkeys. *Am. J. Trop. Med. Hyg.* **7**, 90–94.

1075. Taliaferro, W. H., and Cannon, P. R. (1936). The cellular reactions during primary infections and superinfections of *Plasmodium brazilianum* in Panamanian monkeys. *J. Infect. Dis.* **59**, 72–125.

1076. Taliaferro, W. H., and Taliaferro, L. G. (1934). Morphology, periodicity and course of infection of *Plasmodium brazilianum* in Panamanian monkeys. *Am. J. Hyg.* **20**, 1–49.

1077. Tanaka, H., Fukui, M., Yamamoto, H., Hayama, S., and Kodera, S. (1962). Studies on the identification of common intestinal parasites of primates. *Bull. Exp. Anim.* **11**, 111–116.

1078. Tang, Z.-Z., and Tang, C.-T. (1982). On a new trematode, *Pithecotrema kelloggi*, gen. and sp. nov. (Lecithodendriidae Odhner). *Wuyi Sci. J.* **2**, 60–64 (in Chinese w/ English summary).

1079. Tanguy, Y. (1937). La piroplasmose du singe. *Ann. Inst. Pasteur, Paris* **59**, 610–623.

1080. Tankersley, W. G., Richter, C. B., and Batson, J. S. (1979). Therapy of filariasis in tamarins. *Lab. Anim. Sci.* **29**, 107–110.

1081. Tantalean, M., Gozalo, A., and Montoya, E. (1990). Notes on some helminth parasites from Peruvian monkeys. *Lab. Primate Newsl.* **29**, 6–8.

1082. Tatalean, V. M. (1976). Contribución al conocimiento de los helmintos de vertebrados del Perú. *Biota* **10**, 437–443.

1083. Tate, C. L., and Rubin, L. F. (1973). Intraocular echinococcosis in a rhesus monkey. *J. Am. Vet. Med. Assoc.* **163**, 636–638.

1084. Taylor, A. E. R. (1959). *Dirofilaria magnilarvatum* Price, 1959 (Nematoda:Filarioidea) from *Macaca irus* Cuvier: II. Microscopical studies on the microfilariae. *J. Parasitol.* **45**, 505–510.

1085. Teare, J. A., and Loomis, M. R. (1982). Epizootic of balantidiasis in lowland gorillas. *J. Am. Vet. Med. Assoc.* **181**, 1345–1347.

1086. Terrell, T. G., and Stookey, J. L. (1972). Chronic eosinophilic myositis in a rhesus monkey infected with sarcosporidiosis. *Pathol. Vet.* **9**, 266–271.

1087. Thatcher, V. E., and Porter, J. A., Jr. (1968). Some helminth parasites of panamanian primates. *Trans. Am. Microsc. Soc.* **87**, 186–196.

1088. Thézé, J. (1916). Rapport sur les travaux de l'Institut d'Hygiene et de Bactériologie, 1914–1915. *Bull. Soc. Pathol. Exot.* **9**, 449–469.

1089. Thienpont, D., Mortelmans, J., and Vercruysse, J. (1962). Contribution à l'étude de la Trihuriose du chimpanzé et de son traitement avec la methyridine. *Ann. Soc. Belge Med. Trop.* **2**, 211–218; cited by Flynn (373).

1090. Thornton, H. (1924). The relationship between the ascarids of man, pig and chimpanzee. *Ann. Trop. Med. Parasitol.* **18**, 99–100.

1091. Tihen, W. S. (1970). *Tetrapetalonema marmosete* in cotton-topped marmosets, *Saguinus oedipus*, from the region of San Marcos, Colombia. *Lab. Anim. Sci.* **20**, 759–762.

1092. Toft, J. D., II (1982). The pathoparasitology of the alimentary tract and pancreas of nonhuman primates: A review. *Vet. Pathol.* **19**, Suppl. 7, 44–92.

1093. Toft, J. D., II (1986). The pathoparasitology of nonhuman primates: A review. *In* "Primates; The Road To Self-Sustaining Populations" (K. Benirschke, ed.), pp. 571–679. Springer-Verlag, New York.

1094. Toft, J. D., II, and Ekstrom, M. E. (1980). Identification of metazoan parasites in tissue sections. *In* "The Comparative Pathology of Zoo Animals" (R. J. Montali and G. Migaki, eds.), pp. 369–378. Smithsonian Institution Press, Washington, DC.

1095. Toft, J. D., II, Schmidt, R. E., and DePaoli, A. (1976). Intestinal polyposis associated with oxyurid parasites in a chimpanzee (*Pan troglodytes*). *J. Med. Primatol.* **5**, 360–364.

1096. Trapido, H., and Work, T. H. (1962). Non-human vertebrates and hosts and disseminators of Kyasanur Forest disease. *Proc. Pac. Sci. Congr., 9th, 1957*, Vol. 17, pp. 85–87.

1097. Trapido, H., Goerdham, M. K., Rajagopalan, P. K., and Rebello, M. J. (1964). Ticks ectoparasitic on monkeys in the Kyasanur Forest disease area of Shimoga District, Mysore State, India. *Am. J. Trop. Med.* **13**, 763–772.

1098. Travassos, L. P., and Vogelsang, E. G. (1929). Sobre um novo Trichostrongylidae parasito de *Maccacus* (sic) *rhesus. Sci. Med. Ital.* **7**, 509–511.

1099. Treadgold, C. H. (1920). On a filaria, *Loa papionis* n. sp. parasitic in *Papio cynocephalus. Parasitology* **12**, 113–115.

1100. Troisier, J., and Deschiens, R. E. (1930). Deux cas d'oxyurose chez le chimpanzé traversée de la paroi intestinale jusgu au peritonine. *Ann. Parasitol.* **8**, 562–565.

1101. Troisier, J., Deschiens, R. E., Limousin, H., and Delorme, M. J. (1928). L'infestation du chimpanzé par un nématode du genre *Hépaticola. Ann. Inst. Pasteur, Paris* **42**, 827–840.

1102. Troisier, J., Deschiens, R. E., Limousin, H., and Delorme, M. J. (1928). L'infestation du chimpanzé par un nématode du genre *Hépaticola. Bull. Soc. Pathol. Exot.* **21**, 211–222.

1103. Tscherner, W. (1981). [*Troglodytella*—infestation of anthropoid ape]. *Erkr. Zootiere* **24**, 229–232 (in German w/ English summary).

1104. Tuggle, B. N., and Beehler, B. A. (1984). The occurrence of *Ptergodermatites nycticebi* (Nematoda:Rictulariidae) in a captive slow loris *Nycticebus coucang. Proc. Helminthol. Soc. Wash.* **51**, 162–163.

1105. Turner, T. R., Lambrecht, F. L., and Jolly, C. J. (1982). *Hepatocystis* parasitemia in wild Kenya vervet monkeys (*Cercopithecus aethiops*). *J. Med. Primatol.* **11**, 191–194.

1106. Tzipori, S. (1983). Cryptosporidiosis in animals and humans. *Microbiol. Rev.* **47**, 84–96.

1107. Uemura, E., Houser, W. D., and Cupp, C. J. (1979). Strongyloidiasis in an infant orangutan (*Pongo pygmaeus*). *J. Med. Primatol.* **8**, 282–288.

1108. Uilenberg, G., and Ribot, J. J. (1965). Note sur la toxoplasmose des lémuriens (Primates:Lemuridae). *Rev. Elev. Med. Vet. Pays Trop.* **18**, 247–248.

1109. Ulrich, C. P., Henrickson, R. V., and Karr, S. L. (1981). An epidemiological survey of wild caught and domestic born rhesus monkeys (*Macaca mulatta*) for *Anatrichosoma* (Nematoda:Trichinellida). *Lab. Anim. Sci.* **31**, 726–727.

1110. Umana A., J. A., Ramirez C., J., Espinal T., C. A., and Sabogal M., E. (1984). Establishment of a colony of nonhuman primates (*Aotus lemurinus griseimembra*) in Colombia. *Bull.—Pan Am. Health Organ.* **18**(3), 221–229.

1111. Urbain, A., and Bullier, P. (1935). Un cas de cénurose conjonctive chez un gelada (*Theropithecus gelada*) (Ruppel). *Bull. Acad. Natl. Med. (Paris)* **8**, 322–324.

1112. Urbain, A., and Nouvel, J. (1944). Petite enzootic de strongyloidose observée sur des singes superieurs: Gibbons à favoris blancs (*Hylobates concolor leucogenis* Ogilby) et chimpanzés (*Pan troglodytes* L.). *Bull. Acad. Vét. Fr.* **17**, 337–341.

1113. Usui, M., and Horii, Y. (1982). A survey on helminth parasites of the Japanese monkey (*Macaca fuscata*). *Bull. Fac. Agric., Miyazaki Univ.* **29**, 269–274 (in Japanese w/ English summary).

1114. Valerio, D. A., Miller, R. L., Innes, J. R. M., Courtney, K. D., Pallotta, A. J., and Guttmacher, R. M. (1969). "*Macaca mulatta*: Management of a Laboratory Breeding Colony." Academic Press, New York.

1115. Van Riper, D. C., Day, P. W., Finey, J., and Prince, J. R. (1966). Intestinal parasites of recently imported chimpanzees. *Lab. Anim. Care* **16**, 360–362.

1116. Van Stee, E. W. (1964). "Some Observations on the Clinical Management of the Chimpanzee," Tech. Doc. Rep. SAM-TDR 64-65. USAF Sch. Aerosp. Med. (AFSC), Brooks Air Force Base, Texas.

1117. Van Thiel, P. H. (1926). On some filariae parasitic in Surinam mammals, with the description of *Filariopsis asper* n. g., n. sp. *Parasitology* **18**, 128.

1118. Van Thiel, P. H., and Wiegand-Bruss, C. J. E. (1945). Présence de *Prosthenorhis spirula* chez les chimpanzés. Son rôle pathogène et son développement. Dans *Blattella germanica. Ann. Parasitol. Hum. Comp.* **20**, 304–320.

1119. Vickers, J. H. (1966). *Hepatocystis kochi* in *Cercopithecus* monkeys. *J. Am. Vet. Med. Assoc.* **149**, 906–908.

1120. Vickers, J. H. (1968). Gastrointestinal diseases of primates. *Curr. Vet. Ther.* **3**, 393–396.

1121. Vickers, J. H. (1969). Diseases of primates affecting the choice of species for toxicologic studies. *Ann. N.Y. Acad. Sci.* **162**, 659–672.

1122. Vickers, J. H., and Penner, L. R. (1968). Cysticercosis in four rhesus brains. *J. Am. Vet. Med. Assoc.* **153**, 868–871.

1123. Visvesvara, G. S., Martinez, A. J., Schuster, F. L., Leitch, G. L., Wallace, S. V., Sawyer, T. K., and Anderson, M. (1990). Leptomyxid ameba, a new agent of amebic meningoencephalitis in humans and animals. *J. Clin. Microbiol.* **28**, 2750–2756.

1124. Visvesvara, G. S., Schuster, F. L., and Martinez, A. J. (1993). *Balamuthia mandrillaris*, n. g., n. sp., agent of amebic meningoencephalitis in humans and other animals. *J. Eukaryotic Microbiol.* **40**, 504–514.

1125. Visvesvara, G. S., Moura, H., Kovacs-Nace, E., Walace, S., and Eberhard, M. L. (1997). Uniform staining of *Cyclospora* oocysts in fecal smears by a modified safranin technique with microwave heating. *J. Clin. Microbiol.* **35**, 730–733.

1126. Vitali, E. (1980). Viral, bacterial, and parasitic diseases of primates in captivity. *Erkr. Zootiere* **22**, 59–64.

1127. Vitzhum, H. (1930). *Pneumonyssus stammeri* ein neur lungenparasit. *Z. Parasitenkd.* **2**, 595–615.

1128. Vogel, H. (1927). Beiträge zue anatomie der gattungen *Dirofilaria* und *Loa. Zentralbl. Bakteriol, Parasitenkd., Infektionskr. Hyg., Abt. I: Orig.* **102**, 81.

1129. Vogel, H., and Vogelsang, E. G. (1930). Neue filarien aus dem orangutan und der ratte. *Zentralbl. Bakteriol., Parasitenkd., Infektionskr. Hyg., Abt. 1: Orig.* **117**, 480–485.

1130. Vogel, P., Miller, C. J., Lowenstine, L., and Lackner, A. A. (1993). Evidence of horizontal transmission of *Pneumocystis carinii* pneumonia in simian immunodeficiency virus-infected rhesus macaques. *J. Infect. Dis.* **168**, 836–843.

1131. Voller, A. (1972). *Plasmodium* and *Hepatocystis. In* "Pathology of Simian Primates" (R. N. T.-W. Fiennes, ed.), Part 2, pp. 57–73. Karger, New York.

1132. Vuylsteke, C., and Rodhain, J. (1938). *Dirofilaria schoutedeni* n. sp. de *Colobus polykomos uelensis. Rev. Zool. Bot. Afr.* **30**, 356.

1133. Wahid, S. (1961). On two new species of genus *Enterobius* Leach, 1853 from a colobus monkey. *J. Helminthol.* **35**, 345–352.

1134. Walker, A. E. (1936). *Cysticercosis cellulosae* in the monkey. A case report. *J. Comp. Pathol.* **49**, 141–145.

1135. Walker, E. L. (1913). Experimental balantidiasis. *Philipp. J. Sci., Sect. B* **8**, 333–339.

1136. Wallace, F. G., Mooney, R. D., and Sanders, A. (1948). *Strongyloides fulleborni* infection in man. *Am. J. Trop. Med.* **28**, 299–302.

1137. Wallace, G. D. (1972). Experimental transmission of *Toxoplasma gondii* by cockroaches. *J. Infect. Dis.* **126**, 545–547.

1138. Wardle, R. A., and McLeod, J. A. (1952). "The Zoology of Tapeworms." University of Minnesota Press, Minneapolis.

1139. Warren, McW. (1970). Simian and anthropoid malarias—their role in human disease. *Lab. Anim. Care* **20**, 368–376.

1140. Warren, McW., and Wharton, R. H. (1963). The vectors of simian malaria: Identity, biology, and geographical distribution. *J. Parasitol.* **49**, 892–904.

1141. Warren, McW., Bennett, G. F., Sandosham, A. A., and Coatney, G. R. (1965). *Plasmodium eylesi* sp. nov., a tertian malaria parasite from the white-handed gibbon, *Hylobates lar. Ann. Trop. Med. Parasitol.* **59**, 500–508.

1142. Warren, McW., Coatney, G. R., and Skinner, J. C. (1966). *Plasmodium jefferyi* sp. n. from *Hylobates lar* in Malaya. *J. Parasitol.* **52**, 9–13.

1143. Warren, McW., Shiroishi, T., and Davis, J. (1968). A *Hepatocystis*-like parasite of the gibbon. *Trans. R. Soc. Trop. Med. Hyg.* **62**, 4.

1144. Webber, W. A. F. (1955). The filarial parasites of primates: A review. I. *Dirofilaria* and *Dipetalonema. Ann. Trop. Med. Parasitol.* **49**, 123–141.

1145. Webber, W. A. F. (1955). The filarial parasites of primates: A review. II. *Loa, Protofilaria* and *Parlitomosa*, with notes on incompletely identified adult and larval forms. *Ann. Trop. Med. Parasitol.* **49**, 235–249.

1146. Webber, W. A. F. (1955). *Dirofilaria aethiops* Webber, 1955, a filarial parasite of monkeys: I. The morphology of the adult worms and microfilariae. *Parasitology* **45**, 369–377.

1147. Webber, W. A. F. (1955). *Dirofilaria aethiops* Webber, 1955, a filarial parasite of monkeys: III. The larval development in mosquitoes. *Parasitology* **45**, 388–400.

1148. Webber, W. A. F., and Hawking, F. (1955). The filarial worms *Dipetalonema digitatum* and *D. gracile* in monkeys. *Parasitology* **45**, 401–408.

1149. Weidman, F. D. (1923). The animal parasites, their incidence and significance. *In* "Disease in Captive Wild Mammals and Birds: Incidence, Description, Comparison" (H. Fox, ed.), pp. 614–659. Lippincott, Philadelphia.

1150. Weidman, F. D. (1923). Certain dermatoses of monkeys and an ape. Pemphigus, scabies, sebaceous cyst, local subcutaneous edema, benign superficial blastomycotic dermatosis and tinea capitis and circinata. *Arch. Dermatol. Syphilol.* **7**, 289–302.

1151. Weinberg, M. (1906). Kystes vermineux du gros intestin chez le chimpanzé et les singes inférieurs. *C. R. Seances Soc. Biol., Ses Fil.* **60**, 446–449.

1152. Weinberg, M. (1907). Du rôle des helminthes, des larves d'helminthes, et des larves d'insectes dan la transmission des microbes pathogènes. *Ann. Inst. Pasteur, Paris* **21**, 417–442, 533–561; cited by Ruch (967).

1153. Weinberg, M. (1908). Oesophagostomose des anthropoides et des singes inférieurs. *Arch. Parasitol.* **13**, 161–203.

1154. Weinman, D. (1970). Trypanosomiasis in macaques and in man in Malaysia. *Southeast Asian J. Trop. Med. Public Health* **1**, 11–18.

1155. Weinman, D. (1972). *Trypanosoma cyclops* n. sp.: A pigmented trypansome from the Malaysian primates *Macaca nemestrina* and *M. ira. Trans. R. Soc. Trop. Med. Hyg.* **66**, 628–636.

1156. Weinman, D., Wallis, R. C., Cheong, W. H., and Mahadevan, S. (1978). Triatomines as experimental vectors of trypanosomes of Asian monkeys. *Am. J. Trop. Med. Hyg.* **27**, 232–237.

1157. Wellde, B. T., Johnson, A. J., Williams, J. S., Langbehn, H. R., and Sadun, E. H. (1971). Hematologic, biochemical, and parasitologic parameters of the night monkey (*Aotus trivirgatus*). *Lab. Anim. Sci.* **21**, 575–580.

1158. Wells, D. J., Demes, P., Pindak, F. F., Mora de Pindak, M., and Gardner, W. A., Jr. (1988). Sialic acid specific lectin from parasitic *Tritrichomonads. Abstr., Annu. Meet., Am. Soc. Microbiol.*, p. 60; cited by Scimeca *et al.* (1010).

1159. Welshman, M. D. (1985). Management of newly imported primates. *Ann. Technol.* **36**, 125–129.

1160. Wenrich, D. H. (1933). A species of *Hexamita* (Protozoa, Flagellata) from the intestine of a monkey (*Macacus rhesus*). *J. Parasitol.* **19**, 225–229.

1161. Wenrich, D. H. (1937). Studies of *Iodamoeba butschlii* (protozoa) with special reference to nuclear structure. *Proc. Am. Philos. Soc.* **77**, 183–205.

1162. Wenrich, D. H., and Nie, D. (1949). The morphology of *Trichomonas wenyoni* (Protozoa, Mastigophora). *J. Morphol.* **85**, 519–531.

1163. Wenyon, C. M. (1926). "Protozoology: A Manual for Medical Men, Veterinarians and Zoologists." 2 vols. Baillière, Tindall and Cox, London.

1164. Werner, H., and Lange, W. (1968). Beobachtungen uber den befall des marmoset-pinche-affchens *Saguinus* (*Oedipomidas*) *oedipus* mit mikrofilarien der species *Dipetalonema marmosetae* Faust 1935. *Zentralbl. Bakteriol., Parasitenkd., Infektionskr. Hyg., Abt. 1: Orig.* **208**, 568–578.

1165. Wharton, R. H. (1957). Studies on filariasis in Malaya: Observations on the development of *Wuchereria malayi* in *Mansonia* (*Mansonoides*) *longipalpis*. *Ann. Trop. Med. Parasitol.* **51**, 278–296.

1166. Wharton, R. H. (1959). *Dirofilaria magnilarvatum* Price, 1959 (Nematoda:Filarioidea) from *Macaca irus* Cuvier: IV. Notes on larval development in *Mansonoides* mosquitoes. *J. Parasitol.* **45**, 513–518.

1167. Whitney, R. A., Jr., and Kruckenberg, J. M. (1967). Pentastomid infection associated with peritonitis in mangabey monkeys. *J. Am. Vet. Med. Assoc.* **151**, 907–908.

1168. Whitney, R. A., Jr., Johnson, D. J., and Cole, W. C. (1967). "The Subhuman Primate: A Guide for the Veterinarian," EASP 100-26. Edgewood Arsenal, Edgewood, Maryland.

1169. Wigglesworth, V. B. (1932). Exhibition of a new species of sucking louse from a chimpanzee. *Proc. Zool. Soc. London* pt. 2, p. 1079.

1170. Williams, C. S. F., Murray, R. E., McGovney, R. M., and Cockrell, B. Y. (1973). Adamantinoma in a spider monkey (*Ateles fusciceps*). *Lab. Anim. Sci.* **23**, 273–275.

1171. Wilson, D. A., Day, P. A., and Brummer, E. G. (1984). Diarrhea associated with *Cryptosporidium* sp. in juvenile macaques. *Vet. Pathol.* **21**, 447–450.

1172. Windle, D. W., Reigle, D. H., and Heckman, M. G. (1970). *Physaloptera tumefaciens* in the stump-tailed macaque (*Macaca arctoides*). *Lab. Anim. Care* **20**, 763–767.

1173. Witenberg, G. G. (1964). Cestodiases. *In* "Zoonoses" (J. van der Hoeden, ed.), pp. 649–707. Am. Elsevier, New York.

1174. Witenberg, G. G. (1964). Acanthocephala infections. *In* "Zoonoses" (J. van der Hoeden, ed.), pp. 708–709. Am. Elsevier, New York.

1175. Wolf, R. H., Lehner, N. D. M., Miller, E. C., and Clarkson, T. B. (1969). The electrocardiogram of the squirrel monkey *Saimiri sciureus*. *J. Appl. Physiol.* **26**, 346–351.

1176. Wong, M. M. (1970). Procedure in laboratory examination of primates with special reference to necropsy technics. *Lab. Anim. Care* **20**, 337–341.

1177. Wong, M. M., and Conrad, H. D. (1972). Parasite nodules in the macaques. *J. Med. Primatol.* **1**, 156–171.

1178. Wong, M. M., and Conrad, H. D. (1978). Prevalence of metzoan parasite infections in five species of Asian macaques. *Lab. Anim. Sci.* **28**, 412–416.

1179. Wong, M. M., and Kozak, W. J. (1974). Spontaneous toxoplasmosis in macaques: A report of four cases. *Lab. Anim. Sci.* **24**, 273–278.

1180. Woodard, J. C. (1968). Acarous (*Pneumonyssus simicola*) arteritis in rhesus monkeys. *J. Am. Vet. Med. Assoc.* **153**, 905–909.

1181. Woolf, A., and Anthoney, T. R. (1982). Dropping out. [Toxoplasmosis]. *Lab. Anim.* **11**(7), 13–14.

1182. Worms, M. J. (1967). Parasites of newly imported animals. *J. Inst. Anim. Technicians* **18**, 39–47.

1183. Yamaguti, S. (1954). Studies on the helminth fauna of Japan. Part 51. Mammalian nematodes. V. *Acta Med. Okayama* **9**, 105–121.

1184. Yamaguti, S. (1958). The digenetic trematodes of vertebrates. *In* "Systema Helminthum" (S. Yamaguti, ed.), Vol. 1, Parts 1 and 2. Wiley (Interscience), New York.

1185. Yamaguti, S. (1959). The cestodes of vertebrates. *In* "Systema Helminthum" (S. Yamaguti, ed.), Vol. 2. Wiley (Interscience), New York.

1186. Yamaguti, S. (1961). The nematodes of vertebrates. *In* "Systema Helminthum" (S. Yamaguti, ed.), Vol. 3, Parts 1 and 2. Wiley (Interscience), New York.

1187. Yamaguti, S., and Hayama, S. (1961). A redescription of *Edesonfilaria malayensis* Yeh, 1960, with remarks on its systematic position. *Proc. Helminthol. Soc. Wash.* **28**, 83–86.

1188. Yamashiroya, H. M., Reed, J. M., Blair, W. H., and Schneider, M. D. (1971). Some clinical and microbiological findings in vervet monkeys (*Cercopithecus aethiops pygerythrus*). *Lab. Anim. Sci.* **21**, 873–883.

1189. Yamashita, J. (1963). Ecological relationships between parasites and primates. I. Helminth parasites and primates. *Primates* **4**, 1–96.

1190. Yeh, L.-S. (1957). On a filarial parasite, *Deraiophoronema freitaslenti* n. sp. from the giant anteater, *Myrmecophaga tridactyla* from British Guiana, and a proposed reclassification of *Dipetalonema* and related genera. *Parasitology* **47**, 196–205.

1191. Yeh, L.-S. (1960). On a new filarioid worm, *Edesonfilaria malayensis* gen. et sp. nov. from the long-tailed macaque (*Macaca irus*). *J. Heminthol.* **34**, 125–128.

1192. Yen, W.-C. (1977). Helminths of birds and wild animals from Listan Prefecture Yunnan Province, China II. Parasitic nematodes of mammals. *Acta Zool. Sin.* **19**, 354–364.

1193. Yokogawa, S. (1941). On the classification of the plasmodia found in the indigenous monkey (black-leg monkey) of Formosa found by us and previously reported. *J. Med. Assoc. Formosa* **40**, 2185–2186.

1194. Yorke, W., and Maplestone, P. A. (1926). "The Nematode Parasites of Vertebrates." Blakiston, Philadelphia.

1195. Yoshimura, K., Hishinuma, Y., and Sato, M. (1969). *Ogmocotyle ailuri* (Price, 1954) in the Taiwanese monkey, *Macaca cyclopis* (Swinhoe, 1862). *J. Parasitol.* **55**, 460.

1196. Young, M. D. (1970). Natural and induced malarias in Western Hemisphere monkeys. *Lab. Anim. Care* **20**, 361–367.

1197. Young, R. J., Fremming, B. D., Benson, R. E., and Harris, M. D. (1957). Care and management of a *Macaca mulatta* monkey colony. *Proc. Anim. Care Panel* **7**, 67–82.

1198. Yue, M. Y., and Jordan, H. E. (1986). Studies of the life cycle of *Pterygodermatites nycticebi* (Monnig, 1920) Quentin, 1969. *J. Parasitol.* **72**, 788–790.

1199. Yue, M. Y., Jensen, J. M., and Jorden, H. E. (1980). Spirurid infections (*Rictularia* sp.) in golden marmosets, *Leontopithecus rosalia* (syn. *Leontideus rosalia*) from the Oklahoma City Zoo. *J. Zool. Anim.* **11**, 77–80.

1200. Yunker, C. E. (1964). Infections of laboratory animals potentially dangerous to man: Ectoparasites and other anthropods with emphasis on mites. *Lab. Anim. Care* **14**, 455–465.

1201. Zajicek, D. (1969). Nematodes of the genus *Physaloptera* Rudolphi 1819 and *Abbreviata* Travassos, 1911 fom monkeys imported to Czechoslovakia. *Zool. Garten, Leipzig* **37**, 127–133.

1202. Zaman, V. (1970). *Sarcocystis* sp. in the slow loris, *Nycticebus coucang*. *Trans. R. Soc. Trop. Med. Hyg.* **64**, 195–196.

1203. Zaman, V. (1972). A trypanosome of the slow loris (*Nycticebus coucang*). *Southeast Asian J. Trop. Med. Public Health* **3**, 22–24.

1204. Zaman, V., and Goh, T. K. (1968). Isolation of *Toxoplasma gondii* from the slow loris, *Nycticebus coucang*. *Ann. Trop. Med. Parasitol.* **62**, 52–53.

1205. Zaman, V., and Goh, T. K. (1970). Isolation of *Toxoplasma gondii* from Malayan tree shrew. *Trans. R. Soc. Trop. Med. Hyg.* **64**, 462.

1206. Zeman, D. H., and Baskin, G. B. (1985). Encephalitozoonosis in squirrel monkeys (*Saimiri sciureus*). *Vet. Pathol.* **22**, 24–31.

1207. Ziemann, H. (1902). Über das vorkommen von *Filaria perstans* und von trypanosomen beim chimpanse. *Arch. Schiffs- Trop.-Hyg.* **6**, 362.

1208. Zumpt, F. (1961). The arthropod parasites of vertebrates in Africa south of the Sahara (Ethiopian region), Vol. 1 (Chelicerata). *Publ. S. Afr. Inst. Med. Res.* **9**, 1–457.

1209. Zumpt, F., and Till, W. M. (1954). The lung and nasal mites of the genus *Pneumonyssus* Banks (Acarina: Laelaptidae) with description of two new species from African primates. *J. Entomol. Soc. S. Afr.* **17**, 195–212.

1210. Zumpt, F., and Till, W. M. (1955). The mange-causing mites of the genus *Psorergates* (Acarina: Myobiidae) with description of a new species from a South African monkey. *Parasitology* **45**, 269–274.

1211. Zwicker, G. M., and Carlton, W. W. (1972). Fluke (*Gastrodiscoides hominus*) infection in a rhesus monkey. *J. Am. Vet. Med. Assoc.* **161**, 702–703.

Chapter 4

Neoplasia/Proliferative Disorders

Richard E. Weller

TABLE I

ANTIGENIC MARKERS USEFUL IN THE DIFFERENTIAL DIAGNOSIS OF TUMORS

Marker	Target
Intermediate filaments	
Prekeratin	Marker for epithelial/myoepithelial cells
Vimentin	Marker for nonmuscle origin mesenchymal cells
Desmin	Marker for muscle differentiation
Actin	Present in many cell types
Myosin	Strong positivity in muscle
Laminin	Basal lamina of smooth muscle and Schwann cells
Neurofilament protein	Neural cells
Glial fibrillary acidic protein	Glial cells
Proteins	
Fibronectin	Mesenchymal marker
Myoglobin	Specific for skeletal muscle
Factor VIII rag	Specific for endothelial cells
Myelin basic protein	Peripheral nerve marker
S-100 protein	Cells of neural crest origin or cells with nerve sheath differentiation
α-$_1$-antitrypsin/ α $_1$-antichymotrypsin	Histiocyte markers
p-Glycoprotein	Marker for drug resistance gene product
p 53	Marker for tumor suppressor gene product
Enzymes	
Lysozyme	Histiocyte marker
Acid phosphatase/alkaline phosphatase	Markers for osseous and chondroid tissue

I. INTRODUCTION

Bland-Sutton reported the first spontaneous tumor in a nonhuman primate in 1885 (Splitter *et al.,* 1973). There are several excellent reviews regarding neoplastic and proliferative disorders in nonhuman primates (Lapin, 1973; McClure, 1979; Lowenstine, 1986; Beniashvili, 1989). Each review has correctly indicated that most information regarding these disorders has come from reports that describe a single or a small number of cases. This situation probably reflects the fact that there have been few prospective studies utilizing primates to determine the pathogenesis or incidence of neoplasia in a defined species or population over an average life span. It may also reflect the relative youth of monkeys used in biomedical research or maintained in primate facilities. The result is a lack of epidemiologic data from which to derive age-specific tumor incidence in a species.

One fact emerging from these reviews, however, suggests that this situation might be changing. In his review, Beniashvili (1989) reported that in 1968 there were only 122 reported cases of spontaneous tumors in monkeys. By 1985, this number had increased to a total of 388 lesions (Lowenstine, 1986). Since then, the number has increased to 783 animals reported from institutions around the world (Beniashvili, 1989). In contrast,

Lapin (1973) listed only 78 cases of spontaneous tumors in his report. This steady increase in the reported number of spontaneous tumors in monkeys may be the result of several factors: (1) increased interest in or awareness of neoplastic diseases in primates; (2) improvements in health care and nutrition resulting in greater longevity; (3) a gradual shift from the use of imported to colony-born animals for research, leading to better data on age, genetic background, and clinical history; and (4) recognition of the importance of nonhuman primates as models for studying immunodeficiency disorders and carcinogenesis in humans.

There also is a significant body of literature describing the results of studies in which many species of nonhuman primates have been exposed to a variety of known or potential carcinogenic agents. These agents have included ionizing and nonionizing radiation, chemicals, and viruses.

Nonhuman primates are important for the study of neoplasia because their evolution is similar to that of humans. The anatomic and functional similarities of a number of physiologic systems suggest that nonhuman primates may respond to carcinogens in a manner similar to humans and that they may have parallel pathologic processes.

The goals of this chapter are (1) to build on the information provided previously by Lapin (1973), McClure (1979), Lowenstine (1986), and Beniashvili (1989) in their excellent reviews of neoplastic and proliferative disorders in nonhuman primates and (2) to provide an overview of information regarding neoplasia in nonhuman primates for veterinary practitioners, laboratory animal veterinarians, and scientists concerned with clinical management of those diseases and the comparative aspects of oncology.

II. CLASSIFICATION OF NEOPLASIA

A neoplasm is a disturbance of growth characterized by excessive, uncontrolled proliferation of cells. Neoplasms are classically divided into two primary groups: benign and malignant. In general, benign tumors are slow growing, remain localized, and usually do not produce significant side effects. Malignant tumors, however, are much more aggressive. If not detected and treated early, they exhibit invasive, destructive growth and may metastasize, resulting in debilitation or death of the patient.

A. Criteria

Classification of neoplasia is based on many different criteria, of which a combination of histogenesis, histological features, and biological behavior is most useful.

1. Histogenesis

Tumors are commonly classified as epithelial or mesenchymal in origin. Thus, a malignant tumor of epithelial origin is classified as a carcinoma, and one of mesenchymal origin as a sarcoma. When tumors are highly anaplastic or undifferentiated, the origin of the neoplastic cells may be nearly impossible to determine without special diagnostic techniques. Difficulties also may exist in classifying tumors from cells of disputed origin, such as melanotic tumors. Careful pathologic interpretation of tumors is important because grading and prognosis are often directly related to the diagnostic subtype. The histologic discrimination of some tumors is often particularly difficult because this process is partly based on subjective criteria. Immunohistochemistry and electron microscopy have become important tools for tumor typing through determination of certain internal structures and secretions of individual neoplastic cells (DuBoulay, 1985; Madewell, 1987). These techniques often allow more precise diagnosis than can be accomplished by assessment of morphological criteria alone. This distinction is of great importance from a clinical perspective as germ cell origin will often influence the biological behavior of a particular neoplasm and choice of treatment. Table I lists some antigen markers useful in making those distinctions among some tumors.

2. Histologic Features

Histologic appearance, which includes the size and shape of the tumors cells, their growth pattern, character of stroma, and degree of cellular differentiation or maturity, is also used to classify tumors. For example, a diagnosis of cystadenoma indicates the presence of neoplastic cells forming papillae within cystic ducts. When there is excessive desmoplastic reaction in a tumor of epithelial origin, the term "scirrhous carcinoma" may be used.

3. Behavior

Neoplasms are classified as benign or malignant based on their apparent or anticipated biologic behavior. A benign tumor closely resembles the parent tissue and grows slowly by expansion. Malignant tumors are less differentiated; exhibit invasive, destructive growth; and usually metastasize. Tumors of intermediate behavior are often referred to as locally malignant. These tumors are usually locally invasive and recur following surgical removal, but rarely metastasize. The longer some tumors are present and the larger they become, the greater the likelihood they may undergo malignant transformation. In some instances, the biologic behavior of a tumor cannot be accurately predicted by its histologic appearance, as is occasionally the case with some melanomas and mast cell tumors.

4. Etiology

Classification by etiology is generally not used because the cause of most tumors is unknown and some cancer-causing agents are capable of including more than one type of tumor.

Nevertheless, it is important to determine the etiology of neoplasms so that exposure to the causative agent can be avoided or minimized.

5. Eponyms

Some tumors are known by the name of the person first describing the neoplasm or identifying the cause. Few eponyms are used for classifying neoplasms in nonhuman primates.

6. Anatomy

Tumors are occasionally named for the anatomic site in which they arise. Examples of these are aortic body tumor, hepatoma, and thymoma.

B. Structure of Tumors

1. Gross Features

Benign tumors arising on or near surfaces tend to protrude above the surface by forming a polyp, which can be sessile with a broad base or pedunculated with a narrow base. The surface may be smooth, as in some polypoid vaginal leiomyomas, or have papillary projections, such as those that occur in some rectal adenomas and squamous papillomas. Benign tumors arising in deeper structures are usually round to ovoid and have a smooth surface. Because of their expansive growth, benign tumors often compress surrounding stroma with the formation of a capsule. These tumors are usually freely movable and not attached to adjacent structures. They may be solid or cystic.

Malignant tumors are usually irregular in shape and have ill-defined borders due to the infiltration of surrounding structures. They often ulcerate and have central necrosis and hemorrhage. Carcinomas are often firm because of stimulation of excessive fibrous tissue stroma or desmoplasia. Carcinomas may be cystic or have papillary projections above a surface, but are usually infiltrative, with poorly defined borders. In general, sarcomas are solid and fleshy and tend to merge more with surrounding tissues.

2. Histologic Features

Growth patterns of cells and their relationship to vascular stroma, as well as the size and shape of neoplastic cells, help to ascertain tumor type and distinguish benign from malignant tumors. Most important in determining the histologic type of tumor is the functional activity and differentiation of the tumor cells, e.g., squamous cell carcinomas produce keratin and osteosarcomas produce osteoid.

a. BENIGN TUMORS. Benign tumor cells closely resemble the cells of origin; however, they may be larger with slightly hyperchromatic nuclei. Margins are well circumscribed or encapsulated. Some benign tumors comprise more than one cell type. An example is mixed mammary tumors in dogs in which there may be ductal epithelium and myeloepithelium as well as bone and cartilage.

b. TUMOR-LIKE AND PRECANCEROUS LESIONS. It is often difficult to differentiate hyperplasia and dysplasia from neoplasia. This confusion often occurs in cases of sebaceous and nodular hyperplasias and mammary gland adenomas. These lesions often progress to neoplasia and are thus often incorrectly diagnosed as malignant neoplasms. Nodular hyperplasia also occurs in the adrenal gland, liver, and pancreas. Atypical epithelial hyperplasia, which usually progresses to carcinoma *in situ* and invasive squamous cell carcinoma, is a lesion often seen in unpigmented areas exposed to ultraviolet radiation.

c. CARCINOMAS. Malignant tumors of glandular epithelium are known as adenocarcinomas, and their histologic appearance can be extremely variable. Well-differentiated types form glands resembling their tissue of origin; however, the glandular lumens often contain papillary projections and are lined by multiple layers of cells that are irregular in size, shape, and staining intensity. The lumens usually contain secretory material, e.g., well-differentiated thyroid carcinomas have colloid. In less differentiated types, neoplastic epithelial cells may form solid clumps or lobules, often with central necrosis. Few areas will resemble the parent tissue. The infiltrating cells may stimulate excessive stromal fibrosis, as seen in some sweat gland, mammary gland, and intestinal carcinomas. Intestinal carcinomas also may produce mucin, with formation of large extracellular "lakes" of mucus. Undifferentiated carcinomas are usually highly cellular and tend to form a solid or medullary pattern, which can make it difficult or impossible to determine the cell of origin.

Carcinomas of nonglandular epithelium arise from squamous epithelium, transitional epithelium, and basal cells. They also exhibit various degrees of differentiation. Squamous cell carcinomas, when well differentiated, have intercellular bridges and nests of keratinized cells. Undifferentiated types are usually pleomorphic, and some may be spindle shaped. Squamous cell carcinoma also can develop from glandular epithelium that has undergone squamous metaplasia, as is sometimes seen in the lung and salivary gland.

d. SARCOMAS. Sarcomas are malignant tumors of mesenchymal or connective tissue cells. They are not histologically classified as hematopoietic tumors because they arise from mesenchymal cells of nonhematopoietic origin. These tumors ordinarily are arranged in diffuse sheets that lack the well-defined supporting stroma seen in epithelial tumors. As in other solid neoplasms, they are recognized by their differentiation and pattern. Thus, fibrosarcomas tend to lay down collagen, osteosarcomas produce osteoid, and hemangiosarcomas form blood vessels. Sarcomas that arise from cells that line surfaces, such as mesothelium and synovium, may exhibit a tubular pattern similar to adenocarcinomas.

e. DEVELOPMENTAL TUMORS. Tumors rarely arise from embryonal cells in developing organs and tissues. Multipotential embryonal cells are capable of differentiating into various tissues, such as skin, glands of all types, cartilage, muscle, and nervous tissue.

f. HEMATOPOIETIC TUMORS. Tumors of the hematopoietic system comprise a spectrum of diseases that must be differentiated from (1) tumors that derive from other organs or other tissue types that frequently metastasize and localize in hematopoietic organs and (2) tumors that originate within a hematopoietic organ but are derived from nonhematopoietic cells within that organ. Hematopoietic tumors arise from mesodermally derived pluipotent hematopoietic stems cells and their progeny (Holmberg, 1985). The two major divisions of the hematopoietic system are the lymphoid and myeloid systems, respectively. Sarcomas of the lymphoid system usually arise in lymphoid and hematopoietic tissues, but can develop in any tissue. Malignant lymphoma, the designation for all lymphoid tumors other than lymphoid leukemia, exhibits various morphologic types and degrees of differentiation, which are important in garding and in predicting response to therapy (Holmberg, 1985). Lymphocytic leukemia, a separate anatomic form of lymphoid system neoplasia, is restricted to those tumors that have, from inception, marked involvement of the blood, bone marrow, liver, spleen, and lymph nodes. The myeloid division of the hematopoietic system includes neoplasms derived from erythroid, granulocytic, monocytic, and megakaryocytic cells series and their progenitors. These are primary diseases of the bone marrow.

C. Grading of Tumors

In many malignant neoplasms, it is possible to estimate the degree, or grade, of malignancy on histologic criteria. A numerical grading, such as that used for many human tumors, has not been clearly established for tumors in nonhuman primates. The usual procedure is to comment that a tumor is of low-grade malignancy or is highly malignant. The factors used for grading malignancy are based on degree of differentiation, cellular and nuclear pleomorphism, number of mitotic figures, stromal invasion, and lymphatic invasion. Thus, the neoplasm that is well differentiated with few mitotic figures and minimal stroma invasion is of low-grade malignancy; the tumor with pleomorphic cells, many mitotic figures, and lymphatic invasion is highly malignant. Some tumors lack a correlation between histologic appearance and biologic behavior. In these cases, although histologic features indicate malignancy, metastasis rarely occurs.

D. Metastasis

Tumor cell metastasis is an extremely complex process governed by many different classes of molecules with each class having a separate function. Metastasis is the result of multiple sequential steps and is a highly organized, nonrandom, and organ-selective process (Yeatman and Nicolson, 1993).

The capacity to metastasize unmistakably differentiates malignant from benign neoplasia, and the metastatic potential of a given tumor greatly influences prognosis. Although metastasis always implies malignancy, it is not true that all cancers inevitably metastasize. Malignant neoplasms such as gliomas of the brain, hemangiopericytomas, and some fibrosarcomas exhibit invasive, destructive growth, yet rarely metastasize. Distant metastasis of primary neoplasms is the main factor that limits the success of antineoplastic therapy. Such metastasis can be regarded as an early or late event in the neoplastic process and may vary considerably with tumor type.

A group of coordinated cellular processes is responsible for metastasis: (1) tumor cells capable of autonomous growth are liberated from the primary tumor, breach the epithelial basement membrane, and gain access to the underlying connective tissue compartment; (2) tumor cells penetrate blood vessels or lymphatics; (3) tumor emboli are released into the circulation; (4) emboli lodge or adhere in capillary beds of distant organs; (5) tumor cells transmigrate the wall of the arresting vessel, infiltrate adjacent tissue, and multiply; and (6) the new tumor becomes vascularized, proliferates, and invades surrounding stroma.

Advances in tumor and molecular biology have permitted the identification of a variety of heterogeneous molecules governing invasion (degradative enzymes, motility factors), adhesion (inegrins, selectins, cahedrins, immunoglobulin-like superfamily, annexins), and growth (paracrine and autocrine growth factors) of tumors cells (Yeatman and Nicolson, 1993; Thiery and Sastre-Garau, 1995). Lodgement and invasion are complex events that are not fully defined. Arrest and lodgement appear to require a thromboembolic event in which the metastatic embolus contacts vascular endothelium and adheres to the wall, with thrombus formation following aggregation of platelets and fibrin to the tumor cell. Invasion may involve (1) formation of collagenases by tumor cells, (2) mechanical disruption of vessel walls, or (3) chemotactic factors.

Cancer cells differ greatly from normal cells. It is now clear that the loss or inactivation of negative regulatory products, such as those produced by metastasis suppressor gene nm23 and tumor suppressor genes, may be just as important as acquisition of positive phenotypic effectors. Some genetic changes cause an imbalance of growth regulation, leading to uncontrolled proliferation. However, unrestrained growth does not, by itself, result in invasion and metastasis. Metastatic characteristics therefore require additional genetic alterations (Aznavoorian et al., 1993). Metastatic cancer cells lack contact inhibition, which normally stops cells from dividing when in contact with adjacent cells. They have increased mobility and decreased cohesiveness. Invasive cancer cells elaborate a battery of hydrolytic enzymes that include proteases and glycosidases capable of degrading basement membrane components. Notable among these enzymes are type IV collagenase, a metalloprotease that specifically cleaves type IV collagen, and heparinase, a glycosidase

that degrades the glycosaminoglycan chains of heparin sulfate proteoglycan. The expression of these enzymes by invasive cells is correlated with their ability to invade tissue *in vivo* (Liotta et al., 1980; Tryggvason et al., 1987). When taken together, these properties allow for infiltrative growth and separation from the site of origin.

Many cancers metastasize nonrandomly to particular distant sites, and their colonization properties cannot be explained by mechanical considerations, such as arrest of tumor cells in the first microcirculatory network encountered. Metastatic cells that show a high propensity to metastasize to certain organs adhere at higher rates to microvessel endothelial cells isolated from these target sites, invade into target tissue at higher rates, and respond better to paracrine growth factors from the target site. These properties depend on multiple tumor cell, host cell, and stromal molecules that are differentially expressed by particular tumor and organ cells and by the extracellular matrix. For example, some of the adhesion molecules involved in tumor cell–endothelial cell adhesion have been identified on both tumor and host cells. Among them are integrins, endogenous lectins, annexins, and other molecules. The invasive properties of particular tumor cells are dependent on the production of degradative enzymes, and subsequent growth of particular tumor cells at certain organ sites is determined, in part, by their responses to organ paracrine growth factors and the organ extracellular matrix. Collectively, these factors appear to determine the organ colonization properties of blood-borne metastatic cells (Nicolson, 1991a,b).

Metastatic patterns depend on the route of metastasis, tumor type, and target organ. This knowledge is important when attempting to prognostically stage a tumor, especially when thoracic radiographs or other diagnostic methods reveal no evidence of gross metastatic disease. Some patterns are described as follows.

1. Local Spread or Invasion

Malignant tumors will invade into normal, surrounding structures. The extent of this invasion can be determined only histologically. What may appear to be a well-circumscribed tumor grossly will show extensive invasion microscopically. Cancer cells normally invade along lines of least resistance, such as fascial planes, and not into hard structures, such as cartilage and bone. Those cancer cells capable of distant metastasis will invade into lymphatics and blood vessels.

2. Lymphatic Metastasis

Normally, carcinomas tend to spread through the lymphatic system. Thin-walled lymphatic vessels appear to offer little resistance to tumor penetration. Once the cancer cells penetrate into the lymphatics, they either detach to become emboli or proliferate as a continuous growth within the vessel. Cancer cell emboli lodge first in the subcapsular sinuses of lymph nodes. After growth within the lymph node, they then spread to the next group of nodes and eventually to the bloodstream via the thoracic duct. Sometimes lymphatic obstruction will occur, resulting in retrograde metastasis.

3. Hematogenous Metastasis

Dissemination through blood vessels, particularly veins, is most characteristic of sarcomas. Some carcinomas will metastasize directly through the bloodstream, as is often seen in thyroid and renal carcinomas. Arterial spread of both sarcomas and carcinomas becomes important when tumor cells reach the left side of the heart. The most common sites of metastasis after vascular invasion are the lung and liver, depending on whether the tumor cells gain access to the systemic venous system or the portal circulatory system.

4. Spread by Implantation

Spread by implantation of cancer cells by mechanical means occurs most commonly in serous cavities. A frequently seen example in humans is direct implantation of ovarian carcinoma from the surface of the ovary to surrounding peritoneal surfaces. Gastrointestinal and transitional cell carcinomas also will occasionally implant on peritoneal surfaces. Cancer cells also may be transplanted by instruments during biopsy or surgery, which may produce tumor implantation in uninvolved tissues, or even in the incision itself.

E. Staging of Cancer

The staging of cancer, which is an attempt to define the extent or spread of neoplastic disease in a patient, is important for proper disease management. In addition to establishing the anatomic site or tissue of origin and the grade of the primary neoplasm, staging also includes the extent of spread to regional lymph nodes and metastasis to distant sites. Staging is critical to formulating a therapeutic plan and determining the prognosis for a patient. It is also important when evaluating therapies because one must compare patients in similar stages of disease so that results in one study can be accurately compared to those in another.

Staging cannot be accomplished on the basis of physical examination alone, but requires the use of all diagnostic methodologies available. Radiology, ultrasonography, computer-assisted tomography, magnetic resonance imaging, biopsy, exploratory surgery, and both gross and histopathology are usually necessary to properly stage a malignant neoplasm. Figure 1 illustrates the T, N, M system of classification for tumors of solid organs, where T denotes the extent of primary tumor, N the condition of the regional lymph nodes, and M the presence of distant metastases. In 1978, an international system for clinical staging was developed by the World Health Organization, in cooperation with the Veterinary Cancer Society, to parallel equivalent

human staging systems as closely as possible, thus increasing the comparative value of cancer in animals to that occurring in humans (Owen, 1980). Although designed primarily for canine and feline tumors, there is every reason to believe that this staging system, with modifications, is equally applicable to nonhuman primates as well, thus increasing the comparative value of studying spontaneous and experimentally induced tumors in the various nonhuman primate species.

III. ETIOLOGY AND EPIDEMIOLOGY

The etiology of neoplasms in nonhuman primates is largely unknown, although several contributory causes have been identified in different species, including genetic factors, ionizing radiation, chemical carcinogens, and viruses.

A. Genetic Factors

A lack of epidemiologic data on neoplastic disease in nonhuman primates, particularly the age-specific incidence of neoplasms, makes it very difficult to point to specific factors that might predispose different species to neoplasms. Although the hereditary cancers of human subjects have been reported to number between 50 and 200 (Moolgavkar and Knudson, 1981), similar diseases in nonhuman primates, such as hereditary retinoblastoma, breast cancer, familial polyposis coli, and Wilms' tumor, have rarely been documented. An example of a possible hereditary cancer in nonhuman primates is the colon cancer observed in cotton-top tamarins (*Saguinus oedipus*) (Petersen and Roth, 1993). These animals have a high prevalence of ulcerative colitis and adenocarcinoma of the colon. However, an investigation by Cheverud *et al.* (1993) of the genetic basis for colon cancer in the species indicated no evidence for heritable variation in cancer experience. One study has suggested that the increased susceptibility of the cotton-top tamarin to these diseases is related to limited major histocompatibility complex (MHC) class I polymorphism in the species (Watkins *et al.*, 1988). MHC class I antigens are believed to play a major role in immune recognition of cancer.

Immune senescence is also thought to be causally related to the increased incidence of tumors observed in aging populations. Limited data are available about changes in immune status across life span in nonhuman primates. Immunologic assays conducted on rhesus monkeys (*Macaca mulatta*) ranging in age from 2 to 36 years revealed significant declines in cellular immune function with age (Ershler *et al.*, 1988). These results suggest that as the age of captive populations and breeding colonies increases, so will the incidence of neoplasia. Such results also point to myriad opportunities for cancer researchers interested in comparative oncology and to challenges for those individuals responsible for medical management of those populations.

<u>**T CATEGORIES:**</u>

T_1: Confined to the organ or origin, usually 2 cm in its largest diameter, localized, mobile.

T_2: Deeply invading, usually 2-5 cm in its largest diameter, localized, mobile, or partially mobile.

T_3: Regionally confined, greater than 4 or 5 cm, but less than 10 cm fixed.

T_4: A massive lesion, greater than 10 cm in diameter, destructive, not confined to the region.

<u>**N CATEGORIES:**</u>

N_0: No evidence of disease in lymph nodes.

N_1: Palpable and movable nodes confined to the nodes receiving direct drainage of the specific site or organ. Mestastases are suggested, based on firmness and size (i.e., 2-3 cm in diameter).

N_2: Firm-to-hard nodes, palpable and partially movable, 3-5 cm in size.

N_3: Fixation is complete.

N_4: Nodes involved beyond the first tation.

N_x: Nodes inaccessible to clinical evaluation.

N_- or N_+: Nodes evaluated histologically and designated as negative or positive depending upon findings.

<u>**M CATEGORIES:**</u>

M_0: No evidence of metastasis.

M_1: Solitary isolated metastasis.

M_2: Multiple metastatic foci.

M_x: No metastatic work-up done.

M_p: = pulmonary metastasis; M_h = hepatic; M_s = skin; M_b = brain, etc.

FINAL CLINICAL STAGE = T____ N____ M____

Fig. 1. World Health Organization staging protocol for solid tumors.

B. Radiation Carcinogenesis

Neoplasms have been produced in nonhuman primates exposed to a wide variety of irradiation. It has been written that Petrov was the first to produce malignant tumors in nonhuman primates with radioactive cancerogens (radium ore, radium bromide) (Lapin, 1973). Most radiation carcinogenesis studies employing nonhuman primates have focused on the potential health effects of irradiation in human subjects engaged in occupations with higher risks for exposure or following an accident or catastrophe in which large amounts of radiation are released into the environment.

1. External Irradiation

Nonhuman primates have been used for some time to study the effects of irradiation; however, reports of radiation-induced neoplasms are infrequent. Studies have been conducted using nonhuman primates to determine the effects of whole body irradiation, as well as the effects of therapeutic measures such as bone marrow transplantation (Van Zwieten *et al.*, 1978). In a study of the effects of simulated space irradiations, 1000 rhesus monkeys were exposed to various types of whole body irradiation using protons, electrons, neutrons, and X-rays (Splitter *et al.*, 1973). The study resulted in the development of 19 tumors.

Thirteen of those tumors were considered to be radiation induced, whereas 6 were considered to be spontaneous. The majority of the radiation-induced tumors were grouped histologically as sarcomas, leukemias, and glioblastomas multiforme. The irradiated monkeys showed certain similarities to those individuals exposed to ionizing radiation in Hiroshima and Nagasaki. For example, the life span period in which the myelogenous leukemias occurred correlated with the life span period of the human exposures. The life span occurrence of brain tumors was also similar to that observed in atomic bomb survivors. Glomangiomas, rare tumors arising from arterial–venous shunts known as neuromyoarterial glomi, have only been reported in whole body-irradiated nonhuman primates (Hubbard et al., 1984; Hubbard and Wood, 1984). The effectiveness of fission neutrons (average dose 3.4 Gy) as carcinogens has been evaluated in rhesus monkeys and rats. Radiation-induced tumors were observed in the bone marrow, mammary glands, and lung. On the basis of the number of animals developing tumors as a function of the total observation period and average absorbed dose, relative biological effectiveness (RBE) values between 4 and 5 were derived at the high dose levels (Broerse et al., 1991). The results of radiation carcinogenesis experiments in animal models indicate that the highest RBE values are obtained for neutrons with energies between 0.5 and 1 MeV (Broerse et al., 1985).

2. Internal Irradiation

A pulmonary fibrosarcoma of bronchial origin was produced in a rhesus monkey 9 years after inhalation of plutonium-239 dioxide (Hahn et al., 1987). Baboon experiments with inhaled plutonium-239 dioxide conducted at the Laboratoire de Toxicologie Experimentale in France resulted in lung tumors in three animals between 107 and 2528 days after exposure (Bair et al., 1980). Primary bone tumors in monkeys also have been produced with bone-seeking radionuclides such as radium and strontium (Casarett et al., 1962; Lapin, 1973).

C. Chemical Carcinogenesis

Nonhuman primates are not commonly used in the study of carcinogenesis. For 32 years, the National Cancer Institute (NCI) has funded a large study to evaluate the relative susceptibility of primates to the effects of several known rodent carcinogens, various cancer chemotherapeutic agents, and several food additives/contaminants such as cyclamate, sacchrin, and aflatoxin (Dalgard et al., 1995). In this program, various carcinogens have been administered, by several routes, to test animals for periods of time from 10 months to 10 years or until tumor is detected, with an additional observation period of 5 years. Many of the studies have employed chemical compounds of two types: polycyclic aromatic hydrocarbons, especially benzo[a]pyrene, and N-nitroso compounds, particularly

diethylnitrosamine (DENA). Many of these compounds are extremely toxic and carcinogenic. They also bind the soluble Ah receptor and are thereby capable of inducing cytochrome P450IA1 through expression of CYP1A1 gene (McLemore et al., 1990). Cytochrome P450IA1-dependent aryl hydrocarbon hydroxylase (AHH) activity, in turn plays a central role in metabolism of these chemicals to their ultimate carcinogenic derivatives (Hankinson et al., 1988). These reactive derivatives bind to DNA, forming DNA adducts, which lead to DNA damage often in the form of point mutations. Individuals with genetically higher levels of AHH activity, or altered CYP1A1 gene expression, may be at increased risk for carcinogen-induced cancer.

Diethylnitrosamine was the most potent and predictable hepatocarcinogen in rhesus (Macaca mulatta), cynomolgus (Macaca fascicularis), and African green (Cercopithecus aethiops) monkeys. N-Methyl-N-nitrosourea (MNU) was the only carcinogen that consistently produced neoplasms in the digestive tract, mostly squamous cell carcinomas of the esophagus (Thorgeirsson et al., 1994). Attempts to produce tumors in nonhuman primates with chemical carcinogens that produce malignant tumors in rodents have met with variable success. Of the classical rodent carcinogens studied, urethane was the only one that produced malignant neoplasms in monkeys (Thorgeirsson et al., 1994). Fungal food contaminants, aflatoxin B_1 (AFB1) and sterigmatocystin (SMT), were found to be potent hepatocarcinogens. Aflatoxin B_1 also induced adenocarcinomas of the pancreas, osteosarcomas, and other tumors (Sieber et al., 1979). Also, the aglycone of cycasin, methylazoxymethanol acetate, induced a variety of neoplasms, but primarily hepatocellular and renal cell carcinomas (Sieber et al., 1980). Among the antineoplastic and immunosuppressive agents, procarbazine was the only unequivocal carcinogen, with a 33% tumor incidence, causing acute nonlymphocytic leukemia in most cases (Seiber et al., 1978). Of three heterocyclic amine mutagens currently being evaluated for carcinogenic activity in nonhuman primates, 2-amino-3-methylimidazo[4,5,f]quinoline (IQ) has proven to be one of the most potent hepatocarcinogens in the history of the NCI project, inducing malignant liver neoplasms in 65% of animals, primarily cynomolgus monkeys, over a 7-year period of exposure (Thorgeirsson et al., 1994; Adamson et al., 1995).

It has been suggested that primates lower in the primate phylogenic scale appear to be more responsive to the carcinogenic effects of polycyclic hydrocarbons (Adamson et al., 1970). This change in reaction to polycyclic hydrocarbons appears in primates at about the level of marmosets; however, the mechanism responsible for the observed increased sensitivity to these chemicals in unknown. Prosimian primates, including tree shrews, lemurs, lorises, and tarsiers, respond more like rodents when exposed to chemical carcinogens (Adamson et al., 1970). The subcutaneous administration of chemicals such as benzo[a]pyrene and methylcholanthrene to prosimians caused fibrosarcomas, and other chemicals produced epidermal and adnexal tumors as well as lipomas. The intraperitoneal administration of DENA to galagos (a prosimian) induced primarily mucoepidermoid carcinoma of the nasal cavity compared to the malignant liver tumors induced in higher primates (Thorgeirsson *et al.*, 1994).

Other reports describing the results of chemical carcinogenesis studies in nonhuman primates include (1) the induction of epidermoid carcinoma of the lung in an owl monkey (*Aotus trivirgatus*) with 7,12-dimethylbenz[*a*]anthracene and *Herpesvirus saimiri* (Giddens, 1974), (2) the induction of liver tumors by AFB1 in tree shrews (Reddy *et al.*, 1976), (3) a review article describing a study of platyrrhine monkeys in which liver tumors were found only in marmosets (*Callithrix* spp.) and tamarins given aflatoxins and hepatitis virus (Lowenstine, 1986), and (4) stomach cancer induced in monkeys following chronic oral administration of *N*-methyl-*N*'-nitro-*N*-nitrosoguanidine (Sharashidze *et al.*, 1989).

D. Oncogenic Viruses

1. DNA-Containing Herpesviruses

a. *HERPES SAIMIRI* AND *H. ATELES*.   These viruses were first isolated from primary kidney cell cultures derived from squirrel monkeys (*Saimiri sciureus*) and spider monkeys (*Ateles* spp.), respectively (Barahona *et al.*, 1976; Reitz, 1987). *Herpes saimiri* and *H. ateles* are indigenous to squirrel monkeys and spider monkeys, respectively. They do not cause disease in the host of origin, even though infection is common in both wild and captive animals. Transmission appears to be horizontal. The virus persists in lymphocytes of healthy infected animals and elicits an antibody response. Inoculation of *H. saimiri* into marmosets, spider monkeys, owl monkeys, and cinnamon ringtail monkeys (*Cebus albifrons*) results in a lymphatic leukemia and lymphoma that is often rapidly fatal (Barahona *et al.*, 1976). The target cell appears to be a T cell. *Herpes ateles* quickly induces lymphoblastic lymphoma and acute leukosis in owl monkeys and marmosets after inoculation. This virus also causes malignant lymphoma when inoculated into howler monkeys (*Alouatta* spp.) (Lowenstine, 1986). Both viruses rapidly induce polyclonal malignancy, suggesting that they contain all information necessary for malignant transformation (Reitz, 1987). A specific region of the *H. saimiri* genome, sequences between 0.0 and 4.0 map units (4.5 kb pairs), is required for oncogenicity (Desrosiers *et al.*, 1986). Two nononcogenic mutants of *H. saimiri* were demonstrated to have deleted DNA sequences in the same portion of the genome. Loss of these sequences did not affect the ability of the virus to grow *ex vivo* or produce persistent viremia in neotropical primates, but infected animals did not develop tumors. One gene in this region, the saimiri transformation-associated protein (STP), is required for immortalization of common marmoset T lymphocytes and its deletion renders the virus nononcogenic (Hunt and Desrosiers, 1994). Introduction of the gene into rodent cells results in their transformation and ability to form invasive tumors in nude mice.

b. EPSTEIN–BARR VIRUS.   A ubiquitous herpesvirus, Epstein–Barr virus (EBV), has been strongly associated with human diseases such as Burkitt's lymphoma, nasopharyngeal carcinoma, and infectious mononucleosis. Epstein–Barr virus was initially found in African Burkitt's lymphoma biopsy cultures, but later studies revealed that EBV is a common human herpesvirus distributed widely in the world (Ishida and Yamamoto, 1987). Epstein–Barr-like viruses are widely distributed in various nonhuman primates. They show high-grade biological similarities to EBV and have cross-reacting antigens (Fellinger *et al.*, 1996).

Two species of neotropical primates, the cotton-top tamarin and the owl monkey, have been experimentally infected with EBV, with 25–40% developing malignant lymphoma. The remainder either developed a benign lymphoproliferative disorder or remained clinically healthy (Daniel *et al.*, 1983). Malignant lymphomas in both species were of B-cell origin. Lymphocytes from other species of neotropical primates have been transformed *ex vivo* by EBV; however, the animals themselves failed to develop lymphoproliferative disease or lymphoma following inoculation with the virus.

Epstein–Barr virus-associated lymphomagenesis has also been described in simian immunodeficiency virus (SIV)-immunosuppressed Old World nonhuman primates. B-cell lymphomas develop frequently in SIV-immunosuppressed macaques associated with an EBV-related simian herpesvirus operationally designated as herpesvirus macaca fascicularis I (HVMFI) (Li *et al.*, 1994; Rezikyan *et al.*, 1995). Infection with an EBV-related herpesvirus has been demonstrated in almost 90% of lymphomas in SIV-infected rhesus monkeys at the German Primate Center (Pingel *et al.*, 1997). Malignant B-cell lymphomas in SIV-infected nonhuman primates can be a model for EBV-associated lymphogenesis in immunodeficiency states (Li *et al.*, 1993). Lapin *et al.* (1985) have detected an EBV-related herpesvirus in baboons and other nonhuman primates at the Sukuhmi primate center that developed hemopoietic malignancies. The virus has considerable restriction map homology to human EBV, particularly in the well-conserved polymerase gene region, which showed 90% homology to human EBV (Schatzl *et al.*, 1993).

2. RNA-Containing Retroviruses

a. GIBBON APE LEUKEMIA VIRUSES (GALVs).   Members of this family of viruses were isolated from lymphoid cell lines established from tissues collected from captive gibbons (*Hylobates* spp.) maintained at several diverse geographical locations. These viruses induce leukemia, lymphoma, and a disease resembling chronic myelogenous leukemia in human subjects. The target cell also appears to be a T cell. Although all strains of GALV have been shown to be closely related to each other, they are distinguishable from each other by differences along the length of their genome (Reitz, 1987). The GALVs are not endogenous to primates and are transmitted from animal to animal by horizontal infection, with the possible inclusion of congenital infection.

b. SIMIAN SARCOMA VIRUS (SSV). The SSV, also called the woolly monkey virus, was actually the first isolate of a GALV. This virus was isolated from a spontaneous fibrosarcoma of a pet woolly monkey (*Lagothrix* spp.) (Theilen *et al.,* 1971). It is able to transform cells *in vitro* and causes fibromas when inoculated into marmosets. Simian sarcoma virus is an acutely transforming retrovirus actually consisting of two viruses: one virus is a defective recombinant virus unable to replicate in the absence of a helper virus and the other virus, simian sarcoma-associated virus (SSAV), is capable of replicating and complementing the replicative defects of SSV (Reitz, 1987). Simian sarcoma-associated virus is closely related to all strains of GALV and is considered a member of the GALV group (Reitz, 1987).

c. SIMIAN T-CELL LYMPHOTROPIC VIRUS TYPE 1 (STLV-I). The STLV-I, a type C retrovirus genetically similar to human T-cell lymphotropic virus type I (HTLV-I), has been linked to the development of lymphomas in gorillas, baboons, and macaques and to the development of leukemia in African green monkeys (Tsujimoto *et al.,* 1985; Gardner *et al.,* 1988; D'iachenko *et al.,* 1990; McCarthy *et al.,* 1990; Jayo *et al.,* 1990; Cremer and Gruber, 1992; Hubbard *et al.,* 1993). In Old World nonhuman primates, seroprevalence of antibodies to STLV-1, which shares 90–95% nucleotide homology with HTLV-1, has been shown to be as high as 60% in feral *Papio cynocephalus anubis,* 50% in *Macaca fuscata,* and 45% in *Papio hamadryas,* increasing to 100% in nonhuman primates with malignant lymphoma (Hubbard *et al.,* 1993). Clinical findings include anemia, generalized lymphadenopathy, hepatosplenomegaly, and leukemia with or without multilobulated neoplastic lymphocytes in peripheral blood.

3. Other Reported Oncogenic Viruses in Nonhuman Primates

a. MASON–PFIZER MONKEY VIRUS (MPMV). The MPMV was isolated from a mammary carcinoma of a rhesus monkey. It is horizontally transmitted and is partly related to the endogenous type D virus of langurs (*Presbytis* spp.), whose DNA contains a provirus closely related to MPMV (Dahlberg, 1988). This virus was thought to be tumorigenic, but extensive efforts to induce tumors with purified MPMV were unsuccessful but the virus did induce thymic atrophy and immunosuppression with opportunistic infections in newborn macaques (Fine *et al.,* 1975). The primary pathology of MPMV appears to be immunosuppression, including lymphadenopathy and thymic atrophy. Subsequent research suggests that MPMV is the prototype of those type-D retroviruses associated with simian acquired immune deficiency syndrome (SAIDS) (Gardner *et al.,* 1988; Cremer and Gruber, 1992).

b. PAPOVAVIRUSES. i. JC virus. The human papovavirus JC has been isolated repeatedly from the brains of patients with rare demyelinating disease, progressive multifocal leukoencephalopathy (Rieth *et al.,* 1980). Owl monkeys and squirrel monkeys inoculated intracerebrally with JC virus developed rapidly progressing, highly malignant cerebral tumors that were glial in nature and usually classified as astrocytomas (Daniel *et al.,* 1983; Miller *et al.,* 1984).

ii. Papillomavirus. A virus resembling papillomavirus has been associated with numerous cutaneous papillomas that were seen in colobus monkeys (*Colobus guereza*). The lesions were confined to the extremities (Rangan *et al.,* 1980). Papillomaviruses also have been associated with a genital malignancy— squamous cell carcinoma of the penis—in a rhesus monkey (Kloster *et al.,* 1988).

c. POXVIRUSES. i. Yaba tumor virus. Yaba monkey tumor virus is a poxvirus that causes benign, cutaneous neoplasms that resemble histiocytomas in nonhuman primates. The virus spreads readily from monkey to monkey under natural or experimental conditions, and the tumors appear within 1–3 weeks after infection. In most cases, the lesions spontaneously regress in about 8 weeks, although experimentally induced disease can progress, causing death of the animal. Yaba virus histiocytomas have been reported in macaques and baboons (Lowenstine, 1986; Beniashvili, 1989).

IV. MECHANISMS OF CARCINOGENESIS

Carcinogenesis involves a complex interplay of hereditary and environment. If there is a unifying principle, it is that carcinogenesis is a multistage process. Most experimental and epidemiologic data are consistent with a two-stage model for pathogenesis of cancer (Moolgavkar and Knudson, 1981). This view is supported in several ways: by the classical initiation– promotion experiments of Berenblum and Shubik (1947); by the occurrence of tumors in two forms, one not inherited and the other inherited in an autosomally dominant fashion; and by the observation that the inheritance of the gene in hereditary neoplasms is not sufficient at the cellular level to give rise to cancer. According to the two-stage model, the first mutational event leads to an improperly controlled proliferation of cells that sustain the event. After the second event has occurred, the cell is committed to developing into a clinically apparent cancer.

Despite the importance of the steps that lead to cancer, until recently neither the number of steps nor their nature was known for any neoplasm. Recent advances in molecular biology have enabled the discovery of the molecular events involved in the development of solid tumors. The development of neoplasia is a multistep process involving the clonal evolution of abnormal cell populations that gain a selective growth advantage over normal cells by accumulating specific alterations in at least two groups of genes: protooncogenes and tumor-suppressor genes. Modern molecular technology has made it possible to identify many of these genetic alterations in human tissue, such as inactivation of both alleles of tumor-suppressor genes in human neoplasms through mutation of one allele and deletion of genetic material containing the other. Alterations of tumor-suppressor genes and protooncogenes and loss of heterozygosity (LOH) at multiple chromosomal loci have been identified in a number of human neoplasms (Mao *et al.,* 1997). This stepwise progression has been most clearly demonstrated for colon cancer in humans (Vogelstein *et al.,* 1988) (Fig. 2) and appears to represent a model of genetic carcinogenesis applicable to other neoplasms as well, regardless of site of origin (Mori *et al.,* 1994; Jones *et al.,* 1995; Thiberville *et al.,* 1995; Louis, 1997; Mao *et al.,* 1997; Todd *et al.,* 1997). For example, human bronchial carcinoma is thought to develop through progressive stages from basal cell hyperplasia to squamous metaplasia, dysplasia, carcinoma *in situ,* and finally invasive carcinoma. Studies have shown that the number of chromosome alterations increases significantly from low-grade to high-grade lesions, showing evidence of accumulation of genetic damage from one stage to another. Molecular follow-up analyses showed that the same genomic alteration can persist in a given dysplastic bronchial area for several months or years and that the persistence or the regression of the molecular abnormality is well correlated with the evolution of disease (Thiberville *et al.,* 1995). The series of genetic changes can include point mutations, chromosomal rearrangements and deletions, LOH, gene amplification, and changes in gene expression. The target genes include dominant-acting cellular oncogenes, putative recessive genes uncovered by deletions, and genes for growth factors and/or their receptors, especially the so-called autocrine growth factors produced by cancer cells themselves. Mutations in the p53 tumor-suppressor gene are the most common genetic alterations identified in human neoplasia and provide a fingerprint of the effects of carcinogen exposure (Mao *et al.,* 1997).

V. DESCRIPTION OF TUMORS

Lowenstine (1986) has pointed out that each group of nonhuman primates has its own pattern of neoplasms based on organ systems most frequently affected. In general, prosimians show a high incidence (>15%) of cutaneous, subcutaneous, hepatic, and pancreatic neoplasms; neotropical primates have a high incidence of gastrointestinal tumors and a moderate incidence (10–15%) of female reproductive tract, endocrine gland, and urinary tract neoplasms; and macaques show a high incidence of hematopoietic neoplasms and cutaneous and subcutaneous tumors and a moderate incidence of female reproductive tract, gastrointestinal tract, and endocrine gland tumors.

A. Tumors of the Skin, Soft Tissues, and Bones

The skin, as the largest organ of the body and the protective covering, often reflects many internal disorders. It protects all other organ systems from various environmental insults, but is also exposed to factors that cause disease and cancer (Strafuss, 1985). Tumors of the skin and subcutis are relatively common in nonhuman primates. The highest incidence has been reported in macaques (Beniashvili, 1989; Lowenstine, 1986). Malignant tumors predominate over benign tumors. A know etiologic agent is Yaba virus, which causes tumors resembling histiocytomas in nonhuman primates. Malignant fibrous histiocytomas have been described in the bonnet monkey (*Macaca radiata*) and baboon (Skavlen *et al.,* 1988). A benign cutaneous mast cell tumor was diagnosed in a rhesus monkey (Colgin and Moeller, 1996), and basal cell tumors in an African green monkey (*Cercopithecus aethiops*) (Moran *et al.,* 1995) and a Japanese macaque (*Macaca fuscata*) (Yanai *et al.,* 1995c). There are also reports of a subcutaneous leiomyosarcoma in a Peruvian squirrel monkey (Brunnert *et al.,* 1990), a rhabdomyosarcoma in a rhesus monkey (Blanchard and Watson, 1988), a subcutaneous atypical lipoma in a female capuchin monkey (Klinger *et al.,* 1993), and myelolipomas in adult Goeldi's monkeys (*Callimico goeldii*) (Narama *et al.,* 1985). A tumor resembling an intradermal nevocellular nevus has been described in a rhesus monkey (Frazier *et al.,* 1993).

Primary bone tumors, however, are fairly rare. This may reflect the relatively small size (i.e., body weight) of most nonhuman primates. The majority of spontaneous bone tumors have been reported in rhesus monkeys, although experimentally induced tumors predominate. In the cases reported, osteosarcomas involving the skull and appendicular skeleton predominate, a single case of extraosseous osteosarcoma has been described in a 10-year-old female rhesus monkey (Gliatto *et al.,* 1990). A unique case of peripheral neuropathy associated with an osteosarcoma has been reported in a Japanese monkey (*M. fuscata*) by Yasuda *et al.* (1990). Other osseous tumors include benign osteomas and fibroosteomas. Bony exostoses have been reported in gorillas, a chondrosarcoma in a squirrel monkey (Chalifoux, 1993), and an enchondroma in a rhesus monkey (Silverman *et al.,* 1994).

B. Tumors of the Cardiovascular System

These are extremely rare and, according to Beniashvili (1989), only one tumor, a myocardial fibrosarcoma of the intraventricular septum in a macaque, has been reported. Neoplasms of vascular tissues also have been described, including a cavernous lymphangioma in a squirrel monkey (King *et al.,* 1993), a renal hemangiosarcoma in a moustached tamarin (*Saguinus mystax*) (Gozalo *et al.,* 1993), and a cavernous hemangioma affecting the ovary in a rhesus monkey (Martin *et al.,* 1970).

C. Tumors of Lymphoid and Hematopoietic Systems

Malignant lymphoma and leukemia have been reported in rhesus monkeys, African green monkeys, and baboons, and have also been reported in several species of neotropical non-

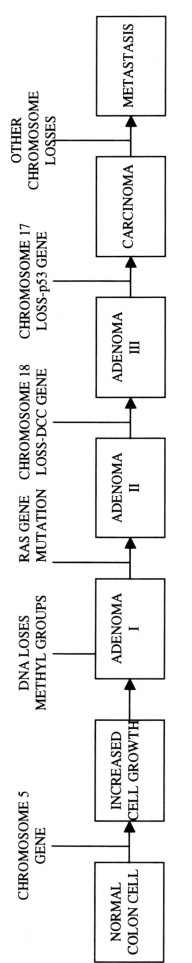

Fig. 2. Diagrammatic representation of the molecular events involved in the multistep process in the development of colonic carcinoma in humans.

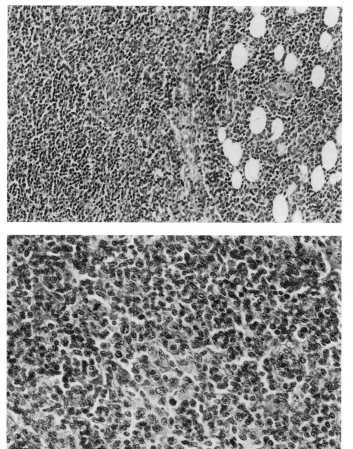

Fig. 3. (Top) Photomicrograph of a portion of a mesenteric lymph node of an owl monkey (*Aotus nancymai*) with experimental *Herpesvirus saimri*-induced lymphoma. The parenchyma as well as the capsule and surrounding adipose tissue of this node have been invaded and replaced by diffuse sheets of neoplastic cells. Magnification: ×175; H & E staining. (Bottom) Higher magnification photomicrograph of a portion of the lymphoma illustrated in A, illustrating the mixed lymphocytic and lymphoblastic nature of the tumor cell infiltrate. Magnification: ×250; H & E staining. (Photographs courtesy of Dr. Norval W. King, Jr.)

TABLE II

SPONTANEOUS MYELOPROLIFERATIVE DISORDERS IN NONHUMAN PRIMATES

Disorder	Species	Reference
Eosinophilic myelocytoma	*Aotus trivirgatus*	Chalifoux and King (1983)
Erythroleukemia	*Pan troglodytes*	McClure *et al.* (1974)
Myeloproliferative disorder	*Saguinus o. oedipus*	Kirkwood and James (1983)
Myeloproliferative disorder	*Aotus* spp.	Matherene *et al.* (1986)
Monocytic leukemia	*Galago c. argentatus*	Holscher *et al.* (1984)
Myeloproliferative disorder	*Cebulla pygmaea*	Lowenstine (1986)
Myelomonocytic leukemia	*Pongo pygmaea*	Gardner *et al.* (1978)
Granulocytic leukemia	*Hylobates lar*	DePaoli *et al.* (1973)
Myelomonocytic leukemia	*Cebus apella*	Bennett *et al.* (1981)

other nonhuman primates (Hubbard *et al.,* 1993; Schatzl *et al.,* 1993). Maxillo-orbital lymphoma (Burkitt's type) has been reported in an infant cynomolgus monkey (Jayo *et al.,* 1988). Acute lymphocytic leukemia has been diagnosed in a 7-month-old Western lowland gorilla (Manning, 1996), and a plasma cell neoplasm was reported in a rhesus monkey (Capozzi *et al.,* 1996).

In contrast to lymphoid leukemias, myeloproliferative disorders appear to be quite infrequent. Spontaneous cases that have appeared in the literature are summarized in Table II.

D. Tumors of the Respiratory Organs

Primary respiratory tract neoplasia is relatively rare in nonhuman primates. In contrast to human subjects, where smoking is clearly the single biggest cause of respiratory tract neoplasia, few risk factors have been clearly identified in nonhuman primates that can be designated primary causes of respiratory carcinogenesis. Nasal cavity tumors of nonhuman primates are rare, although an interesting group of neoplasms, cited by Lowenstine (1986) in her review, documents the incidence of carcinomas of the nasal and oral cavities and pharynx in common marmosets. This observation was intriguing given the association between EBV and nasopharyngeal carcinoma in human subjects. Although no antibodies to the virus were detected in one of the studies cited (McIntosh *et al.,* 1985), the prevalence of these neoplasms in common marmosets warrants further study. A highly aggressive, malignant, intranasal tumor diagnosed as a carcinosarcoma has been described in a male bonnet macaque (Slayter, 1988).

human primates. Most occur in a setting of immune deficiency or dysregulation and are associated with an EBV-like virus. Epstein–Barr virus-associated lymphogenesis in SIV-induced immunosuppressed nonhuman primates has been well described by scientists at the Karolinska Institute (Feichtinger *et al.,* 1992; Rezikyan *et al.,* 1995) and others (Levine, 1994). Experimental infection of cotton-top tamarins and owl monkeys with lymphocyte-transforming doses of EBV has been shown to result in malignant B-cell lymphomas (Levine, 1994). Malignant lymphoma also has been reported in several neotropical primates species, as either spontaneous disease or related to oncogenic herpesvirus infection (Fig. 3). A herpes-associated lymphoma was diagnosed in a slow loris (*Nycitcebus coucang*) (Stetter *et al.,* 1993). Additionally, STLV-1 has been implicated as an etiologic agent of viral lymphogenesis in baboons and

Primary lung cancer in nonhuman primates is even rarer. A malignant mesothelioma involving the pleural cavity has been reported in an olive baboon (*Papio anubis*) (Fortman *et al.*, 1993). Miller (1994) has described a bronchiolar–alveolar adenoma in a rhesus monkey, which was the first reported case of a spontaneous primary pulmonary adenoma in a macaque.

E. Tumors of the Digestive System

Tumors of the digestive system reported in primates have been associated most commonly with the oral cavity, stomach, and colon. Squamous cell carcinomas of the tongue, buccal pouch, and gingiva are the most frequently reported tumors of the oral cavity. Zhang *et al.* (1992) have described esophageal cancer in Chinese rhesus monkeys. The survey for this review also identified a surgically excised ameloblastic odontoma in a cynomolgus monkey (Banks *et al.*, 1988), two cases of oral squamous cell carcinoma in capuchin monkeys (Grana *et al.*, 1992), two cases of oral squamous cell carcinoma in squirrel monkeys (Sasseville *et al.*, 1993; Morris, 1994), and an odontoameloblastoma in a snow monkey (*Macaca fuscata*) (Yanai *et al.*, 1995a). Gastric neoplasia represents one of the largest groups of spontaneous neoplasms in nonhuman primates, although most tumors of the stomach have been classified as adenopapillomas. Invasion of the stomach by the nematode *Nochtia nochti* has been postulated as one of the etiologic agents responsible for development of these lesions. Malignant tumors of the stomach are uncommon, although malignant lymphoma has been described in rhesus monkeys, African green monkeys, and baboons (Lowenstine, 1986). In addition, gastric stromal tumors have been reported in two female rhesus monkeys (Banerjee *et al.*, 1991), and a malignant rhabdoid tumor in the gastric wall was described in an aged orangutan (*Pongo pygmaeus*) (Schauer *et al.*, 1994).

Adenocarcinomas of the small bowel and colon have been described in several species; the highest incidence of colonic neoplasia has been reported in the cotton-top tamarin (Brack, 1988). As many as 60% of captive cotton-top tamarins spontaneously develop ulcerative colitis and 15% of these animal develop adenocarcinoma of the colon (Moore *et al.*, 1988). Colonic carcinoma in the cotton-top tamarin is often multifocal, arises from flat mucosa, is not preceded by adenomas, and lacks preinvasive (dysplastic) lesions (Fig. 4). Cecal adenocarcinomas were observed in a squirrel monkey (Lenz, 1994) and a white-handed gibbon (*Hylobates lar*) (Yanai *et al.*, 1995b). Diverticulosis and colonic leiomyosarcoma have been reported in an aged rhesus monkey (Bunton and Bacmeister, 1989), and a rectal adenocarcinoma in a capped langur (*Presbytis pileata*) (Yanai *et al.*, 1994). An abdominal leiomyosarcoma measuring 10 to 12 cm in diameter was found in the abdomen of a 2-year-old, male rhesus monkey (Bradfield *et al.*, 1995).

Neoplasms of the liver and exocrine pancreas are among the more common malignancies reported in prosimians. These tumors have included hepatocellular carcinomas, cholangiocarcinoma, hepatomas, pancreatic adenocarcinomas, and pancreatic carcinoids. A hepatocellular carcinoma associated with chronic *Schistosoma mansoni* infection has been reported in a 12-year-old chimpanzee (*Pan troglodytes*) (Abe *et al.*, 1993). A hepatocellular carcinoma has also been observed in two species of squirrel monkey, *Saimiri boliviensis* (Borda *et al.*, 1996) and *Saimiri sciureus* (Morris and Abdi, 1996), and a lemur (*Varecia variegata rubra* × *variegata*) (Wohlsein *et al.*, 1996). Myelolipomas of the liver and adrenal gland have been observed in the common marmoset (Kakinuma *et al.*, 1994).

F. Tumors of the Urogenital System

Reports describing spontaneous tumors of the urinary tract have dealt primarily with the kidney. Bilateral undifferentiated renal sarcomas were found in one case (Chrisp *et al.*, 1985). In recent years, a renal papillary adenoma has been observed in a cotton-top tamarin (Brack, 1985), a tubulopapillary renal carcinoma in a baboon (Witt *et al.*, 1989), and a spontaneous renal lymphosarcoma in a juvenile cynomolgus monkey that tested negative for simian immunodeficiency virus (SIV), STLV-1, and SRV-5 (see Section VII,A) (Anderson *et al.*, 1994). Spontaneous tumors of other parts of the urinary tract are less frequent.

Uterine and ovarian tumors appear to be somewhat common. Uterine tumors have included choriocarcinoma, leiomyoma, adenocarcinoma, cervical papilloma, and cervical carcinoma (Kollias, 1979). Two reports describe uterine leiomyomas and endometrial polyps in an aged spider monkey (Binhazim *et al.*, 1989), and endometrial carcinoma in a Celebese black macaque (*Macaca nigra*) (Shaw *et al.*, 1989). Ovarian tumors described in nonhuman primates include teratoma (Scott *et al.*, 1975; Rohovsky, 1977; Baskin *et al.*, 1982), adenocarcinoma (Bunton and Lollini, 1983), dysgerminoma (Holmberg *et al.*, 1978), and cystadenoma (Martin *et al.*, 1970).

Tumors of the male reproductive system appear to be uncommon and are reported less frequently than those of the female reproductive system. Of the reported male reproductive tumors, testicular neoplasia, primarily seminoma, appears to be the most common (Gozalo *et al.*, 1992). A Sertoli cell tumor has been reported in a cotton-top tamarin (Watkins and Warren, 1992), and a bilateral seminoma in an African green monkey (Minoia and Bufo, 1982). A Leydig cell tumor was described in a western lowland gorilla by Karesh *et al.* (1988). Benign adenoma of the prostate in baboons (Lapin, 1982) and rhesus monkeys (McEntee *et al.*, 1996) and prostatic carcinoma in a rhesus monkey have also been reported (Hubbard *et al.*, 1985).

G. Tumors of the Nervous System

Tumors of the nervous system are rarely reported in nonhuman primates and usually involve the brain, spinal cord, and

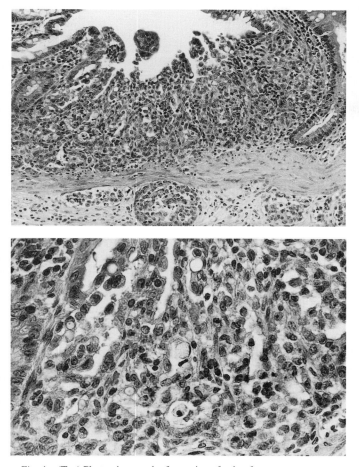

Fig. 4. (Top) Photomicrograph of a section of colon from a cotton-top tamarin (*Saguinus oedipus*) in which there is a focus of adenocarcinoma arising in the flat mucosa. The neoplastic cells are also present within several lymphatic vessels in the submucosa. A number of the tumor cells are of the "signet ring" type and contain large droplets of mucin in their cytoplasm. Magnification: ×250; H & E staining. (Bottom) Higher magnification photomicrograph of a portion of the tumor shown in A, illustrating the pleomorphic and occasional "signet ring" configuration of the tumor cells. Magnification: ×850; H & E staining. (Photographs courtesy of Dr. Norval W. King, Jr.)

peripheral nerves. Nervous system neoplasms found in the survey conducted for this review included an intestinal schwannoma (neurilemmoma) in a rhesus monkey (Barbolt and Egy, 1990); a neurohypophyseal astrocytoma (pituicytoma), also in a rhesus monkey (HogenEsch *et al.*, 1992); an astrocytoma in a cynomolgus monkey (Yanai *et al.*, 1992); an SV-40 associated astrocytoma in a pig-tailed macaque (*Macaca nemestrina*) (Hurley *et al.*, 1993); and an oligodendroglioma in an owl monkey (R. E. Weller, G. E. Dogle and C. A. Malaga, unpublished data).

H. Tumors of the Endocrine System

For the most part, endocrine tumors tend to be benign and nonfunctional in most nonhuman primate species. They have

been reported most commonly in macaques, although a more recent publication describes neoplasms arising from the endocrine system in New World nonhuman primates (Dias *et al.*, 1996). One finding of interest is that some animals have presented with multiple endocrine tumors that resemble the multiple endocrine neoplasia (MEN) syndrome. For example, multiple endocrine neoplasms, composed of a thyroid chief cell adenoma, a pheochromocytoma, and an islet cell adenoma, have been diagnosed in a mantled howler monkey (Lowenstine, 1986). Multiple endocrine neoplasia syndrome is categorized into two main classes (types I and II) and has been described in humans, dogs, cattle, and a golden hamster (Orsher and Eigenmann, 1985). MEN-I is characterized by benign tumors of the parathyroid and pituitary glands, and by either benign or malignant tumors of the pancreas. MEN-II is characterized by the simultaneous occurrence of a medullary thyroid carcinoma and bilateral pheochromocytoma. Finding multiple primary endocrine tumors in nonhuman primates suggests that such tumors may be causally related or that a predisposition to neoplasia exists within individuals of a given species.

Mammary neoplasia has been primarily described in macaques, although infrequent cases have been reported in other species. Malignant tumors occur more frequently than benign and tend to be fairly aggressive clinically, with metastasis to regional lymph nodes, lungs, liver, and kidneys. Breast cancer with cerebral metastases has been reported in a Sumatran orangutan (*Pongo pygameus abelii*) (Bryant *et al.*, 1991).

VI. TREATMENT AND PROGNOSIS

Very little has been written regarding the clinical management of either spontaneous or experimentally induced neoplasms in nonhuman primates, despite the fact that most primate neoplasms are nearly identical to those found in human subjects (Adamson *et al.*, 1974; Muchmore and Socha, 1976). Given this similarity, it appears reasonable to assume that the methods for diagnosing and treating neoplasia in humans and domestic animals are directly applicable to treating neoplasia in nonhuman primates. For example, a 7-month-old western lowland gorilla with acute lymphocytic leukemia was treated by a pediatric oncologist from Children's Hospital of Oklahoma with the same chemotherapeutic protocol used to treat children with the same illness (Manning, 1996). With the current emphasis on captive breeding and obtaining maximum benefit from existing populations of nonhuman primates, it is important to be able to recognize and treat neoplastic diseases in order to improve the animals' quality of life, more effectively utilize existing populations, and avoid depleting wild populations of potentially endangered species that are important to biomedical research. One strategy for reducing the risk of neoplasia in nonhuman primates is to prevent or minimize exposure to known etiologic agents. Knowledge gained from working with those viruses that

Battelle Primate Facility

Location: Building No._____ Room No. _____ Cage No. _____

Genus and Species:_____ Common Name:_____

Animal Identification Number:_____

Sex: Male   Female   Date of Birth:____/____/____   Age:_____
                                             mm dd   yy   months

Instructions: Circle correct response for sections B through H. Key is at bottom of page.

1. Exam Date:_____/_____/_____
                mm   dd   yy

2. Status: R Routine   I Injured   C Clinical   Q Quarantine   T Terminal
               S Sick   E Estrus   P Pregnant   X On Study   O Other

3. Exam Method: A Anesthetized   U Unanesthetized
    If anesthetized: Drug_____   Dose_____
    Route of administration: O Oral   I Intraocular   M Intramuscular
                               T Topical   V Intravenous   S Subcuteanous

A.   General Condition

      1. Attitude: A Alert   W Weak   L Lethargic
                         C Collapsed Conscious   U Unconscious/Comatose
      2. Nutritional Status: N Normal   O Obese   T Thin   C Cachectic
      3. Hydration: N Normal   D Dehydrated (< 5%)   F 5%
                        S 6%   E 8%   T 10%
      4. Weight, gm_____
      5. Crown-rump Length, cm_____
      6. Photo Taken: Y Yes   N No

B.   General External Exam

      1. Conformation: N A NE _____
      2. Skin: N A NE _____
      3. Hair Coat: N A NE _____
      4. Musculoskeletal System: N A NE _____
      5. External Palpation: N A NE _____
      6. External Lymph Nodes: N A NE _____

C.   Thorax: Cardivascular and Respiratory Systems

      1. Mucous Membranes: N A NE _____
      2. Heart Rate: N Increased Decreased NE _____
      3. Pulse Character: N A NE _____
      4. Capillary Refill Time: N A NE _____
      5. EKG: N A NE _____
      6. Respiration Rate: N A NE _____
      7. Auscultation of the Thorax: N A NE _____

                   Key: N-Normal   A-Abnormal   NE-Not Examined

Fig. 5.   Example of the physical examination form used at the Battelle Primate Facility.

TABLE III

COMMON LABORATORY TESTS USED IN DIAGNOSING AND STAGING CANCER

Test	Diagnosis	Staging	Sensitivity	Specificity	Predictive value in diagnosis of symptomatic patients
Routine blood/urine studies	Useful	Not useful	Fair–good	Fair–poor	Low
Routine X-rays	Useful	May be used selectively	Good–excellent	Good	Medium
Special imaging technologies	Useful	Useful	Good–excellent	Good	High
Radionuclide studies	Not useful	Useful	Good	Poor	Low
Biochemical markers	May be used selectively	Good	Good–excellent	Good–excellent	High
Genomic markers	Useful	Good	Good–excellent	Good	High

cause immunosuppression in human subjects and nonhuman primates offers hope in this regard. For example, a vaccine that protected pig-tailed macaques from STLV-I infection has been reported (Dezzutti *et al.,* 1990), as have reports on the prevention of EBV-induced lymphoma in cotton-top tamarins using virus envelope glycoprotein gp340 (Morgan *et al.,* 1988a,b).

A. Diagnosis

Once an animal is recognized with a sign that might signify neoplastic disease, the animal is introduced into the clinical realm of differential diagnosis (Madewell, 1987). The goal is to identify and localize the neoplasm. The diagnostic process begins with a thorough, general physical examination (Hornbuckle, 1988) consisting of several parts. First is a "hands-off" observation of the animal to assess its condition, attitude, conformation, nutritional status, and movements. Depending on the size of the animal, this observation can be done while the animal is either in its cage or in the examination room. Next comes the systemic, "hands-on" inspection, which should be conducted in such a way to minimize stress and the possibility of physical injury to the animals as well as animal care personnel.

The examiner should establish a routine procedure for physical examination in order to ensure that all accessible systems, organs, structures, and orifices of the animal are examined. Development of this routine is often facilitated by use of a physical examination form, as shown in Fig. 5 (Weller *et al.,* 1991). The emphasis and time spent on certain areas of the examination are determined from the history and initial visual observations. Routinely recorded observations should include body weight, rectal temperature, respiratory rate, mucous membrane color, capillary refill time, and hydration status. Examination should always include careful palpation and inspection of those regional lymph nodes that drain the anatomical area in which the suspected neoplasm is located.

Results of the physical examination are used to plan a problem-oriented diagnostic approach for eliminating other differential considerations and obtaining a specific diagnosis. Verification of the initial impression involves ordering selected

laboratory studies: the sensitivity, specificity, and predictive values of these studies must be known or estimated. Efficient diagnosis refers to selection of tests that yield the greatest information with the least cost and risk. Table III presents an overview of commonly used laboratory tests in cancer diagnosis and staging, as well as an evaluation of the sensitivity and specificity of those methods evaluated in one study (Kahn, 1983). The accuracy of the diagnostic approach is enhanced by the availability of new technologies such as clinicopathologic determinations, cytology, endoscopy, and imaging modalities. For example, a technique for catheterization and cystoscopic examination of the urinary bladder has been described for the cynomolgus monkey (Bahnson *et al.,* 1988). This could facilitate earlier diagnosis of diseases affecting the urogenital system in the species.

1. Laboratory Findings

Abnormalities in nonhuman primates with neoplastic disease may be detectable by routine hematology, serum biochemistry, and urinalysis. Anemia, leukopenia, leukocytosis, platelet abnormalities, coagulopathies, hypercalcemia, hypoproteinemia, hyperproteinemia, hypoglycemia, increased serum enzyme activity, isosthenuria, hematuria, and abnormal urine sediment have been associated with a variety of neoplasms. A problem-oriented diagnostic approach, identification of inciting cause, and consideration of pathogenesis are critical to effective management of these paraneoplastic signs.

2. Biopsy Techniques

A biopsy sample is obtained by some method of surgical removal, such as excision, aspiration, imprint, scraping, or wash. Biopsies are performed to diagnose disease, monitor response to therapy, and obtain living cells for studies such as tissue culture. Biopsies should not be performed unless there is a clear expectation of informative result and unless the expected result outweighs the risk of the procedure. Ultrasound-guided biopsy is a safe and useful tool for obtaining samples from deeper tissues and organs. The complete process for taking biopsies and preparing specimens has been summarized in several reviews (Osborne, 1974; Madewell, 1987; Carter and Valli, 1990).

3. Cytologic Diagnosis

Although the definitive diagnosis for most neoplasms requires histologic evaluation of excised tumor masses, cytology is a useful adjunct to histopathology. For some neoplasms, the diagnosis may be more readily based on cytology. Several tumors, including lymphoma, mast cell tumor, histiocytoma, melanoma, and epithelial and mesenchymal tumors of the skin, have cytologic characteristics that make them amenable to cytologic diagnosis. Samples for cytologic evaluation can be collected from many body sites. In general, sampling techniques involve collection of abnormal fluid by fine-needle aspiration from body cavities or collection of cells from solid tissue masses by fine-needle aspiration, impression smears, or tissue scrapings. Cytodiagnosis often can be facilitated through the use of monoclonal antibodies, immunohistochemical techniques, cytochemical stains, and flow cytometry. For example, immunohistochemistry was used to facilitate diagnosis of an intradermal nevocellular nevus in a rhesus monkey (Frazier *et al.*, 1993) and a cecal adenocarcinoma in a white-handed gibbon (Yanai *et al.*, 1995b). The techniques used in sample collection and processing for cytologic examination have been described in numerous references (Perman *et al.*, 1979; Valli, 1984; Allen and Prasse, 1986; Wellman, 1990).

4. Imaging Methods

Imaging methods such as routine X-rays, computer-assisted tomography, magnetic resonance imaging, positron emission tomography, and radionuclide scans can provide useful information for diagnosing and staging neoplasms. Scintigraphic imaging using radiolabeled monoclonal antibodies has been used to diagnose colorectal neoplasia in cotton-top tamarins (Crook and Clapp, 1993).

B. Treatment

Clinical management of a nonhuman primate with neoplasia may require one or more of several traditional anticancer treatments employed in human and veterinary oncology. These options include surgery, radiation therapy, chemotherapy, immunotherapy (biological response modification), hyperthermia, cryotherapy, phototherapy, and combined modalities (chemoimmunotherapy, hyperthermia combined with chemotherapy, hyperthermia combined with radiation therapy). However, nonhuman primate clinicians could take advantage of the many novel and experimental anticancer therapies being evaluated in nonhuman primates.

The concept of neoplasia as a systemic disease affects the treatment of cancer. Therapy must be designed to simultane-

ously treat local disease, metastatic disease, paraneoplastic syndromes, and the secondary physiologic effects of cancer. At times it may be more important to treat the systemic consequences of the cancer, such as paraneoplastic syndromes, before instituting specific anticancer therapy.

1. Paraneoplastic Syndromes

Disorders associated with neoplasia that are unrelated to the size, location, metastases, or physiologic activities of the mature tissue of origin are considered paraneoplastic and secondary to the tumor. Paraneoplastic disorders (PNDs) occur in approximately 75% of human cancer patients; the true incidence of PNDs in animal cancer patients is unknown. The PND, which may present as signs or specific syndromes, may precede tumor diagnosis by weeks, months, or even years. Various types of PNDs, singly or in multiples, may be associated with either benign or malignant tumors and may involve almost every organ system directly or indirectly. Often overlooked in the presence of neoplasia, PNDs constitute significant clinical entities in animals with neoplasms. They may cause morbidity and moratality in affected individuals, with effects more severe than those caused by the associated neoplasm. Accurate clinical evaluation of these disorders is important in differential diagnosis and treatment, for failure to realize that neoplasia can produce many clinical signs similar to other diseases may lead to incorrect diagnosis and delay therapy. Early recognition of the etiology underlying the PND is essential to selecting the proper therapeutic approach and maximizing the patient's chances for remission and survival. The presence of these disorders may complicate or rule out the preferred therapy in some cases, as the addition of cytotoxic drugs may worsen the existing PND, predisposing the animal to a variety of complications. Appropriate management of the PND may be of more immediate importance than treatment of the neoplasm. The study and recognition of PNDs may be valuable for a number of reasons: to facilitate early diagnosis of the neoplasm, for the observed abnormalities may represent tumor cell markers; to allow assessment of premalignant states; to aid in the search for metastases; to help quantify and monitor response to therapy; to aid in the evaluation of recurrence or progression of the neoplasm; to aid in identifying specific pathophysiologic processes by which cancer produces systemic effects; and to provide insight into the study of malignant transformation. Recognition of PNDs is relevant to the diagnosis and treatment of many problems in veterinary cancer medicine. With increasing emphasis on diagnosis and treatment of neoplasms in nonhuman primates, PNDs will be identified with greater frequency and will assume greater importance in the management of those patients (Weller, 1985).

Peripheral neuropathy, an uncommon PND, associated with an osteosarcoma, has been reported in a Japanese monkey (Yasuda *et al.*, 1990), and PNDs observed in domestic animals with neoplastic disease have been described (Weller, 1982;

Ogilvie, 1989). Weight loss, characterized as anorexia or cachexia, is one of the most common and important PNDs encountered in patients with neoplasia. Cancer cachexia is a complex syndrome that occurs despite adequate nutrition. It affects a large percentage of animals with cancer even before any clinical signs are seen. This PND results in alterations in carbohydrate, lipid, and protein metabolism that, if left untreated, decrease the animal's quality of life and lead to poorer responses to anticancer therapy (Weller, 1988).

2. Anticancer Therapeutics

Historically, it would appear that surgery alone has been the primary method for treating neoplasms in nonhuman primates (Banks *et al.*, 1988; Wissman and Parsons, 1992; Brown and Swenson, 1995; Meehan *et al.*, 1995), although blood transfusion therapy (Muchmore and Socha, 1976), chemotherapy (Adamson *et al.*, 1974; Bennett and Dunker, 1995; Manning, 1996), and other modalities have been used infrequently. All conventional and experimental therapeutic regimens employed in treating neoplasia in humans and domestic animals can be used to treat nonhuman primates species. Most are well-established methods for treatment of neoplasia in small animals, and their rational use requires a basic grasp of the mechanisms that govern their biological effects and potential complications.

Anticancer treatment modalities are discussed briefly here, but to describe the principles and applications of each modality is beyond the scope of this chapter.

a. SURGERY. Surgery can be used alone or in combination with other anticancer treatments to cure, control, palliate, or diagnose neoplasia. Cure is the optimal goal of oncologic surgery; however, in general, cure occurs only when the tumor is benign or well localized. Surgery can also potentiate the efficacy of chemotherapy, radiation therapy, hyperthermia, and therapy with biological response modifiers by decreasing the number of cells to be treated (Ogilvie, 1992).

b. CHEMOTHERAPY. Anticancer chemotherapy has become routine in veterinary medicine. The reliance on this modality to treat companion animals can be attributed to several factors, including (1) an increase in the demand by pet owners for state-of-the-art therapy for their pets with cancer; (2) convincing evidence that, for some malignancies, chemotherapy is effective in tumor control; and (3) proof that chemotherapy can control metastatic disease. Anticancer chemotherapy in veterinary medicine has evolved from the use of single agents, which produce only limited remissions, to the concept of combination chemotherapy. Three basic principles underlie the design of combination chemotherapy protocols:

1. The fraction of tumor cells killed by one drug is independent of the fraction killed by another drug.
2. Drugs with different mechanisms of action should be chosen so that the antitumor effects will be additive.

3. Because different classes of drugs have different toxicities, the toxic effects will not be additive.

For convenience, anticancer drugs are grouped into six categories: alkylating agents, antimetabolites, antitumor antibiotics, plant alkaloids, hormones, and miscellaneous drugs. Usually, drugs within the same category share similar chemical structures and mechanisms of action. The usefulness of most chemotherapeutic agents depends on their therapeutic-to-toxic ratio (therapeutic index). Anticancer chemotherapy is limited when tumor cells develop drug resistance, especially to multiple drugs. However, tumor resistance to one drug of a class does not necessarily imply resistance to other drugs in the same class.

c. IMMUNOTHERAPY. Much of what used to be called immunotherapy is now included in the term "biological response modifiers" (BRMs). The field of biological response modification is progressing very rapidly. A BRM is defined as an agent or approach that modifies the biological response of the host to tumor cells to result in therapeutic effects (MacEwen, 1990). The goal of BRM therapy is to stimulate the immune system of the animal to recognize tumor cells or to increase the ability of the immune system to kill tumor cells. This therapy is usually used as an adjuvant therapy to definitive primary therapy.

d. RADIATION THERAPY. The role of radiation therapy in managing neoplasia in animals is undergoing refinement due to advances in technology, radiation biology, and clinical application. Historically, radiation therapy was considered only when a tumor was beyond or had failed surgical resection. This strategy was largely a consequence of unavailability and expense of treatment as well as limited tumor response data. Current efforts in veterinary radiation oncology are focusing on optimizing treatment delivery. Accurate delivery of radiation and real-time dosimetry are essential. Radiation therapy can be used as either a primary or adjuvant modality and should be considered fundamental in planning the treatment of many solid tumors (Thrall and Dewhirst, 1989).

Two general classes of radiation therapy are available to treat neoplasms in animals. Telotherapy uses X-ray-producing machines or radioactive compounds (cobalt-60 and cesium-137) that administer radiation at some distance from the patient; brachytherapy is a form of radiation therapy in which radioactive sources (cobalt-60 and cesium-137 needles, radon-222 seeds) are placed in or on the tumor (Ogilvie, 1992). Combined modality therapy (surgery, radiation, chemotherapy, and hyperthermia) should help in reducing local tissue side effects of radiation alone and in increasing local tumor control.

e. HYPERTHERMIA. Observations that neoplastic cells are sensitive to temperature change led to the use of cryosurgery and hyperthermia to induce tumoricidal activity. Hyperthermia, one of the newer areas of research in veterinary oncology, can be used locally or systemically. This therapy seems to be most effective when combined with other modalities, particularly radiation or chemotherapy (Page *et al.,* 1987; Thompson *et al.,* 1987).

f. PHOTODYNAMIC THERAPY.   This therapy uses photosensitizing chemicals activated with proper wavelengths of light to cause a photochemical reaction that subsequently kills surrounding tissue. Tumors seem to preferentially concentrate the photosensitizing agents after they are administered parenterally to the animal. Fiber-optic cables are generally used to deliver the light generated by argon lasers, associated with a dye laser, to the tumor (Ogilvie, 1992).

3. Management of Complications of Anticancer Therapy

The use of anticancer therapies in nonhuman primates may result in significant side effects and toxicities, such as alopecia, nausea, diarrhea, anemia, neutropenia, thrombocytopenia, and sepsis. Toxic side effects of anticancer drugs have been classified as immediate, early, delayed, and late. Immediate side effects are those that occur within the first 24 hr. Early side effects have their onset within days or weeks. Delayed effects occur within weeks to months after drug administration. Finally, late effects become evident months to years later. The clinician must be concerned with the incidence, predictability, severity, and reversibility of potential side effects. These factors vary with the drug, dose, route of administration, and with the simultaneous use of other drugs. Several host factors, such as species, age, nutrition, and preexisting diseases, also must be considered.

Toxicities attributed to, for example, anticancer chemotherapy in animals include hypersensitivity reactions, dermatologic toxicity, cardiotoxicity, pulmonary toxicity, gastrointestinal toxicity, hepato- and nephrotoxicity, hematologic toxicity, neurotoxicity, acute tumor lysis syndrome, and second malignancies associated with chemotherapeutic agents. It is important that the clinician be able to recognize and manage such complications should they occur. A comprehensive review of potential complications is beyond the scope of this chapter; the reader is referred to Giger and Gorman (1984) and Couto (1990).

VII. LESIONS THAT STIMULATE NEOPLASMS

A. Lymphoproliferative Disorders

Like neoplasms of the lymphoid and hematopoietic systems, benign lymphoproliferative disorders in nonhuman primates occur in a setting of immunosuppression or dysregulation associated with the presence of either DNA- or RNA-containing viruses. Type D retroviruses have been identified as one of the causative agents of naturally occurring infectious immunodeficiency disease in several species of macaques at different primate centers in the United States. The disease was similar to human acquired immune deficiency syndrome (AIDS) and was called simian AIDS, or SAIDS. SAIDS retroviruses (SRVs) are

an important cause of spontaneous SAIDS at these primate centers (Gardner *et al.,* 1988; Hunt and Desrosiers, 1994; Gardner, 1996). Another immunosuppressive retrovirus, distinct from type D retrovirus, but with morphological and antigenic similarities to human immunodeficiency virus (HIV), was isolated from four species of immunodeficient macaques as well as healthy African green monkeys and sooty mangabeys (*Cercocebus torquatus*). This disease was designated simian immunodeficiency virus (SIV) and classified as a lentivirus (Gardner *et al.,* 1988; Cremer and Gruber, 1992; Hunt and Desrosiers, 1994; Gardner, 1996). In addition to immunosuppression and opportunistic infections, clinical findings in nonhuman primates infected with SRVs or SIV often include a progressive generalized lymphadenopathy syndrome. In the early stages of disease, lymph node changes are characterized histologically by marked follicular hyperplasia and a reduced paracortex comprised predominately of T8-positive cells. In nonhuman primates with more advanced disease, lymph nodes show follicular involution of follicle/germinal centers due to follicular dendritic cell destruction, corresponding to the degree of immunodeficiency, followed by marked depletion of T and B lymphocytes (Chalifoux *et al.,* 1984; Muller *et al.,* 1991; Kaaya *et al.,* 1993). Other clinical findings can include splenomegaly, widespread visceral mononuclear cell infiltration, bone marrow hyperplasia, and hematologic abnormalities (Baskin *et al.,* 1988; Chalifoux *et al.,* 1986, 1987). Whether these changes are "premalignant/prodromal" and represent one stage on the pathway to malignancy is unclear (Meyer *et al.,* 1985).

B. Retroperitoneal Fibromatosis: Mesenchymoproliferative Disorders

A peculiar fibroproliferative syndrome called retroperitoneal fibromatosis (RF) has been observed in several species of macaques. It is characterized by the rapid proliferation of spindle cell accompanying inflammatory cell infiltrates, fibroblasts, and endothelial cells subjacent to the pleura and peritoneum. In the early, proliferative phase of the disease, most of the fibroblast-like cells contain factor VIII-related antigen (Giddens *et al.,* 1985). Immunocytochemistry results suggest that the RF spindle cells are derived from vascular smooth muscle cells (Tsai *et al.,* 1997). Two syndromes have been recognized: (1) localized, in which only solitary fibroproliferative nodules are observed; and (2) progressive, in which the disease occurs throughout the pleural and abdominal cavities. A subcutaneous syndrome also has been described (Giddens *et al.,* 1985). The disease is associated with type D retrovirus-induced simian immunodeficiency syndrome (SRV-2) (Marx and Lowenstine, 1987; Tsai *et al.,* 1990; Cremer and Gruber, 1992) and two homologs of the Kaposi's sarcoma-associated herpesvirus (human herpesvirus 8) (Schalling *et al.,* 1995; Kemeny *et al.,* 1997; Rose *et al.,* 1997) and may be useful as a model for AIDS-associated Kaposi's sarcoma. Other evidence suggests that SRV-2 converts endothelial cells to RF and also increases interleukin-6 messenger RNA and protein production; interleukin-6 presumably serves as an autocrine growth factor (Roodman *et al.,* 1991).

C. Endometriosis

Endometriosis is a condition in which normal endometrial epithelium and stroma, under the influence of estrogen, grow outside the endrometrial cavity. This condition is thought to be due to retrograde flow of endometrium during menstruation, with metastasis via hematogenous and lymphatic routes, and is seen most commonly on the peritoneal and pelvic serosal surfaces via direct implantation. One report has described metastatic lesions in lymph nodes in addition to foci on the serosal wall of pelvic organs, and invasion of the mucosal layer of the intestine (Saegusa *et al.,* 1989). It has been hypothesized, from these observations, that endometriosis might behave like a malignant neoplasm. The etiology of endometriosis is not known. Spontaneous endometriosis in nonhuman primates has been reported in rhesus, pig-tailed, cynomolgus, African green monkeys, DeBrazza's monkeys, and baboons. Endometriosis has also been observed in female rhesus monkeys exposed to whole-body doses of ionizing radiation in the form of single-energy protons, mixed-energy protons, X-rays, and electrons (Fanton and Golden, 1991), and some chronically exposed to dioxin for a period of 4 years (Rier *et al.,* 1993). Of all the macaque species, endometriosis has been reported most commonly in the rhesus following cesarean section or other pelvic surgery (Rippy *et al.,* 1996). The reported incidence ranges from 20 to 43% in infertile female macaques (Rippy *et al.,* 1996). The ages of affected nonhuman primates range from 11 to 23 years of age (Ami *et al.,* 1993). Exposure to three or more estradiol implants or one or more hysterotomies appear to be significant risk factors (Hadfield *et al.,* 1997). Clinical signs vary with the location of the ectopic implants, and differential diagnosis requires either a biopsy or a response to antiestrogenic therapy. It has been suggested that immuosuppression might increase the progression of endometriosis in baboons with spontaneous disease (D'Hooghe *et al.,* 1995). Bilateral salpingo-oophorectomy alone or combined with a total hysterectomy may partially or completely resolve the disorder in some cases. In one study, survival of female macaques following surgical treatment of endometriosis was unaffected by choice of surgical approach (Fanton *et al.,* 1986). Postoperative survival rates at 1 and 5 years for rhesus monkeys recovering from surgery were 48 and 36%, respectively (Fanton and Golden, 1991). A report by Mann *et al.* (1986) indicated that either continuous infusion of a gonadotropin-releasing hormone agonist or administration of levonorgestrel is effective for treating endometriosis in nonhuman primates.

D. Gastric Mucosal Response to *Nochtia nochti*

For a discussion of this response see Section V,E.

E. "Luteomas"

The ovaries of female cebids appear to have a developmental phase in which there is massive proliferation of interstitial cells that could be mistaken for ovarian neoplasia (Lowenstine, 1986).

F. Metabolic Bone Disease

Bone disorders presenting as fibrous osteodystrophy can exhibit clinical features resembling primary bone tumors (Wallach and Boever, 1983; Fowler, 1987). The disease is a response to hypocalcemia resulting from dietary deficiency of vitamin D_3 and protein, minimal exposure to sunlight, or renal secondary hyperparathyroidism (Junge *et al.,* 1992) and is primarily a disease of New World nonhuman primates. Lesions usually develop on facial bones, although one case involving the left humerus of a woolly monkey has been reported (Smith *et al.,* 1978).

REFERENCES

Abe, K., Kagei, N., Teramura, Y., and Ejima, H. (1993). Hepatocellular carcinoma associated with chronic *Schistosoma mansoni* infection in a chimpanzee. *J. Med. Primatol.* **22,** 237–239.

Adamson, R. H., Cooper, R. W., and O'Gara, R. W. (1970). Carcinogen-induced tumors in primative primates. *J. Natl. Cancer Inst. U.S.)* **45,** 555–560.

Adamson, R. H., Ablashi, D. V., Cicmanec, J. L., and Dalgard, D. L. (1974). Chemotherapy of *Herpesvirus saimiri* induced lymphoma-leukemia in the owl monkey. *J. Med. Primatol.* **3,** 68–72.

Adamson, R. H., Farb, A., Virmani, R., Synderwine, E. G., Thorgeirsson, S. S., Takayama, S., Sugimura, T., Dalgard, D. W., and Thorgeirsson, U. P. (1995). Studies on the carcinogenic and myocardial effects of 2-amino-3-methylimidazo [4,5-f] quinoline (IQ) in nonhuman primates. *Princess Takamatsu Symp.* **23,** 260–267.

Allen, S. W., and Prasse, K. W. (1986). Cytologic diagnosis of neoplasia and perioperative implementation. *Compend. Contin. Educ. Pract. Vet.* **72,** 71.

Ami, Y., Suzaki, Y., and Goto, N. (1993). Endometriosis in cynomolgus monkeys retired from breeding. *J. Vet. Med. Sci.* **55,** 7–11.

Anderson, W. I., Inhelder, J. L., and King, N. W., Jr. (1994). Spontaneous renal lymphosarcoma in a juvenile cynomolgus monkey (*Macaca fascicularis*). *J. Med. Primatol.* **23,** 56–57.

Aznavoorian, S., Murphy, A. N., Stetler-Stevenson, W. G., and Liotta, L. A. (1993). Molecular aspects of tumor cell invasion and metastasis. *Cancer (Philadelphia)* **71,** 1368–1383.

Bahnson, R. R., Ballou, B. T., Ernstoff, M. S., Schwentker, F. N., and Hakala, T. R. (1988). A technique for catheterization and cystoscopic evaluation of cynomolgus monkey urinary bladders. *Lab. Anim. Sci.* **38,** 731–733.

Bair, W. J., Metivier, H., and Park, J. F. (1980). Comparison of early mortality in baboons and dogs after inhalation of $^{239}PuO_2$. *Radiat. Res.* **82,** 588–610.

Banerjee, M., Lowenstine, L. J., and Munn, R. J. (1991). Gastric stromal tumors in two rhesus macaques (*Macaca mulatta*). *Vet. Pathol.* **28,** 30–36.

Banks, R. E., Davis, J. A., Bach, D. E., and Beattie, R. J. (1988). Surgical excision of an ameloblastic odontoma in a cynomolgus monkey (*Macaca fascicularis*). *Lab. Anim. Sci.* **38,** 316–319.

Barahona, H., Melendez, L. V., Hunt, R. D., and Daniel, M. D. (1976). The owl monkey (*Aotus trivirgatus*) as an animal model for viral diseases and oncologic studies. *Lab. Anim. Sci.* **26,** (Part II), 1104–1112.

Barbolt, T. A., and Egy, M. A. (1990). Intestinal schwannoma in a rhesus monkey. *J. Comp. Pathol.* 103, 471–475.

Baskin, G. B., Soike, K., Jirge, S. K., and Wolf, R. W. (1982). Ovarian teratoma in an African green monkey (*Cercopithecus aethiops*). *Vet. Pathol.* 19, 219–221.

Baskin, G. B., Murphey-Corb, M., Watson, E. A., and Martin, L. N. (1988). Necropsy findings in rhesus monkeys experimentally infected with cultured simian immunodeficiency virus (SIV)/delta. *Vet. Pathol.* 25, 456–467.

Beniashvili, D. S. (1989). An overview of the world literature on spontaneous tumors in nonhuman primates. *J. Med. Primatol.* 18, 423–437.

Bennett, A. R., and Dunker, F. H. (1995). Clinical management of lymphoma in a black and white colobus monkey (*Colobus guereza*). *Proc. Annu. J. Conf. AAZV [Am. Assoc. Zoo Vet.]/WDA[Wildl. Dis. Assoc.]/AAWV [Am. Assoc. Wildl. Vet.]* pp. 351–353.

Bennett, B. T., Beluhan, F. Z., and Sarpel, S. C. (1981). Acute myelomonocytic leukemia in a capuchin monkey (*Cebus apella*). *Lab. Anim. Sci.* 31, 519–521.

Berenblum, I., and Shubik, P. (1947). A new, quantitative, approach to the study of the stages of chemical carcinogenesis in the mouse's skin. *Br. J. Cancer* 1, 383–391.

Binhazim, A. A., Chapman, W. L., and Isaac, W. (1989). Multiple spontaneous lesions in an aged spider monkey. *Lab. Anim. Sci.* 39, 355–357.

Blanchard, J. L., and Watson, E. A. (1988). Spontaneous rhabdomyosarcoma in a rhesus monkey. *J. Comp. Pathol.* 99, 109–113.

Borda, J. T., Ruiz, J. C., and Sanchez-Negrette, M. (1996). Spontaneous hepatocellular carcinoma in *Saimiri boliviensis. Vet. Pathol.* 33, 724–726.

Brack, M. (1985). Renal papillary adenoma in a cotton-topped tamarin (*Saguinus oedipus*). *Lab. Anim.* 19, 132–133.

Brack, M. (1988). Intestinal carcinomas in two tamarins (*Saguinus fuscicollis, Saguinus oedipus*) of the German Primate Centre. *Lab. Anim.* 22, 114–147.

Bradfield, J. F., Strausbauch, P. H., Vore, S. J., and Pryor, W. H. (1995). Abdominal leiomyosarcoma in a rhesus macaque. *Contemp. Top. Lab. Anim. Sci.* 34, 70–73.

Broerse, J. J., Hennen, L. A., and van Zwieten, M. J. (1985). Radiation carcinogenesis in experimental animals and its implications for radiation protection. *Int. J. Radiat. Biol. Relat. Stud. Phys., Chem. Med.* 48, 167–187.

Broerse, J. J., van Bekkum, D. W., Zoetelief, J., and Zurcher, C. (1991). Relative biological effectiveness for neutron carcinogenesis in monkeys and rats. *Radiat. Res.* 128, S128–S135.

Brown, B. G., and Swenson, R. B. (1995). Medical management: Part D. Surgical management. *In* "Nonhuman Primates in Biomedical Research" (B. T. Bennett, C. R. Abee, and R. Hendrickson, eds.), pp. 297–304. Academic Press, San Diego, CA.

Brunnert, S. R., Herron, A. J., and Altman, N. H. (1990). Subcutaneous leiomyosarcoma in a Peruvian squirrel monkey (*Saimiri sciureus*). *Vet. Pathol.* 27, 126–128.

Bryant, W. M., Gardner, J. J., Schluter, J. J., and Wood, G. (1991). Breast cancer with metastasis to the brain in a Sumatran orangutan. *Proc. Annu. Meet., Am. Assoc. Zoo Vet., Annu. Proc.,* pp. 169–169.

Bunton, T. E., and Bacmeister, C. X. (1989). Diverticulosis and colonic leiomyosarcoma in an aged rhesus macaque. *Vet. Pathol.* 26, 351–352.

Bunton, T. E., and Lollini, L. (1983). Ovarian adenocarcinoma in a bonnet monkey: Histologic and ultrastructural features. *J. Med. Primatol.* 12, 106–111.

Capozzi, D. K., Klein, E. C., and Wagner, R. A. (1996). Plasma cell neoplasia in a rhesus monkey and a brief review of related dysplasias in man and nonhuman primates. *Contemp. Top. Lab. Anim. Sci.* 35, 80–83.

Carter, R. F., and Valli, V. E. O. (1990). Taking a biopsy. *Vet. Clin. North Am.: Small Anim. Pract.* 20, 939–968.

Casarett, G. W., Tuttle, L. W., and Baxter, R. C. (1962). Pathology of imbibed ⁹⁰Sr in rats and monkeys. *In* "Some Aspects of Internal Irradiation" (T. F. Dougherty, W. S. S. Jee, C. W. Mays, and B. J. Stover, eds.), pp. 329–339. Pergamon, New York.

Chalifoux, L. V. (1993). Chondrosarcoma in a squirrel monkey. *In* "Nonhuman Primates II" (T. C. Jones and U. Mohr, eds.), pp. 128–131. Springer-Verlag, Berlin.

Chalifoux, L. V., and King, N. V. (1983). Eosinophilic myelocytoma in an owl monkey (*Aotus trivirgatus*). *Lab. Anim. Sci.* 33, 189–191.

Chalifoux, L. V., King, N. W., and Letvin, N. L. (1984). Morphologic changes in lymph nodes of macaques with an immunodeficiency syndrome. *Lab. Invest.* 51, 22–26.

Chalifoux, L. V., King, N. W., Daniel, M. D., Kannagi, M., Desrosiers, R. C., Sehgal, P. K., Waldron, L. M., Hunt, R. D., and Letvin, N. L. (1986). Lymphoproliferative syndrome in an immunodeficient rhesus monkey naturally infected with an HTLV-III virus (STLV-III). *Lab. Invest.* 55, 43–50.

Chalifoux, L. V., Ringler, D. J., King, N. W., Sehgal, P. K., Desrosiers, R. C., Daniel, M. D., and Letvin, N. L. (1987). Lymphadenopathy in macaques experimentally infected with the simian immunodeficiency virus (SIV). *Am. J. Pathol.* 128, 104–110.

Cheverud, J. M., Tardif, S., Henke, M. A., and Clapp, N. K. (1993). Genetic epidemiology of colon cancer in the cotton-top tamarin (*Saguinus oedipus*). *Hum. Biol.* 65, 1005–1012.

Chrisp, C. E., Cary, C., Rush, H. G., and Cohen, B. J. (1985). Bilateral undifferentiated renal sarcomas in a rhesus monkey. *Vet. Pathol.* 22, 516–517.

Colgin, L. M. A., and Moeller, R. B. (1996). Benign cutaneous mast cell tumor in a rhesus monkey. *Lab. Anim. Sci.* 46, 123–124.

Couto, C. G. (1990). Management of complications of cancer chemotherapy. *Vet. Clin. North Am.: Small Anim. Pract.* 20, 1037–1053.

Cremer, K. J., and Gruber, J. (1992). Animal models of retrovirus-associated malignancies. *Vet. Pathol.* 29, 572–578.

Crook, J. E., and Clapp, N. K. (1993). Scintigraphic imaging of tamarin colorectal carcinoma with radiolabeled monoclonal antibodies. *In* "A Primate Model for the Study of Colitis and Colonic Carcinoma: The Cotton-Top Tamarin, *Saguinus oedipus*" (N. K. Clapp, ed.), pp. 309–316. CRC Press, Boca Raton, FL.

Dahlberg, J. E. (1988). An overview of retrovirus replication and classification. *Adv. Vet. Sci. Comp. Med.* 32, 1–35.

Dalgard, D. W., Thorgeirsson, U. P., and Adamson, R. H. (1995). Laparoscopy as a means of monitoring live tumor induction in nonhuman primates. *Princess Takamatsu Symp.* 23, 268–273.

Daniel, M. D., King, N. W., and Hunt, R. D. (1983). Nonhuman primate models of human viral disease. *In* "Nonhuman Primate Models for Human Diseases" (W. R. Dukelow, ed.), pp. 45–47. CRC Press, Boca Raton, FL.

DePaoli, A., Johnson, D. O., and Noll, N. W. (1973). Granulocytic leukemia in whitehanded gibbons. *J. Am. Vet. Med. Assoc.* 163, 624–628.

Desrosiers, R. C., Silva, D. P., Waldron, L. M., and Letvin, N. L. (1986). Nononcogenic deletion mutants of herpesvirus saimiri are defective for in vitro immortalization. *J. Virol.* 57, 701–705.

Dezzutti, C. S., Frazier, D. E., Huff, L. Y., Stromberg, P. C., and Olsen, R. G. (1990). Subunit vaccine protects *Macaca nemestrina* (pig-tailed macaque) against simian T-cell lymphotropic virus type I challenge. *Cancer Res.* 50, 5687S–5691S.

D'Hooghe, T. M., Bambra, C. S., Raeymaekers, B. M., De Jonge, I., Hill, J. A., and Koninckx, P. R. 91995). The effects of immunosuppression on development and progression of endometriosis in baboons (*Papio anubis*). *Fertil. Steril.* 64, 172–178.

D'iachenko, A. G., Kondzhariia, I. G., Indzhiaa, E. V., Lapin, B. A., Iakovleva, L. A., Rudaia, L. D., and Dzhalagoniia, B. L. (1990). Monoclonal integration of simian T-cell leukemia virus in hamadryas with malignant lymphoma. *Eksp. Onkol.* 12, 15–18.

Dias, J. L. C., Montali, R. J., Strandberg, J. D., Johnson, L. K., and Wolff, M. J. (1996). Endocrine neoplasia in New World primates. *J. Med. Primatol.* 25, 34–41.

DuBoulay, C. E. H. (1985). Immunohistochemistry of soft tissue tumors: A review. *J. Pathol.* 146, 77–94.

Ershler, W. B., Coe, C. L., Gravenstein, S., Schultz, K. T., Klopp, R. G., Meyer, M., and Houser, W. D. (1988). Aging and immunity in nonhuman primates:

I. Effects of age and gender on cellular immune function in rhesus monkeys (*Macaca mulatta*). *Am. J. Primatol.* **15**, 181–188.

Fanton, J. W., and Golden, J. G. (1991). Radiation-induced endometriosis in *Macaca mulatta*. *Radiat. Res.* **126**, 141–146.

Fanton, J. W., Yochmowitz, M. G., Wood, D. H., and Salmon, Y. L. (1986). Surgical treatment of endometriosis in 50 rhesus monkeys. *Am. J. Vet. Res.* **47**, 1602–1604.

Feichtinger, H., Kaaya, E., Putkonen, P., Li, S.-L., Ekman, M., Gendelman, R., Biberfeld, G., and Biberfeld, P. (1992). Malignant lymphoma associated with human AIDS and with SIV-induced immunodeficiency in macaques. *AIDS Res. Hum. Retroviruses* **8**, 339–348.

Fellinger, J., Rietschel, W., and Czerny, C.-P. (1996). Prevalence of Epstein–Barr virus (EBV) antibodies in primate stocks of zoological gardens. *J. Med. Primatol.* **25**, 327–332.

Fine, D. L., Landdon, J. C., Pienta, R. J., Kubicek, M. T., Valerio, M. G., Loeb, W. F., and Chopra, H. C. (1975). Responses of infant rhesus monkeys to inoculation with Mason-Pfizer monkey virus materials. *J. Natl. Cancer Inst. (U.S.)* **54**, 651–658.

Fortman, J. D., Manaligod, J. R., and Bennett, B. T. (1993). Malignant mesothelioma in an olive baboon (*Papio anubis*). *Lab. Anim. Sci.* **43**, 503–505.

Fowler, M. E. (1987). Zoo animals and wildlife. *In* "Veterinary Cancer Medicine" (G. H. Theilen and B. R. Madewell, eds.), 2nd ed., pp. 649–662. Lea & Febiger, Philadelphia.

Frazier, K. S., Herron, A. J., Hines, M. E., and Altman, N. H. (1993). Immunohistochemical and morphologic features of an intradermal nevocellular nevus (benign intradermal junctional melanocytoma) in a rhesus monkey (*Macaca mulatta*). *Vet. Pathol.* **30**, 306–308.

Gardner, M. B. (1996). The history of simian AIDS. *J. Med. Primatol.* **25**, 148–157.

Gardner, M. B., Esra, G., Cain, M. J., Rossman, S., and Johnson, C. (1978). Myelomonocytic leukemia in an orangutan. *Vet. Pathol.* **15**, 667–670.

Gardner, M. B., Luciw, P., Lerche, N., and Marx, P. (1988). Nonhuman primate retrovirus isolates and AIDS. *Adv. Vet. Sci. Comp. Med.* **32**, 171–226.

Giddens, W. E. (1974). Inoculation of owl monkeys (*Aotus trivirgatus*) with 7, 12-dimethylbenz(a)anthracene and *Herpesvirus saimiri*. Induction of epidermoid carcinoma in the lung. *In* "Experimental Lung Cancer" (E. Karbe and J. F. Park, eds.), pp. 280–291. Springer-Verlag, New York.

Giddens, W. E., Tsai, C. C., Morton, W. R., Ochs, H. D., Knitter, G. H., and Blakley, G. A. (1985). Retroperitoneal fibromatosis and acquired immunodeficiency syndrome in macaques. Pathologic observations and transmissions studies. *Am. J. Pathol.* **119**, 253–263.

Giger, U., and Gorman, N. T. (1984). Oncologic emergencies in small animals. Part I. Chemotherapy related hematologic emergencies. *Compend. Contin. Educ. Pract. Vet.* **6**, 689–698.

Gliatto, J. M., Bree, M. P., and Mello, N. K. (1990). Extraosseous osteosarcoma in a nonhuman primate (*Macaca mulatta*). *J. Med. Primatol.* **19**, 507–513.

Gozalo, A., Nolan, T., and Montoya, E. (1992). Spontaneous seminoma in an owl monkey in captivity. *J. Med. Primatol.* **21**, 39–41.

Gozalo, A., Chavera, A., Dagle, G. E., Montoya, E., and Weller, R. E. (1993). Primary renal hemangiosarcoma in a moustached tamarin. *J. Med. Primatol.* **22**, 431–432.

Grana, D., Mareso, E., and Gomez, E. (1992). Oral squamous cell carcinoma in capuchin monkeys (*Cebus apella*). Report of two cases. *J. Med. Primatol.* **21**, 384–386.

Hadfield, R. M., Yudkin, P. L., Coe, C. L., Scheffler, J., Uno, H., Barlow, D. H., Kemnitz, J. W., and Kennedy, S. H. (1997). Risk factors for endometriosis in the rhesus monkey (*Macaca mulatta*): A case-control study. *Hum. Reprod. Update* **3**, 109–115.

Hahn, F. F., Brooks, A. L., and McWhinney, J. A. (1987). A primary pulmonary sarcoma in a rhesus monkey after inhalation of plutonium dioxide. *Radiat. Res.* **112**, 391–397.

Hankinson, O., Bannister, R. M., Carramanzana, N., Chu, F. F., Hoffman, E. C., Reyes, H., Sander, F., and Watson, A. J. (1988). Genetic and molecular analysis of chtochrome P-450IA1 induction in a mouse hepatoma cell line.

In "Multilevel Health Effects Research: From Molecules to Man" (J. F. Park and R. A. Pelroy, eds.), pp. 335–342. Battelle Press, Columbus, OH.

HogenEsch, H., Broerse, J. J., and Zurcher, C. (1992). Neurohypophyseal astrocytoma (pituicytoma) in a rhesus monkey (*Macaca mulatta*). *Vet. Pathol.* **29**, 359–361.

Holmberg, C. A. (1985). Classification of hematopoietic system neoplasia in the dog. *Vet. Clin. North Am.: Small Anim. Pract.* **15**, 697–707.

Holmberg, C. A., Sesline, D., and Osburn, B. (1978). Dysgerminoma in a rhesus monkey: morphologic and biological features. *J. Med. Primatol.* **7**, 53–58.

Holscher, M. A., Sly, D. L., Cousar, J. B., Glick, A. D., and Casagrande, V. A. (1984). Monocytic leukemia in a greater bushbaby (*Galago crassicaudatus argentatus*). *Lab. Anim. Sci.* **34**, 619–620.

Hornbuckle, W. E. (1988). General physical examination of the cat and dog. *In* "Handbook of Small Animal Practice" (R. V. Morgan, ed.), pp. 3–11. Churchill-Livingstone, New York.

Hubbard, G. B., and Wood, D. H. (1984). Glomangiomas in four irradiated *Macaca mulatta*. *Vet. Pathol.* **21**, 609–610.

Hubbard, G. B., Fanton, J. W., Harvey, R. C., and Wood, D. H. (1984). Paralysis due to a glomangioma in a *Macaca mulatta*. *Lab. Anim. Sci.* **34**, 614–615.

Hubbard, G. B., Eason, R. L., and Wood, D. H. (1985). Prostatic carcinoma in a rhesus monkey (*Macaca mulatta*). *Vet. Pathol.* **22**, 88–90.

Hubbard, G. B., Mone, J. P., Allan, J. S., Davis, K. J., III, Leland, M. M., Banks, P. M., and Smir, B. (1993). Spontaneously generated non-Hodgkin's lymphoma in twenty-seven simian T-cell leukemia virus type-1 antibody-positive baboons (*Papio* species). *Lab. Anim. Sci.* **43**, 301–309.

Hunt, R. D., and Desrosiers, R. C. (1994). Study of spontaneous infectious diseases of primates: Contributions of the regional primate research centers program to conservation and new scientific opportunities. *Am. J. Primatol.* **34**, 3–10.

Hurley, J., Ilyinski, P., Simon, M., Horvath, C., Pauley, D., Hesterberg, P., Desrosiers, R., and Ringler, D. (1993). An SV-40 associated malignant astrocytoma in an SIV-infected macaque. *Vet. Pathol.* **30**, 454 (abstr.).

Ishida, T., and Yamamoto, K. (1987). Survey of nonhuman primates for antibodies reactive with Epstein–Barr virus (EBV) antigens and susceptibility of their lymphocytes for immortalization with EBV. *J. Med. Primatol.* **16**, 359–371.

Jayo, M. J., Jayo, J. M., Jerome, C. P., Krugner-Higby, L., and Reynolds, G. D. (1988). Maxilloorbital lymphoma (Burkitt's-type) in an infant *Macaca fascicularis*. *Lab. Anim. Sci.* **38**, 722–726.

Jayo, M. J., Laber-Laird, K., Bullock, B. C., Tulli, H. M., and Reynolds, G. M. (1990). T-cell lymphosarcoma in a female African green monkey (*Cercopithecus aethiops*). *Lab. Anim. Sci.* **40**, 37–41.

Jones, K. A., Brown, M. A., and Solomon, E. (1995). Molecular genetics of sporadic and familial breast cancer. *Cancer Surv.* **25**, 315–334.

Junge, R. E., Mehren, K. G., Meehan, T. P., Gilula, L., Gannon, F., Finkel, G., and Whyte, M. P. (1992). Hypertrophic osteoarthropathy and renal disease in three black lemurs (*Lemur macaco*). *Proc. Annu. Meet. Am. Assoc. Zoo Vet.* pp. 324–330.

Kaaya, E., Li, S. L., Feichtinger, H., Stahmer, I., Putkonen, P., Mandache, E., Mgaya, E., Biberfeld, G., and Biberfeld, P. (1993). Accessory cells and macrophages in the histopathology of SIV sm-infected synomolgus monkeys. *Res. Virol.* **144**, 81–92.

Kahn, S. B. (1983). Cancer diagnosis. *In* "Concepts in Cancer Medicine" (S. B. Kahn, ed.), pp. 267–287. Grune & Stratton, New York.

Kakinuma, C., Harada, T., Watanabe, M., and Shibutani, Y. (1994). Spontaneous adrenal and hepatic myelolipomas in the common marmoset. *Toxicol. Pathol.* **22**, 440–445.

Karesh, W. B., Burton, M. S., Russell, R. G., and Burns, M. W. (1988). Leydig cell tumor in a Western lowland gorilla (*Gorilla gorilla gorilla*). *J. Zoo Anim. Med.* **19**, 51–54.

Kemeny, L., Gyulai, R., Kiss, M., Nagy, F., and Dobozy, A. (1997). Kaposi's sarcoma-associated herpesvirus/human herpesvirus-8: A new virus in human pathology. *J. Am. Acad. Dermatol.* **37**, 107–113.

King, C. S., Streett, J. W., and Brownstein, D. G. (1993). Cavernous lymphangioma in a squirrel monkey. *Lab. Anim. Sci.* **43**, 252–254.

Kirkwood, J. K., and James, M. P. (1983). Myeloproliferative disease in a cotton-top tamarin (*Saguinus oedipus oedipus*). *Lab. Anim.* **17**, 70–73.

Klinger, M. M., Levee, E. M., and Scholes, J. V. (1993). Giant fatty tumor in a *Cebus apella*. *J. Med. Primatol.* **22**, 435–436.

Kloster, B. E., Manias, D. A., Ostrow, R. S., Shaver, M. K., McPherson, S. W., Rangen, S. R., Uno, H., and Faras, A. J. (1988). Molecular cloning and characterization of the DNA of two papillomaviruses from monkeys. *Virology* **166**, 30–40.

Kollias, G. V. (1979). Tumors in zoo animals and wildlife. *In* "Veterinary Cancer Medicine" (G. H. Theilen and B. R. Madewell, eds.), pp. 407–423. Lea & Febiger, Philadelphia.

Lapin, B. A. (1973). The importance of monkeys for the study of malignant tumors in man. *In* "Nonhuman Primates and Medical Research" (G. H. Bourne, ed.), pp. 213–224. Academic Press, New York.

Lapin, B. A. (1982). Use of nonhuman primates in cancer research. *J. Med. Primatol.* **11**, 327–341.

Lapin, B. A., Timanovskaja, V., and Yakovleva, L. (1985). Herpesvirus HVMA: A new representative in the group of the EBV-like B-lymphotrophic herpesviruses of primates. *Hematol. Blood Transfus.* **29**, 312–313.

Lenz, B. (1994). Metastasizing adenocarcinoma of the cecum in a squirrel monkey (*Saimiri sciureus*). *Vet. Pathol.* **31**, 276–278.

Levine, A. M. (1994). Lymphoma complicating immunodeficiency disorders. *Ann. Oncol.* **5**, 29–35.

Li, S. L., Feichtinger, H., Kaaya, E., Migliorini, P., Putkonen, P., Biberfeld, G., Middeldorp, J. M., Biberfeld, P., and Ernberg, I. (1993). Expression of Epstein–Barr-virus-related nuclear antigens and B-cell markers in lymphomas of SIV-immunosuppressed monkeys. *Int. J. Cancer* **55**, 609–615.

Li, S. L., Biberfeld, P., and Ernberg, I. (1994). DNA of lymphoma-associated herpesvirus (HVMF1) in SIV-infected monkeys (*Macaca fascicularis*) shows homologies to EBNA-1, -2 and -5 genes. *Int. J. Cancer* **59**, 287–295.

Liotta, L. A., Tryggvason, K., Garbisa, S., Hart, I., Foltz, C. M., and Shafie, S. (1980). Metastatic potential correlates with enzymatic degradation of basement membrane collagen. *Nature (London)* **284**, 67–68.

Louis, D. N. (1997). A molecular genetic model of astrocytoma histopathology. *Brain Pathol.* **7**, 755–764.

Lowenstine, L. J. (1986). Neoplasms and proliferative disorders in nonhuman primates. *In* "Primates: The Road to Self-Sustaining Populations" (K. Benirschke, ed.), pp. 781–814. Springer-Verlag, New York.

MacEwen, E. G. (1990). Biological response modifiers: The future of cancer therapy? *Vet. Clin. North Am.* **20**, 1055–1073.

Madewell, B. R. (1987). Cancer diagnosis. *In* "Veterinary Cancer Medicine" (G. H. Theilen and B. R. Madewell, eds.) 2nd ed., pp. 3–12. Lea & Febiger, Philadelphia.

Mann, D. R., Collins, D. C., Smith, M. M., Kessler, M J., and Gould, K. G. (1986). Treatment of endometriosis in monkeys: Effectiveness of continuous infusion of a gonadotropin-releasing hormone agonist compared to treatment with a progestational steroid. *J. Clin. Endocrinol. Metab.* **63**, 1277–1283.

Manning, A. (1996). Leukemia strikes zoo's baby gorilla. *USA Today*, January 16, Sect. D, p. 1.

Mao, L., Lee, J. S., Kurie, J. M., Fan, Y. H., Lippman, S. M., Lee, J. J., Ro, J. Y., Broxson, A., Yu, R., Morice, R. C., Kemp, B. L., Khuri, F. R., Walsh, G. L., Hittelman, W. N., and Hong, W. K. (1997). Clonal genetic alterations in the lungs of current and former smokers. *J. Natl. Cancer Inst.* **89**, 857–862.

Martin, C. B., Jr., Misenhimer, H. R., and Ramsey, E. M. (1970). Ovarian tumors in rhesus monkeys (*Macaca mulata*): Report of three cases. *Lab. Anim. Care* **20**, 686–692.

Marx, P. A., and Lowenstine, L. J. (1987). Mesenchymal neoplasms associated with type D retroviruses in macaques. *Cancer Surv.* **6**, 101–115.

Matherne, C. M., Gibson, S. V., Kelley, S. T., and Wagner, J. E. (1986). Myeloproliferative syndrome in two owl monkeys. *Lab. Anim. Sci.* **36**, 551 (abstr.).

McCarthy, T. J., Kennedy, J. L., Blakeslee, J. R., and Bennett, B. T. (1990). Spontaneous malignant lymphoma and leukemia in a simian T-lymphotropic virus type I (STLV-I) antibody positive olive baboon. *Lab. Anim. Sci.* **40**, 79–81.

McClure, H. M. (1979). Neoplastic diseases of nonhuman primates: Literature review and observations in an autopsy series of 2176 animals. *In* "The Comparative Pathology of Zoo Animals" (R. Montali and G. Migaki, eds.), pp. 549–565. Smithsonian Institution Press, Washington, DC.

McClure, H. M., Keeling, M. E., Custer, R. P., Marshak, R. P., Abt, D. A., and Ferrer, J. F. (1974). Erythroleukemia in two infant chimpanzees fed milk from cows naturally infected with bovine C-type virus. *Cancer Res.* **34**, 2745–2757.

McEntee, M. F., Epstein, J. I., Syring, R., Tierney, L. A., and Strandberg, J. D. (1996). Characterization of prostatic basal cell hyperplasia and neoplasia in aged macaques: Comparative pathology in human and nonhuman primates. *Prostate* **29**, 51–59.

McIntosh, G. H., Giesecke, R., Wilson, D. F., and Goss, A. N. (1985). Spontaneous nasopharyngeal malignancies in the common marmoset. *Vet. Pathol.* **22**, 86–88.

McLemore, T. L., Adelberg, S., Liu, M. C., McMahon, N. A., Yu, S. J., Hubbard, W. C., Czerwinski, M., Wood, T. G., Storeng, R., Lubet, R. A., Eggleston, J. C., Body, M. R., and Hines, R. N. (1990). Expression of CYP1A1 gene in patients with lung cancer: Evidence for cigarette smoke-induced gene expression in normal lung tissue and for altered gene regulation in primary lung carcinomas. *J. Natl. Cancer Inst.* **82**, 1333–1339.

Meehan, T. P., Zdziarski, J. M., Briggs, M. B., Anderson, D. B., Zelby, A. S., Grigg-Damberger, M., Thomas, C., Murnane, R. D., and Walsh, T. M. (1995). Surgical removal of an intracranial tumor in a western lowland gorilla. *Proc. Annu. Jt. Conf. AAZV [Am. Assoc. Zoo Vet.]/WDA[Wildl. Dis. Assoc.]/AAWV [Am. Assoc. Wildl. Vet.]*, pp. 255–256.

Meyer, P. R., Ormerod, L. D., Osborn, K. G., Lowenstine, L. J., Hendrickson, R. V., Modlin, R. L., Smith, R. E., Gardner, M. B., and Taylor, C. R. (1985). An immunopathologic evaluation of lymph nodes from monkeys to man with acquired immune deficiency syndrome and related conditions. *Hematol. Oncol.* **3**, 199–210.

Miller, G. F. (1994). Bronchiolar-alveolar adenoma in a rhesus monkey (*Macaca mulatta*). *Vet. Pathol.* **31**, 388–390.

Miller, N. R., McKeever, P. E., London, W. T., Padgett, B. L., Walker, D. L., and Wallen, W. C. (1984). Brain tumors of owl monkeys inoculated with JC virus contain the JC virus genome. *J. Virol.* **49**, 848–856.

Minoia, P., and Bufo, P. (1982). Bilateral seminoma in a *Cercopithecus aethiops*. *Acta Med. Vet.* **28**, 599–605.

Moolgavkar, S. H., and Knudson, A. G. (1981). Mutation and cancer: A model for human carcinogenesis. *JNCI, J. Natl. Cancer Inst.* **66**, 1037–1052.

Moore, R., King, N., and Alroy, J. (1988). Differences in cellular glycoconjugates of quiescent, inflamed, and neoplastic colonic epithelium in solitis and cancer-prone tamarins. *Am. J. Pathol.* **131**, 484–489.

Moran, J. L., Duncan, D. E., and Rowell, T. J. (1995). Basal cell tumor in an African green monkey (*Cercopithecus aethiops*). *Contemp. Top. Lab. Anim. Sci.* **34**, 70 (abstr.).

Mori, T., Yanagisawa, A., Kato, Y., Miura, K., Nishihira, T., Mori, S., and Nakamura, Y. (1994). Accumulation of genetic alterations during esophageal carcinogenesis. *Hum. Mol. Genet.* **3**, 1969–1971.

Morgan, A. J., Finerty, S., Lovgren, K., Scullion, F. T., and Morein, B. (1988a). Prevention of Epstein–Barr (EB) virus-induced lymphoma in cotton-top tamarins by vaccination with the EB virus envelope glycoprotein gp340 incorporated into immune-stimulating complexes. *J. Gen. Virol.* **69**, 2093–2096.

Morgan, A. J., Mackett, M., Finerty, S., Arrand, J. R., Scullion, F. T., and Epstein, M. A. (1988b). Recombinant vaccinia virus expressing Epstein–Barr virus glycoprotein gp340 protects cotton-top tamarins against EB virus-induced malignant lymphoma. *J. Med. Virol.* **25**, 668–675.

Morris, T. H. (1994). A further case of squamous cell carcinoma in the oral cavity of a squirrel monkey. *J. Med. Primatol.* **23**, 317–318.

Morris, T. H., and Abdi, M. M. (1996). Hepatocellular carcinoma in a squirrel monkey (*Saimiri sciureus*). *J. Med. Primatol.* **25**, 137–139.

Muchmore, E., and Socha, W. W. (1976). Blood transfusion therapy for leukemic chimpanzees. *Lab. Primate Newsl.* **15**, 13–15.

Muller, J. G., Stahl-Hennig, C., Rethwilm, A., Kneitz, C., Kerkau, T., Schmauser, B., Schindler, C., Krenn, V., terMeulen, V., and Muller-Hermelink, H. K. (1991). Morphological alterations of lymph nodes and thymus during the early course of SIV infection in rhesus monkeys. *Verh. Dtsch. Ges. Pathol.* **75**, 102–107.

Narama, I., Nagatani, M., Tsuchitani, M., and Inagaki, H. (1985). Myelolipomas in adult Goeldi's monkeys (*Callimico goeldii*). *Nippon Juigaku Zasshi* **47**, 549–555.

Nicolson, G. L. (1991a). Molecular mechanisms of cancer metastasis: Tumor and host properties and the role of oncogenes and supressor genes. *Curr. Opin. Oncol.* **3**, 75–92.

Nicolson, G. L. (1991b). Tumor and host molecules important in the organ preference of metastasis. *Semin. Cancer Biol.* **2**, 143–154.

Ogilvie, G. K. (1989). Paraneoplastic syndromes. *In* "Clinical Veterinary Oncology" (S. J. Withrow and E. G. MacEwen, eds.), pp. 29–40. Lippincott, Philadelphia.

Ogilvie, G. K. (1992). Principles of oncology. *In* "Handbook of Small Animal Practice" (R. V. Morgan, ed.) 2nd ed., pp. 799–811. Churchill-Livingstone, New York.

Orsher, R. J., and Eigenmann, J. E. (1985). Endocrine tumors. *Vet. Clin. North Am: Small Anim. Pract.* **15**, 643–658.

Osborne, C. A. (1974). Biopsy techniques. *Vet. Clin. North Am.* **4**.

Owen, L. N., ed. (1980). "TNM Classification of Tumours in Domestic Animals," 1st ed. World Health Organi. Geneva.

Page, R. L., Thrall, D. E., Dewhirst, M. W., and Meyer, R. E. (1987). Wholebody hyperthermia: Rationale and potential use for cancer treatment. *J. Vet. Intern. Med.* **1**, 110–120.

Perman, V., Alsaker, A. D., and Riis, R. C. (1979). "Cytology of the Dog and Cat." Am. Anim. Hosp. Assoc., South Bend, IN.

Petersen, G. M., and Roth, M.-P. (1993). Genetic epidemiology of colon cancer. *In* "A Primate Model for the Study of Colitis and Colonic Carcinoma: The Cotton-Top Tamarin, *Saguinus oedipus*" (N. K. Clapp, ed.), pp. 187–198. CRC Press, Boca Raton, FL.

Pingel, S., Hannig, H., Matz-Rensing, K., Kaup, F. J., Hunsmann, G., and Bodemer, W. (1997). Detection of Epstein–Barr virus small RNAs EBER1 and EBER2 in lymphomas of SIV-infected rhesus monkeys by *in situ* hybridization. *Int. J. Cancer* **72**, 160–165.

Rangan, S. R. S., Gutter, A., Baskin, G. B., and Anderson, D. (1980). Virus associated papillomas in colobus monkeys (*Colobus guereza*). *Lab. Anim. Sci.* **30**, 885–889.

Reddy, J. K. Svoboda, D. J., and Rao, M. S. (1976). Induction of liver tumors by aflatoxin B1 in the tree shrew (*Tupaia glis*), a nonhuman primate. *Cancer Res.* **36**, 151–160.

Reitz, M. S., Jr. (1987). Hematopoietic neoplasms, sarcomas and related conditions: Part X. Primates (nonhuman and human). *In* "Veterinary Cancer Medicine" (G. H. Theilen and B. R. Madewell, eds.), 2nd ed., pp. 465–470. Lea & Febiger, Philadelphia.

Rezikyan, S., Kaaya, E. E., Ekman, M., Voevodin, A. F., Feichtinger, H., Putkonen, P., Castanos-Velez, E., Biberfeld, G., and Biberfeld, P. (1995). B-cell lymphomagenesis in SIV-immunosuppressed cynomolgus monkeys. *Int. J. Cancer* **61**, 574–579.

Rier, S. E., Martin, D. C., Bowman, R. E., Dmowski, W. P., and Becker, J. L. (1993). Endometriosis in rhesus monkeys (*Macaca mulatta*) following chronic exposure to 2,3,7,8-tetracholorodibenzo-p-dioxin. *Fundam. Appl. Toxicol.* **21**, 433–441.

Rieth, K. G., Di Chiro, G., London, W. T., Sever, J. L., Houff, S. A., Kornblith, P. L., McKeever, P. E., Buonomo, C., Padgett, B. L., and Walker, D. L. (1980). Experimental glioma in primates: A computed tomography model. *J. Comput. Assist. Tomogr.* **4**, 285–290.

Rippy, M. K., Lee, D. R., Pearson, S. L., Bernal, J. C., and Kuehl, T. J. (1996). Identification of rhesus macaques with spontaneous endometriosis. *J. Med. Primatol.* **25**, 346–355.

Rohovsky, M. W. (1977). Benign ovarian teratomas in two rhesus monkeys (*Macaca mulata*). *Lab. Anim. Sci.* **27**, 280–281.

Roodman, S. T., Woon, M. D., Hoffman, J. W., Theodorakis, P., and Tsai, C. C. (1991). Interleukin-6 and retroperitoneal fibromatosis from SRV-2 infected macaques with simian AIDS. *J. Med. Primatol.* **20**, 201–205.

Rose, T. M., Strand, K. B., Schultz, E. R., Schaefer, G., Rankin, G. W., Jr. Thouless, M. E., Tsai, C.-C., and Bosch, M. L. (1997). Identification of two homologs of the Kaposi's sarcoma-associated herpesvirus (human herpesvirus 8) in retroperitoneal fibromatosis of different macaque species. *J. Virol.* **71**, 4138–4144.

Saegusa, J., Tanoika, Y., and Koizumi, H. (1989). Massive endometriosis in two rhesus monkeys. *Jikken Dobutsu* **38**, 275–278.

Sasseville, V. G., Pauley, D. R., Spaulding, G. L., Chalifoux, L. V., Lee-Parritz, D., and Simon, M. A. (1993). A spontaneous squamous cell carcinoma of the oral cavity in a squirrel monkey (*Saimiri sciureus*). *J. Med. Primatol.* **22**, 272–275.

Schalling, M., Ekman, M., Kaaya, E. E., Linde, A., and Biberfeld, P. (1995). A role for a new herpes virus (KSHV) in different forms of Kaposi's sarcoma. *Nat. Med.* **1**, 707–708.

Schatzl, H., Tschikobava, M., Rose, D., Voevodin, A., Nitschko, H., Sieger, E., Busch, U., von der Helm, K., and Lapin, B. (1993). The Sukhumi primate monkey model for viral lymphomogenesis: High incidence of lymphomas with presence of STLV-I and EBV-like virus. *Leukemia* **7**, S86–S92.

Schauer, G., Moll, R., Walter, J. H., Rumplet, H. J., and Goltenboth, R. (1994). Malignant rhabdoid tumor in the gastric wall of an aged orangutan (*Pongo pygmaeus*). *Vet. Pathol.* **31**, 510–517.

Scott, W. J., Fradkin, R., and Wilson, J. G. (1975). Ovarian teratoma in a rhesus monkey. *J. Med. Primatol.* **4**, 204–206.

Sharashidze, L. K., Beniashvili, D. S., Sherenesheva, N. I., and Turkiia, N. G. (1989). The induction of stomach cancer in monkeys with N-methyl-N'-nitro-N-nitrosoguanidine. *Vopr. Onkol.* **35**, 335–338.

Shaw, D. P., Overend, M. F., and Grina, L. A. (1989). Endometrial carcinoma in a Celebese black macaque (*Macaca nigra*). *Vet. Pathol.* **26**, 451–452.

Sieber, S. M., Correa, P., Dalgard, D. W., and Adamson, R. H. (1978). Carcinogenic and other adverse effects of procarbazine in nonhuman primates. *Cancer Res.* **38**, 2125–2134.

Sieber, S. M., Correa, P., Dalgard, D. W., and Adamson, R. H. (1979). Induction of osteogenic sarcomas and tumors of the hepatobiliary system in nonhuman primates with aflatoxin B1. *Cancer Res.* **39**, 4545–4554.

Sieber, S. M., Correa, P., Dalgard, D. W., McIntire, K. R., and Adamson, R. H. (1980). Carcinogenicity and hepatotoxicity of cycasin and its aglycone methylazoxymethanol acetate in nonhuman primates. *JNCI, J. Natl. Cancer Inst.* **65**, 177–189.

Silverman, J., Weisbrode, S. E., Myer, C. W., Biller, D. S., and Kerpsack, S. J. (1994). Enchondroma in a rhesus monkey. *J. Am. Vet. Med. Assoc.* **204**, 786–788.

Skavlen, P. A., Speers, W. C., Peterson, R. R., Stevens, J. O., and Reite, M. L. (1988). Malignant fibrous histiocytoma in a bonnet macaque (*Macaca radiata*). *Lab. Anim. Sci.* **38**, 310–311.

Slayter, M. V. (1988). Nasal cavity carcinosarcoma in a bonnet macaque (*Macaca radiata*). *J. Med. Primatol.* **17**, 49–56.

Smith, K., Dillingham, L., and Giddens, W. E. (1978). Metabolic bone disease resembling osteosarcoma in a wooly monkey. *Lab. Anim. Sci.* **28**, 451–456.

Splitter, G. A., Kirk, J. H., and Casey, H. W. (1973). Radiation-related and spontaneous tumors in primates. *In* "Radionuclide Carcinogenesis" (C. L. Sanders, R. H. Busch, J. E. Ballou, and D. D. Mahlum, eds.), pp. 55–89. U.S. At. Energy Comm., Oak Ridge, TN.

Stetter, M. D., Worley, M. R., and Ruiz, B. (1993). Herpes associated lymphoma in a slow loris (*Nycticebus coucang*). *Proc. Annu. Meet., Am. Assoc. Zoo Vet.*, pp. 120–122.

Strafuss, A. C. (1985). Skin tumors. *Vet. Clin. North Am.: Small Anim. Pract.* **15**, 473–492.

Theilen, G. H., Gould, D., Fowler, M., and Dungworth, D. L. (1971). C-type virus in tumor tissue of a woolly monkey (*Lagothrix* spp.) with fibrosarcoma. *J. Natl. Cancer Inst. (U.S.)* **47**, 881–889.

Thiberville, L., Payne, P., Vielkinds, J., LeRiche, J., Horsman, D., Nouvet, G., Palcic, B., and Lam, S. (1995). Evidence of cumulative gene losses with progression of premalignant epithelial lesions to carcinoma of the bronchus. *Cancer Res.* **55**, 5133–5139.

Thiery, J. P., and Sastre-Garau, X. (1995). Metastatic process. *Rev. Prat.* **45**, 1909–1919.

Thompson, J. M., Gorman, N. T., and Bleehen, N. M. (1987). Hyperthermia and radiation in the management of canine tumors. *J. Small Anim. Pract.* **28**, 457–477.

Thorgeirsson, U. P., Dalgard, D. W., Reeves, J., and Adamson, R. H. (1994). Tumor incidence in a chemical carcinogenesis study of nonhuman primates. *Regul. Toxicol. Pharmacol.* **19**, 130–151.

Thrall, D. E., and Dewhirst, M. W. (1989). Radiation therapy. *In* "Clinical Veterinary Oncology" (S. J. Withrow and E. G. MacEwen, eds.), pp. 79–91. Lippincott, Philadelphia.

Todd, R., Donoff, R. B., and Wong, D. T. (1997). The molecular biology of oral carcinogenesis: toward a tumor progression model. *J. Oral Maxillofacial Surg.* **55**, 613–623.

Tryggvason, K., Hoyhta, M., and Salo, T. (1987). Proteolytic degradation of extracellular matrix in tumor invasion. *Biochim. Biophys. Acta* **907**, 191–217.

Tsai, C. C., Tsai, C. C., Roodman, S. T., and Woon, M. D. (1990). Mesenchymoproliferative disorders (MDP) in simian AIDS associated with SRV-2 infection. *J. Med. Primatol.* **19**, 189–202.

Tsai, C. C., Wu, H., and Meng, F. (1997). Immunocytochemistry of Kaposi's sarcoma-like tumor cells from pigtailed macaques with simian AIDS. *J. Med. Primatol.* **24**, 43–48.

Tsujimoto, H., Seiki, M., Nakamura, H., Watanabe, T., Sakakibara, I., Sasagawa, A., Honjo, S., Hayami, M., and Yoshida, M. (1985). Adult T-cell leukemia-like disease in a monkey naturally infected with simian retrovirus related to human T-cell leukemia virus type I. *Jpn. J. Cancer Res.* **76**, 911–914.

Valli, V. E. O. (1988). Techniques in veterinary cytopathology. *Semin. Vet. Med. Surg. Small Anim.* **3**, 85–93.

Van Zwieten, M. J., Zurcher, C., and Hollander, C. F. (1978). Longevity studies in rhesus monkeys after x-ray and neutron irradiation. *In* "Late Biological Effects of Ionizing Radiation," Vol. 2, pp. 165–179. IAEA, Vienna.

Vogelstein, B., Fearon, E. R., Hamilton, S. R., Kern, S. E., Preisinger, A. C., Leppert, M., Nakamura, Y., White, R., Smits, A. M., and Bos, J. L. (1988). Genetic alteration during colorectal tumor development. *N. Engl. J. Med.* **319**, 525–532.

Wallach, J. D., and Boever, W. J. (1983). "Diseases of Exotic Animals: Medical and Surgical Management." Saunders, Philadelphia.

Watkins, D. I., Hodi, F. S., and Letvin, N. L. (1988). A primate species with limited major histocompatibility complex class I polymorphism. *Proc. Natl. Acad. Sci. U.S.A.* **85**, 7714–7718.

Watkins, P. E., and Warren, B. F. (1992). Sertoli cell tumor in the cotton-top tamarin. *J. Pathol.* **167**, 130A.

Weller, R. E. (1982). Paraneoplastic disorders in companion animals. *Compend. Contin. Educ. Pract. Vet.* **4**, 423–428.

Weller, R. E. (1985). Paraneoplastic disorders in dogs with hematopoietic tumors. *Vet. Clin. North Am.: Small Anim. Pract.* **15**, 805–816.

Weller, R. E. (1988). Paraneoplastic syndromes. *In* "Handbook of Small Animal Practice" (R. V. Morgan, ed.), pp. 819–827. Churchill-Livingstone, New York.

Weller, R. E., Wierman, E. L., Malaga, C. A., and LeMieux, T. P. (1991). Battelle primate facility. *J. Med. Primatol.* **20**, 133–137.

Wellman, M. L. (1990). The cytologic diagnosis of neoplasia. *Vet. Clin. North Am.: Small Anim. Pract.* **20**, 919–938.

Wissman, M., and Parsons, B. (1992). Surgical removal of a lipoma-like mass in a lemur (*Lemur fulvus fulvus*). *J. Small Exotic Anim. Med.* **2**, 8–12.

Witt, C. J., Bacmeister, C. X., and Bunton, T. E. (1989). A tubulopapillary renal carcinoma and a renal calculus in a baboon. *Lab. Anim. Sci.* **39**, 443–445.

Wohlsein, P., Petzold, D. R., and Brandt, H.-P. (1996). Hepatocellular carcinoma in a lemur (*Varecia variegata rubra x variegata*): A case report. *Dtsch. Tieraerztl. Wochensch.* **103**, 180–183.

Yanai, T., Teranishi, M., Manabe, S., Takaoka, M., Yamoto, T., Matsunuma, N., and Goto, N. (1992). Astrocytoma in a cynomolgus monkey (*Macaca fascicularis*). *Vet. Pathol.* **29**, 569–571.

Yanai, T., Hosoi, M., Masegi, T., Ueda, K., Iwasaki, T., Kimura, N., Katou, A., and Kotera, S. (1994). Adenocarcinoma of the rectum in a capped langur (*Presbytis pileata*). *J. Med. Primatol.* **23**, 410–412.

Yanai, T., Masegi, T., Tomita, A., Kudo, T., Yamazoe, K., Iwasaki, T., Kimura, N., Katou, A., Kotera, S., and Ueda, K. (1995a). Odontoameloblastoma in a Japanese monkey (*Macaca fuscata*). *Vet. Pathol.* **32**, 57–59.

Yanai, T., Masegi, T., Hosoi, M., Iwasaki, T., Yamazoe, K., Ueda, K., and Chiba, T. (1995b). Immunohistochemical and morphologic features of a cecal adenocarcinoma in a white-handed gibbon. *Vet. Pathol.* **32**, 60–63.

Yanai, T., Wakabayashi, S., Masegi, T., Iwasaki, T., Yamazoe, K., Ishikawa, K., and Ueda, K. (1995c). Basal cell tumor in a Japanese macaque (*Macaca fuscata*). *Vet. Pathol.* **32**, 318–320.

Yasuda, H., Taniguchi, T., and Shigeta, Y. (1990). Peripheral neuropathy associated with osteosarcoma in a Japanese monkey. *Jikken Dobutsu* **39**, 285–289.

Yeatman, T. J., and Nicolson, G. L. (1993). Molecular basis of tumor progression: Mechanisms of organ-specific tumor metastasis. *Semin. Surg, Oncol.* **9**, 256–263.

Zhang, H.-X., Zhang, H.-L., Zhu, D.-M., Zhao, X.-B., and Hou, B.-H. (1992). Esophageal cancer in rhesus monkeys from the Taihang mountain area: A preliminary report. *Chin. J. Oncol.* **14**, 411–413.

Chapter 5

Environmental Hazards

Ann S. Line

I. INTRODUCTION

Captive primates live in microenvironments defined by their caging or housing systems, which are further influenced by additional factors or elements of the larger macroenvironment. Environmental factors encompass all the circumstances and conditions that act on an individual or group of animals to determine its form and survival. From the perspective of the research animal facility as an extension of the research laboratory, environmental factors represent variables that may influence the reliability of research data. From a clinical perspective, nearly every element encountered in the environment has the potential to cause injury. Environmental surveillance is necessary for risk assessment. Understanding the age-related and species-specific behaviors of primates is especially important in defining a safe and healthy environment. Specific knowledge of primate anatomy and physiology helps ensure appropriate medical intervention in the event of environmental injury.

II. HAZARDS ASSOCIATED WITH CAGE DESIGN OR CONDITION

A. General Considerations

All materials planned for use in new construction or renovation should be evaluated for animal exposure risks as structures housing primates will be explored and may be reconfigured by the inhabitants. Nonhuman primates often use oral exploration and may mouth or ingest nonfood items. In outdoor enclosures or enclosures with indoor plantings, available plant materials should be surveyed for toxicity. Routine maintenance should not be overlooked, as the risk of ingestion may vary with the integrity of contact surfaces.

B. Examples of Toxicity Associated with Ingestion or Contact

A commonly cited example of toxin exposure in captive primates involves the inadvertent poisonings that occurred at primate centers across the United States in the 1970s. Before their manufacture was banned due to public health concerns, various polyhalogenated, polycyclic aromatic hydrocarbon compounds (PHPAHs) were used in the electrical utility industry and as extenders for paints and insecticides. Although a source of the toxicant was not found during investigations of spontaneous poisonings at the Oregon Regional Primate Research Center, a concrete sealant was implicated. Later analysis of stored tissues confirmed the presence of polychlorinated biphenyls. In the rhesus macaque model, poisonings with PHPAHs can be fatal. Signs of toxicity to this class of compounds include characteristic epidermal and gastric mucosal metaplasias, severe wasting, and bone marrow supression (McNulty, 1993). Fortunately, none of these compounds, including polybrominated biphenyls, have been incorporated into commercial products in the United States for over a decade. Therefore, PHPAH toxicities in captive primates are unlikely to be contemporary concerns.

A second example of inadvertent poisonings describes conditions of exposure in which captive primates may play a more active role. Primates with access to surfaces coated with leaded paint, which was still in use prior to 1950, showed a predilection for oral ingestion similar to that seen in young children. The incidence of lead poisoning or plumbism in one large zoo reportedly dropped from an estimated 10% (with a mortality near 40%) to zero following the removal of leaded paint from the cages (Zook, 1993). Chronic poisoning by inorganic lead results in aberrant hemoglobin synthesis and a microcytic, hypochromic anemia. Signs of acute neurologic dysfunction can include apparent blindness and seizures. Companion animals exposed to toxic lead levels may show gastrointestinal signs and possible hysteria, aggression, nervousness, vocalizing, tremors, seizures, blindness, and dementia (Meric, 1992). For pet animals, accessible lead-containing products include linoleum, rug padding, old lead-based paints, putty, caulking, or roofing materials, used motor oil, golf balls, fishing sinkers, pellets, and lead shot. It is hoped that captive primates would rarely have access to these materials. The toxic dose of lead required to experimentally poison primates varies with the source, route, diet, age, and species. Younger animals absorb a higher fraction of ingested lead than adults and are at greater risk for poisoning. However, cumulative lead ingestion in adult rhesus monkeys has resulted in an acute moribund state marked by anemia, nephropathy, or sudden death. A history of exposure, onset of characteristic signs, complete blood count changes, and an elevated blood lead level may aid in diagnosis. Lead exposure in pregnancy causes placental lesions, abortion, or congenital encephalopathy in neonates. Lead poisoning of young primates produces permanent cognitive deficits.

Clearly, inadvertent exposure to hazardous substances can have serious health implications for research primate populations. In certain circumstances, both animal exposure and public health issues could be relevant. Additional information on hazardous materials toxicology can be found in the current veterinary and medical literature (Sullivan and Krieger, 1992).

C. Surveillance for Physical Hazards

Health surveillance should be especially vigilant during the introduction of animals to a new facility. Cages need to be secure in order to prevent escape or injury. This is particularly true where juvenile primates are concerned. Young primates are generally more active and manipulative than adults, and are strong enough to force their way into small openings or to climb seemingly insurmountable walls. In one facility, juvenile long-tailed macaques used the heads of sheet metal screws on the wall of a corral as handholds to climb out of the enclosure. An extra strip of metal, fastened with rivets, was installed over the screws and solved the problem. Cages should be free of sharp edges that could cause puncture wounds or lacerations. It is also important to regularly inspect doors, chutes, perches, and other parts of the cage to make sure there are no defects caused by the primates themselves. The size of the opening between bars should be small enough to prevent the occupants from pushing an arm between the bars. Juvenile monkeys can entrap an arm at the elbow while attempting to reach food crumbs in the cage pan. Developing limb edema makes it impossible for the animal to pull its arm back into the cage. Depending on the type of housing, entrapment could result in exposure and/or water deprivation. Rescue requires sedation, followed by lubrication and extraction or, in some cases, cutting the cage to free the limb.

D. Environmental Enrichment Devices

Environmental enrichment devices may also present unforeseen hazards. Decisions concerning material selection and design should consider the species of primate, age of individuals, and observed behaviors. Short lengths of almond wood branches placed in the cages of adult rhesus macaques at the California Primate Research Center were chewed and manipulated, but no adverse effects were associated with this exposure to a natural substrate (Line *et al.,* 1991). Other materials may be less benign. Fragments of materials such as polypropylene rope may become gastrointestinal foreign bodies if unbraided and ingested. Tires may be chewed to expose fine wires that can produce gastrointestinal perforation and peritonitis if ingested (Etheridge and O'Malley, 1996). Sleeves of flexible polyvinyl chloride (PVC) tubing are recommended to sheath hanging chains and to prevent the snagging risk of open links. When feasible, the use of shorter chains or ropes may reduce the risk of entanglement.

Hanging ropes, chains, or cables could potentially present a risk of strangulation or near-hanging injury. With cervical entrapment and compression, unconsciousness can occur within 15 sec, with brain cell death ensuing within 4–5 min. With immediate rescue, response to initial resuscitation efforts and an early return of spontaneous respirations after transport to an emergency department have been described as positive prognostic indicators in children with similar injuries. Children have survived near-hanging injuries with good neurologic outcome despite presentation with an initial pH of less than 7.2, apnea or agonal respiratory patterns, and pulmonary compromise requiring mechanical ventilation (Digeronimo and Mayes, 1994). Although cervical dislocations and vertebral fractures are reportedly rare in children with these injuries, damage to the thyroid cartilage or hyoid bone can occur. These children are considered at high risk to develop cerebral edema. Therapeutic measures, including controlled hyperventilation, fluid restriction, and other supportive measures to limit intracranial pressure, are recommended. In cases of near-hanging injury in animals, airway or cerebral edema, seizures, respiratory compromise, and pulmonary infiltrates consistent with aspiration pneumonia or adult respiratory distress syndrome should be anticipated. These animals may need ventilatory support.

E. Shelters within Outdoor Enclosures

The extent to which some health problems of captive primates can be directly attributed to the cage environment should be an ongoing area of concern. For outdoor cages in areas subject to inclement weather, several precautions regarding shelter should be kept in mind. Adequate space within sheltered areas of the cage must be provided for all group members to access the shelters. Multiple shelter locations are appropriate as dominant group members sometimes exclude subordinates from a shelter. If radiant lamps are used to provide supplemental heat, the bulbs must be positioned and shielded to ensure that the animals cannot sit too close. Full-thickness skin burns may result if animals sit stationary in front of the lamps for hours. In cold ambient temperatures, the conductivity of the material used for flooring (as in a stainless steel cage) or for perches will influence heat loss of the animal in contact with it.

III. COLD-RELATED INJURIES

A. Hypothermia

Accidental hypothermia describes an unintentional decline in the core body temperature following environmental exposure as heat dissipation exceeds heat production. The potential for injury in a cold environment depends on the ambient temperature and the additional convection losses as cool air carries away body heat (the wind chill factor), as well as any conductive losses if the animal is wet (water chill). As core temperature falls, the compensatory physiologic responses to minimize heat loss through radiation, conduction, convection, respiration, and evaporation begin to fail. Hypothermia is a predictable complication of prolonged exposure to severe cold and windy conditions. However, hypothermia can also develop at temperatures well above freezing. Various risk factors contribute to decreased thermostability. Small size, age extremes, insufficient fuel (malnutrition or hypoglycemia), trauma, sepsis and other disease states, and inactivity or immobility are predisposing factors that may be encountered in primate populations. Lack of adaptation to cold conditions must also be considered. In humans, the clinical manifestations of these changes show substantial individual variability. Nonhuman primates show similar physiologic variance. For instance, skin temperatures in cynomolgus macaques subjected to cold reportedly show a greater decline and a slower rate of rewarming than those of Japanese, rhesus, stump-tail, or Formosan macaques (Okada *et al.,* 1975).

The physiologic effects of profound hypothermia have been studied in a baboon model of central nervous system (CNS) cooling as a surgical adjunct (McCormick *et al.,* 1994). Brain temperatures lagged behind core body temperatures measured with an esophageal thermometer during cooling and rewarming. Although cerebral oxygen extraction dropped progressively at brain temperatures below 20° C (68° F), measurable cerebral oxygen extraction continued at 2° C (35.6° F). However, at any given brain temperature, oxygen consumption was considerably greater during rewarming than cooling. Accelerated cerebral oxygen metabolism during rewarming may reflect the process of reestablishing the energy-dependent ionic gradients, across cellular and organelle membranes in the neuronal and glial cells, which are essential for a return to normal function. Cerebral lactate production occurred predominately during the rewarming phase, reflecting anaerobic metabolism resulting from an oxygen availability consumption mismatch. Damage to plasma proteins and formed blood elements was expected with cooling to less than 15° C (59° F) and produced a clinically obvious coagulopathy on rewarming despite administration of stored whole blood collected during cooling.

Vasoconstriction, ventilation–perfusion mismatch, and increased blood viscosity all contribute to poor tissue oxygenation. Below 32° C (89.6° F), the heart is more susceptible to arrhythmias and ventricular fibrillation resulting from hypoxia, hypovolemia, and mechanical jostling (Besson, 1996). Human patients with temperatures less than 26.7° C (80° F) usually present unconscious, with bradycardia, hypotension, slow and shallow respiration, and miotic pupils. Coma, areflexia, and lack of pupillary response ensue as temperatures fall below 25° C (77° F). During studies employing radio frequency energy for rewarming, anesthetized rhesus monkeys were cooled to the point of cardiovascular collapse (at 20° C; 68° F) but were successfully resuscitated (Olsen, 1987, 1988). The response to medications declines with falling core temperature; liver function is impaired and protein binding increased. Drug therapy and electric cardioversion may be futile until the core temperature reaches the range of 28° C (82.4° F) (Lee-Paritz and Pavletic, 1992) to above 30° C (>86° F) (Besson, 1996). Human medical protocols suggest that resuscitation continue and pronouncement of death be delayed until resuscitation fails following rewarming to a core temperature of 36° C (96.8° F) (Besson, 1996; Petersdorf, 1994).

Hypothermic humans and animals are predisposed to coagulopathies, which may occur despite deceptively normal prothrombin time (PT) and partial thromboplastin time (PTT), if the tests are run at 37° C. Cold also directly inhibits the enzymatic reactions of the coagulation cascade (Danzl and Pozos, 1994a). Platelet function is impaired as the production of thromboxane B_2 by platelets is temperature dependent. Cold-induced thrombocytopenia may result from direct bone marrow suppression and hepatosplenic sequestration. Hypercoagulability also occurs and could result in thromboembolism.

Treatment priorities include oxygenation, fluid resuscitation, gentle handling, and thermal stabilization (Danzl and Pozos, 1994b). Fluids for intravenous administration may be warmed and delivered at 38° C (100.4° F), as hemolysis may occur when blood is subjected to temperatures above 40° C (104° F) (McCullough, 1995). Cardiac monitoring and measurement of blood gases and serum electrolytes will help direct therapy. Blood pressure monitoring will detect persistent hypotension or pressure declines resulting in oliguria. A pediatric radiant warmer unit makes an ideal workstation. The heat output of the overhead lamp can be manually adjusted as needed or operated on a servomechanism with the temperature of the animal recorded by skin probe. Air- or water-circulating heating pads are helpful for surface rewarming in mild to moderate hypothermia. However, surface-only warming may carry the risk of peripheral vasodilation and potential vascular collapse (Haskins, 1995). Active core warming (via gastric, peritoneal, or thoracic lavage) is indicated for animals with rectal temperatures below 30° C (86° F) or for those showing severe physiologic dis-

equilibrium. Core rewarming preferentially warms the internal organs, including the heart, which decreases myocardial irritability and helps restore normal cardiac function. Positive outcomes have been reported following the core rewarming of companion animals with gastric gavage of saline warmed to 40–45° C (104–108° F) (Haskins, 1995). In the author's experience, adverse cardiac effects associated with stimulation during gastric lavage have not proved to be a problem in macaques treated with this technique, provided tube placement is gentle. Peritoneal dialysis (with fluids warmed to 45° C) (108° F) has been recommended for companion animals but has not been used by this author. Finally, although hemodialysis machines are not currently available to most primate clinicians, portable hemodialysis units may find future applications in veterinary medicine. Hemodialysis provides greater heat delivery than peritoneal lavage and avoids arrhythmias seen in human patients during pleural lavage (Murray and Fellner, 1994; Hernandez et al., 1993).

Rapid acceleration of the rate of rewarming alone does not appear to improve the survival of human patients with spontaneously perfusing cardiac rhythms (Danzl and Pozos, 1994a). Many acutely hypothermic primates have been successfully resuscitated to recover with apparently normal mental and motor function. Varying degrees of cognitive impairment and a persistent acral neuropathy have been reported in human patients following extreme hypothermia (Antretter et al., 1994).

B. Frostbite

Skin injury due to cold exposure follows local cooling of the skin due to vasoconstriction. Uninterrupted cooling progresses to freezing of tissues. In nonhuman primates, the ears, digits, and tail are particularly susceptible. It is important to remember that water conducts heat away from the body 25 times faster than still air (Grant et al., 1994b). Therefore, exposure to standing water, slush, or snow can quickly exacerbate cold injury.

Cold injury may be recognized in primates species by painful reactions similar to the tingling and burning sensations described by human patients during rewarming following frostbite or incipient frostbite (frostnip). Thirty of 43 cynomolgus monkeys in a group reportedly suffered frostbite during 25 min outside on a cold and snowy day (Laber-Laird et al., 1988). Signs of acute discomfort of their distal extremities (with rubbing and self-biting) were observed upon returning indoors. Frostbite lesions include edema, blistering of the skin, and focal necrosis. Injuries may be inapparent until the damaged tissue sloughs several days later. In the most severe cases, gangrene results in loss of the affected body part.

Treatment priorities include transfer of the animal to a warm environment and warming of the affected area (Grant et al., 1994b; Haskins, 1995). Warm water submersion should be performed with care. Warming following thaw can cause further damage. Areas of frostbitten tissue should be protected from any friction or compression, as massage of tissues containing ice crystals could exacerbate the injury. Opioid analgesia may be required to control pain during rewarming. Cage rest and soft protective bandages also help minimize discomfort and enhance healing.

IV. HEAT-RELATED INJURIES

A. Hyperthermia

Disorders causing elevated temperature and thermoregulatory failure result in hyperthermia when heat production (or retention) exceeds heat dissipation. Exertional hyperthermia in animals or humans can be a consequence of intense exercise on a hot day, especially if the temperature exceeds 28° C (82.4° F) (Walker and Vance, 1996). This was demonstrated in a male Japanese macaque when his summer escape from an outdoor corral resulted in exertional hyperthermia. When recaptured after a brief chase, he was weak and disoriented, had a rectal temperature above 40° C (104° F), and had myoglobinuria. Human patients showing heat stroke present with elevated core temperatures, hyperventilation, hypotension, tachycardia, and altered consciousness. Pulmonary edema, disseminated intravascular coagulation (DIC), and cardiovascular abnormalities are common after initial cooling and stabilization. Acute renal failure, caused by a combination of direct thermal injury, hypotension, shock from cardiovascular collapse, and rhabdomyolysis, occurs in up to 35% of human patients with heat stroke (Ayres and Keenan, 1995). Terminal events include shock, myocardial ischemia, cardiac arrhythmias, and neurologic dysfunction. Splanchnic ischemia may impair the gut mucosal barrier, rendering the patient susceptible to endotoxemia and ultimately multiple organ failure (Zuckerman *et al.,* 1994).

Treatment priorities include oxygenation, rapid cooling, intravenous hydration with room temperature fluids, correction of electrolyte and acid–base abnormalities, and careful cardiovascular monitoring. Heat dissipates by four mechanisms: conduction, radiation, convection (with vasodilation), or evaporation. Evaporative heat loss is the most efficient, producing cooling rates that are two to three times as rapid as those produced by immersion in ice water, which relies on conduction (Slovis, 1994). Sponging the animal with tepid water and then using electric fans or hand-held hair dryers (set on cool) is preferable to immersion and allows continuous close monitoring. Centrally active antipyretic agents are effective in fever but not hyperthermia (Simon, 1993). Ice packs can be applied along the trunk as long as shivering, generating additional heat from muscle, is not induced. Alcohol sponge baths are no longer recommended due to the risk of acute alcohol intoxication (Salzberg, 1994). Because core temperature continues to decline after surface cooling ceases, active cooling should continue only until the temperature reaches 39–39.4° C (102.2–103° F). Intraperitoneal, gastric, or colonic irrigation with cool saline may be considered in severe cases (Haskins, 1995; Weiss, 1993; Zuckerman *et al.,* 1994).

Dehydration attenuates the expected increase in skin blood flow during environmental heating. At core temperatures of 39.5–39.8° C (103.1–103.6° F), hindlimb blood flow in chronically instrumented baboons was unaffected by induced hyperosmolality but decreased in response to dehydration produced by 65–69 hr of water deprivation and by furosemide treatment, resulting in an extracellular fluid volume deficit (Proppe, 1990; Ryan and Proppe, 1990a,b).

Depending on the species of primate, physiologic compensatory mechanisms may act to a greater or lesser degree to maintain plasma volume during thermal dehydration. Hamadryas baboons lost 10% of their body mass, 12.5% of their total body water space, but only 4% of their plasma volume after 2 days when experimentally water deprived at high ambient temperature. Hematocrit, hemoglobin concentration, blood viscosity, and blood pressure were unchanged in the face of thermal dehydration, although total protein and albumin levels and colloid osmotic pressure were higher than in hydrated baboons (Zurovsky *et al.,* 1984). Although weight loss would be evident, primates highly adapted to desert environments may show few changes on screening hematology.

Although the neurologic effects rarely produce lasting harm in human cases of hyperthermia, persistent peripheral neuropathies are possible sequelae. Also, there may be an association between hyperthermia during pregnancy and fetal malformations or spontaneous abortions (Ayres and Keenan, 1995). Experimental induction of elevated maternal core temperatures during organogenesis in *Macaca radiata* and *Callithrix jacchus* resulted in developmental abnormalities and intrauterine death (Hendrickx and Binkerd, 1983).

B. Thermal Burns

Fortunately, catastrophic facility fires are uncommon occurrences. However, heat lamp and heating pad burns occasionally occur in veterinary medical centers despite careful precautions. Other circumstances may inadvertently facilitate chemical or thermal injuries. For instance, a predisposition to burns has been noted in human surgical preparation with mechanical abrasion of the skin from scrubbing and from pooling of a prep agent under a torso or tourniquet. Blister formation, skin sloughing, and eschar development have been reported in human neonates when isopropyl alcohol pledgets were substituted for conducting paste beneath limb electrodes (Ayres and Keenan, 1995).

Burns can be classified by severity based on degree, percentage of the body square area *(BSA)*, region involved, and mechanism of injury. The wound area is measured and its area calculated and divided by the total body surface area. Alternatively, the area of the burn can be estimated by comparison to the palmar surface of the hand. Minor burns involve less than 15% *BAS*. Moderate burns involve 15–25% BSA. Major burns involve 25% *BSA* with functionally significant injury to hands, feet, face, perineum, electrical, inhalation, or other concurrent injury or preexisting medical conditions. Any burns involving infants or geriatric animals should be considered critical injuries.

Initial management is based on burn severity. Priority is given to resuscitation (airway/breathing/circulation), evaluation for inhalation injury, protection of burns from contamination, initial fluid resuscitation, possible tetanus prophylaxis, and adequate analgesia. Cooling within 30 min of injury may limit tissue damage and provide some analgesia. Minor first-degree (superficial, partial thickness) and second-degree burns (partial thickness with blisters) can be treated with applications of gauze soaked in cold sterile saline (Hummel *et al.,* 1991). More extensive (full-thickness, third-degree) burns may be associated with general hypothermia, which would be a contraindication for cool applications. With severe thermal injury, inflammatory mediators are released that compromise the fatty acid portion of the cell membrane, disrupting its function and causing it to leak fluid and proteins, resulting in edema. Fluid balance may be tenuous and central venous pressure monitoring may be indicated. Intravenous lactated Ringer's solution should be given to maintain a urine output of at least 1 ml/kg/hr. Serum protein, albumin, and osmolality measurements will be necessary for assessing the need for colloid therapy (Rudloff and Kirby, 1994; Grant *et al.,* 1994a).

Use of prophylactic antibiotics has not been shown to prevent infection or the development of cellulitis in human burn patients. References suggest that fluoroquinolones may be useful in the management of burn sepsis in veterinary patients (Bistner and Ford, 1995). At some burn centers, ibuprofen is utilized for analgesia and for helping suppress the inflammatory response. Narcotic agonists and agonist–antagonists may be necessary for adequate pain control. Sterile saline or a dilute chlorhexidine solution may be used for initial irrigation cleansing. Burns can then be coated with a topical burn medication, such as silver sulfadiazine cream (Silvadene, Hoechst Marion Roussel, Inc. Kansas City, MO), and bandaged with dry sterile dressings. Alternatively, the burn area can be covered with treated gauze (xeroform, Sherwood Medical St. Louis, MO) or a semisynthetic occlusive dressing before bandaging. After 24 hr the dressing may be removed by soaking in cool water, if necessary, and the wound assessed for further debridement. Saline cleansing should precede daily bandage replacement. Aloe vera preparations applied topically have been reported to assist in maintaining a patent dermal vasculature in partial thickness burns through an antiprostaglandin and antithromboxane effect (Bistner and Ford, 1995). Some burn wounds are best treated by excision with primary closure. More extensive burns will necessitate the use of autografts, zenografts, or other synthetic materials (Argenta and Morykwas, 1996; Line *et al.,* 1996; Morykwas, 1994). Early and adequate nutritional support is essential to support healing and recovery.

C. Electrical Burns

1. Low Voltage Injury

Episodes of electric shock are associated with a wide spectrum of injury. At low voltages (less than 100 V) the low frequency alternating current range, such as that used in household or commercial applications, is three times more dangerous than direct current (Dimick, 1994). Brief exposure to low intensity current may produce only mind aversive stimulation or cause instantaneous sudden death resulting from ventricular fibrillation or ventricular standstill, depending on the path of the current. Exposure to electric shock may occur because of defective equipment. Unexpected cage escape might also allow a primate to contact an unprotected outlet or gain access to wiring. When in use, extension cords must always be out of reach of caged primates. Signs of electric shock can include acute onset of dyspnea, with moist rales, due to a centroneurogenically mediated increase in peripheral vascular resistance resulting in pulmonary edema. Localized burns may occur on limbs or lips and tongue. Evolution of tissue injury and vascular necrosis are usually complete within 7–10 days.

Treatment priorities include oxygenation, treatment of pulmonary edema with diuretic administration and bronchodilator therapy, and local wound care. Following significant current exposure, multisystem involvement is common. The full extent of injury may not be appreciated initially. Electrical shock during pregnancy may be harmful because the amnionic fluid effectively conducts current to the fetus. Women experience increased risk of spontaneous abortion and fetal demise. Surviving infants have an increased risk of growth retardation and postnatal complications (Fontanarosa, 1996).

2. High Voltage Injury

At high voltages (above 600 V), high frequency alternating or direct currents are equally lethal. Aggressive life support is appropriate based on reports of successful resuscitation in human victims of high voltage electrical injury without permanent neurologic damage after prolonged cessation of vital functions (Dimick, 1994). Blunt trauma and skeletal injury should be ruled out. Fluid therapy may be indicated, especially if fluid losses into damaged tissues result in hypovolemia. Myoglobinuria and acute tubular necrosis from hemochromogen deposition and hypovolemia represent serious complications.

In the primate forelimb, high voltage electrical injury produces characteristic injury in skin, muscles, blood vessels, and nerves (Zelt *et al.,* 1988). Tissue with high fluid and electrolyte content conduct current more readily. Severe tissue damage occurs at regions of decreased cross-sectional areas where highly resistant tissue (such as bone) result in icreased heat production. Vascular damage is prominent, with segmental narrowing and pruning of the large vascular trunks, and nutrient arteries are decreased in the affected areas. Nerve conduction may be permanently interrupted.

D. Lightning Strike

Lightning strike differs from exposure to manmade electricity in that the magnitude of energy is greater (3 to 200 million V), the duration of exposure is shorter, and the current pathway is different. Direct strike of an animal could occur by direct contact should a tree or metal pole become part of a current path. Side flash or splash injury describes direct strike of a tree, light pole, or building which then splashes to affect an adjacent individual or group. Usual triage strategies are reversed in the case of a witnessed lightning strike. Victims who appear dead are treated before conscious survivors. Urgent intervention is necessary for respiratory arrest in order to avoid hypoxic cardiac arrest. Also, because ocular autonomic disturbances may occur after lightning strike, dilated and unresponsive pupils are not assessed as a sign of brain death (Fontanarosa, 1996). First- and second-degree cutaneous burns have occurred in rain-soaked human victims when high temperatures in the lightning current converted skin surface moisture to steam. Immediate neurologic sequelae include loss of consciousness, seizures, and vision loss. The term keraunoparalysis describes a transient flaccid paralysis that usually involves the lower extremities and is common in human victims following lightning strike. Long-term sequelae could include paralysis, paraesthesias, neuralgias, and cognitive dysfunction. In contrast to electrocution, lightning strike is not usually associated with renal involvement.

V. EXPOSURE TO OTHER TOXINS

A. Fire Atmospheres

Exposures to fire atmospheres initiate a complex sequence of pulmonary and pathophysiologic events. Fire can burn the skin and body tissues, heat can alter the regulatory mechanisms of the body, and smoke can damage the eyes and airways.

The volume and composition of inhaled material influence the severity of the pulmonary manifestations of inhalation injury. Decreased alveolar oxygen tension and hypoxia may result from a lowered concentration of oxygen as it is consumed during combustion. High concentrations of carbon dioxide can produce severe acidosis. Exposure to carbon monoxide (CO), as it too is released as a basic by-product of combustion, results in the formation of carboxyhemoglobin with the displacement of oxygen from hemoglobin. Building materials and furnishings contain plastics, rubber, and other synthetics that release toxic fumes when they become overheated or burn. Hydrogen cyanide gas can be liberated during a fire by pyrolysis of wool, silk, nylons, polyurethanes, and polyacrylonitriles. Long-tailed macaques became rapidly incapacitated when exposed in the laboratory to atmospheres containing either mixed pyrolysis products of polyacrylonitrile or low levels of hydrogen cyanide gas. Loss of consciousness occurred in 1–5 min. Termination

of gas exposure was followed by rapid recovery (Purser *et al.,* 1984). Incomplete products of combustion can enter the bronchi and bronchioles and combine with mucus to produce toxic acids and alkalis. Hot vapors can damage the upper airways to the level of the larynx, with the risk of laryngeal edema and airway obstruction. The complex geometry of the nasal vestibule and the distribution of nasal lesions following inhalation exposure have been studied in the rhesus monkey using acrylic molds of the nasal airways (Morgan *et al.,* 1991).

Smaller primates would be expected to manifest earlier symptoms of increased ambient carbon monoxide because they have increased metabolic demand as do human infants and pets. The percentage of carboxyhemoglobin (HbCO) in the blood depends on the amount of carbon monoxide in the inspired air and the time length of exposure. Carboxyhemoglobin concentrations of 40–80% in the blood result in cyanosis, nausea, collapse, respiratory failure, and death (Clancy and Litovitz, 1995). Blood carboxyhemoglobin levels of zero were recorded in controls and 40–48% in anesthetized baboons after induction of a moderate smoke injury. Carboxyhemoglobin levels had dropped to 10 or less after 1 hr of spontaneous respiration in 100% oxygen (Cioffi et al., 1993). This represents the optimal therapeutic approach, as the half-life of HbCO is 4 hr in room air and 30 min in 100% oxygen. Following carbon monoxide exposure, mild to moderate acidosis should not be aggressively treated because hydrogen ions shift the oxygen dissociation curve to the right, enhancing oxygen delivery to the tissues. A conscious animal without severe respiratory difficulty can be treated with high flow oxygen by mask or placed in an oxygen cage with humidified oxygen. Supplemental oxygen should continue until HbCO levels fall below 10%. With more severe signs, anesthesia, tracheal intubation, and mechanical ventilatory assistance will be necessary. Fluid therapy will assist in metabolism and clearance of some toxins, such as cyanide. Normal arterial blood gas values do not rule out the possibility of CO toxicity. Oxygen saturation determined by pulse oximetry may be overestimated by high HbCO concentrations (Ayres and Keenan, 1995).

Heat damage may affect the mucus membranes of the upper respiratory tract, including the larynx, leading to laryngeal edema within several hours. Severe mucosal damage is suggested by evidence of singed facial hair or oral lesions. Progressive edema or upper airway compromise may necessitate endrotracheal or tracheostomy tube placement and ventilator assistance. Adult baboons subjected to moderate smoke injury under controlled conditions were ventilated for 7 days with either conventional volume ventilation or modes of high-frequency ventilation (Cioffi et al., 1993). Although ventilatory support was tailored to the same physiologic end points and hemodynamics did not vary, the end points were achieved only with conventional volume ventilation (CON) and a high-frequency flow interruption (HFFI) mode. In this study, animals treated with the high-frequency mode had significantly less parenchymal damage and evidence of barotrauma than those treated with CON. Reduced mortality associated with prophylactic use of HFFI has been reported in human patients with bronchoscopically diagnosed inhalation injury requiring ventilatory support. Management strategies for smoke inhalation injury are the subject of ongoing research efforts.

Severe lung changes (edema, atelectasis, pleural effusion, and pneumonia) may not develop until 16–24 hr following an inhalation insult. The injured airway may be colonized by bacteria, especially if an endrotracheal tube is present. This necessitates strict aseptic technique during suctioning and tube care. Culture specimens should provide the basis for antimicrobial therapy. Prophylactic antibiotics are not routinely recommended in human or companion animal cases, as use will only lead to selection and overgrowth of resistant organisms. It has also been well demonstrated that the early use of high-dose corticosteroids in the presence of a body burn increases rather than decreases the morbidity and mortality associated with smoke inhalation (Robinson *et al.,* 1982). Neurologic dysfunction that persists after resuscitation, treatment of hypovolemia, and reversal of CO toxicity may reflect the effects of the initial hypoxic insult.

B. Insect Bites and Stings

Insect and arachnid hypersensitivity syndromes have been described in both humans and animals (Griffin, 1993). Severe systemic reactions to stinging insects are known to occur in dogs and cats (Cowell *et al.,* 1991; Neuman *et al.,* 1983). Unless the stinging episode is observed, local reactions with significant swelling may be difficult to differentiate from cellulitis, which is uncommon after an insect sting. Toxic reactions could follow many simultaneous stings. Progression of signs with edema of the upper airways, circulatory collapse with shock and hypotension, and bronchospasm may be life threatening.

The two major subgroups of insects of the order Hymenoptera that sting are the vespids (including yellow jacket, hornet, and wasp) and apids (including the honeybee and bumblebee). Stings from yellow jackets are common in most parts of the United States, reflecting exposure that occurs because these insects nest in the ground and are disturbed by lawn mowing and other outdoor activities. Honeybees and bumblebees are generally docile and sting only when provoked. When the honeybee stings, the multiple barbs on the stinger imbed in tissue and death of the insect follows detachment of the stinging apparatus. Few barbs are present on the stingers of vespids, so multiple stings can be inflicted.

The venom of Africanized honeybees (or killer bees), currently found in Texas, Arizona, and California, is no more allergic or toxic than that of the European honeybee found throughout the United States. However, killer bees are more aggressive and massive stinging incidents have led to human death from venom toxicity (Reisman, 1994).

At least 18 allergens and 55 different enzymes have been identified in whole bee venom. Primary allergens are phospho-

lipase A_2, acid phosphatase, hyaluronidase, melitten, and an unidentified allergen (Ag-1). Other venom components include histamine, dopamine, noradrenaline, amino acids, and volatile substances (Fowler, 1993).

The fire ant, *Solenopsis invicta,* is a nonwinged hymenopteran currently found in the southeast and south central United States, especially along the Gulf coast. The fire ant is characterized by a tendency to swarm if provoked and to attack in great numbers. It too inflicts multiple stings, but will bite and hold on with its jaws as it repositions its abdominal stinger in a circular sweep. On human and nonhuman primate skin, a sterile pustule develops at the site of the sting within 6–24 hr (Saluzzo, 1996; R. P. Bohm, Jr., personal communication, 1996).

Other than analgesics and possibly cold compresses if applied early, little treatment is necessary for uncomplicated local reactions. Mild allergic responses will usually resolve in 1–6 hr without treatment. Antihistamines (such as diphenhydramine at 1 mg/kg IM) may help alleviate urticaria and itching. Treatment of toxic reactions or anaphylaxis includes administration of epinephrine in a 1:1000 dilution (1 mg/ml) at a dose of 0.01 mg/kg IM or SQ (to a maximum dose of 0.2 to 0.5 ml) along with emergency life support efforts. Animals surviving the first 5 min of an anaphylactic reaction have a good prognosis (Thompson, 1995).

Because insect stings may go unnoticed, especially in primates housed outdoors, little information is available concerning the incidence of unusual adverse reactions following insect venom exposure in nonhuman primate species. In humans, sequelae or reactions occurring in a temporal relation to insect stings have been reported, including vasculitis, nephrosis, neuritis, encephalitis, and serum sickness. The onset may be within several days to several weeks following the stinging episode and signs may persist for some time (Reisman, 1994).

C. Spider Bites

At least 60 species of spiders in the United States have been associated with medically significant bites in humans. Venomous spiders are found worldwide, and the clinical signs following bite exposure are reported to be highly variable. Admittedly, diagnosis of a spider bite would be difficult without direct observation of a spider–animal interaction. Some knowledge of bite reactions is warranted, however, considering that spiders may be transported from one area or country to another in packing containers, upholstered furniture, or produce. In exceptional circumstances, captive animals could conceivably receive nonnative spider bites (Fowler, 1993).

The two most important species of venomous spiders in the United States are widow spiders (*Latrodectus* spp.) and recluse spiders (*Loxosceles* spp.). Drop for drop, venom of the common black widow spider of the southern United States has been estimated to be 15 times more toxic than rattlesnake venom. A potent neurotoxin causes the release of neurotransmitters, such as noradrenaline and acetylcholine, with progression to paralysis. Animal exposure to widow spiders may occur readily because they inhabit fields, soil crevices, and vegetation. Bites to dogs are fairly frequent, and fatalities in both dogs and cats have been reported. In dogs, envenomation results in initial hyperesthesia, hypertension, muscle fasciculations, and intense excitability. Abdominal muscle rigidity (without tenderness) has been described, as have tonic–clonic convulsions. Death can follow in hours or within several days. Domestic cats, which are extremely sensitive to the toxin, show severe paralytic signs early, along with salivation, diarrhea, and vomiting. Equine origin antivenom is available (Lyovac, Merck & Co, Inc. West Point, PA); pretreatment with antihistamines is recommended. In the absence of antivenom, cardiac monitoring during a slow intravenous infusion of 10% calcium gluconate has been recommended (Bistner and Ford, 1995; Nicholson, 1995).

Recluse spiders inhabit the southern United States, from Texas to Florida, and the midwest. They are shy and nocturnal, frequently found in undisturbed storage areas and around rubbish. The bite is reportedly painless. In dogs and cats, systemic signs rarely reported include hemolysis, thrombocytopenia, fever, weakness, joint pain, and possibly death. Within several days, an indolent ulcer appears at the bite site and may take several months to heal. Treatment is aimed at debridement and general wound care.

The Sydney (Australia) funnel web spider *(Atrax robusta)* is reputed to be the most dangerous Australian spider. It is found in the vicinity of Sydney, Australia. It is included here because the pathophysiology observed in nonhuman primates exposed to the venom closely parallels the responses seen in humans and companion animals. Although the bite of a funnel web spider can kill a human, it is not necessarily lethal to rabbits, guinea pigs, dogs, cats, or nonhuman primates. Humans show muscle fasciculations, hypertension, tachycardia, excessive salivation and lacrimation, respiratory failure, and coma. Signs of envenomation are associated with the release of endogenous catecholamines. The response of anesthetized dogs and cats to intravenous funnel web spider venom includes transient hypertension, tachycardia, and increased cerebrospinal fluid pressure (Fowler, 1993). Studies in primates confirmed similar responses to the administration of atraxin, an isolated neurotoxin from the venom gland, and to whole, milked male funnel web spider venom. Respiratory disturbances (dyspnea and apnea) and profound alterations in the heart rate and blood pressure followed intravenous atraxin doses of 70–80 μg/kg body weight. Skeletal muscle fasciculations, salivation, lacrimation, and elevated body temperatures were also noted at these dosages (Mylecharane *et al.,* 1984). Treatment is directed at supportive and local wound care.

D. Snake Bites

Three groups of venomous snakes inhabit North America (Fowler, 1993; Bistner and Ford, 1995). Of these, the pit vipers (family Crotalidae) are considered the major dangerous species.

The pit viper group includes the water (cottonmouth) moccasin, the copperhead, and numerous species of rattlesnakes. In contrast to the copperhead, which rarely causes serious bites, the water (cottonmouth) moccasin reportedly can cause moderate to severe animal envenomations. The coral snake group (Elapidae) includes the eastern coral snake, Texas coral snake, and the Sonoran coral snake. Coral snakes are reported to pose little risk to animals due to their small size and secretive behavior; however, series of bites to dogs have been reported. The last group contains typical snakes of the family Colubridae. Several species in this group previously considered to be nonpoisonous have been shown to actually envenomate on biting (Bistner and Ford, 1995). Bites from other truly nonpoisonous snakes may appear as superficial scratches with little local reaction and probably often go unnoticed.

Primates exposed to snake venoms show similar pathophysiologic responses to those reported in humans and companion animals. Elapid venoms are less complex than crotalid venoms, which contain a high percentage of nonneurotoxin proteins, including proteolytic enzymes, hemorrhagic toxins, and myotoxins. In dogs and cats, local reactions to a crotalid snake bite with envenomation include erythema and rapidly developing edema. Signs are nonspecific and include nausea, vomiting, diarrhea, abnormal gait, incoordination, and respiratory distress. Dyspnea may develop if swelling obstructs the airway. Hypovolemic shock is common in smaller animals. Hemolytic anemia, thrombocytopenia, and a urinary hemoglobin:myoglobin ratio greater than four may be seen (Bailey and Garland, 1992). Although characteristic clinical pathology has not been reported for primate exposures, a saline wet preparation has been used to identify echinocytosis of red blood cells and support a clinical diagnosis of rattlesnake envenomation in dogs (Wingfield *et al.,* 1994).

The responses of anesthetized beagle dogs and adults rhesus monkeys to intravenous venoms from a variety of poisonous snakes have been compared in the laboratory (Vick, 1994). Venom from snakes of the family Viperidae produced death of the macaques within about 3 hr. Extensive tissue destruction and necrosis at the site of the bite were noted. Clotting factors, fibrinogen, and platelet counts were decreased and moderate hemolysis of the formed elements occurred. Only moderate hemolysis was seen following administration of Elapidae venom, and death followed at an average of 1.7 hr, primarily due to respiratory paralysis. Both viper and elapid venoms produced significant changes in heat rate and blood pressure, with electrocardiographic changes consisting of extrasystoles, arrhythmias, premature ventricular contractions, and depressed S-T segments.

Treatment recommendations for pit viper envenomation in companion animals describe basic supportive care during the collection of baseline laboratory samples. Intravenous or subcutaneous administration of diphenhydramine follows, as a pretreatment for antivenom administration. Antivenom is given only if signs of envenomation occur (Fowler, 1993). If so, intravenous equine origin Crotalidae antivenom (Wyeth Laboratories, Inc. Marietta, PA) is given slowly (to prevent complement reaction to foreign proteins), while monitoring for anaphylaxis. A minimum of one vial is recommended but additional vials may be necessary at intervals of 30 to 60 min, depending on patient size and clinical response. Corticosteroids have not been found beneficial and may enhance toxicity. Local cryotherapy or ice packs are likewise not recommended. Broad-spectrum antibiotics are recommended by various authors; tetanus antitoxin is optional (Bistner and Ford, 1995; Nicholson, 1995).

Cases of coral snake envenomation in the dog show a relative absence of local tissue reaction as the venom lacks significant proteolytic activity (as compared with crotalids). Neurotoxins predominate in coral snake venom. Coral snake bite wounds may be very small and resemble scratches or abrasions. There may be a delayed onset of clinical signs (of several hours). Dogs have shown signs of lethargy, weakness, hemolysis, hemoglobinuria, and rare cardiac dysrhythmias (with ventricular tachycardia most common). Coral snake envenomation is included in the differential diagnosis when an animal within the geographic range (in the southern United States) presents with acute onset quadriplegia, especially when accompanied by hemolysis and hemoglobinuria. Pharyngeal paralysis may be recognized due to difficulty swallowing and predispose to aspiration. Bulbar paralysis with respiratory collapse is the primary cause of death.

The approach to treatment of an elapid bite is similar to that for crotalid bites. An equine origin Elapidae antivenom (Wyeth) is available for the treatment of envenomations, except those from the Arizona (Sonoran) coral snake. Ventilatory assistance is recommended in respiratory failure with hypoxemia ($pO_2 < 60$ mm Hg) and hypercarbia ($pCO_2 > 50$ mm Hg). With ventilatory support the respiratory paralysis usually subsides within 48–72 hr. Broad-spectrum antibiotics may be reserved for those cases with aspiration pneumonia (Kremer and Schaer, 1995; Rowat et al., 1994).

Acute renal failure may follow certain poisonous snake bites in human and nonhuman primates. Circulatory insufficiency, intravascular hemolysis, and myoglobinemia contribute to vascular constriction and renal ischemia with resultant tubular and cortical necrosis. The injected dose, as well as the potency of the venom, may affect the systemic manifestations seen. Investigators reported hypotension, hemorrhage, severe hypocomplementemia, intravascular hemolysis, and disseminated intravascular coagulation in rhesus monkeys exposed to lethal and sublethal doses of viperidae venoms (Chugh et al., 1984). Monkeys given lethal doses of venom developed hypotensive shock, DIC, and hemolysis and died within 24 hr. No renal functional changes or lesions were observed. In contrast, monkeys given sublethal doses of the Viperidae venom showed significant elevations in serum creatinine levels after 48 hr and histopathologic renal lesions were observed in a majority of the animals. These findings emphasize the need to maintain adequate renal perfusion throughout the course of treatment and to serially monitor laboratory parameters of renal function.

REFERENCES

Antretter, H., Dapunt, O. E., and Mueller, L. C. (1994). Accidental hypothermia. *N. Engl. J. Med.* **300**, 219.

Argenta, L. C., and Morykwas, M. J. (1996). New concepts in wound healing. *In* "Recent Advances in Plastic Surgery" (I. T. Jackson, ed.), Vol. 5. pp. 13–16. Churchill-Livingstone, Edinburgh.

Ayres, S. M., and Keenan, R. L. (1995). The hyperthermic syndromes. *In* "Textbook of Critical Care" (S. M. Ayres, A. Grenvik, P. R. Holbrook, and W. C. Shoemaker, eds.), pp. 1520–1523. Saunders, Philadelphia.

Bailey, E. M., and Garland, T. (1992). Toxicologic emergencies. *In* "Veterinary Emergency and Critical Care" (R. J. Murtaugh and P. M. Kaplan, eds.), pp. 427–452. Mosby, St. Louis, MO.

Besson, H. A. (1996). Hypothermia. *In* "Emergency Medicine" (J. E. Tintinalli, E. Ruiz, and R. L. Krone, eds.), pp. 846–850. McGraw-Hill, New York.

Bistner, S. I., and Ford, R. B., eds. (1995). "Kirk and Bistner's Handbook of Veterinary Procedures and Emergency Treatment." Saunders, Philadelphia.

Chugh, K. S., Pal, Y., Chakravarty, R. N., Datta, B. N., Mehta, R., Saakhuja, V., Mandal, A. K., and Sommers, S. C. (1984). Acute renal failure following poisonous snakebite. *Am. J. Kidney Dis.* **4**, 30–38.

Cioffi, W. G., deLemos, R. A., Coalson, J. J., Gerstmann, D. A., and Pruitt, B. A. (1993). Decreased pulmonary damage in primates with inhalation injury treated with high frequency ventilation. *Ann. Surg.* **218**, 328–335.

Clancy, C., and Lovitz, T. L. (1995). Poisoning. *In* "Textbook of Critical Care" (W. C. Shoemaker, S. M. Ayres, A. Grenvik, and P. R. Holbrook, eds.), pp. 1186–1210. Saunders, Philadelphia.

Cowell, A. K., Cowell, R. L., Tyler, R. D., and Nieves, M. A. (1991). Severe systemic reactions to Hymenoptera stings in three dogs. *J. Am. Vet. Med. Assoc.* **198**, 1014.

Danzl, D. F., and Pozos, R. S. (1994a). Accidental hypothermia. *N. Engl. J. Med.* **331**, 1756–1760.

Danzl, D. F., and Pozos, R. S. (1994b). Accidental hypothermia. *N. Engl. J. Med.* **332**, 1035.

Digeronimo, R. J., and Mayes, T. C. (1994). Near-hanging injury in childhood: A literature review and report of three cases. *Pediatri. Emerg. Care* **10**, 150–156.

Dimick, A. R. (1994). Electrical injuries. *In* "Harrison's Principles of Internal Medicine" (K. J. Isselbacher, J. B. Martin, E. Braunwald, A. S. Fauci, J. D. Wilson, and D. L. Kasper, eds.), 13th ed., Vol. 2, pp. 2480–2482. McGraw-Hill, New York.

Etheridge, M. S., and O'Malley, J. (1996). Diarrhea and peritonitis due to traumatic perforation of the stomach of a rhesus macaque (hardware disease). *Contemp. Top. Lab. Anim. Sci.* **3**, 57–59.

Fontanarosa, P. B. (1996). Electrical and lightning injuries. *In* "Emergency Medicine" (J. E. Tintinalli, E. Ruiz, and R. L. Krone, eds.), pp. 905–914. McGraw-Hill, New York.

Fowler, M. E. (1993). "Veterinary Zootoxicology." CRC Press, Boca Raton, FL.

Grant, H. D., Murray, R. H., and Bergeron, J. D. (1994a). Burns and hazardous materials. *In* "Brady Emergency Care" (G. Bizjak et al., eds.), pp. 536–559. Prentice Hall, Englewood Cliffs, NJ.

Grant, H. D., Murray, R. H., and Bergeron, J.D. (1994b). Heat, cold, water, and ice. *In* "Brady Emergency Care" (G. Bizjak et al., eds.), pp. 561–583. Prentice Hall, Englewood Cliffs, NJ.

Griffin, C. E. (1993). Insect and arachnid hypersensitivity. *In* "Current Veterinary Dermatology: The Science and Art of Therapy" (C. E. Griffin, K. W. Kwochka, and J. M. MacDonald, eds.), pp. 133–137. Mosby, St. Louis, MO.

Haskins, S. C. (1995). Thermoregulation, hypothermia, hyperthermia. *In* "Textbook of Veterinary Internal Medicine" (S. J. Ettinger and E. C. Feldman, eds.), Vol. 1 4th edition, pp. 26–30. Saunders, Philadelphia.

Hendrickx, A. G., and Binkerd, P. E. (1983). Teratology and birth defects. *In* "Primate Models for Human Diseases" (W. R. Dukelow, ed.), pp. 131–158. CRC Press, Boca Raton, FL.

Hernandez, E., Praga, M., and Alcazar, J. M. (1993). Hemodialysis for treatment of accidental hypothermia. *Nephron* **63**, 214–216.

Hummel, R. P., Monafo, W. W., and Stair, T. O. (1991). Sophisticated care for small burns. *Patient Care* **10**, 107–120.

Kremer, K. A., and Schaer, M. (1995). Coral snake *(Micrurus fulvius fulvius)* envenomation in five dogs: Present and earlier findings. *J. Emerg. Med. Crit. Care* **5**, 9–15.

Laber-Laird, K., McDole, G., and Jerome C. (1988). Unexpected frostbite in cynomolgus macaques after a short exposure to snow. *Lab. Anim. Sci.* **38**, 325–326.

Lee-Paritz, D. E., and Pavletic, M. M. (1992). Physical and chemical injuries: Heatstroke, hypothermia, burns, and frostbite. *In* "Veterinary Emergency and Critical Care Medicine" (R. J. Murtaugh and P. M. Kaplan, eds.), pp. 194–212. Mosby, St. Louis, MO.

Line, A. S., Morykwas, M. J., and Line, S. W. (1996). Use of cultured human epidermal xenografts for wound treatment in nonhuman primates. *J. Zoo Wildl. Med.* **26**, 517–524.

Line, S. W., Morgan, K. N., and Markowitz, H. (1991). Simple toys do not alter the behavior of aged rhesus monkeys. *Zoo Biol.* **10**, 473–484.

McCormick, F. W., Zamramski, J. M., McCormick, J., and Kurbat, J. (1994). The influence of profound hypothermia and rewarming on primate cerebral oxygen metabolism. *Adv. Exp. Med. Biol.* **345**, 597–602.

McCullough, J. (1995). Transfusion medicine. *In* "Blood: Principles and Practice of Hematology" (R. I. Handin and T. P. Stossel, eds.), 1997–2006. Lippincott, Philadelphia.

McNulty, W. P. (1993). Epidermal and gastric mucosal metaplasias caused by polychlorinated biphenyls, dibenzo-p-dioxins and dibenzofurans in rhesus monkeys. *In* "Monographs on the Pathology of Laboratory Animals: Nonhuman Primates" (T. C. Jones, U. Mohr, and R. D. Hunt, eds.), Vol. 1, pp. 155–163. Springer-Verlag, Berlin and New York.

Meric, S. M. (1992). Neuromuscular disorders. *In* "Essentials of Small Animal Internal Medicine" (R. W. Nelson and C. G. Couto, eds.), pp. 752–763. Mosby, St. Louis, MO.

Morgan, K. T., Kimbell, J. S., Monticello, T. M., Patra, A. L., and Fleishman, A. (1991). Studies of inspiratory airflow patterns in the nasal passages of the F344 rat and rhesus monkey using nasal molds: Relevance to formaldehyde toxicity. *Toxicol. Appl. Pharmacol.* **110**, 223–240.

Morykwas, M. J. (1994). Synthetic and biologic skin replacements. *In* "Problems in General Surgery; Biomaterials; AIDS and the General Surgeon" (B. Klitzman and A. M. Davis, eds.), Vol. 2, pp. 192–208. J. B. Lippincott Co., Philadelphia, PA.

Murray, P. T., and Fellner, S. K. (1994). Efficacy of hemodialysis in rewarming accidental hypothermia victims. *Nephrology* **5**, 422.

Mylecharane, E. J., Spence, I., and Gregson, R. P. (1984). In vivo actions of atraxin, a protein neurotoxin from the venom glands of the funnel web spider *(Atrax robustus)*. *Comp. Biochem. Physiol.* **79**, 395–399.

Neuman, M. G., Ishay, J. S., and Eshchar, J. (1983). Hornet *Vespa orientalis* venom sac extract causes hepatic injury in cats. *Comp. Biochem. Physiol.* **74**, 469.

Nicholson, S. S. (1995). Toxicology. *In* "Textbook of Veterinary Internal Medicine" (S. J. Ettinger and E. C. Feldman, eds.), Vol. 1 4th ed., pp. 312–326. Saunders, Philadelphia.

Okada, M., Tokura, H., and Kondo, S. (1975). Finger skin temperature responses during ice water immersion. *In* "Contemporary Primatology" (S. Kondo, M. Kawai, and A. Ehara, eds.), pp. 193–200. Karger, Basel.

Olsen, R. G. (1987). Rewarming of the hypothermic rhesus monkey with electromagnetic radiation. *Bioelectromagnetics (N.Y.)* **8**, 183–193.

Olsen, R. G. (1988). Reduced temperature afterdrop in rhesus monkeys with radio frequency rewarming. *Aviat. Space Environ. Med.* **59**, 78–80.

Petersdorf, R. G. (1994). Hypothermia and hyperthermia. *In* "Harrison's Principles of Internal Medicine" (K. J. Isselbacher, J. B. Martin, E. Braunwald,

A. S. Fauci, J. D. Wilson, and D. L. Kasper, eds.), 13th ed., Vol. 2, p. 2473. McGraw-Hill, New York.

Proppe, D. W. (1990). Effects of hyperosmolality and diuretics on heat-induced limb vasodilation in baboons. *Am. J. Physiol.* **258**, 309–317.

Purser, D. A., Grimshaw, P., and Berrill, K. R. (1984). Intoxication by cyanide in fires: A study in monkeys using polyacrylonitrile. *Arch. Environ. Health* **39**, 394–400.

Reisman, R. E. (1994). Insect stings *N. Engl. J. Med.* **331**, 523–527.

Robinson, N., Hudson, L., and Rum, M. (1982). Steroid therapy following isolated smoke inhalation injury. *J. Trauma* **22**, 876–880.

Rowat, S., Laing, G., Smith, D. C., Theakston, D., and Landon, J. (1994). A new antivenom to treat eastern coral snake *(Micrurus fulvius fulvius)* envenoming. *Toxicon* **32**, 185–190.

Rudloff, E., and Kirby, R. (1994). Hypovolemic shock and resuscitation. *Vet. Clin. North Am.: Small Anim. Pract.* **24**, 1026–1033.

Ryan, K. L., and Proppe, D. W. (1990a). Effect of water or saline intake on heat-induced limb vasodilation in dehydrated baboons. *Am. J. Physiol.* **258**, 318–324.

Ryan, K. L., and Proppe, D. W. (1990b). Effects of compartmental fluid repletion on heat-induced limb vasodilation in dehydrated baboons. *Am. J. Physiol.* **259**, 1139–1147.

Saluzzo, R. F. (1996). Insect and spider bites. *In* "Emergency Medicine" (J. E. Tintinalli, E. Ruiz, and R. L. Krone, eds.), pp. 856–864. McGraw-Hill, New York.

Salzberg, M. R. (1994). Hyperthermia. *N. Engl. J. Med.* **330**, 218.

Simon, H. B. (1993). Hyperthermia. *N. Engl. J. Med.* **329**, 483–487.

Slovis, C. M. (1994). Hyperthermia. *N. Engl. J. Med.* **330**, 218.

Sullivan, J. B., and Krieger, G. R., eds. (1992). "Hazardous Materials Technology: Clinical Principles of Environmental Health." Williams & Wilkins, Baltimore.

Thompson, J. P. (1995). Immunologic disease. *In* "Textbook of Veterinary Internal Medicine" (S. J. Ettinger and E. C. Feldman, eds.), 4th ed. Vol. 2, pp. 2003–2029. Saunders, Philadelphia.

Vick, J. A. (1994). Medical studies of poisonous land and sea snakes. *J. Clin. Pharmacol.* **34**, 709–712.

Walker, J. S., and Vance, M. V. (1996). Heat emergencies. *In* "Emergency Medicine" (J. E. Tintinalli, E. Ruiz, and R. L. Krone, eds.), pp. 850–856. McGraw-Hill, New York.

Weiss, E. A. (1993). Hyperthermia. *In* "Emergency Medicine: A Comprehensive Review" (T. C. Kravis, C. G. Warner, and L. M. Jacobs, eds.), 3rd ed. pp. 653–659. Raven Press, New York.

Wingfield, W. E., Brown, D. E., and Meyer, D. J. (1994). Echinocytosis associated with rattlesnake envenomation in dogs. *In* "Proceedings of the Fourth International Veterinary Emergency and Critical Care Symposium" (J. E. Rush, ed.), p. 718. Omnipress, Madison, WI.

Zelt, R. G., Daniel, R. K., Ballard, P. A., Brissette, Y., and Heroux, P. (1988). High-voltage electrical injury: Chronic wound evolution. *Plast. Reconstr. Surg.* **82**, 1027–1041.

Zook, B. C. (1993). Lead poisoning in nonhuman primates. *In* "Monographs on the Pathology of Laboratory Animals: Nonhuman Primates" (T. C. Hunt, U. Mohr, and R. D. Hunt, eds.), Vol. 1, pp. 163–169. Springer-Verlag, Berlin and New York.

Zuckerman, G. B., Conway, E. E., and Singer, L. (1994). Hemorrhagic shock and encephalopathy syndrome and heatstroke: A physiologic comparison of two entities. *Pediatr. Emerg. Care* **10**, 172–177.

Zurovsky, G. B., Shkolnik, A., and Ovadia, M. (1984). Conservation of blood plasma fluids in Hamadryas baboons after thermal dehydration. *J. Appl. Physiol.* **57**, 768–771.

Chapter 6

Cardiovascular and Lymphoreticular Systems

Milton April and James C. Keith, Jr.

I. INTRODUCTION

One of the great events in medicine came in 1628 when William Harvey published his book (Exercitatio Anatomica de Motu Cordis et Sanguinis in Animalibus) that showed for the first time that the circulation of the blood was through proper function of the heart. Until the work of Harvey was published, it was generally believed that the circulation of the blood was a simple ebb and flow in the arteries and veins. He developed the first complete theory of circulation of blood using animals. This was probably the most important single discovery at that point in medical history and certainly had a more far-reaching effect in medicine as time passed.

The cardiovascular and lymphoreticular systems in nonhuman primate species have been intensely studied through experimental manipulations and investigations primarily because these animals have the closest phylogenetic and physiologic relationship to humans. In this chapter, the most relevant topics concerning the cardiovascular and lymphoreticular systems of nonhuman primates are addressed with discussion relating to important spontaneous pathophysiologic syndromes affecting specific areas of the system.

Major features of cardiovascular and lymphoreticular pathophysiology will be described using an anatomical approach. Emphasis will be placed on etiology, basic pathophysiologic mechanisms, and clinical signs.

II. HEMATOLOGY

A. Examination

Because examination and analysis of blood samples acquired from nonhuman primates comprise the most common of all clinical procedures performed in primate medicine, it is essential that proper blood-sampling techniques and expedient handling of laboratory samples be employed. It is also critical that reference values be available to enable the clinician or the researcher to distinguish between normal and pathologic conditions. A considerable number of reports are available in the literature with respect to hematologic and blood chemistry values of rhesus monkeys (*Macaca mulatta*) primarily because they are reported on most frequently. McClure (1975) conducted a limited number of studies at the Yerkes Regional Primate Research Center. He coupled these data with an excellent review of the literature with respect to similar data reported from other laboratories. Compiled within this study are reference tables on hematologic values, blood chemistry, and cerebrospinal fluid data.

Lilly (1995) published an important set of hematology data from 45 2-year-old rhesus female macaques randomly captured from a large production colony. Although this information was part of a doctorate thesis designed to show several clinical and behavioral parameters, noteworthy hematological and immunological data were derived. Included in the dissertation were significant tables illustrating current hematologic and immunologic profiles.

Hainsey *et al.* (1993) have produced an excellent report on the clinical hematology parameters of normal baboons and chimpanzees. In addition to an expanded hematologic profile, including red blood cell distribution width and mean platelet volume, and a more comprehensive chemical profile of 28 individual tests, additional data collected included values for coagulation profiles, arterial blood gases, serum protein electrophoresis, and urine osmolalities. Samples for evaluation were obtained from clinically normal sedated adult baboons (*Papio* sp.) and chimpanzees (*Pan troglodytes*) and were processed

TABLE I

Erythrocyte Numbers in Unanesthetized Monkeys [a]

Species	Erythrocytes ($10^6/mm^3$)	No. of Animals	Ref.
Callithrix jacchus, common marmoset	4.6	27	Felton *et al.* (1984)
Common marmoset	5.65 ± 1.0 [b]	61 males	Yarbrough *et al.* (1984)
Common marmoset	5.74 ± 1.1	33 females	Yarbrough *et al.* (1984)
Common marmoset	5.07 ± 0.78	46 juvenile males	Yarbrough *et al.* (1984)
Common marmoset	5.04 ± 0.65	32 juvenile females	Yarbrough *et al.* (1984)
Leontopithecus rosalia, golden tamarins	5.70	162	Bush *et al.* (1982)
Aotus nancymai, owl monkey	6.1 ± 0.6 6.3 ± 0.5	124 females 130 males	Malaga *et al.* (1990) Malaga *et al.* (1990)
Saimiri sciureus, Bolivian squirrel monkey	7.26	38 males	Kakoma *et al.* (1987)

[a] Means.
[b] Means $\pm$ SD.

conventionally according to Good Laboratory Practices Act standards. The evaluation of large and stable defined populations of baboons and chimpanzees offered an excellent opportunity to obtain reliable basic clinical laboratory data for these animals. The information in this report should be valuable to investigators and clinicians responsible for research and clinical care of baboons and chimpanzees.

B. Hematopoiesis

1. Erythrocytes

Erythrocytes are normally derived from stem cells in the bone marrow of all nonhuman primates. Table I displays comparative characteristics of erythrocyte numbers across several species of smaller nonhuman primates sampled while being physically restrained.

The majority of procedures performed in larger nonhuman primate species require the use of ketamine hydrochloride for obvious clinical purposes of providing safe and relatively innocuous chemical restraint. Loomis *et al.* (1980) compared blood samples from awake, physically restrained rhesus monkeys to those under the influence of ketamine used for restraint. The hematocrit appeared to decrease significantly 20 min after ketamine administration, but not after 10 min when compared to samples obtained from animals that were physically restrained. Porter (1982) compared erythrocyte counts over a

TABLE II
HEMOGLOBIN VALUES IN UNANESTHETIZED MONKEYS[a]

Species	Hemoglobin (g/dl)	No. of Animals	Ref.
Saguinus labiatus, tamarin	14.2 ± 1.3	24 sex unknown	Gutteridge *et al.* (1986)
Leontopithecus rosalia, golden tamarins	15.4 ± 1.6	72 males	Bush *et al.* (1982)
	14.8 ± 1.3	61 females	Bush *et al.* (1982)
Saimiri sciureus, squirrel monkey	14.25 ± 0.11	38 sex unknown	Kakoma *et al.* (1987)
Aotus nancymai, owl monkey	16.1 ± 1.8	124 females	Malaga *et al.* (1990
	16.5 ± 1.3	130 males	Malaga *et al.* (1990)
Callithrix jacchus	16.1 ± 3.5	61 males	Yarbrough *et al.* (1984)
Common marmoset	15.0 ± 1.8	33 females	Yarbrough *et al.* (1984)
Common marmoset	13.9 ± 1.3	46 juvenile males	Yarbrough *et al.* (1984)
Common marmoset	13.6 ± 1.3	32 juvenile females	Yarbrough *et al.* (1984)

[a] Means ± SD.

40-min period following ketamine administration in rhesus monkeys and found no differences after the onset of chemical immobilization.

Hemoglobin values for small physically restrained nonhuman primates are shown in Table II. Erythrocyte and hemoglobin values for several larger species are reported during chemical restraint in Table III. As is the case in humans, almost all species of nonhuman primates exhibit sex differences with females exhibiting markedly lower hemoglobin concentration values than males (Hack and Gleiser, 1982; Brizzee *et al.,* 1988; Malaga *et al.,* 1990; Yarbrough *et al.,* 1984). However, Melville *et al.* (1967) failed to find this difference.

Iron metabolism is of critical importance in the formation of the heme groups of hemoglobin. Transferrin is the protein that binds with iron in the gastrointestinal system, transports it to the bone marrow, and is largely responsible for making iron available for heme synthesis. Smith (1982) demonstrated that polymorphism of transferrin exists in rhesus monkeys and suggested that homozygosity for transferrin C provided maximum delivery of iron for heme synthesis.

Human ABO blood groups, simian blood group antigens, and their corresponding isoantibodies are present in nonhuman primates (Socha, 1980; Terao *et al.,* 1988; Socha *et al.,* 1982). However, as in most animal species other than humans, transfusion with large volumes of untyped blood does not result in life-threatening transfusion reactions. Socha *et al.* (1982) reported that repeated transfusions of untyped blood in rhesus monkeys and baboons (*Papio* sp.) resulted in decreased eryth-

rocyte life spans. However, in emergency situations, untyped blood can be used to initially stabilize the animal.

Nonhuman primates play a vital role in the research of transfusion medicine, blood storage research, and the related experimental studies that foster clinical and scientific data. Although transfusions and blood research are an obvious part of clinical medicine, nonhuman primates play an important role as animal models for certain human diseases. Historically, nonhuman primates have been extremely important and have contributed significantly as laboratory animal models for research with tissue transplantation, blood storage methods, hemoglobin synthesis, and new blood typing techniques. Red and white blood cell groups were reviewed in a special issue of the *Journal of Medical Primatology* (January 1993).

Cissik *et al.* (1986) reported blood gas, cardiopulmonary, and urine electrolyte reference values in 13 clinically normal baboons (*Papio cynocephalus*). Reference values were established for urine sodium and potassium; respiratory rates; arterial and mixed venous blood gases; adult and fetal heart rates; hematocrit; plasma sodium and potassium; cardiac output; and arterial, pulmonary artery, central venous, and pulmonary wedge pressures.

2. Leukocytes

Leukocyte counts have been reported for a variety of species after sample collection with and without the use of chemical restraint. Table IV contains values obtained in animals under physical restraint and under ketamine hydrochloride. Porter (1982) and Loomis *et al.* (1980) reported markedly lower neutrophil numbers under chemical restraint with ketamine. They suggested that the lower numbers of neutrophils may be due to the factor of lowered "stress" and anxiety under chemical restraint. Reinhardt *et al.* (1990) reported that 14 female rhesus monkeys sampled repeatedly in their home cages had no significant increase in plasma cortisol, whereas females sampled in restraint cages had 50% increases in cortisol beginning with the second blood sample.

Lymphocytes have been quantitated, both in terms of absolute numbers and in terms of the subpopulations present in the peripheral blood (Wright *et al.,* 1982; Smit *et al.,* 1988; Eichberg *et al.,* 1988; Mendelow *et al.,* 1980). Percentages of T and B lymphocytes were similar among gorillas, (*Gorilla* sp.), orangutans (*Pongo pygmaeus*), and chimpanzees (*Pan troglodytes*) (Wright *et al.,* 1982), and their respective T and B lymphocyte levels closely resembled those found in humans. Mendelow *et al.* (1980) reported similar results for baboons.

Although the baboon lymphocyte reponse was initially thought to be only one-tenth of that of human lymphocytes when subjected to the mixed lymphocyte response test, Smit *et al.* (1988) demonstrated that with slight test modifications, baboon T and B lymphocyte cellular responses are in fact comparable to those of human lymphocytes.

Eichberg *et al.* (1988) observed that the T-cell subset ratios in chimpanzees were correlated with the age of the animal. The ratio of helper cells to suppressor cells decreased with age, most

TABLE III

ERYTHROCYTE AND HEMOGLOBIN VALUES IN ANESTHETIZED MONKEYS[a]

Species	Hb (g/dl)	Erythrocytes (10^6/mm³)	No. of Animals	Ref.
Pan troglodytes, chimpanzee	13.0 ± 1.5	5.1 ± 0.6	186 samples from 54	Vie *et al.* (1989)
Papio sp.	12.6 ± 0.9	4.97 ± 0.28	43 juveniles	Hack and Gleiser (1982)
Baboon	11.7 ± 0.7	4.55 ± 0.38	16 adult females	Hack and Gleiser (1982)
Baboon	13.4 ± 1.0	5.06 ± 0.38	16 adult males	Hack and Gleiser (1982)
Macaca mulatta, rhesus monkey	12.9 ± 1.8	5.02 ± 0.55	580 samples from 60	McClure (1975)
M. mulatta	14.4 ± 1.21	—	104 adult males	Valerio *et al.* (1969)
M. mulatta	13.5 ± 0.91	—	77 adult females	Valerio *et al.* (1969)
M. arctoides, stump-tail macaques	11.2^b	—	36 male and 56 female adults	de Neff *et al.* (1987)

[a] Means $\pm$ SD.
[b] Mean.

likely because both the helper cell population decreased and the suppressor cell number increased. The ratio was approximately 1:1 after chimpanzees reached 12 years of age, whereas the ratio in humans was 2:1.

3. Thrombocytes and Coagulation Factors

Platelet counts have been determined for several species of monkeys, but few specific studies of platelet life span and function have been reported. Juvenile marmosets (*Saguinus* sp.) reported by Yarbrough *et al.* (1984) appeared to have higher platelet counts than adult animals.

Various blood coagulation parameters have been reported for owl monkeys (*Aotus* sp.) (Mrema *et al.,* 1984), rhesus monkeys (Schiffer *et al.,* 1984), and baboons (Kelly and Gleiser, 1986). Most of the values are similar to those reported for humans, and a summary is presented in Table V.

Few studies have been conducted on platelet function in nonhuman primates. Platelets are of critical importance in the normal physiologic process of hemostasis as they are the first line of defense in maintaining the structural integrity of the injured blood vessel by forming the initial hemostatic barrier to further blood loss. When platelets are activated, adhesion and aggregation of platelets occur at the site of vascular injury. The irreversible phase of platelet aggregation is mediated by thromboxane production, a derivative of arachidonic acid via the cyclooxygenase and thromboxane synthetase enzyme systems found in platelets. An excellent review of comparative hemostasis has been published by Lewis (1996).

Dhawan *et al.* (1990) studied platelet reactivity and thromboxane production in normal and hypercholesterolemic atherosclerotic rhesus monkeys. Although control animals were fed only a standard monkey diet for the 1-year study, their platelet thromboxane generation capacity increased 4-fold during the study period. Thus, even normal adult rhesus monkeys seemed to exhibit increased platelet activity while being maintained in a typical laboratory setting. Monkeys fed a high cholesterol type diet exhibited more than a 5.5-fold increase in thromboxane production and a 12% increase in platelet aggregation in response to typical agonists such as ADP and collagen.

C. Anemias

Many pathologic conditions will produce anemia in nonhuman primates. Marmosets develop a wasting syndrome (Chalifoux *et al.,* 1982) that is accompanied by anemia. Nutritional deficiency (Baskin *et al.,* 1983) and injury to the red blood cells generated by lack of antioxidants or increased lipid peroxides that mitigate this type of reaction (oxidative stress) have been suggested as possible causes (Gutterridge *et al.,* 1986). Blood researchers have been able to demonstrate erythrocyte membrane susceptibility and red blood cell damage due to conditions relating to oxidative stress. A large portion of marmosets exhibit Heinz bodies in their erythrocytes. Although the presence of Heinz bodies has been associated with anemias (oxidative stress) in humans, Omorphos *et al.* (1989) found that affected marmoset erythrocytes did not have increased rates of membrane lipid peroxidation. However, erythrocyte membrane fluidity was increased, suggesting that the membranes might be more susceptible to shear stress in the flowing blood.

Causes of nutritional deficiency anemias in nonhuman primates have been reviewed (Wixson and Griffith, 1986). Table VI shows that the most common types of anemias result from spontaneous and/or experimentally induced nutritional deficiencies. Some researchers (Baskin *et al.,* 1983; Draper and Saari, 1969; Bieri and Poukka Evats, 1972) have suggested that vitamin E and selenium deficiency may be important in the wasting syndrome of marmosets, but general therapy with vitamin E orally or parenterally has not demonstrated clinical improvement. Megaloblastic anemia has been reported in a chimpanzee reared on an all-milk diet. In this case, it was surmised that the anemia was probably induced by vitamin B_{12} and folic acid deficiency as the animal also manifested central nervous system dysfunction.

TABLE IV

LEUKOCYTE NUMBERS IN AWAKE AND ANESTHETIZED SIMIANS

Species and Number	Total leukocytes (10^3/mm^3)	Segments (%)	Lymphocytes (%)	Monocytes (%)	Eosinophils (%)	Basophils (%)	Ref.
Macaca mulatta 104 males	10.3 ± 2.8[a]	32.9 ± 1.4	58 ± 1.4	4.2 ± 0.2	4.1 ± 0.3	0.4 ± 0.06	Valerio *et al.* (1969)
M. mulatta 77 females	10.3 ± 3.1[a]	38.7 ± 1.4	52.1 ± 1.3	3.2 ± 0.3	5.4 ± 0.4	0.5 ± 0.08	Valerio *et al.* (1969)
M. mulatta	8.0 ± 0.5[a,c]	33 ± 2.3	61.3 ± 4.9	—	—	—	Loomis *et al.* (1980)
M. mulatta 61 male and female	8.2 ± 3.3[a,c]	37.3 ± 9.6	58.8 ± 15	2.15 ± 2.2	2.56 ± 2.7	0.2 ± 0.5	McClure and Guiland (1975)
Saimiri sciureus 38 males	8.0 ± 0.4[a]	34.8 ± 2.1	58 ± 2.1	3.5 ± 0.5	—	—	Kakoma *et al.* (1987)
Aotus nancymai 254 male and female	9.9 ± 3.3[b]	28.2 ± 17.4	62.5 ± 2.9	3.5 ± 3	4.7 ± 5.4	1.5 ± 1.6	Malaga *et al* (1990)
Callithrix jacchua							
61 males, adult	8.1 ± 3.2[b]	43 ± 16	51 ± 16	3.3 ± 2.9	0.4 ± 1.0	0.8 ± 1.3	Yarbrough *et al.* (1984)
33 females, adult	7.4 ± 2.8[b]	54 ± 15	40 ± 14	3.6 ± 2.8	0.5 ± 0.9	1.5 ± 2.1	Yarbrough *et al.* (1984)
46 males, juvenile	9.3 ± 3.7[b]	46 ± 14	50 ± 16	1.1 ± 1.2	0.6 ± 1.0	0.8 ± 1.2	Yarbrough *et al.* (1984)
32 females, juvenile	9.1 ± 3.4[b]	47 ± 17	51 ± 17	1.0 ± 1.0	0.3 ± 0.7	1.0 ± 0.9	Yarbrough *et al.* (1984)
Leontopithecus rosalia 170 male and female	7.13 ± 2.8[b]	62 ± 35.2	30.4 ± 16	2.2 ± 2.5	4.2 ± 5.6	1.1 ± 2.0	Bush *et al.* (1982)
Papio sp.							
16 males	10.9 ± 4.0[b,c]	54 ± 20	42 ± 20	1.0 ± 1.2	2.0 ± 1.7	0.1 ± 0.3	Hack and Gleiser (1982)
16 females	10.8 ± 3.0[b,c]	64 ± 21	33 ± 19	1.0 ± 1.1	1.0 ± 0.9	0.1 ± 0.3	Hack and Gleiser (1982)
43 juveniles, male and female	7.6 ± 2.7[b,c]	44 ± 13	53 ± 13	0.5 ± 0.7	1.6 ± 1.9	0.1 ± 0.2	Hack and Gleiser (1982)

[a] Means ± SE.
[b] Means ± SD.
[c] Anesthetized.

Microcytic, hypochromic anemia is associated with simian acquired immunodeficiency syndrome (MacKenzie *et al.,* 1986). This would be expected as most monkeys affected by this syndrome become iron deficient, probably due to malnutrition (vomiting and diarrhea).

Malaria can cause severe anemia in nonhuman primates. Various species of the malaria protozoan will infect nonhuman primates, but *Plasmodium* sp. are the most common infestations documented (Donovan *et al.,* 1983). Naturally occurring malaria is manifested as a macrocytic, normochromic anemia (Donovan *et al.,* 1983) in cynomolgus monkeys (*Macaca fascicularis*). However, acute cases of the disease have been reported that present a severe microcytic anemia (Stokes *et al.,* 1983). Some effect on the bone marrow is postulated and immunologic factors may contribute to the anemia (Smith *et al.,* 1972).

Marmosets infected with *Plasmodium knowlesi* and Epstein–Barr virus developed severe normocytic, normochromic anemia that persisted until therapy with chloroquine phosphate was commenced (Felton *et al.,* 1984). Adams *et al.* (1984) reported hemobartonellosis in a domestic breeding colony of squirrel monkeys (*Saimiri sciureus*). A moderate normocytic, normochromic anemia was present in one clinically affected monkey. Examination of a Wright–Giemsa-stained blood smear revealed punctate basophilic stippling of several erythrocytes. The animal was treated supportively with multiple B vitamins, and 14 days later the hemogram of the animal was normal. Immunosuppression or splenectomy has been associated with the recrudescence of latent infections of hemobartonellosis.

The common occurrences of moderate to severe anemias in squirrel monkeys and cynomolgus monkeys may reflect their high levels of hemolytic complement (Rommel *et al.,* 1980; Rosenberg *et al.,* 1982; McMahan, 1982). However, marmosets do not develop anemia as rapidly or to the same extent as do other nonhuman primate species; this is perhaps due to the fact that their levels of hemolytic complement are very low (Rommel *et al.,* 1980).

D. Leukemias

Leukemias of hematopoietic origin have been reported in nonhuman primates. Lymphocytic leukemias or lymphomas are the most common neoplasms documented in nonhuman primates (McCarthy *et al.,* 1990), with a high percentage probably associated with simian T-lymphotropic virus type 1 (STLV-1), a type of C retrovirus.

TABLE V

Coagulation Parameters[a]

Species and number	Platelet count ($\times 10^3$/mm^3)	APTT[b] (sec)	PT[c] (sec)	ACT[d]	Ref.
Callithrix jacchus					
60 males	281 ± 101	—	—	—	Yarbrough *et al.* (1984)
33 females	281 ± 121	—	—	—	Yarbrough *et al.* (1984)
46 juvenile males	344 ± 154	—	—	—	Yarbrough *et al.* (1984)
32 juvenile females	328 ± 123	—	—	—	Yarbrough *et al.* (1984)
Saimiri sciureus	521.6 ± 10.5[e]	—	—	—	Kakoma *et al.* (1987)
38 male and female					
Aotus nancymai					
124 females	452 ± 130	—	—	—	Malaga *et al.* (1990)
130 males	411 ± 104	—	—	—	Malage *et al.* (1990)
A. tirvirgatus	—	19.6 ± 1.8	—	—	Mrema *et al.* (1984)
28 male and female					
Macaca mulatta					
30 males	—	—	—	94 ± 10	Schiffer *et al.* (1984)
30 females	—	—	—	98 ± 11	Schiffer *et al.* (1984)
Papio sp.					
16 males	334 ± 73	—	—	—	Hack and Gleiser (1982)
16 females	333 ± 136	—	—	—	Hack and Gleiser (1982)
43 juveniles	399 ± 76	—	—	—	Hack and Gleiser (1982)
Papio sp.					
20 males	—	32.5 ± 1.7	13 ± 0.7	—	Kelly and Gleiser (1986)
21 females	—	31.0 ± 2.1	12.5 ± 0.9	—	Kelly and Gleiser (1986)
20 juveniles	—	33.5 ± 2.1	12.5 ± 0.4	—	Kelly and Gleiser (1986)

[a] Means ± SD.
[b] Activated clotting time.
[c] Means ± SE.
[d] Activated partial thromboplastin time.
[e] Prothrombin time.

A report describing a spontaneously generated non-Hodgkin's lymphoma in baboons (Hubbard *et al.,* 1993) implies that leukemia/lymphoma in Old World monkeys is closely related to human T-cell leukemia virus type 1 (HTLV-1), the etiologic agent of adult T-cell leukemia/lymphoma in humans. Clinical signs and laboratory findings in nonhuman primates are variable, but generally include lethargy, low body weight, anemia, dyspnea, lymphadenopathy, hepatosplenomegaly, pneumonia, nodular skin lesions, and leukemia with or without multilobulated lymphocytes in peripheral blood.

The same report suggests that transmission of STLV-1 in baboons is probably similar to the transmission of HTLV-1 in humans as indicated by the increasing seropositivity associated with the age of the baboon, sex predilection, and lack of infection in infants. This means transmission is exogenic, perinatal, sexual, and parenteral, including blood transfusion and blood vectors. In humans infected with HTLV-1, the virus is typically latent for several years, with the only evidence of infection being antibody titers. It is believed that reactivation of the virus, perhaps by antigenic stimulation of the host T cell, results in reexpression of the virus and subsequent malignant transfor-mation. The results of Hubbard *et al.* (1993) strongly implicate such a mechanism in the development of T-cell malignant lymphoma in the baboon and perhaps other nonhuman primates.

TABLE VI

Anemias Caused by Nutritional Deficiencies

Nutrient	Type of anemia	Ref.
Iron	Microcytic, hypochromic	Huser (1970)
Niacin	Normocytic	Tappan (1952)
Vitamin B$_6$	Microcytic, hypochromic	Wixson & Griffith (1986)
Pantothenic acid	Normocytic	Wixson & Griffith (1986)
Riboflavin	Normocytic, normochromic	Wixson & Griffith (1986)
Vitamin B$_{12}$	Macrocytic, hypochromic	May *et al.* (1952)
Folic acid	Megaloblastic	Wixson and Griffith (1986)

Malignant lymphomas and Hodgkin's disease have been reported in baboons (Gleiser *et al.*, 1984; McCarthy *et al.*, 1990), cynomolgus monkeys (Joax *et al.*, 1988), and African green monkeys (*Cercopithecus aethiops*) (Jayo *et al.*, 1990).

B-cell non-Hodgkin's lymphomas, while common in African children, are rarely reported in African nonhuman primates. However, Jayo *et al.* (1988) have reported a maxillo-orbital lymphoma (Burkitt's type) in an infant cynomolgus monkey. Although sera of the mother were positive for Epstein–Barr virus, the primate facility was contaminated with polychlorinated biphenyls that may have caused immunosuppression. Therefore, the cause in this case could not be positively established.

Although acute leukemias caused by granulocytic or monocytic cell lines are common in humans, they have been reported infrequently in nonhuman primates. DePaoli *et al.* (1973) reported granulocytic leukemia in six white-handed gibbons (*Hylobates lar*) maintained in captivity. Bennett *et al.* (1981) described acute myelomonocytic leukemia in a capuchin monkey (*Cebus apella*) that first showed clinical signs 2 weeks after giving birth and died 1 day after becoming clinically ill. A similar case of monocytic leukemia was reported in a greater bushbaby (*Galago* sp.) that died suddenly (Holscher *et al.*, 1984). In both cases, multiple organ infiltration with neoplastic mononuclear cells was observed. Finally, eosinophilic myelocytoma (Chalifoux and King, 1983) has been reported in an owl monkey that died suddenly. Multiple organ infiltration and an anterior mediastinal mass were noted at necropsy.

III. THE HEART

Disorders of the cardiovascular system and the heart of nonhuman primates have been reviewed previously (McNulty and Malinow, 1972; Ruch, 1959; Lapin and Yakovleva, 1963). In stark contrast to humans, nonhuman primates seem to enjoy a much lower incidence of spontaneous cardiac and arterial disease. This may be due to the facts that most nonhuman primates eat a very different diet than humans, their life span is markedly shorter, or to a relatively small number of postmortem examinations performed on nonhuman primates as compared to humans. Hubbard *et al.* (1991) reported that the primary causes of death in chimpanzees at their research institute since 1982 were heart diseases. Heart lesions included myocarditis, necrosis, fibrosis, and mineralization. The main categories of causes of death in order of importance from that time were cardiovascular, followed by trauma, respiratory, and gastrointestinal. Bond *et al.* (1980) reported myocardial infarction in primates with atherosclerosis. Levin and Carey (1986) reported congestive heart failure and pneumonia in a baboon during a routine health evaluation. Physically, the baboon appeared healthy, but had a 5-year history of hypertension that had been induced by stenosing its left renal artery. One month before the discovery of the leukocytosis, polyethylene catheters had been implanted in

the internal iliac artery and common iliac vein as part of the tethering procedure to monitor blood pressure.

A. Electrocardiography

The electrocardiograms (ECGs) of many species of nonhuman primates have been reported previously. Tables VII and VIII display comparative values for the typical ECG parameters that are recorded, and Fig. 1 displays typical lead II electrocardiograms recorded in right lateral or supine (dorsal) recumbency.

The electrical activation sequence of the nonhuman primate heart is very similar to that of humans. Nonhuman primates have the same ventricular activation scheme as human and are classified as category A animals (Hamlin and Smith, 1965). The ventricular activation sequence is displayed in Fig. 2. Therefore, it is very easy to use the nonhuman primate ECG to gather data that can help determine relative chamber enlargements and changes in myocardial mass.

Routine electrocardiography can also be used to determine the origin of rhythm disturbances in nonhuman primates. Hayes (1986) described the diagnosis of ventricular tachycardia in a baboon. The animal was initially stabilized with intravenous lidocaine hydrochloride, and then electroconversion was used to abolish the ventricular rhythm and reestablish a normal sinus rhythm. Long-term medical management with quinidine hydrochloride was then instituted.

Experimentally induced atrial arrhythmias can be diagnosed in nonhuman primates (Klein *et al.*, 1974; Randall and Hasson, 1981), but spontaneous atrial or supraventricular arrhythmias remain to be described in nonhuman primates.

Complete and incomplete left and right bundle branch blocks were described in mature nonhuman primates, along with descriptions of local disorders of the electrical conduction system of the myocardium in rhesus monkeys by Bristow and Malinow (1965). Hugo *et al.* (1988) reported a 2:1 atrioventricular (AV) block in a baboon anesthetized with ketamine and pentobarbital. The block progressed to a complete AV block and was abolished with atropine administration. Gonder (1978) described a left anterior fascicular conduction block in a 2-week-old rhesus macaque. Bundle branch blocks appear to cause no impairment of growth and development, but they can mimic ECG signs of right and left ventricular hypertrophy. Because of this, thoracic radiographs should be obtained, and the amplitude of the R wave in leads II and AVR should be carefully evaluated to rule out ventricular hypertrophy.

As is the case in humans, changes in the Q wave, notching of the QRS complex, and elevation of the S-T segment can be used to diagnose old or recent/evolving myocardial infarctions (Groover *et al.*, 1963).

It is recommended that electrocardiography should become a routine ancillary test for evaluation of the heart in nonhuman primates. However, it is only one part of the total clinical as-

TABLE VII

ECG INTERVALS AND DURATIONS[a]

Species	P wave duration	P-R interval	QRS duration	QT interval	Ref.
Saimiri sciureus, squirrel monkey 268 male and female	30 ± 5	50 ± 7	30 ± 4	150 ± 22	Wolf *et al.* (1969)
Cebus apella, capuchin monkey 18 male and female	35	65	35	150	Szabuniewicz *et al.* (1971)
Cercopithecus aethiops African green monkeys 46 male and female	41 ± 9	85 ± 17	42 ± 5	209 ± 30	Bellinger *et al.* (1980)
Saimiri sciureus,[b] squirrel monkey 100 male and female	30 ± 10	60 ± 10	20 ± 10	150 ± 10	Gonder *et al.* (1980)
C. aethiops,[b] African green monkeys 100 male and female	30 ± 10	90 ± 10	30 ± 10	190 ± 30	Gonder *et al.* (1980)
C. apella,[b] capuchin monkey 13 male and female	30 ± 10	80 ± 10	20 ± 10	150 ± 10	Gonder *et al.* (1980)
Erythrocebus patas,[b] patas monkey 50 male and female	40 ± 10	110 ± 10	30 ± 10	210 ± 20	Gonder *et al.* (1980)
Macaca fascicularis,[b] cynomolgus macaque 100 male and female	30 ± 10	80 ± 10	30 ± 10	190 ± 20	Gonder *et al.* (1980)
M. mulatta, rhesus monkey 25 male and female	40 ± 10	90 ± 10	30 ± 10	200 ± 20	Gonder *et al.* (1980)
M. fascicularis,[b] cynomolgus macaque 33 males	36 ± 8	82 ± 10	42 ± 9	222 ± 24	Verlangieri *et al.* (1985)
M. arctoides,[b] stump-tail macaque 7 males	30 ± 6	71 ± 7	30 ± 6	233 ± 17	Verlangieri *et al.* (1985)
Papio sp. baboon 150 male and female	40 ± 20	70 ± 20	30 ± 20	160 ± 30	Osborne and Roberts (1972)

[a] Data in milliseconds; means ± SD.
[b] Immobilized with ketamine.

sessment, which must also include history, signalment, physical exams, blood sampling, and radiography.

Among physiological conditions that temporarily increase the heart rate are muscular exercise, emotional excitement, and high environmental temperature. The heart rate also increases somewhat during digestion and is lowered during sleep. Pathological conditions that cause an increase in cardiac rate are hemorrhage, surgical shock, hyperthyroidism, fever (an increase of 10 beats per 1°F rise in temperature), and certain cardiac arrhythmias, e.g., paroxysmal tachycardia and atrial fibrillation.

B. Disease of the Coronary Vessels

Coronary artery disease accounts for hundreds of thousands of deaths in humans yearly around the world by causing myocardial infarction or abrupt coronary death. The nonhuman primate has been used extensively in studies of experimentally induced coronary artery disease to study the progression and sex-related differences in this devastating syndrome (Kaplan *et al.,* 1982; Kransch and Hollander, 1968; Clarkson *et al.,* 1984; Clarkson and Klumpp, 1990).

Although coronary atherosclerosis, myointimal thickening with associated lipid deposition, occurs when the nonhuman

primate is manipulated by dietary intervention or social stress (Kaplan *et al.,* 1983), the incidence of spontaneous coronary artery atherosclerosis remains markedly lower than that reported for humans. The most common lesion reported is arteriosclerosis, myointimal fibrous thickening of the coronary artery without lipid disposition (Chakravarti *et al.,* 1976). The lesions tend to affect the epicardial branches of the coronary arteries in the larger nonhuman primate species and the smaller intramural coronary vessels in smaller species of nonhuman primates (Stout, 1968; Chawla *et al.,* 1967; Malinow and Storvick, 1968).

C. Diseases of the Myocardium

1. Ischemic Heart Disease

Occlusive coronary artery disease is relatively rare in nonhuman primates when fed a chow diet; however, isolated cases have been reported. Congestive heart failure has been reported in a gorilla (Robinson and Benirschke, 1980) that subsequently died despite medical therapy. Necropsy revealed long-standing diffuse myocardial fibrosis, probably due to hypertension-induced coronary arterial stenosis caused by chronic nephritis. Acute myocardial infarction and death occurred in a rhesus

TABLE VIII

ECG Parameters[a]

Species	P wave (mV)	Q wave (mV)	R wave (mv)	T wave (mV)	MEA[b] (°c)	HR (bpm)	Ref.
Saimiri sciureus, squirrel monkey 268 male and female	0.19 ± 0.06	—	1.73 ± 0.78	—	62 ± 27	248 ± 38	Wolf *et al.* (1969)
Cercopithecus aethiops, African green monkeys 46 male and female	0.18 ± 0.11	0.0 − 0.3	0.7 − 2.5	0.1 − 0.5	61 ± 3	162 ± 5	Bellinger *et al.* (1980)
S. sciureus, squirrel monkey 100 male and female	0.17 ± 0.05	—	0.9 ± 0.01	—	56 ± 22	250 ± 44	Gonder *et al.* (1980)
C. aethiops,[c] African green monkeys 100 male and female	0.19 ± 0.09	—	1.2 ± 0.6	—	47 ± 27	181 ± 41	Gonder *et al.* (1980)
Cebus apella,[c] capuchin monkey 13 male and female	0.35 ± 0.12	—	0.9 ± 0.3	—	58 ± 31	230 ± 27	Gonder *et al.* (1980)
Erythrocebus patas,[c] patas monkey 50 male and female	0.21 ± 0.10	—	1.4 ± 0.3	—	75 ± 15	152 ± 24	Gonder *et al.* (1980)
Macaca fascicularis,[c] cynomolgus macaque 100 male and female	0.16 ± 0.05	—	0.7 ± 0.3	—	65 ± 22	203 ± 29	Gonder *et al.* (1980)
M. mulatta,[c] rhesus monkey 25 male and female	0.20 ± 0.05	—	0.8 ± 0.3	—	69 ± 16	178 ± 29	Gonder *et al.* (1980)
M. fascicularis,[c] cynomolgus macaque 33 males	0.06 ± 0.02	—	0.3 ± 0.2	—	48 ± 24	152 ± 21	Verlangieri *et al.* (1985)
M. arctoides,[c] stump-tail macaque 7 males	0.02 ± 0.07	—	0.23 ± 0.16	—	57 ± 29	149 ± 14	Verlangieri *et al.* (1985)
Papio sp., baboon 150 male and female	0.16 ± 0.3	0.0 − 0.63	0.0 + 1.04	0 ± 3.53	48 ± 85	230 ± 46	Osborne and Roberts (1972)

[a]Means ± SD.
[b]Mean electrical axis of the ventricles in the frontal plane.
[c]Immobilized with ketamine.

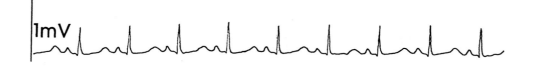

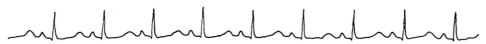

Fig. 1.   Lead II electrocardiograms of (top) right lateral and (bottom) dorsal recumbancy.

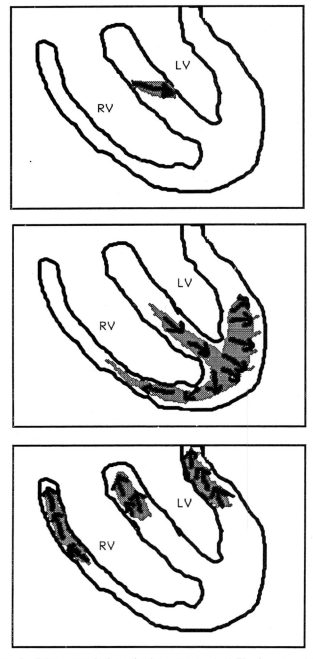

Fig. 2. Primate ventricular activation sequence. (top) The first area of the ventricular myocardium to begin depolarization after the Purkinje system has been activated is the right middle portion of the interventricular septum. The wave of depolarization spreads across the septum in a leftward and slightly dorsal direction. If the wave front has less of a dorsal direction, a small positive deflection is seen. A strong dorsal vector results in a negative potential, the Q wave. (middle) After the middle septum activates, the ventral septum and the left and right ventricular free walls depolarize, resulting in the R wave. (bottom) The final portion of the ventricular depolarization involves the basilar portions of the septum and left and right ventricular free walls. This electrical event is usually represented by the S wave. However, it may not be seen if the basilar myocardial mass is small.

monkey (Gonder *et al.,* 1982), diffuse myocardial fibrosis and congestive heart failure secondary to coronary artery disease was reported in an adult male chimpanzee (Hansen *et al.,* 1984), and congestive heart failure occurred in a hypertensive baboon (Levin and Carey, 1986).

Myocardial necrosis and subsequent fibrosis seen with ischemic heart disease are the result of two factors. First, occlusive coronary artery disease can produce anoxia, which will lead to cell death. The other phenomenon is reduced blood flow followed by periods of reperfusion. Reperfusion injury has been postulated to be mediated by reactive oxygen species (oxygen- "free radicals") that are generated and can cause cell damage. The pigment, lipofuscin, thought to be produced by oxygen- free radicals, is produced continually as the heart ages and increases in nonhuman primates as the animals reach sexual maturity (Nakano *et al.,* 1990).

2. Myocarditis

Inflammation of the myocardium may occur in response to bacterial, viral, or parasitic infections. Regional myocarditis caused by repeated catecholamine release is thought to occur in almost all facility-maintained nonhuman primates. An excessive catecholamine release results in intense brief vasoconstriction and, at the same time, increases myocardial contractility. These two phenomena produce repeated bouts of ischemia/ reperfusion, leading to regional myocardial necrosis, and a mild inflammatory reaction ensues.

Trypanosomiasis-induced myocarditis has been demonstrated in capuchin monkeys (Bullock *et al.,* 1967) and in a Celebes black macaque (*Macaca nigra*) (Olson and Skinner, 1986). Nonhuman primates may be infected years previously and only under stress does the infection reassert itself. Marmosets can be spontaneously infected with *Angiostrongylus costaricensis,* a naturally occurring nematode of Central American rodents. Sly *et al.* (1986) described myocarditis caused by eggs and larvae of this parasite.

Encephalomyocarditis virus (EMCV) was reported to have caused the death of 85 baboons in an epizootic episode that extended over a 7-month period (Hubbard *et al.,* 1992). Acute death was the most common history. Clinical disease was characterized by labored breathing associated with acute congestive heart failure. The most significant histologic lesion was a non-supportive necrotizing myocarditis. Other inflammatory cardio-vascular type conditions have been reported by Schmidt (1978) in an extensive compilation of systemic diseases seen in chimpanzees.

Experimental infection with the encephalomyocarditis virus will also cause severe necrotizing myocarditis in African green and squirrel monkeys (Blanchard *et al.,* 1987). This virus is a member of the family of Picornaviridae and is of the same family (coxsackie B virus) that also produces myocarditis in nonhuman primates (Sun *et al.,* 1967).

3. Cardiomyopathy

Idiopathic-dilated cardiomyopathy is infrequently described in nonhuman primates. Although hypertrophic cardiac disease (HCD) in nonhuman primates is similar to lesions found in humans, many HCD cases go unrecognized clinically because of the vague signs and lack of specific diagnostic criteria (Roger *et al.*, 1986). Gozalo *et al.* (1992) reported two cases of spontaneous cardiomyopathy in owl monkeys and attributes this disease to important causes of death in captive breeding colonies. The specific lesion in these monkeys was concentric hypertrophic cardiomyopathy. Although routine electrocardiography can be used to diagnose this disease, it is typically diagnosed at necropsy by measurement of myocardial thickness.

Jackson *et al.* (1996) reported a case of cardiac hypertrophy in a tamarin (*Saguinus mystax*). The myocardial fiber hypertrophy was most prominent in the areas of myofiber disorganization with infiltration of inflammatory cells. The clinical signs were related to suspected aortic thrombosis. However, cardiac lesions in the heart were consistent with left ventricular hypertrophy due to hypertrophic cardiomyopathy and volume/pressure overload. Hypertrophic cardiomyopathy has been reported in humans, primates, cats, dogs, and pigs and has been studied in humans more extensively than in any other species. The relationship of hypertension to renal and cardiomyopathic diseases in the tamarin has not been established, and there are no normative blood pressure data currently published for the species.

A type of cardiomyopathy associated with vitamin E deficiency has also been reported in Gelada baboons (Liu *et al.*, 1984). Typical myocardial lesions included myocytolysis, vacuolization of myocardial cells, replacement fibrosis, and hypertrophy of surviving myocytes. Vitamin E supplementation was instituted following confirmation of low serum vitamin E levels in affected animals. Vitamin E functions as a cellular antioxidant, and decreased levels are associated with oxidative injury and cell damage.

D. Valvular Heart Disease

Spontaneous degeneration of the valves of the heart has been termed endocardiosis. This lesion is known to occur in humans and dogs. Schmidt (1970) described two cases of left atrioventricular valvular endocardiosis in rhesus monkeys. The lesion, composed of collagen fibers and acid mucopolysaccharide, leads to valvular incompetence and subsequent congestive heart failure.

Roberts and Innes (1966) reported two cases of valvular disease in rhesus monkeys. One was described as endocardiosis, whereas the second case appeared to have infectious endocarditis of the mitral and aortic valves. Cantrell *et al.* (1986) reported mitral endocarditis produced by endometritis following intrauterine fetal demise and abortion in a rhesus monkey. Right atrioventricular valvular endocarditis caused by *Staphylococcus* sp. was described by Wood *et al.* (1978).

Mitral valve prolapse has been well described in humans. Swindle *et al.* (1985) described the syndrome of mitral valve prolapse in a colony of rhesus monkeys, where almost 20% of the colony was affected. After a review, the breeding records indicated that this malady appeared to be a dominant genetic trait. Murmurs and systolic clicks were audible on clinical examination in affected animals, and several died from congestive heart failure.

E. Diseases of the Pericardium

Acute purulent pericarditis has been reported in association with severe myocarditis (Raina *et al.*, 1971), and pericardial effusion was also present. Bacterial culture yielded *Streptococcus* as the infectious agent. Pericardial effusion has also been documented in severe congestive heart failure (Levin and Carey, 1986).

F. Congenital Defects of the Heart

Congenital defects of the heart are reported in nonhuman primates. The most common defects reported include ventricular septal defect, patent ductus arteriosus, and atrial septal defect (Jerome, 1987).

Confirmation of ventricular septal defects has been accomplished in a gorilla using *in vivo* oximetry and two-dimensional echocardiography (Machado *et al.*, 1989) and in a rhesus monkey using echocardiography and cardiac angiography (Swindle *et al.*, 1986).

IV. DISEASES OF THE GREAT VESSELS

A. Atherosclerosis

Atherosclerosis is defined as a pathologic process of large arteries in which there are local accumulations of cells, lipids, and fibrous tissue within the tunica intima. It is a progressive condition characterized by degeneration and hardening of the arterial walls (arteriosclerosis). As the disease progresses there is often necrosis with ulceration and resulting thrombosis. Thrombosis (formation of thrombi within the lumen of the blood vessel) produces the clinical event, often resulting in occlusion of the vessel. Since the mid-1970s, considerable effort has been devoted toward developing the nonhuman primate as an animal model for atherosclerosis research. Many of these studies were prompted because of the relative significance of the same disease in humans, in that induced atherosclerosis in nonhuman primates resembles the syndrome in humans more closely than in other experimental animals. A good review of this topic is presented by Taylor (1965). Also, excellent review articles are available that summarize the findings in several nonhuman primates (Clarkson and Klumpp, 1990; Kalter, 1980; Kaplan *et al.,* 1983; Chakravarti *et al.,* 1976; Dieter, 1968; Scott *et al.,* 1967).

Ample evidence shows that atherosclerosis occurs in many different species of nonhuman primates. There have been numerous experiments of induced atherosclerosis as well as case reports of spontaneous atherosclerosis. In all cases the pathologic lesions are relatively the same except for variations in reporting methods. It could be assumed that atherosclerosis is more common in captive animals, but this is probably due to the fact that they live longer, eat prepared diets, and are more likely to be examined after death. It has been fairly well concluded that there is essentially no clinical difference between the spontaneous disease and the experimentally induced disease. Although atherosclerosis appears morphologically similar in most nonhuman primates, the susceptibility from species to species appears to be different.

Among nonhuman primates characterized as responders and nonresponders to diet, several different metabolic processes are influenced by dietary cholesterol and fat. This variability in response may be the primary reason that there is no consensus about the differential mechanisms underlying the hyperlipoproteinemic effects of dietary cholesterol and saturated fat. It is generally assumed that dietary cholesterol influences the serum cholesterol concentration by increasing the amount of cholesterol absorbed, but variations in the degree of suppression of cholesterol synthesis and in the capacity to increase cholesterol or bile acid excretion rates also have been implicated. Although the type of dietary fat has a small influence on cholesterol absorption, there is no agreement about whether the effects of saturated vs unsaturated fat on plasma lipoproteins are mediated by mechanisms similar to those of cholesterol (Mott *et al.,* 1992).

The occurrence of spontaneous atherosclerosis in nonhuman primates has been well documented through clinical observation and pathologic description in both Old World and New World species (Bhardwaj *et al.,* 1983; Chakravarti and Kukreja, 1981; DiGiacomo *et al.,* 1978; Henderson *et al.,* 1970; Stout, 1968; Chawla *et al.,* 1967; Middleton *et al.,* 1963). Although the pathological conditions of the naturally occurring disease are relatively similar, there is no conclusive evidence that one nonhuman primate species has definite predilection for atherosclerosis over another. Baboons, rhesus monkeys, squirrel monkeys, cynomolgus monkeys, and African green monkeys are mentioned most frequently in the literature, with the cynomolgus monkey overtaking the baboon as the predominate nonhuman primate animal model of study.

Reports of atherosclerosis in anthropoids are rare. McClure (1971) reported on several cases in the "Comparative Pathology of Chimpanzees" where there were focal coronary and cerebral artery plaques and diffuse lesions in the aorta, but atherosclerosis is considered to be of minor clinical significance in the chimpanzee. One reference reported that coronary atherosclerosis was associated with death in a gorilla (Gray and O'Neal, 1981); but as in the chimpanzee, the condition is infre-

quent and grossly visible lesions of the coronary vessels are rare (Strong and McGill, 1965; Clarkson, 1965).

B. Aneurysm, Stroke, Vasculitis

Spontaneous vascular lesions in the nonhuman primate are observed relatively frequently but are usually seen secondary to primary diseases such as atherosclerosis or to neoplasms invading soft tissue in or around major vessels. It is interesting to note that a number of references in the literature relate many of the lesions to similar clinical entities that are commonly seen in humans. However, there are an insufficient number of definitive references and characterized studies to draw significant related conclusions about the relative incidence of the conditions in nonhuman primates. Enough clinical observations have been documented in nonhuman primates to confirm the importance of this occurrence and to establish spontaneous vascular lesions for consideration in differential diagnosis lists. This is particularly true for captive bred primates maintained in biomedical facilities over a long period of time.

Spontaneous vascular lesions occur in both Old World and New World nonhuman primates with a similar prevalence. Vascular endothelial damage may result from inflammation, infection, endocarditis, or aberrant parasite migration. Many reported vascular lesions typically seen at necropsy include aortic aneurysm, often ones that are arteriosclerotic and dissecting in nature. The anatomical characteristics and location closely resemble those observed in human autopsies (Anderson, 1971; Wyngaarden, 1982). The arteries most often affected in decreasing order of frequency are the aorta, popliteal, femoral, carotid, subclavian, and brachycephalic (Gould and Guttman, 1968). A retrospective study of aneurysms in squirrel monkeys indicated that incidence and type of lesion mimic those of the human (Strickland and Bond, 1983). Atherosclerosis may predispose to the formation of aneurysms. However, this does not appear to be a frequent sequel to experimental atherosclerosis in the squirrel monkey (Boorman *et al.,* 1976; Middleton *et al.,* 1963).

There are differences in the reported prevalence of naturally occurring arterial lesions among Old World nonhuman primate species. The cynomolgus monkey (*M. fascicularis*) appears to be the most susceptible to spontaneous arteriosclerotic lesions, even in their natural habitat of West Malaysia (Prathap and Lau, 1972). The baboon appears to have the next highest prevalence of arteriosclerosis (McGill *et al.,* 1960). Studies of arteries from control rhesus monkeys have suggested that spontaneous lesions are uncommon in that species (Taylor *et al.,* 1962). One reference reports the death of a gorilla caused by a dissecting aneurysm and subsequent cardiac tamponade (Hruban *et al.,* 1986). Aortic dissection is a common cause of death in humans and is usually associated with atherosclerosis, hypertension, and inflammation (Larson and Edmonds, 1984). Only one case of cerebral infarction has been reported in a squirrel monkey but this animal was on an atherogenic diet (Bullock, 1979).

Sex differential may play a possible role in coronary heart disease as reported by Sheridan *et al.* (1989) whereas studies have demonstrated receptors for dihydrotestosterone in the myocardium and smooth muscle cells of arteries from a number of primate species. Further, McGill (1989) has indicated that sex steroid hormone receptors in the cardiovascular system have an impact on cardiovascular disease. Biochemical analyses suggest that sex steroid hormone receptor content and distribution are sexually dimorphic and are modulated by sex steroid hormones. Some aspects of cellular metabolism of these tissues may be subject to local modulation by sex steroid hormones.

C. Thrombosis/Emboli

Thrombosis is a pathologic manifestation of hemostasis that occurs due to a defect (injury) in the vessel wall, stasis of blood flow, and increased coagulability of the blood. The abnormal thrombotic mass can cause occlusion of the vessel lumen; if dislodged from the defect on the vessel wall and carried by the flowing blood, it becomes an embolus. The embolus can then lodge in a smaller vessel at a distant site and produce obstruction to blood flow (ischemia).

Spontaneously occurring thrombi are more than likely associated with many natural diseases but are infrequently reported in the literature. According to Suter and Fox (1995), diseases such as idiopathic hypertension, primary cardiomyopathic disease, or inherited hypertrophic cardiomyopathy can contribute to thrombus formation. Vascular endothelial or vascular wall disorders, sluggish blood flow, or conditions leading to a hypercoagulable state also may advance thrombosis and thromboembolism.

Bacterial endocarditis has been reported more frequently in the rhesus monkey primarily because of the greater number of this particular nonhuman primate used in research. Several publications have also included a chimpanzee (Douglas *et al.*, 1970), a howler monkey (*Alouatta* sp.) (Maruffo and Malinow, 1966), and an African green monkey (Wood *et al.*, 1978). The source of infections for the most part are speculative. Complicating factors of endocarditis associated with thrombosis and embolization include hemodynamic and immunologic interactions. Most valvular heart lesions develop subsequent embolic lesions in the lungs or systemic infections produce secondary heart involvement. The most commonly reported bacteria are *Staphylococcus* or *Streptococcus* species as mentioned previously in Section III, C. Parasitic vasculitis and pulmonary embolization have been reported in cynomolgus (Kornegay *et al.*, 1986) and rhesus monkeys (Baskin and Eberhard, 1982).

Cerebral venous thrombosis was reported in four rhesus monkeys with severe gastrointestinal disease (Sheffield *et al.*, 1981). This syndrome has been associated with severe gastrointestinal disorders in humans.

V. HYPERTENSION

A. Measurement of Blood Pressure

Systemic hypertension is one of the leading risk factors for the development of heart disease in humans. For this reason, experimental studies of nonhuman primates have been conducted (McGill *et al.*, 1961; Hayreh *et al.*, 1989). Although a relationship among hypertension, atherosclerosis, and stroke is well documented in humans, this relationship has yet to be established in nonhuman primates (Kannell *et al.*, 1979). Prusty *et al.* (1988) reported two cases of spontaneous stroke in cynomolgus monkeys that were part of a larger group of 16 on a pharmacologic regimen designed to reduce elevated blood pressure. These two animals showed severe cerebrovascular atherosclerosis and a marked reduction in blood pressure, suggesting that antihypertension medication played a role in their pathogenesis, possibly predisposing stenotic cerebral vessels to the development of occlusive thrombi. Whatever the mechanism, the occurrence of strokes in both humans and monkeys in this setting underscores the potential hazard of excessive treatment of hypertension in the presence of severe atherosclerosis. Current therapy in humans includes bypass or endarterectomy of accessible stenotic vessel segments, coupled with anticoagulant therapy and antihypertensive agents. Earlier studies utilized direct arterial pressure measurement, whereas more recent studies have used auscultatory or oscillatory methods (Mitchell *et al.*, 1982). The oscillometric technique can be easily performed and does not require the placement of a microphone or transducer. The pulsations transmitted from the artery to an inflated cuff are conveyed to a microprocessor in the oscillograph apparatus. Mitchell *et al.* (1982) reported that values recorded from conscious animals were highly correlated to direct intraarterial values. Gavellas *et al.* (1987) reported ease in recording arterial blood pressures in conscious baboons using the oscillometric method. In humans, nonhuman primates, and rodents, cerebral blood flow is autoregulated over a wide range of mean arterial blood pressures. At the lower limit of autoregulation, cerebral blood flow decreases, and at its upper limit it increases. With arterial hypertension, both the upper and the lower limits of autoregulation are set at higher mean arterial blood pressures (Reed and Devons, 1985).

Coelho *et al.* (1991) reported on the effects of social environment on blood pressure and heart rates of baboons. Baboons were tested in individual housing, housing with social companions, and housing with social strangers to evaluate if environmental differences would produce different mean arterial blood pressure and heart rate responses. Housing with social strangers resulted in both elevated blood pressure and elevated heart rate, relative to the social companion condition. Responses observed during this study demonstrated the sensitivity of blood pressure and heart rates to variation in social environment.

B. Types of Hypertension

1. Essential Hypertension

Although several types of experimentally induced hypertension have been reported, only two cases of spontaneous hypertension have been reported in the nonhuman primate. Modi *et al.* (1975) detailed hypertension in wild-caught rhesus monkeys, and Gidde *et al.* (1987) described spontaneous hypertension in woolly monkeys (*Lagothrix* sp.) that subsequently died of congestive heart failure, renal failure, or cerebral vascular accident. These monkeys were affected with arteriolar nephrosclerosis. Despite the renal lesions, the renin levels in these animals remained normal, and thus the hypertension was essential hypertension, idiopathic in nature.

Eichberg and Shade (1987) found that during routine physical examination (under ketamine sedation), blood pressure measurements from 140 male and 170 female chimpanzees (derived over a period of 3 years) increased with age. This information constitutes a useful management tool, identifies essential hypertension in chimpanzees, and suggests that chimpanzees could be used as models for hypertension research.

2. Renovascular Hypertension

Although spontaneous atherosclerosis of the renal arteries has been reported (Chawla *et al.*, 1967; Hamerton, 1937, 1938), no changes in blood pressure were documented. Therefore, the existence of renovascular hypertension in nonhuman primates remains to be established.

3. Pulmonary Hypertension

Weesner and Kaplan (1987) reported extensive pulmonary vascular disease with hypertension in a colony of stump-tail macaques.

VI. LYMPHORETICULAR SYSTEM

The lymphatic system is charged with two main functions. The system of lymphatic vessels drains the interstitial tissues and returns excess tissue fluid to the venous system. Situated along the course of these vessels are large accumulations of lymphoid cells, the lymph nodes. These lymph nodes and the B and T lymphocytes residing therein are essential to providing the body with an adequate immunological defense system.

In addition to the peripheral lymph nodes, other important lymphatic organs include the spleen, thymus, and fixed reticuloendothelial system (RES) cells: the Kupffer cells in the liver and the RES cells of the bone marrow.

A. Peripheral Lymphadenopathy

Generalized peripheral lymphadenopathy is the commonly reported disorder in nonhuman primates, aside from lymphoma and the leukemias previously discussed (Valerio *et al.*, 1969). Lymphatic obstruction may occur when any lesion impedes the normal lymphatic flow. Most types of edema in nonhuman primates are associated with neoplastic lesions or inflammatory lesions that obstruct lymphatics.

Gooteratne (1972) studied the distribution of the lymphatic system by lymphangiography and reported the dominant role of the inguinal lymph nodes in the rhesus monkey. Sapin and Kharin (1981) described the morphology of the lymphatics in rhesus monkeys and baboons. Their study emphasized the structural features of the lymph nodes.

B. Lymphangitis

Zhang *et al.* (1990) described a fulminating lymphangitis caused by *Enterobius* sp. (pinworms) in a chimpanzee. The parasites, whose normal location should be the lumen of the large intestine, were thought to have gained entry to the lymphatic and venous systems via an intestinal ulcer. Other disorders of the lymphatic system, such as lymphangitis, chylothorax, and congenital and acquired lymph edema, have not been reported in nonhuman primates.

REFERENCES

Adams, M. R., Lewis, J. C., and Bullock, B. C. (1984). Hemobartonellosis in squirrel monkeys (*Saimiri sciureus*) in a domestic breeding colony: Case report and preliminary study. *Lab. Anim. Sci.* **34**, 82–85.

Atta, A. G., and Vanace, P. W. (1960). Electrocardiographic studies in the *Macaca mulatta* monkey. *Ann. N.Y. Acad. Sci.* **85**, 811–819.

Baskin, G. B., and Eberhard, M. L. (1982). *Dirofilaria immitis* infection in a rhesus monkey. *Lab. Anim. Sci.* **32**(4), 401–402.

Baskin, G. B., Wolf, R. H., Worth, C. L., Soike, K., Gibson, S. V., and Bieri, J. G. (1983). Anemia, steatitis and muscle necrosis in marmosets (*Saguinus labiatus*). *Lab. Anim. Sci.* **33**, 74–80.

Belkanija, G. S., and Tatojan, S. H. (1976). Electrocardiographic analysis of orthostatic reactions in rhesus monkeys. *Z. Versuchstierkd.* **18**, 247–263.

Bellinger, D., Green, A. W., and Corbett, W. T. (1980). Electrocardiographic studies in African green monkeys (*Cercopithecus aethiops*). *Lab. Anim. Sci.* **30**, 854–859.

Bennett, B. T., Beluhan, F. Z., and Sarpel, S. C. (1981). Acute myelomonocytic leukemia in a capuchin monkey (*Cebus apella*). *Lab. Anim. Sci.* **31**, 519–521.

Bhardwaj, P. R., Jindai, G. D., Dhaeni, J. B., and Brulkar, G. B. (1983). Impedance cardiography in valvular diseases of the heart. *Indian Heart J.* **35**(1), 46–49.

Bieri, J. G., and Poukka Evats, R. H. (1972). Vitamin E nutrition in the rhesus monkey. *Proc. Soc. Exp. Biol. Med.* **140**, 1162–1165.

Blanchard, J. L., Soike, K., and Baskin, G. B. (1987). Encephalomyocarditis virus infection in African green and squirrel monkeys: Comparison of pathologic effects. *Lab. Anim. Sci.* **37**(5), 635–639.

Bond, *et al.* (1980). Myocardial infarction in primates with atherosclerosis. *Am. J. Pathol.* **101,** 675–692.

Boorman, G. A., Silverman, S., and Anderson, J. H. (1976). Spontaneous dissecting aortic aneurysm in a squirrel monkey (*Saimiri sciureus*). *Lab. Anim. Sci.* **26,** 942–947.

Bristow, J. D., and Malinow, M. R. (1965). Spontaneous bundle branch block in rhesus monkeys. *Circ. Res.* **16,** 210–220.

Brizzee, K. R., Ordy, J. M., Dunlap, W. P., Kendrick, R., and Wengenack, T. M. (1988). Phenotype and age differences in blood gas characteristics, electrolytes, hemoglobin, plasma glucose and cortisol in female squirrel monkeys. *Lab. Anim. Sci.* **38,** 200–202.

Bullock, B. C. (1974). Atherosclerosis in pigeons and squirrel monkeys. *Adv. Cardiol.* **13,** 134–140.

Bullock, B. C., Wolf, R. H., and Clarkson, T. B. (1967). Myocarditis associated with trypanosomiasis in a cebus monkey (*Cebus albifrons*). *J. Am. Vet. Med. Assoc.* **151,** 920–922.

Bullock, B. C., Clarkson, T. B., Lehner, N. D. *et al.* (1969). Atherosclerosis in cebus albifrons monkeys (clinical and pathologic studies). *Exp. Med. Pathol.* **10,** 39–62.

Bush, M., Custer, R. S., Whitla, J. C., and Smith, E. E. (1982). Hematologic values of captive golden lion tamarins (*Leontopithecus rosalia*): Variations with sex, age and health status. *Lab. Anim. Sci.* **32,** 294–297.

Bustow, J. D., and Malinow, M. R. (1965). Spontaneous bundle branch block in rhesus monkeys. *Circ. Res.* **16,** 210–220.

Cantrell, C., Baskin, G., and Garcia, R. (1986). Endometritis and valvular endocarditis in a rhesus monkey. *J. Am. Vet. Med. Assoc.* **189,** 1221–1222.

Chakravarti, R. N., and Kukreja, R. S. (1981). Naturally occurring athero-arteriosclerosis in rhesus monkeys. *Indian J. Med. Res.* **73,** 603–609.

Chakravarti, R. N., Kumar, N., Singh, S. P. *et al.* (1975). In vivo thrombolysis. An experimental model in the rhesus monkey. *Atherosclerosis (Shannon, Irel.)* **21**(3), 349–359.

Chakravarti, R. N., Mohan, A. P., and Komal, H. S. (1976). Atherosclerosis in *Macaca mulatta:* Histopathological, morphometric, and histochemical studies in aorta and coronary arteries of spontaneous and induced atherosclerosis. *Exp. Mol. Pathol.* **25,** 390–401.

Chalifoux, L. V., and King, N. W. (1983). Eosinophilic myelocytoma in an owl monkey (*Aotis trivirgatus*). *Lab. Anim. Sci.* **33,** 189–191.

Chalifoux, L. V., Bronson, R. T., Excajadillo, A., and McKenna, S. (1982). An analysis of the association of gastroenteric lesions with chronic wasting syndrome of marmosets. *Vet. Pathol.* **19**(57), 141–162.

Chapman, W. L., Jr. (1968). Neoplasia in nonhuman primates. *J. Am. Vet. Med. Assoc.* **153,** 872–878.

Chawla, K. K., Murthy, C. D. S., Chakravarti, R. N., and Chhuttani, P. N. (1967). Arteriosclerosis and thrombosis in wild rhesus monkeys. *Am. Heart J.* **73,** 85–91.

Cissik, J. H., Hankins, G. D., Hauth, J. C., and Kuehl, T. J. (1986). Blood gas, cardiopulmonary, and urine electrolyte reference values in the pregnant yellow baboon (*Papio cynocephalus*). *Am. J. Primatol.* **11,** 277–284.

Clarkson, T. B. (1965). Spontaneous atherosclerosis in subhuman primates. *In* "Comparative Atherosclerosis" (J. C. Roberts and R. Straus, eds.), pp. 211–214. Harper & Row, New York.

Clarkson, T. B., and Klumpp, S. A. (1990). The contribution of nonhuman primates to understanding coronary artery atherosclerosis in humans. *IL. Nw,* **32,** 4–8.

Clarkson, T. B., Kaplan, J. R., and Adams, M. R. (1984). The role of individual differences in lipoprotein, artery wall, gender, and behavioral responses in the development of atherosclerosis. *Ann. N.Y. Acad. Sci.* **xx,** 28–45.

Coelho, A. M., Carey, K. D., and Shade, R. E. (1991). Assessing the effects of social environment on blood pressure and heart rates of baboons. *Am. J. Primatol.* **23,** 257–267.

Cupp, C. J., and Uemural, E. (1981). Body and organ weights in relation to age and sex in *Macaca mulatta. J. Med. Primatol.* **10,** 110–123.

DePaoli, A., Johnsen, D. O., and Noll, W. W. (1973). Granulocytic leukemia in whitehanded gibbons. *J. Am. Vet. Med. Assoc.* **163,** 624–628.

Dhawan, V., Sharda, N., Majumdar, S., Ganguly, N. K., and Chakravarti, R. N. (1990). Platelet aggregability and serum thromboxane levels in hyperchlolesterolaemic atherosclerotic monkeys. *Med. Sci. Res.* **18,** 149–151.

DiGiacomo, R. F., Gibbs, C. J., Jr., and Gardner, P. C. (1978). Pulmonary arteriosclerosis and thrombosis in a cynamolgus macaque. *J. Am. Vet. Med. Assoc.* **173**(9), 1205–1207.

Donovan, J. C., Stokes, W. S., Montrey, R. D., and Rozmiarek, H. (1983). Hematologic characterization of naturally occurring malaria (*Plasmodium inui*) in cynomolgus monkeys (*Macaca fascicularis*). *Lab. Anim. Sci.* **33,** 86–89.

Douglas, J. D., Schmidt, R. E., and Prine, J. R. (1970). Vegetative endocarditis in a chimpanzee. *J. Am. Vet. Med. Assoc.* **157,** 736–741.

Draper, H. H., and Saari, C. A. (1969). A simplified hemolipis test for vitamin E deficiency. *J. Nutr.* **98,** 390–394.

Eichberg, J. W., and Shade, R. E. (1987). Normal blood pressure in chimpanzees. *J. Med. Primatol.* **16,** 317–321.

Eichberg, J. W., Montiel, M. M., Morale, B. A., King, D. E., Chanh, T. C., Kennedy, R. C., and Dressman, G. R. (1988). *Lab. Anim. Sci.* **38,** 197.

Felton, S. C., Hoffman, C., Kreier, J. P., and Glaser, R. (1984). Hematologic and immunologic responses in common marmosets (*Callithrix jacchus*) infected with plasmodium knowlesi and Epstein-Barr virus. *Lab. Anim. Sci.* **34,** 164–168.

Gleiser, C. A., Carey, K. D., and Heberling, R. L. (1984). Malignant lymphoma and Hodgkin's disease in baboons (*Papio* sp.). *Lab. Anim. Sci.* **34,** 286–289.

Gonder, J. C. (1978). Left anterior fascicular block in an infant rhesus macaque. *J. Am. Vet. Med. Assoc.* **173,** 1232–1234.

Gonder, J. C., Gard, E. A., and Lott, N. E. (1980). Electrocardiograms of nine species of nonhuman primates sedated with ketamine. *Am. J. Vet. Res.* **41,** 972–975.

Gonder, J. C., Houser, W. D., Uno, H., and Poff, B. C. (1982). Myocardial infarction in a rhesus macaque. *J. Am. Vet. Med. Assoc.* **181**(11), 1427–1428.

Gooteratne, B. W. (1972). The lymphatic system in rhesus monkeys (*Macaca mulatta*) outlined by lower limb lymphography. *Acta Anat.* **81,** 602–608.

Gould, L. (1967). The rule of 6. *JAMA, J. Am. Med. Assoc.* **202,** 915–927.

Gould, L., and Guttman, A. B. (1968). Recurrent mitral stenosis in the adult—The contributory role of rheumatic endocarditis. *Dis. Chest* **54,** 146–150.

Gozalo, A., Doyle, G. E., Montoya, E., Weller, R. E., and Malaga, C. A. (1992). Spontaneous cardiomyopathy and nephropathy in the owl monkey (*Aotus* sp.) in captivity. *J. Med. Primatol.* **21,** 279–284.

Gray, R., and O'Neal, R. M. (1981). Sudden death associated with atherosclerosis in a gorilla. *J. Am. Vet. Med. Assoc.* **179,** 1306–1307.

Groover, M. E., Seljeskog, E. L., Haglin, J. J. *et al.* (1963). Myocardial infarction in the Kenya baboon without demonstrable atherosclerosis. *Angiology* **14,** 409–416.

Gutteridge, J. M. C., Taffs, L. F., Hawkey, C. M., and Rice-Evans, C. (1986). Susceptibility of Tamarin (*Saguinus labiatus*) red blood cell membrane lipids to oxidative stress: Implications for wasting marmoset syndrome. *Lab. Anim.* **20,** 140–147.

Hack, C. A., and Gleiser, C. A. (1982). Hematologic and serum chemical reference values for adult and juvenile baboons (*Papio* sp.). *Lab. Anim. Sci.* **32,** 502–505.

Hainsey, B. M., Hubbard, G. B., Leland, M. M., and Brasky, K. M. (1993). Clinical parameters of the normal baboons (*Papio* species) and chimpanzees (*Pan troglodytes*). *Lab. Anim. Sci.* **43,** 236–243.

Hamlin, R. L., and Smith, C. R. (1965). Categorization of common domestic mammals based upon their ventricular activation process. *Ann. N. Y. Acad. Sci.* **127,** 195–203.

Hamlin, R. L., Robinson, F. R., and Smith, C. R. (1961). Electrocardiogram and vectorcardiogram of *Macaca mulatta* in various postures. *Am. J. Physiol.* **201,** 1083–1089.

Hansen, J. F., Alford, P. L., and Keeling, M. E. (1984). Diffuse myocardial fibrosis and congestive heart failure in an adult male chimpanzee. *Vet. Pathol.* **21,** 529–531.

Hayes, R. S. (1986). Tachyrhythmia in a baboon: A case report. *J. Med. Primatol.* **15**, 367–372.

Hayreh, S. S., Servais, G. E., and Virdi, P. S. (1989). Macular lesions in malignant arterial hypertension. *Ophthalmologica* **198**(4), 230–246.

Henderson, J. D., Irv-Webster, W. S., Bullock, B. C. *et al.* (1970). Naturally occurring lesions seen at necropsy in eight wooly monkeys (*Lagothrix* sp.). *Lab. Anim. Care* **20**, 1087–1097.

Holscher, M. A., Sly, D. L., Cousar, J. B., Glick, A. D., and Casagrande, V, A. (1984). Monocytic leukemia in a greater bushbaby (*Galago crassicaudatus argentatus*). *Lab. Anim. Sci.* **34**, 619–620.

Hruban, Z., Meehan, T., Wolff, P., Wollman, R. L., and Glagou, S. (1986). Aortic dissection in a gorilla. *J. Med. Primatol.* **15**(4), 287–293.

Hubbard, G. B., Lee, D. R., and Eichberg, J. W. (1991). Diseases and pathology of chimpanzees at the Southwest Foundation for Biomedical Research. *Am. J. Primatol.* **24** (Part II), 273–282.

Hubbard, G. B., Soike, K. F., Butler, T. M. *et al.* (1992). An encephalomyocarditis virus epizootic in a baboon colony. *Lab. Anim. Sci.* **42**, 233–239.

Hubbard, G. B., Mone, J. P. *et al.* (1993). Spontaneously generated non-Hodgkin's lymphoma in twenty-seven simian T-cell leukemia virus type 1 antibody-positive baboons (*Papio* species). *Lab. Anim. Sci.* **43**, 301–309.

Hugo, N., Kilian, J. G., Dormehl, I. C., and Van Gelder, A. L. (1988). Atrioventricular block in a baboon (*Papio ursinus*). *J. Med. Primatol.* **17**, 135–144.

Jayo, M. J., Jayo, J. M., Jerome, C. P., Krugner-Higby, L., and Reynolds, G. D. (1988). Maxilla-orbital lymphoma (Burkitt's-Type) in an infant *Macaca fascicularis. Lab. Anim. Sci.* **38**, 722–726.

Jayo, M. J., Laber-Laird, K., Bullock, B. C., Tulli, H. M., and Reynolds, G. M. (1990). T-cell lymphosarcoma in a female African green monkey (*Cercopithecus aethiops*). *Lab. Anim. Sci.* **40**, 37–41.

Jerome, C. P. (1987). Congenital malformations and twinning in a breeding colony of old world monkeys. *Lab. Anim. Sci.* **37**, 624–630.

Joax, N. K., Petrali, J. P., and Joax, J. P. (1988). Lymphoma of the pharynx and abdominal wall in two cynomolgus monkeys. *Lab. Anim. Sci.* **38**, 198–200.

Kakoma, I., James, M. A., Jackson, W., Montealegre, F., Bennett, G., Carpunky, P., and Ristic, M. (1987). Distribution, characteristics and relationships between hematologic variables of healthy Bolivian squirrel monkeys. *Lab. Anim. Sci.* **37**, 352–353.

Kalter, S. S. (1980). "The Use of Nonhuman Primates in Cardiovascular Diseases," Southwest Foundation Symposium. University of Texas Press, Austin and London.

Kannell, W. B., Wolf, P. A., Verter, J., and McNamara, M. (1979). Epidemiological assessment of the role of blood pressure in stroke." *JAMA, J. Am. Med. Assoc.* **214**, 301–310.

Kaplan, J. R., Manvick, S. B. *et al.* (1982). Social status, environment, and atherosclerosis in cynomolgus monkeys. *Atheroscler. Thromb.* **2**, 359–368.

Kaplan, J. R., Manuck, S. B. *et al.* (1983). Social stress and atherosclerosis in normocholesterolemic monkeys. *Science* **220**, 733–735.

Kelly, C. A., and Gleiser, C. A. (1986). Selected coagulation reference values for adult and juvenile baboons. *Lab. Anim. Sci.* **36**, 173–175.

Klein, H. O., Sullivan, T. A., and Hoffman, B. F. (1974). Ectopratrial rhythms in the primate. *Am. Heart J.* **87**, 750–656.

Kornegay, R. W., Giddens, W. E., Jr., Morton, W. R., and Knitter, G. H. (1986). Verminous vasculitis, pneumonia, and pulmonary infection in a cynomolgus monkey after treatment with ivermectin. *Lab. Anim. Sci.* **36**(1), 45–47.

Kransch, D. M., and Hollander, W. (1968). Occlusive atherosclerotic disease of the coronary arteries in monkeys (*Macaca iris*) induced by diet. *Exp. Mol. Pathol.* **9**, 1–22.

Kupper, J. L., Kessler, M. J., Clayton, J. D., and Brown, R. J. (1981). Establishment of normal electrocardiographic values for a colony of rhesus monkeys (*Macaca mulatta*) under sedated and unsedated conditions. *J. Med. Primatol.* **10**, 329–335.

Lapin, B. A. (1962). Spontaneous diseases of monkeys and possibility of their use as models of important human diseases. *Vestn. Akad. med. Nauk. SSSR* **17**(11), 82–89.

Lapin, B. A., and Yakovleva, L. A. (1963). "Comparative Pathology in Monkeys," pp. 144–162. Thomas, Springfield, IL.

Larsen, V. P. (1962). Preventive factor in cardiovascular disease—Clinical application of present knowledge of atherosclerosis. *Jpn. Heart J.* **3**, 151–153.

Levin, J. L., and Carey, K. D. (1986). Congestive heart failure and pneumonia in a baboon. *J. Am. Vet. Med. Assoc.* **189**(9), 1226–1227.

Lewis, J. H. (1996). "The Primates: Comparative Hemostasis in Vertebrates," pp. 154–166. Plenum, New York.

Lilly, A. A. (1995). Behavioral and biological markers of stress susceptibility in adolescent female rhesus macaques experiencing separation from natal social groups Doctoral Dissertation, Rutgers University, New Brunswick, Nd. *Diss. Abstr. Int.* **57**, 0745.

Liu, S., Dolensek, E. P., Tappe, J. P., Stover, J., and Adams, C. R. (1984). Cardiomyopathy associated with vitamin E deficiency in seven gelada baboons. *J. Am. Vet. Med. Assoc.* **185**(1), 1347–1350.

Loomis, M. R., Henrickson, R. V., and Anderson, J. H. (1980). Effects of ketamine hydrochloride on the hemogram of rhesus monkeys (*Macaca mulatta*). *Lab. Anim. Sci.* **30**, 851–853.

Machado, C., Mihm, F. G., and Noe, C. (1989). Diagnosis of a ventricular septal defect in a gorilla using in vivo oximetry. *J. Zoo Wildl. Med.* **20**(2), 199–202.

MacKenzie, M., Lowenstine, L., Lalchandani, R., Lerche, N., Osborn, K., Spinner, A., Bleviss, M., Hendrickson, R., and Gardner, M. (1986). Hematologic abnormalities in simian acquired immune deficiency syndrome. *Lab. Anim. Sci.* **36**, 14–19.

Malaga, C. A., Weller, R. E., Buschbom, R. L., and Ragan, H. A. (1990). Hematology of the wild caught karyotype 1 owl monkey (*Aotus nancymai*). *Lab. Anim. Sci.* **40**, 204–206.

Malinow, M. R. (1966). An electrocardiographic study of *Macaca mulatta. Folia Primatol.* **4**, 51–65.

Malinow, M. R., and Storvick, C. A. (1968). Spontaneous coronary lesions in Howler monkeys (*Alouatta caraya*). *J. Atheroscler. Res.* **8**, 421–431.

Maruffo, C. A., and Malinow, M. R. (1966). Dissecting aneurysm of aorta in howler monkey (*Alouatta caraya*). *J. Pathol. Bacteriol.* **92**, 567–570.

McCarthy, T. J., Kennedy, J. L., Blakeslee, Jr., and Bennett, B. T. (1990). Spontaneous malignant lymphoma and leukemia in a simian T-lymphotropic virus type I (STLV-I) antibody positive olive baboon. *Lab. Anim. Sci.* **40**, 79–81.

McClure, H. M. (1975). Hematologic, blood chemistry, and cerebrospinal fluid data for the rhesus monkey. In "The Rhesus Monkey" (G. H. Bourne, ed.), pp. 409–429. Academic Press, New York.

McClure, H. M., and Guiland, W. B. (1975). "Comparative Pathology of the Chimpanzee," Vol. 4, pp. 221–226. Karger, Basel, 1971).

McGill, H. C., Jr. (1989). "Sex Steriod Hormone Receptors in the Cardiovascular System," Symp. Spec. Rep. pp. 64–68. Wyeth-Ayerst Laboratories.

McGill, H. C., Jr., Strong, J. P., Holman, R. L., and Werthessen, N. T. (1960). Arterial lesions in the Kenya baboon. *Circ. Res.* **8**, 670–679.

McGill, H. C., Jr., Frank, M. H., and Gier, J. C. (1961). Ascitic lesions in hypertensive monkeys. *Arch. Pathol.* **71**, 96–102.

McMahan, M. R. (1982). Complement components C3, C4, and BF in six nonhuman primate species. *Lab. Anim. Sci.* **32**, 57–59.

Melville, G. S., Jr., Whitcomb, W. H., and Martinez, R. S. (1967). Hematology of the *Macaca mulatta* monkey. *Lab. Anim. Care* **17**, 189–198.

Mendelow, B., Grobicki, D., de la Hunt, M., Marcus, F., and Metz, J. (1980). Normal cellular and humoral immunologic parameters in the baboon (*Papio ursinus*) compared to human standards. *Lab. Anim. Sci.* **30**, 1018–1021.

Middleton, C. C., Rosal, J., Clarkson, T. B., Lofland, H. B., and Prichard, R. W. (1963). Atherosclerosis in the squirrel monkey, naturally occurring lesions of the aorta and coronary arteries. *Arch. Pathol.* **78**, 16–23.

Mitchell, D. S., Graham, J. R., and Castracane, V. D. (1982). Operant elevation of blood pressure in unrestrained olive baboons (*Papio cynocephalus anubis*). *Am. J. Primatol.* **3**(1–4), 229–238.

Modi, K. K., Suri, R. K., and Chakravarti, R. N. (1975). An experimental model of aortic coarctation in rhesus monkeys. *Indian J. Med. Res.* **67**, 773–780.

Mott, G. E., Jackson, E. M. *et al.* (1992). Dietary cholesterol and type of fat differentially affect cholesterol metabolism and atherosclerosis in baboons. *Am. Inst. Nutr.* 1397–1406.

Mrema, J. E. K., Johnson, G. S., Kelley, S. T., and Green, T. J. (1984). Activated partial thromboplastin time of owl monkey *(Aotus tribirgatus)* plasma. *Lab. Anim. Sci.* **34**, 295–298.

Nakano, M., Mizuno, T., and Gotah, S. (1990). Accumulation of cardae lipofuscin in mammals: Correlation between sexual maturation and first appearance of lipofuscin. *Mech. Ageing Dev.* **52**(1), 93–106.

Ochsner, A. J. (1977). Cardiovascular and respiratory responses to ketamine hydrochloride in the rhesus monkey *(Macaca mulatta). Lab. Anim. Sci.* **27**, 69–71.

Olson, L. C., and Skinner, S. F. (1986). Encephalitis associated with *Trypanosoma cruzi* in a celebes black macaque. *J. Lab. Anim. Sci.* **36**, 667–670.

Omorphos, S. C., Rice-Evans, C., and Harkey, C. (1989). Heinz bodies do not modify the membrane characteristics of common marmoset *(Callithrix jacchus)* erythrocytes. *Lab. Anim.* **23**, 66–69.

Osborne, B. E., and Roberts, C. N. (1972). The elecrocardiogram (ECG) of the baboon *(Papio* spp.). *Lab. Anim.* **6**, 127–133.

Porter, W. P. (1982). Hematologic and other effects of ketamine and ketamineacepromazine in rhesus monkeys *(Macaca mulatta). Lab. Anim. Sci.* **32**, 373–375.

Prathap, K., and Lau, K. S. (1972). Spontaneous and experimental arterial lesions in the Malaysian long-tailed monkey. *J. Med. Primatol.,* (Part III), 343–349.

Prusty, S., Kenyen, T., Moss, M., and Hollander, W. (1988). Occurance of stroke in a nonhuman primate model of cardiovascular disease. *Stroke* **19**(1), 84–90.

Raina, S. N., Chakravarti, R. N., and Berry, J. N. (1971). Diseases in the heart in wild rhesus monkey. *Indian Med. J.* **12**, 483–489.

Randall, D. C., and Hasson, D. N. (1981). Cardiac arrhyhmias in the monkey during classically conditioned fear and excitement. *Pavlovian J. Biol. Sci.* **16**, 97–107.

Reed, G., and Devons (1985). Cerebral blood flow autoregulation and hypertension (Southwest Internal Medicine Conference). *Am. J. Med. Sci.* **289**, 37–44.

Reinhardt, V., Cowley, D., Scheffler, J. *et al.* (1990). Cortisol response of female rhesus monkeys to venipuncture in homecage versus venipuncture in restraint apparatus. *J. Med. Primatol.* **19**, 601–606.

Roberts, W. C., and Innes, J. R. M. (1966). Valvular heart disease in the monkey. *Am. Heart J.* **72**, (2), 206–213.

Robinson, P. T., and Benirschke, K. (1980). Congestive heart failure and nephritis in an adult gorilla. *J. Am. Vet. Med. Assoc.* **177**, (9), 937–938.

Roger, R. F., Hartley, L. H., Ringler, D. J., and Nicolas, R. J. (1986). Hypertrophic cardiomyopathy in owl monkeys *(Aotus trivirgatus)*; clinical diagnosis and clinicopathologic correlations. *Lab. Anim. Sci. J.* **36**, 561–563.

Rommel, F. A., Bendure, D. W., and Kalter, S. S. (1980). Hemolytic complement in nonhuman primates. *Lab. Anim. Sci.* **30**, 1926–1029.

Rosenberg, L. T., Coe, C. L., and Levine, S. (1982). Complement levels in the squirrel monkey *(Saimiri sciureus). Lab. Anim. Sci.* **32**, 371–372.

Sapin, M. R., and Kharin, G. M. (1981). Morphology of the lymphatic organs in some species of monkeys. *Folia Morphol.* **29**, 404–114.

Schiffer, S. P., Gillett, C. S., and Ringler, D. H. (1984). Activated coagulation time for rhesus monkeys *(Macaca mulatta). Lab. Anim. Sci.* **34**, 191–193.

Schmidt, R. E. (1970). Endocardiosis in rhesus monkeys. *Primates* **2**, 177–180.

Schmidt, R. E., (1978). Systemic pathology of chimpanzees. *J. Med. Primatol.* **7**, 274–318.

Scott, R. E., Morrison, E. S., Jarmolych, J. *et al.* (1967). Experimental atherosclerosis in rhesus monkeys—Gross and light microscopy features and lipid values in serum and aorta. *Exp. Mol. Pathol.* **7**, 11–33.

Sheffield, W. D., Squire, R. A., and Strandberg, J. D. (1981) Central venous thrombosis in the rhesus monkey. *Vet. Pathol.* **18**(3), 326–334.

Sheridan, P. J., McGill, H. C., Jr. *et al.* (1989). Heart contains receptors for dihydrotestosterone but not testosterone: Possible role in the sex differential in coronary heart disease. *Anat. Rec.* **223**, 414–419.

Simonson, E. (1974). Principles and pitfalls in establishing normal electrocardiographic limits. *Annu. J. Cardiol.* **33**, 271–276.

Sly, D. L., Toft, J. D. *et al.* (1986). Spontaneous occurrence of *Angiostrongylus costaricensis* in marmosets *(Saguinun mystax). Lab. Anim. Sci.* **32**, 286–288.

Smit, J. A., Stark, J. H., and Myburgh, J. A. (1988). Improved technique for the mixed lymphocyte response in the Chacma baboon. *Lab. Anim.* **22**, 212–216.

Smith, D. G. (1982). Iron binding and transferrin polymorphism in rhesus monkeys *(Macaca mulatta). Lab. Anim. Sci.* **32**, 153–156.

Smith, H. A., Hunt, T. C., and Jones, R. D. (1972). "Diseases Due to Protozoa," *Vet. Pathol.* Lea & Febiger, Philadelphia.

Socha, W. W. (1980). Blood groups of apes and monkeys: Current status and practical applications. *Lab. Anim. Sci.* **30**, 698–702.

Socha, W. W., Rowe, A. W., Lenny, L. L., Lasano, S. G., and Moor-Jankowski, J. (1982). Transfusion of incompatible blood in rhesus monkeys and baboons. *Lab. Anim. Sci.* **32**, 48–56.

Stokes, W. S., Donovan, J. C., Montrey, R. D., Thompson, W. L., Wannemacher, R. W., Jr., and Rosmiarek, H. (1983). Acute clinical malaria *(Plasmodium inui)* in a cynomolgus monkey *(Macaca fascicularis). Lab. Anim. Sci.* **33**, 81–85.

Stout, C. (1968). Atherosclerosis in captive subhuman primates: Findings in sixty-two individuals, twenty-five species. *In* "Use of Nonhuman Primates in Drug Evaluation" (H. Vagtborg, ed.), pp. 494–504. University of Texas Press, Austin.

Strickland, H. L., and Bond, G. M. (1983). Aneurysms in a large colony of squirrel monkeys *(Saimiri sciureus). Lab. Anim. Sci.* **33**, 589–592.

Strong, J. P., and McGill, H. C., Jr. (1965). Spontaneous arterial lesions in baboons. *In* "The Baboon in Medical Research" (H. Vagtborg, ed.), Vol. 1, pp. 471–483. University of Texas Press, Austin.

Sun, S. C., Burch, G. E., Sohal, R. S. *et al.* (1967). Coxsackie virus B4 pancarditis in cynomolgus monkeys resembling rheumatic heart lesions. *Br. J. Exp. Pathol.* **48**, 655–661.

Suter, P. F., and Fox, P. R. (1995). Peripheral vascular disease. *In* "Textbook of Veterinary Internal Medicine" (S. J. Ettinger and E. C. Feldman, eds.), 4th ed., pp. 1068–1067. Saunders, Philadelphia.

Swindle, M. M., Blum, J. R., Lima, S. D., and Weiss, J. L. (1985). Spontaneous mitral valve prolapse in a breeding colony of rhesus monkeys. *Circulation* **71**(1), 146–153.

Swindle, M. M., Kan, J. S., Adams, R. J., Starr, F. L., III, Samphilipo, M. A., Jr., and Porter, W. P. (1986). Ventricular septal defect in a rhesus monkey. *Lab. Anim. Sci.* **36**(6), 693–695.

Taylor, C. B. (1965). Experimentally induced arteriosclerosis in nonhuman primates. *In* "Comparative Atherosclerosis" (J. C. Roberts and R. Straus, eds.), pp. 215–243. Harper & Row, New York.

Taylor, C. B., Cox, G. E., Manalo-Estrella, P., Southworth, J., Patton, R. E., and Cathcait, C. (1962). Atherosclerosis in rhesus monkeys. II. Arterial lesions associated with hypercholesteremia induced by dietary fat and cholesterol. *Arch. Pathol.* **74**, 16–34.

Terao, A., Hiyaoka, A., Cho, F., and Honjo, S. (1988). The simian-type M and the human-type ABO blood groups in the Arican green monkey *(Cercopithecus aethiops)*: Their inheritance, distribution and significance for the management of a breeding colony. *Lab. Anim.* **22**, 347–354.

Toback, J. M., Clark, J. C., and Moorman, W. J. (1978). The electrocardiogram of *Macaca facsicularis. Lab. Anim. Sci.* **28**, 182–185.

Tsai, C., Giddens, W. E., Jr., Morton, W. R., Rosenkranz, S. L., Ochs, H. D., and Benveniste, R. E. (1985). Retroperitoneal fibromatosis and acquired immunodeficiency syndrome in macaques: Epidemiologic studies. *Lab. Anim. Sci.* **35**, 460–464.

Verlangieri, A. J., DePriest, J. C., and Kapeghian, J. C. (1985). Normal, serum biochemical, hematological and EKG parameters in anesthetized adult male *Macaca fascicularis* and *Macaca arctoides. Lab. Anim. Sci.* **35**, 63–66.

Vie, J. C., Cooper, R. W., Dupont, A., and Fassassi-Jarreton, A. (1989). Megaloblastic anemia in a handreared chimpanzee. *Lab. Anim. Sci.* **39,** 613–615.

Weesner, K. M., and Kaplan, K. (1987). Hemodynamic and echocardiographic evaluation of the stumptailed macaque: A potential nonhuman primate model for pulmonary vascular disease. *J. Med. Primatol.* **16,** 185–202.

Wixson, S. K., and Griffith, J. W. (1986). Nutritional deficiency anemias in nonhuman primates. *Lab. Anim. Sci.* **36,** 231–236.

Wolf, R. H., Lehner, N. D. M., Miller, E. C., and Clarkson, T. B. (1969). Electrocardiogram of the squirrel monkey (*Saimire sciureus*). *J. Appl. Physiol.* **26,** 246–351.

Wood, L. L., Bond, M. G., and Bullock, B. C. (1978). Bacterial endocarditis with obstruction in an african monkey. *Lab. Anim. Sci.* **28,** 85–80.

Wright, J. Johnson, D. R., Peterson, D. A., Wolfe, L. G., Deinhardt, F. W., and Maschgan, E. R. (1982). Serology and lymphocyte surface markers of great apes maintained in a zoo. *J. Med. Primatol.* **11,** 67–76.

Yarbrough, L. W., Tollett, J. L., Montrey, R. D., and Beattie, R. J. (1984). Serum biochemical, hematological and body measurement data for common marmosets (*Callithrix jacchus jacchus*). *Lab. Anim. Sci.* **34,** 276–280.

Zhang, G. W., Ji, X. R., and McManus, D. P. (1990). The presence of pinworms (*Erterobius* sp.) in the mesenteric lymph nodes, liver and lungs of a chimpanzee, *Pan troglodytes. J. Helminthol.* **64**(1), 29–34.

Chapter 7

Respiratory Diseases

Kent G. Osborn and Linda J. Lowenstine

NONHUMAN PRIMATES IN BIOMEDICAL RESEARCH: DISEASES

263

I. INTRODUCTION

The respiratory system is one of the most commonly affected systems in reports describing nonhuman primate disease, pathology, and/or clinical management. Such general papers include data pertaining to prosimians (Brockman *et al.,* 1988; Feeser and White, 1992; Kohn and Haines, 1982), New World primates (Abee, 1985; Baer, 1994; Chalmers *et al.,* 1983; Chapman *et al.,* 1973; J. B. Deinhardt *et al.,* 1967; Gozalo and Montoya, 1990, 1992; Kalter, 1985; Lehner, 1984; Nelson *et al.,* 1966; Potkay, 1992; Richter, 1984; Tucker, 1984; Valverde *et al.,* 1993; Weller, 1994), Old World primates (Adang *et al.,* 1987; Courtenay, 1988; Ensley, 1981; Henrickson, 1984; Janssen, 1993; Keeling and Wolf, 1975; Kim and Kalter, 1975a; Munson and Montali, 1990; Schmidt, 1978), or primates in general (Benirschke, 1983; Fiennes *et al.,* 1972; Griner, 1983; Lapin and Yakovleva, 1963; Martin, 1978; Padovan and Cantrell, 1983; Schmidt *et al.,* 1986; Wallach and Boever, 1983). Tables I and II summarize the magnitude and support the importance of respiratory disease in nonhuman primates. Respiratory system structure itself is highly complex. It has evolved to meet a variety of physiologic demands in which the basic physical requirement is intimate contact between large volumes of air and blood. Such contact brings with it a high potential for respiratory system exposure to a myriad of potentially damaging agents carried in the air or blood. An understanding of general respiratory system structure, function, and disease, as well as associated diagnostic approaches and reported respiratory problems in nonhuman primates, is essential for any individual involved in primate medicine.

II. RESPIRATORY SYSTEM STRUCTURE AND FUNCTION

An overview of general respiratory system structure and function can provide a foundation for understanding respiratory vulnerability and response to injury, as well as associated diagnostic and therapeutic methods. Good resources can be found in a comparative lung anatomy monograph by Parent (1992) and in pathology texts (Cotran *et al.,* 1994; Dungworth, 1993; Kobzik and Schoen, 1994; Stookey and Moe, 1978), including a specific primate pathology monograph (Scott, 1992a,b). Additional sources include papers by Boatman *et al.* (1979) and Boyden (1976).

A. Structural and Functional Features of the Respiratory System

1. Upper Respiratory System

The upper respiratory system includes the nasal cavities, nasopharynx, pharynx, larynx, trachea, and bronchi. In a number of primate species, laryngeal diverticula, also called air sacs, are also present (Hill, 1960; Hilloowala, 1971; Swindler and Wood, 1973). A report by Harkema (1991) discusses comparative nasal airway anatomy, including that of primates. Upper respiratory tract function includes air exchange and filtration, separation of food and liquids from the air stream as it enters the tracheobronchial tree, vocalization, and senses of taste, smell, and hearing. This section addresses anatomy and function related to respiratory disorders.

The nasal cavities are bone-encased airways divided by the nasal septum and include osseous and cartilaginous structures, the turbinates. Nasal cavity mucosa includes four conspicuous, distinct epithelial types: stratified squamous epithelium (SE), transitional epithelium (TE), ciliated pseudostratified respiratory epithelium (RE), and olfactory epithelium (OE), as well as a recently described fifth form: lymphoepithelium (LE), which overlies nasal-associated lymphoid tissue (NALT). Respiratory epithelium (RE) includes ciliated, mucous, nonciliated columnar, cuboidal, and basal cells. Olfactory epithelium (OE) is composed of olfactory sensory cells, sustentacular cells, and basal cells. Most of the nasal mucosa epithelial lining is composed of RE, which has many similarities, structurally and in response to injury, to tracheal and bronchial epithelium. Lamina proprial serous, mucus, and mixed tubuloalveolar glands contribute to nasal secretions. The paranasal sinuses are continuous with the nasal cavity and have similar mucosal lining as in the nasal cavity.

The nasopharynx is also supported by surrounding bony structures, with a submucosal layer of striated muscle and two layers of fascia. It is lined by RE, with zones of SE. Lymphoid nodules are present throughout the nasopharyngeal submucosa. The Eustachian (auditory) tubes extend from the nasopharynx to the middle ears and are similarly lined by RE.

Laryngeal, tracheal and bronchial patency is maintained by hyaline cartilage plates and rings. Spaces between the cartilage are made up of fibroelastic membranes, termed the annular tracheal ligament. The ends of incomplete tracheal rings are joined

TABLE I

DIFFERENTIAL DIAGNOSIS OF PRIMATE RESPIRATORY DISEASE: GENERAL DISEASES/SYNDROMES

Disease/lesion	Etiology	Clinical signs		Reported species	Comments
		Respiratory	Other		
Rhinitis, nasal polyposis, and sinusitis	Viruses, allergens, irritant volatile gases, dust, very low atmospheric humidity, certain parasites	Sneezing, nasal discharge, epistaxis, open mouth breathing, occasional cough	Facial swelling, epiphora	Macaques, chimpanzees	
Epistaxis	Trauma, *Branhamella catarrhalis,* see rhinitis/sinusitis	Nasal hemorrhage	—	Macaques	*Branhamella catarrhalis* zoonotic
Nasal cavity foreign body		Sneezing, unilateral nasal discharge, gagging, and retching	None noted in published reports	Macaques, chimpanzees	
Trachiobronchial foreign body		Paroxysmal nonproductive coughing or respiratory distress	Fever, anorexia, depression, and weight loss	Macaques, chimpanzees	
Cleft palate	Congenital anomaly	Nasal regurgitation	Trouble nursing		Susceptible to secondary bacterial or fungal rhinitis and aspiration pneumonia
Air sacculitis	*Klebsiella pneumoniae,* gram-negative and gram-positive enteric organisms	Nasal discharge, intermittent cough, rapid, shallow breathing patterns	Cervical swelling, halitosis, lethargy, anorexia	Owl monkeys, pig-tail macaques, baboons, chimpanzees, pygmy chimpanzees, gorillas, orangutans	Aspiration and secondary pneumonia
Asthma	(1) Extrinsic asthma: extrinsic antigen (2) Intrinsic asthma: respiratory tract infection and inhaled irritants	Dyspnea, coughing, and wheezing; nonproductive cough or exertional dyspnea	None noted in published reports	*Macaca fascicularis,* chimpanzees	(1) May be precipitated by cold, stress or exercise (2) Chronic disease sequelae may include emphysema, chronic bronchitis or pneumonia, or cor pulmonale and heart failure

by smooth muscle, the trachealis. It is not unusual for tracheal ring ossification to occur in older animals. The laryngeal mucosa includes SE from the vestibule to the oral margin of the vocal cords, whereas the posterior lumen is lined by RE. Laryngeal diverticula, the air sacs, which are thought by many to function as a resonating or amplifying apparatus for phonation, are lined by stratified cuboidal and ciliated pseudostratified columnar epithelium. The air sacs pass over the external surfaces of the trachea, thyroids, salivary glands, skeletal muscle in the neck region, and, in some species (orangutans and gorillas), even extend over the clavicles and into the axilla. The air sac opening in monkeys is usually single, on the midline at the base of the epiglottis. In orangutans, there are paired openings directed laterally from the lateral ventricles (Fig. 1). The air sac adventitia is quite vascular and includes abundant adipose tissue

and nerves. The trachea and bronchi are lined by pseudostratified epithelium that includes ciliated, mucous, and nonciliated cells. Nonciliated cells include serous, basal, and neuroendocrine cells. The tracheal and bronchial mucosa also includes lymphocytes, globular leukocytes, and intraepithelial nerve fibers. The submucosa contains connective tissue, blood vessels, lymph channels, nerves, glands, and occasional focal or diffuse lymphocyte infiltrates.

A stereotypic pattern of repair follows injury to the tracheobronchial epithelium. Normal RE exists in a state of low-level turnover. Ciliated cells are terminally differentiated, with little or no regenerative capacity. When epithelial injury occurs, the ciliated cells are sloughed and replaced by nonciliated cell types, primarily mucous cells and nonciliated cells, with basal cells providing a smaller contribution. The mucous and non-

TABLE I—*Continued*

DIFFERENTIAL DIAGNOSIS OF PRIMATE RESPIRATORY DISEASE: GENERAL DISEASES/SYNDROMES

Disease/lesion	Etiology	Clinical signs		Reported species	Comments
		Respiratory	Other		
Neonatal respiratory distress syndrome	Pulmonary surfactant deficiency	Tachypnea, dyspnea	tachycardia, cyanosis	*Macaca nemistrina*	Mechanical ventilation and oxygen toxicity can give rise to a subacute or chronic condition called bronchopulmonary dysplasia
Pulmonary edema	Left-sided or bilateral cardiac failure (cardiogenic edema), hypervolemia, acute brain injury, corrosive gases (including 80–100% oxygen), systemic toxins, endotoxins, and shock-like states	Tachypnea, dyspnea	tachycardia, cyanosis		
Pulmonary thrombosis and embolism	Bacterial emboli, fat emboli, hypercoagulation states, endothelial damage, tumor emboli	Often clinically inapparent; dyspnea, tachypnea	tachycardia	*Macaca fascicularis*	Types of emboli bring with them a variety of possible sequelae
Adult respiratory distress syndrome	Sepsis syndrome, gastric content aspiration, toxic fumes inhalation, oxygen toxicity, near drowning, pulmonary contusion, drugs including heroin, salicylate, and paraquat, pneumonitis (bacterial, viral), pancreatitis, multiple transfusions, fat embolism, amniotic fluid embolism	Respiratory insufficiency	Cyanosis, tachycardia and severe arterial hypoxemia that is not responsive to oxygen therapy		
Diaphragmatic hernia	Congenital, trauma	Low-grade respiratory signs, possibly associated with exercise or posture (recumbency)	Episodic gastrointestinal distress	Baboons, chimpanzees, rhesus monkeys, squirrel monkeys, golden lion tamarins	Presence of subclinical hernia may be unmasked by the development of secondary problems (see text)

ciliated cells regenerate themselves and undergo differentiation into ciliated cells and other epithelial types.

Approximately 50% of total airway resistance occurs in the nasal cavities. The nasal mucosa functions to warm and humidify inspired air, as it includes a large surface area and has extensive submucosal vascular plexuses, particularly in the turbinates and nasal septum. Nasal plexus hyperemia can cause a significant decrease in nasal airway caliber, resulting in increased airflow resistance. Of the remaining airflow resistance, approximately 80% is present in the first four to seven bronchial tree divisions, in which airflow is rapid. Relatively small amounts of bronchoconstriction or air wall edema and inflammation can cause large increases in overall respiratory resistance and ascultable airway sounds.

A key upper respiratory tract function involves the removal of larger particles and water-soluble gases via the mucous lining. Depending on the material, this occurs via inertial impaction, gravitational sedimentation, diffusion, or a combination of these. Inertial impaction occurs primarily in the nasal passages and pharynx at points of air stream change in direction and turbulence. Gravitational sedimentation and diffusion take place primarily in the lower respiratory system and are discussed later in relation to the vulnerability and formation of certain lesions in those areas. Virtually all particles greater than 10 μm in diameter are deposited above the nasopharynx, as are a large percentage of inhaled particles smaller than 10 μm. This deposition is associated with initial replication of many viral and bacterial agents in the upper respiratory epithelium and

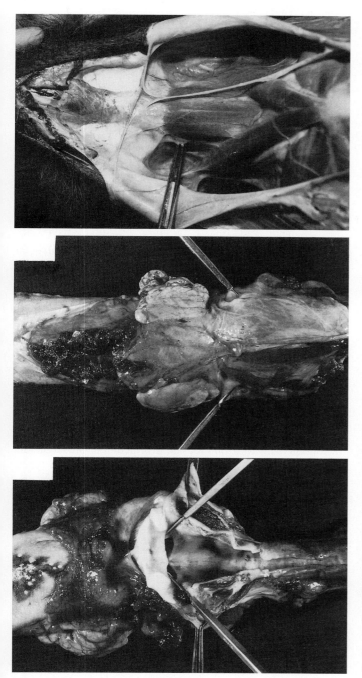

Fig. 1. Cervical air sacs, orangutan (*Pongo pygmaeus*). (top) Orangutan cervical air sacs, ventral view *in situ*. Right external ostium indicated with forceps. Note extension of air sac space over clavicles and shoulders. (middle) Orangutan larynx, ventral view. Probes indicate position of external ostea that connect the larynx to the cervical air sacs. (bottom) Orangutan larynx, dorsal view. Probes indicate position of lateral vestibules, connection point leading to the cervical air sacs.

lymphoid tissue before they spread systemically or are redistributed into the lower respiratory tract after nebulization and inspiration.

The mucociliary blanket consists of a mucus layer with physical properties of viscoelastic gel, which lies over a watery sol into which the cilia project and beat. The gel–sol mucus layer is derived from surface mucous cells and submucosal glands that include both serous and mucous secretory cells. The mucociliary blanket moves toward the pharynx at a velocity of 5 to 15 mm/min. These secretions and deposited materials are subsequently cleared when they are swallowed after they reach the pharynx. When circumstances result in airway secretion volume that is greater than can be cleared by normal mucociliary clearance, coughing is an important mechanism that aids in the movement of this additional material. Well-developed lymphoid tissue in the tonsillar and dorsal nasopharyngeal regions provides the opportunity for immune response to the variety of antigens deposited there, but also provides a route for primary infection by organisms such as *Mycobacterium paratuberculosis* and *Brucella* spp. (Dungworth, 1993). The transport and deposition of particles from the mucociliary blanket provide a mode of spread for diseases such as tuberculosis and a variety of helminth eggs and larvae. Normal mucociliary function depends on intact, functional ciliated epithelium and the normal viscous properties and quantity of secretions. Problems with one or more of these can predispose to infection.

Additional activity of the tracheobronchial mucosa includes the metabolism of a number of endogenous and xenobiotic compounds, the synthesis and secretion of neutral endopeptidase, interferon, lysozyme and lactoferrin, and the synthesis and secretion of immunoglobulins (Ig), primarily IgA, by nasal and bronchial associated lymphoid tissue (NALT and BALT). Clara cells (nonciliated epithelia cells) have high cytochrome P450 monooxygenase activity, which can activate a number of xenobiotic compounds into pulmonary toxins. Tracheobronchial epithelial cells metabolize arachidonic acid to eicosanoids, including prostaglandin E_2 and hydroxyeicosatetraenoic acid (12-HETE), which may regulate local smooth muscle tone and vascular flow. Neutral endopeptidase is an enzymatic regulator of airway neuropeptides such as substance P and neurokinin A, which in turn can stimulate increased vascular permeability and airway smooth muscle contraction. Following injury and interaction with cytokines, bronchial epithelial cells can also upregulate the expression of intercellular adhesion molecule-1. Intracellular adhesion molecule-1 promotes adhesion and migration of circulating neutrophils and monocytes into airways during an inflammatory reaction. Interferon is a nonspecific compound that can help limit local viral infection, whereas lysozyme and lactoferrin have selective antibacterial activity. The presence of pathogen-specific secretory IgA on the respiratory mucosa is one of the most important components of immunity to respiratory pathogens. Finally, normal bacterial flora in the nose and nasopharynx are important in that they specifically adhere to receptors on cilia and epithelial surfaces, preventing adherence and colonization by more virulent organisms.

2. Lower Respiratory System

The lungs make up the lower respiratory system. They are generally divided into multiple lobes on each side, with differences in lung lobation among the different primate groups (Scott, 1992a,b). The right lung in prosimians, New World monkeys, and many Old World species has four lobes, except for a few prosimians and Cebidae, which have three right lobes as well as the great apes, which lack the accessory (azygous) lobe. The left lung of smaller and more primitive species consists of two lobes, whereas the larger Old World species generally have three and great apes generally have two. An interesting exception to this lobation is the orangutan, which has a single lung lobe on each side. An important anatomic variation of note is the right superior bronchus site of origin. In some species (e.g., orangutan and bonobo), it branches from the trachea proximal to the main tracheal bifurcation at the carina, increasing the possibility for accidental obstruction during tracheal intubation, leading to atelectasis of the right cranial lung lobe (Robinson and Janssen, 1980). The bronchi progressively branch and decrease in diameter, eventually becoming bronchioles, the last generation of which is termed the terminal bronchiole. The branching airways are accompanied by a double arterial supply, the pulmonary and bronchial arteries. Bronchioles are distinguished from bronchi by the absence of cartilage and submucosal glands within their walls. Each terminal bronchiole opens to the functional unit for gas exchange, the acinus. An individual acinus includes respiratory bronchioles, alveolar ducts, alveolar sacs, alveoli, and associated blood vessels.

With no cartilage in the bronchiole walls, bronchiole patency is dependent on the attachment of interalveolar septa to a thin connective tissue layer in the bronchiolar wall. As lung volume increases, the radially arranged interalveolar septa pull on the bronchiolar wall, with a resulting maximal bronchiolar luminal diameter during maximum volume. This process is reversed with expiration, such that small bronchioles may collapse at low volume. Airflow out of the pulmonary acinus supplied by the collapsed bronchiole ceases without sufficient collateral ventilation. The thin walls, collapsibility, and small diameter of bronchioles make them much more susceptible than bronchi to pathologic processes occurring in the surrounding alveolar parenchyma. Similarly, inflammatory processes originating in bronchioles are likely to spread to adjacent alveoli. The small lumens increase the likelihood for bronchioles to become obstructed by inflammatory exudate. Although the resistance to airflow in individual bronchioles is high, the total cross-sectional area of all bronchiolar generations is considerably larger than that of the bronchi. Consequently, pathologic processes that affect small numbers of bronchioles can be clinically inapparent with regard to signs of airway obstruction. Clinically apparent disease usually occurs only when a large percentage of bronchioles are affected.

Proximal generation bronchioles are generally lined by epithelium similar to that in the distal bronchi. Distal, small caliber bronchioles are lined by simple columnar to cuboidal epithelial lining that is made up almost entirely of ciliated cells and nonciliated bronchiolar (Clara) cells. The nonciliated cells have regenerative capacity as described earlier with regard to respiratory epithelial response to injury. Clara cells have a high concentration of cytochrome P450 monooxygenase enzyme systems, making them particularly sensitive to toxic injury by xenobiotic compounds.

The alveolar parenchyma includes capillary endothelium, type I and type II alveolar epithelial cells, and alveolar macrophages, as well as fibroblasts and other interstitial cells. Covering approximately 93% of the alveolar surface, type I alveolar epithelial cells are squamous cells across which gas exchange occurs. They are vulnerable to injury by a variety of agents, with little ability to adapt to injury. Injured type I cells usually quickly slough from the basement membrane. Type II alveolar cells are cuboidal cells, making up approximately 7% of the alveolar septum surface area. They have a number of key functions, including pulmonary surfactant production, differentiation to type I cells during normal turnover, and rapid proliferation to cover the exposed alveolar basement membrane in response to type I cell damage and loss. Type II cells also synthesize a variety of matrix components, including fibronectin, type IV collagen, and proteoglycans. They also metabolize arachidonic acid to form eicosanoids, including prostaglandin E_2, which influences the function of other alveolar cell types. Finally, type II cells can express major histocompatibility complex (MHC) I receptors and function as antigen-presenting cells.

The lungs represent the largest capillary bed in the body. Alveolar capillary endothelial cells are the initial permeability barriers between capillary lumen and pulmonary interstitium, with important transport functions for solutes, water, and gases. Among their many metabolic functions are uptake and clearance of serotonin, norepinephrine, prostaglandins E and F, bradykinin, hormones, and drugs. Endothelial cells have angiotensin-converting enzyme activity, converting angiotensin I to angiotensin II. They are sensitive to toxic damage by xenobiotic compounds, due to cytochrome P450 monooxygenase activity. Endothelial cells upregulate cell adhesion molecules when exposed to a number of mediators, including leukotriene B_4, as well as cytokines such as tumor necrosis factor and interleukins 1–8. This facilitates attachment and migration of neutrophils and other leukocytes into the interstitium and alveoli.

Alveolar fibroblasts are connective tissue cells with heterogenous morphology and varying protein synthetic activity, contractile function, and cell and matrix interactions. The alveolar interstitial matrix includes elastic and collagen types I, III, IV, V, and VI, with a predominance of types I and III. Other pulmonary fibroblast products include laminin, fibronectin, glycosaminoglycans, and proteoglycans. This admixture of intercellular matrix components contributes to lung mechanical properties.

Four types of macrophage populations are present in the lungs. These include alveolar macrophages, interstitial macrophages, pulmonary intravascular macrophages (which are not present in all species), and dendritic cells. Alveolar macrophages are a key pulmonary defense against agents that reach the alveoli after bypassing upper respiratory tract defenses. Derived from blood monocytes, alveolar macrophages undergo a maturation step in the interstitium before they migrate into the alveolar lumen, except in inflammatory states, during which they migrate directly into the alveolus. The wide variety of alveolar macrophage functions starts with phagocytosis and killing of infectious agents and degradation of other phagocytosed particles. They also have a key role in inflammatory, immune, and repair process control, mediated through their release of cytokines and a variety of regulatory molecules. Among the macrophage-produced cytokines are interleukin-1, tumor necrosis factor, interferon α and γ, and histamine releasing factor. Inflammatory mediators released by alveolar macrophages include leukotriene B_4 and C_4, platelet-activating factor, and thromboxane A_2. Macrophage-associated control and regulation of repair processes come through the release of cytokines such as transforming growth factor β and α, fibroblast growth factor, insulin-like growth factor, and platelet-derived growth factor. Finally, alveolar macrophages have a role in cellular and humoral immune responses as antigen-presenting cells.

Dendritic cells are present in the alveolar interstitium and airway lamina propria. They are bone marrow-derived leukocytes with enhanced antigen-presenting capacity. These cells lack phagolysosomes, have a very irregular, folded nucleus, and numerous long, irregular dendritic processes. They normally express high levels of MHC class I and II molecules and common leukocyte antigen. They lack many of the cytoplasmic surface markers of mononuclear phagocytes and do not efficiently phagocytize particles. Pulmonary intravascular macrophages (PIM) are unique mononuclear phagocytes that have been found in the lung of certain species, including cattle, sheep, pigs, goats, cats, and humans. They are present in alveolar capillary lumens as large mature macrophages, attached to endothelium via membrane adhesive complexes. These highly phagocytic cells play a role in the clearance of circulating bacteria and particles as they pass through the pulmonary circulation. They release a variety of inflammatory mediators in association with this clearance process, thus contributing to acute pulmonary inflammation.

Inspired particles that are not removed in the upper respiratory tract are deposited in the lower respiratory tract via gravitational settlement and diffusion. Gravitational settlement is proportional to particle size and density and generally occurs in the relatively still air of the most distal parts of the respiratory system. Diffusion involves particles less than 0.3 μm in diameter and requires minimal flow as occurs in the alveoli. With decreasing size of particles (less than 10 μm), an increasing proportion pass into the deep lung. Many of these are subsequently exhaled; however, droplet nuclei and other irritant or infectious particles approximately 1–2 μm in diameter tend to deposit at the bronchiolar–alveolar junction. This phenomenon is associated with the sudden drop of the air stream linear velocity to zero at this point, due to the abrupt increase in the airspace cross-sectional area. It is a major factor in the apparent vulnerability of the bronchiolar–alveolar junction to damage by inhaled irritants.

Alveolar macrophage phagocytosis is the key to alveolar defense against small-sized particles. Although phagocytosis can occur within a relatively short time (e.g., 4 hr after alveolar deposition of bacteria), the physical removal of particulates from alveoli is inefficient compared to particles deposited on the mucociliary blanket. Depending on particle physical nature and irritant characteristics, it can take several days to months or longer for 50% clearance of particles. Macrophage-phagocytosed particles are either inactivated or sequestered as the macrophages move toward the bronchioles and onto the mucociliary blanket. If not phagocytized, particles within the alveoli tend to be cleared with the alveolar lining liquid as it moves centripetally to the bronchioles or it may penetrate the pulmonary interstitium. The latter tends to occur more with increased particulate load. Interstitial penetration is generally by endocytosis across alveolar type I epithelial cells. Particles within the interstitium are removed with lymph flow and are phagocytosed by interstitial macrophages. Peribronchiolar and perivascular clusters of particle-laden macrophages are associated with lymphatics, with some eventually moving to local lymph nodes.

The alveolar-lining liquid contains a variety of factors that are important for helping to maintain alveolar sterility and to protect against tissue damage. Immunoglobulin G is the primary immunoglobulin in the liquid. Both IgG and surfactant are important opsonizing factors that enhance phagocytosis by alveolar macrophages. Lysozyme, lactoferrin, and complement are additional factors with roles in pathogen control. Catalase and the glutathione peroxidase system, which help protect against reactive oxygen radical-associated injury, and α_1-antitrypsin, which contributes to protection against acute lung injury and development of alveolar emphysema, are important humoral components of the pulmonary-lining liquid.

3. Pulmonary Circulatory and Lymphatic Systems

The pulmonary circulation receives the entire output of the right ventricle via the pulmonary artery. It is a low pressure system made up of densely anastomosing capillaries in the alveolar septa. The bronchial artery, originating from the aorta, is the second blood source in the dual pulmonary blood supply. The pulmonary artery carries systemic venous blood to the pulmonary parenchyma for gaseous exchange in the alveolar capillaries. The pulmonary arteries generally run parallel to the bronchi and bronchioles, with a similar branching pattern. With their origin in the aorta, the bronchial arteries supply oxygenated blood to the airways and supporting pulmonary connective tissue, including the pulmonary artery vasa vasorum. Bronchial artery branches are closely associated with bronchial and bronchiolar walls. Venous drainage of the lungs occurs primarily through the pulmonary veins, with just a small amount of blood returning through the bronchial veins. Normal pulmonary and cardiac function are closely interdependent. This is evident with the observation that cardiovascular diseases can result in impaired respiratory function in association with pulmonary edema and congestion, whereas chronic pulmonary diseases that interfere with pulmonary blood flow can affect normal heart function and systemic circulation.

The dual supply, extensive anastomosis and function as a capillary bed through which the entire right ventricle output flows, provides a mechanism for efficient filtration and trapping of emboli while minimizing the potential damage due to vascular obstruction. Common emboli include bacteria, fungi, protozoa, endogenous fat, normal cells (e.g., megakaryocytes), or abnormal cells (usually neoplastic). Other emboli can include fragments of thrombi, helminth parasites for which the respiratory system is a natural or accidental habitat, and even parasitic ova. Rare emboli that may be found in the lung circulation include epidermal fragments and hair inadvertently introduced into the blood during injections or intervertebral disk nucleus pulposis fragments. This blood filter function of the pulmonary circulation can be both beneficial and a source for additional problems. The trapping of emboli serves to prevent them from reaching the systemic circulation and causing infarction in major organs such as heart, brain, and kidneys. Problems can occur as it serves to set up the lungs themselves as sites of spreading infection, tumor metastasis, and pulmonary thromboembolism.

Pulmonary lymphatic drainage occurs through a subpleural network as well as through perivascular and peribronchial lymph channels. The lymph flow is centripetal, eventually draining through hilar (tracheobronchial) lymph nodes. In addition, direct lymphatic connections are known to exist between lower lung lobes and the diaphragmatic and coeliac lymph nodes in humans. Such connections could provide a potential route for the extension of pathologic processes between the thorax and the abdomen. Lymphatic channels are not demonstrable in alveolar septa.

III. APPROACH TO THE PATIENT WITH RESPIRATORY DISEASE

A. Signs of Respiratory System Disease

1. Sneezing and Nasal Discharge

Sneezing and nasal discharge are primary signs of sinus, nasal, and nasopharyngeal disorders. The approach to the veteri-

nary patient with sneezing and nasal discharge is reviewed by McKiernan (1995). With persistent disease, sneezing may decrease, whereas nasal discharge may increase in volume and change character.

Sneezing is an involuntary airway reflex that is an important protective respiratory system defense mechanism. Among the many primary causes of sneezing are congenital anomalies (e.g., cleft palate, cilial defects), inflammatory conditions (e.g., allergy), and infections (e.g., virus, bacteria, fungi, parasites). Other direct causes include mechanical and chemical stimuli (e.g., foreign bodies, environmental dusts, odors, or pollutants) and simple trauma.

Nasal secretions normally are cleared via the mucociliary apparatus toward the nasopharynx. When material appears at the external nares (nasal discharge), it can be due to excessive secretion production and/or decreased clearance ability (e.g., due to obstruction). Extranasal disease can cause nasal discharge as well, as noted later.

The character of the nasal discharge provides important clues about the primary medical condition. The type of discharge can be serous, mucoid, mucopurulent, purulent, blood-tinged, overtly bloody (epistaxis), and/or may include food particles. Most nasal and sinus diseases start with a serous discharge, but with persistence of the primary cause can progress to mucoid, then mucopurulent, then purulent. The presence of blood can be associated with a number of conditions, including focal irritation/inflammation, erosion or ulceration, mucosal capillary trauma associated with violent sneezing, or as part of a systemic disease such as coagulopathy or thrombocytopenia. Whether the discharge is initially unilateral or bilateral can help in suggesting the type of disease process. For example, a unilateral discharge could be associated with upper arcade dental disease, nasal foreign body, nasal tumor, or mycotic infection or parasites. When a nasal discharge is bilateral from the start, it may suggest viral or bacterial infection, allergy, environmental agents (e.g., dust, smoke), or extranasal disease (such as pneumonia, esophageal stricture, megaesophagus, and cricopharyngeal disorders).

2. Dyspnea and Tachypnea

Dyspnea is the presence of labored or difficult breathing. The assessment of respiratory rate, rhythm, and character is used to determine whether an inappropriate degree of breathing effort is present. Dyspnea is further characterized as exertional, paroxysmal (suddenly recurring or intensified), or continuous, with differences due to the cause and extent of the abnormality. Tachypnea, an increased rate of breathing, is not necessarily an indication of respiratory disease, as it occurs in a number of normal physiological states, such as exercise, hyperthermia, or anxiety. Orthopnea indicates difficulty breathing while recumbent, such that orthopnic animals tend to maintain an upright position. The cardinal importance of normal respiratory function to homeostasis is reflected in the occurrence of dyspnea and tachypnea when any of a number of systems are involved, including respiratory, cardiovascular, hematologic, and nervous systems, as well as certain metabolic disorders. The general approach to the dyspneic veterinary patient is reviewed by Turnwald (1995).

A variety of disorders associated with dyspnea involve airway obstruction at one or more sites, with the obstruction source potentially being within the lumen, within the airway wall, or externally compressing the airway. Obstruction above the thoracic inlet tends to result in increased inspiratory effort, whereas lower airway obstruction is often associated with increased expiratory effort. In either case, obstructive disease may include tachypnea. A second set of dyspnea-associated disorders functionally limit normal lung expansion and can include pulmonary parenchymal disease, as well as disorders of the pleural space, diaphragm, peritoneum, or peripheral nerves. Such disorders, termed restrictive respiratory disorders, often are associated with rapid, shallow breathing patterns. Some conditions can have both obstructive and restrictive elements.

Among the dyspnea-associated problems that are not primary respiratory disorders are certain nervous system, anemia-associated, and metabolic disorders. Nervous system disorders include brain disease, spinal cord, and peripheral nerve disorders. The respiratory effect of brain disease varies with the anatomic distribution of the lesion. Tachypnea may be present, and breathing depth may be more or less than normal. An increase in breathing rate and depth occurs as respiratory compensation for a variety of disorders that result in metabolic acidosis. The level of anemia-associated hypoxia that leads to dyspnea varies among individuals and in association with the rate of onset of anemia, with acute onset hypoxia more often causing respiratory changes than slower onset disorders. As with compensation for metabolic acidosis, breathing rate and depth are generally increased in anemia-associated dyspnea.

3. Cough

Excess secretions and foreign bodies can be cleared from the tracheobronchial tree by coughing, which involves explosive expiratory effort. Coughing can be reflexive or voluntary. Cough is triggered by foreign materials and inflammation-associated stimulation of airway cough receptor nerves. The end result of the cough sequence is an intratracheal air flow rate that approaches the speed of sound, producing efficient shearing forces and subsequent movement of material up the airways to the pharynx.

B. Diagnostic Procedures in Respiratory Disease

A diagnostic plan always should start with a good history and physical examination. Radiographic imaging is the third common information source upon which the differential diagnostic list for respiratory disease is initially established. The results of these primary steps can help suggest a logical progression for further diagnostic workup, with varying degrees of invasiveness and need for equipment and technical support and ability. Decisions made in further pursuing the diagnostic plan must take into account variable sensitivity and specificity of each procedure and their associated interpretation problems and diagnostic value.

1. Physical Examination and History

History and signalment can give useful diagnostic clues due to the prevalence of certain disorders in association with the background of an animal. Congenital conditions, e.g., cleft palate, pectus excavatum, and diaphragmatic hernia, are more likely to be associated with clinical signs in young animals. Middle-aged or older animals are more likely to have neoplastic or chronic disorders (e.g., chronic dental disease as a cause of nasal disease). Husbandry associated conditions include environment (indoor vs outdoor housing), with differing potential for air pollutant, allergen, or foreign body exposure, trauma, and so on, and geographic origin and history, which can indicate potential for exposure to various mycotic organisms (e.g., coccidioidomycosis, histoplasmosis, blastomycosis). A previous medical history can reveal problems (trauma, surgery, dental disease, allergy, etc.) that could subsequently have led to the current presenting problem. Differential diagnosis can be refined with information about vaccination history (e.g., measles vaccination) and response to previous medical treatments (e.g., antibiotic responsiveness can occur with tooth abscesses or foreign bodies but generally not in association with neoplastic disease or mycotic infection) can help as well in forming a diagnosis. Other important information can include the duration and progression of signs such as nasal discharge or dyspnea (e.g., unilateral vs bilateral nasal discharge, changes in discharge character), evidence of exercise intolerance, and the involvement of other body systems (e.g., mouth, eyes, regional lymph nodes).

A comprehensive physical examination of a patient with respiratory signs involves observation, palpation, auscultation, and, at times, percussion. The physical examination should assess the animal in general, with particular emphasis on the upper and lower respiratory tracts and the cardiovascular system, as respiratory and cardiovascular disorders can frequently lead to similar signs. Elements of observation include the presence of discharges, deformities, or other lesions and the presence of sneezing or coughing. The breathing pattern character (rate and rhythm, effort during inspiration and expiration) and the intensity and quality of respiratory sounds (wheezing, crackles) are additional important factors to note. Features of importance regarding nasal discharge include discharge characteristics and whether it is unilateral or bilateral. Open mouth breathing in an otherwise calm, unstressed animal may be a sign of bilateral nasal obstruction, complete nasopharyngeal obstruction, or severe lower respiratory tract disease. Cyanosis occurs in severely affected animals. General systemic signs such as weight loss, anorexia, and depression can occur at the same time and may be the only sign(s). Hypoxia and acute hypercapnea can be associated with disturbances in mentation and even coma.

Important aspects of the physical examination of animals with other evidence of nasal involvement include assessment of nasal airflow, presence of possible bony or other palpable changes, and examination of mouth, regional lymph nodes, and eyes. Airflow assessment techniques can include visually comparing the size of condensation formed by airflow out of either nostril onto a smooth cool surface such as a glass slide or ophthalmoscope base and/or listening to or feeling the airflow out of each nostril while the other one is occluded. The nasal, sinus, and oral regions should be palpated for evidence of distortion or swelling. Percussion and transillumination can be additional helpful techniques for the evaluation of possible sinus filling. A careful oral examination is essential for the assessment of possible nasal cavity problems. This would include examination of the hard palate (defects, swellings), soft palate (ventral depression associated with nasopharyngeal swelling), oral mucosa in general (trauma, erosions, ulcers, plaques, petechia/purpura), and tonsils, teeth, and periodontia. Local lymph nodes (submandibular, retropharyngeal) may be enlarged in association with neoplasia and/or chronic inflammation/infection. Ocular examination findings that can relate to rhinitis include conjunctivitis and, to a lesser extent, chorioretinitis.

For assessment of dyspneic animals, thoracic auscultation is crucial. This would include evaluation of thoracic pulmonary and heart sounds, as well as respiratory sounds directly over the trachea, larynx, and nose. The latter steps can help localize the site of a lesion, with sounds generally more intense near their site of origin. Swollen cervical lymph nodes or other cervical soft tissue structures can be the cause of tracheal narrowing and associated respiratory difficulty.

Laboratory tests (CBC, serum chemistry, urinalysis, and more specific tests such as a coagulation panel) are an important aspect of the overall workup of an animal. Results can be useful for indicating the presence of such systemic disorders as bacterial infection (pneumonia), anemia, thrombocytopenia, coagulopathy, or metabolic acidosis associated with renal failure or diabetes.

2. Radiography and Other Imaging Techniques

Radiography is a generally available diagnostic technique that can provide valuable information for localizing and initially characterizing respiratory system lesions (Silverman, 1975). It also often provides clues for the selection of subsequent diagnostic procedures. Positioning can be very important, with the most useful views being those that can help differentiate which side is affected, while minimizing the overlap of structures of interest. For nasal radiographs, such features as loss of symmetry, increases or decreases in nasal cavity density, bone abnor-

malities, and the presence of foreign bodies are some of the more frequently occurring changes with nasal disease. Tracheal radiographs are evaluated for variation in diameter and course. At times, contrast studies are needed in cases of suspected tracheal rupture or fracture or to help visualize suspected radiolucent foreign bodies. Thoracic radiographs are generally made with the animal in erect position, with exposure timed to coincide with near peak inspiration. Use of the lateral decubitus position may be helpful for revealing small pleural effusions not evident with the upright position. Many pulmonary diseases can have a variety of possible radiographic patterns, with no pattern specific enough to establish a diagnosis, but particular patterns can more often be associated with certain diseases (Gillett et al., 1984; Goldberg et al., 1991; Karesh et al., 1990; Marcella and Wright, 1985; Odkvist and Schauman, 1980; Rawlings and Splitter, 1973; Robinson and Bush, 1981; Silverman et al., 1975, 1976; Stills and Rader, 1982; Wolff et al., 1989).

Certain other special imaging techniques can be helpful (Friedman, 1994). Computed tomography (CT) and magnetic resonance imaging (MRI) can provide additional detail for skull internal structure in particular and are becoming more available at regional diagnostic facilities. Computed tomography can be particularly useful in determining the extent of a problem, including whether it has extended into epidural areas or the brain itself (Cambre, 1986). For thoracic imaging, CT is useful for characterizing pleural disease (e.g., differentiating fluid from tumor); with contrast injections, differentiating tissue masses from vascular structures; and identifying small parenchymal nodules. Magnetic resonance imaging remains largely an investigational technique for pulmonary disease imaging, with potential to provide fine definition of mediastinal and pleural lesions. Early use of these highly sensitive techniques is somewhat compromised because little base line information is available to indicate how many "normal" individuals have the small, previously undetected parenchymal lesions, and it is not yet known how to differentiate the specific type of lesion (e.g., is it neoplastic?). Pulmonary scintigraphy provides the opportunity to further differentiate and locate various disease processes (e.g., inflammation, neoplasia), using radionucleotides with affinity for certain cells types (Karesh et al., 1990).

3. Skin and Serologic Tests

Skin tests for specific antigens are available, including tuberculosis, coccidioidomycosis, histoplasmosis, blastomycosis, trichinosis, toxoplasmosis, and aspergillosis. Tuberculosis skin testing is commonly used with nonhuman primates as an important part of preventive medicine programs (Henrickson, 1984; Southers and Ford, 1995). Tuberculin testing of nonhuman primates provides a good example of the potential variability in sensitivity and specificity when performing skin tests in general (Chaparas et al., 1975; Dillehay and Huerkamp, 1990; Kaufmann and Anderson, 1978; Kuhn and Selin, 1978; McLaughlin and

Marrs, 1978; Wells *et al.,* 1990). As with skin testing antigens, a number of potentially useful serologic tests have been developed that include a variety of infectious agents that involve the respiratory system. Using appropriate serologic tests can help avoid the use of more extensive/invasive diagnostic procedures. Sensitivity, specificity, and the specific types of available serologic tests [e.g., enzyme-linked immunosorbent assay (ELISA), agar gel immunodiffusion, indirect immunofluorescence, latex agglutination] vary within institutions, however, requiring close interaction with the responsible laboratory for test result interpretation.

4. Endoscopy

Rhinoscopy and bronchoscopy provide the opportunity for direct visualization of the areas, biopsy of suggestive or obvious lesions, removal of foreign bodies, and regional lavage, brushing, or even biopsy of the lung for culture and cytology. For anterior rhinoscopy, a variety of equipment can be used, from an otoscope to a rigid pediatric arthroscope, to a flexible fiberoptic endoscope (FOE). Flexible fiber-optic technology has tremendously improved the ability to perform these procedures (McKiernan, 1995; Moser, 1994; Muggenburg *et al.,* 1982; Strumpf *et al.,* 1979). The flexible FOE is composed of fiber-optic bundles that provide both illumination and visualization pathways. One or more small channels traverse the FOE, through which instruments can be passed, fluids delivered, and suction applied. An FOE is most useful for posterior rhinoscopy, although a dental mirror may provide some visualization of the nasopharynx. The major contraindication for endoscopic examination, particularly in the lower respiratory system, is lack of experience, which both reduces the diagnostic and therapeutic potential and increases the risks (e.g., hypoxia, laryngospasm, and bronchospasm, pneumothorax, and biopsy-associated hemorrhage).

Pleuroscopy, thoracoscopy, and mediastinoscopy are procedures that can yield important information and samples (Moser, 1994). These techniques can involve the use of rigid or flexible devices. As with rhinoscopy and bronchoscopy, operator experience is a key to minimizing risks and maximizing diagnostic and therapeutic potential.

5. Nasal Flushing, Transtracheal Aspiration, Bronchioalveolar Lavage, and Thoracentesis

Forceful nasal flushing with saline can yield samples useful for the cytological assessment of nasal cavity cytology. Transtracheal aspiration (TTA) is a useful technique for sampling the lungs and lower airways for cytology and culture, avoiding the potential contamination of the pharyngeal flora (Dysko and Hoskins, 1995; Moser, 1994). In this technique, a 17- or 19-gauge intravenous catheter and needle set are aseptically placed into the tracheal lumen through the skin and between

tracheal cartilage rings. Once in the lumen, the needle is withdrawn, and a sample of sterile saline is introduced via the catheter then immediately aspirated back into the same syringe. Approximately 4 ml is often recovered from an initial instillation of 10 to 15 ml (Stills *et al.,* 1979).

Bronchioalveolar lavage can be practiced with a FOE (Gundel *et al.,* 1992). It is generally performed by lightly wedging a FOE into a distal airway, gently irrigating the airway with saline, and then retrieving the fluid for cytology and possible culture. Thoracentesis should be performed to sample pleural fluid for all pleural effusions of uncertain etiology and can be indicated for relief of effusion-associated symptons as well (Dysko and Hoskins, 1995).

6. Cytology, Microbiology, and Biopsy

Fluid samples obtained in any of the previously mentioned techniques should be examined in a variety of ways. Examination should include cytology and bacterial examination (Wright-type, Gram, and possibly acid fast stain). Samples should minimally be saved in transport medium (refrigerate) for possible culture, which would be indicated if evidence of inflammation is found in the cytology sample. Culture techniques would be based on the cytology and physical examination findings, including aerobic culture minimally, but also potentially anaerobic (e.g., with an inflammatory pleural effusion) or mycobacterial culture (e.g., granulomatous inflammation with or without acid fast organisms). Pharyngeal and nasal cultures are often of questionable use due to the potential to reflect airway colonization without actually indicating the microbial disease cause.

A variety of biopsy techniques are used for respiratory system sampling. With nasal cavity lesions (McKiernan, 1995), these can include the use of plastic catheters (e.g., shortened urinary catheters) cut to a sharp tip to obtain a core samples, endoscopic cup forceps used to obtain a pinch biopsy, or more invasive procedures such as nasal and sinus trephination or rhinotomy. For lung biopsy, techniques including both closed and open approaches are used. Closed biopsies are obtained via a fiber-optic endoscope (transbronchial) or a percutaneous cutting needle. Using a FOE provides the opportunity for multiple biopsies in one procedure; however, care must be taken when sampling close to the pleural surface. Even though performed with fluoroscopic or CT guidance, the cutting needle techniques have a relatively high potential for complications due to pneumothorax and/or bleeding. Open lung biopsy approaches include thoracotomy and, to a lesser extent, thoracoscopic techniques. These procedures are relatively safe regarding complications and allow direct visualization of the optimum biopsy site and the opportunity to obtain a sample of adequate size. All specimens obtained via biopsy should be processed for pathologic examination and should be cultured. Imprint cytology from biopsy material can be useful in the diagnosis of neoplastic and some infection-associated lesions (e.g., *Penicillium, Cryptococcus, Herpesvirus*). Final diagnosis should, nevertheless, generally be based on histopathologic findings.

7. Gas Exchange Assessment

The most definitive measure of gas exchange between alveolar spaces and blood is arterial PaO_2 and $PaCO_2$. Blood gas analysis, including arterial and/or venous oxygen, carbon dioxide, and pH, as well as total serum carbon dioxide and bicarbonate concentrations, can give additional information regarding the extent of hypoxemia and acidosis. These data are more easily obtained than is generally thought and can provide important information for the assessment and supportive treatment of seriously ill animals (Rosenberg, 1995). In comparing arterial and venous blood gas levels, venous samples provide a great deal of useful information, with greater ease in sample procurement. Differences in arterial and venous sample pH and PCO_2 levels are magnified in animals with hypovolemia or other systemic circulatory disturbances (King and Hendricks, 1995).

Pulse oximetry provides an indirect measure of hemoglobin oxygen saturation percent (SaO_2) as well as pulse rate, using a technique involving absorption of two wavelengths of light by hemoglobin in pulsatile blood in a skin or mucosal fold. Differential absorption of the two light wavelengths by oxygenated and nonoxygenated hemoglobin allows calculation of the percent of hemoglobin that is saturated with oxygen. It is important to be aware of certain issues when interpreting pulse oxymetry data (Weinberger and Drazen, 1994). First, the oxyhemoglobin saturation curve becomes flat above arterial PaO_2 60 mm Hg (corresponding to an $SaO_2 = 90\%$), such that the oximeter is relatively insensitive to changes in PaO_2 above this level. The curve position and relationship between PaO_2 and SaO_2 can also change in relation to temperature, pH, and the erythrocyte concentration of 2,3-diphosphoglyceric acid (2,3-DPG). Second, low tissue perfusion can make the oximeter signal less reliable or even unobtainable. Third, the two wavelengths of light do not detect other forms of hemoglobin, such as carboxyhemoglobin and methemoglobin, such that SaO_2 determined by the pulse oximeter in the presence of significant amounts of either of these hemoglobin forms is unreliable. Finally, the often-used goal of $SaO_2 \geq 90\%$ does not reflect CO_2 elimination and thus does not ensure that $PaCO_2$ levels are clinically acceptable.

8. Other Pulmonary Function Testing

Some commonly used pulmonary function tests in human medicine, e.g., spirometry for quantification of respiratory rate, tidal volume, and lung compliance, are not generally clinically useful due to difficulties involving the need for anesthesia in most animals as compared to the need for voluntary maneuvers from human patients in order to obtain these data. In certain research situations, however, including toxicology and infectious disease research, some such tests are carried out under

controlled circumstances. Reports available in the literature regarding such work include those by Besch *et al.* (1996), Binns *et al.* (1972), and Liu and DeLauter (1977).

9. Postmortem Assessment

Thorough gross examination of the entire respiratory tract is necessary for the recognition and appropriate sampling of lesions as well as of unaffected tissue. Postmortem examination of the lungs can include varying degrees of complexity (Tyler *et al.*, 1985), depending on the diagnostic and/or research needs. The presence of discrete lesions, characteristics of airway mucus coat, and the presence of airway edema or hemorrhage should be noted, as well as the characteristics of the lung parenchyma (color and consistency, including the presence of consolidation, atelectasis, or scarring). Tissue may be taken for microbial studies. Removal of the lungs prior to fixation is important for overall assessment and sampling of the unfixed tissue, including microbiology sample selection.

Tyler *et al.* (1985) describe a variety of fixatives and fixation techniques for lungs, each with its own advantages and disadvantages. This includes a discussion of fixation by immersion versus intratracheal infusion versus vascular perfusion fixation via the pulmonary artery. Neutral-buffered formalin is the standard fixative for light microscopic assessment. For electron microscopy, a variety of other fixatives are more suitable, generally containing paraformaldehyde, glutaraldehyde, or mixtures of the two, with phosphate or cacodylate buffer (e.g., Karnovsky's fixative). Fixation of tissue slices by immersion generally provides adequate samples for the assessment of microscopic morphology. Infusion of fixative via the airways provides for the rapid fixation of larger volumes of tissue, and the expanded air spaces allow for the easier interpretation of lesion orientation and alveolar epithelial and interstitial changes. Tracheal perfusion fixation disadvantages include the possibility that cellular exudates and inhaled particles may be translocated to other areas in the lung during the infusion process. With generalized disease processes, the use of immersion fixation of lung slices for some samples, combined with inflation via airways for other lobes, can provide a good compromise.

IV. UPPER AIRWAY DISEASES

A. Nose, Nasal Sinuses, Nasopharynx, and Trachea

1. Rhinitis, Nasal Polyposis, and Sinusitis

Normal nasopharyngeal microflora plays an important protective role against potential pathogens by excluding adherence to and subsequent colonization of the mucosa by more virulent organisms. This adherence is specific, via bacterial adhesins to sugar-containing epithelial surface-binding sites. In circumstances of mucosal injury, the usually nonpathogenic normal flora occasionally can produce problems itself. Mucosal injury can also compromise the attachment sites for normal flora, providing an opportunity for attachment and colonization by pathogenic organisms. Immune compromise, as with certain systemic immunodeficiency or nonspecific stress-associated immune dysfunction, can contribute to immune dysfunction in the nasal cavity and subsequent infection. Finally, prolonged antibiotic therapy can adversely affect normal bacterial flora populations, promoting conditions for opportunistic organisms, including funguses.

Viruses are the primary agents of nasal mucosal damage. Allergens are also a relatively common problem. Other injurious agents include irritant volatile gases, dust, and very low atmospheric humidity as well as certain parasites. Rhinitis generally results from an interaction between viruses or other injurious agents and bacteria or fungi.

Rhinitis can be differentiated according to time course and in relation to morphology. Time course differentiation is referred to simply as acute or chronic. Morphologic differentiation includes such categories as serous, catarrhal (mucous), purulent, ulcerative, pseudomembranous, hemorrhagic, or granulomatous inflammation. The course of acute rhinitis generally includes an initial serous response, which can progress to catarrhal then purulent inflammation. The presence of pseudomembranous, ulcerative, or hemorrhagic inflammation indicates very severe mucosal damage. A hallmark of chronic rhinitis is proliferative change, although atrophy is also a potential manifestation. Rhinitis can lead to a number of potential complications, the most common of which is sinusitis. Bronchopneumonia associated with the aspiration of nasal exudate can also occur. Finally, intracranial lesions such as thrombophlebitis, abscess, or meningitis can occur due to reflux blood flow via the diploic veins, which are valveless.

The mucosa of serous rhinitis is swollen and variably hyperemic. The swelling is associated with mild respiratory discomfort and subsequent sneezing and snuffling. Thin, clear seromucin secretion is present. Microscopically, the secretion contains small numbers of leukocytes and epithelial cells. There is mucosal epithelial cell hydropic degeneration and cilia loss, and goblet cells and submucosal glands are hyperactive. The lamina propria has edema and mild inflammatory cell infiltration. With time (hours to a few days), changes in glandular secretion and early bacterial infection lead to more severe hyperemia, edema, and swelling. Epithelial cell desquamation and increased leukocyte emigration result in a catarrhal to purulent discharge. Both epithelial regeneration and ulceration may be present. Acute rhinitis is often self-limiting, with treatment directed at palliative measures, such as the use of oral nasal decongestants and/or antihistamine preparations. In the case of allergic rhinitis, environmental management to control allergen exposure and allergen desensitization are also potential measures for control/prevention. Finally, if possible (e.g., with a well-trained Great Ape), topical corticosteroid sprays are available and potentially very effective.

Chronic rhinitis follows repeated attacks of acute rhinitis, whatever the cause, and generally is complicated by superimposed bacterial infection. This is probably the result of multiple interacting factors, including the compromise of local defense mechanisms, further infection by usually nonpathogenic flora, and self-sustaining inflammation caused by interactions of the infiltrating mixed inflammatory cells and associated inflammatory mediators and cytokines. Chronic rhinitis can result in atrophic rhinitis, which is characterized by foul odor and epistaxis with nasal obstruction, and results in the presence of crusting, debris, and necrosis of normal tissues and turbinates. Causes include various types of infection, as well as granulomatous diseases such as Wegener's granulomatosis. Treatment requires management of the underlying disease and can include the use of saline nasal douches.

Nasal polyp formation occurs in association with chronic or recurrent inflammation (e.g., allergic rhinitis). The polyps, which are sessile or with increased size, pedunculated, may be localized or diffusely distributed. They are covered by a variable-appearing mucosa, which may be hyperplastic, metaplastic, or ulcerated. The subepithelial tissue is edematous and contains mixed inflammatory cells, which can include neutrophils, eosinophils, plasma cells, and lymphocytes. Subepithelial fibrosis occurs with time. Polyps may impair nasal cavity air flow and slow or obstruct sinus drainage. Treatment includes surgical removal and treatment of the underlying cause for inflammation (e.g., allergic rhinitis).

Allergic rhinitis has been reported in an adult female chimpanzee (Halpern et al., 1989; Dumonceaux et al., 1995) and in Japanese macaques (Sakaguchi et al., 1992). The report of pollinosis in Japanese macaques (Sakaguchi et al., 1992) describes specific serum IgE to allergens from Japanese cedar trees and refers to reports indicating pollinosis in both wild and captive Japanese macaques throughout Japan. The tested monkeys had clinical signs of sneezing, rhinorrhea, pruritus, and epiphora. The chimpanzee had a long history of upper respiratory tract allergic disease, first confirmed and treated after a 12-year history of clinical signs. Seasonal (March through fall) signs included nasal discharge, impacted nares, open mouth breathing, facial swelling, bilateral epiphora, and an occasional cough. Annual tuberculin tests were negative, and previous hematology, serum chemistry, throat cultures, and thoracic radiographs had no significant abnormalities. A variety of antibiotic regimes produced equivocal results. Initial symptomatic treatment with prednisolone, followed by use of the oral antihistamine terfenadine, 60 mg twice daily, reduced the severity of upper respiratory disease. Both intradermal skin testing and serum IgE (IgE FAST-plus: fluorescent allergosorbent test) allergy tests indicated specific allergies to a number of species of local trees and grasses. Signs recurred within 5 years, with increased severity and persistence. Switch to a second antihistamine, loratidine, 10 mg orally once a day, produced only a temporary response. A purulent nasal discharge initially improved with oral cephalexin, 500 mg b.i.d., but then recurred and was unresponsive to an additional antibiotic regimen. Further workup at that time revealed the presence of multiple bilateral nasal polyps. These polyps, plus purulent material and plant fibers resembling hay, were removed from the nasal cavities. The animal was subsequently started on an oral desensitization regimen, similar to investigational techniques for humans (Korzeniowska-Zuk, 1992; Sjövall, 1990). The combination of endoscopic surgery and immunotherapy eliminated clinical signs during the initial part of the subsequent allergy season, at the time of the report (Dumonceaux *et al.,* 1995).

Additional reports of nasal polyposis in chimpanzees exist (Jacobs *et al.,* 1984; Nichols, 1939). In the report by Jacobs *et al.* (1984), the cause for the polyposis in a 15-year-old female chimpanzee did not appear to be allergy related, as suggestive signs of allergic respiratory tract disease had not been observed and radioallergosorbent test (RAST) results were negative for the presence of IgE to common aeroallergens. The polyps were first diagnosed when the animal was 10 years old during evaluation for a purulent nasal discharge. Left untreated, the animal appeared to tolerate the polyps over the next 5 years, with apparent increasing nasal obstruction to the point that continuous open mouth breathing was necessary. At that time she successfully delivered her second infant and subsequently was sedated prior to transport to a new local. During sedation, respiratory tract compromise occurred, with subsequent cardiac and respiratory arrest and death.

Sinusitis usually is preceded by acute or chronic rhinitis, but occasionally arises in association with tooth root abscesses that extend into the maxillary sinuses. Edema associated with nasal mucosal inflammation contributes to the potential conditions for sinusitis by impeding sinus secretion outflow. Mucocele is the condition in which mucous secretions accumulate without bacterial invasion. When the accumulated material is purulent exudate, the condition is termed sinus empyema. The associated bacterial flora in empyema usually consists of normal mixed oral microflora. Fungi cause particularly severe forms of chronic sinusitis, such as mucormycosis, which is particularly prevalent in individuals suffering from diabetes-associated ketoacidosis. Sinusitis often is clinically inapparent unless it has caused facial deformity or a fistula in the overlying skin. The sinus proximity to the brain carries with it increased potential for severe complications, including local osteomyelitis and spread into the cranium and brain. Sinusitis treatment is directed at the primary disease cause (e.g., tooth root abscess, foreign body) and associated infection when present (antibiotics, antifungal therapy) but may also require surgical curettage and drainage.

A case of ethmoiditis/sinusitis has been reported in an 8-month-old mother-raised orangutan (*Pongo pygmaeus*) (Cambre, 1986). The animal presented initially with bilateral exophthalmos and supraorbital swelling, then developed weight loss, depression, and lack of vigor. Physical examination included aspiration of the swellings, which yielded caseous suppurative material with rare gram-negative rods. *Escherichia coli* was isolated in pure

culture. The response to antibiotic therapy was equivocal, so a CAT scan was performed. This revealed evidence of bilateral ethmoiditis, left maxillary sinusitis, bilateral extraconal intraorbital infection, and apparent epidural inflammation. Surgical debridement and drainage was performed, followed by a 6-week period of intravenous antibiotic therapy to treat a mixed bacterial infection. Microscopic appearance of the tissues was compatible with chronic inflammation of the ethmoids, sinus mucosa, bone, and dura. The animal recovered completely, with CAT scan-confirmed resolution, and was returned to his parents after 4 months of separation.

2. Epistaxis

Epistaxis in individual animals is most commonly caused by trauma. A variety of other causes and associated conditions exist, including allergic rhinitis, sinusitis, nasal polyps, and a number of infections, such as acute viral infections, typhoid fever, nasal diphtheria, pertussis, and malaria. Severe bleeding may occur with congenital vascular anomalies and with thrombocytopenia, clotting factor deficiency, hypertension, and renal failure.

Epistaxis in nonhuman primates has been reported in association with both benign and very severe infections. In particular, viruses such as simian hemorrhagic fever virus and filoviruses can cause generalized bleeding disorders and may present with epistaxis and nasal discharge. [Centers for Disease Control (CDC), 1990]. Occasional outbreaks of acute, self-limiting epistaxis have been reported in groups of cynomolgus macaques (*Macaca fascicularis*), termed "bloody-nose syndrome" (Cooper and Baskerville, 1976; Olson and Palotay, 1983; Vande Woude and Luzarraga, 1991).

Clinical signs among the three reports of bloody-nose syndrome included epistaxis, nasal discharge, sneezing, and eyelid swelling. One report (Olson and Palotay, 1983) also noted palpebral bullae, whereas another (Vande Woude and Luzarraga, 1991) included wheezing. In all three reported outbreaks, *Branhamella catarrhalis* (formerly *Neisseria catarrhalis*) was isolated from a number of animals. The latest report (Vande Woude and Luzarraga, 1991) included transmission studies that supported the role of *B. catarrhalis* as an upper respiratory pathogen in cynomolgus macaques, with a syndrome similar to previously reported bloody-nose syndrome. Antibiotic therapy (penicillin) in that report resulted in diminished clinical signs within 24 hr, although it was noted that some β-lactamase-resistant strains have been noted in the human literature. Other factors are thought to contribute to the severity of clinical disease, including concurrent viral or bacterial disease, stress (e.g., recent transport), and/or low humidity. Although no apparent human infection was noted among animal care staff in any of the three reports, *B. catarrhalis* is a recognized human respiratory pathogen, supporting the potential for zoonotic transmission of this organism. In a similar note, human *B. catarrhalis*-associated disease has a similar fall/winter seasonality as has been noted in reports of bloody-nose syndrome in macaques.

3. Foreign Body

In the veterinary literature, most intranasal foreign bodies are of plant origin, deposited as a result of inhalation. Other foreign bodies may enter the nasal cavity via palatine defects. Initial signs suggesting intranasal foreign body include sudden onset vigorous and persistent sneezing. Unilateral nasal discharge and obstruction can be suggestive of a foreign body presence. If the foreign body is dislodged, mild inflammation may still be present for several days. With time, if the foreign body remains in place, sneezing may subside, and the clinical presentation is characterized by the presence of chronic nasal discharge with potential complications such as bacterial and possible fungal infection. A foreign body in the posterior nasal cavity may result in nasopharyngeal drainage that causes gagging and retching. Vegetative foreign bodies are not apparent with radiology. Rhinoscopy provides the opportunity for both recognition and removal of foreign body material. Occasionally, rhinotomy may be necessary.

Signs associated with trachiobronchial foreign body can vary depending on the degree of airway obstruction, lodging site, the length of time it has been present, and the irritant/inflammation-producing potential of the object. Often there is initial acute, severe, paroxysmal nonproductive coughing or respiratory distress. If the initial period of coughing and respiratory distress is missed, a relatively long period of time may pass, during which an occasional cough or slight wheezing may be apparent. At some point, relatively nonspecific systemic signs may occur, including fever, anorexia, depression, and weight loss, which are generally associated with the presence of pneumonia. Radiography of the thorax and neck may reveal soft tissue or mineral density, but this is relatively uncommon. With time, an inflammation-associated tissue response, including localized bronchial or parenchymal densities, may become more apparent. Definitive diagnosis is generally made with bronchoscopy. If animals with recurrent pneumonia are examined with radiography early after antibiotic initiation and within 1 week of completion of treatment, focal radiodense areas may indicate the site of foreign body lodging. Plant-associated (e.g., grass awn) foreign bodies can be particularly troublesome due to increased difficulty in their detection and their potential for migration. Tissue migration can lead to such complications as bronchopulmonary abscess, pneumothorax, pyothorax, discospondylitis, or signs due to penetration of other organs. Treatment consists of foreign body removal and appropriate antibiotic therapy for secondary bacterial infection. Bronchoscopic removal is generally preferred, although a surgical approach may be necessary in some cases.

Marcella and Wright (1985) reported on the intratracheal presence of a 1 × 1-cm rock in an adult female rhesus monkey (*Macaca mulatta*). The animal presented with an occasional dry, nonproductive cough that had increased in frequency over a 2-week period. Radiographs revealed an irregularly shaped radiodense object at the tracheal bifurcation. Using a flexible bronchoscope, the object was identified as a triangular, wedge-shaped rock and removed. Coughing decreased immediately after the procedure and ceased 1 week after bronchoscopy.

In another report (Odkvist and Schauman, 1980), a 15-year-old multiparous female chimpanzee initially was noted to have signs of fatigue and malaise, with reduced appetite, rapid weight loss, episodes of apparent pain, and cough. A few months later, she had a spontaneous abortion during the third month of pregnancy. Subsequent medical workup included thoracic radiography, which revealed a radiopaque foreign body in the right main stem bronchus. With bronchoscopy, the right bronchus at the carina was observed to have swollen mucosa with overlying crusts and contained a dark foreign body covered with pus. Removal of the crusts and suction made it possible to identify a firmly embedded metallic foreign body, which was extracted. The foreign body consisted of two pieces of 3-cm-long wire resembling fencing material. The animal recovered without complication.

4. Developmental Anomalies

a. CLEFT PALATE. Cleft palate occurs alone or with other defects, related to the need for integration of a number of embryonic processes for the development of normal facies and oral cavity. The palate is formed, except for a small rostral contribution from the frontonasal process, from bilateral ingrowth of the maxillary process lateral palatine shelves, which fuse with each other and with the nasal septum. Failure of this fusion generally results in a central, unilateral, or bilateral defect in the hard and/or soft palate. With regard to respiratory function and problems, neonates with palatine defects commonly have trouble nursing, show nasal regurgitation, and are susceptible to secondary bacterial or fungal rhinitis and aspiration pneumonia. Treatment is via corrective surgery. Reports of cleft palate in nonhuman primates are summarized by Wilson (1978), including cleft palate in two marmosets (Hill 1953–1955, Kraus and Garrett, 1968) and cleft lip and palate in a rhesus monkey (Swindler and Merrill, 1971).

5. Neoplasia

Respiratory system tumors are relatively infrequent in nonhuman primates (Beniashvili, 1989; Lowenstine, 1986). Nasopharyngeal tumors of various kinds have been described, with epithelial tumors occurring most frequently. Of particular note is the apparent propensity for nasal, nasopharyngeal, and oral carcinoma in marmosets (Baskerville *et al.*, 1984; Betton, 1984; McIntosh *et al.*, 1985). This high rate of occurrence has been suspected to be associated with the presence of underlying oncogenic virus infection, as occurs in Epstein–Barr virus (EBV)-associated nasopharyngeal carcinomas of humans. McIntosh *et al.* (1985) looked for but were unable to detect EBV antibodies in their study. The initial presentation of these animals is facial swelling with or without nasal discharge and visual impairment. These signs are relatively common in marmosets, usually related to abscesses of the upper canine, but, at least in marmosets, nasal carcinoma is also important to keep high on the differential diagnostic list. Tumors in marmosets appear to have a high potential for pulmonary metastasis.

Among other primate species, two reports not included in the reviews by Beniashvili (1989) and Lowenstine (1986) also include epithelial tumors, including nasal papillary adenocarcinoma in a Taiwan macaque (*M. cyclopis*) (Brown *et al.,* 1977) and a nasal cavity carcinosarcoma in a bonnet macaque (*M. radiata*) (Slayter, 1988). The bonnet macaque presented with unilateral left lower eyelid swelling, epiphora, and nasal discharge. The Taiwanese macaque presented with left maxilla swelling. Biopsy was used for diagnosis in both animals. The tumor recurred after attempted surgical excision in the Taiwanese macaque. Both animals were euthanized. In each case, pulmonary metastasis had occurred. Based on radiographic monitoring of the Taiwanese macaque, metastasis was a late development, with metastatic nodules not detected until 1 year after the initial diagnosis was made.

B. Larynx and Air Sacs

1. Air Sacculitis

Laryngeal air sacs are present in many primate species and are reported sites of infection for owl monkeys (Giles *et al.,* 1974), pig-tailed macaques (Brown and Swenson, 1995), baboons (Gross, 1978; Lewis *et al.,* 1975), chimpanzees (Strobert and Swenson, 1979), pygmy chimpanzees (Brown and Swenson, 1995), gorillas (Hastings, 1991), and orangutans (Cambre *et al.,* 1980; Clifford *et al.,* 1977; Guilloud and McClure, 1969; McManamon *et al.,* 1994). The report by Hastings (1991) details the recognition and successful treatment of air sac infection in a wild, free-ranging mountain gorilla (*Gorilla gorilla beringei*). The potential complications of this infection, including fatal bronchopneumonia and sepsis, make it extremely important to monitor animals for signs of air sac infection and to promptly treat such infections when they occur.

Nonspecific clinical signs for airsacculitis include halitosis, lethargy, and anorexia, as well as such respiratory signs as nasal discharge, intermittent cough, and rapid, shallow breathing patterns. The latter signs tend to occur with progressive disease and are indications of lower respiratory system involvement. At times the only sign is the presence of cervical swelling, corresponding to air sac swelling. The variable consistency of air sac exudate (liquid to consolidated and tenacious) can make diagnosis by palpation and ballottement extremely difficult in some cases. Radiography may reveal an air–liquid interface in the air sac. For problematic cases, endoscopy, aspiration (with or without irrigation), and ultrasound have been useful for confirmation of airsacculitis.

Although the owl monkey report (Giles *et al.,* 1974) found *Klebsiella pneumoniae* to be a primary cause of airsacculitis in that species, reports of airsacculitis in other primate species have characterized the infections as mixed, including gram-negative and gram-positive enteric organisms (*Proteus vulgaris, P. morganii, Pseudomonas aeruginosa, Escherichia coli,* streptococci, *Staphylococcus* spp., *Aerobacter cloacae,* etc.). Sensitivity testing is essential for optimal therapy. McManamon *et al.* (1994) note that chronically infected air sacs may be compartmentalized, with different bacterial populations in different compartments, and recommend separate cultures of each compartment.

The goal of treatment is to clear infection, prevent aspiration and secondary pneumonia, and prevent recurrence (Brown and Swenson, 1995). Infection severity and time course, as well as primate species, are important variables in the choice and effectiveness of the treatment technique. System antibiotics alone or in combination with simple exudate aspiration are not effective in the treatment of even simple air sac infection. The presence of secondary pulmonary infection is an important indication for systemic antibiotic use. A 1- to 2-week period of repeated closed irrigation and drainage with saline, followed each time with local antibiotic instillation, can be effective for mild infection. Gross (1978) describes the effectiveness of surgical air sac ablation in a baboon. This is much more difficult, if not impossible, in great apes, in which the air sacs extend into the axillary region and, in male orangutans, even around the mandible toward the ears and cheeks. Severe or persistent infections require open drainage. Successful control of chronic, progressive air sac infection in animals has been achieved using intermittent reevaluation, drainage, and antibiotic therapy in some animals and with permanent air sac marsupialization in others. Chronic air sac marsupialization prevents extensive exudate accumulation, but chronic aspiration of small amounts of exudate can continue, leading to chronic pulmonary infection or immune complex glomerulonephritis. Brown and Swenson (1995) and McManamon *et al.* (1994) briefly describe a promising technique to eliminate the occurrence of secondary pneumonia in orangutans with chronic or recurrent airsacculitis through surgical closure of the paired ostea between the trachea and air sacs.

V. LOWER RESPIRATORY TRACT DISEASES

A. Bronchi and Bronchiolar Disease

1. Asthma

Asthma is a disease in which episodic, reversible bronchoconstriction occurs in response to any of a variety of stimuli. This generalized bronchoconstriction results in the clinical hallmarks of asthma, including dyspnea, coughing, and wheezing.

A less common presentation of asthma involves intermittent episodes of nonproductive cough or exertional dyspnea. Most asthmatics are asymptomatic between attacks; however, a subset of individuals with chronic disease may develop emphysema, chronic bronchitis or pneumonia, or cor pulmonale and heart failure.

A classification for asthma generally includes two basic types: extrinsic and intrinsic. Extrinsic asthma is associated with a type I hypersensitivity reaction induced by exposure to an extrinsic antigen. Subclassification of extrinsic asthma includes atopic asthma, which is precipitated by specific allergens; occupational asthma, which is precipitated by chemical challenge; and allergic bronchopulmonary aspergillosis, which is associated with the *Aspergillus* colonization of airways followed by development of *Aspergillus*-specific IgE. Intrinsic asthma is associated with such precipitating factors as respiratory tract infection and inhaled irritants. All types of asthma may be precipitated by cold, stress, or exercise, and patients with one form may also be likely to experience asthma associated with another form.

Specific clinical diagnosis of asthma is based on pulmonary function testing that demonstrates reversible airway obstruction or increased airway responsiveness. In human medicine, reversible airway obstruction is determined by measuring the 1-sec forced expiratory volume (FEV_1), with reversible airway obstruction defined as a 15% or greater increase in FEV_1 following two puffs of a β-adrenergic agonist. Increased airway responsiveness can be diagnosed by demonstrating increased airway responsiveness to challenge with histamine, methacholine, or isocapnic hyperventilation of cold air. In veterinary medicine, techniques to test lung compliance and resistance are being used experimentally for the assessment of airway obstruction in a variety of conditions (King and Hendricks, 1995). For allergy-associated asthma, nonspecific tests that support the possibility of hypersensitivity-associated disease include blood eosinophil count and quantitative serum IgE levels, as well as skin testing and serum IgE (IgE FAST-plus: fluorescent allergosorbent test) tests for various specific antigens. Radiographs that demonstrate hyperinflation are also not in themselves diagnostic.

Gross morphologic changes with asthma include the presence of lung hyperinflation, often with small areas of atelectasis. Bronchi and bronchioles are occluded by thick, tenacious mucous plugs. Microscopically, numerous eosinophils and Charcot–Leyden crystals are present. The latter are crystalloid collections made up of eosinophil membrane protein. The mucous plugs contain whorls of shed epithelium. Other findings include bronchial epithelium basement membrane thickening, bronchial wall edema, and an inflammatory infiltrate that includes 5–50% eosinophils, submucosal gland, and bronchial smooth muscle hypertrophy. With time, emphysematous changes may occur, and bronchitis may be present due to secondary bacterial infection.

The most successful method for treating asthma is through environmental modification, eliminating specific agents that cause the condition, such as the type of bedding material used with an animal. In addition, desensitization, as described earlier for allergic rhinitis, provides an additional possibility for specific treatment. Nonspecific treatment is directed toward relieving bronchoconstriction and reducing airway inflammation. To control severe inflammation, systemic corticosteroids are used. Drugs used for bronchodilation include oral albuterol, aminophylline, and theophylline. Topical (inhalant) drug preparations are used in human practice for chronic asthma control and prevention. These include bronchodilators (e.g., albuterol), corticosteroids (e.g., beclomethasone), and mast cell stabilizers (e.g., cromolyn sodium).

Asthma has been recognized in chimpanzees (Janssen, 1993) and has been experimentally induced and studied in susceptible cynomolgus macaques (*Macaca fascicularis*) (Gundel et al., 1992). Inhalant allergy and asthma in chimpanzees and pygmy chimpanzees have been characterized by nonspecific chronic respiratory disease with an increased susceptibility to bacterial pneumonia, often with associated problems, including rhinitis and chronic sinusitis. Treatment for such animals is reported to include long-term antibiotic therapy to eliminate chronic infections and antihistamines or bronchodilators for dyspneic episodes. Experimental work with cynomolgus macaques involved exposure of animals to inhaled *Ascaris suum* extract as part of a study of the pathogenesis of the acute- and late-phase bronchoconstriction recognized in human asthmatics. Some animals exhibited an acute bronchoconstriction in response to the allergen, as well as the less common (among human asthmatics) delayed bronchoconstriction, providing a valuable model for the pathogenesis factors for the delayed response.

B. Lungs

1. Atelectasis and Fetal Distress

Atelectasis refers to incomplete lung expansion (congenital/neonatal atelectasis) or to collapse of a previously inflated lung (acquired atelectasis). Complete atelectasis occurs in lungs of stillborn animals (fetal atelectasis), as they have never been aerated. The fleshy, dark reddish blue lungs do not float. Alveoli are lined by rounded epithelial cells, and alveolar lumens contain fluid, sloughed epithelial cells from aspirated amniotic fluid, and sometimes bright yellow meconium particles. Andrews (1974) describes how careful assessment of the alveolar lumen components can provide important evidence of the circumstances of fetal death, including fetal distress and possible placentitis. Large numbers of squamous cells in alveolar lumens (small numbers are normal in the term fetus), especially if meconium is also present, are evidence of amniotic fluid aspiration during exaggerated respiratory movements of the distressed fetus.

Patchy congenital atelectasis in neonates may be associated with incomplete expansion and/or acquired atelectasis of a briefly aerated lung. Incomplete expansion can be associated with weak respiratory movement due to general debilitation or central nervous system damage. Other possible causes include laryngeal dysfunction, airway obstruction, and lung or related thoracic structure anomalies. The gross appearance of the areas of patchy atelectasis is of dark red areas of variable size that are depressed below the surface of the surrounding aerated lung. These areas are flabby rather than consolidated as with inflamed lung. Microscopically, the alveolar walls are closely apposed, with only small amounts of fluid, epithelial debris, and alveolar macrophages present.

The presence of extensive neonatal atelectasis is a feature of neonatal respiratory distress syndrome (RDS). The fundamental defect in RDS is a deficiency of pulmonary surfactant, often associated with inadequate surfactant production by type II epithelial cells due to their immaturity or to more specific metabolic derangement of their surfactant synthesis, such as might occur with fetal hypothyroidism and possibly hypoadrenocorticism. The high levels of insulin in diabetic mothers can counteract the effects of endogenous corticosteroids, which are particularly important for the induction of surfactant formation in the fetal lung, resulting in a higher risk for RDS in the infants of diabetic mothers. Other factors can contribute to RDS, such as fetal asphyxia, decreased pulmonary arterial blood flow, amniotic fluid aspiration, and inhibition of surfactant by fibrinogen, other edema fluid constituents, or components in aspirated amniotic fluid, particularly meconium. An additional contributing factor comes with the need for oxygen therapy and mechanical ventilation in these patients. High concentrations of oxygen for prolonged periods can cause toxic pulmonary changes. In particular, mechanical ventilation and oxygen toxicity can give rise to a subacute or chronic condition called bronchopulmonary dysplasia (BPD). Fetal and neonatal atelectasis, as well as RDS, are reported as causes of perinatal and neonatal death in infant *Macaca nemistrina* (Morton *et al.,* 1979). Primates also provide experimental models of RDS and BPD (Coalson, 1988; Coalson *et al.,* 1982; Escobedo *et al.,* 1982), as well as meconium aspiration as a cause of RDS (Block *et al.,* 1981; Carey, 1988).

Affected lungs in RDS are largely atelectic. They are heavy, fleshy, often edematous, and generally sink in fixative. Cream-colored or red foam is often present in airways and exudes from cut surfaces. Characteristic microscopic changes include alveolar septal congestion, variably collapsed or fluid-filled alveoli, and the presence of acidophilic hyaline membranes that line terminal bronchioles, alveolar ducts, and random, usually proximal, alveoli. Focal hemorrhage and interstitial edema are also common. Persistent respiratory distress occurs with BPD. Bronchopulmonary dysplasia-associated pathology changes include epithelial hyperplasia and squamous metaplasia in large airways, plus thickened alveolar walls, with peribronchial and interstitial fibrosis.

Treatment of RDS must approach the basic defect, inadequate pulmonary exchange of O_2 and CO_2, as well as deal with secondary problems of metabolic acidosis and circulatory insufficiency. This requires close monitoring of heart and respiratory rates, blood gases, and pH, as well as provision of general support to maintain blood glucose levels, blood pressure, and temperature. It is necessary to provide increased oxygen levels, often with respiratory assistance via mechanical ventilation. For immature lungs, it is now possible to provide exogenous surfactant intratracheally, a measure that is extremely helpful in allowing a minimization of the degree and time of mechanical ventilation assistance. Minimizing mechanical ventilation can help avoid potential problems, including barotrauma, oxygen toxicity, nosocomial pneumonia, tracheal stenosis, and deconditioning of respiratory muscles. The added complication of meconium aspiration, with associated inflammation and neutralization of surfactant, has led to further intervention, including pulmonary lavage with surfactant solutions to wash out inflammatory products and replace affected surfactant, as well as the use of extracorporeal membrane oxygenation (ECMO). Techniques for the latter procedures are currently experimental.

Acquired atelectasis most commonly occurs due to airway obstruction, as would occur with the presence of exudate, parasites, aspirated foreign material, granulomas, or tumors. Compression can also cause atelectasis, as with pleural or intrapulmonary space-occupying lesions. Examples of space-occupying lesions include hydrothorax, hemothorax, pneumothorax, exudative pleuritis, and mediastinal and pulmonary tumors. Apparent massive atelectasis occurs when animals die while being maintained with 80–100% oxygen while in intensive care. This occurs when the oxygen is rapidly absorbed into tissues, such that the lungs are devoid of gas at the time they are examined postmortem. Recognition and treatment of the primary problem can lead to the resolution of acquired atelectasis.

2. Circulatory Disturbances

A variety of circulatory disturbances can affect the lungs, including problems involving pulmonary vessels or the heart, as well as pulmonary vascular changes secondary to primary pulmonary disease. Functionally, the most important consequence of these problems is hypoxemia due to ventilation/perfusion mismatching. Attenuation of alveolar capillaries associated with emphysema or pulmonary fibrosis can lead to pulmonary ischemia. Pulmonary arterial obstruction actually tends to lead to pulmonary congestion due to the presence of the dual pulmonary blood supply (pulmonary and bronchial arteries) and extensive collateral circulation. Active hyperemia is a component of acute inflammation and occurs with a variety of problems that cause acute pulmonary injury. Pulmonary congestion occurs with multiple problems, including left-sided or bilateral cardiac failure, and conditions that lead to the redistribution of blood from systemic to pulmonary circulation. Such redistribution commonly occurs terminally and can also be caused by acute hypothalamic damage.

a. PULMONARY EDEMA. Pulmonary edema is a very common pulmonary abnormality associated with increased capillary hydrostatic pressure, increased air–blood barrier permeability, or a combination of both. Pulmonary edema is most often due to increased microvascular hydrostatic pressure, as occurs in association with left-sided or bilateral cardiac failure (cardiogenic edema) and also can occur with hypervolemia, as with excessive fluid therapy. Acute brain injury can lead to pulmonary edema (neurogenic edema) due to increased microvascular pressure associated with catecholamine release-caused pulmonary hypertension followed by increased capillary permeability.

Damage to alveolar type I epithelium and capillary endothelium leads to rapid-onset edema with a higher protein concentration than in cardiogenic forms. Among the agents that cause such damage are corrosive gases (including 80–100% oxygen), systemic toxins, endotoxins, and shock-like states. Many of the toxic or shock-like states that lead to pulmonary injury-associated edema can cause abnormalities associated with acute interstitial pneumonia.

b. PULMONARY THROMBOEMBOLISM. As a capillary bed through which the entire right ventricular output flows, the pulmonary circulation is situated to catch emboli originating in the systemic venous circulation. Various possible types of emboli bring with them a number of possible outcomes. Bacterial emboli can cause acute pulmonary edema and interstitial pneumonia. Infected thrombi can generate septic emboli, which can cause thromboembolism, arteritis, multiple abscessation, and sometimes suppurative pneumonia. Tumor emboli can lead to metastatic neoplastic foci. Fat emboli can occur in association with bone fracture and with hepatocyte rupture in severe hepatic lipidosis, lodging in pulmonary capillaries and appearing as a large empty capillary distention in paraffin-embedded sections. An incidental finding associated with intravenous injections is hair emboli. This has been described by Kast (1994).

Pulmonary thrombosis can occur with blood stasis, in hypercoagulation states, or in association with endothelial damage. Pulmonary embolism and endarteritis can also predispose to thrombosis. DiGiacomo *et al.,* (1978) report a case of pulmonary arteriosclerosis and thrombosis in a cynomolgus macaque (*Macaca fascicularis*). The animal was found dead. A saddle thrombus was present at the initial bifurcation of the pulmonary artery, with complete occlusion of the left pulmonary artery. Microscopic examination revealed generalized pulmonary arteriosclerosis, with intimal and medial thickening (endothelial hyperplasia, subendothelial fibrosis, and medial smooth muscle hyperplasia). Cause and pathogenesis for this condition were not determined. A similar case has been reported by Ulland (1968).

3. Lung Inflammation

Pulmonary inflammation varies according to the type of initiating agent and the agent entry route, distribution, and persistence. A useful morphologic classification that gives clues regarding pathogenesis and possible etiology focuses on the initial site of involvement and pattern of spread. Three catego-

ries in this classification scheme are bronchopneumonia, lobar pneumonia, and interstitial pneumonia.

Initiation of inflammation by agents arriving via an aerogenous route generally results in bronchopneumonia, usually originating at the bronchioalveolar junction, often as an extension of bronchial inflammation. Such inflammation often is located in cranioventral lung regions. Bacteria are the major causes of clinically significant bronchopneumonia, often in association with predisposing factors such as viral infection or severe stress. Lobar pneumonia is basically similar to bronchopneumonia, with the key differentiation being the presence of extensive consolidation with uniform parenchymal involvement as opposed to a recognizable bronchiolar orientation.

Interstitial pneumonia is characterized by diffuse or patchy damage to alveolar septa. Inflammatory features generally include an early exudative response, followed by proliferative and fibrotic responses. The acute injury is caused by or associated with such conditions as severe viral pneumonia, chemical lung injury, acute pancreatitis, shock, and septicemia. It is generally associated with a hematogenous exposure route, although aerogenous exposure to very high concentrations of toxic gases can also produce severe diffuse damage. Pneumoconioses involve a chronic progressive process that starts with aerogenous exposure; however, they often are not clinically apparent until after the initially terminal bronchiole-oriented process of granulomatous inflammation or fibrosis has spread into adjacent parenchyma. An exception to the often diffuse nature of hematogenous exposure occurs with chemicals that are not themselves toxic, but which are metabolized into toxic metabolites by localized cells such as Clara cells, which in turn are the only cells that are injured.

Pulmonary abscesses occur in association with focal residues of severe suppurative inflammation or with septic emboli. Those arising from suppurative pneumonia often are oriented cranioventrally, whereas hematogenous sources often lead to multiple, widely distributed abscesses. Direct traumatic penetration of the lung and aspiration of foreign bodies such as plant awns are also recognized causes of pulmonary abscess.

4. Adult Respiratory Distress Syndrome

Adult respiratory distress syndrome (ARDS) is a term that is applied to acute, diffuse infiltrative lung disease, with severe life-threatening respiratory insufficiency, tachycardia, cyanosis, and severe arterial hypoxemia that is not responsive to oxygen therapy. Severe pulmonary edema is generally present, lung compliance is decreased, and a diffuse alveolar infiltrative pattern is apparent in thoracic radiographs. Adult respiratory distress syndrome is associated with a variety of etiologic agents, including (1) gastric content aspiration; (2) inhalation of toxic fumes; (3) oxygen toxicity; (4) near drowning; (5) pulmonary contusion; (6) drugs including heroin, salicylate, and paraquat; (7) pneumonitis (bacterial, viral); (8) sepsis syndrome; (9) pancreatitis; (10) multiple transfusions; (11) fat embolism; and

(12) amniotic fluid embolism. Nonhuman primates have been important models for ARDS, particularly with regard to pathophysiologic mechanisms (Balis *et al.*, 1974; Campbell *et al.*, 1984; Drake *et al.*, 1993; Hangen *et al.*, 1987; Holcroft *et al.*, 1977; Revak *et al.*, 1985; Schlag *et al.*, 1992; Taylor *et al.*, 1994). In addition to diffuse pulmonary damage, secondary compromising of pulmonary surfactant also generally occurs. The complexity of ARDS pathophysiology contrasts with neonatal respiratory distress syndrome, in which the primary problem involves inadequate pulmonary surfactant production associated with lung immaturity, along with the highly compliant nature of the infant chest wall. Despite the variety to potential causes, ARDS clinical characteristics, pathophysiologic derangement, and general supportive measures are similar. Untreated ARDS is almost uniformly fatal. With the current level of treatment, prognosis is still poor, with a mortality in humans of 50–60%. Treatment includes mechanical ventilatory support and identification and treatment of the primary problem. For sepsis-associated ARDS, identification of the source of infection and responsible organism(s) is necessary. Abscess surgical drainage is extremely important. Treatment of the pulmonary injury focused on the variety of possible bacterial products, and factors involved in the injury and inflammatory process have been proposed and are subjects of clinical trials, but no single clear-cut strategy exists. These strategies include use of such things as antibodies to endotoxin and a variety of chemokines, as well as the administration of exogenous surfactant. Such methods hold promise to further reduce the mortality rate associated with this syndrome.

5. Neoplasia

Reviews of neoplasia in nonhuman primates note a low relative prevalence of primary pulmonary tumors (Beniashvili, 1989; Giddens and Dillingham, 1971; Lowenstine, 1986). All of the reported spontaneous lung tumors are malignant epithelial tumors. A single bronchial fibrosarcoma has been reported in a rhesus monkey (*Macaca mulatta*) that died due to pulmonary fibrosis 9 years following experimental inhalation of plutonium-239 (Hahn *et al.*, 1987).

Among descriptions of experimental induction of pulmonary neoplasia is the occurrence of pulmonary epidermoid carcinoma in an owl monkey (*Aotus trivirgatus*) that had been inoculated intratracheally 350 days earlier with 7,12-dimethylbenz[*a*]anthracene (DMBA) and *Herpesvirus saimiri* (Giddens, 1974). Allen *et al.* (1970) described an 18-year-old rhesus monkey with multiple small carcinoids (bronchial adenomas) in the lung, associated with exposure to 1100 roentgens of X-irradiation between the ages of 2 and 6 years. Death in this animal, which also had four other unrelated tumors in other areas of the body, was due to the effects of severe diarrhea. Finally, squamous (epidermoid) carcinoma of the lung occurred in two of six galagos (*Galago crassicaudatus panengiensis*) that received a weekly intratracheal instillation of 3–15 mg of benzo[*a*]pyrene combined with an equal weight of powdered ferric oxide over a 67- to 69-week period (Crocker *et al.*, 1970).

Among the reports of spontaneous primary pulmonary tumors in nonhuman primates are multiple peripheral carcinoid tumors in the lungs of a rhesus monkey (Giddens and Dillingham, 1971); a bronchial adenoma in a lion-tail macaque (*M. silenus*) (Griner, 1983); a bronchioloalveolar neoplasm of a possible type II alveolar epithelium origin in a bonnet macaque (*M. radiata*) (Nicholls and Schwartz, 1980); a bronchogenic squamous cell carcinoma in a Sykes monkey (*Cercopithecus mitis stuhlmani*) (Suleman *et al.*, 1984); and a clear cell carcinoma in a pig-tailed macaque (*M. nemestrina*) (Tsai and Giddens, 1985). An additional report describes squamous cell carcinoma of the prepuce and penis of a rhesus monkey with metastasis to the lungs (Hubbard *et al.*, 1983).

VI. DISORDERS OF THE DIAPHRAGM, PLEURA, AND THE MEDIASTINUM

Bauer and Woodfield (1995) provide a detailed review of the variety of problems in veterinary medicine associated with the diaphragm, pleura, and mediastinum.

A. Diaphragm

The most common disorder of the diaphragm is diaphragmatic hernia. This term refers to disorders in which abdominal viscera encroach on or enter the thoracic cavity via a diaphragmatic defect. The abdominal viscera may be free in the pleural space or be contained within a hernial sac. The herniation can occur at any level and may be congenital or acquired. Reports of congenital diaphragmatic hernia are summarized by Wilson (1978), including cases in a baboon fetus (Hendrickx and Gasser, 1967), a chimpanzee (McClure, 1972), a rhesus monkey (Dalgard, 1969), and a squirrel monkey. A more recent report by Montali (1993) documents the occurrence of congenital retrosternal diaphragmatic defects in golden lion tamarins (*Leontopithecus rosalia*).

Diaphragmatic hernia may present as an acute, subacute, or chronic disorder. A vague history of episodic gastrointestinal distress may be present. There may be low-grade respiratory signs, possibly associated with exercise or posture (recumbency). Signs may be progressive and intensify over time. The presence of a subclinical hernia may be unmasked by the development of secondary problems, including (1) gastric dilatation of a herniated stomach, with subsequent lung compression and dyspnea; (2) intrathoracic splenic torsion; (3) intrathoracic bowel obstruction; and (4) cholangitis or cholangiohepatitis secondary to liver lobe incarceration. Definitive diagnosis is difficult, with radiography being the most useful technique, particularly contrast studies (barium swallow, contrast pleurography, contrast peritoneography, etc.). Treatment involves surgical correction.

B. Pleura

The pleura consists of a membrane of mesothelial origin. It makes up the surface of the chest wall, mediastinum, and lung. The pleural cavity is a potential space that contains a few milliliters of fluid, which provide lubrication during respiratory motion. This fluid is serum like, with a total protein level of 0.3–4.1 g per deciliter.

Apparent respiratory difficulty is the most common sign occurring with pleural effusion. The primary problem causing pleural effusion may contribute to other signs, including cough or fever. Diagnostic techniques range in invasiveness and potential diagnostic yield. Generally, more invasive techniques are needed for specific diagnosis. The clinical situation helps dictate whether the early use of invasive diagnostic procedures is appropriate, with a more serious clinical condition supporting the earlier use of invasive techniques.

A variety of problems can produce pleural effusion. Congestive heart failure, both right sided and biventricular, is a major cause. This condition can coexist with other disorders, including neoplasia, parapneumonic effusion, and pulmonary embolism or thrombosis. Pleural tumors are usually metastatic tumors, although spontaneous malignant mesothelioma has been reported in an adult female olive baboon (*Papio anubis*) (Fortman *et al.*, 1993). Pleural tumors generally produce effusion via the obstruction of pleural lymphatics, although other secondary mechanisms may also contribute to or cause the effusion. Pleural effusions may occur as a secondary effect of pneumonia (parapneumonic effusion), characterized as serous or hemorrhagic, sterile effusions. Empyema, or pyothorax, is the accumulation of infected exudate within the pleural space. Three routes for thoracic invasion of microbial agents include (1) hematogenous or lymphatic; (2) spread from an adjacent structure, e.g., severely affected lung, ruptured esophagus, or mediastinitis; or (3) direct introduction via penetrating trauma, foreign bodies, thoracentesis, or surgery. An example of the second route has been reported for an African green monkey (Stills and Rader, 1982). The occurrence of empyema is a medical emergency and should be treated immediately, including the use of tube thoracostomy to achieve effective drainage.

C. Mediastinum

The mediastinum is the central portion of the thoracic cavity. It contains all of the structures of the cranial and caudal thoracic cavity, including esophagus, trachea, thymus, lymph nodes, nerves, and major blood vessels. Signs of mediastinal disease are often nonspecific and vary in association with lesion size, location, pathologic consequences, and peripheral vascular signs. Space-occupying effects can produce obstruction of the vena cava, with associated edema and swelling. Respiratory signs may occur in relation to airway or pulmonary parenchymal compression. Signs of upper airway obstruction, changes in vocalization, and stridor may be the primary clinical signs.

VII. VIRAL DISEASES

In the human primate, respiratory viral infections in the form of the "flu" and the "common cold" are familiar and annoying conditions caused by agents of several genera, including rhinoviruses (Picornaviridae; Rhinovirinae), adenoviruses, paramyxoviruses [including respiratory syncytial virus and paramyxoviruses 1, 2, 3 (also called parainfluenza viruses 1, 2, and 3)], and orthomyxoviruses (influenza A and B) (see Table II). Nonhuman primates are also susceptible to many of these infections, although only in chimpanzees (*Pan troglodytes* and *P. paniscus*) are colds a common and regular problem. Much of the work on the natural history of simian respiratory viral infections dates from the 1960s and 1970s, although nonhuman primates are still used as animal models in the study of influenza.

A. Paramyxoviruses

1. Respiratory Syncytial Virus/Chimpanzee Coryza Agent

Several species of nonhuman primates can be infected experimentally with RSV, including *Cebus* spp., *Saimiri* spp., *M. mulatta*, and *P. troglodytes*. Only the chimpanzee, however, develops clinical illness (Belshe *et al.*, 1977). Chimpanzees are often naturally infected and were the species from which this agent was initially isolated in 1956 (Morris *et al.*, 1956). In one serosurvey, 100% of the chimpanzees tested had antibodies (Kalter, 1983). Other great apes (*Gorilla gorilla gorilla, G. Gorilla beringi, Pongo pygmaeus,* and *Pan paniscus*) are also often seropositive, but the association with clinical disease is uncertain (L. J. Lowenstine, unpublished).

Signs most commonly reported in chimpanzees are rhinorrhea or coryza (hence the name chimpanzee coryza agent), coughing, and sneezing. Initial infections in very young animals may lead to lower respiratory tract involvement, principally bronchitis. In older animals or individuals that have been previously exposed, the infection is limited to the upper respiratory tract. As in humans, reinfection appears to be common. The disease is usually self-limiting, but can predispose to pneumococcosis, pertussis, or other bacterial infections (Gustavsson *et al.*, 1990). Clinical diagnosis relies on demonstration of a rising antibody titer, or virus isolation.

Lesions of RSV infection in nonhuman primates have not been described in the literature, presumably because of the relatively self-limiting nature of the infection.

2. Paramyxovirus-1 (Parainfluenza-1), PMV-2, and PMV-3

The susceptibility of many nonhuman primates, including callitricids, cebids, cercopithicines, and pongids, has been established by virologic and serologic studies and by experimental inoculation. Outbreaks of PI-1 or Sendai-like virus have been reported in marmosets associated with fatal pneumonia (Flecknell *et al.*, 1983; Murphy *et al.*, 1972). In one outbreak in

TABLE 2

DIFFERENTIAL DIAGNOSIS OF PRIMATE RESPIRATORY DISEASE: INFECTIOUS DISEASES

Etiology	Disease	Clinical signs		Reported species	Comments, including zoonotic potential
		Respiratory	Other		
Virus disease					
Respiratory syncytial virus	Chimpanzee coryza	Rhinorrhea, cough, sneezing	Fever	Chimpanzee	(1) Infections in very young animals may lead to lower respiratory tract involvement, principally bronchitis; can predispose to pneumococcosis, pertussis, or other bacterial infections (2) Zoonotic potential: risk of human to nonhuman primate infection. Minimal risk to humans
paramyxovirus-1 (parainfluenza-1), PMV-2, and PMV-3		Upper respiratory signs: mild serous or occasionally purulent nasal exudate	Systemic illness and death (associated with severe interstitial pneumonia)	Marmosets, chimpanzees, gorillas, orangutans	(1) Predisposes to pneumo-coccosis, pertussis, or other bacterial infections (2) Zoonotic potential: risk of human to nonhuman primate infection. Minimal risk to humans
Measles (rubeola)	Measles	Rhinorrhea, cough	Maculopapular rash, fever, conjunctivitis, depression, dehydration, facial edema	New World and Old World monkeys and apes	(1) Gastrointestinal lesions or immunosuppression rather than respiratory disease can be the most important sequela (2) Zoonotic potential: risk of human to nonhuman primate infection plus monkey to human transmission
Influenza A and B	Influenza	Rhinorrhea, dyspnea, tachypnea, cough, sneezing	Depression, fever, lethargy, anorexia	Capuchins, squirrel monkeys, owl monkeys, macaques, baboons, gibbons, chimpanzees	(1) Most reports are for experimental infection. Gibbon infection was a spontaneous outbreak (2) Sequela can include pneumococcal super-infection with lethal outcome (3) Zoonotic potential: risk of human to nonhuman primate infection. Minimal risk to humans
Adenoviruses		Nasal discharge, cough tachypnea	Conjunctivitis, and erythema, skin rash, facial edema, cyanosis, diarrhea	Macaques	(1) Histology: bronchiolar and alveolar epithelium necrosis and enlarged nuclei filled with amphophilic to basophilic inclusions (2) Zoonotic potential: risk of human to nonhuman primate infection. Minimal risk to humans

TABLE 2—*Continued*

DIFFERENTIAL DIAGNOSIS OF PRIMATE RESPIRATORY DISEASE: INFECTIOUS DISEASES

Etiology	Disease	Clinical signs		Reported species	Comments, including zoonotic potential
		Respiratory	Other		
Herpesvirus simiae		Purulent nasal exudate	Oral ulcers, splenomegaly, hepatomegaly	Bonnet monkeys	(1) Histology: Hemorrhagic interstitial pneumonia (2) Endemic simian type D retrovirus infection (SRV-1) also present in the affected population (3) Zoonotic potential: infection in humans can be fatal
Herpesvirus SA8		Not noted in published reports	None noted in published reports	Baboons	Histology: necrotizing bronchiolitis and interstitial pneumonia
Varicella-zoster-like herpesviruses		Not noted in published reports	Vesicular rash	Macaques, African green monkeys, patas monkeys, great apes	(1) Histology: pulmonary edema and alveolar septa necrosis with marked fibrin exudation (2) Zoonotic potential: risk of human to nonhuman primate infection. Minimal risk to humans
Rhinoviruses		Sneezing, rhinorea, often clinically inapparent	Not noted in published reports	Chimpanzees	(1) Experimental inoculation in other species has been unsuccessful (2) Zoonotic potential: risk of human to nonhuman primate infection. Minimal risk to humans
Simian immunodeficiency virus (SIV)	Retroviral giant cell pneumonia	Generally no specific respiratory signs	Anorexia, weight loss, inactivity	Macaques	(1) Histology: histologic examination reveals thickening of alveolar septa, marked exudation of macrophages, lesser amounts of proteinaceous material, and large numbers of syncytial giant cells (2) Lentiviruses of cercopithecine monkeys are indigenous to African monkeys of the genera *Cercopithecus, Cercocebus,* and *Papio (Mandrillus)*. Very low pathogenicity in African species (3) Zoonotic potential: rare reports of human seroconversion; no associated human disease reported, closely related to HIV-2
Bacterial diseases *Mycobacterium tuberculosis,* and *M. bovis*	Tuberculosis	Usually clinically inapparent, cough with pulmonary parenchymal loss, dyspnea with advanced disease	Low-grade fever, weakness, weight loss	New World and Old World monkeys and apes	Zoonotic potential: risk of human to nonhuman primate infection. Usual subclinical nature plus potential disease severity make this a disease routinely screened for in nonhuman primate populations and associated humans

Etiology	Disease	Clinical signs		Reported species	Comments, including zoonotic potential
		Respiratory	Other		
Streptococcus pneumoniae	Pneumococcal infection	Cough, dyspnea	Anorexia, weakness, facial edema	Macaques, great apes	(1) Lesions include lobar pneumonia, bronchopneumonia, empyema, and upper respiratory infection (middle ear, sinuses) as well as severe meningitis or brain abscesses (2) Clinical disease associated with the presence of other predisposing problems, such as stress, inclement weather, or viral respiratory infections (3) Zoonotic potential: risk of human to nonhuman primate infection. Minimal risk to humans
Klebsiella pneumoniae		Nasal discharge, congestion	Fever, anorexia, weight loss, unexpected death without clinical signs	Macaques, chimpanzees	(1) Lesions include pneumonia (lobular or lobar), urinary tract infection, and miscellaneous septic lesions, including sinusitis, meningitis, and otitis (2) Zoonotic potential: risk of human to nonhuman primate infection. Minimal risk to humans
Bordetella pertussis	Whooping cough	Coughing, sneezing, nasal discharge	Peripheral lymphocytosis, malaise, weight loss, mild fever, subcutaneous emphysema, convulsions	Chimpanzees	(1) Zoonotic potential: risk of human to nonhuman primate infection. Minimal risk to humans
B. bronchiseptica		Bilateral mucopurulent nasal discharge, occasional dyspnea	Torticollis, seizures, mild fever, sudden death	Prosimians, New World primates, Old World primates	(1) Generally, cases have occurred in association with potentially weakened pulmonary defenses (stress, virus, age, etc.) (2) Zoonotic potential: common part of respiratory mucosa microflora. Minimal risk to humans
Nocardia sp.	Nocardiosis	Productive cough	Fever	Macaques, orangutans	(1) Signs associated with pulmonary nocardiosis are often nonspecific and even subclinical until late in the disease course (2) Zoonotic potential: not transmitted between individual animals or humans. Can be found as a primary infection, but often is noted as an apparent opportunist

TABLE 2—*Continued*

DIFFERENTIAL DIAGNOSIS OF PRIMATE RESPIRATORY DISEASE: INFECTIOUS DISEASES

Etiology	Disease	Clinical signs		Reported species	Comments, including zoonotic potential
		Respiratory	Other		
Pasteurella multocida or *P. hemolytica*	Pasteurellosis	Dyspnea	Anorexia, lethargy	Goeldi's monkeys, owl monkeys, patas monkeys	(1) Predisposing factors include stress induced by such factors as transportation, crowding, climatic changes, or respiratory viral infections (2) Zoonotic potential: common part of respiratory mucosa microflora. Minimal risk to humans
Mycotic diseases					
Coccidioides immitis	Coccidioidomycosis	Often clinically inapparent, cough, dyspnea	Fever, weakness, weight loss, convulsions, urine retention, diarrhea	Ring-tailed lemurs, macaques, baboons, gorilla	Zoonotic potential when handling infected tissue, via parenteral inoculation or inspiration of aerosolized infectious material
Histoplasma capsulatum	Histoplasmosis	Similar to coccidioidomycosis	Similar to coccidioidomycosis	Squirrel monkeys, de Brazza's monkeys	Zoonotic potential when handling infected tissue, via parenteral inoculation or inspiration of aerosolized infectious material
Cryptococcus neoformans	Cryptococcosis	Dyspnea	Neurologic signs, depression, death without prior clinical signs		Clinical signs usually inapparent and when present, nonspecific. Meningitis is a very common complication
Pneumocystis carinii		Dyspnea, nonproductive cough	Fever, anorexia	Marmosets, owl monkeys, macaques, chimpanzees	(1) Associated with SIV infection in macaques (2) Zoonotic potential: considered an opportunist in immune-compromised hosts. Risk to humans minimal. Epidemiologic and experimental data support the occurrence of airborne, possible horizontal, transmission in humans and animals, including nonhuman primates
Parasitic diseases					
Toxoplasma gondii	Toxoplasmosis	Found acutely moribund with audible rales and fluid, blood, or foam coming from the nares and mouth	Anorexia and lethargy, diarrhea	Prosimians, New World and Old World monkeys	New World monkeys and prosimians in which infection is most devastating and in which it has occurred in outbreak form
Taenia sp.	Cysticercosis	Usually incidental findings at necropsy	Not reported	Red-ruffed lemurs	Should be included in the differential diagnosis for space-occupying lesions
Echinococcus sp.	Hydatidosis, echinococcosis	Usually incidental findings at necropsy	Not reported	Baboons	Should be included in the differential diagnosis for space-occupying lesions
Mesocestoides sp.	Tetyrathyridiosis	Usually incidental findings at necropsy	Not reported	Cynomolgus monkeys	Should be included in the differential diagnosis for space-occupying lesions

Etiology	Disease	Clinical signs		Reported species	Comments, including zoonotic potential
		Respiratory	Other		
Filaroides sp. *Filariopsis* sp.	Pulmonary nematodiasis	Generally clinically inapparent, occasional coughing, pulmonary hemorrhage	Not reported	Marmosets, squirrel monkeys, cebus monkeys, howler monkeys, cynomolgus monkeys	
Anatrichosoma cutaneum or *A. cynomolgi*	Nasal nematodiasis	Usually subclinical	Not reported	Rhesus monkeys, cynomolgus monkeys, patas monkeys, vervets, talapoin monkeys, mangabeys, baboons	
Dinobdella ferox, Limnatus africana	Nasal annelids	May be asymptomatic, epistaxis, asphyxiation	Restlessness, anemia, weakness, sometimes death		Clinical problems relate to numbers of leeches present
Pneumonyssus sp., *Pneumonyssoides* sp.	Pulmonary acariasis	Usually subclinical, severe infections may have associated cough and dyspnea	Not reported	Woolly monkeys, howler monkeys, macaques, douc langurs, proboscis monkeys, chimpanzees	Complications of lung mite infection include pneumothorax and pulmonary arteritis
Rhinophaga sp.	Nasal acariasis	Not reported	Not reported	Rhesus monkeys, baboons, orangutans	

common marmosets (*Callithrix jacchus*) there was high morbidity (69/91) and low mortality (10/69) (Flecknell *et al.,* 1983; Sutherland *et al.,* 1986). Clinical signs included upper respiratory signs of mild serous or occasionally purulent nasal exudate or systemic illness and death. In animals that died or were euthanized, the main finding was diffuse pulmonary consolidation and edema with histologic evidence of acute interstitial pneumonia. Histopathologic lesions were not well described. The upper respiratory tracts were contaminated with hemolytic *E. coli, Staphylococcus aureus, Klebsiella pneumoniae* and *Neisseria* spp., but only 1 of 8 animals necropsied had bacteria in the lungs and this isolate was *K. pneumoniae.*

Fatal pneumonia due to PMV (PI)-3 has also been reported in marmosets (F. Deinhardt *et al.,* 1967) and patas monkeys (*Erythrocebus patas*) (Churchill, 1963). Parainfluenza type 3 has been incriminated in predisposing chimpanzees to serious pneumococcal pneumonia (Jones *et al.,* 1984).

Serologic evidence for PMV-1, -2 and -3 exposure has been found in many species of primates, but seems most common in great apes. Among 31 gorillas and chimpanzees tested for paramyxoviruses as part of battery screening, the seroprevalence was 0 for PMV-1, 39% for PMV-2, and 52% for PMV-3 (Kalter

and Heberling, 1990). Orangutans are also susceptible (L. J. Lowenstine, unpublished). It is likely that these often represent anthropozoonoses, as infection in the human population is very high. In the great apes this infection is usually self-limiting.

3. Measles (Rubeola)

The measles virus is broadly infective for nonhuman primates, including New World and Old World monkeys and apes. Little work has been done in prosimians. The portal of entry of this highly contagious zoonotic virus is generally considered to be respiratory, but the disease is systemic. Gastrointestinal lesions or immunosuppression, rather than respiratory disease, is often the most important sequela to the infection. In New World monkeys there may be no respiratory involvement at all.

Clinical signs in macaques include conjunctivitis, rhinorrhea, rash, depression, and dehydration. Animals may be leukopenic. Diagnosis is based on serology, virus isolation (from lymphocytes), immunostaining of conjunctival smears or other cytologic material, and histopathology. Morbidity is high and mortality is variable. It is highest in New World monkeys, Asian colobines, and young animals.

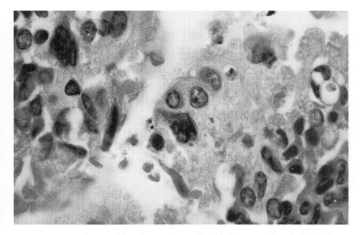

Fig. 2. Measles. Multinucleate giant cell with intracytoplasmic inclusions, air sac, mountain gorilla (*Gorilla gorilla*).

Lesions in the respiratory tract are a bronchointerstitial pneumonia typically centered on the small bronchioles or respiratory ducts. There is a desquamation of bronchiolar epithelium and alveolar lining cells along with an increase in bronchoalveolar macrophages. Indistinct intranuclear and cytoplasmic inclusion bodies and multinucleated giant cells (Fig. 2) may occur, especially as type II pneumocyte hyperplasia ensues (Lowenstine, 1993b). The laryngeal air sacs may also be involved. Secondary bacterial infections and superimposed bronchopneumonia may occur.

B. Orthomyxoviruses: Influenza Viruses

That both influenza A and B have been described in nonhuman primates is not surprising given the wide host range of these viruses (Renegar, 1992). What is surprising is the relatively few reports of active disease. Serologic screening of primate colonies and collections has revealed that exposure to influenza A is more common than exposure to influenza B (Kalter and Heberling, 1990).

Much of our knowledge of the effects of flu viruses in nonhuman primates comes from experimental inoculations that have been carried out in New World monkeys (*Cebus* spp., *Saimiri* sp., and *Aotus* sp.), Old World monkeys (*Macaca mulatta, M. fascicularis, Papio* spp.), and apes (*Hylobates* sp. and *Pan troglodytes*). Squirrel monkeys are one of the animal models of choice for vaccine and therapeutic studies (Renegar, 1992); they and capuchins have also been used for pathogenesis studies. In capuchins, the severity of disease varied with the route of inoculation (intratracheal more severe than intranasal) and strain of virus (A/Victoria/3/75 more pathogenic than A/New Jersey/76). The incubation period was 3–5 days, although virus could be recovered on day 1. Clinical signs included depression and dyspnea in the worse cases and rhinorrhea in the

less severely affected animals. Radiographic evidence of pneumonia was more evident on lateral than anterior–posterior projections and was most evident in middle and lower (caudal) lobes. Pathologic findings in animals killed at days 4 to 6 included gross evidence of tracheal hyperemia and patchy pulmonary consolidation. Histologically there was a loss of ciliated cells, erosion, hemorrhage, and mononuclear inflammation in tracheal and bronchial epithelium accompanied by squamous metaplasia. Extension into the parenchyma was characterized by thickening of alveolar septa by mononuclear cells and exudation of fibrin. Upper repiratory lesions were limited by mild submucosal inflammation (Grizzard *et al.,* 1978).

A study in squirrel monkeys highlighted the significance of pneumococcal superinfection in causing lethal outcomes in influenza virus infections (Berendt *et al.,* 1975). Clinical signs of "flu" in these monkeys were fever, coryza, tachypnea, dyspnea, coughing or sneezing, lethargy, and anorexia. Signs were least severe in animals inoculated with *Streptococcus pneumoniae* alone and most severe in animals sequentially infected with influenza virus and *S. pneumoniae,* and although mortalities occurred in all groups, they were most numerous in the dually infected animals. Lesions in the virus-infected animals were similar to those described in capuchins with the exception of the presence of neutrophils (postinoculation day 6). In sequentially infected animals the lungs were grossly consolidated with pleural exudate. Histologically the pneumonia was fibrinopurulent and necrotizing.

There is one well-documented outbreak of influenza A in a colony of gibbons (*Hylobates lar lar*) in southeast Asia in which morbidity was about 30% and mortality about 10% (Johnsen *et al.,* 1971). This outbreak was initiated by experimental inoculation but spread to involve uninoculated contact animals. Clinical signs reported were anorexia, depression, serous to suppurative nasal exudate, coughing, and gastrointestinal signs. In many animals the signs were short-lived and self-limiting. Two of the animals that died had no premonitory upper respiratory signs.

Gross lesions in the gibbons included posterior consolidation, congestion, and edema. Microscopically, the lungs of animals without secondary bacterial infections had evidence of bronchointerstitial pneumonia centered on small bronchioles. Sloughing of epithelium was evident and in one animal was accompanied by early proliferative bronchiolitis. Exudation of erythrocytes, fibrin, and alveolar macrophages was evident in the parenchyma. The presence of marked neutrophilic exudation was associated with secondary bacterial pathogens.

C. Adenoviruses

Adenoviruses have been readily isolated from many species of nonhuman primates; however, clinical disease is less common (Espana, 1974). Conjunctivitis and rhinitis have been described in patas monkeys and macaques infected with SV17, macaques infected by SV15, and chimpanzees infected with SV32. Pneumonias in macaques have been associated with SV11, SV15, SV20, and SV37. "Pneumoenteritis" has been described in African green monkeys and baboons infected with V404 and V340. Adenoviral pneumonia has also been described in a juvenile chimpanzee (Butchin *et al.,* 1992). Adenoviral pneumonia may be secondary to recrudescence of latent infection in the face of immunosuppression caused by retroviruses (King, 1993a; Lowenstine, 1993a).

Clinical signs depend on the host and strain of virus. Many of the reports have been in juvenile or infant monkeys. Acute respiratory infections in macaques with signs of skin rash, conjunctivitis, facial edema and erythema, nasal discharge, and cough were attributed to adenoviruses based on isolation of SV15 and SV32 and histologic evidence of necrotizing pneumonia with basophilic inclusions in which adenovirus-like particles were identified by electron microscopy (Espana, 1971, 1974). In another report (Boyce *et al.,* 1978), clinical signs in infant rhesus included tachypnea, cough, and cyanosis unresponsive to oxygen. Gross lesions in neonatal monkeys were limited to the lungs and consisted of consolidation, gray discoloration, and failure to collapse. There was necrosis of bronchiolar and alveolar epithelium and enlarged nuclei filled with amphophilic to basophilic inclusions. Cowdry type A eosinophilic inclusions were less common. Exudate consisted of necrotic cellular debris, fibrin, alveolar macrophages, and low numbers of neutrophils. The diagnosis was based on electron microscopy.

D. Herpesviruses

Simian alphaherpesviruses are associated with systemic disease during which the lungs may become involved. Pneumonic involvement as a primary "complaint" is less common, but has been reported.

1. Herpesvirus simiae

An outbreak of respiratory herpesvirus infection was described in bonnet monkeys (*Macaca radiata*) (Espana, 1973). Clinical signs included purulent nasal exudate. No oral ulcers were observed. Morbidity was 50% and about 50% of affected animals died. Grossly the lungs were consolidated and foci of hemorrhage were observed. There was also splenomegaly and hepatomegaly with multifocal necrosis. Histologic lesions were those of a hemorrhagic interstitial pneumonia. Inclusion bodies were seen in the livers. The virus was subsequently determined to be *Herpesvirus simiae.* In retrospect, this colony of bonnet monkeys was found to have an endemic simian type D retrovirus infection (SRV-1) (L. J. Lowenstine, unpublished data). Periodic epizootics of herpesvirus infections were seen subsequent to the original report and respiratory disease was often a manifestation, although oral ulcers and encephalitis were seen as well.

2. Herpesvirus SA8

Herpesviral pneumonia was reported in two zoo-born perinatal Gelada baboons (*Theropithecus gelada*). The animals had died without clinical signs having been recognized. Gross lesions included large areas of pulmonary consolidation and pulmonary hemorrhage. Necrotizing bronchiolitis and interstitial pneumonia was present with many basophilic Cowdry type A inclusion bodies. Similar inclusions were also seen in brain, kidney, and spleen. Herpesviral particles were demonstrated by electron microscopy and the infection was suspected, although not proven, to be SA8.

Herpesviral tracheobronchopneumonia has been produced experimentally in newborn yellow baboons (*Papio cynocephalus*) inoculated intratracheally. Clinical disease was not described but terminal illness developed within 2 days of inoculation. Tracheal and bronchial epithelium was affected initially followed by bronchiolar involvement and spread to the parenchyma. Lesions were hemorrhagic and necrotizing.

3. Varicella-Zoster-like Herpesviruses

Several simian varicella-zoster-like viruses have been isolated. Macaques are the hosts for many of these agents, and fatal disease has been seen in naturally and experimentally infected African primates, including African green monkeys and patas monkeys. Intratracheal inoculation produced systemic disease with viremia and a vesicular rash. Pulmonary lesions included edema and petechial hemorrhages. Histologically, pulmonary edema and necrosis of alveolar septa with marked fibrin exudation was seen (Dueland *et al.,* 1992).

E. Rhinoviruses: Picorniviridae, Rhinovirinae

The susceptibility of chimpanzees to natural and experimental infection with human rhinoviruses has been documented (Dick and Dick, 1974), but the infection is often clinically inapparent or mild. Attempts at experimental inoculation in other species have been limited but unsuccessful. Species inoculated included *Papio doguera, P. hamadryas, Theropithecus gelada, Macaca mulatta, M. arctoides, Cercopithecus aethiops, Erythrocebus patas, Cebus albifrons,* and *Saimiri sciureus.* Gibbons (*Hylobates lar*) proved somewhat susceptible. Based on serosurveys, natural infection of chimpanzees with human rhinoviruses is considered to be rare. Clinical signs and lesions have not been described.

F. Retroviruses

Several different retrovirus infections have been described in nonhuman primates. Of the exogenous or pathogenic retroviruses, only infections with simian type D retroviruses (SRV) and simian immunodeficiency viruses (SIV) have been associ-

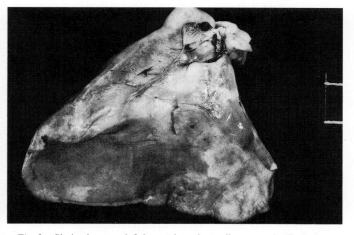

Fig. 3. Simian immunodeficiency virus giant cell pneumonia. Typical gross "styrofoam"-like lung appearance.

ated with respiratory tract lesions. In infections with SRV the lesions encountered are due to secondary opportunistic infections (Lowenstine, 1993a). Similar infections may also be seen in SIV-infected animals; however, SIV also causes a primary retroviral pneumonia in macaques (Baskerville *et al.,* 1992; King, 1993a).

1. Simian Immunodeficiency Virus

Lentiviruses of cercopithecine monkeys are indigenous to African monkeys of the genera *Cercopithecus, Cercocebus,* and *Papio (Mandrillus).* The viruses are of very low pathogenicity in African species. In Asian macaques, however, these viruses cause devastating disease characterized by immune dysfunction, wasting, opportunistic infections, and primary retroviral pneumonia and encephalitis. Historically, many macaques were infected by accidental iatrogenic exposure, by direct contact with African species, and through exposure to other infected macaques (Lowenstine *et al.,* 1986). Currently in most vivaria, natural SIV infection of macaques is rare to nonexistent (Daniel *et al.,* 1984). However, macaques are commonly experimentally infected as models for human HIV infection.

Primary retroviral pneumonia is a common finding in experimentally infected rhesus (Baskerville *et al.,* 1992; Baskin *et al.,* 1989; King, 1993a). Clinical signs are nonspecific, including anorexia, weight loss, and inactivity. Grossly the lungs fail to collapse and are diffusely or patchily discolored tan to cream or yellow, sometimes with pleural opacification. They are spongy to slightly firm on palpation with minimal free exudate on cut surface (Fig. 3).

Histologic examination reveals thickening of alveolar septa, marked exudation of macrophages, lesser amounts of proteinaceous material, and large numbers of syncytial giant cells. The pneumonia is readily differentiated from measles giant cell pneumonia by the absence of inclusion bodies in the SIV pneu-

monia giant cells and the diffuse alveolar involvement as opposed to the measles orientation around small bronchioles (i.e., no necrotizing bronchiolitis).

VIII. BACTERIAL DISEASES AND AGENTS

A. Tuberculosis

Tuberculosis is a disease of major concern in primate colonies, both for its potential devastating effect on captive primate populations (Henrickson, 1984; Lehner, 1984; Renquist and Whitney, 1978) and for its zoonotic potential (Dannenberg, 1978). Although most notably a problem among Old World primates, it occurs naturally in New World monkeys as well (Hessler and Moreland, 1968; Leathers and Hamm, 1976). The disease is generally associated with infection by the organisms *Mycobacterium tuberculosis* and *M. bovis* (Hessler and Moreland, 1968; Kaufmann and Anderson, 1978; McLaughlin, 1978; Renner and Bartholomew, 1974; Tarara *et al.,* 1985; Thoen *et al.,* 1977; Ward *et al.,* 1985; Wolf *et al.,* 1988); however, a number of other *Mycobacterium* species have occasionally been reported in association with clinical disease (King, 1993b). Nontuberculous mycobacterial infection is also recognized in nonhuman primates, usually associated with agents belonging to the *Mycobacterium avium-intracellulare* complex, but also reported in association with *M. paratuberculosis.* Surveillance and diagnostic techniques for tuberculosis are important preventive health procedures for captive primate colonies (Kaufmann and Anderson, 1978; Kuhn and Selin, 1978; McLaughlin and Marrs, 1978; Montali and Hirschel, 1990; Renquist and Whitney, 1978; Southers and Ford, 1995). Interpretation of surveillance results can vary for individual animals, depending on the state of disease or *Mycobacterium* exposure, and has been a particular problem with orangutans (Calle *et al.,* 1989; Chaparas *et al.,* 1975; Dillehay and Huerkamp, 1990; Kaufmann and Anderson, 1978; Kuhn and Selin, 1978; McLaughlin and Marrs, 1978; Wells *et al.,* 1990). For orangutans, a high rate of positive tuberculin reaction (60% of those tuberculin tested) generally has been associated with exposure to a variety of nontuberculous *Mycobacterium* species, including *M. fortuitum, M. terrae, M. nonchromogenicum, M. avium,* and *M. cheloni* (Calle *et al.,* 1989; Wells *et al.,* 1990), with no evidence of mycobacterial disease.

Mycobacteria are aerobic, slightly curved or straight, occasionally beaded, rod-shaped bacilli that stain poorly with Gram's stain, but stain positively with acid fast staining (e.g., Ziehl–Nielson stain, Fite–Faraco stain). Culture of these organisms requires special media and techniques to destroy contaminating nonacid fast bacteria. Tuberculosis is extremely rare in natural populations of nonhuman primates that are remotely situated away from human populations. Infection in captive populations is generally thought to be related to the transmission of disease from humans to animals (Cappucci *et al.,* 1972). Tuberculosis is a particularly contagious and potentially fulminant disease in macaques, especially in rhesus monkeys (King, 1993b). Strict quarantine procedures and routine tuberculin testing of nonhuman primates and animal care personnel have contributed to a marked reduction in the occurrence of tuberculosis in captive nonhuman primate populations.

Transmission of tuberculosis occurs most commonly via respiratory exposure to infected aerosols, although ingestion of infected materials and subsequent gastrointestinal infection is also a recognized infection route. Disease pathogenesis, reviewed by Dannenberg (1978) and King (1993b), involves phagocytosis of organisms by tissue-resident macrophages. Variability in macrophage ability to kill the organisms exists, leading to diverse possibilities for infection outcome and lesion morphology. When organisms are able to survive phagocytosis and replicate intracellularly, the macrophage is eventually killed. Successful intracellular killing of mycobacteria by macrophages leads to processing of the agent and antigen presentation for immune response by T lymphocytes. The T cells, as well as peripheral blood monocytes, are recruited to the infection site by various macrophage-derived cytokines. Further activation of mononuclear phagocytes occurs in these sites in response to mycobacterial products and cytokines released by the reactive lymphocytes. The activated macrophages phagocytize the bacteria and tend to transform into immobile epitheliod cells, forming epithelioid granuloma. A subset of macrophages remain mobile and may eventually move to regional lymph nodes and other tissues, where, if intracellular killing has not been complete, the infection process and associated inflammatory response continue. Additional processes that contribute to the classical morphology of tuberculous lesions include fusion of macrophages to form multinucleate Langhans-type giant cells and promotion of potentially encapsulating fibrosis by various mediators.

A spectra of possible gross lesions are recognized in nonhuman primates with tuberculosis. Lesions may be inapparent or may include widely disseminated, 1.0–10.0 cm, yellow-white, focal to confluent granulomas affecting all major organs. Large granulomas in the lung may be cavitary, a result of drainage of caseous exudate into adjacent airways. Among the most commonly affected organs are lungs, tracheobronchial lymph nodes, spleen, liver, kidney, intestine, and mesenteric nodes.

Microscopic variation may also exist as influenced by the time course and extent of disease. Early lesions may be widely scattered microscopic granulomas made up of circumscribed collections of epithelioid cells and an occasional Langhans' giant cell. Some of these lesions may include central neutrophil aggregates. Such small lesions may initially be confined to lung or intestinal tract, in association with the initial route of infection. The tubercle is the ''classic'' lesion of advanced tuberculosis. It includes a central core of acellular necrotic debris, surrounded by a zone of epithelioid cells and scattered Langhans-type, multinucleate, giant cells. At times the core is calcified. The tubercle periphery is generally made up of variable amounts of fibrous connective tissue and infiltrating lymphocytes. Acid fast special stains usually reveal acid fast bacilli in the epithelioid and multinucleate giant cells, although there are instances in which many tissue sections must be examined in order to find tubercle bacilli.

Differential diagnosis of microscopic lesions seen with tuberculosis includes other granulomatous disease, including certain foreign bodies (e.g., kaolin), mycotic, protozoan, and parasitic organisms. Definitive diagnosis is with identification of a specific mycobacterium species from the lesions, using such techniques as isolation and/or polymerase chain reaction (PCR). Although the lack of positive culture results would prevent the ability to designate a particular mycobacterium species, the presence of acid fast bacilli in granuloma or tubercle microscopic sections confirms the diagnosis of tuberculosis. Among the lesions assessed for differential diagnosis, those caused by *Nocardia* can be confused, particularly because of the partial acid fast nature of *Nocardia*; however, *Nocardia* organisms stain gram positive and are beaded and branching, making differentiation relatively easy.

When tuberculosis is diagnosed in a population of animals, it is extremely important that the outbreak be controlled. All animal movement within the colony should be halted, and animals previously housed in the same room with the infected animal(s) should be located. These animals should be tested biweekly with tuberculin for a minimum of five consecutive negative tests. This is necessary because detecting infected animals early postinfection can be difficult. The nature of the tuberculin skin test, which measures delayed-type hypersensitivity, is not sensitive under conditions of recent infection and generally does not become positive until at least a short time after the infected animal has begun to shed organisms (Clarke, 1968; Henrickson, 1984).

When screening animals in quarantine, or as part of an ongoing preventive health program (Southers and Ford, 1995), positive test results may occur. Some of these results may be equivocal. In such cases, or in cases such as those involving potentially false-positive reactions in orangutans, additional tests may be performed. In the meantime, no animals should be moved into or out of the group. Additional tests can include differential skin tests with a panel of tuberculins, usually including avian tuberculin, as well as a variety of other procedures including gastric and bronchial lavage with cytology and culture, as well as thoracic radiography.

The combination of the high level of risk to a colony and the difficulty in achieving successful treatment often results in the decision to euthanize positive-reacting animals. This makes it possible to eliminate the potential for infection spread. In some cases, usually involving the value of the individual animal, treatment is carried out. The potential for emergence of drug-resistant mutants has led to the routine use of at least two effective drugs (Daniel, 1994). Prolonged courses of drug therapy are always necessary due to the long generation time of myco-

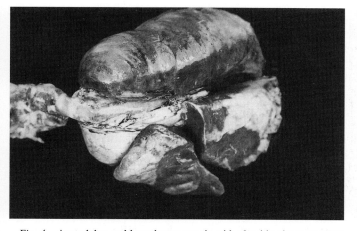

Fig. 4. Acute lobar and bronchopneumonia with pleuritis, rhesus monkey (*Macaca mulatta*), etiology: *Streptococcus pneumonia.*

bacteria and their extended periods of metabolic inactivity. The most effective available treatment regimen for humans involves regimens that include isoniazid and rifampin for 9 to 12 months, with a favorable outcome in 99% of patients (Daniel, 1994). Drug toxicity is an important factor in the choice of therapeutic agents. Drug-associated hepatitis is of greatest concern. Serum enzymes and other blood tests predicting liver disease are not helpful as monitors of toxicity and are not recommended (Daniel, 1994). Discontinuation of medication at the onset of jaundice generally leads to the resolution of drug-associated hepatitis.

Reports of treatment in nonhuman primates document the use of a multiple drug regime such as isoniazid, rifampin, and ethambutol (Wolf *et al.,* 1988) or streptomycin and isoniazid (Ward *et al.,* 1985) over a period that minimally lasts 9 to 12 months, and up to 30 months in one report included in a summary by Wolf *et al.* (1988). Treatment must be carried out in conjunction with culture and sensitivity testing, as supported by the failure of combined isoniazid and *p*-aminosalicylic acid therapy to resolve tuberculosis in orangutans due to drug resistance of the particular organism (Haberle, 1970). Ward *et al.* (1985) used a treatment period of 6 months, and 1 animal out of 195 exposed animals (48 became tuberculin reactive) subsequently developed tuberculosis. If animals are being treated, it is important to be aware that the tuberculin reaction can be masked when animals are undergoing chemotherapy (Clarke and Schmidt, 1969; Dillehay and Huerkamp, 1990).

B. Pneumococcal Infection

Streptococcus pneumoniae is found in nasal secretions of up to 60% of normal human adults during winter months. This gram-positive coccus is the cause of 90–95% of lobar pneumonia in humans. In addition, it is also a cause of broncho-

pneumonia, empyema, and upper respiratory infection (middle ear, sinuses), as well as severe meningitis or brain abscesses. Severe infections can lead to pneumococcal bacteremia. Similarly, it has been reported to cause up to 95% of pneumonia cases in one report of nonhuman primate respiratory disease (Fiennes and Dzhikidze, 1972). The presence of large numbers of paired gram-positive cocci in exudate smears supports the diagnosis of *S. pneumonia* infection. Outbreaks of *S. pneumoniae*-associated respiratory disease in nonhuman primates (Fig. 4) are associated with the presence of other predisposing problems, such as stress, inclement weather, or viral respiratory infections. Jones *et al.* (1984) describe the association between parainfluenza type 3 virus infection and invasive *S. pneumoniae* infection. *Streptococcus pneumoniae* is sensitive to penicillin, such that use of long-acting penicillin during an outbreak can decrease morbidity during an outbreak. Valuable populations of vulnerable animals may benefit from immunization with pneumococcal polysaccharide (CDC, 1989).

C. *Klebsiella pneumoniae*

Klebsiella pneumoniae is a common enterobacterium that causes a disease spectrum that includes severe pneumonia (lobular or lobar), urinary tract infection, and miscellaneous septic lesions, including sinusitis, meningitis, and otitis. In humans it is an unusual part of pharyngeal and oral microflora, but is recognized in up to 20% of hospital patients. Lung infections arise. Pneumonia in *K. pneumoniae* infections is generally a bronchopneumonia, with a tendency for abscess formation and pleuritis. The exudate associated with *Klebsiella* is typically gelatinous. In hematoxylin and eosin (H&E) and Gram-stained sections, the organism has a characteristic evenly spread distribution and a thick clear capsule. Although often associated with acute pneumonia, the pneumonia may be followed by persistent, chronic infection, including chronic bronchitis, bronchiectasis, and pulmonary abscess. *Klebsiella pneumonia* speticemia may occur in association with localized infection.

Eichberg (1985) reports an outbreak of *K. pneumoniae* infection in a group of nursery-housed infant chimpanzees. The disease began with nasal discharge. Two animals died, including one that had no recognized signs of clinical illness. The first animal that died had congestion, fever, anorexia, and weight loss along with the nasal discharge. Treatment with tetracyeline was unsuccessful. Postmortem lesions in the animal were restricted to the lungs, including consolidation and pleural adhesions. Microscopic lesions were of diffuse severe bronchopneumonia. Gross lesions in the second animal included multifocal subepicardial hemorrhage and mild pulmonary edema, with scattered multifocal yellow-gray lesions in all lobes and scattered subpleural petechiae. Histologic examination revealed lesions compatible with septicemia, including moderate to severe pneumonia. Culture in each case yielded pure cultures of *K. pneumoniae,* for which gentamycin was the drug of choice.

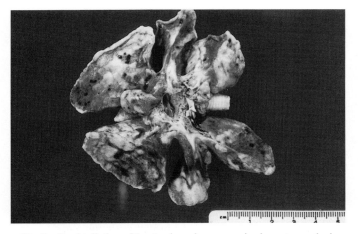

Fig. 5.   *Bordetella bronchiseptica* bronchopneumonia plus cytomegalovirus interstitial pneumonia, rhesus monkey (*Macaca mulatta*). The macaque had primary simian retrovirus-1 infection. Cytomegalovirus-associated lesions include hilar edema and multifocal hemorrhage.

Other animals were treated with gentamycin and the disease was rapidly cleared. Based on findings that many normal adult chimpanzees had positive throat and rectal cultures for *K. pneumoniae*, it was presumed that very young chimpanzees were immunologically compromised and at risk for clinical disease. Following this outbreak, strict husbandry and nursery management procedures were instituted, including restricted access, routine sanitation procedures of equipment and nursery enclosures, and use of protective clothing by nursery caretakers.

Fox and Rohovsky (1975) present two cases of *K. pneumonia* infection in rhesus monkeys. The animals were involved in experimental work that included use of an atherogenic diet. Each case had meningitis, one had severe bronchopneumonia, and the other's lesions were compatible with septicemia, including pneumonia. Other reports of *K. pneumonia* in nonhuman primates were reviewed, and the occurrence of high mortality and frequent multiple drug resistance in the isolated organisms was discussed. Rapid identification and antibiotic sensitivity are keys for sucessful treatment in *K. pneumonia* outbreaks.

D. *Bordetella*

1. *Bordetella bronchiseptica*

Bordetella bronchiseptica is an obligate parasite of the upper respiratory tract of a number of animal species, including primates. It is the documented cause of pneumonia and upper respiratory disease in prosimians (Kohn and Haines, 1977), New World primates (Baskerville *et al.,* 1983), and Old World primates (Graves, 1970; Klein *et al.,* 1987). Generally, these cases have occurred in association with potentially weakened pulmonary defenses (stress, virus, age, etc.) (Fig. 5).

Kohn and Haines (1977) described the occurrence of *B. bronchiseptica* interstitial pneumonia, pleuritis, middle ear infection, and meningitis in lesser bushbabies (*Galago senegalensis*) within 1 week of arrival. The first animal presented with torticollis and later developed seizures. Necropsy findings included middle ear infection, meningitis, and interstitial pneumonia. A second animal died unexpectedly the day following this necropsy and a third animal died 12 days later. Both animals had severe pulmonary consolidation and one also had severe fibrinopurulent pericarditis and pleuritis. Microscopic examination of the lungs in all animals revealed a mixed inflammatory infiltrate with an interstitial distribution, without apparent bronchial involvement.

Bordetella bronchiseptica-associated disease is documented by Baskerville *et al.* (1983) in a colony of marmosets that had initially been established as *B. bronchiseptica* free. Bilateral mucopurulent nasal discharge was noted in animals of all ages. Cough was not recognized, and animals often remained bright and alert, with occasional signs of dyspnea when handled. Affected animals had mild fever. Over a 3-month period, 16 animals died out of a total colony size of 156 animals. Fifteen of the deaths occurred in animals less than 12 months old, whereas the other death occurred in a 5-year-old animal. Deaths occurred suddenly, with typical gross lesions consisting of pneumonia and pleuritis and two animals with pericarditis. Microscopic lung lesions were coalescing acute purulent bronchopneumonia. Animals were treated with oxytetracycline, with clinical recovery in adults after several days. Despite clinical recovery, *B. bronchiseptica* was still present in the nasopharynx of these animals 8 weeks later. Nasal cultures of the entire colony yielded positive cultures for *B. bronchiseptica* in 71 of the 156 animals. The fulminant disease in the young animals, as evidenced by the rapid onset of clinical signs then death, was deemed to have made treatment initiation too late to alter their disease course.

Graves (1970) reports the occurrence of fatal *B. bronchiseptica* pneumonia in a group of six African green monkeys (*Cercopithecus aethiops*) over a 6-month period after the arrival of a total of 25 animals. In experimental studies of simian type D retrovirus serotype 1 (SRV-1) infection in rhesus monkeys (*Macaca mulatta*), *B. bronchiseptica* pneumonia occurred in 3 out of 22 animals that died with simian AIDS (K. G. Osborn, unpublished data). *Bordetella bronchiseptica* pneumonia had not otherwise been a recognized problem at the California Regional Primate Research Center.

2. *Bordetella pertussis*

Whooping cough is an acute, highly communicable respiratory disease caused by *Bordetella pertussis,* a small pleomorphic gram-negative coccobacillus. The organism has a strong tropism for bronchial epithelial brush border, to which it attaches and grows in tangled colonies without tissue invasion. The characteristic lesions and signs (enhanced cough reflex, peripheral lymphocytosis, malaise, weight loss, mild fever) are thought to be related to exotoxin production. These signs persist as long as the toxin is present within cells, even after the bacteria are gone. Immune protection and recovery are based on the production of secretory IgA, which inhibits bacterial adhesion and this subsequent proliferation. The disease has a 7- to 10-day incubation period, at the end of which there is a "catarrhal" period of coughing and sneezing, followed by the onset of the characteristic violent paroxysmal coughing. Occasional complicating problems that can occur include subcutaneous emphysema and convulsions associated with hypoxia and constant coughing. Lesions of established whooping cough are of laryngotracheobronchitis. In severe cases this can include bronchial mucosal erosion, hyperemia, and copious mucopurulent exudate. Mucosal lymph follicles and peribronchial lymph nodes are enlarged and hypercellular, paralleling the marked peripheral lymphocytosis seen in complete blood count data. Immunization has traditionally been provided as part of the DPT (diphtheria, pertussis, tetanus) vaccination; however, complications in both humans and in at least one infant chimpanzee (Southers and Ford, 1995) associated with the pertussis component have raised a cautionary note to the routine use of DPT. A DT vaccine is now available and could be considered as an alternative in conjunction with policies regarding immunization for employees and that prevent potential contact with children.

An epizootic of whooping cough has been described in a group of zoo chimpanzees (*Pan troglodytes*) (Gustavsson *et al.*, 1990). Clinical signs and epidemiologic data were compared to an outbreak of respiratory syncitial virus infection that occurred in the same group earlier in the same year. During the whooping cough outbreak, which started in early August, animals exhibited cough and some exhibited nasal catarrh. Following this period, animals developed drawn-out paroxysmal coughing fits and associated dyspnea. The coughing gradually decreased and eventually ceased during September.

E. Nocardiosis

Nocardiosis is an infrequent disease in nonhuman primates that must be differentiated from cases of tuberculosis. Nocardiae are found worldwide as soil-dwelling saphrophytic organisms. They are gram-positive, weakly acid fast-positive, long, filamentous (1 μm diameter) aerobic organisms that frequently aggregate in branching chains, growing extracellularly in tissue. Culture requirements are less exacting than *Mycobacterium* sp., as they grow in common culture media and under aerobic conditions.

Nocardial infection occurs in a variety of species, including humans and nonhuman primates (Klumpp and McClure, 1993). The disease is not transmitted among individual animals or humans. It can be found as a primary infection, but often is noted as an apparent opportunist, occurring in cases of chronic illness or with other states that may have associated immune

dysfunction. In humans, it appears as pulmonary or skin infection. Cases reported in nonhuman primates also include extrapulmonary infection with lesion distribution supporting the likelihood of an oral infection route (Liebenberg and Giddens, 1985).

Clinical signs associated with pulmonary nocardiosis are often nonspecific and even subclinical until late in the disease course. Fever and productive cough occur. Late dissemination may occur, including such sequelae as meningitis and cerebral abscess. Nocardia may not be suspected until after more common bacteria have been excluded and the response to antibiotics has proved unsuccessful. Antimicrobial testing for *Nocardia* species may not be clinically relevant, such that choice of effective antibiotic should generally be based on published clinical experience. Recommended treatment most often includes the use of long-term sulfonamide or minocycline. In addition to sulfonamides and minocycline, most aminoglycosides, fusidic acid, and some newly developed β-lactam antibiotics are active against most *Nocardia* strains (Filice, 1994). Increased efficacy has been suggested when sulfonamide is combined with streptomycin or trimethoprim (Liebenberg and Giddens, 1985). It is unknown whether combination therapy is actually more effective than single agent therapy (Filice, 1994). The potential for increased efficacy must be weighed against the increased risk for toxicity.

Pulmonary lesions often include multinodular to diffuse consolidation, as well as abscess and cavitary lesion formation. Pleural involvement may also occur, including fibrinous pleuritis or empyema. Nodules and abscesses may also occur in peritoneum, liver, kidney, brain, and subcutis. Microscopically, lesions frequently contain central areas of necrotic debris, bacteria, and neutrophils. Granulation or fibrous connective tissue often surrounds this lesion center, with a mixed inflammatory infiltrate that includes neutrophils, lymphocytes, plasma cells, macrophages, epithelioid cells, and multinucleate giant cells. Bacteria are generally not readily apparent with H&E staining but can generally be localized with either Gram or methenamine silver stain. An exception to inapparent bacterial presence occurs when they occasionally form large colonies, often termed "sulfur granules." This feature has resulted in the potential for misdiagnosis of nocardiosis as actinomycosis, actinobacillosis, or botryomycosis. The difficulties that can occur with microscopic differential diagnosis make definitive diagnosis dependent on isolation and identification of the organism.

Pulmonary nocardiosis in an outdoor housed adult male orangutan (*Pongo pygmaeus*) was associated with a history of recurrent upper respiratory infection signs over a 22-month period (McClure *et al.*, 1976). The episodes were considered to be not severe enough to warrant examination and treatment. A terminal episode occurred in which the animal was found lethargic and severely dyspneic, with epistaxis. Gross lesions included extensive chronic pneumonia and pleuritis, as well as air sac infection. Microscopic lesions were similar to those generally described with nocardiosis, including the presence of occasional granules made up of bacteria. Brown and Brenn stains revealed gram-positive, branched filamentous organisms. These were acid fast negative with a variety of acid fast stains, leading to an initial diagnosis of actinomycosis. Microbiology resulted in culture of *Nocardia asteroides*.

F. Pasteurellosis

Pasteurellae are strict animal parasites, generally inhabiting the nasopharyngeal and oral mucous membranes. Pasteurellosis can be caused by *Pasteurella multocida* or *P. hemolytica*. It may occur as peracute or acute septicemia, or may be less acute, and causes signs associated with the primary organ of infection. It often occurs when local and systemic defense mechanisms are impaired. Predisposing factors include stress induced by such factors as transportation, crowding, and climatic changes or by the damaging effects of respiratory viral infections.

Reported cases in nonhuman primates include outbreaks in Goeldi's monkeys (*Callimico goeldii*) (Duncan *et al.*, 1995) and owl monkeys (*Aotus trivirgatus*) (Benjamin and Lang, 1971), as well as a case in a patas monkey (*Erythrocebus patas*) (Okoh and Ocholi, 1986). Possible predisposing conditions included the presence of lingual gongylonemiasis in the Goeldi's monkeys, recent acquisition and transport of the owl monkeys, and the onset of cold, rainy seasonal weather for the patas monkey. The Goeldi's monkeys had a clinical history of a long-term increase in salivation, with no other signs prior to the death of three out of four animals over an 8-hr period. The owl monkeys were received in poor condition and were anorexic and lethargic, with one animal found dead 3 days after arrival and two more animals dead 3 days later. Respiratory difficulty had been noted in the patas monkey for 2 weeks prior to her death, during which she appeared to improve with penicillin–streptomycin therapy. Lesions in all three supported the occurrence of acute bacteremia, with pulmonary involvement that included the presence of fibrinopurulent interstitial inflammation associated with fibrinous thrombi and bacteria in pulmonary vessels. *Pasteurella multocida* was isolated from the Goeldi's monkeys and the owl monkeys, whereas *P. hemolytica* was isolated from the patas monkey.

IX. MYCOTIC DISEASES

A. Coccidioidomycosis

Coccidioides immitis is a dimorphic fungus that grows as a saprophyte in endemic geographic areas, including arid regions of California, Arizona, and Texas, as well as in similarly arid portions of northern Mexico, Central America, and South America. It naturally infects a variety of wild rodent species (Pappagianis, 1985), and high concentrations of the fungus may be found in rodent burrows. Vegetative growth occurs in these

areas after rains, with dispersion of spores (arthroconidia) by the wind after the soil dries. Other activity that disturbs the contaminated soil, such as construction or agricultural, also can increase the possibility of spreading the infective spores. Very severe dust storms have resulted in epizootics of disease, and cases may occur in areas geographically associated with, but not normally recognized as, endemic sites of *C. immitis* growth, as the windblown spores arrive from many miles away.

Coccidioidmycosis is primarily a respiratory disease, with inhalation of arthrospores as the mode of infection. It is not transmitted via the respiratory route from animal to animal. The tissue form is not generally considered to be pathogenic, although ingestion of infected mouse cadavers by other mice, rats, or hamsters has produced infection (Pappagianis, 1985). This latter finding supports the use of caution when handling diagnostic or postmortem material to avoid parenteral exposure or aerosolization and possible inhalation. Over time, it is likely that many animals and humans in endemic areas are exposed and possibly infected, with relatively few clinically apparent cases. When present, clinical signs in those with pulmonary disease may include fever and cough, and in humans have been noted to include pleuritic pain and hypersensitivity-type skin lesions (erythema nodosum, erythema multiforme). In a small percentage of individuals, more generalized disease occurs, with signs such as continued fever, chills, night sweats, weakness, and weight loss. Diagnostic workup can include radiology (Silverman *et al.*, 1975), as well as serology, biopsy, and culture (Pappagianis, 1985). Treatment involves the use of antimycotic agents, such as amphotericin B, ketoconazole, and fluconazole (Bennett, 1994a; Graybill *et al.*, 1985, 1990; Pappagianis, 1985).

Gross pulmonary lesions include focal gray-white foci of consolidation as well as more diffuse consolidation. Local lymph node enlargement may also occur. When disseminated disease is present, there is more diffuse pulmonary involvement, with multifocal involvement of other tissues, including lymph nodes, spleen, bones, liver, meninges, and adrenals. The host inflammatory reaction depends on the phase of the organism that is present. Inflammation in acute and fulminant lesions includes a marked neutrophilic response, which generally occurs in response to arthroconidia and endospores. A granulomatous reaction takes place in response to the presence of the classical tissue-phase stage of *C. immitis* growth; the thick-walled spherule (sporangium), which measures 10 to 70 μm in diameter and has a thick, double-contoured wall. Endospores are produced in large numbers within the spherules and generally are 2–5 μm in diameter. They are released into the tissues when a spherule ruptures. The presence of all phases of fungus growth within an infection site can lead to a lesion morphology that includes foci of neutrophilic aggregation in association with endospores, as well as extensive fibrosis with epithelioid cells, giant cells, lymphocytes, and neutrophils, often in association with spherules. When infection is well contained by the host, the granulomatous response predominates, and numbers of organisms are small, making detection and etiologic diagnosis more difficult.

There are multiple reports of coccidioidomycosis occurring in nonhuman primates (Pappagianis, 1985). In each reported case, as well as in more recent reports (Bellini *et al.,* 1991; Burton *et al.,* 1986; Graybill *et al.,* 1990), the affected animals either resided in endemic areas or had originated from endemic areas. The report by Burton *et al.* (1986) describes coccidioidomycosis in a ring-tailed lemur (*Lemur catta*) that had been relocated to a zoo in Oklahoma from a zoo in Phoenix. The initial clinical problem of that animal was unilateral corneal opacity, followed 3 months later by convulsions, urine retention, and diarrhea. Within a week the condition of the animal continued to deteriorate, with dyspnea and radiologically apparent pleural effusion. Exploratory laparotomy revealed peritonitis as well, and the animal was subsequently euthanized. Pathological workup revealed the presence of multifocal granulomatous inflammation in multiple tissues including the retina, lungs, liver, kidney, and chest wall associated with thick-walled spherules compatible with *C. immitis* infection. Culture and serology confirmed the diagnosis.

Graybill *et al.,* (1990) document the occurrence of coccidioidomycosis in a free-ranging group of more than 200 Japanese macaques (*Macaca fuscata*) in Dilley, Texas. The report further deals with the use of fluconazole in efforts to treat animals with coccidioidomycosis. Four gravely ill monkeys died within 1 month of starting treatment, whereas eight animals showed rapid improvement with an oral regimen of approximately 2–3 mg/kg/day, given as caramel candy into which the drug had been mixed. Therapy was successful when given over a prolonged period of time (minimum of 13 months in this group); however, at the time of publication, only one animal in this group of eight had actually had treatment discontinued without a recurrence of clinical disease. Two animals that had therapy interrupted at 2 months relapsed, then showed improvement again after resumption of therapy. The deaths of two other monkeys that had initially responded to therapy were directly related to a temporary interruption of the fluconazole supply. The authors discuss the potential benefit of higher doses and provide a review that includes initially mixed results in human trials. Finally, they reference earlier work that demonstrated great effectiveness of a liposomal preparation of amphotericin B, which could be administered just once or twice weekly and produced remission in treated animals (Graybill *et al.,* 1985), but which could not be used in the field situation in which the free-ranging macaques were involved.

B. Histoplasmosis

Histoplasmosis, caused by *Histoplasma capsulatum,* is a mycotic disease with a number of similarities to coccidioidomycosis, including (1) the occurrence of granulomatous pulmonary disease that can resemble tuberculosis, (2) fungus species characteristics that include thermal dimorphism (hyphae with spores at room temperatures, yeast-type growth at body temperature), and (3) a tendency for geographic localization (Ohio and Mississippi rivers and the Caribbean for *Histoplasma* and United States southwest and far west plus Mexico for *Coccidioides*). Histoplasmosis occurs generally by ingestion or inhalation of contaminated dust, which is often associated with pigeon, chicken, or bat feces-contaminated areas. *Histoplasma* exists in the infected individual as an intracellular parasite of the monocyte–macrophage system, with subsequent potential for dissemination throughout the reticuloendothelial system. Diagnosis can be made with a delayed-type hypersensitivity skin test or by morphologic identification in affected tissue specimens. Treatment is as for other systemic mycotic infections.

There are few reports of histoplasmosis in nonhuman primates (Migaki, 1986). Systemic histoplasmosis occurred in a de Brazza's monkey (*Cercopithecus neglectus*) in Kenya (Frank, 1968), with extensive renal involvement and less affected liver and lungs. Bergeland *et al.* (1970) report a squirrel monkey with *Histoplasma*-associated granulomatous pneumonia, hepatitis, and splenitis. The animal died 2 months after being purchased from a Minneapolis pet shop. Disseminated histoplasmosis has been reported as an opportunistic infection in an SIV-infected rhesus monkey (Baskin, 1991a).

C. Cryptococcosis

Cryptococcus neoformans is a yeast-like fungus that is found in soil throughout the world and occurs in particularly high frequency in old pigeon nests and droppings. Cryptococcosis generally occurs as an opportunistic primary respiratory infection via inhalation, more often affecting the nasal passages than the lungs. The pulmonary infection frequently remains mild or subclinical while the fungus spreads to other organs, including the central nervous system, skin, liver, spleen, adrenals, and bones. Meningitis is a very common complication in human cases. In humans the disease usually occurs as an opportunistic infection, but infection in normal individuals also occurs, often in association with overwhelming exposure.

Clinical signs of cryptococcosis are usually inapparent and, when present, nonspecific. Most infected humans present with meningoencephalitis and associated symptoms, including headache, nausea, staggering gait, dementia, irritability, confusion, and blurred vision (Bennett, 1994b). Reports of nonhuman primates have included signs such as marked depression in an Allen's swamp monkey (*Allenopithecus nigroviridis*) (Barrie and Stadler, 1990) and a lion-tailed macaque (*Macaca silenus*) (Miller and Boever, 1983), death without prior clinical signs, dyspnea, and/or neurologic signs in tree and elephant shrews (Tell *et al.,* 1993), seizures several days before death in a purple-faced langur (*Presbytis senex vetulus*) (Migaki, 1986), and a mandibular mass in a squirrel monkey (Roussilhon *et al.,* 1987).

Diagnosis of pulmonary cryptococcosis can be suggested with radiography (Feigin, 1983) or computerized tomography (Barrie and Stadler, 1990), but requires biopsy or culture for confirmation. The radiographic appearance and microscopic morphology can vary depending on the immune function of the host (Feigin, 1983; Samuelson and von Lichetenberg, 1994). In immunocompromised patients, gelatinous fungal masses may exist with no/minimal associated inflammation. Inflammatory infiltrates even in immune competent patients may often contain relatively few cells, consisting of a mixture of macrophages, lymphocytes, and plasma cells, although granulomatous inflammation with epithelioid and giant cells occurs as well, particularly in lung lesions. In section and cytologic specimens, the yeast has a characteristic very wide capsule. The capsule remains unstained in H&E-stained sections and stains positively with periodic acid–Schiff (PAS), mucicarmine, or alcian blue. Use of India ink in cytologic specimens is a negative staining technique that reveals the distinctive thick capsule as a clear halo around the yeast.

Cryptococcosis treatment in humans and nonhuman primates has included the use of amphotericin B alone or in combination with flucytosine and fluconazole alone or combined with flucytosine (Barrie and Stadler, 1990; Bennett, 1994b; Roussilhon et al., 1987). Barrie and Stadler (1990) describe marked improvement in response when fluconazole was substituted for amphotericin B. One of the tree shrews described by Tell et al., (1993) was treated with fluconazole alone, with clinical improvement within 5 days of therapy initiation. For the tree shrew colony in which 11 deaths occurred in addition to the animal that apparently recovered, preventive husbandry measures were undertaken, including complete disinfection of the enclosures, substitution of sterilized wood shavings for previously used leaf/pine bark mulch substrate in the tree shrew enclosure, and removal of birds and a lizard from the mixed species enclosures.

D. *Pneumocystis carinii*

Pneumocystis carinii is an important opportunistic respiratory pathogen, the environmental sources of which are as yet unknown. Analysis of ribosomal RNA gene sequences, mitochondrial proteins, major enzymes (thymidylate synthase, dihydrofolate reductase), and cell wall components (include glucans) provides evidence that *P. carinii* is a fungus rather than its previous classification as a protozoan. This is further supported by the effectiveness of drugs that inhibit 1,3-β-glucan synthesis in fungi when used in the treatment of *P. carinii* in animal models (Walzer, 1994). Most normal children are seropositive to the organism by the time they are 3 to 4 years old. In humans, *P. carinii* pneumonia occurs in premature or malnourished infants, children with primary immunodeficiency diseases, patients receiving immunosuppressive therapy, and people with AIDS. Epidemiologic and experimental data support the occurrence of airborne, possibly horizontal transmission in humans and animals, including nonhuman primates (Vogel et al., 1993; Walzer, 1994).

Clinical signs associated with *P. carinii* pneumonia in humans and nonhuman primates include dyspnea, fever, anorexia, and nonproductive cough (Chandler et al., 1976; Walzer, 1994). Radiographic findings often include bilateral diffuse pulmonary infiltrates. Because the clinical and radiographic findings are nonspecific, etiologic diagnosis depends on identification of the organism itself. Bronchoalveolar lavage fluid is the key material for demonstration of the organism, which is generally made apparent using such traditional stains as methenamine silver, toluidine blue, or cresyl echt violet, which stain the cell wall. Specific immunostaining or molecular probe techniques are also available. The typical microscopic lesion is a diffuse or patchy pneumonia. Alveolar spaces contain variable amounts of amphophilic, foamy amorphous material that resembles proteinaceous edema fluid, which is composed of *Pneumocystis* and cellular debris. Variable degrees of interstitial thickening are often present due to edema, minimal to mild mixed inflammatory cell infiltrates, and fibrosis. Type II pneumocyte hyperplasia may also be present.

Two major drugs are used in the treatment of *P. carinii* pneumonia: trimethoprim–sulfamethoxazole (TMP–SMX) and pentamidine isethionate. The treatment success rate in affected humans is similar for both drugs, 70 to 80%. TMP–SMX is administered orally or intravenously in three or four divided doses, whereas pentamidine is given in a single slow intravenous infusion once per day. A combined use of TMP–SMX and pentamidine has not proven to be more effective than either agent used along (Walzer, 1994). TMP–SMX, while well tolerated in non-AIDS patients, has associated serious adverse effects in over half of AIDS patients. Pentamidine is a toxic drug for all recipients. A number of alternative regimes show promise for effective use with fewer side effects, including TMP–SMX and dapsone combination, clindamaycin, and primaquine. Drugs undergoing clinical evaluation include trimetrexate, 566C80 (a hydroxynaphthoquinone), and eflornithine (a polyamine inhibitor).

Spontaneous *P. carinii* infection has been reported in nonhuman primates, including endemic infection in a marmoset colony (Richter et al., 1978), infection in two aged owl monkeys (*Aotus trivirgatus*) and two young chimpanzees (*Pan troglodytes*) (Chandler et al., 1976), and infection in macaques (Matsumoto et al., 1987). Richter et al. (1978) describe a retrospective survey of lungs from 441 marmosets for the occurrence of *Pneumocystis*. Fifty of the animals had histologically detected *Pneumocystis*, with just two animals that were thought to have associated clinical disease. The most affected age groups were the 7- to 12-month age group and aged animals (approximately 4 years plus). In the report by Chandler et al. (1976), one of the owl monkeys had no concurrent disease, whereas the other had been experimentally inoculated with *Treponema pallidum* 44 months before death. The chimpanzees in the same report each had an underlying myeloproliferative malignant neoplasm (erythroleukemia, McClure *et al.*, 1974). A retrospective survey of macaque necropsies by Matsumoto *et al.* (1987) revealed low rates (7.7%) of *Pneumocystis* in Japanese macaques (*M. fuscata fuscata*), 4 out of 52; crab-eating macaques (*M. fascicularis*), 1 out of 13; and none detected among 35 rhesus monkeys (*M. mulatta*). All of the affected animals were relatively young (four juveniles, 7 to 22 months, and one young adult). Of the infected macaques, just 2 of the Japanese monkeys were felt to have clinically significant *Pneumocystis* infections, one was 16 months old and the other apparently an infant (body weight listed at 490 g).

Other reports of *P. carinii* in nonhuman primates include descriptions of the lesion and a relatively high rate of infection among macaques infected with SIV (Baskerville *et al.*, 1991; Furuta *et al.*, 1993: Vogel *et al.*, 1993). Furuta *et al.* (1993) found *Pneumocystis* pneumonia in three of five SIV-infected rhesus monkeys (*M. mulatta*) and suggest that this represents reactivation of latent *Pneumocystis* infection. In the report by Vogel *et al.* (1993), 44 of 85 terminally ill, SIV-infected rhesus monkeys and 2 of 22 SIV-infected animals in earlier stages of SIV infection had detectable *P. carinii*. Clinically significant *P. carinii* infection increased from 0 in the first 2 years of SIV infection to >50% during the fourth year of virus infection. Epidemiologic data strongly supported the horizontal transmission of *Pneumocystis* cases in this report as opposed to reactivation of latent infection. Description of the lesions included the orientation of *P. carinii* infection centered on terminal airways in 59% of the infected animals.

X. PROTOZOAN DISEASES

A. Toxoplasmosis

Toxoplasma gondii is a protozoan parasite of the Apicomplexa subphylum, which also includes coccidia. Like other apicomplexans, toxoplasma often has a two-host life cycle. The only known definitive hosts are members of the cat family (Felidae). Intermediate hosts include essentially all other warm-blooded animals, including nonhuman primates. Sexual reproduction of the parasite takes place in the intestinal tract of the felid and unsporulated oocysts are shed in the feces. Sporulation takes place in the environment, and it is the sporulated oocytes that are infectious. Intermediate and definitive hosts become infected by ingesting the sporulated oocytes or by ingesting an infected definitive or intermediate host in which tissue cysts (bradyzoites) are present.

Laboratory-housed primates may become infected through contamination of feed stuffs with cat feces, infected food items that might be offered (e.g., raw ground meat, especially horse meat or sheep heart), or vermin, especially mice that might be caught and eaten (Anderson and McClure, 1993). Paratinic

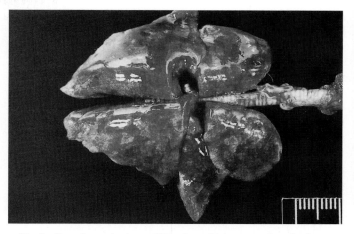

Fig. 6. Toxoplasmosis. Acute diffuse interstitial pneumonia and pulmonary edema, cotton-top tamarin (*Saguinus oedipus*).

hosts such as cockroaches that might transport infective oocysts have not been definitively described in outbreaks of toxoplasmosis, but have been implicated in transmission of the related apicomplexan *Sarcocystis falcatula* (Clubb and Frenkel, 1992).

Among nonhuman primates, infection has been documented in prosimians, New World monkeys, and Old World monkeys (Anderson and McClure, 1993), but it is the New World monkeys and prosimians in which infection is most devastating and in which it has occurred in outbreak form. In New World monkeys, especially the cebids such as squirrel monkeys (*Saimiri*) (Anderson and McClure, 1982; Cunningham *et al.*, 1992), capuchins (*Cebus*), and woolly monkeys (*Lagothrix*), toxoplasmosis is manifest as severe respiratory distress or as sudden death. Animals may be found acutely moribund with audible rales and fluid, blood, or foam coming from the nares and mouth. There may be nonspecific premonitory signs of anorexia and lethargy. Diarrhea may also be present. In Old World monkeys, the infection is often self-limiting, inapparent, and may be seen in the context of immune suppression (Lowenstine *et al.*, 1992).

Gross lesions include marked pulmonary congestion and edema (Fig. 6), white or bloody froth in the trachea, and hilar (tracheobronchial) lymphadenopathy. The lungs fail to collapse when the pluck is removed. Mesenteric lymphadenopathy, overt enteritis, and other lesions reflecting the systemic and fulminating nature of the infection may also be seen.

Histologically, the catholic tropism of the organism becomes apparent. The tachyzoites excyst in the small intestine where they cause intestinal necrosis and are swept into the systemic circulation via lymphatics and blood vessels. Necrosis of pancreas and mesenteric lymph nodes are common. Hepatic and splenic multifocal acute necrosis result from dissemination via the portal circulation. Necrosis of the lung capillaries and endothelial cells results in the profound pulmonary edema. In animals that survive a few days, type II pneumocyte hyperplasia may be evident. Cerebral edema and necrosis have also been reported. Individual tachyzoites can be seen in histologic section, but are best demonstrated in impression smears. Tissue cysts with bradyzoites can be found in areas of acute necrosis. If the primate is less severely affected, bradyzoite tissue cysts can be found in heart and skeletal muscle and brain.

The organisms are PAS negative, but with a PAS-positive cyst margin. They are gram negative. Differential diagnosis in a nonhuman primate would include microsporidiosis which may also be found in nervous tissue and possibly *Neospora* spp. which have been recognized to experimentally infect nonhuman primate (rhesus) infants (Barr *et al.,* 1994). Definitive diagnosis can be made in tissue section and confirmed by immunohistochemistry or electron microscopy.

Treatment in fulminating cases is often futile as the infection is widely disseminated by the time clinical signs are noted. The treatment of choice in human patients (Kasper, 1994), is pyramethamine plus sulfadiazine in a prolonged course (4–6 weeks), which is effective only against the tachyzoite stage. Toxicity is relatively common in humans. Possible substitute drugs for sulfadiazine include dapsone (diaminodiphenyl sulfone), clindamycin, spiramycin, or clarithromycin. The agent hydroxynaphthoquinone (BW566C80) is thought to be effective against bradyzoite-containing cysts and has provided prolonged remission of toxoplasmosis in an experimental model.

XI. METAZOAN PARASITES

Toft (1986) provides a comprehensive and useful review of parasites in nonhuman primates. Metazoan parasites found in respiratory system include (larval) cestodes, nematodes (metastrongylids), annelids (leeches), and arthropods (mites), as detailed later.

A. Cestodes

Nonhuman primates can be intermediate hosts for several cestode species. Of those associated with the respiratory system, these are most commonly "bladder"-type larvae of taeniid cestodes, including the genera *Taenia* (cysticercosis) and *Echinococcus* (hydatid cyst), although there is one report of tetrahyhridial larvae resembling *Mesocestoides* sp. (Guillot and Green, 1992). The presence of such larvae generally causes no clinical signs or ill effects and are usually incidental findings at necropsy. However, cyst location, number, size, death, and/or rupture may lead to significant clinical problems. Such infection should be included in the differential diagnosis for space-occupying lesions recognized in wild and/or free-ranging nonhuman primates. The zoonotic risks associated with such larvae increase the importance of recognition of this as a potential problem.

1. Cysticercosis

Cysticercosis cysts occur in herbivorous or omnivorous animals. The adult tapeworms (genus *Taenia*) parasitize a variety of carnivorous and omnivorous birds and mammals. The oval, translucent cysts contain a single invaginated scolex with four suckers. The cysts have been found in the abdominal and thoracic cavities, muscle, subcutaneous tissue, and central nervous system. Viable cysts generally have little or no associated host reaction, although clinical problems may be associated with the space-occupying effect of the cyst. Inflammation occurs in association with cyst death. Diagnosis depends on finding the characteristic bladder-shaped structure in the tissues, with species identification based on the scolex hook size and structure.

Wolff *et al.* (1989) report the presence of cysticercus pneumonitis and pleuritis in a red-ruffed lemur. The condition was initially recognized with fully body radiographs taken during quarantine screening procedures. A mineralized density and a soft tissue density were recognized in the left ventrocaudal thorax and left dorsocaudal lung, respectively. Exploratory thoracotomy revealed an extrapleural bilobed firm mass in the left ventral pleural space, attached via fibrous adhesions to the left caudal lung lobe, and a 1.0-cm encapsulated nodule within the dorsal margin of the left caudal lung lobe. These were excised. An intact cysticercus with armed scolex and a larval remnant with associated mixed inflammation (eosinophils, plasma cells, neutrophils) were found with microscopic examination of the pulmonary nodule. The extrapleural mass contained degenerate remnants of calcified larval cestodes and fibrinous exudate. The animal recovered uneventfully and was later released from quarantine.

2. Hydatidosis

Hydatidosis, or echinoccocosis, results from infection by the larval stage of *Echinococcus* sp. cestodes. Adult *Echinococcus* is a parasite in the small intestine of caniid species. The larval stage has been found in a wide variety of species, including various wild and domestic herbivores, as well as nonhuman primates and humans. Hydatid cysts are large, unilocular cysts. They are usually spherical. The cyst wall inner layer is composed of germinal epithelium from which multiple brood capsules develop. Multiple scolices develop for the wall of each brood capsule. Hydatid cysts may be located in the abdominal cavity, liver, lungs, subcutis, or throughout the body. Death due to anaphylactic shock has been reported several times associated with hydatid cyst rupture. Free scolices from ruptured cysts will produce additional cysts. Diagnosis of hydatid disease includes imaging studies, as with radiology or ultrasonography, as well as serological tests such as the Casoni intradermal skin test and indirect hemagglutination (Goldberg *et al.,* 1991). Species identification is based on morphology of the detached scolices in the cyst fluid or on cyst wall morphology.

Echinococcosis in a wild-caught baboon (*Papio anubis*) has been reported by Goldberg *et al.* (1991). The condition was discovered using thoracic radiography during quarantine screening, which revealed multiple fluid-filled cysts in the thoracic cavity. The animal was clinically normal, with normal hematology and serum biochemistry profiles. Indirect hemagglutination testing for *Echinococcus* was negative, a finding that occurs in approximately 50% of human patients with isolated pulmonary *Echinococcus* lesions. The animal was euthanized due to the interference the lesions would have in the intended research study, and necropsy confirmed the presence of *Echinococcus granulosus* cysts on the pleural surface of the left caudal and right middle lung lobes. Although treatment was not carried out with this animal, the report discusses the potential therapeutic approaches in similar cases, which include the use of chemotherapy and/or surgery. Generally, surgical procedures involving resection, enucleation, or evacuation of echinococcal cysts are the recommended treatments for human disease. During such surgery, scolicidal agents (e.g., silver nitrate, hypertonic saline) have been injected into the cyst to help reduce the risks of accidental spillage of cysts and the subsequent spread of the condition. Promising chemotherapeutic approaches involve the use of benzimidazole carbamate compounds over extended periods (e.g., 1 month; Morris *et al.*, 1985, cited in Bryan and Schantz, 1989).

3. Tetyrathyridiosis

Infection by larval stages of the cestode genus *Mesocestoides* produces a condition referred to as tetrathyridiosis. Adult *Mesocestoides* infect various bird species and domestic and wild mammalian carnivores. The larva, or tetrathyridum, has been found in the coelom or peritoneum of vertebrates, including snakes, mice, dogs, and cats, as well as in nonhuman primates. Guillot and Green (1992) report the presence of multiple *Mesocestoides* sp. tetrathyridia-like larvae in the lungs of a cynomolgus monkey (*Macaca fascicularis*) that died due to respiratory arrest within several hours following recovery from a surgical procedure. The animal had been apparently clinically healthy up to the time it died. Multiple 1- to 3-mm-diameter cysts were recognized in all lung lobes during necropsy.

B. Nematodes

1. Pulmonary Nematodiasis

Pulmonary nematodiasis, due to infection with metastrongylid lungworms of the genera *Filaroides* and *Filariopsis,* has been recognized commonly in New World monkeys (marmosets, squirrel monkeys, cebus monkeys, and howler monkeys) (Toft 1986) (Fig. 7). Lung lesions have been much less commonly associated with nematodes within pulmonary vascular lumens, including the occurrence of filarioid nematode-associated ver-

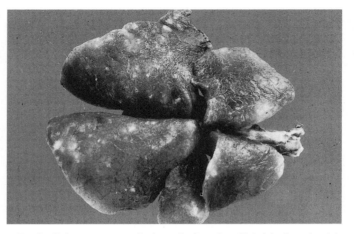

Fig. 7. Pulmonary nematodiasis, squirrel monkey (*Saimiri sciureus*), etiology: *Filuroides gordius.*

minous vasculitis in a cynomolgus monkey (*Macaca fascicularis*) following recent ivermectin treatment (Kornegay *et al.,* 1986), *Dirofilaria immitis* in rhesus monkeys (Baskin, 1991b), and intravascular pinworms (*Enterobius* sp.) in a chimpanzee (*Pan troglodytes*) with fatal enterobiasis (Zhang *et al.,* 1990).

The very slender and fragile adults of metastrongylid lungworms are located in terminal bronchioles, respiratory bronchioles, and alveoli. Larvae are produced by the viviparous female, are coughed up, swallowed by the host, and passed in the feces. The rest of the life cycle is not known (Toft, 1986). Infection is generally clinically inapparent, although occasional coughing and even pulmonary hemorrhage have been reported (Wolff, 1993). Antemortem diagnosis is made by finding larvae in nasopharyngeal mucus or in feces. Various drugs used for treatment include fenbendazole, albendazole, or levamisole (Wolff, 1993).

Gross lesions are small, elevated, subpleural, pink to gray, sometimes hyperpigmented, nodules. Microscopically, some alveolar septal loss is present, and epithelial changes, including atrophy and/or hyperplasia, as well as focal bronchiolar squamous metaplasia, occur. Localized chronic mixed inflammation is also often present, with mild interstitial fibrosis (Brack *et al.,* 1974).

In the report by Kornegay *et al.* (1986), an apparently healthy cynomolgus monkey died 2 hr after routine inhalation anesthesia and femoral catheter implantation. Seventeen days before the surgery the animal had been treated with ivermectin for gastrointestinal parasites prior to quarantine release. Gross necropsy findings included patchy raised areas of pulmonary hemorrhage and consolidation. Filarioid nematodes (*Edesonfilaria malayensis*) were present in pulmonary blood vessels and in multifocal cysts on visceral and parietal pleural surfaces, as well as in the urinary bladder wall. Microscopically, there were verminous vasculitis, pulmonary infarcts, and pneumonia. The

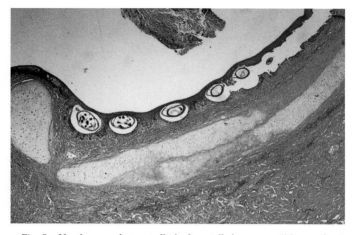

Fig. 8. Nasal mucosal nematodiasis, long-tailed macaque (*Macaca fascicularis*), etiology: *Anatrichosoma* sp.

condition of the parasites themselves was compatible with parasite death due to the earlier drug treatment. The report postulates that parasitic emboli led to pulmonary infarction and severe inflammation and that this condition contributed to death following anesthesia due to pulmonary function compromise.

Zhang *et al.* (1990) describe a case of fatal enterobiasis in a 5-year-old chimpanzee from the Qingdao Zoo in China. The animal became clinically ill, with anorexia and diarrhea. Fecal examination noted erythrocytes and inflammatory cells, and the animal was treated with ampicillin, dexamethasone, and other unnamed drugs over a 14-day period, at which time it died. Numerous pinworms were noted in the bloody stool before death. Death was associated with disseminated intravascular coagulation. In addition to extremely large numbers of pinworms (*Enterobius* sp.) in the colon, which also contained multifocal ulcers to which worms were attached, pinworms were found microscopically in the mesenteric lymph nodes and lymphatic vessels, hepatic veins, and pulmonary vessels.

2. Nasal Nematodiasis

Nasal mucosal nematodiasis, due to infection with anatrichosomatid nematodes *Anatrichosoma cutaneum* or *A. cynomolgi*, occurs in both Asian and African Old World nonhuman primates, including rhesus monkeys, cynomolgus monkeys, patas monkeys, vervets, talapoin monkeys, mangabeys, and baboons (Toft, 1986). The adults are small and slender, with the males lying in the lamina propria and the females in the stratified squamous epithelium of the nasal mucosal epithelium (Fig. 8). The bipolar, embryonated eggs are laid in tunnels within the stratified epithelium and are shed, either in nasal secretions or in the feces after being swallowed.

Infection is usually subclinical. Diagnosis is made via use of nasal mucosal scrapings or swabs, which contain the characteristic eggs (Conrad and Wong, 1973). Postmortem microscopy

of nasal mucosal sections may reveal adult worms. Microscopic lesions include mucosal epithelial parakeratotic hyperplasia, with underlying mixed inflammation (neutrophils, histiocytes, and lesser numbers of eosinophils and lymphocytes) (Stookey and Moe, 1978). The life cycle and transmission method are not known.

C. Annelids

The leech, *Dinobdella ferox,* is distributed throughout southern Asia and is a frequent parasite of the nasal cavities of macaques in this region (Pryor *et al.,* 1970; Toft, 1986). A similar leech, *Limnatus africana,* occurs in Africa. The life cycle of *D. ferox* is direct. The hermaphroditic adults lay eggs attached in a cocoon to objects on the surface of the water. The immature leeches hatch out and remain at the pond surface, gaining entry through the host oral or nasal cavity as the host drinks. The leeches attach to the upper respiratory tract mucosa (nasal passages, nasopharynx, larynx) and suck blood for a period of a few days to many weeks. During this period they grow and mature, then detach and drop out through the nostrils. Adult leeches are not parasitic.

Clinical problems relate to numbers of leeches present. Infection involving few parasites may be asymptomatic; however, heavy infection is associated with restlessness, epistaxis, anemia, weakness, asphyxiation, and sometimes death. Microscopic lesions contain mild, focal, chronic inflammation, with increased mucus production. Recognition and identification of the parasite in its typical anatomic location within the host are the bases for diagnosis. Treatment (Stookey and Moe, 1978) involves removal of the leeches. In military dogs in Southeast Asia, nasopharyngeal leech infestation was a significant problem. These animals were treated by flushing the nares with 15 to 20% alcohol while under anesthesia, with an endotracheal tube in place. The flushing continued until all of the leeches were detached and washed out into the oral cavity.

D. Arthropods

Respiratory acariasis in nonhuman primates includes the occurrence of pulmonary acariasis and of nasal acariasis, as reviewed by Kim (1980) and Toft (1986).

1. Pulmonary Acariasis

A number of species of lung mites, genus *Pneumonyssus*, cause pulmonary acariasis in Old World monkeys and great apes, and a similar species, *Pneumonyssoides* sp., causes similar infection in some New World monkeys, including woolly monkeys and howler monkeys. In association with their widespread use in biomedical research, most reports regarding this condition describe *Pneumonyssus simicola* infection in macaques. *Pneumonyssus simicola* occurs in up to 100% of wild or imported rhesus monkeys (*Macaca mulatta*). Transmission appears to require close association with infected animals. Raising newborns away from infected animals can prevent infection.

In rhesus monkeys, pulmonary acariasis is usually a subclinical infection, although it may predispose to secondary infection due to bronchiolar epithelial changes and impaired mucociliary clearance (Kim, 1980). Severe infections may have associated cough and dyspnea, but animals with heavy infections may exhibit no signs prior to finding infection during necropsy (Stookey and Moe, 1978). Tracheobronchiolar lavage is the most useful technique for antemortem diagnosis (Furman *et al.,* 1974; Joseph *et al.,* 1984), although false-negative results may occur. Treatment with a single subcutaneous dose of ivermectin (200 mg/kg) was effective in killing lung mites in infected rhesus monkeys (Joseph *et al.,* 1984), with a progressive decrease in mite-associated inflammatory changes following treatment.

Gross lung mite lesions are discrete, ovoid, pale yellow to gray/tan cystic foci, usually only a few millimeters in diameter. The lesions are present throughout the lung parenchyma (Fig. 9a). They have a small central lumen, which often contains one or more mites. Fibrinous or fibrous adhesions are often present between visceral and parietal pleura. Microscopically, the lesions consist of dilated, thickened bronchioles with epithelial erosion or loss, often with sections of mite within the lumen, and with a surrounding zone of mixed inflammatory cells (lymphocytes, eosinophils, and macrophages) (Fig. 9b). The macrophages frequently contain characteristic birefringent crystalline golden brown to black pigment. The pigment is thought to be a product of the mite. The pathology of lung mite infection in baboons and chimpanzees is similar to that described for the rhesus monkey (Kim and Kalter, 1975a,b; McClure and Guilloud, 1971).

Reported complications of lung mite infection in rhesus monkeys include pneumothorax (Rawlings and Splitter, 1973) and pulmonary arteritis (Woodard, 1968). Massive infections and resulting death have been reported for other primate species, including the douc langur (*Pygathrix nemaeus nemaeus*), proboscis monkey (*Nasalis larvatus orintalis*) (Robinson and Bush, 1918), and pig-tailed macaque (*macaca nemestrina*) (Stone and Hughes, 1969).

2. Nasal Acariasis

Nasal mites of the genus *Rhinophaga* have been described from the upper skull and olfactory mucosa of Old World monkeys (rhesus monkeys, baboons, *Cercopithecus* sp.) and great apes (orangutan) (Toft, 1986). Mucosal polyps in the maxillary sinuses of the chacma baboon (*Papio ursinus*) are associated with *Rhinophaga papinosis* infection (McConnell, 1977). A very long mite, *Rhinophaga elongata,* also is found in the nasal mucosa of chacma baboons, with its anterior end embedded deeply in a raised nodule. *Rhinopaga dinolti* occurs in the lungs and nasal cavities of rhesus monkeys, but without reported lesions (Toft, 1986). Pneumonitis and excessive mucus pro-

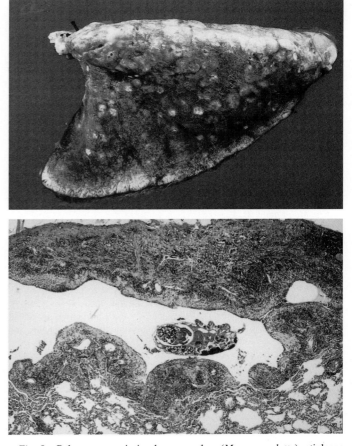

Fig. 9. Pulmonary acariasis, rhesus monkey (*Macaca mulatta*), etiology: *Pneumonyssus simicola.* (Top) Left caudal lung lobe, multifocal mite-associated nodules apparent on the pleural surface. (Bottom) Microscopic section of lung mite-associated bulla. Extensive mixed inflammation surrounds lumen, in which an adult female mite with an internal larval mite is present.

duction are associated with the presence of *Rhinophaga cercopitheci* in several guenon species (*Cercopithecus ascanius, C. mitis*) (Toft, 1986).

ACKNOWLEDGMENT

We thank Jackie Pritchard and the Primate Information Center at the Washington Regional Primate Research Center for carrying out a comprehensive literature search.

REFERENCES

Abee, C. R. (1985). Medical care and management of the squirrel monkey. *In* "Handbook of Squirrel Monkey Research" (L. A. Rosenblum and C. L. Coe, eds.), pp. 447–488. Plenum, New York.

Adang, O. M. J., Wensing, J. A. b., and Van Hooff, J. A. R. A. M. (1987). The Arnhem Zoo colony of chimpanzees (*Pan troglodytes*): Development and management techniques. *Int. Zoo Yearb.* **26**, 236–248.

Allen, J. R., Houser, W. D., and Carstens, L. A. (1970). Multiple tumors in a *Macaca mulatta* monkey. *Arch. Pathol.* **90**, 167–175.

Anderson, D. C., and McClure, H. M. (1982). Acute disseminated fatal toxoplasmosis in a squirrel monkey. *J. Am. Vet. Med. Assoc.* **181**, 1363–1366.

Anderson, D. C., and McClure, H. M. (1993). Toxoplasmosis. *In* "Monographs on Pathology of Laboratory Animals" (T. C. Jones, U. Mohr, and R. D. Hunt, eds.), Vol. 1, pp. 63–69. Springer-Verlag, Berlin and New York.

Andrews, E. J. (1974). Pulmonary pathology in stillborn nonhuman primates. *J. Am. Vet. Med. Assoc.* **164**, 715–718.

Baer, J. F. (1994). Husbandry and medical management of the owl monkey. *In* "Aotus: The Owl Monkey" (J. F. Baer, R. E. Weller, and I. Kakoma, eds.), pp. 133–164. Academic Press, San Diego, CA.

Balis, J. U., Gerber, L. I., Rappaport, E. S., and Neville, W. E. (1974). Mechanisms of blood vascular reactions of the primate lung to acute endotoxemia. *Exp. Mol. Pathol.* **21**, 123–137.

Barr, B. C., Conrad, P. A., Sverlow, K. W., Tarantal, A. G., and Hendrickx, A. G. (1994). Experimental fetal and transplacental *Neospora* infection in the nonhuman primate. *Lab. Invest.* **71**, 236–242.

Barrie, M. T., and Stadler, C. K. (1990). Antemortem diagnosis and treatment of cryptococcosis in an Allen's swamp monkey (*Allenopithecus nigroviridis*). *Proc. Annu. Meet., Am. Assoc. Zoo Vet. 1990*, p. 274.

Baskerville, A., Dowsett, A. B., Cook, R. W., Dennis, M. J., Cranage, M. P., and Greenaway, P. J. (1991). *Pneumocystis carinii* pneumonia in simian immunodeficiency virus infection: Immunohistological and scanning and transmission electron microscopical studies. *J. Pathol.* **164**, 175–184.

Baskerville, A., Ramsay, A. D., Addis, B. J., Dennis, M. J., Cook, R. W., Cranage, M. P., and Greenaway, P. J. (1992). Interstitial pneumonia in simian immunodeficiency virus infection. *J. Pathol.* **167**, 241–247.

Baskerville, M., Wood, M., and Baskerville, A. (1983). An outbreak of *Bordetella bronchiseptica* pneumonia in a colony of common marmosets (*Callithrix jacchus*). *Lab. Anim.* **17**, 350–355.

Baskerville, M., Baskerville, A., and Manktelow, B. W. (1984). Undifferentiated carcinoma of the nasal tissues in the common marmoset. *J. Comp. Pathol.* **94**, 329–338.

Baskin, G., Murphey-Corb, M., and Martin, L. (1989). Lentivirus-induced pneumonia in rhesus monkeys infected with SIV. *Lab. Invest.* **60**, 7A.

Baskin, G. B. (1991a). Disseminated histoplasmosis in a SIV-infected rhesus monkey. *J. Med. Primatol.* **20**, 251–253.

Baskin, G. B. (1991b). *Dirofilaria immitis* infection in a rhesus monkey (*Macaca mulatta*). *Lab. Anim. Sci.* **32**, 401–402.

Bauer, T., and Woodfield, J. A. (1995). Mediastinal, pleural, and extrapleural diseases. *In* "Textbook of Veterinary Internal Medicine: Diseases of the Dog and Cat" (S. J. Ettinger and E. C. Feldman, eds.), pp. 812–842. Saunders, Philadelphia.

Bellini, S., Hubbard, G. B., and Kaufman, L. (1991). Spontaneous fatal coccidioidomycosis in a native-born hybrid baboon (*Papio cynocephalus anubis/ Papio cynocephalus cynocephalus*). *Lab. Anim. Sci.* **41**, 509–511.

Belshe, R. B., Richardson, L. S., London, W. T., Sly, D. L., Lorfeld, J. H., Camargo, E., Prevar, D. A., and Chanock, R. M. (1977). Experimental respiratory syncytial virus infection of four species of primates. *J. Med. Virol.* **1**, 157–162.

Beniashvili, D. S. (1989). An overview of the world literature on spontaneous tumors in nonhuman primates. *J. Med. Primatol.* **18**, 423–437.

Benirschke, K. (1983). Occurrence of spontaneous diseases. *In* "Viral and Immunological Diseases in Nonhuman Primates" (S. S. Kalter, ed.), pp. 17–30. Liss, New York.

Benjamin, S. A., and Lang, M. C. (1971). Acute pasteurellosis in owl monkeys (*Aotus trivirgatus*). *Lab. Anim. Sci.* **21**, 258–262.

Bennett, J. E. (1994a). Diagnosis and therapy of fungal infections. *In* "Harrison's Principles of Internal Medicine" (K. J. Isselbacher, J. B. Martin, E. Braunwald, A. S. Fauci, J. D. Wilson, and D. L. Kasper, eds.), 13th ed., pp. 854–856. McGraw-Hill, New York.

Bennett, J. E. (1994b). Cryptococcosis. *In* "Harrison's Principles of Internal Medicine" (K. J. Isselbacher, J. B. Martin, E. Braunwald, A. S. Fauci, J. D. Wilson, and D. L. Kasper, eds.), 13th ed., pp. 859–860. McGraw-Hill, New York.

Berendt, R. F., Long, G. G., and Walker, J. S. (1975). Influenza alone and in sequence with pneumonia due to *Streptococcus pneumoniae* in the squirrel monkey. *J. Infect. Dis.* **132**, 689–693.

Bergeland, M. E., Barnes, D. M., and Kaplan, W. (1970). Spontaneous histoplasmosis in a squirrel monkey. *Primate Zoonosis Surveillance Report 1*, **January-February 1970**, 10–11. CDC, Atlanta.

Besch, T. K., Ruble, D. L., Gibbs, P. H., and Pitt, M. L. M. (1996). Steady-state minute volume determination by body-only plethysmography in juvenile rhesus monkeys. *Lab. Anim. Sci.* **46**, 539–544.

Betton, G. R. (1984). Spontaneous neoplasms of the marmoset. Oral and nasopharyngeal squamous cell carcinomas. *Vet. Pathol.* **21**, 193–197.

Binns, R., Clark, G. C., and Simpson, C. R. (1972). Lung function and blood gas characteristics in the rhesus monkey. *Lab. Anim.* **6**, 189–198.

Block, M. F., Kallenberger, D. A., Kern, J. D., and Nerveux, R. D. (1981). In utero meconium aspiration by the baboon fetus. *Obstet. Gynecol.* **57**, 37–40.

Boatman, E. S., Arce, P., Luchtel, D., Pump, K. K., and Martin, C. J. (1979). Pulmonary function, morphology and morphometrics. *In* "Aging in Nonhuman Primates" (D. M. Bowden, ed.), pp. 292–313. Van Nostrand-Reinhold, New York.

Boyce, J. T., Giddens, W. E., and Valerio, M. (1978). Simian adenoviral pneumonia. *Am. J. Pathol.* **91**, 259–276.

Boyden, E. A. (1976). The development of the lung in the pigtail monkey. (*Macaca nemestrina*, L.). *Anat. Rec.* **186**, 15–37.

Brack, M., Boncyk, L. H., and Kalter, S. S. (1974). *Filaroides cebus* (Gebauer, 1933) parasitism and respiratory infection in *Cebus apella*. *J. Med. Primatol.* **3**, 164–173.

Brockman, D. K., Willis, M. S., and Karesh, W. B. (1988). Management and husbandry of ruffed lemurs, *Varecia variegata*, at the San Diego Zoo. III. Medical considerations and population management. *Zoo Biol.* **7**, 253–262.

Brown, B. G., and Swenson, R. B. (1995). Surgical management. *In* "Nonhuman Primates in Biomedical Research: Biology and Management" (B. T. Bennet, C. R. Abee, and R. Henrickson, eds.), pp. 297–304. Academic Press, San Diego, CA.

Brown, R. J., Cole, W. C., Berg, H. S., Chiang, H. S., Chang, C. P., and Banknieder, A. R. (1977). Nasal adenocarcinoma in a Taiwan macaque. *Vet. Pathol.* **14**, 294–296.

Bryan, R. T., and Schantz, P. M. (1989). Echinococcosis (hydatid disease). *J. Am. Vet. Med. Assoc.* **195**, 1214–1217.

Burton, M., Morton, R. J., Ramsay, E., and Stair, E. L. (1986). Coccidioidomycosis in a ring-tailed lemur. *J. Am. Vet. Med. Assoc.* **189**, 1209–1211.

Butchin, R., Letcher, J., Weisenberg, E., and Snook, S. (1992). Presumptive adenoviral pneumonia in a juvenile chimpanzee (*Pan troglodytes*). *Proc. Annu. Meet., Am. Assoc. Zoo Vet., 1992*, pp. 386–387.

Calle, P. P., Thoen, C. O., and Roskop, M. L. (1989). Tuberculin skin test responses, mycobacteriologic examinations of gastric lavage, and serum enzyme-linked immunosorbent assays in orangutans (*Pongo pygmaeus*). *J. Zoo Wildl. Med.* **20**, 307–314.

Cambre, R. C. (1986). Ethmoiditis/sinusitis with intracranial extension in a baby orangutan. *Proc. Annu. Meet., Am. Assoc. Zoo Vet., 1986*, p. 182.

Cambre, R. C., Wilson, H. L., Spraker, T. R., and Favara, B. E. (1980). Fatal airsacculitis and pneumonia, with abortion, in an orangutan. *J. Am. Vet. Med. Assoc.* **177**, 822–824.

Campbell, G. D., Coalson, J. J., and Johanson, W. G., Jr. (1984). The effect of bacterial superinfection on lung function after diffuse alveolar damage. *Am. Rev. Respir. Dis.* **129**, 974–978.

Cappucci, D. T., Jr., O'Shea, L. J., and Smith, G. D. (1972). An epidemiologic account of tuberculosis transmitted from man to monkey. *Am. Rev. Respir. Dis.* **106**, 819–823.

Carey, J. C. (1988). Baboon model for aspiration. *In* "Nonhuman Primates in Perinatal Research" (Y. W. Brans and T. J. Kuehl, eds.), pp. 333–336. Wiley, New York.

Centers for Disease Control (CDC) (1989). Pneumococcal polysaccharide. *Morbid. Mortal. Wkly. Rep.* **38,** 64–76.

Centers for Disease Control (CDC) (1990). Ebola-related filovirus infection in non-human primates and interim guidelines for handling nonhuman primates during transit and quarantine. *Morbid. Mortal. Wkly. Rep.* **39,** 1–3.

Chalmers, D. T., Murgatroyd, L. B., and Wadsworth, P. F. (1983). A survey of the pathology of marmosets (*Callithrix jacchus*) derived from a marmoset breeding unit. *Lab. Anim.* **17,** 270–279.

Chandler, F. W., McClure, H. M., Campbell, W. G., Jr., and Watts, J. C. (1976). Pulmonary pneumocystosis in nonhuman primates. *Arch. Pathol. Lab. Med.* **100,** 163–167.

Chaparas, S. D., Good, R. C., and Janicki, B. W. (1975). Tuberculin-induced lymphocyte transformation and skin reactivity in monkeys vaccinated or not vaccinated with bacille Calmette-Guerin, then challenged with virulent *Mycobacterium tuberculosis*. *Am. Rev. Respir. Dis.* **112,** 43–47.

Chapman, W. J., Jr., Crowell, W. A., and Isaac, W. (1973). Spontaneous lesions seen at necropsy in 7 owl monkeys (*Aotus trivirgatus*). *Lab. Anim. Sci.* **23,** 434–442.

Churchill, A. E. (1963). The isolation of Parainfluenza 3 virus from fatal cases of pneumonia in *Erythrocebus patas* monkeys. *Br. J. Exp. Pathol.* **44,** 529–537.

Clarke, G. L. (1968). The relationship of hypersensitivity of shedding of *Mycobacterium tuberculosis* in experimentally infected *Macaca mulatta*. *Am. Rev. Respir. Dis.* **98,** 416–423.

Clarke, G. L., and Schmidt, J. P. (1969). Effect of prophylactic isoniazid on early developing experimental tuberculosis in *Macaca mulatta*. *Am. Rev. Respir. Dis.* **100,** 224–227.

Clifford, D. H., Yang Yoo, S., Fazekas, S., and Hardin, C. J. (1977). Surgical drainage of a submandibular air sac in an orangutan. *J. Am. Vet. Med. Assoc.* **171,** 862–865.

Clubb, S. L., and Frenkel, J. K. (1992). *Sarcocystis falcutala* of opossums: Transmission by cockroaches with fatal pulmonary disease in psittacine birds. *J. Parasitol.* **78,** 116–124.

Coalson, J. J. (1988). Pathology of perinatal lung disease. *In* "Nonhuman Primates in Perinatal Research" (Y. W. Brans and T. J. Kuehl, eds.), pp. 285–298. Wiley, New York.

Coalson, J. J., Kuehl, T. J., Escobedo, M. B., Hilliard, J. L., Smith, F., Meredith, K., Null, D. M., Jr., Walsh, W., Johnson, D., and Robotham, J. L. (1982). A baboon model of bronchopulmonary dysplasia. II. Pathologic features. *Exp. Mol. Pathol.* **37,** 335–350.

Conrad, H. D., and Wong, M. M. (1973). Studies of *Anatrichosoma* (nematoda: trichinellida) with descriptions of *Anatrichosoma rhina* sp. n. and *Anatricosoma nacepobi* sp. n. from the nasal mucosa of *Macaca mulatta*. *J. Helminthol.* **47,** 289–302.

Cooper, J. E., and Baskerville, A. (1976). An outbreak of epistaxis in cynomolgus monkeys (*Macaca fascicularis*). *Vet. Rec.* **99,** 438–439.

Cotran, R. S., Kumar, V., and Robbins, S. L. (1994). Head and neck. *In* "Pathologic Basis of Disease" (R. S. Cotran, V. Kumar, and S. L. Robbins, eds.), 5th ed., pp. 735–753. Saunders, Philadelphia.

Courtenay, J. (1988). Infant mortality in mother-reared captive chimpanzees at Taronga Zoo, Sydney. *Zoo Biol.* **7,** 61–68.

Crocker, T. T., Chase, J. E., Wells, S. A., and Nunes, L. L. (1970). Preliminary report on experimental carcinoma of the lung in hamsters and in a primate. *In* "Morphology of Experimental Respiratory Carcinogenesis," Symp. No. 21, pp. 317–328. Atomic Energy Commission, Oak Ridge, TN.

Cunningham, A. A., Buxton, D., and Thomson, K. M. (1992). An epidemic of toxoplasmosis in a captive colony of squirrel monkeys (*Saimiri sciureus*). *J. Comp. Pathol.* **107,** 207–219.

Dalgard, D. W. (1969). Herniation of a hepatic lobe into the right thorax of a rhesus monkey (*Macaca mulatta*). An incidental report. *Lab. Anim. Care* **19,** 109–110.

Daniel, M. D., Letvin, N. L., Sehgal, P., Schmidt, D. K., Sikva, P., Solomon, K. R., Hodi, S. F., Ringler, D. J., Hunt, R. D., King, N. W., and Desrosiers, R. C. (1984). Prevalence of antibodies to three retroviruses in a captive colony of macaque monkeys. *Int. J. Cancer* **31,** 608–610.

Daniel, T. M. (1994). Tuberculosis. *In* "Harrison's Principles of Internal Medicine" (K. J. Isselbacher, J. B. Martin, E. Braunwald, A. S. Fauci, J. D. Wilson, and D. L. Kasper, eds.), 13th ed., pp. 710–718. McGraw-Hill, New York.

Dannenberg, A. M., Jr. (1978). Pathogenesis of pulmonary tuberculosis in man and animals: Protection of personnel against tuberculosis. *In* "Mycobacterial Infections of Zoo Animals" (R. J. Montali, ed.), pp. 65–75. Smithsonian Institution Press, Washington, DC.

Deinhardt, F., Holmes, A. W., Devine, J., Deinhardt, J. (1967). Marmosets as laboratory animals. IV. The microbiology of laboratory kept marmosets. *Lab. Anim. Care* **17,** 48–70.

Deinhardt, J. B., Devine, J., Passovoy, M., Pohlman, R., and Deinhardt, F. (1967). Marmosets as laboratory animals. I. Care of marmosets in the laboratory, pathology and outline of statistical evaluation of data. *Lab. Anim. Care* **17,** 11–29.

Dick, E. C., and Dick, C. R. (1974). Natural and experimental infections of nonhuman primates with respiratory viruses. *Lab. Anim. Sci.* **24,** 177–181.

DiGiacomo, R. F., Gibbs, C. J., Jr., and Gajdusek, D. C. (1978). Pulmonary arteriosclerosis and thrombosis in a cynomolgus macaque. *J. Am. Vet. Med. Assoc.* **173,** 1205–1207.

Dillehay, D. L., and Huerkamp, M. J. (1990). Tuberculosis in a tuberculin-negative rhesus monkey on chemoprophylaxis. *J. Zoo Wildl. Med.* **21,** 480–484.

Drake, T. A., Cheng, J., Chang, A., and Taylor, F. B., Jr. (1993). Expression of tissue factor, thrombomodulin, and E-selectin in baboons with lethal *Escherichia coli* sepsis. *Am. J. Pathol.* **142,** 1458–1470.

Dueland, A. N., Martin, J. R., Devlin, M. E., Wellish, M., Mahalingam, R., Cohrs, R., Soike, K. F., and Gilden, D. H. (1992). Acute simian varicella infection: Clinical, laboratory, pathologic and virologic features. *Lab. Invest.* **66,** 762–773.

Dumonceaux, G. A., Phillips, L. G., Lamberski, N., Clutter, D., and Nagy, S. M., Jr. (1995). Treatment of bilateral nasal polyposis and chronic refractory inhalant allergic rhinitis in a chimpanzee (*Pan troglodytes*). *Proc. Annu. Jt. Conf. AAZV WDA AAWV, 1995,* pp. 269–270.

Duncan, M., Tell, L., Gardiner, C. H., and Montali, R. J. (1995). Lingual gongylonemiasis and pasteurellosis in Goeldi's monkeys (*Calliimico goeldii*). *J. Zoo Wildl. Med.* **26,** 102–108.

Dungworth, D. L. (1993). The respiratory system. *In* "Pathology of Domestic Animals" (K. V. F. Judd, P. C. Kennedy, and N. Palmer, eds.), 4th ed., Vol. 2, pp. 539–699. Academic Press, San Diego, CA.

Dysko, R. C., and Hoskins, D. E. (1995). Collection of biological samples and therapy administration. *In* "Nonhuman Primates in Biomedical Research: Biology and Management" (B. T. Bennet, C. R. Abee, and R. Henrickson, eds.), pp. 270–286. Academic Press, San Diego, CA.

Eichberg, J. W. (1985). Changes in infant chimpanzee husbandry in response to a *Klebsiella pneumoniae* outbreak. *In* "Clinical Management of Infant Great Apes" (C. E. Graham and J. A. Bowen, eds.), pp. 43–45. Liss, New York.

Ensley, P. K. (1981). Nursery raising orangutans: Medical problems encountered at the San Diego Zoo. *Proc. Annu. Meet., Am. Assoc. Zoo Vet., 1981,* pp. 50–54.

Escobedo, M. B., Hilliard, J. L., Smith, F., Meredith, K., Walsh, W., Johnson, D., Coalson, J. J., Kuehl, T. J., Null, N. M., Jr., and Robotham, R. L. (1982). A baboon model of bronchopulmonary dysplasia. I. Clinical features. *Exp. Mol. Pathol.* **37,** 323–334.

Espana, C. (1971). Review of some outbreaks of viral disease in captive nonhuman primates. *Lab. Anim. Sci.* **21,** 1023–1031.

Espana, C. (1973). *Herpesvirus simiae* infection in *Macaca radiata*. *Am. J. Phys. Anthropol.* **38,** 447–454.

Espana, C. (1974). Viral epizootics in captive nonhuman primates. *Lab. Anim. Sci.* **24**, 167–176.

Feeser, P., and White, F. (1992). Medical management of *Lemur catta, Varecia variegata,* and *Propithecus verreauxi* in natural habitat enclosures. *Proc. Annu. Meet., Am. Assoc. Zoo Vet., 1992,* pp. 320–323.

Feigin, D. S. (1983). Pulmonary cryptococcosis: Radiologic-pathologic correlates of its three forms. *AJR, Am. J. Roentgenol.* **141**, 1263–1272.

Fiennes, R. N. T.-W.-, and Dzhikidze, E. K. (1972). Respiratory pathogens and other organisms. *In* "Pathology of Simian Primates" (R. N. T.-W.-Fiennes, ed.), Part 2, pp. 277–282. Karger, Basel.

Fiennes, R. N. T.-W.-, Lapin, B. A., Dzhikidze, E. K., and Yakovleva, L. A. (1972). The respiratory and alimentary systems. *In* "Pathology of Simian Primates" (R. N. T.-W.-Fiennes, ed.), Part 1, pp. 671–710. Karger, Basel.

Filice, G. A. (1994). Nocardiosis. *In* "Harrison's Principles of Internal Medicine" (K. J. Isselbacher, J. B. Martin, E. Braunwald, A. S. Fauci, J. D. Wilson, and D. L. Kasper, eds.), 13th ed., pp. 696–699. McGraw-Hill, New York.

Flecknell, P. A., Parry, R., Needham, J. R., Ridley, R. M., Baker, H. F., and Bowes, P. (1983). Respiratory disease associated with parainfluenza type I (Sendai) virus in a colony of marmosets (*Callithrix jacchus*). *Lab. Anim.* **17**, 111–113.

Fortman, J. D., Manaligod, J. R., and Bennett, B. T. (1993). Malignant mesothelioma in an olive baboon (*Papio anubis*). *Lab. Anim. Sci.* **43**, 503–505.

Fox, J. G., and Rohovsky, M. W. (1975). Meningitis caused by *Klebsiella* spp. in two rhesus monkeys. *J. Am. Vet. Med. Assoc.* **167**, 634–636.

Frank. H. (1968). Systemissche Histoplasmose bei einem afrikanischen Affen. *Dtsch. Tieraerztl. Wochenschr.* **75**, 371–374.

Friedman, P. J. (1994). Imaging in pulmonary disease. *In* "Harrison's Principles of Internal Medicine" (K. J. Isselbacher, J. B. Martin, E. Braunwald, A. S. Fauci, J. D. Wilson, and D. L. Kasper, eds.), 13th ed., pp. 1159–1163. McGraw-Hill, New York.

Furman, D. P., Bonasch, H., Springsteen, R., Stiller, D., and Rahlmann, D. F. (1974). Studies on the biology of the lung mite, *Pneumonyssus simicola* Banks (Acarina: Halarachnidae) and diagnosis of infestation in macaques. *Lab. Anim. Sci.* **24**, 622–629.

Furuta, T., Fujita, M., Mukai, R., Sakakibara, I., Sata, T., Miki, K., Hayami, M., Kojima, S., and Yoshikawa, Y. (1993). Severe pulmonary pneumocystosis in simian acquired immunodeficiency syndrome by simian immunodeficiency virus: Its characterization by the polymerase-chain-reaction method and failure of experimental transmission to immunodeficient animals. *Parasitol. Res.* **79**, 624–628.

Giddens, W. E., Jr. (1974). Inoculation of owl monkeys (*Aotus trivirgatus*) with 7,12-dimethylbenz (A) anthracene and *Herpesvirus saimiri:* Induction of epidermoid carcinoma in the lung. *In* "Experimental Lung Cancer: Carcinogenesis and Bioassays" (E. Karbe and J. F. Park, eds.), pp. 280–291. Springer-Verlag, Berlin.

Giddens, W. E., Jr., and Dillingham, L. A. (1971). Primary tumors of the lung in nonhuman primates. Literature review and report of peripheral carcinoid tumors of the lung in a rhesus monkey. *Vet. Pathol.* **8**, 467–478.

Giles, R. C., Jr., Hildebrandt, P. K., and Tate, C. (1974). Klebsiella air sacculitis in the owl monkey (*Aotus trivirgatus*). *Lab. Anim. Sci.* **24**, 610–616.

Gillett, C. S., Ringler, D. H., and Pond, C. L. (1984). Pneumatocele in a pigtailed macaque (*Macaca nemestrina*). *Lab. Anim. Sci.* **34**, 91–93.

Goldberg, G. P., Fortman, J. D., Beluhan, F. Z., and Bennet, B. T. (1991). Pulmonary *Echinococcus granulosus* in a baboon (*Papio anubis*). *Lab. Anim. Sci.* **41**, 177–180.

Gozalo, A., and Montoya, E. (1990). Mortality causes of owl monkeys (*Aotus nancymae* and *Aotus vociferans*) in captivity. *J. Med. Primatol.* **19**, 69–72.

Gozalo, A., and Montoya, E. (1992). Mortality causes of moustached tamarin (*Saguinus mystax*) in captivity. *J. Med. Primatol.* **21**, 35–38.

Graves, I. L. (1970). Agglutinating antibodies for *Bordetella bronchiseptica* in sera before, during and after an epizootic of pneumonia in caged monkeys. *Lab. Anim. Care* **20**, 246–250.

Graybill, J. R., Craven, P. C., Clark, L., Taylor, R. L., Johnson, J. E., and Vaden, P. (1985). Treatment of coccidioidomycosis with liposome-associated amphotericin B in three Japanese macaques. *In* "Coccidioidomycosis: Proceedings of the Fourth International Conference" (H. Einstein and A. Catanzaro, eds.), pp. 292–305. National Foundation for Infectious Diseases, Washington, DC.

Graybill, J. R., Griffith, L., and Sun, S. H. (1990). Fluconazole therapy for coccidioidomycosis in Japanese macaques. *Rev. Infect. Dis.* **12**, S286–S290.

Griner, L. A. (1983). Primates. *In* "Pathology of Zoo Znimals," pp. 316–381. Zoological Society of San Diego, San Diego, CA.

Grizzard, M. B., London, W. T., Sly, D. L., Murphy, B. R., James, W. D., Parnell, W. P., and Chanock, R. M. (1978). Experimental production of respiratory tract disease in cebus monkeys after intratracheal or intranasal infection with influenza A/Victoria/3/75 or influenza A/New Jersey/76 virus. *Infect. Immun.* **21**, 201–205.

Gross, G. S. (1978). Medical and surgical approach to laryngeal air sacculitis in a baboon caused by *Pasteurella multocida. Lab. Anim. Sci.* **28**, 737–741.

Guillot, L. M., and Green, L. C. (1992). Pulmonary cestodiasis in a cynomolgus monkey (*Macaca fascicularis*). *Lab. Anim. Sci.* **42**, 158–160.

Guilloud, N. B., and McClure, H. M. (1969). Air sac infection in the orangutan (*Pongo pygmaeus*). *In* "Proceedings of the Second International Congress of Primatology" (H. O. Hofer, ed.), Vol. 3, pp. 143–144. Karger, Basel.

Gundel, R. H., Wegner, C. D., and Letts, L. G. (1992). Antigen-induced acute and late-phase responses in primates. *Am. Rev. Respir. Dis.* **146**, 369–373.

Gustavsson, O. E. A., Roken, B. O., and Serrander, R. (1990). An epizootic of whooping cough among chimpanzees in a zoo. *Folia Primatol.* **55**, 45–50.

Haberle, A. J. (1970). Tuberculosis in an orangutan. *J. Zoo Anim. Med.* **1**, 10–15.

Hahn, F. F., Brooks, A. L., and McWhinney, J. A. (1987). A primary pulmonary sarcoma in a rhesus monkey after inhalation of plutonium dioxide. *Radiat. Res.* **112**, 391–397.

Halpern, G. M., Gershwin, L. J., Gonzales, G., and Fowler, M. E. (1989). Diagnosis of inhalant allergy in a chimpanzee using *in vivo* and *in vitro* tests. *Allergol. Immunopathol.* **17**, 271–276.

Hangen, D. H., Bloom, R. J., Stevens, J. H., O'Hanley, P., Ranchod, M., Collins, J., and Raffin, T. A. (1987). Adult respiratory distress syndrome: A live *E. coli* septic primate model. *Am. J. Pathol.* **126**, 396–400.

Harkema, J. R. (1991). Comparative aspects of nasal airway anatomy: Relevance to inhalation toxicology. *Toxicol. Pathol.* **19**, 321–336.

Hastings, B. E. (1991). The veterinary management of a laryngeal air sac infection in a free-ranging mountain gorilla. *J. Med. Primatol.* **20**, 361–364.

Hendrickx, A. G., and Gasser, R. F. (1967). A description of a diaphragmatic hernia in sixteen week baboon fetus (*Papio* sp.). *Folia Primatol.* **7**, 66–77.

Henrickson, R. V. (1984). Biology and disease of old world primates. *In* "Laboratory Animal Medicine" (J. G. Fox, B. J. Cohen, and F. M. Loew, eds.), pp. 301–321. Academic Press, Orlando, FL.

Hessler, J. R., and Moreland, A. F. (1968). Pulmonary tuberculosis in a squirrel monkey (*Saimiri sciureus*). *J. Am. Vet. Med. Assoc.* **153**, 923–927.

Hill, W. C. O. (1953–1955). Report of the Society's prosector for the year 1953. *Proc. Zool. Soc. London* **124**, 303–311.

Hill, W. C. O. (1960). "Primates Comparative Anatomy and Taxonomy. IV. Cebidae, Part A." Interscience, New York.

Hilloowala, R. A. (1971). The laryngeal air sacs and air spaces in certain primates. *Anat. Rec.* **169**, 340.

Holcroft, J. W., Blaisdell, F. W., Trunkey, D. D., and Lim, R. C. (1977). Intravascular coagulation and pulmonary edema in the septic baboon. *J. Surg. Res.* **22**, 209–220.

Hubbard, G. B., Wood, D. H., and Fanton, J. W. (1983). Squamous cell carcinoma with metastasis in a rhesus monkey (*Macaca mulatta*). *Lab. Anim. Sci.* **33**, 469–472.

Jacobs, R. L., Lux, G. K., Speilvogel, R. L., Eichberg, J. W., and Gleiser, C. A. (1984). Nasal polyposis in a chimpanzee. *J. Allergy Clin. Immunol.* **74**, 61–63.

Janssen, D. L. (1993). Diseases of great apes. *In* "Zoo and Wild Animal Medicine" (M. E. Fowler, ed.), Curr. Ther., Vol. 3, pp. 334–338. Saunders, Philadelphia.

Johnsen, D. O., Wooding, W. L., Tanticharoenyos, P., and Karnjanaprakorn, C. (1971). An epizootic of A₂/Hong Kong/68 influenza in gibbons. *J. Infect. Dis.* **123**, 365–370.

Jones, E. E., Alford, P. L., Reingold, A. L., Russell, H., Keeling, M. E., and Broome, C. V. (1984). Predisposition to invasive pneumococcal illness following parainfluenza type 3 virus infection in chimpanzees. *J. Am. Vet. Med. Assoc.* **185**, 1351–1353.

Joseph, B. E., Wilson, D. W., Henrickson, R. V., Robinson, P. T., and Benirschke, K. (1984). Treatment of pulmonary acariasis in rhesus macaques with ivermectin. *Lab. Anim. Sci.* **34**, 360–364.

Kalter, S. S. (1983). Primate viruses—their significance. *In* "Monographs in Primatology" (S. S. Kalter, ed.), Vol. 2, pp. 67–89. Liss, New York.

Kalter, S. S. (1985). Immunology and pathology of the squirrel monkey. *In* "Handbook of Squirrel Monkey Research" (L. A. Rosenblum and C. L. Coe, eds.), pp. 379–445. Plenum, New York.

Kalter, S. S., and Heberling, R. L. (1990). Viral battery testing in nonhuman primate colony managment. *Lab. Anim. Sci.* **40**, 21–23.

Karesh, W. B., Liddel, R. M., and Sirotta, P. (1990). Clinical challenge: Case 1. *J. Zoo Wildl. Med.* **21**, 241–242.

Kasper, L. H. (1994). *Toxoplasma* infection and toxoplasmosis. *In* "Harrison's Principles of Internal Medicine" (K. J. Isselbacher, J. B. Martin, E. Braunwald, A. S. Fauci, J. D. Wilson, and D. L. Kasper, eds.), pp. 903–908. McGraw-Hill, New York.

Kast, A. (1994). Pulmonary hair embolism in monkeys. *Exp. Toxicol. Pathol.* **46**, 183–188.

Kaufmann, A. F., and Anderson, D. C. (1978). Tuberculosis control in nonhuman primate colonies. *In* "Mycobacterial Infections of Zoo Animals" (R. J. Montali, ed.), pp. 227–234. Smithsonian Institution Press, Washington, DC.

Keeling, M. E., and Wolf, R. H. (1975). Medical management of the rhesus monkey. *In* "The Rhesus Monkey" (G. H. Bourne, ed.), pp. 12–96. Academic Press, London.

Kim, J. C. S. (1980). Pulmonary acariasis in old world monkeys: A review. *In* "The Comparative Pathology of Zoo Animals" (R. J. Montali and G. Migaki, eds.), pp. 383–394. Smithsonian Institution Press, Washington, DC.

Kim, J. C. S., and Kalter, S. S. (1975a). A review of 105 necropsies in captive baboons (*Papio cynocephalus*). *Lab. Anim.* **9**, 233–239.

Kim, J. C. S., and Kalter, S. S. (1975b). Pathology of pulmonary acariasis in baboons (*Papio* sp.). *J. Med. Primatol.* **4**, 70.

King, L. G., and Hendricks, J. C. (1995). Clinical pulmonary function tests. *In* "Textbook of Veterinary Internal Medicine: Diseases of the Dog and Cat" (S. J. Ettinger and E. C. Feldman, eds.), pp. 738–754. Saunders, Philadelphia.

King, N. W., Jr. (1993a). Simian immunodeficiency virus infection. *In* "Monographs on the Pathology of Laboratory Animals: Nonhuman Primates" (T. C. Jones, U. Mohr, and R. D. Hunt, eds.), Vol. 1, pp. 5–20. Springer-Verlag, Berlin and New York.

King, N. W., Jr. (1993b). Tuberculosis. *In* "Monographs on the Pathology of Laboratory Animals: Nonhuman Primates" (T. C. Jones, U. Mohr, and R. D. Hunt, eds.), Vol. 1, pp. 141–148. Springer-Verlag, Berlin and New York.

Klein, H. J., Hall, W. C., and Pouch, W. J. (1987). Characterization of an outbreak of *Bordetella bronchiseptica* in a group of African green monkeys (*Cercopithecus aethiops*). *Lab. Anim. Sci.* **37**, 524.

Klumpp, S. A., and McClure, H. M. (1993). Nocardiosis, lung. *In* "Monographs on the Pathology of Laboratory Animals: Nonhuman Primates" (T. C. Jones, U. Mohr, and R. D. Hunt, eds.), Vol. 2, pp. 99–103. Springer-Verlag, Berlin and New York.

Kobzik, L., and Schoen, F. J. (1994). The lung. *In* "Pathologic Basis of Disease" (R. S. Cotran, V. Kumar, and S. L. Robbins, eds.), 5th ed., pp. 673–734. Saunders, Philadelphia.

Kohn, D. F., and Haines, D. E. (1977). *Bordetella bronchiseptica* infection in the lesser bushbaby (*Galago senegalensis*). *Lab. Anim. Sci.* **27**, 279–280.

Kohn, D. F., and Haines, D. E. (1982). Diseases of the prosimii: A review. *In* "The Lesser Bushbaby (Galago) as an Animal Model: Selected Topics" (D. E. Haines, ed.), pp. 285–301. CRC Press, Boca Raton, FL.

Kornegay, R. W., Giddens, W. E., Jr., Morton, W. R., and Knitter, G. H. (1986). Verminous vasculitis, pneumonia and pulmonary infarction in a cynomolgus monkey after treatment with ivermectin. *Lab. Anim. Sci.* **36**, 45–47.

Korzeniowska-Zuk, E. (1992). [Studies on the possibility of desensitization of patients sensitive to plant pollens and house dust by an oral route.] *Pneumonol. Alergol. Pol.* **60**, 32–38.

Kraus, B. S., and Garrett, W. S. (1968). Cleft palate in a marmosets: Report of a case. *Cleft Palate. J. Am. Vet. Med. Assoc.* **5**, 340–345.

Kuhn, U. S. G., III, and Selin, M. J. (1978). Tuberculin testing in great apes. *In* "Mycobacterial Infections of Zoo Animals" (R. J. Montali, ed.), pp. 129–134. Smithsonian Institution Press, Washington, DC.

Lapin, B. A., and Yakovleva, L. A. (1963). "Comparative Pathology in Monkeys." Thomas, Springfield, IL.

Leathers, C. W., and Hamm, T. E. (1976). Naturally occurring tuberculosis in a squirrel monkey and a *Cebus* monkey. *J. Am. Vet. Med. Assoc.* **169**, 909–911.

Lehner, N. D. M. (1984). Biology and disease of cebidae. *In* "Laboratory Animal Medicine" (J. G. Fox, B. J. Cohen, and F. M. Loew, eds.), pp. 321–353. Academic Press, Orlando, FL.

Lewis, J. C., Montgomery, C. A., and Hildebrandt, P. K. (1975). Airsacculitis in the baboon. *J. Am. Vet. Med. Assoc.* **167**, 662–664.

Liebenberg, S. P., and Giddens, W. E., Jr. (1985). Disseminated nocardiosis in three macaque monkeys. *Lab. Anim. Sci.* **35**, 162–166.

Liu, C. T., and DeLauter, R. D. (1977). Pulmonary functions in conscious and anesthetized rhesus macaques. *Am. J. Vet. Res.* **38**, 1843–1848.

Lowenstine, L. J. (1986). Neoplasms and proliferative disorders in nonhuman primates. *In* "Primates: The Road to Self-Sustaining Populations" (K. Benirschke, ed.), pp. 781–814. Springer-Verlag, Berlin and New York.

Lowenstine, L. J. (1993a). Type D retrovirus infection, macaques. *In* "Monographs on the Pathology of Laboratory Animals: Nonhuman Primates" (T. C. Jones, U. Mohr, and R. D. Hunt, eds.), Vol. 1, pp. 20–32. Springer-Verlag, Berlin and New York.

Lowenstine, L. J. (1993b). Measles virus infection, nonhuman primates. *In* "Monographs on the Pathology of Laboratory Animals: Nonhuman Primates" (T. C. Jones, U. Mohr, and R. D. Hunt, eds.), Vol. 1, pp. 108–118. Springer-Verlag, Berlin and New York.

Lowenstine, L. J., Pederson, N. C., Higgins, J., Pallis, K. C., Uyeda, A., Marx, P., Lerche, N., Munn, R. J., and Gardner, M. B. (1986). Seroepidemiologic survey of captive old-world primates for antibodies to human and simian retroviruses, and isolation of a lentivirus from sooty mangabeys (*Cercocebus atys*). *Int. J. Cancer* **38**, 563–574.

Lowenstine, L. J., Lerche, N. W., Yee, J. A., Uyeda, A., Jennings, M. B., Munn, R. J., McClure, H. M., Anderson, D. C., Fultz, P. N., and Gardner, M. B. (1992). Evidence for a lentiviral etiology in an epizootic of immune deficiency and lymphoma in stump-tailed macaques (*Macaca arctoides*). *J. Med. Primatol.* **21**, 1–14.

Marcella, K. L., and Wright, E. M. (1985). A tracheal foreign body in a rhesus monkey. *Compend. Contin. Educ. Pract. Vet.* **7** 1048, 1049.

Martin, D. P. (1978). Primates. *In* "Zoo and Wild Animal Medicine" (M. E. Fowler, ed.), Curr. Ther., Vol. 3, pp. 525–552. Saunders, Philadelphia.

Matsumoto, Y., Yamada, M., Tegoshi, T., Yoshida, Y., Gotoh, S., Suzuki, J., and Matsubayashi, K. (1987). *Pneumocystis* infection in macaque monkeys: *Macaca fuscata fuscata* and *Macaca fascicularis*. *Parasitol. Res.* **73**, 324–327.

McClure, H. M. (1972). Animal model for human disease. Down's syndrome (mongolism, trisomy 21). *Am. J. Pathol.* **67**, 413–416.

McClure, H. M., and Guilloud, N. B. (1971). Comparative pathology of the chimpanzee. *In* "The Chimpanzee, Vol. 4. Behavior, Growth and Pathology of Chimpanzees (G. H. Bourne, ed.), pp. 103–272. University Park Press, Baltimore.

McClure, H. M., Keeling, M. E., Custer, R. P., Marshak, R. R., Abt, D. A., and Ferrer, J. F. (1974). Erythroleukemia in two infant chimpanzees fed milk from cows naturally infected with the bovine C-type virus. *Cancer Res.* **34**, 2745–2757.

McClure, H. M., Chang, J., Kaplan, W., and Brown, J. M. (1976). Pulmonary nocardiosis in an orangutan. *J. Am. Vet. Med. Assoc.* **169**, 943–945.

McConnell, E. E. (1977). Parasitic diseases observed in free-ranging and captive baboons. *Comp. Pathol. Bull.* **9**, 2.

McIntosh, G., Ciegecke, R., and Wilson, D. (1985). Spontaneous nasopharyngeal malignancies in the common marmoset. *Vet. Pathol.* **22**, 86–88.

McKiernan, B. C. (1995). Sneezing and nasal discharge. *In* "Textbook of Veterinary Internal Medicine: Diseases of the Dog and Cat" (S. J. Ettinger and E. C. Feldman, eds.), pp. 79–85. Saunders, Philadelphia.

McLaughlin, R. M. (1978). *Mycobacterium bovis* in nonhuman primates. *In* "Mycobacterial Infections of Zoo Animals" (R. J. Montali, ed.), pp. 151–156. Smithsonian Institution Press, Washington, DC.

McLaughlin, R. M., and Marrs, G. E. (1978). Tuberculin testing in nonhuman primates: OT vs. PPD. *In* "Mycobacterial Infections of Zoo Animals" (R. J. Montali, ed.), pp. 123–128. Smithsonian Institution Press, Washington, DC.

McManamon, R., Swenson, R. B., and Lowenstine, L. J. (1994). Update on diagnostic and therapeutic approaches to airsacculitis in orangutans. *Proc. Annu. Meet., Am. Assoc. Zoo Vet., 1994*, pp. 219–220.

Migaki, G. (1986). Mycotic infections in nonhuman primates. *In* "Primates: The Road to Self-Sustaining Populations" (K. Benirschke, ed.), pp. 557–570. Springer-Verlag, Berlin and New York.

Miller, R. E., and Boever, W. J. (1983). Cryptococcosis in a lion-tailed macaque (*Macaca silenus*). *J. Zoo Anim. Med.* **14**, 110–114.

Montali, R. J. (1993). Congenital retrosternal diaphragmatic defects, golden lion tamarins *In* "Monographs on the Pathology of Laboratory Animals: Nonhuman Primates" (T. C. Jones, U. Mohr, and R. D. Hunt, eds.), Vol. 2, pp. 132–133. Springer-Verlag, Berlin and New York.

Montali, R. J., and Hirschel, P. G. (1990). Survey of tuberculin testing practices at zoos. *Proc. Annu. Meet., Am. Assoc. Zoo Vet., 1990*, pp. 105–109.

Morris, D. L., Clarkson, M. S., Stallbaumer, M. F., Pritchard, J., Jones, R. S., and Chinnery, J. B. (1985). Albendazole treatment of pulmonary hydatid cysts in naturally infected sheep: A study with relevance to man. *Thorax* **40**, 453–458.

Morris, J. A., Blount, R. E., Jr., and Savage, R. E. (1956). Recovery of cytopathogenic agent from chimpanzees with coryza. *Proc. Soc. Exp. Biol. Med.* **92**, 544–549.

Morton, W. R., Giddens, W. E., Jr., and Boyce, J. T. (1979). Survey of neonatal and infant disease in *Macaca nemestrina*. *In* "Nursery Care of Nonhuman Primates" (G. C. Ruppenthal, ed.), pp. 227–235. Plenum, New York.

Moser, K. M. (1994). Diagnostic procedures in respiratory diseases. *In* "Harrison's Principles of Internal Medicine" (K. J. Isselbacher, J. B. Martin, E. Braunwald, A. S. Fauci, J. D. Wilson, and D. L. Kasper, eds.), pp. 1163–1167. McGraw-Hill, New York.

Muggenburg, B. A., Hahn, F. F., Bowen, J. A., and Bice, D. E. (1982). Flexible fiberoptic bronchoscopy of chimpanzees. *Lab. Anim. Sci.* **32**, 534–537.

Munson, L., and Montali, R. J. (1990). Pathology and diseases of great apes at the National Zoological Park. *Zoo Biol.* **9**, 99–105.

Murphy, B. L., Maynard, J. E., Krushak, D. H., and Berquist, K. R. (1972). Microbial flora of imported marmosets: Viruses and enteric bacteria. *Lab. Anim. Sci.* **22**, 339–343.

Nelson, B., Cosgrove, G. E., and Gengozian, N. (1966). Disease of an imported primate *Tamarinus nigricollis*. *Lab. Anim. Care* **16**, 255–275.

Nicholls, J., and Schwartz, L. W. (1980). A spontaneous bronchiolo-alveolar neoplasm in a nonhuman primate. *Vet. Pathol.* **17**, 630–634.

Nichols, R. E. (1939). Nasal polypus in a chimpanzee *J. Am. Vet. Med. Assoc.* **47**, 56.

Odkvist, L. M., and Schauman, P. (1980). A bronchial foreign body in a chimpanzee. *J. Small Anim. Pract.* **21**, 347–350.

Okoh, A. E. J., and Ocholi, R. A. (1986). A fatal case of Pasteurellosis in a Patas monkey in Jos Zoo, Nigeria. *J. Zoo Anim. Med.* **17**, 55–56.

Olson, L. C., and Palotay, J. L. (1983). Epistaxis and bullae in cynomolgus macaques (*Macaca fascicularis*). *Lab. Anim. Sci.* **33**, 377–379.

Padovan, D., and Cantrell, C. (1983). Causes of death of infant rhesus and squirrel monkeys. *J. Am. Vet. Med. Assoc.* **183**, 1182–1184.

Pappagianis, D. (1985). Coccidioidomycosis. *In* "Models in Dermatology" (H. I. Maibach and N. J. Lowe, eds.), Vol. 1, pp. 98–104. Karger, Basel.

Parent, R. (1992). "Comparative Anatomy of the Normal Lung." CRC Press, Boca Raton, FL.

Potkay, S. (1992). Diseases of the Callitrichidae: A review. *J. Med. Primatol.* **21**, 189–236.

Pryor, W. H., Bergner, J. F., and Raulston, G. L. (1970). Leech (*Dinobdella ferox*) infection of a Taiwan monkey (*Macaca cyclopis*). *J. Am. Vet. Med. Assoc.* **157**, 1926–1927.

Rawlings, C. A., and Splitter, G. A. (1973). Pneumothorax associated with lung mite lesions in a rhesus monkey. *Lab. Anim. Sci.* **23**, 259–261.

Renegar, K. B. (1992). Influenza virus infections and immunity: A review of human and animal models. *Lab. Anim. Sci.* **42**, 222–232.

Renner, M., and Bartholomew, W. R. (1974). Mycobacteriologic data from two outbreaks of bovine tuberculosis in nonhuman primates. *Am. Rev. Respir. Dis.* **109**, 11–16.

Renquist, D. M., and Whitney, R. A. (1978). Tuberculosis in nonhuman primates—An overview. *In* "Mycobacterial Infections of Zoo Animals" (R. J. Montali, ed.), pp. 9–16. Smithsonian Institution Press, Washington, DC.

Revak, S. D., Rice, C. L., Schraufstetter, I. U., Halsey, W. A., Bohl, B. P., Clancy, R. M., and Cochrane, C. G. (1985). Experimental pulmonary inflammatory injury in the monkey. *J. Clin. Invest.* **76**, 1182–1192.

Richter, C. B. (1984). Biology and disease of callitrichidae. *In* "Laboratory Animal Medicine" (J. G. Fox, B. J. Cohen, and F. M. Loew, eds.), pp. 353–383. Academic Press, Orlando, FL.

Richter, C. B., Humason, G. L., and Godbold, J. H., Jr. (1978). Endemic *Pneumocystis carinii* in a marmoset colony. *J. Comp. Pathol.* **88**, 171–180.

Robinson, P. T., and Bush, M. (1981). Clinical and pathologic aspects of pulmonary acariasis in douc langur and proboscis monkeys. *Zool. Garten* **51**, 161–169.

Robinson, P. T., and Janssen, D. L. (1980). Iatrogenic anesthetic emergencies in nondomestic animals: Three case reports. *J. Am. Anim. Hosp. Assoc.* **16**, 279–282.

Rosenberg, D. P. (1995). Critical care. *In* "Nonhuman Primates in Biomedical Research: Biology and Management" (B. T. Bennet, C. R. Abee, and R. Henrickson, eds.), pp. 316–334. Academic Press, San Diego, CA.

Roussilhon, C., Postal, J.-M., and Ravisse, P. (1987). Spontaneous cryptococcosis of a squirrel monkey (*Saimiri scureus*) in French Guyana. *J. Med. Primatol.* **16**, 39–47.

Sakaguchi, M., Inouye, S., Imaoka, K., Miyazawa, H., Hashimoto, M., Nigi, H., Nakamura, S., Gotoh, S., Minezawa, M., Fujimoto, K., Honjo, S., Taniguchi, Y., and Ando, S. (1992). Measurement of serum IgE antibodies against Japanese cedar pollen (*Cryptomeria japonica*) in Japanese monkeys (*Macaca fuscata*) with pollinosis. *J. Med. Primatol.* **21**, 323–327.

Samuelson, J., and von Lichtenberg, F. (1994). Infectious diseases. *In* "Pathologic Basis of Disease" (R. S. Cotran, V. Kumar, and S. L. Robbins, eds.), 5th ed., pp. 305–377. Saunders, Philadelphia.

Schlag, G., Redl, H., van Vuuren, C. J. J., and Davies, J. (1992). Hyperdynamic sepsis in baboons: II. Relation of organ damage to severity of sepsis evaluated by a newly developed morphological scoring system. *Circ. Shock* **38**, 253–263.

Schmidt, R. E. (1978). Systemic pathology of chimpanzees. *J. Med. Primatol.* **7**, 274–318.

Schmidt, R. E., Hubbard, G. B., and Fletcher, K. C. (1986). Systematic survey of lesions from animals in a zoologic collection: III. Respiratory system. *J. Zoo Anim. Med.* **17**, 17–23.

Scott, G. B. D. (1992a). "Comparative Primate Pathology." Oxford University Press, Oxford.

Scott, G. B. D. (1992b). The respiratory system. *In* "Comparative Primate Pathology," pp. 120–135. Oxford University Press, Oxford.

Silverman, S. (1975). Diagnostic radiology: Its utilization in nonhuman primate medicine. *Lab. Anim. Sci.* **25**, 748–752.

Silverman, S., Henrickson, R., Wisloh, A., and Hoffman, R. (1975). What is your diagnosis? *J. Am. Vet. Med. Assoc.* **167**, 669–670.

Silverman, S., Poulos, P. W., and Suter, P. F. (1976). Cavitary pulmonary lesions in animals. *J. Am. Vet. Radiol. Soc.* **17**, 134–146.

Sjövall, P. (1990). Oral hyposensitization in allergic contact dermatitis. *Semin. Dermatol.* **9**, 206–209.

Slayter, M. V. (1988). Nasal cavity carcinosarcoma in a bonnet macaque (*Macaca radiata*). *J. Med. Primatol.* **17**, 49–56.

Southers, J. L., and Ford, E. W. (1995). Medical management. *In* "Nonhuman Primates in Biomedical Research: Biology and Management" (B. T. Bennet, C. R. Abee, and R. Henrickson, eds.), pp. 257–270. Academic Press, San Diego, CA.

Stills, H. F., Jr., Balady, M. A., and Liebenberg, S. P. (1979). A comparison of bacterial flora isolated by transtracheal aspiration and pharyngeal swabs in *Macaca fascicularis*. *Lab. Anim. Sci.* **29**, 229–233.

Stills, H. F., Jr., and Rader, W. R. (1982). What is your diagnosis? *J. Am. Vet. Med. Assoc.* **180**, 949–950.

Stone, W. B., and Hughes, J. A. (1969). Massive pulmonary acariasis in the pig-tail macaque. *Bull. Wildl. Dis. Assoc.* **5**, 20.

Stookey, J. L., and Moe, J. B. (1978). The respiratory system. *In* "Pathology of Laboratory Animals" (K. Benirschke, F. M. Garner, and T. C. Jones, eds.), Vol. 1, pp. 71–113. Springer-Verlag, New York.

Strobert, E. A., and Swenson, R. B. (1979). Treatment regimen for air sacculitis in the chimpanzee (*Pan troglodytes*). *Lab. Anim. Sci.* **29**, 387–388.

Strumpf, I. J., Bacher, J. D., and Gadek, J. E. (1979). Flexible fiberoptic bronchoscopy of the rhesus monkey. *Lab. Anim. Sci.* **29**, 785–788.

Suleman, M. A., Tarara, R., Mandalia, K. M., and Weiss, M. (1984). A spontaneous bronchogenic carcinoma in a Sykes monkey (*Cercopithecus mitis stuhlmani*). *J. Med. Primatol.* **13**, 153–157.

Sutherland, S. D., Almeida, J. D., Gardner, P. S., Skarpa, M., and Stanton, J. (1986). Rapid diagnosis and management of parainfluenza I virus infection in common marmosets (*Callithrix jacchus*). *Lab. Animals* **20**, 121–126.

Swindler, D. R., and Merrill, O. M. (1971). Spontaneous cleft lip and palate in a living nonhuman primate, *Macaca mulatta*. *Am. J. Phys. Anthropol.* **34**, 435–439.

Swindler, D. R., and Wood, C. D. (1973). "An Atlas of Primate Gross Anatomy. Baboon, Chimpanzee, and Man." University of Washington Press, Seattle.

Tarara, R., Suleman, M. A., Sapolsky, R., Wabomba, M. J., and Else, J. G. (1985). Tuberculosis in wild olive baboons, *Papio cynocephalus anubis* (Lesson), in Kenya. *J. Wildl. Dis.* **21**, 137–140.

Taylor, G. B., Jr., Kosanke, S., Randolph, M., Emerson, T., Hinshaw, L., Catlett, R., Blick, K., and Edgington, T. S. (1994). Retrospective description and experimental reconstitution of three different responses of the baboon to lethal *E. coli*. *Circ. Shock* **42**, 92–103.

Tell, L., Nichols, D., and Bush, M. (1993). Cryptococcosis in tree shrews (*Tupaia tana* and *Tupaia minor*) and elephant shrews (*Macroscelides proboscides*). *Proc. Annu. Meet., Am. Assoc. Zoo Vet., 1993*, pp. 49–50.

Thoen, C. O., Beluhan, F. Z., Himes, E. M., Capek, V., and Bennet, T. (1977). *Mycobacterium bovis* infection in baboons (*Papio papio*). *Arch. Pathol. Lab. Med.* **101**, 291–293.

Toft, J. D., II (1986). The pathoparasitology of nonhuman primates: A review. *In* "Primates: The Road to Self-Sustaining Populations" (K. Benirschke, ed.), pp. 571–679. Springer-Verlag, Berlin and New York.

Tsai, C.-C., and Giddens, W. E., Jr. (1985). Clear cell carcinoma of the lung in a pigtailed macaque. *Lab. Anim. Sci.* **35**, 85–88.

Tucker, M. J. (1984). Observations on the pathology of the respiratory system in the ICI marmoset (*Callothrix jacchus*). *In* "Symposium on Marmoset Pathology," pp. 50–53.

Turnwald, G. H. (1995). Dyspnea and tachypnea. *In* "Textbook of Veterinary Internal Medicine: Diseases of the Dog and Cat" (S. J. Ettinger and E. C. Feldman, eds.), pp. 61–64. Saunders, Philadelphia.

Tyler, W. S., Dungworth, D. L., Plopper, C. G., Hyde, D. M., and Tyler, N. K. (1985). Structural evaluation of the respiratory system. *Fundam. Appl. Toxicol.* **5**, 405–422.

Ulland, B. M. (1968). Chronic occlusive thrombosis of the pulmonary trunk and main right pulmonary artery in a four-year-old *Macaca mulatta*. **124**, 245–247.

Valverde, C. R., Pettan-Brewer, K. C. B., Lerche, N., and Lowenstine, L. J. (1993). A 20 year retrospective study of causes of mortality in a colony of titi monkeys (*Callicebus* spp.). *Proc. Annu. Meet., Am. Assoc. Zoo Vet., 1993*, pp. 208–213.

VandeWoude, S. J., and Luzarraga, M. B. (1991). The role of *Branhamella catarrhalis* in the "bloody-nose syndrome" of cynomolgus macaques. *Lab. Anim. Sci.* **41**, 401–406.

Vogel, A. P., Miller, C. J., Lowenstine, L. J., and Lackner, A. A. (1993). Evidence of horizontal transmission of *Pneumocystis carinii* pneumonia in simian immunodeficiency virus-infected rhesus macaques. *J. Infect. Dis.* **168**, 836–843.

Wallach, J. D., and Boever, W. J. (1983). Primates. *In* "Diseases of Exotic Animals. Medical and Surgical Management," pp. 1–133. Saunders, Philadelphia.

Walzer, P. D. (1994). *Pneumocystis carinii* pneumonia. *In* "Harrison's Principles of Internal Medicine" (K. J. Isselbacher, J. B. Martin, E. Braunwald, A. S. Fauci, J. D. Wilson, and D. L. Kasper, eds.), 13th ed., pp. 908–910. McGraw-Hill, New York.

Ward, G. S., Elwell, M. R., Tingpalapong, M., and Pomsdhit, J. (1985). Use of streptomycin and isoniazid during a tuberculosis epizootic in a rhesus and cynomolgus breeding colony. *Lab. Anim. Sci.* **35**, 395–399.

Weinberger, S. E., and Drazen, J. M. (1994). Disturbances of respiratory function. *In* "Harrison's Principles of Internal Medicine" (K. J. Isselbacher, J. B. Martin, E. Braunwald, A. S. Fauci, J. D. Wilson, and D. L. Kasper, eds.), 13th ed., Vol. 2, pp. 1152–1159. McGraw-Hill, New York.

Weller, R. E. (1994). Infectious and noninfectious diseases of owl monkeys. *In* "Aotus: The Owl Monkey" (J. F. Baer, R. E. Weller, and I. Kakoma, eds.), pp. 177–215. Academic Press, San Diego, CA.

Wells, S. K., Sargent, E. L., and Andrews, M. E. (1990). Tuberculosis and tuberculin testing in orangutans (*Pongo pygmaeus*). *Proc. Annu. Meet., Am. Assoc. Zoo Vet., 1990*, pp. 110–114.

Wilson, J. G. (1978). Developmental abnormalities. Nonhuman primates. *In* "Pathology of Laboratory Animals" (K. Benirschke, F. M. Garner, and T. C. Jones, eds.), Vol. 2, pp. 1911–1917. Springer-Verlag, New York.

Wolf, R. H., Gibson, S. V., Watson, E. A., and Baskin, G. B. (1988). Multidrug chemotherapy of tuberculosis in rhesus monkeys. *Lab. Anim. Sci.* **38**, 25–33.

Wolff, M., Bush, M., Montali, R., and Gardiner, C. H. (1989). Clinical challenge: Case 2. *J. Zoo Wildl. Med.* **20**, 383–385.

Wolff, P. L. (1993). Parasites of New World primates. *In* "Zoo and Wild Animal Medicine" (M. E. Fowler, ed.), Curr. Ther., Vol. 3, pp. 378–389. Saunders, Philadelphia.

Woodard, J. C. (1968). Acarous (*Pneumonyssus simicola*) arteritis in rhesus monkeys. *J. Am. Vet. Med. Assoc.* **153**, 905–909.

Zhang, G.-W., Ruiji, X., and McManus, D. P. (1990). The presence of pinworms (*Enterobius* sp.) in the mesenteric lymph nodes, liver and lungs of a chimpanzee, *Pan troglodytes*. *J. Helminthol.* **64**, 29–34.

Chapter 8

Urogenital System

Elizabeth W. Ford, Jeffrey A. Roberts, and Janice L. Southers

PART A. URINARY SYSTEM

Jeffrey A. Roberts, Elizabeth W. Ford,
and Janice L. Southers

I. ANATOMY

The urogenital system of the nonhuman primate has basic functional similarity to those of other mammalian species and represents an area susceptible to not only primary but also a wide range of secondary complications.

A. Kidney

The structure of the kidney is similar across the primate order with the exceptions of humans and the genus *Ateles*. Generally, the bean-shaped, retroperitoneal kidney is located on either side of the descending aorta and is a uniform, unipapillate organ with a single pyramidal structure from the cortex into the medulla. In contrast to this usual arrangement, *Homo* and *Ateles* have a multipyramidal, multipapillate kidney with a primary cortex projecting to the renal pelvis. Physiological studies have shown that the functional capability of the kidney in *Homo* and *Ateles* is very similar to that observed in other primate species (Straus and Arcadi, 1958; Goodman *et al.,* 1977). However, the proportions of renal cortex and medulla differ in these groups, with humans showing a thinner cortex in contrast to relatively equivalent-sized structures in cattarhine primates (Tischer, 1975; Straus and Arcadi, 1958). The medulla is relatively small in three species of macaques: the rhesus macaque (*Macaca mulatta*), the cynomolgus macaque (*M. fascicularis*), and the stump-tailed macaque (*M. speciosa*). The importance of this anatomical variation is that the length of the loop of Henle has long been thought to relate to urine concentrating ability. Nevertheless, the concentrating ability of cattarrhine primates is

very similar to that found in the genus *Homo*. In rhesus macaques, the maximal urine osmolality observed after 48 hr of fluid deprivation was 1412 $\pm$ 151 mOsm/kg of H_2O, which is very close to the maximal urine osomolality found in humans (1000 $\pm$ 200 mOsm/kg H_2O) (Tischer *et al.,* 1972; Tischer, 1975). Knowing these values is, of course, important for clinical medicine but is also a valuable baseline for monitoring experimental protocols involving water deprivation, which may be compounded by chronic inflammatory conditions.

The microscopic anatomy of the kidney is similar in nonhuman primates to that of humans and other laboratory animals (Tischer, 1975). The renal glomerulus consists of (1) a network of capillaries lined by endothelial cells, (2) an interstitium of mesangial cells with mesangial matrix material, and (3) visceral and parietal epithelial cells and their associated basement membrane. Renal glomeruli are also anatomically similar across the order, although ultrastructural studies may show some variation (Brack and Weber, 1994). Electron microscopy and immunohistochemistry show indications of increased mesangial cell activity in callitrichids, which may be related to structural differences or to the effects of chronic damage (Brack and Weber, 1994).

The proximal tubule has three separate segments with distinctive histologic differences. The first segment is composed of tall columnar cells with a well-developed brush border, prominent mitochondria, and a dramatic transition from the squamous epithelial cells of Bowman's capsule. These cells in the proximal tubule then progress to low columnar shapes with a shorter brush border and fewer mitochondria. The final part of the proximal tubule or pars recta has cuboidal cells with a distinct brush border. These cells have fewer organelles and have a gradual transition to the thin descending loop of Henle (Tischer, 1975). The inner medulla of the rhesus kidney is poorly developed and lacks a well-defined loop of Henle. The loop of Henle is very short and its turn is characterized by tubular epithelium of the thick limb of Henle (Tischer, 1975).

The distal tubule is composed of three segments, including the pars recta of the distal tubule, the macula densa, and the pars convoluta or distal convoluted tubule. The tubule begins as cuboidal cells and contains abundant mitochondria. The tubule ascends into the cortex and contacts the renal corpuscle of its origin. The point of contact of the tubule with the corpuscle results in the macula densa with tall columnar cells. These cells have apically located nuclei and masses of secretory or absorbative organelles located away from the lumen. These structures, along with the myoepitheliod cells and juxtaglomeruler cells, form the juxtaglomerular apparatus which is involved in sensing pressure and solute changes to control renal perfusion. The anatomy of this structure in primates is very similar to that of humans and other laboratory animals. The distal convoluted tubule extends from the macula densa to the cortical collecting duct where there is a transition to cuboidal epithelial cells of somewhat greater height than those in the pars recta (Tischer, 1975). The collecting duct is divided into four sections: the collecting duct to the medullary ray, the collecting tubule in the medullary ray, the outer medullary segment, and the inner medullary segment. These sections resemble their human counterparts, except for the inner medullary segment, which is extremely abbreviated in length. Ducts descending from the outer medulla toward the inner medulla form the ducts of Belleni, which have a modified type of transitional epithelium and collect urine from multiple nephrons within the kidney.

B. Ureter, Bladder, and Urethra

The histology of the ureter, bladder, and urethra in nonhuman primates is very similar to that found in humans. The cell layers are primarily transitional cells to the distal urethra, which is composed of stratified or pseudostratified columnar epithelium, except for the distal segment that converts to squamous epithelium (Roberts, 1972). Bladder muscle consists of smooth muscle fibers with the ureter surrounded by two layers of smooth muscle; a circular and a longitudinal layer.

II. CLINICAL ASSESSMENT

A. Urological Examination

A complete physical examination in the nonhuman primate must include assessment of the urinary system. Numerous references in the literature report vague clinical presentations preceding euthanasia, followed by gross and histologic presentation of significant pathologic changes in the urinary system (Gozalo and Montoya, 1990; Stills and Bullock, 1981; Chapman *et al.*, 1973). Failure to correlate specific clinical pathology results with detailed anatomic pathology hampers understanding of the pathogenesis of disease and the development of potential therapies.

It is important that the clinician who is responsible for laboratory animals be familiar with dysfunctions of the urinary system not only from the perspective of treating spontaneous disease, but also for managing the complications associated with experimental protocols.

The importance of the renal system is such that its functional reserve capacity allows up to 75% of the renal parynchema to be destroyed before homeostasis is disrupted (Brenner *et al.*, 1987). Once disrupted, the sequelae from renal dysfunction is severe and widespread. Therefore, all available diagnostic techniques should be used as early in the disease process as possible for the clinician to achieve successful intervention and therapy for nonhuman primates.

The first step in examination of the urinary system is collection of the urine sample. In primates, as in other species, this can be accomplished in a variety of ways (Rahlman *et al.*, 1976). Free catch is possible in most species, when animals are trained to respond to the presence of a caretaker at specific times during the day to allow placement of a container for collection of freely voided urine (Dysko and Hoskins, 1995). This method is frequently used in monitoring reproductive hormones in primate species. Alternative methods are catheterization and cystocentesis, which are described in this series in "Nonhuman Primates in Biomedical Research: Volume I, Biology and Management, Collection of Biological Samples and Therapy Administration."

The method of sample collection dictates the range of diagnostic procedures that may be performed on the sample. Ideally for microbial culture, a sample collected aseptically by cystocentesis or catheterization is required.

An initial examination of urine would include an assessment of pH, protein, glucose, ketones, occult blood, and bilirubin. Urinary pH has a wide range, from pH 4.5 to 8, in humans, and with the varied diets found in the primates this represents a narrow spectrum. Protein may be evaluated by heat and an acetic acid dipstick test (Bili-Labstix, Miles Inc., Elkhart, IN). However, a single positive test is not diagnostic for any disease process and should be followed with additional assessments of urine protein content and then interpreted in light of other characteristics such as urine concentration.

When significant proteinuria is present, electrophoresis of the sample is used to identify the specific protein fractions. The presence of proteinuria may be indicative of renal disease associated with increased glomerular filtration of protein, reduced tubular resorption of protein, and the addition of protein to urine in the renal tubules. Overall protein loss can be determined from 24-hr urine collections or from single samples with the amount of urinary protein excretion coupled to urine creatinine assessment (Weller *et al.*, 1991).

Determination of serum and urine osmolality can be very valuable in the management of fluid therapy in volume-depleted or dehydrated animals (Rosenberg, 1995). Anuric or oligouric animals should be monitored very closely during fluid therapy to assess urine production and levels of normal renal function. Urine reference values for rhesus macaques are shown

TABLE A.I

PRIMATE REFERENCE VALUES FOR URINALYSIS [a]

Parameter	Unit	Mean	Mean ± 2 [b]	Minimum	Maximum
Specific gravity		1.018	1.000–1.038	1.003	1.035
pH	pH units	6.4	4.2–8.6	5.0	8.5
Protein	mg/dl	1	0–3	0	4
Glucose	mg/dl	0	0	0	0
Ketone	mg/dl	0	0–1	0	4
Bilirubin		0	0	0	0
Occult blood		0	0–2	0	3
White blood cells	/hpf	0	0	0	0
Red blood cells	/hpf	2	0–29	0	100
Epithelial cells		1	0–3	0	4
Crystals		1	0–4	0	4
Nova pH	pH units	6.474	4.574–8.374	2.340	7.872
Nova sodium	mM/liter	20	0–44	7	69
Nova potassium	mM/liter	28.9	3.9–53.9	4.4	50.4
Osmolality	mOsm/kg	47	2–92	23	138

[a] Outdoor rhesus monkeys ($n = 131$).

[b] Mean ± standard deviation.

in Table A.I. These were collected from 131 animals housed outdoors at the California Regional Primate Research Center (A. Spinner, personal communication, 1995).

Analysis of serum chemistry is also critical for the successful management of renal disease. The most common values assessed are blood urea nitrogen (BUN) and creatinine. Blood urea nitrogen is easily measured with dipsticks, and these values can serve as rough indicators of trends in case management. However, because elevations in BUN are common in prerenal conditions, BUN values should be combined with assessment of creatinine values to have a better assessment of renal involvement (Rosenberg, 1995). Moreover, it is important to remember that neither BUN nor creatinine values reflect kidney damage until approximately 75% of the renal parenchyma is damaged (Brenner et al., 1987).

The kidney represents a highly complex and sophisticated filtration system capable of secretion, resorption, and many other active processes requiring sophisticated measurements for thorough assessment. The renal functions of nonhuman primates are more like those of humans than any other laboratory animal species (Roberts, 1972). The first step in assessing kidney function is to measure the glomerular filtration rate (GFR), usually by determining the removal rate of substances such as inulin or creatinine from the blood over a set period of time (Tischer, 1975). Inulin clearance in young rhesus monkeys has been established as 3.30 ± SD 0.69 ml/min/kg body weight and creatinine as 4.30 ± 0.9 ml/min/kg body weight, giving a ratio of creatinine to inulin clearance of 1.30 (Tischer, 1975). This ratio compares well with that from a study in awake baboons in which the creatinine/inulin ratio was found to range from 1.16 ± 0.03 to 1.56 ± 0.04, depending on the level of serum creatinine (Gavellas et al., 1987). These ratios show that

primates, like rats and humans, excrete creatinine through the glomeruli but also through the tubules (Gavellas et al., 1987). Therefore, measurement of creatinine clearance overestimates GFR, which may lead to overestimates of 50% in individuals with high levels of serum creatinine (Gavellas et al., 1987). Renal plasma flow can be assessed by measurement of p-aminohippurate (PAH) clearance by the kidney. Measurements of 8.06 ± 1.22 ml/min/kg body weight in the rhesus macaque agree quite closely with human values of 9 ml/min/kg body weight in 70-kg adult humans (Tischer, 1975).

Data on sodium and water resorption are limited. Water resorption is limited in the proximal tubule or loop of Henle, although significant amounts of sodium are resorbed in the ascending limb. During water restriction, water resorption also occurs in the distal tubule, and the collecting duct can then resorb a major portion of remaining water (Tischer, 1975). As mentioned previously, the maximum urine concentrating ability in rhesus and squirrel monkeys (Roberts, 1972) is similar to that seen in humans, although the inner medulla is significantly decreased in size. In a 48-hr period, fluid deprivation in rhesus monkeys resulted in a greater maximum urine concentration than did the administration of exogenous vasopression. Maximum urine osmolality (U_{max}) was 1087 ± 310 mOsm/kg/H_2O versus a U_{max} of only 711 ± 157 mOsm/kg H_2O with exogenous vasopression administration (Tischer, 1975).

B. Physical Examination, Cystoscopy, and Ultrasound

A complete examination of the renal system includes thorough palpation of both kidneys and the abdomen. Marked asymmetry, atrophy, or absence of an organ can provide imme-

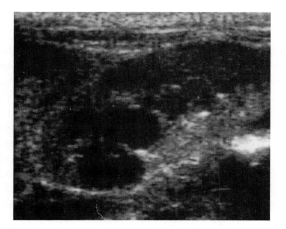

Fig. A.1. A sonogram depicting renal cysts in a macaque.

diate insight into the nature of abnormal function. Cystoscopy has been used in macaques to assess tumors, bladder masses, and cellular changes in the bladder wall and may be a helpful tool in establishing therapy (Bahnson *et al.,* 1988). At the same time, the availability of a diagnostic ultrasound unit is invaluable in evaluating the presence of renal hypertrophy, hydroureter, renal cysts, or cystic calculi (Fig. A.1) (James *et al.,* 1976). Contrast radiography may also provide important diagnostic information with respect to renal function and possible disease states. Anatomical relationships and assessments of possible herniations can be made with positive contrast peritoneography (James *et al.,* 1975).

III. RENAL DISEASE

A. Glomerulonephritis

The glomerulus represents a key link in the chain of renal function. In the process of filtering the blood for metabolites and waste products, the functional integrity of the glomerulus is critical to the successful functioning of more distal elements of the nephron, such as the proximal convoluted tubules, loop of Henle, and distal tubules. A reduced GFR affects resorption and secretion in the medulla, and disruption of capillary integrity in the glomerular tufts results in protein passage and the presence of cellular material in the postglomerular system with accompanying pathology.

Diseases of the glomeruli can have a primary or secondary source, with secondary disturbances being more common (Anderson and Klein, 1993). Inflammatory problems may be caused by an infection or, more commonly, by a disruption of capillary integrity from immune complex formation. These disorders may take one of three forms (Scott, 1992). Small immune complexes appear to pass through the glomerular wall and bind to the outer

wall of the basement membrane. Complement is activated but does not seem to initiate acute damage, with probable dilution occurring in the glomerular filtrate. Eventually, long-term thickening of the basement membrane can result in membranous glomerulonephritis, a condition seen in humans and also nonhuman primates, and which can lead to nephrotic syndrome with globulin, albumin, and red blood cells in the urine.

Intermediate-size immune complexes formed in the plasma can disrupt basement membranes in glomerular tufts with swelling and proliferation of mesangial and endothelial cells. This is probably secondary to the damage that follows complement fixation and results in leakage of protein and cellular material into Bowman's space.

The formation of large immune complex deposits on the glomerular capillary endothelium results in phagocytosis by mesangial cells. Large numbers of such complexes, over time, promote mesangial and endothelial cell proliferation once again followed by disruption of the capillary endothelium and leakage of protein and cells into the glomerular filtrate.

Glomerulonephritis in nonhuman primates is most frequently associated with infectious agents that cause chronic antigen–antibody formation, which in turn damage the glomerular structure. Spontaneous glomerulonephritis has been reported in the bush baby (*Galago* sp.), the pig-tailed macaque (*Macaca nemestrina*), the cynomolgus macaque, and the owl monkey (*Aotus trivirgatus*) (Burkholder, 1981; Boyce *et al.,* 1981; Poskitt *et al.,* 1974). However, many of these reports describe animals caught in the wild afflicted with chronic parasitism or poorly maintained captive populations that have suffered from long-term catheterization or inadequate environmental conditions. Specific lesions in these cases cover a wide spectrum, including mesangio proliferative, diffuse proliferative, and sclerotic (Boyce *et al.,* 1981; Burkholder, 1981). Typically, the "inflammatory" nature of these lesions is characterized not by the infiltration of leukocytes but rather by an increase in the numbers of mesangial cells and the surrounding matrix. Immunostaining of these tissues also shows that they contain antigen–IgM complexes as well as the third component of complement (Boyce *et al.,* 1981; Burkholder, 1981). In a survey describing renal disease, 4 out of 10 aged pig-tailed macaques had mesangioproliferative glomerulonephritis and 6 individuals had some evidence of proteinuria. Granular IgM deposits were evident in all 5 of the animals stained for immunofluorescence, but this outcome did not correlate well with glomerulopathy (Giddens *et al.,* 1979). The link between infection and the development of glomerulonephritis is well established, e.g., as a sequelae of streptococcal infections in rhesus macaque, chronic *Staphylococcus aureus* infections in baboons (*Papio* sp.), and *Plasmodium* sp. in rhesus macaque and owl monkeys (Markowitz, 1969). Immunostaining in these cases commonly shows deposits of IgG, IgM, IgA, and several components of complement (Leary *et al.,* 1981; Nimri and Lamners, 1994). Clinical pathology assays typically reveal proteinuria with or without a decrease in total serum protein levels (Leary *et al.,* 1981). Animals with chronic glomerulonephritis may develop subcutaneous edema, particularly in dependent portions of the body, associated with marked hypoproteinemia and hypoalbuminemia. Albumin/globulin ratios become substantially altered, which are seen as a drop in albumin and an increase in IgG and IgM. Progressive increases in BUN and serum creatinine may also occur as more and more renal parenchyma becomes affected (Boyce *et al.,* 1981). A severe case of glomerulonephritis led to uremia in a female chimpanzee (*Pan troglylodytes*) following the death of her infant from *Diplococcus pneumoniae* (Schmidt and Butler, 1973). Her BUN was elevated and necropsy revealed lesions in the gastric tract, pericarditis, oral ulcers, arteritis, and a vascular lesion in the choroid of the eye. This picture is very similar to that of lesions seen with uremia in humans (Schmidt and Butler, 1973). Chronic glomerulonephritis can also lead to nephrotic syndrome with the increased premeability of glomerular capillaries to plasma protein. The sequence may entail fibrosis of the glomerulus and dilation of tubules in the medulla and cortex as they fill with proteinaceous and hemoglobinuric casts (Hunt and Blake, 1993). Severe nephrotic syndrome was associated with glomerulonephritis in a rhesus macaque that had been catheterized for 9 months. This animal developed severe submandibular edema (Feldman and Bree, 1969). Clinical pathology values showed a mild elevation of BUN to 40 mg/ml and a urine-specific gravity of 1.020 with approximately 300 mg/100 ml of protein. The animal was euthanized, and at necropsy both kidneys were swollen, soft, and pale. Glomeruli were enlarged and hypercellular with nonspecific degenerative changes of the tubular epithelium. The diagnosis was subacute proliferative glomerulonephritis. The edema that accompanies nephrotic syndrome is a combination of both osmotic and vascular changes. Reduced glomerular filtration increases the sodium concentration, while at the same time, the increased permeability permits excessive protein loss. The increased sodium levels activate aldosterone secretion, which results in moderate sodium and water retention, further increasing physiologic problems. Particularly important to note is that the edematous component of the nephrotic syndrome does not result from hypoproteinemia alone (Feldman and Bree, 1969).

Glomerular damage may also be associated with systemic trauma from muscle-crushing injuries producing rhabdomyolysis, myoglobinemia, and subsequent renal failure. The release of myoglobin not only directly damages the glomerulus and impairs filtration, it also precipitates in the tubules, causing obstruction and possible acute necrosis of tubule epithelial cells when absorbed (Seibold *et al.,* 1971; Bicknese, 1990; Rosenberg, 1995). Prompt administration of fluids is indicated if there is any concern about extensive muscle trauma. Clinical pathology values may be unremarkable or may show elevated serum creatinine kinase, dark urine with granular casts in the sediments, and a positive reaction for blood on Bili-Labstix, Miles Inc., Elkhart, IN). Immunodiffusion can be used to confirm the presence of myoglobin. Serum chemistry tests may show hyperkalemia, hyperphosphatemia, hypocalcemia, hyperuremia, and elevated lactate dehydrogenase (LDH) (Bickese, 1990).

B. Interstitial Nephritis

Interstitial nephritis is a lesion that may be seen in nonhuman primate populations with or without accompanying renal pathology. The lesion is characterized by the multifocal interstitial infiltration of lymphocytes and plasma cells into the parenchyma, followed by fibrosis and eventual mineralization (Giddens *et al.,* 1981; Brack and Rothe, 1981). Interstitial nephritis was listed as the most frequently observed lesion in a survey of lesions seen at necropsy in a collection of zoo primates (Hubbard *et al.,* 1987). In a survey of spontaneous renal lesions in 150 wild-caught rhesus macaques, two young males had focal interstitial infiltrates of lymphocytes, mononuclear histocytes, and occasional plasma cells. These lesions were without accompanying clinical signs and did not affect the adjacent tubules or related structures (Kaur *et al.,* 1968). A review of anemia and nephritis in the owl monkey described interstitial nephritis in addition to the more commonly recognized glomerular pathology. Although the two diseases often appear together, they do occur separately in some animals with periglomerular infiltration by lymphocytes, eosinophils, and plasma cells (Chalifoux *et al.,* 1981). These lesions may also progress to diffuse or linear sclerosis of renal parenchyma. Finally, a strong correlation exists between the presence of interstitial nephritis and anemia (Chalifoux *et al.,* 1981). Elsewhere, chronic tubulo-interstitial nephritis has been associated with protein malnutrition and "wasting disease" in another New World species, *Callithrix jacchus,* the common marmoset (Brack and Rothe, 1981). In addition to other organic and renal changes, these animals had lymphocytes infiltrating the tubular interstitium along with extensive interstitial fibrosis. A survey of 113 necropsied prosimians from a zoo populations revealed 22 with renal pathology. Of these, 4 had interstitial nephritis leading to fibrosis with tubular atrophy and cysts. Some glomerular changes were observed and were believed to be secondary to the primary interstitial lesion (Boraski, 1981). Nephritis and congestive heart failure were observed in a 30-year-old male gorilla that died after several weeks of therapy. Urinalysis revealed a moderate amount of albumin with waxy, granular casts. The creatinine level was elevated and, on necropsy, the kidney contained an old infarct with diffuse interstitial scarring as well as tubular degeneration (Robinson and Benirschke, 1980).

C. Suppurative Nephritis and Pyelonephritis

Probably the most common renal disease caused by bacteria is pyelonephritis and secondary suppurative nephritis, although this state is infrequently reported in the primate literature. For example, one survey of renal pathology in samples from 590 necropsies from a large primate facility placed the incidence of chronic pyelonephritis at only 0.65% (Roberts *et al.,* 1972).

Bacterial or other infections may occur by one of two routes: a hematogenous source or the urogenital tract. However, the incidence of iatrogenic infections by either route is an important reason to practice strict sterile procedure when placing catheters. Clinical signs of such infections may include depression and/or anorexia, leading to a lack of responsiveness. Pyuria and bacilliuria may be evident on urine examination. The most common bacteria isolated are of the coliform group (Scott, 1992). In wild rhesus macaques, three young males with pyelonephritis had focal destruction of the renal tubules, which contained clumps of inflammatory cells and granular eosinophilic material. Pure *Escherichia coli* was cultured from the urine of one animal (Kaur *et al.,* 1968). Similarly, urine from a gorilla with severe acute pyelonephritis grew not only *E. coli,* but also *Klebsiella* sp., *Staphylococcus aureus,* and *Enterococcus* sp. (O'Neill *et al.,* 1978). These bacterial species and *Proteus mirabilis* are also considered to be causes of acute pyelonephritis in the squirrel monkey, rhesus, and stump-tailed macaque (*Macaca arctoides*). Additionally, *Pseudomonas aeruginosa* was reported as the causative organism in the death of a rhesus macaque and an orangutan (*Pongo pygmaeus*) (Roberts *et al.,* 1972). *Corynebacterium pseudotuberculosis* and *Pseudomonas* sp. are other causes of suppurative nephritis in chimpanzees (*Pan troglodytes*) (Migaki *et al.,* 1979). Histologic analysis of an animal infected with *Pseudomonas* sp. showed multiple abcesses throughout the renal cortex and medulla, although the pelvis was not affected. This outcome and the predominance of lesions in the renal cortex indicate a likely hematogenous spread. An interesting note is that the authors associated the onset of this clinical state with a prior adenoviral infection in the chimpanzee colony (Migaki *et al.,* 1979).

Animals with miliary tuberculosis infections, *Mycobacterium tuberculosis,* may also develop renal lesions in a secondary form as tubercle bacteria are filtered by the bloodstream (Roberts *et al.,* 1972; Scott, 1992). Because reports of bacterial infections in the lower urinary tract are uncommon in nonhuman primates, such infections most likely spread via the hematogenous route. On necropsy, pyelonephritis of a blood-borne origin is visible as red streaks in the periphery of the renal cortex but may be gray or yellow if gross suppuration is present (Scott, 1992). Yet another source of severe renal damage was septic embolic nephritis observed in chronically catheterized animals (Heidel *et al.,* 1981).

Research into vesicoureteral reflux and pyelonephritis in humans has utilized the rhesus macaque as a model of disease. Although the incidence of vesicoureteral reflux is high at birth, the condition ceases by 3 years of age in the macaque. Experimental infections of the bladder and ureter with a P-fimbrinated *E. coli* resulted in endotoxin release, but the absence of peristalsis or ureteral dilation limited the entry of bacteria into the renal parenchyma. The outcome of untreated, granulocytic aggregation and capillary obstruction was renal ischemia and damage associated with free radical release (Roberts, 1992). However, combined therapy with a third-generation cephalosporin (cefonicid) at 15 mg/kg/day IM for 10 days and a xanthine oxidase inhibitor (allopurinol) at 200 mg/kg/day for 10 days has been successful in eliminating infections and in limiting renal damage if administered within 72 hr (Roberts *et al.,* 1990). Leukocytosis may be present, although fever is variable.

D. Parasitic Nephritis

A variety of parasitic diseases can affect the renal system either asymptomatically or with clinical manifestations that may be difficult to diagnose. *Schistosoma haematobium* can be associated with renal pathology and the presence of ova in the bladder of affected monkeys. This infection has been found in several species, including African green monkeys (*Cercopithecus aethiops*), rhesus macaques, capuchin *Cebus* sp. Talopoin, *Miopithecus* sp., and baboons (*Papio* sp.). Thickening of the bladder may result from chronic infection in the presence of ova (Sturrock, 1986).

An excellent review of parasitology by Toft (1986) presents systemic lesions found in different primate taxa. *Toxoplasma gondii* is associated with lesions of the kidney in prosimians, New World monkeys, Old World monkeys, and the great apes. In contrast, *Encephalitozoon cuniculi* has been reported only in New World species, primarily squirrel monkeys and titi monkeys (*Callicebus moloch*). This obligate intracellular protozoan may produce nephritis and can be isolated from the urine. Parasitic infection may also result in secondary renal pathology as a result of lesions within the peritoneal cavity. Hydatid disease and infections with *Echinococcus granulosus* have been associated with hydroureter and hydronephrosis in bush babies, ring-tailed lemur (*Lemur catta*), and rhesus macaques (Palotay and Uno, 1975).

E. Nephrosis

Tubular nephrosis progressing to necrosis may be a sequelae to numerous clinical problems in nonhuman primates. The "fatal fasting" syndrome observed in obese macaques is associated with changes in multiple organs, including the liver and kidney. Affected animals present with anorexia and lethargy. Clinical pathology values show elevated creatinine levels, and urinalysis may reveal elevations of ketones, protein, and glucose. At necropsy, animals have diffuse, pale-tan kidneys with fatty changes in the epithelium of the renal tubules. Vacuolation of the proximal renal tubular epithelium may be moderate to severe (Gliatto and Bronson, 1993). Eosinophilic proteinaceous material appears in the collecting ducts, and the animals are subject to multifocal tubular necrosis (Laber-Laird *et al.,* 1987). In another case, tubular lipidosis afflicted pig-tailed macaques (*Macaca nemestrina*) that appeared to be suffering from a fatal fasting-type syndrome (Giddens *et al.,* 1981). Nephrosis was reported in two wild-caught female rhesus macaques whose epithelial cells lining the convoluted tubules had pyknotic degeneration and chromatolysis of the nuclei. The lumen of the tubule contained epithelial debris and the urine contained albumin, degenerating white blood cells, and hyaline and fatty casts (Kaur *et al.,* 1968).

Iatrogenic tubular nephrosis may be a consequence of antibiotic therapy in a fluid volume-depleted macaque. In administering certain classes of antibiotic compounds, such as aminoglycosides, it is essential that adequate renal function be assessed first. Animals with anuria or oliguria should be started on fluid therapy and their urine output monitored closely. A good description of analyzing fluid therapy is found in Rosenberg (1995).

In a large population of pig-tailed macaques (*Macaca nemestrina*), a retrospective survey of 674 necropsies demonstrated tubular nephrosis in 22.6% of the adults (Giddens *et al.*, 1981). This was the most common lesion found and most frequently involved the proximal convoluted tubules. The tubular epithelium showed a loss of the brush border, flattening to a low cuboidal pattern, and an increase in the lumen. The lumen was filled with proteinaceous material as well as casts and cell debris, yet many epithelial cells displayed regenerative features, including prominent nucleoli and mitotic figures. The authors attributed the severe changes observed to treatment with gentomycin and related antibiotics without adequate concern for the potential nephrotoxicity of these compounds.

Tubular nephrosis may also follow shock related to trauma or septicemia. Vasoconstriction can lead to extensive damage of the tubular basement membrane in the terminal region of the proximal convoluted tubule and in all of the distal convoluted tubule (Giddens *et al.*, 1981). Related oxalate nephrosis was observed in wild-caught animals in which crystals were present in tubular lumens of both the cortex and the medulla. Tubular epithelium adjacent to crystals showed evidence of damage and necrosis. Unfortunately, the source of these oxalate crystals was never determined (Giddens *et al.*, 1981). Myoglobin and urate crystals have also caused tubular obstruction and necrosis in rhabdomyolysis or Meyer–Betz disease (Bicknese, 1990; Brack, 1981). These changes were in addition to the primary glomerular damage mentioned earlier. In other instances, renal tubular damage may be a sequelae to malaria infection and an addition to glomerulopathy. For example, *Plasmodium falciparum* infection of the owl monkey (*Aotus trivirgatus*) and squirrel monkey produced cellular debris in the collecting ducts and fat in the proximal tubules (Aikawa *et al.*, 1988a,b).

F. Renal Amyloidosis

Amyloidosis is a disease with varied clinical presentations, characterized by the extracellular deposition of amyloid protein fibrils. These deposits are visible at necropsy after staining with Congo red, which appears as green biorefringence under polarized light. Amyloidosis is classified into five main groups: primary amyloidosis, amyloidosis associated with multiple myeloma, secondary amyloidosis associated with infectious or inflammatory disease processes, amyloid associated with neoplastic disease, and familial amyloidosis (Slattum *et al.*, 1989b). Amyloidosis secondary to an infectious or inflammatory process is the most prominent type reported in nonhuman primates.

Amyloid deposited around the capillaries can increase permeability, leading to proteinuria and ultimately to the nephrotic syndrome. In this situation, the glomerular capillaries become narrowed, eventually causing secondary tubular ischemia, atrophy, and fibrosis (Scott, 1992). Eventually, these lesions may progress until chronic renal failure occurs. In a review of amyloidosis in 248 pig-tailed macaques (*Macaca nemestrina*), renal lesions were relatively uncommon and involved primarily the interstitial peritubular tissue with only rare involvement of the glomeruli (Slattum *et al.*, 1989b). Epidemiological studies of this population confirmed the relationship of secondary amyloidosis to infection or inflammatory processes. A significant association was found between amyloidosis and diarrheal disease as well as infections with the type D retrovirus, which also produced retroperitoneal fibrosis, a neoplastic-like disorder (Slattum *et al.*, 1989a). Insular amyloidosis and diabetes mellitus in a De Brazza's guenon (*Cercopithecus neglectus*) resulted in secondary systemic amyloidosis with renal involvement as one element. Renal lesions included severe focal glomerulosclerosis, deposition of amyloid in the basement membrane, interstitial fibrotic tubular proteinaceous casts, and tubular cystic dilation (Tham *et al.*, 1992). Blanchard (1993) reviews amyloidosis in nonhuman primates with an emphasis on pathology.

G. Vascular Lesions

A characteristic of diabetes mellitus is the increased permeability of vascular endothelium throughout the body. The high volume of blood flow through the glomerular capillaries makes them particularly susceptible to damage resulting in increased GFR and renal size in insulin-dependent diabetes mellitus (Scott, 1992; Jonasson *et al.*, 1985). The basement membrane increases in thickness, leading to a change in intrarenal hemodynamics and hyperfiltration. Proteinuria occurs with secondary mesangial cell damage, increased cell proliferation, and matrix deposition, which can produce diabetic glomerulosclerosis (Jonasson *et al.*, 1985). Insulin-dependent diabetes mellitus can occur spontaneously in the adult macaque or may be induced with streptozotocin, alloxan, or total pancreatectomy (Yosuda *et al.*, 1988).

Arteriolar nephrosclerosis may begin as a sequela to spontaneous hypertension in the woolly monkey (*Lagothrix lagotricha*) (Giddens *et al.*, 1987). A survey of 38 woolly monkeys that died revealed that 26 of the animals had lesions of the small muscular arterioles. In those with mild disease, the region looked normal grossly with small amounts of hyaline deposited beneath the intima. In moderately severe cases, the kidneys were pale, granular, and shrunken with pits and depressions. Hyaline deposits were more extensive, sometimes occluding the vessel lumen. Animals with severe disease had multiple renal lesions, including glomerulosclerosis, tubular atrophy, interstitial fibrosis, and interstitial lymphocyte infiltration (Giddens *et al.*, 1987). In the survey, all animals over 4 years of age were affected, as shown by blood pressure measurements denoting hypertension of 194 ± 20 mm Hg. Because clinical pathology data revealed no underlying cause for hypertension, this disease appeared to represent hypertension associated with the aging process.

IV. UROLITHIASIS AND RENAL CALCIFICATION

A. Urinary Calculi

Urinary tract calculi are infrequent, but have been reported in several species of nonhuman primates. In humans, renal calculi fall into three main groups: uric acid stones that are a combination of uric acid and urates, calcium oxalate stones, and triple phosphate stones containing a mixture of magnesium, ammonium, and calcium (Scott, 1992). The first two types form in acid urine, sometimes together. The third type of stone forms in alkaline urine and may be deposited on preexisting calculus in the urinary tract. The exact way in which urinary calculi form is debatable, but stone formation is usually considered to require foreign bodies that serve as a nidus (Drach and Boyce, 1972). A close relationship often exists among urinary obstruction, calculi, and infection, although oxalate or phosphate crystals present in the urine may act as nuclei for stone formation (Scott, 1992; Drach and Boyce, 1972).

Urinary stones have been reported in a male golden-bellied managabey (*Cercocebus torquatus*), squirrel monkeys, cynomolgus and rhesus macaques, a Taiwan macaque (*Macaca cyclopis*), and a proboscis monkey (*Nasalis pygathrix*) (Scott, 1992; Pryor *et al.,* 1969; Resnick *et al.,* 1978; Stephens *et al.,* 1979). Uroliths can block the urinary tract, yielding severe effects on the rest of the urinary system. A cynomolgus macaque, with severe depression and anorexia, was euthanized for humane reasons. On necropsy, the animal had a 2.0 × 1.4 × 0.9-cm calculus in the bladder. Analysis by X-ray diffraction identified the calculus as a calcium carbonate crystal (Renlund *et al.,* 1986). The primary lesion was a markedly thickened bladder wall that enclosed the calculus. A 6-year-old female cynomolgus macaque presented with a severely debilitated condition and the following clinical signs: diarrhea, dehydration, hypothermia, hypoproteinemia, hypokalemia, and anemia. The animal had either undergone a subcapsular hemorrhage or abcessation in both kidneys. Both ureters were grossly distended, with the right ureter containing white floccullant material. Additionally, a teardrop-shaped urolith had lodged in the trigone area of the bladder. The stone was composed of calcium carbonate and some plant-like material (Lees *et al.,* 1995). Another adult female cynomolgus macaque died suddenly when one of three cystic calculi lodged in her urethra (Stephens *et al.,* 1979). The stones were 1–2.5 cm in diameter and were composed of oxalates, phosphates, carbonates, ammonium salts, magnesium and calcium. Renal lesions included those of chronic interstial and glomerular nephritis and hyperplasia of the transitional epithelium of the bladder.

B. Nephrocalcinosis

Nephrocalcinosis has been described in squirrel monkeys, both spontaneously formed and experimentally induced (Roberts, 1972; Drach and Boyce, 1972). Deposits of calcium in renal papilla form lesions referred to as Randall's plaques and represent interstitial nephrocalcinosis. These plaques are thought to be precursors to stone formation in humans. Although clumps of calcified conglomerates of necrotic tissue have been found in the renal tubules of squirrel monkeys, no evidence of stone formation was apparent (Drach and Boyce, 1972). One rhesus macaque manifested patchy necrosis and early calcinosis of the convoluted tubules, although glomeruli and remaining interstitial tissue appeared normal (Kaur *et al.,* 1968).

Rickets and osteomalacia have been reported in several species of New World primates fed a diet containing only vitamin D_2 and/or not receiving exposure to ultraviolet light (Clarkson *et al.,* 1970). The consequences may be secondary hyperparathyroidism with hypocalcemia and simultaneous excess production of parathyroid hormone. This situation may also occur with diets high in phosphorus and low in calcium, leading to soft tissue mineralization, impaired locomotion, an increased alkaline phosphatase level, and poor skeletal mineralization (Tomson *et al.,* 1980). In addition to this nutritional form of secondary hyperparathyroidism, a similar condition may occur with chronic renal failure when serum phosphate levels increase as the renal GFR drops below 25% of normal, decreasing the serum calcium concentration and the ability of the kidney to synthesize the active metabolite of vitamin D (Brenner *et al.,* 1987). All these syndromes may result in severe changes of soft and boney tissues, including mineralization of the kidney. Nephrolithiasis was associated with osteomalacia in a capuchin monkey (*Cebus* sp.), with large yellow-gray discolored kidneys (Ruch, 1959). Nutritional secondary hyperparathyroidism has also been reported in Japanese macaques (*Macaca fuscata*) and in ring-tailed lemurs (*Lemur catta*). No disruption of renal function was reported with either occurrence (Snyder *et al.,* 1980; Tomson *et al.,* 1980).

V. CYSTITIS

Reports of cystitis separate from infection of more proximal portions of the renal tract are infrequent. However, clinicians at the California Regional Primate Research Center have detected six cases of cystitis of an unusual nature since 1991. The animals were diagnosed with gross hematuria and, upon urinalysis, had pronounced eosinophilic cystitis but without elevated peripheral eosinophilia (C. Valverde, personal communication,

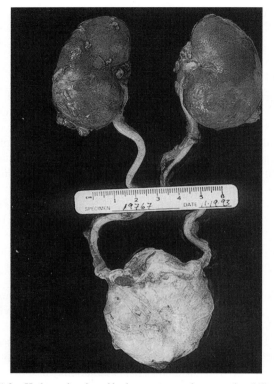

Fig. A.2.   Hydronephrosis and hydroureter secondary to eosinophilic cystitis of unknown etiology.

1995). Although these animals presented with eosinophilic cystitis, they had secondary involvement of the ureter and kidney with hydroureter and hydornephrosis (Fig. A.2). Biopsies showed a pronounced mixed cellular infiltrate composed predominately of eosinophils in the bladder mucosa without any etiologic agent. Eosinophilic cystitis is also reported as an idiopathic condition in humans (DeVries and Freiha, 1990) and also in animals experimentally infected with simian immunodeficiency virus (SIV) as well as normal uninfected animals. Administration of systemic corticosteroids appears to have little effect, although intravesicular administration has provided some benefit. Some cases resolved spontaneously within several months (C. Valverde, personal communication, 1995).

VI. CONGENITAL MALFORMATIONS

A wide variety of congenital malformations have been reported in the nonhuman primate. Some changes seen late in life may actually be acquired and not represent true congenital defects. These may be secondary to disease conditions such as pyelonephritis and glomerulnephritis, which can precipitate tubule damage (Scott, 1992). True congenital polycystic renal disease occurs anytime during infancy or adult life. Adults do

not manifest the disorder until late in life, when they may develop hypertension or uremia (Scott, 1992). Cysts may present as single defects or multiple structures. Infants with this disease may have hepatic cysts as well as the hypertensive or uremic status typical of this disorder. In humans this disease is passed by an autosomal recessive mode of inheritance (Sakakibara and Honjo, 1990). Typically, kidneys are extremely enlarged due to a failure of fusion of the upper renal tubules and the collecting tubule, leading to distortion and enlargement of the renal tubule with eosinophilic material (Scott, 1992; Baskin *et al.,* 1981). There are two reports of infantile polycystic renal disease in nonhuman primates. The first was in a male stillborn cynomolgus macaque and the other in a 3-day-old male rhesus macaque that died acutely (Baskin *et al.,* 1981).

Adult polycystic disease in humans is a dominant inherited disease in contrast to the infantile form. The adult form of polycystic renal disease has been reported in squirrel monkeys, pig-tailed macaques (*Macaca nemestrina*), titi monkeys (*Calicebus moloch*), and baboons (*Papio* sp.). These animals had milder disease with smaller cysts than those described elsewhere (Kessler *et al.,* 1984). A severe form of adult polycycstic disease has been observed in a 16-year-old male rhesus macaque found comatose. Clinical pathology values indicated uremia with a BUN of 300 mg/dl and a serum creatine of 15.0 mg/dl. The animal was humanely euthanized, and complete necropsy showed significant distortion of the renal parenchyma, with the left kidney two to three times the normal size and a large cyst (4.0 cm in diameter in the right kidney). The cyst was filled with clear yellow serosanguinous fluid, which yielded *E. coli* and *P. aeruginosa* in the left kidney. Other pathological changes observed in the kidneys included interstitial fibrosis and accumulated lymphocytes, histiocytes, and eosinophils (Kessler *et al.,* 1984).

Nonhuman primates also have other congenital defects, including renal aplasia. In humans, agenesis usually occurs in the left kidney, with the ureter also being absent (Scott, 1992). Nevertheless, a case report of renal aplasia in a baboon (*Papio anubis*) involved the right kidney and ureter with apparent compensation by the remaining left organ. The animal was used for a drug study to test a potentially nephrotoxic compound, but showed no evidence of impaired renal function compared to other normal animals (McCraw *et al.,* 1973). Two male African green monkeys (*Cercopithecus aethiops*) were identified with "horseshoe" kidneys, i.e., cases of renal fusion, in a necropsy survey of 503 vervets (Seier *et al.,* 1990). Unilateral renal aplasia was reported elsewhere in a nonhuman primate, although the affected kidney was not mentioned. The kidneys were fused at their caudal pole, but the remainder of the renal tissue appeared normal. Renal pelvises and ureters were separate and renal function appeared normal in both animals. In contrast, this condition in humans is often associated with complications such as calculus and hydronephrosis, often requiring surgery (Seier *et al.,* 1990). The incidence of horseshoe kidneys in humans is estimated as 1 in every 400–500 births. Renal anomalies have also been reported in langurs (*Presbytis* sp.), howler monkeys (*Alouatta* sp.), and ring-tailed lemurs (*Lemur catta*) (Chalifoux, 1986). Renal ectopia was noted in a female squirrel monkey (Chalifoux, 1986). The squirrel monkey anomaly was an incidental finding at necropsy, with the left kidney located posterior to the bifurcation of the aorta and between the common iliac arteries. A male owl monkey (*Aotus trivirgatus*) similarly afflicted was euthanized due to end stage kidney disease with severe glomerulonephritis. Both kidneys were fused to the right of the midline with an abnormal shape to the renal mass. In neither case did the abnormal placement and fusion of the kidney appear to affect overall health. The glomerulonephritis in the owl monkey appeared to be unrelated to the anomaly (Chalifoux, 1986).

Of 150 wild-caught rhesus macaques, 3 animals had congenital anomalies, including a right-sided double ureter, idiopathic renal ectasia, or patchy cystic dilatation of the renal tubules, and 1 animal had a unilateral cystic kidney (Kaur *et al.,* 1968).

Congenital conditions may include external genitalia as well as the other malformations listed. Hypospadias in a male rhesus macaque involved the midshaft of the penis (Harrison, 1976). Similarly, in humans, 25% of such defects are associated with genetic anomalies such as cryptorchidism, an enlarged prostatic utricle, and a bifid scrotum (Harrison, 1976). Histological examination of the penis indicated that the abnormality was congenital, not attributable to trauma. Persistent cloaca was reported in a 15-year-old female cynomolgus macaque (Lewis *et al.,* 1978). Persistent cloaca involves impaired development of the urorectal septum, agenesis of some tissue, and developmental arrest leading to a common excretory passageway for fecal, urinary, and reproductive products. The affected animal also had cysts in the right ovary and in both kidneys (Lewis *et al.,* 1978).

VII. NEOPLASTIC DISEASE

Although a great many tumors affect the urinary system, unfortunately few, if any, reports on this subject include population-based data. Animals with neoplasia should be assessed for viral status regarding potentially oncogenic agents such as herpes saimiri or simian T-cell lymphotropic virus I, as these agents may be associated with neoplastic disease in nonhuman primates (Lowenstine, 1986). Benign renal tumors, which are usually incidental findings at necropsy, should be carefully classified. Examples in one publication included small discrete adenomas from renal epithelium and fibromas or hematomas derived from mesenchymal structures (Scott, 1992). A survey of 17 cases of primary renal tumors revealed four adenomas, one adenoleiomyofibromatous hamartoma, and one transitional cell papillomatous hyperplastic kidney (Jones and Casey, 1981). A cortical adenoma with spindle-shaped cells and mitotic figures was observed in a 9-year-old female rhesus ma-

caque that was examined as part of a group of 150 animals (Kaur *et al.,* 1968). Another survey of 1065 nonhuman primate necropsies representing nine species included a papillary renal cell adenoma and one papillary renal cell adenocarcinoma (Seibold and Wolf, 1973). Malignant tumors are prominent in the literature on renal neoplasia of nonhuman primates, and these growths can present as adenomas or carcinomas derived from renal epithelium (Scott, 1992). Tumors develop in many animals 15 years of age or older, just as 70–80% of all renal cancers in humans are renal cell carcinomas and occur between 50 and 70 years of age (Scott, 1992). Neoplasia may be unilateral or bilateral, affecting both renal bodies.

Documented malignant neoplasms of the renal system include a spontaneous renal lymphosarcoma in a juvenile cynomolgus macaque (Anderson *et al.,* 1994). Sheets of plump cells with indistinct borders and scant amphophilic cytoplasm had infiltrated the renal mass, but mitosis was uncommon. Tumor tissue was also present in the adrenal medulla, prostate, seminal vesicle, myocardium, and pulmonary interstitium. Serological tests for the common simian retroviruses were negative. Another publication described a primary renal hemangiosarcoma in a moustached tamarin (*Saguinius mystax*) that died of chronic colitis (Gozalo *et al.,* 1993). A malignant tumor of endothelial cells, the tumor was detected as a small reddish zone in the renal cortex of one kidney. On histologic examination, nuclei of neoplastic cells were ovoid and hyperchromatic with few mitotic figures. An adult male baboon (*Papio* sp.) reportedly suffered severe abdominal distention and pain after 3 years in captivity. Following unsuccessful therapy, the baboon was euthanized and found to have a large renal tubulopapillary carcinoma with a 1-cm-diameter urolith composed of magnesium and carbonate lodged at the entrance of the ureter (Witt *et al.,* 1989). The majority of neoplastic cells formed tubular structures with cell debris and proteinaceous fluid. These cells were anaplastic with indistinct margins and occasional multinucleation. Another renal tumor, an adenocarcinoma, occurred in an owl monkey (*Aotus trivirgatus*) that died of severe bloody diarrhea (Brown *et al.,* 1975). The mass was an incidental finding with cells containing considerable cytoplasm and irregular nuclei. The tumor was encapsulated by surrounding renal parenchyma. The previously mentioned survey of 17 nonhuman primate necropsies included 10 cases of renal carcinoma and 1 case of nephroblastoma (Jones and Casey, 1981). The carcinomas had three distinct histologic growth patterns: papillary, tubular, and solid. These carcinomas could be found separately or in combination. The cells were generally large and pleomorphic with abundant cytoplasm, except in spindle cells. None of the carcinomas metastasized. The nephroblastoma was unusual in that it occurred in an adult male cotton-top tamarin (*Saguinus oedipus*). This renal embryonic tumor is rare, particularly in adults. In humans, it typically occurs within the first 3 months of life and signals a very poor prognosis (Scott, 1992). This picture more closely agrees with that of a malignant nephroblastoma identified in a 4-month-old female long-tailed macaque that had numerous pulmonary metastasis to the lungs. The tumor itself was a large grayish-yellow mass in the right kidney. The cells were a mixed population scattered throughout a loose fibrous stroma (Bennett *et al.,* 1982). Beniashvili (1995) presents an excellent overview of neoplasia in nonhuman primates, including a section on tumors of the urinary tract. He reviews many of the renal neoplasms cited here and also an adenocarcinoma, a reticulosarcoma, and a hypernephroma in *Cacajao* sp., *Papio anubis,* and *Cebus apella.*

The range of diseases affecting the urinary system of nonhuman primates closely parallels their counterparts in humans. These disorders are well represented in terms of gross and microscopic pathology in the literature. It is now the responsibility of those who monitor and treat laboratory animals to utilize all available diagnostic tools for the documentation of antemortem manifestations as well.

REFERENCES

Aikawa, M., Jacobs, G., Whiteley, H. E. Igarashi, I., and Ristic, M. (1988a). Glomerulopathy in squirrel monkeys with acute *Plasmodium falciparum* infection. *Am. J. Trop. Med. Hyg.* **38,** 7–14.

Aikawa, M., Broderson, J. R., Igarashi, I., Jacobs, G., Pappaioanou, M., Collins, W. E., and Campbell, C. C. (1988b). An atlas of renal disease in *Aotus* monkeys with experimental *Plasmodial* infection. *Am. Inst. Biol. Sci.*

Anderson, S. T., and Klein, E. C. (1993). Systemic lupus erythematosus in a rhesus macaque. *Arthritis Rheum.* **36,** 1739–1742.

Anderson, W. I., Inhelder, J. L., and King, N. W., Jr. (1994). Spontaneous renal lymphosarcoma in a juvenile cynomolgus monkey (*Macaca fascicularis*). *J. Med. Primatol.* **23,** 56–57.

Bahnson, R. R., Ballou, B. T., Ernstoff, M. S., Schwentker, F. N., and Hakala, T. R. (1988). A technique for catheterization and cystoscopic evaluation of cynomolgus monkey urinary bladders. *Lab. Anim. Sci.* **38,** 731–733.

Baskin, G. B., Roberts, J. A., and McAfee, R. D. (1981). Infantile polycystic renal disease in a rhesus monkey (*Macaca mulatta*). *Lab. Anim. Sci.* **31,** 181–183.

Beniashvili, D. S. (1995). Tumors of the genitourinary system. *In* "Experimental Tumors in Monkeys," pp. 87–89. CRC Press, Boca Raton, FL.

Bennett, B. T., Beluhan, F. Z., and Welsh, T. J. (1982). Malignant nephroblastoma in *Macaca fascicularis. Lab. Anim. Sci.* **32,** 403–404.

Bicknese, E. J. (1990). Rhabdomyolysis in macaques. *Proc. Annu. Meet., Am. Assoc. Zoo Vet. 1990,* pp. 316–318.

Blanchard, J. L. (1993). Generalized amyloidosis, nonhuman primates. *In* "Monographs on the Pathology of Laboratory Animals: Nonhuman Primates" (T. C. Jones, U. Mohr, and R. D. Hunt, eds.), Vol. 1, pp. 194–197. Springer-Verlag, Berlin and New York.

Boraski, E. A. (1981). Renal disease in prosimians. *Vet. Pathol.* **18,** Suppl. 6, 1–5.

Boyce, J. T., Giddens, W. E., Jr., and Seifert, R. (1981). Spontaneous mesangioproliferative glomerulonephritis in pigtailed macaques (*Macaca nemestrina*). *Vet. Pathol.* **18,** Suppl. 6, 82–88.

Brack, M. (1981). Renal pathology in captive baboons (*Papio cynocephalus*). *Vet. Pathol.* **18,** Suppl. 6, 55–58.

Brack, M., and Rothe, H. (1981). Chronic tubulointerstitial nephritis and wasting disease in marmosets (*Callithrix jacchus*). *Vet. Pathol.* **18,** Suppl. 6, 45–54.

Brack, M., and Weber, M. (1994). Ultrastructural and immunohistochemical studies in callitrichid renal glomeruli. *J. Med. Primatol.* **23,** 325–332.

Brenner, B. M., Hostettner, T. H., and Hebert, S. C. (1987). Disturbances of renal function. *In* "Principles of Internal Medicine" (E. Braunwald, K. J. Isselbacher, R. G. Petersdorf, J. D. Wilson, J. B. Martin, and A. S. Fauci, eds.), pp. 1143–1149. McGraw-Hill, New York.

Brown, R. J., Cole, W. C., Chang, C. P., and Hsu, S. H. (1975). Renal adenocarcinoma in an owl monkey (*Aotus trivirgatus*). *J. Med. Primatol.* **4,** 62–64.

Burkholder, P. M. (1981). Glomerular disease in captive galagos. *Vet. Pathol.* **18,** Suppl. 6, 6–22.

Chalifoux, L. V. (1986). Crossed renal ectopia in a squirrel monkey (*Saimiri scureus*) and an owl monkey (*Aotus trivirgatus*). *J. Med. Primatol.* **15,** 235–239.

Chalifoux, L. V., Bronson, R. T., Sehgal, P., Blake, B. J., and King, N. W. (1981). Nephritis and hemolytic anemia in owl monkeys (*Aotus trivirgatus*). *Vet. Pathol.* **18,** Suppl. 6, 23–37.

Chapman, W. L., Jr., Crowell, W. A., and Isaac, W. (1973). Spontaneous lesions seen at necropsy in 7 owl monkeys (*Aotus trivirgatus*). *Lab. Anim. Sci.* **23**(3), 434–442.

Clarkson, T. B., Bullock, B. C., Lehner, N. D. M., and Manning, P. J. (1970). Rickets and osteomalacia. *In* "Feeding and Nutrition of Nonhuman Primates" (R. S. Harris, ed.), pp. 244–245. Academic Press, New York.

DeVries, C. R., and Freiha, F. S. (1990). Hemorrhagic cystitis: A review. *J. Urol.* **143,** 1–9.

Drach, G. W., and Boyce, W. H. (1972). Nephrocalcinosis as a source for renal stone nuclei. Observation on humans and squirrel monkeys and on hyperparathyroidism in the squirrel monkey. *J. Urol.* **107,** 897–904.

Dysko, R. C., and Hoskins, D. E. (1995). Medical management. Part B. Collection of biological samples and therapy administration. *In* "Nonhuman Primates in Biomedical Research: Biology and Management" (B. T. Bennett, C. R. Abee, and R. Henrickson, eds.), pp. 270–283. Academic Press, San Diego, CA.

Feldman, D. B., and Bree, M. M. (1969). The nephrotic syndrome associated with glomerulonephritis in a rhesus monkey (*Macaca mulatta*). *J. Am. Vet. Med. Assoc.* **155,** 1249–1252.

Gavellas, G., Disbrow, M. R., Hwang, K. H., Hinkle, D. K., and Bourgoignie, J. J. (1987). Glomerular filtration rate and blood pressure monitoring in awake baboons. *Lab. Anim. Sci.* **37,** 657–662.

Giddens, W. E., Jr., Seifert, R. A., and Boyce, J. T. (1979). Renal disease. *In* "Aging in Nonhuman Primates" (D. M. Bowden, ed.), pp. 324–334. Van Nostrand-Reinhold, New York.

Giddens, W. E., Jr., Boyce, J. T., Blakley, G. A., and Morton, W. R. (1981). Renal disease in the pig-tailed macaque (*Macaca nemestrina*). *Vet. Pathol.* **18,** Suppl. 6, 70–81.

Giddens, W. E., Combs, C. A., Smith, O. A., and Klein, E. C. (1987). Spontaneous hypertension and its sequelae in Woolly monkeys (*Lagothrix lagotricha*). *Lab. Anim. Sci.* **37,** 750–756.

Gliatto, J. M., and Bronson, R. T. (1993). Fatal fasting syndrome of obese macaques. *In* "Monographs on the Pathology of Laboratory Animals: Nonhuman Primates" (T. C. Jones, U. Mohr, and R. D. Hunt, eds.), Vol. 1, pp. 198–202. Springer-Verlag, Berlin and New York.

Goodman, J. R., Wolf, R. H., and Roberts, J. A. (1977). The unique kidney of the spider monkey (*Ateles geoffroyi*). *J. Med. Primatol.* **6,** 232–236.

Gozalo, A., and Montoya, E. (1990). Mortality causes of owl monkeys (*Aotus nancymae* and *Aotus vociferans*) in captivity. *J. Med. Primatol.* **19,** 69–72.

Gozalo, A., Chavera, A., Dagle, G. E., Montoya, E., and Weller, R. E. (1993). Primary renal hemangiosarcoma in a moustached tamarin. *J. Med. Primatol.* **22,** 431–432.

Harrison, R. M. (1976). Hypospadias in a male rhesus monkey. *J. Med. Primatol.* **5,** 60–63.

Heidel, J. R., Giddens, W. E., Jr., and Boyce, J. T. (1981). Renal pathology of catheterized baboons (*Papio cynocephalus*). *Vet. Pathol.* **18,** Suppl. 6, 59–69.

Hubbard, G. B., Schmidt, R. E., and Fletcher, K. C. (1987). Systematic survey of lesions from animals in a zoologic collection. *J. Zoo Anim. Med.* **18**, 14–46.

Hunt, R. D., and Blake, B. J. (1993). Glomerulonephritis, owl monkeys. *In* "Monographs on the Pathology of Laboratory Animals: Nonhuman Primates" (T. C. Jones, U. Mohr, and R. D. Hunt, eds.), Vol. 2, pp. 143–147. Springer-Verlag, Berlin and New York.

James, A. E., Jr., Heller, R. M., Jr., Bush, M., Gray, C. W., and Oh, K. S. (1975). Positive contrast peritoneography and herniography in primate animals with special reference to indirect inquinal hernias. *J. Med. Primatol.* **4**, 114–119.

James, A. E., Jr., Brayton, J. B., Novak, G., Wight, D., Shehan, T. K., Bush, R. M., and Sanders, R. C. (1976). The use of diagnostic ultrasound in evaluation of the abdomen in primates with emphasis on the rhesus monkey (*Macaca mulatta*). *J. Med. Primatol.* **5**, 160–175.

Jonasson, O., Jones, C. W., Bauman, A., John, E., Manaligod, J., and Tso, M. O. M. (1985). The pathophysiology of experimental insulin-deficient diabetes in the monkey. Implications for pancreatic transplantation. *Ann. Surg.* **201**, 27–39.

Jones, S. R., and Casey, H. W. (1981). Primary renal tumors in nonhuman primates. *Vet. Pathol.* **18**, Suppl. 6, 89–104.

Kaur, J., Chakravarti, R. N., Chugh, K. S., and Chuttani, P. N. (1968). Spontaneously occurring renal diseases in wild rhesus monkeys. *J. Pathol. Bacteriol.* **95**, 31–36.

Kessler, M. J., Roberts, J. A., and London, W. T. (1984). Adult polycystic kidney disease in a rhesus monkey (*Macaca mulatta*). *J. Med. Primatol.* **13**, 147–152.

Laber-Laird, K. E., Jokinen, M. P., and Lehner, N. D. M. (1987). Fatal fatty liver-kidney syndrome in obese monkeys. *Lab. Anim. Sci.* **37**, 205–209.

Leary, S. L., Sheffield, W. D., and Strandberg, J. D. (1981). Immune complex glomerulonephritis in baboons (*Papio cynocephalus*) with indwelling intravascular catheters. *Lab. Anim. Sci.* **31**, 416–420.

Lees, C. J., Carlson, C. S., and O'Sullivan, M. G. (1995). Urinary calculus caused by plant material in a cynomolgus monkey. *Lab. Anim. Sci.* **45**, 441–442.

Lewis, R. W., Palazzo, M. C., and Kim, J. C. S. (1978). Persistent cloaca in a cynomolgus monkey (*Macaca fascicularis*). *J. Med. Primatol.* **7**, 237–241.

Lowenstine, L. J. (1986). Neoplasms and proliferative disorders in nonhuman primates. *In* "Primates: The Road to Self-Sustaining Populations" (K. Benirschke, ed.), pp. 781–814. Springer-Verlag, Berlin and New York.

Markowitz, A. S. (1969). Streptococcal-related glomerulonephritis in the rhesus monkey. *Transplant. Proc.* **1**, 985–991.

McCraw, A. P., Rotheram, K., Sim, A. K., and Warwick, M. H. (1973). Unilateral renal aplasia in the baboon. *J. Med. Primatol.* **2**, 249–251.

Migaki, G., Asher, D. M., Casey, H. W., Locke, L. N., Gibbs, C. J., Jr., and Gajdusek, C. (1979). Fatal suppurative nephritis caused by *Pseudomonas* in a chimpanzee. *J. Am. Vet. Med. Assoc.* **175**, 957–959.

Nimri, L. F., and Lanners, N. H. (1994). Immune complexes and nephropathies associated with *Plasmodium inui* infection in the rhesus monkey. *Am. J. Trop. Med. Hyg.* **51**, 183–189.

O'Neill, W. M., Jr., Hammar, S. P., Ramirez, G., Bloomer, H. A., and Moore, J. G. (1978). Acute pyelonephritis in an adult gorilla (*Gorilla gorilla*). *Lab. Anim. Sci.* **28**, 100–101.

Palotay, J. L., and Uno, H. (1975). Hydatid disease in four nonhuman primates. *J. Am. Vet. Med. Assoc.* **167**, 615–618.

Poskitt, T. R., Fortwengler, H. P. Jr., Bobrow, J. C., and Roth, G. J. (1974). Naturally occurring immune-complex glomerulonephritis in monkeys (*Macaca irus*). Light, immunofluorescence and electron microscopic studies. *Am. J. Pathol.* **76**, 145–160.

Pryor, W. H., Jr., Chang, C.-P., and Raulston, G.L. (1969). Urolithiasis in a Taiwan monkey (*Macaca cyclopis*). A literature review and case report. *Lab. Anim. Care* **19**, 862–865.

Rahlmann, D. F., Mains, R. C., and Kodama, A. M. (1976). A urine collection device for use with the male pigtail macaque (*Macaca nemestrina*). *Lab. Anim. Sci.* **26**, 829–831.

Renlund, R. C., McGill, G. E., and Cheng, P. T. (1986). Calcite urolith in a cynomolgus monkey. *Lab. Anim. Sci.* **36**(5), 536–537.

Resnick, M. I., Oliver, J., and Drach, G. W. (1978). Intranephronic calculosis in the Brazilian squirrel monkey. *Invest. Urol.* **15**, 295–298.

Roberts, J. A. (1972). The urinary system. *In* "Pathology of Simian Primates" (R. N. T.-W.-Fienes, ed.), Part 1, pp. 821–840. Karger, Basel.

Roberts, J. A. (1992). Vesicoureteral reflux and pyelonephritis in the monkey: Review. *J. Urol.* **148**, 1721–1725.

Roberts, J. A., Clayton, J. D., and Seibold, H. R. (1972). The natural incidence of pyelonephritis in the nonhuman primate. *Invest. Urol.* **9**, 276–281.

Roberts, J. A., Kaack, M. B., and Baskin, G. (1990). Treatment of experimental pyelonephritis in the monkey. *J. Urol.* **143**, 150–154.

Robinson, P. T., and Benirschke, K. (1980). Congestive heart failure and nephritis in an adult gorilla. *J. Am. Vet. Med. Assoc.* **177**, 937–938.

Rosenberg, D. P. (1995). Medical management. Part F. Critical care. *In* "Nonhuman Primates in Biomedical Research: Biology and Management" (B. T. Bennett, C. R. Abee, and R. Henrickson, eds.), pp. 316–334. Academic Press, San Diego, CA.

Ruch, T. C. (1959). Diseases of the endocrine, reproductive, and urinary systems. Urinary system. *In* "Diseases of Laboratory Primates" (T. C. Ruch, ed.), pp. 463–471. Saunders, Philadelphia.

Sakakibara, I., and Honjo, S. (1990). Spontaneously occurring congenital polycystic kidney in a cynomolgus monkey (*Macaca fascicularis*). *J. Med. Primatol.* **19**, 501–506.

Schmidt, R. E., and Butler, T. M. (1973). Glomerulonephritis and uremia in a chimpanzee. *J. Med. Primatol.* **2**, 144–154.

Scott, G. B. D. (1992). The urinary system. *In* "Comparative Primate Pathology," pp. 216–232. Oxford University Press, Oxford.

Seibold, H. R., and Wolf, R. H. (1973). Neoplasms and proliferative lesions in 1065 nonhuman primate necropsies. *Lab. Anim. Sci.* **23**, 533–539.

Seibold, H. R., Roberts, J. A., and Wolf, R. H. (1971). Idiopathic muscle necrosis with apparent myoglobinuria in *Macaca arctoides*. *Lab. Anim. Sci.* **21**, 242–246.

Seier, J. V., Fincham, J. E., and Taljaard, J. J. F. (1990). Horseshoe kidneys in vervet monkeys. *J. Med. Primatol.* **19**, 595–599.

Slattum, M. M., Rosenkranz, S. L., DiGiacomo, R. F., Tsai, C.-C., and Giddens, W. E., Jr. (1989a). Amyloidosis in pigtailed macaques (*Macaca nemestrina*): Epidemiologic aspects. *Lab. Anim. Sci.* **39**, 560–566.

Slattum, M. M., Tsai, C. C., DiGiacomo, R. F., and Giddens, W. E., Jr. (1989b). Amyloidosis in pigtailed macaques (*Macaca nemestrina*): Pathologic aspects. *Lab. Anim. Sci.* **39**, 567–570.

Snyder, S. B., Omdahl, J. L., Law, D. H., and Froelich, J. W. (1980). Osteomalacia and nutritional secondary hyperparathyroidism in a semi-free-ranging troop of Japanese monkeys. *In* "The Comparative Pathology of Zoo Animals" (R. J. Montali and G. Migaki, eds.), pp. 51–57. Smithsonian Institution Press, Washington, DC.

Stephens, E. C., Middleton, C. C., and Thompson, L. J. (1979). Urinary cystic calculi in a cynomolgus monkey (*Macaca fascicularis*): A case report. *Lab. Anim. Sci.* **29**, 797–799.

Stills, H. F., Jr., and Bullock, B. C. (1981). Renal disease in squirrel monkeys (*Saimiri scureus*). *Vet. Pathol.* **18**, Suppl. 6, 38–44.

Straus, W. L., Jr., and Arcadi, J. A. (1958). Urinary system. *In* "Primatologia. Handbook of Primatology" (H. O. Hofer, A. H. Schultz, and D. Starck, eds.), Vol. 3, Part 1, pp. 507–541. Karger, Basel.

Sturrock, R. F. (1986). A review of the use of primates in studying human schistosomiasis. *J. Med. Primatol.* **15**, 267–279.

Tham, V. L., Schultz, D. J., and Randall, K. M. (1992). Amyloidosis and suspect diabetes mellitus in a De Brazza's guenon (*Cercopithecus neglectus*). *J. Zoo Wildl. Med.* **23**, 353–356.

Tischer, C. C. (1975). Structure and function of the rhesus kidney. *In* "The Rhesus Monkey" (G. H. Bourne, ed.), Vol. 1, pp. 107–143. Academic Press, New York.

Tischer, C. C., Schrier, R. W., and McNeil, J. S. (1972). Nature of urine concentrating mechanism in the macaque monkey. *Am. J. Physiol.* **223**, 1128–1137.

Toft, J. D. (1986). The pathoparasitology of nonhuman primates: A review. *In* "Primates: The Road to Self-Sustaining Populations" (K. Benirschke, ed.), pp. 571–580. Springer-Verlag, Berlin and New York.

Tomson, F. N., Keller, G. L., and Knapk, F. B. (1980). Nutritional secondary hyperparathyroidism in a group of lemurs. *In* "The Comparative Pathology of Zoo Animals" (R. J. Montali and G. Migaki, eds.), pp. 59–64. Smithsonian Institution Press, Washington, DC.

Weller, R. E., Malaga, C. A., Buschbom, R. L., Baer, J. F., and Ragan, H. A. (1991). Protein concentration in urine of normal owl monkeys. *J. Med. Primatol.* **20**, 365–369.

Witt, C. J., Bacmeister, C. X., and Bunton, T. E. (1989). A tubulopapillary renal carcinoma and a renal calculus in a baboon. *Lab. Anim. Sci.* **39**, 443–445.

Yasuda, M., Takaoka, M., Fujiwara, T., and Mori, M. (1988). Occurrence of spontaneous diabetes mellitus in a cynomolgus monkey (*Macaca fascicularis*) and impaired glucose tolerance in its descendants. *J. Med. Primatol.* **17**, 319–332.

PART B. GENITAL SYSTEM

Elizabeth W. Ford, Jeffrey A. Roberts,
and Janice L. Southers

I. GENITAL SYSTEM: FEMALE, NONPREGNANT

A. Introduction

The purpose of this section is to describe disorders and diseases of the genital system in nonhuman primates and to provide information on diagnosis and treatment. The authors will first review conditions that affect the female, nonpregnant animal followed by those of the pregnant female and finally those of the male. For an extensive review of normal reproductive biology and breeding of prosimians and New World species and the more common Old World species and great apes, readers are directed to a previous volume in this series: "Nonhuman Primates in Biomedical Research: Biology and Management." In that volume, Chapter 9 emphasizes current knowledge about the reproductive cycle of both sexes (Hendrickx and Dukelow, 1995a), and Chapter 14 covers the breadth of information that has been accumulated on breeding nonhuman primates (Hendrickx and Dukelow, 1995b).

Diagnosis and treatment of genital disorders in these valuable laboratory animals are essential for providing humane care and efficient management. Despite the many nonhuman primates used for breeding, relatively little has been reported in the literature about their genital diseases. This lapse probably reflects the young, healthy population used in research and a lack of systematic gathering of data, as well as a lack of familiarity with this complex organ system and its dysfunctions.

Physiologically, the reproductive systems of human and nonhuman primates are so similar that, as expected, their disease states are similar. Because routine examination of nonhuman primates fairly often reveals lesions of the genital tract, it is prudent to review the published literature on their diseases pre-

ceding examination. Although spontaneous diseases of laboratory animals are often reported as isolated incidences, a large volume of information is available from the experimental literature and cumulative reviews. For example, a wide spectrum of gynecological pathologic findings is reported in a review of 63 rhesus monkeys, *Macaca mulatta* (DiGiacomo, 1977). An earlier review describes reproductive system disorders of numerous nonhuman primate species, both female and male, maintained in captivity and in the wild (Ruch, 1959).

All genital sites are susceptible to both infectious organisms and neoplastic conditions. An overview of the literature on infectious agents reveals a plethora of pathogenic organisms that seek these sites. Specific agents will be discussed by the anatomical locations they prefer. As to spontaneous urogenital tumors in nonhuman primates, no age- or species-specific incidence is obvious (Beniashvili, 1989, 1995), which probably reflects the selection criteria for nonhuman primates in research, not necessarily the true incidence. As nonhuman primates are held in captivity longer, the incidence of neoplasms increases. No attempt is made here to provide a comprehensive review of neoplasms of the genital tract; therefore, only those neoplasms that are clinically relevant are described. The reader is directed to the following reviews for additional information: Beniashvili (1989, 1995) and McClure (1980).

The lower genital tract (i.e., vulva, vagina, cervix) is particularly susceptible to trauma, sexually transmitted diseases, and incursions of foreign bodies. Sexually transmitted diseases have been attributed to simian immunodeficiency virus (SIVagm), simian agent 8 (SA8), and herpes simiae (B virus) (Phillips-Conroy *et al.,* 1994; Levin *et al.,* 1988; Simon *et al.,* 1993). Seropositivity for SIVagm paralleled patterns of sexual activity in wild African green monkeys, (*Cercopithecus aethiops*), and was nearly universal in females of reproductive age as well as many adult males. This evidence supports the sexual mode of transmission of SIVagm. Levin *et al.* (1988) reported an outbreak of SA8 at the Southwest Foundation for Biomedical Research in an outdoor field corral where most adult and adolescent baboons (*Papio* sp.) of both sexes had genital lesions. The lesion type and frequency at this center and elsewhere suggest a sexual mode of transmission.

The upper genital tract (i.e., uterus, oviducts, ovaries) is subject to ascending infection from lower genital tract sites. Some agents preferentially infect certain sites and give rise to characteristic symptoms. Several of these infections can produce severe disease in both adults and their newborns infected *in utero.* Either colonization of abnormal organisms or a marked increase in quantities of normal flora can produce infection, resulting in clinical disease.

B. Normal Flora

Normal aerobic and anaerobic bacterial flora of the genital tract of 37 female rhesus macaques have been described. Samples from the vagina and uterus identified *Streptococcus viridans,* coagulase negative *Staphylococcus, Mobiluncus curtisii, Corynebacterium renale, Peptostreptococcus anaerobius,* and *Gardnerella*-like organisms as the most common bacteria (Doyle *et al.,* 1991). Normal vaginal microbial flora of 8 female baboons (*Papio cynocephalus*) included *Bacteroids* sp., *Corynebacterium,* group D *Streptococcus,* and *Lactobacillis* isolated from 47.5% of the animals and *Mycoplasma* isolated from 44.7% of the animals (Skangalis *et al.,* 1979). The mean number of organisms isolated from each animal was nine. In the Senegal bush baby (*Galago* sp.), normal vaginal flora were *Staphylococcus aureus, S. epidermis,* and *Proteus mirabilis* (Butler, 1970). Finally, the most common vaginal isolates from pig-tailed macaques (*Macaca nemestrina*) were *Bacteroides* and *Fusobacterium* (Johnson *et al.,* 1985).

Species specificity probably also plays a role in susceptibility to particular infectious agents. In an experimental study, 10 pig-tailed macaques (*M. nemestrina*) were inoculated with *Gardnerella vaginalis* and became infected, i.e., *Gardnerella* could be cultured from their vaginal samples for 11–39 days. However, four tamarins (*Saguinus labiatus*) and three chimpanzees (*Pan troglodytes*) were also intravaginally inoculated with this agent but not successfully colonized (Johnson *et al.,* 1985).

When an animal becomes infected, the agent must be identified unequivocally because the selection of effective therapy depends on a correct specific diagnosis. Antibiotic therapy eliminates at least part of the natural vaginal flora, thereby promoting periurethral colonization with enterobacteria. In an experimental study with rhesus monkeys, nine animals were treated with amoxicillin. The vaginal mucosa of all nine animals spontaneously colonized with an adhering *Escherichia coli* normally present in the feces (Herthelius-Elman *et al.,* 1992; Herthelius *et al.,* 1989b). Subsequent studies revealed that vaginal colonization with *E. coli* was eliminated by the administration of normal flora and *Lactobacillus* (Herthelius *et al.,* 1989a). Similarly, the vaginal mucosa of cynomolgus monkeys that had been resistant to persistent colonization by pyelonephritogenic *E. coli* became susceptible after the administration of amoxicillin.

II. GYNECOLOGICAL ASSESSMENT

A. History

Examination of the reproductive organs should begin with a general review of the health of each animal to gather baseline information. This would include family history of genetic disorders, endocrine or metabolic disease, cardiovascular disease, hematological disorders, renal disorders, and gastrointestinal or neurological disorders if known. Knowing the assignment of the animal to prior research projects may also provide important insight into specific health problems.

In addition to this general information, specific facts regarding the female menstrual cycle are valuable, including interval, length, and quantity of menstrual flow (indicated as absent/scant to abundant with or without blood clots). Additional information may be deduced from the health record. For example, it is unlikely that the animal would have a history of dysmenorrhea; however, the record may indicate cyclical anorexia, depression or listlessness, vomiting, or diarrhea. The cyclical nature of abnormalities may correspond to the menstrual cycle.

For animals of breeding age, a review of the reproductive behavior is an essential component of history-taking. Infertility may be due to unsuccessful breeding, inability to conceive, or early pregnancy loss. The behavior of the female when placed with a proven male breeder is important information when evaluating infertility. If copulation occurs, infertility due to inappropriate breeding behavior can be ruled out. If pregnancy is confirmed, then unsuccessful breeding and inability to conceive can be ruled out. Important information for the investigation of abortion includes estimated gestational age and examination of the conceptus and placenta, if available. If death is perinatal, examination of the lungs to determine whether they were inflated would provide information on the ability of the mother to care for an infant.

B. Physical Examination

The behavior, general appearance, and activity of all animals should be carefully observed prior to immobilization for physical examination and collection of laboratory samples. Examination of nonhuman primates for assessment of reproductive function has been described previously (Van Pelt, 1974). In addition, Van Pelt (1974) describes findings associated with genital tract cysts, ovarian cysts, mucocoele, endometriosis, genital tract tuberculosis, and hyperinvolution of the uterus in nonpregnant females.

Inspection of the perineal area may identify areas of sex skin trauma. This skin changes in consistency with menstrual cycles and, in some nonhuman primates, e.g., baboons, can become turgid, friable, and easily damaged (Fig. B.1). Repair of lacerations is difficult because the tissue does not hold sutures well. In addition, this area is difficult to keep clean and free from infection. The best treatment is to clean the wounds well, suture only very large lacerations, and monitor frequently. As the sex skin decreases in size in parallel with the menstrual cycle, the wounds heal.

Nonhuman primates can be examined most effectively if immobilized. A complete physical examination, including laboratory tests, should be performed. The examination should include an appraisal of general appearance to evaluate skeletal abnormalities of the head, neck, thorax, lumbar, and pelvic areas. Deformities may be present that will affect reproduction secondarily. In one example, bonnet macaques (*Macaca radiata*) had a high incidence of neonatal

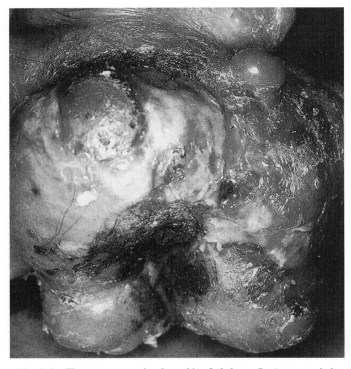

Fig. B.1. The tumescent perineal sex skin of a baboon, *Papio cynocephalus.* Multiple abrasions and lacerations are characteristic of this friable tissue.

method using the rectum has been reported (Hartman, 1932; Van Pelt, 1974). A good description, including a diagram, is found in Hendrickx and Dukelow (1995b). Briefly, a gloved and lubricated middle finger of the dominant hand is gently inserted into the rectum, allowing the sphincter to relax. The other hand, placed on the lower abdomen, directs with gentle counterpressure the reproductive organs toward the finger in the rectum. The end of the finger can be moved about freely. The general dimensions and content of the pelvic cavity are noted with a sweeping movement of the palpating finger. The uterine cervix, which is easily identified as a firm rounded structure palpated midventrally against the pelvis, differs in size and shape in different macaque species. The entire outline of the nonpregnant uterine fundus is easy to identify. The bimanual technique can outline its position, size, shape, consistency, and degree of mobility. A distinction must be made between the tactile impression of the size of uterine structures gained from palpation, with the actual size of the same organ. Considerable

deaths eventually attributed to rudimentary nipples (Sesline *et al.,* 1983).

1. Vulva, Vagina, and Cervix

The pelvic examination begins with perineum and external genitalia and then proceeds to a search for evidence of developmental anomalies, discharge, odors, skin texture, or color changes. The external urethral orifice can be examined with the aid of a small nasal speculum.

Vaginal examination can be accomplished in most medium-sized nonhuman primates with an appropriately sized speculum and good light source (Fig. B.2). The speculum blade should be inserted obliquely through the introitus, immediately rotated to the horizontal plane, and then slowly opened after reaching the vaginal apex. After the vaginal walls and cervix are inspected for lesions, any vaginal discharge is assessed for volume, color, consistency, and odor. The endocervical discharge is also examined and sampled for cervical or vaginal cytology, cultures, and direct microscopic examination. Before the speculum is removed, the cervix should be evaluated for ectropion, erosion, infection, discharge, laceration, polyps, ulceration, and tumors.

2. Bimanual Examination of the Uterus and Ovaries

Direct vaginal palpation is usually not possible due to the small size of this area in most nonhuman primates. A bimanual

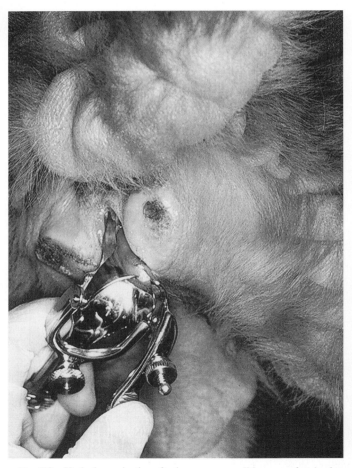

Fig. B.2. Vaginal examination of a rhesus macaque (*Macaca mulatta*) using a speculum. The pelvis of the animal can be elevated to aid examination. Note the turgid folds of sex skin from the base of the tail down the backs of the legs in this animal.

experience is required to determine the actual size. The width of the uterus may be compared to the width of the palpating finger for reference.

Although the authors have not been able to reliably palpate the ovaries, others reportedly routinely palpated them on either side of the uterus in the rhesus monkey (Mahoney, 1975). The right ovary is usually situated quite close to the uterus with a short uterovarian ligament, whereas the left ovary, with its usual longer attachment, may not be identifiable. Bimanual rectal palpation of the ovaries as a means of detecting ovulation was compared to the more invasive technique of laparotomy and the less reliable vaginal cytology and evaluation of cervical mucous (Mahoney, 1975).

C. Diagnostic Procedures

A variety of specific diagnostic procedures may aid in identifying genital system problems. The most direct procedure is visualization with a speculum in macaques or larger sized species described earlier in section II,B,1. Additionally, biopsy, cytology, and culture of the vagina and external cervix may aid in identifying such infectious agents as bacteria, viruses, parasites, or neoplastic changes of these organs.

A method of flushing the uterus for the recovery of fertilized ova in baboons has been described (Goodeaux et al., 1990). The technique involves transcervical cannulation, which may be difficult due to the tortuous cervical canal of some species of nonhuman primates. This technique may be used to sample the contents of the uterus or as a therapeutic measure to flush the uterus.

Reproductive serum hormone profiles may aid in the diagnosis of disorders related to the ovary. Serum hormone profiles were successful in determining the timing of pregnancy and identifying early pregnancy loss in the squirrel monkey, *Saimiri sciureus* (Diamond et al., 1985). A thorough review of reproductive endocrinology is provided by Hendrickx and Dukelow (1995a).

Hysterosalpingography has been described in both cynomolgus macaques and squirrel monkeys. The contrast media was delivered with some difficulty through the cervical os in the cynomolgus macaques (Parmley et al., 1983). The related approach in squirrel monkeys was transabdominal and was helpful for pinpointing the cause of infertility associated with dysfunction of the oviducts and abnormalities of the oviducts and uterine cavity. This procedure, hysterosalpingography, identified three animals with evidence of obstruction at the uterotubal junction that could not be identified by laparoscopy (Abbee and Aksel, 1983).

Biopsy of the uterine corpus is possible with biopsy forceps either directly by laparoscopy or laparatomy or percutaneously. A quick, simple percutaneous technique that allows repeat full-thickness (endometrium, myometrium, serosa) biopsies of the uterine fundus has been described (Olson and Sternfeld, 1987).

By far the most valuable diagnostic tool in this context is the ultrasound evaluation of pelvic contents. The equipment is expensive and requires both familiarity and expertise, but the procedure is noninvasive and can be repeated often without detrimental effects. This tool is useful in maintaining a healthy colony and in indentifying potential models of human disease. Normal anatomical and pathological changes of the uterus and adnexal tissues in rhesus and cynomolgus macaques have been reported (Tarantal, 1992; James et al., 1976). Endometrial thickness, reflectivity, and appearance of the endometrial–myometrial interface are used to diagnose the endometrial cycle stage in normal menstrual cycles. This method correlates well with serum estradiol, progesterone, and cycle day (Foster et al., 1992).

III. DISORDERS AND DISEASES

A. Vulva and Vagina

The vulvar skin is of ectodermal origin and is subject to diseases that are common to the skin elsewhere and to infectious processes that are more specific to the area. Lesions of the vulva and vaginal wall may include inflammatory lesions (candidiasis), viral lesions [*Herpesvirus hominis* (HHV2), simian agent 8, molluscum contagiosum, papillomavirus], ulcerative lesions (*Chlamydia*), traumatic lesions, and hyperkeratotic lesions such as those resulting from chronic irritation associated with prolapse, neoplasia, and cystic lesions.

Vaginal foreign bodies are observed occasionally. Figure B.3 depicts grass and stones that were incidental findings at necropsy in a rhesus macaque (*Macaca mulatta*). The material was packed in the vagina of the animal and posed no obvious health problems, but obviously would have had an effect on reproductive efficiency.

1. Bacterial Diseases

Vaginal infections are one of the most common gynecologic problems in nonhuman primates. A review of infertility cases at the National Institute for Neurological Disease and Stroke (NINDS) revealed that the probable cause in 15 of the females was subacute vaginitis (DiGiacomo, 1977). Known causes of bacterial vaginitis are *E. coli* and coagulative-positive *Staphylococcus* (Doyle et al., 1991). Clinical signs of infection vary with the agent, but may include increased vaginal discharge, vulvar irritation and pruritus, external dysuria, and a foul odor.

Mycoplasma and *Ureaplasma* are responsible for vaginal infections, spontaneous abortion, and infertility in humans. These organisms probably play a similar role in nonhuman primates. In one report, *Mycoplasma* caused vaginal infection in 8 of 23 (34.8%) chimpanzees (*Pan troglodytes*) studied (Swenson and O'Leary, 1977). Elsewhere, experimental inoculation of *Mycoplasma hominis* and *M. fermentans* into the upper genital tracts

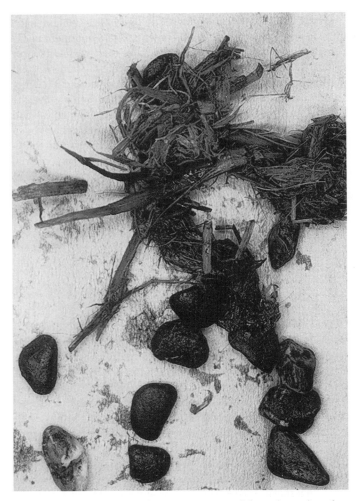

Fig. B.3. Bits of grass and stone were removed from the vagina of an outdoor-housed rhesus macaque (*Macaca mulatta*). The cause of this behavior is unknown.

of African green monkeys (*Cercopithecus aethiops*) produced parametritis and salpingitis. Dissemination was by the blood vessels and lymphatics to the parametria and to the outer layers of the oviducts (Moller and Freundt, 1983). Tetracycline has been effective in treating *Mycoplasma* infections.

2. Viral Diseases

Viruses infect the vulva and vagina of nonhuman primates. Simon *et al.* (1993) described a case of disseminated *Herpes simiae* in a cynomolgus macaque following dystocia. Uterine inertia secondary to peritonitis may have contributed to the dystocia. During the cesarean section, the uterine wall was noted to be thin and friable, with multiple areas of acute necrosis. Aside from the reproductive tract, lesions were also noted on the liver, intestine, pancreas, adrenals, and lungs.

The characteristic appearance of *Herpesvirus hominis* type 2 (human *Herpesvirus hominis* 2; HHV2) is multiple vesicles surrounded by a diffuse area of inflammation and edema. Cervical and vaginal lesions are usually associated with leukorrhea and occasional abnormal bleeding. After the disease runs its course, the lesions heal spontaneously but often reappear sporadically. Naturally occurring HHV2 infection of two pygmy chimpanzees (*Pan paniscus*) caused ulcerated and pustulovesicular lesions on the inner labial fold (McClure, 1980). Hunt (1993) reviews herpesviruses of nonhuman primates.

Thirty-five *Cebus albifrons* primates were experimentally inoculated intravaginally with HHV2. Latent infections occurred in 69% of the adolescents and in 42% of the adults. Compared to animals in this study that developed acute infections, latently infected animals were easier to infect, shed virus longer, and generally had more severe lesions consisting of vesicles, ulcers, and crusting of the vulva, vagina, and occasionally the cervix (Reeves *et al.*, 1981). Marmosets infected with HHV2 exhibited extensive lesions of the genital tract, i.e., ulcers of the vulva and vagina, which became necrotic and hemorrhagic. In some animals, a purulent vaginal exudate resulted from necrosis of the cervix. These animals died from the infection. Baboons appeared to be resistant to attempts at experimental infection with this virus (Felsburg *et al.*, 1973).

Simian Agent 8, a neurotropic herpes virus much like *Herpesvirus hominis* 2 was responsible for a naturally occurring outbreak at the Southwest Foundation for Biomedical Research (Levin *et al.*, 1988). The clinical signs observed were genital and oral lesions in both adult and juvenile male and female baboons. The lesions on the female began as patches of erythema, turning to papules and vesicles. These fragile vesicles ruptured easily, leading to ulcerations on the vulva, anus, and perineal tissue. Healing resulted in scar formation of the vulva and perineum that was sometimes severe enough to cause vaginal introital stenosis. These animals were poor breeders and were predisposed to urinary tract infections. Singleton *et al.*, (1995) described reconstructive surgery that was successful in returning these animals to the breeding colony. Depo-Provera (50 mg intramuscular) was used to arrest the estrus cycle in order to reduce swelling to allow adequate visualization for surgical exposure of the vagina.

Venereal papilloma has been reported in a colobus monkey (*Colobus guereza*) (O'Banion *et al.*, 1987). In addition, several cases of polyposis or papillomatosis found at necropsy but not associated with clinical signs were reported by Ruch (1959). Papillomavirus has been associated with neoplasia in humans, i.e., 85% of malignant and premalignant cervical and vulvar lesions contain papillomavirus DNA. Genital warts should be treated if possible, although treatment may not be successful because many lesions are not visible or accessible. In humans, a variety of cytotoxic agents are used for this purpose in addition to liquid nitrogen, electrocauterization, or surgical excision.

3. Parasitic Disease

Trichomonas vaginalis has been reported to survive and thrive in the human and nonhuman primate vagina, although no gross pathological lesions have been identified that could be attributed to the protozoa (Kraemer and Vera Cruz, 1972).

4. Neoplasia

An example of spontaneous squamous cell carcinoma of the vulva with metastasis of the inguinal lymph node and lung was described in a female cynomolgus macaque (Morin *et al.,* 1980). The primary tumor presented as a pedunculated mass at the mucocutaneous junction of the left labia anterior to the clitoris. The mass was hemorrhagic and ulcerated. The lymph nodes were bilaterally enlarged and the animal presented with a normocytic, hypochromic anemia. Surgical excision has been the mainstay of therapy for this neoplasm.

In utero exposure to diethylstilbesterol (DES) resulted in a clear cell carcinoma associated with vaginal adenosis in *Cebus apella* (Johnson *et al.,* 1981). The occurrence of neoplasia, associated with exogenous estrogen administration, illustrates the importance of hormonal influence on neoplasia.

B. Uterine Cervix

The cervix (Latin for neck) is a narrow, cylindrical extension of the uterus. The lower intravaginal portion is a free segment that projects into the vault of the vagina and is covered with a mucous membrane. The cervical canal extends from the external os through the internal os, where it joins the uterine cavity. Cervical shapes vary considerably in macaques, and their cervical canals usually run a tortuous course; the stump-tailed macaque (*Macaca actoides*) is an exception (Davis and Schneider, 1975). For a comparison of uterine anatomy in four species of nonhuman primates, see Hendrickx and Dukelow (1995b).

Prolapse of the cervix due to loose pelvic-supporting ligaments is occasionally reported. The usual presentation is slight prolapse of the vagina and possibly the cervix in a multiparous female during late pregnancy. Progressively more genital tissue becomes visible at the introitus (Fig. B.4). The condition usually resolves after pregnancy but recurs with future pregnancies. In time, the vagina and/or cervix can become chronically prolapsed with thickening and fissures that bleed easily. Surgical repair of genital prolapse in rhesus monkeys has been described (Adams *et al.,* 1985).

1. Cervicitis

The most common cause of acute cervicitis in nonhuman primates is an infection caused by streptococci, staphylococci, or enterococci as an extension of a vaginal infection (Doyle *et al.,* 1991). The cervix and the rest of the vaginal vault are often red, swollen, and edematous. Diagnosis is made by assessing appropriate cytological smears and cultures and sensitivities derived from the cervical discharge. Treatment consists of appropriate antibiotic therapy.

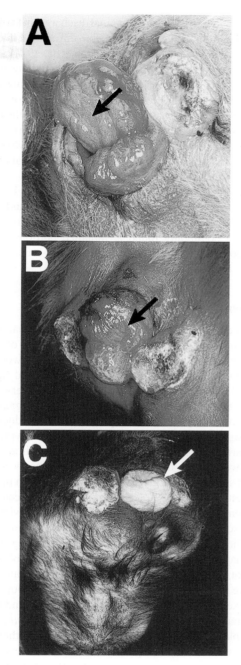

Fig. B.4. Various presentations of genital prolapse in macaque species. A prolapse can be recent, as evidenced by moist, glistening, often hemorrhagic tissue (A) or as a more dry, thickened chronic condition (B and C).

Subacute chronic inflammation of the squamocolumnar junction has been reported in 11 rhesus macaques (DiGiacomo, 1977). The extent of endocervical involvement compared with exocervical involvement appears to have some relation to the infecting agent in women and other primates. The cervix that harbors a chronic infection offers no constant picture that may be regarded as characteristic. The most common clinical manifestation is cervical erosion with a vaginal discharge that is usually yellowish white, thick, and tenacious. The differential diagnosis should include malignant neoplasia (London *et al.,* 1974).

Complete blockage or stenosis of the cervix may result from chronic infections. These conditions are usually asymptomatic, but may cause abnormal genital bleeding, dysmenorrhea, or infertility. Total stenosis may also cause distention of the uterine cavity with blood (hematometra), fluid (hydrometra), or exudate (pyometra). Manifestations can be confused with those from adnexal masses of ovarian origin as the uterus often feels cystic on bimanual palpation.

Simian immunodeficiency virus-infected cells are known to localize in the submucosa of the cervix and vagina and also in the vaginal epithelium. Simian immunodeficiency virus-infected cells are most commonly found at inflamed portions of these sites. Therefore, the mechanism of SIV transmission potentially relies on this location (Miller *et al.,* 1992a,b).

2. Cervical Polyps

Cervical polyps usually arise from the cervical canal. Microscopically, these polyps are a hyperplastic condition of the endocervical endothelium, as has been reported in two rhesus macaques (DiGiacomo, 1977). Treatment consists of ligation, excision, and destruction of the base with electrocautery. Tissue should be examined microscopically to rule out malignancy.

Foci of apparently abnormal proliferation of endocervical glands, designated adenomatous hyperplasia or atypical hyperplasia, are frequently found in surgical specimens from women. However, no definite neoplastic potential has been established when such enlarged glands appear in nonhuman primates. Seventy-eight reproductive tracts from mature, wild-caught cynomolgus females were examined histologically for evidence of dysplastic squamous epithelium of the cervix and vagina. Eleven of these animals showed dysplasia, indicating that this condition may be a naturally occurring phenomenon of the species. It is not yet known whether all nonhuman primate female reproductive tracts show a prevalence of dysplasia, but caution should be exercised in interpretation of dysplasia found in nonhuman primates on reproductive studies (Hertig *et al.,* 1983). Foci of dysplasia at the junction of the squamous epithelium of the exocervix and columnar epithelium of the endocervix were reported in rhesus macaques. Also reported was carcinoma at the tip of the cervical fold, just before the cervical os (DiGiacomo, 1977).

C. Uterine Corpus

1. Endometrium

Growth and development of the endometrium reflect hormonal changes and are best observed during the different phases of the menstrual cycle. The endometrium may also reflect abnormal endocrine states and is responsive to the exogenous ad-

ministration of hormones, occasionally resulting in pathologic conditions.

a. ENDOMETRITIS.   Lymphocytes and neutrophils normally appear in the endometrium in the second half of the menstrual cycle; however, their presence does not necessarily constitute endometritis. The appearance of plasma cells, however, represents an immune response, usually to foreign antigen, i.e., pathogenic organisms. Endometritis can present as an acute or chronic problem. Adhesions may be a consequence, leading to cessation of menses and to infertility. If endometritis causes obstruction of the cervical canal, the uterine cavity may become distended by exudate or blood. As an example, pyometra in a 15-year-old rhesus macaque was described as an enlarged and-fluctuant uterus containing a large quantity of yellow-brown fluid. The animal was depressed with a high white blood cell count and degenerative shift (Strozier *et al.,* 1972). *Escherichia coli* was identified as the etiologic agent. In another case, *Actinomyces* and *Staphylococcus* sp. were identified as the etiologic agents (Lang and Benjamin, 1969). A retrospective view of cases at the California Primate Research Center identified *E. coli* and coagulase-positive *Staphylococcus* as the most common isolates from animals with endometritis (Doyle *et al.,* 1991).

b. ENDOMETRIAL HYPERPLASIA.   One of the most controversial subjects in gynecology for the past several decades has been the definition of biologic activity and treatment of endometrial hyperplasia. Hyperplasia represents part of the spectrum that is a continuum that begins as benign changes and becomes neoplastic, i.e., adenocarcinoma. There appear to be two separate and biologically unrelated diseases of the endometrium: hyperplasia and neoplasia. The important feature that distinguishes one from the other is the degree of cytologic atypia. However, endometrial hyperplasia and adenocarcinoma found together in a 15-year-old rhesus macaque (*Macaca mulatta*) illustrate the continuum in a single animal (Strozier *et al.,* 1972). Chalifoux (1993c) reviews endometrial adenocarcinoma in the squirrel monkey with an emphasis on pathology.

c. ENDOMETRIAL POLYPS.   Endometrial polyps, which are sessile or pedunculated projections of the endometrium, develop as solitary or multiple soft tumors, frequently composed of hyperplastic endometrium. It is difficult to determine which symptoms actually result from endometrial polyps because they are frequently associated with leiomyomas of the uterus and endometrial hyperplasia. These polyps are usually asymptomatic but may cause nonspecific abnormal uterine bleeding. A pedunculated mass in the uterine lumen of a 32-year-old spider monkey (*Ateles sp.*) was characterized as cystic adenomatous hyperplasia of the endometrial stroma, but this female showed no clinical signs (Binhazim *et al.,* 1989). In another report, a polyp originating from the right oviduct and extending into the uterus of a rhesus macaque was identified as an endometrial cystadenoma (Ruch, 1959). A review of infertility cases identified nine animals (14%) with endometrial polyps but could not establish whether they were the primary cause of infertility (DiGiacomo, 1977).

2. Myometrium

a. LEIOMYOMAS. Leiomyomas are well-circumscribed, but nonencapsulated, benign uterine tumors composed primarily of smooth muscle but with some fibrous connective tissue. Myomas are classified according to location, with intramural tumors being the most common. Usually multiple and of various sizes, they distort the contour of the uterus. Most myomas do not produce symptoms other than possibly abnormal bleeding patterns, although the pressure they exert on the urinary bladder may produce incontinence. Constipation can result from their pressure on the rectum, and extremely large tumors may cause edema or varicosity of the legs. Distortion of the abdomen with or without infertility as the tumors fill the uterine cavity may also be a problem. Necrosis from torsion or twisting of a pedunculated myoma may be associated with pain, tenderness, fever, and leukocytosis. During pregnancy, if these tumors increase in size due to edema and degeneration, the risk of spontaneous abortion increases. In late pregnancy, fetal malpresentation, uterine inertia or mechanical dystocia, and postpartum hemorrhage may be produced by the myoma. These tumors occur in a number of nonhuman primates, including the chimpanzee, *Pan troglodytes* (Schmidt, 1978; DiGiacomo, 1977). A leiomyoma projecting from the serosal surface of the uterus, consisting of interlacing bundles of smooth muscle fibers, often intersecting at right angles, was reported in a 32-year-old spider monkey, *Ateles* (Binhazim *et al.*, 1989). The central area of one mass was necrotic, and mitotic figures were rare.

Tumors are palpated as firm, irregular nodules arising from the pelvis and extending into the lower abdomen. Bimanual pelvic examination followed by ultrasound is the most revealing diagnostic approach (Tarantal, 1992). Hysterectomy or removal of the tumor can alleviate significant symptoms.

b. ADENOMYOSIS. Adenomyosis is a benign disease of the uterus characterized by areas of endometrial glands and stroma within the myometrium. Adenomyoma refers to a localized tumor-like mass composed of hyperplastic smooth muscle admixed with foci of endometrium. This structure is not a tumor but rather a hyperplastic growth, either localized or diffuse. Although the clinical signs of growth are nonspecific, they may include abnormal bleeding, a tender uterus, and dysmenorrhea. A focus of heterotropic endometrial glands characteristic of adenomyosis was reported in a spider monkey (Binhazin *et al.*, 1989). Another publication cited 21 rhesus macaques with adenomyosis (DiGiacomo, 1977).

A case of adenomyosis was diagnosed in a pig-tailed macaque (*Macaca nemestrina*), although she exhibited no clinical signs. Her condition was identified during a prestudy magnetic resonance imaging (MRI) screening, at which time the uterus

occupied 25.3 cm³, a substantial enlargement, and was grossly distorted and asymmetric with patchy high signal features in the myometrium (Waterton *et al.*, 1993). Treatment with a pure estrogen agonist, which removed the endogenous estrogen drive, was beneficial in reducing the size of the lesion.

Estrogenic compounds can be carcinogenic in lower mammals, and uterine tumors have been noted to occur in women following estrogen therapy. Seven of 10 squirrel monkeys on an experimental protocol exhibited malignant uterine mesotheliomas after prolonged treatment with DES. They had large, irregular, nodular outgrowths of the uterine corpus and numerous small white nodules present throughout the mesentary. Three of the animals showed early proliferative lesions of the uterine serosa (McClure and Graham, 1973). Ovariohysterectomy is the treatment of choice for mesotheliomas in women.

D. Oviduct, Broad Ligament, and Ovary

1. Salpingitis

Salpingitis occurs when the uterus and the oviduct are infected by organisms that are usually confined to the cervix and vagina. Acute, primary salpingitis is an infection that results when the pathological organism that causes cervicitus invades the oviduct. Salpingitis can also begin as a perisalpingitis secondary to intraabdominal infection, but this type of infection is much less common. Inflammation of the oviduct can impair fertility if scarring and adhesions form an obstruction. A case of salpingitis was reported in a pig-tail macaque (*Macaca nemestrina*) as a result of infection with *Chlamydia trachomatos* (Cappuccio, 1994).

2. Cysts

a. PAROVARIAN CYSTS. A variety of cysts and tumors arise in the pelvic-supporting structures of primates. These lesions are usually benign and originate from peritoneal inclusions or embryonic remnants. Cysts of the broad ligament are of mesonephric or paramesonephric origin. They may be intraligamentous or pedunculated. Pedunculated cysts of the broad ligament are common and are referred to as hydatids of Morgagni. They are also referred to as parovarian cysts because of their location. Malignant change is rare. For the most part, they can be ignored unless they become twisted on the pedicle or stalk. This can cause rupture and hemorrhage requiring surgical removal.

Routine necropsy of a squirrel monkey revealed a small, fluid-filled, hydatid cyst of Morgagni. This cyst lay between the peritoneal surfaces of the mesovarium and mesosalpinx and was attached to the oviduct by a narrow, cord-like pedicle (Brown and Kupper, 1972). Parovarian cysts were the most frequently found growths of this type in the rhesus macaque. They varied greatly in size, were single or multiple, and were associated with one or both ovaries (DiGiacomo, 1977).

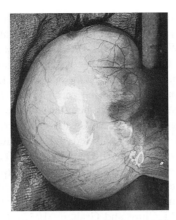

Fig. B.5. An example of an ovarian follicular cyst. These are usually incidental findings.

b. FOLLICULAR CYSTS.   Mature or atretic follicles that become distended with pale, straw-colored fluid frequently occupy the ovary (Fig. B. 5). Follicular cysts result from a failure of ovulation, after which the follicles continue to grow. Usually multiple and occurring in both ovaries, they rarely produce symptoms but resolve on their own within a few months. Follicular cysts identified in eight rhesus monkeys were not associated with overt signs but were in a population of animals examined for infertility (DiGiacomo, 1977).

c. LUTEAL CYSTS.   In the absence of pregnancy, the corpus luteum normally collapses and is eventually replaced by hyaline connective tissue to form the corpus albicans. Occasionally the corpus luteum becomes cystic as a result of unusual continued growth or hemorrhage into the lumen. Symptoms are related to the size or to complications due to torsion, rupture, or hemorrhage. The condition may simulate ectopic pregnancy, and continued hormone production may cause amenorrhea and subsequent irregular uterine bleeding. More commonly, the cyst produces no symptoms and undergoes regression spontaneously. Two rhesus macaques with corpus luteal cysts were described (DiGiacomo, 1977).

3. Neoplasia

Early diagnosis of ovarian cancer is difficult because symptoms are often vague or nonexistent until the neoplasm has attained a large size and metastasized. Radiographs are of value in the diagnosis of ovarian neoplasms because they may reveal calcification, i.e., teeth, within a benign cystic teratoma. Ultrasound is important in differentiating cystic from solid tumors and uterine from adnexal masses. Percutaneous fine-needle aspiration, with sonographic guidance, is an accurate method of diagnosing a variety of tumors. However, it should not be used for the diagnosis of ovarian tumors because such neoplasms must be surgically excised, regardless of the results of aspira-

tion. In addition, there is some risk that a cystic neoplasm may rupture when aspirated.

a. BENIGN OVARIAN TERATOMA.   Benign cystic teratomas, also called dermoid cysts, are relatively common. They are derived from primordial germ cells and are composed of any combination of well-differentiated ectodermal, mesodermal, and endodermal elements. The tumors are almost always benign. In the unusual case of malignancy, the malignant element is usually squamous epithelium. Benign ovarian teratomas found in two rhesus monkeys at necropsy failed to produce clinical symptoms in either instance. A radiograph of one monkey revealed a circumscribed mass in the lower quadrant of the abdomen with scattered areas of calcification. On palpation, the 5.0 × 5.0 × 3.0-cm mass could be moved easily within the abdominal cavity and, because of its postion, was thought to be associated with the genital tract. The mass contained foul, dark brown, viscous material and a large amount of hair (Rohovksy *et al.*, 1977). In the other monkey, one ovary contained a focus of well-differentiated, mature cartilage and multiple cystic spaces lined by low cuboidal to tall columnar epithelium. There were no clinical symptoms except infertility, as evident after the female was repeatedly placed with proven breeder males and failed to conceive (Eydelloth and Swindle, 1983). An additional benign ovarian teratoma was identified in a rhesus monkey during an embryectomy on the 32nd gestational day. As the uterus was manipulated for surgery, the right ovary was observed to be noticeably enlarged to 2.6 × 1.8 cm with a number of hairs protruding into the interior. Microscopic examination revealed a preponderance of structures characteristic of skin (Scott *et al.*, 1975). Similar cases of a benign cystic teratoma in a rhesus macaque (Martin *et al.*, 1970) and in an African green monkey (*Cercopithecus aethiops*) were also reported (Baskin *et al.*, 1980). The subject of benign ovarian teratomas in nonhuman primates with an emphasis on pathology is detailed in a review by Chalifoux (1993a).

Several other benign neoplasms were reported in the literature, including a papillary serous cystadenoma and a cavernous hemangioma in a rhesus macaque (Martin *et al.*, 1970). In addition, an arrenoblastoma and a fibrothecoma, two other benign ovarian neoplasms, have been observed in the chimpanzee, *Pan troglodytes* (Graham and McClure, 1977).

b. SERTOLI–LEYDIG TUMOR.   Sertoli–Leydig tumors are relatively rare. They are characteristically androgenic, and virilization usually occurs, although some tumors fail to produce hormones or produce them at a level insufficient to cause symptoms. However, estrogen made by the Sertoli cell component of the tumor or peripheral conversion of androgenic hormones may cause estrogenic manifestations. A Sertoli–Leydic cell tumor, an endometrial polyp, and adenomatous hyperplasia located at necropsy in a 38-year-old female chimpanzee (*Pan troglodytes*) (Graham and McClure, 1976) resembled a type I Sertoli–Leydig cell tumor. The lesion was located within the medulla of the ovary near the hilus, but was contiguous to the cortical tissue. Extensive follicular atresia and thecal hypertrophy, possibly a result of hyperestrinism, were also noted. The excessive estrogenic secretion may have originated in the hypertrophic thecal tissue instead of in the tumor.

c. DYSGERMINOMA.   Dysgerminoma, the most common malignant germ cell tumor of the ovary in women, is a solid fleshy tumor with a smooth exterior. An example of a malignant dysgerminoma in a rhesus monkey was observed in an animal follwed for 31 months after surgical removal of a primary ovarian tumor. Although the well-circumscribed and encapsulated primary lesion was easily removed surgically, the histological features of malignancy, including the high mitotic index and undifferentiated cell type, suggested a poor prognosis. Metastatic lesions were removed 24 to 28 months after excision of the primary tumor, and the animal was euthanized 31 months after removal of the primary tumor (Holmberg *et al.,* 1978).

d. OVARIAN CARCINOMA.   Most epithelial tumors are derived ultimately from the ovarian surface epithelium, a specialized type of mesothelium. An ovarian adenocarcinoma was identified arising from the left ovary at necropsy in a 10-year-old female bonnet monkey, *Macaca radiata*. Despite the fact that no metastatic foci were seen in other organs, the multifocal lack of cellular organization, stratification of the epithelial cells, cellular pleomorphism, and invasion of the adjacent stroma and capsule of the tumor led to the diagnosis of malignancy (Bunton and Lollini, 1983). Previously, a 2×6-mm pedunculated tumor had been found at necropsy in a 4-year-old female Barbary ape, *Macaca sylvana* (Wagner and Carey, 1976). The ovarian carcinoma was attached to the left ovary near the junction of the ovary and oviduct. Scattered throughout the omentum, mesentery, and serosal surface of the abdominal cavity were numerous round, slightly raised, yellow-gray nodules 1–5 mm in diameter. Many of the lesions, most abundantly in the caudal portion of the abdominal cavity, had coalesced. The neoplasm can spread by directly invading the adjacent tissue or by way of peritoneal fluid either through blood vessels or lymphatics. Transcelomic metastasis may be responsible for the secondary growth of certain abdominal neoplasms and appears to be the mechanism of spread in this case. Tumors of the ovaries and oviducts commonly disseminate by this route in women.

E. Mammary Gland

1. Mastitis

Although an infrequently recognized disease problem in primate breeding colonies, mastitis may complicate lactation. Both coagulase-positive *Staphylococcus aureus* and hemolytic *Streptococci* sp. have been isolated from sites of mastitis in nonhuman primates. With the usual form of puerperal mastitis, a localized area of inflammation and tenderness accompany slight elevations of temperatue and white blood cell count. A report

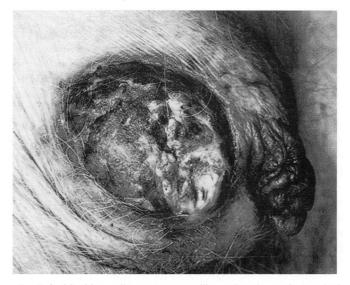

Fig. B.6.   Mastitis usually presents as swelling and erythema of one or both glands in a female that is reluctant to allow the infant to nurse. It may also progress to an abscess or more serious necrotic lesion as depicted.

of mastitis in a 7-year-old bonnet macaque (*Macaca radiata*) with a 4-month-old nursing infant revealed *Corynebacterium ulcerans* as the etiologic agent (Fox and Frost, 1974). The swollen right mammary gland of the macaque yielded milk that was thick in consistency and contained flecks of purulent debris. In this case, *C. ulcerans* was able to form necrotizing toxins. The mastitis was successfully treated with prompt and sustained antibiotics. Usual treatment consists of continuation of breast feeding or emptying the gland and the use of appropriate antibiotics. If there is no response, a breast abscess may be suspected (Fig. B. 6), which requires open drainage and hot packs in addition to antibiotics. Adequate drainage should be established under general anesthesia. If possible, the generous incision should be circumareolar and, if drainage cannot be maintained, a Penrose drain should be considered.

2. Mammary Neoplasia

An intraductal mammary carcinoma was reported in a rhesus macaque. There were essentially no clinical signs or gross lesions noted at necropsy. In this particular case it was diagnosed histologically in conjunction with another incidental finding, ovarian teratoma. Eydelloth and Swindle (1983) describe this case and review the literature.

IV. ENDOMETRIOSIS

Endometriosis is one of the most common reproductive disorders in Old World nonhuman primates. The literature is replete with case reports involving rhesus and cynomolgus macaques (Ami *et al.,* 1993; Fanton *et al.,* 1986a; McCann and Myers, 1970). In addition, isolated case reports have been published for other nonhuman primate species, such as *Macaca nemestrina* (DiGiacomo *et al.,* 1977), *Papio hamadryas* (DaRif *et al.,* 1984; Shalev *et al.,* 1992), and *P. doguera* (Folse and Stout, 1978). The nonhuman primate has been proposed as a naturally occurring model of this disease in humans (MacKenzie and Casey, 1975), and the condition has been induced experimentally in macaques through endometrial autografts to the peritoneal cavity (Schenken *et al.,* 1987).

Endometriosis has been defined clinically as the presence of both endometrial glands and stroma outside the uterine cavity and musculature. It is associated with a variety of symptoms, most commonly pain and infertility. However, the disease may be entirely asymptomatic, even in advanced cases, as evidenced by the number of reports of incidental findings at necropsy. Although some symptoms may be strongly suggestive of endometriosis, none are diagnostic of the disorder.

Suggestive clinical signs of endometriosis in nonhuman primates are cyclical anorexia, depression, and possibly the absence of feces lasting several days (Fanton and Hubbard, 1983; Lindberg and Busch, 1984; Schaerdel, 1986). Clinical and pathologic findings from 70 rhesus monkeys with confirmed cases of endometriosis were documented (Fanton *et al.,* 1986a). The disease was classified as minimal (14%), moderate (20%), and massive (66%). Clinical examination indicated palpable masses in the abdomens and pelvic cavities of most of these animals: 29% exhibited constipation, 39% anorexia, 17% irregular menses, and 38% radiographic evidence of soft tissue masses. Pathologic findings were intraabdominal endometrial cyst formation (73%) and adhesions involving the ureters (51%), colon (66%), urinary bladder (50%), and ovaries (81%). Other nonspecific clinical signs included abdominal distention (Folse and Stout, 1978; Schiffer *et al.,* 1984) and weight loss (Strozier *et al.,* 1972). Physical examination may reveal discrete movable cysts (Schiffer *et al.,* 1984) or diffuse omental, peritoneal, and intestinal adhesions between adjacent abdominal and pelvic viscera (DiGiacomo *et al.,* 1977) or a large firm mass encompassing the uterus, cervix, urinary bladder, distal end of each ureter, and colon (Strozier *et al.,* 1972). Aspiration of cysts usually yields a chocolate-colored fluid, hence the name "chocolate cyst" (Fig. B. 7).

Pelvic pain is the most common symptom in women. In nonhuman primates, this may manifest as abdominal discomfort or prostation, and some animals so-affected have died during menstrual periods (MacKenzie and Casey, 1975).

Infertility is frequent when endometriosis distorts the relationship among pelvic organs or obstructs the oviducts. A review of 21 cynomolgus macaques with endometriosis stated that their fertility was impaired, mediated collectively by luteinized unruptured follicles, luteal phase defects, and pelvic adhesions (Schenken *et al.,* 1984a,b).

Dysfunctional uterine bleeding has often been linked to endometriosis; however, there is no evidence that endometriosis

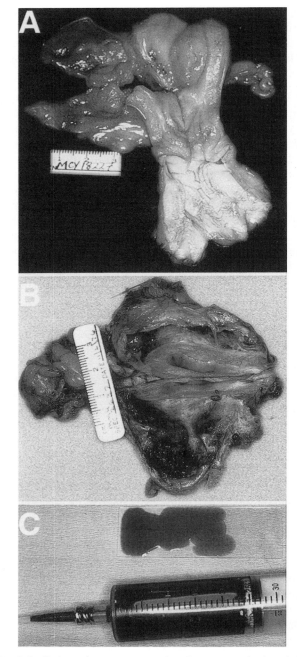

Fig. B.7. Endometriomas encompassing the uterus and adnexal tissue (A and B). Characteristic "chocolate fluid" found in most endometriomas (C).

is a cause of such bleeding. Schaerdel (1986) described an adult rhesus monkey with recurring abnormal menstrual cycles consisting of prolonged bleeding for 8–10 days coupled with inappetence and mild anemia (PCV=28–30). In another report, an animal was recumbent with hypothermia and had a markedly distended abdomen. At necropsy, a small amount of blood was visible in the vulva, and 700 ml of unclotted blood was removed from the abdomen (Schiffer *et al.,* 1984).

Endometriosis has been found in virtually every part of the body, although it is most frequently observed in the pelvis. Such a range of locations may produce a variety of uncommon, site-specific symptoms. For example, an unexpected death resulted from a large bowel infarction caused by fibrous adhesions from endometriosis (Schaerdel, 1986). At necropsy there was a distinct line of demarcation and the bowel was distended with gas. Another report (DaRif *et al.,* 1984) described rectal fistulas and chronic supperative peritonitis in a baboon (*Papio hamadryas*) stemming from endometrial tissue in the rectal wall that had penetrated the rectal mucosa. As a result, bacterial contamination led to the formation of a fistulous tract. Not uncommonly, endometrial adhesions in the abdomen impinge on the pelvic ureters, creating hydroureter and, in severe cases, hydronephrosis of one or both kidneys.

Understanding the pathogenesis of endometriosis requires examination of histiogenesis, etiology, and factors critical to growth and maintenance. Three major theories are accepted regarding the histogenic origins of endometriosis. Originally, coelomic metaplasia was considered to be the cause. Next, ectopic transplantation of the endometrium was thought to be responsible. Finally, the induction hypothesis of endometriosis, a combination of the theories of coelomic metaplasia and transplantation, proposes that unidentified substances released from shed endometrium cause undifferentiated mesenchyme to form endometriosis. However, in addition to histiogenesis, other etiologic factors are necessary for the development of endometriosis.

Retrograde menstruation as the major mechanism for transplantation or induction is the theory most consistent with clinical observations. Frequent X-rays, ovarian steroids, and uterine surgery that may seed the abdomen with endometrial tissue have been examined as risk factors (Bertens *et al.,* 1982). When a colony of rhesus monkeys previously exposed to radiation was reviewed (Fanton and Golden, 1991), the incidence of endometriosis in animals that had received radiation was 53%, whereas in nonirradiated controls it was only 26%. In a group of 35 rhesus macaques, 9 were identified with endometriosis. The group with the highest incidence of endometriosis (5/8) had received ovarian steroids after hysterotomy. Animals with frequent uterine surgeries had the least incidence (1/18) and ovarian steroids alone accounted for 2/6. Ami (1993) evaluated 27 female cynomolgus macaques for endometriosis but found no significant difference in incidence between groups that had and had not undergone cesarean sections. The interval since the last pregnancy was significantly longer in affected animals than in those not affected. This is probably attributable both to the protective effects of pregnancy against progression of the disease and to some causal relationship between endometriosis and infertility.

Still other factors involved in the development of this disease are the amount of retrograde menstruation, the capacity to remove this debris, a defective immune response to the ectopic tissue, or the presence of an unknown factor critical to implantation. Finally, once endometriosis is initiated, maintenance may be a limiting step. Previously, growth and maintenance were thought to be estrogen dependent. However, studies now suggest that the process is much more complex, involving growth factors and protooncogenes.

Three approaches have been used to diagnose endometriosis: serum testing, imaging techniques, and surgical examination of the peritoneal cavity. A number of different serum markers have been evaluated but have failed to demonstrate sufficient sensitivity or specificity for clinical utility. Imaging techniques, ultrasound (US), and MRI have been used to define the size, shape, and location of pelvic abnormalities. Although highly suggestive, the appearance of lesions is not pathognomonic. Magnetic resonance imaging has a sensitivity of 64% and a specificity of 60%, whereas US has a sensitivity of 11%. Palpation of fluctuant cysts primarily in the lower abdomen and ultrasound-aided aspiration of a brownish fluid are the most efficacious methods for diagnosing endometriosis. Direct visualization at the time of surgery, by laparoscopy or laparotomy, is also helpful in establishing a definitive diagnosis.

Medical strategies for combating endometriosis have generally attempted to alter the menstrual cycles of the female. One of the drugs used for this purpose is danazol, an isoxazol derivative of 17-α-ethyltestosterone. This drug acts by attenuating the midcycle luteinizing hormone surge, inhibiting multiple enzymes in the steroidogenic pathway, and increasing free serum testosterone. The resulting state is one of chronic anovulation with hyperandrogenism. In the rhesus monkey, danazol induces short luteal phases and decreases progesterone production due to a direct effect at the gonadal level. Danazol at doses of 400–800 mg daily to the point of amenorrhea (usually 2–6 months) has been used successfully at the California Primate Research Center to treat endometriosis.

Leuprolide, a gonadotropin-releasing hormone agonist that halts menstrual cycles, was used successfully in an aged rhesus macaque (Moody *et al.,* 1991). The animal presented with a 7-cm abdominal mass adhered to the uterus and bladder. Leuprolide was chosen over danazol as therapy because fewer side effects have been reported. Dramatic clinical improvement was obtained with 0.5 mg SC SID administered for 6 months. Side effects, which mimic menopause, were treated with pentazocine (Talwin, Sanofi Winthrop, Ny, Ny) and acetaminophen.

Progestional agents, primarily medroxyprogesterone, are also used to treat endometriosis. They act by producing an initial decidualization of endometrial tissue, followed by eventual atrophy. After medroxyprogesterone (Depo-Provera; 40 mg/month) was used as a treatment for endometriosis (McCarthy *et al.,* 1989), the recipient developed pyometra secondary to cystic gland hyperplasia and bacterial infection. The animal presented with a large, firm abdominal mass and hemopurulent vaginal discharge originating from the cervix. Subsequent treatment consisted of appropriate antibiotics and transcervical flushing.

Oral contraceptives have also been used to mimic the pseudopregnant state. Pregnancy exerts a beneficial effect on endometriosis. An experimental model utilized endometrial or

TABLE B.I

ALGORITHM FOR EVALUATION OF AMENORRHEA IN NONHUMAN PRIMATES

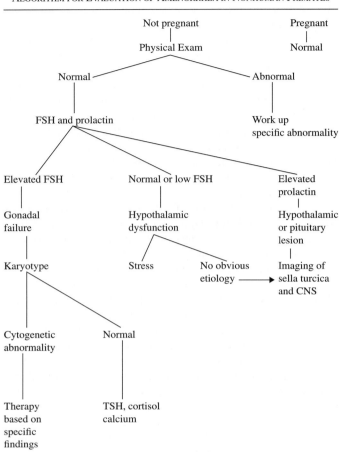

TABLE B.II

DEFINITION OF ABNORMAL UTERINE BLEEDING

Term	Definition
Oligomenorrhea:	Bleeding at intervals of greater than 40 days that usually is irregular
Polymenorrhea:	Bleeding at intervals of less than 22 days that may be regular or irregular
Menorrhagia:	Bleeding that is excessive in both amount and duration at regular intervals
Metrorrhagia:	Bleeding of usually normal amount but at irregular intervals
Menometrorrhagia:	Bleeding that is excessive in amount, is prolonged in duration, and may occur at regular or irregular intervals
Hypomenorrhea:	Regular uterine bleeding in decreased amount
Intermenstrual bleeding:	Bleeding that occurs between what is otherwise regular menstrual bleeding
Dysmenorrhea:	Painful menstruation that may present as an isolated disorder or in association with other conditions

adipose autografts placed in the peritoneal cavity to induce endometriosis and to evaluate the related effects of pregnancy. Pregnant animals with minimal to mild endometriosis underwent complete remission and those with moderate disease had a significant improvement but not complete remission. Endometriosis progressed unchecked in the nonpregnant animals (Schenken *et al.,* 1987).

The ability to eliminate endometriotic lesions by surgery is undocumented but is believed to be quite substantial. However, thoroughness is dependent on recognition of all forms of the disease. The rate of recurrence following surgery can be significant. Definitive treatment consists of hysterectomy with salpingo-oophorectomy (Fanton *et al.,* 1986b).

Another therapeutic approach uses adjunctive medical treatment to control the pain. Nonsteroidal anti-inflammatory agents have been used with success. The most effective regime is to administer the agent prior to the onset of the menstrual cycle and continue for the entire cycle.

V. DISORDERS OF MENSTRUATION

A. Amenorrhea

Menstrual dysfunction is a symptom of some underlying abnormality of the reproductive system. The abnormality may be developmental, endocrinologic, or acquired as the result of an anatomic lesion. Disorders in menstruation can be separated into two categories: the absence of menstruation (amenorrhea) and abnormal uterine bleeding. Amenorrhea is further classified as primary, if menarche fails to occur, and secondary, if menses cease for at least 6 months in a postmenarchal animal. Amenorrhea can result from a hypothalamic or pituitary dysfunction, ovarian failure, or anatomic abnormality. Table B.I provides an algorithm for diagnosis and treatment of amenorrhea in the nonhuman primate (Brumsted and Riddick, 1994).

B. Abnormal Uterine Bleeding

Abnormal uterine bleeding, whether too little or too much, reflects a significant change in the pattern of bleeding that must be characterized accurately because therapy is dependent on specific etiologies. Table B.II provides definitions that are helpful in describing and characterizing abnormal uterine bleeding in the nonpregnant animal (Severino, 1995). Numerous menstrual disorders have been recognized in nonhuman primates (Van Pelt, 1974). To evaluate the underlying pathophysiologic conditions and institute effective therapy, a complete understanding of the normal anatomy, embryology, and endocrinology of the reproductive tract is required. Problems with menstruation in nonhuman primates rarely receive thorough workups to the point of definitive diagnosis. Instead, such animals are usually assigned to studies not related to reproduction and are treated for clinical signs that may interfere with good health, e.g., menorrhagia. Table B.III provides an algorithm for the diagnosis and treatment of abnormal uterine bleeding in the nonhuman primate (Brumsted and Riddick, 1994).

Blood loss due to menstrual flow in Old World species is both a cause and effect of iron deficiency. In the presence of iron deficiency, endometrial spiral arterioles do not contract adequately, thereby prolonging the period of heavy menstrual flow, leading to excessive blood loss. Iron deficiency, therefore, may lead to menorrhagia which, in turn, produces a more severe iron deficiency. The vicious cycle thus created is alleviated by iron therapy (Wixson and Griffith, 1986). Daily oral vitamins with iron are effective for treatment/prevention.

C. Dysmenorrhea

Dysmenorrhea, or painful menstruation, may present as an isolated disorder or in association with other conditions. One cause of primary dysmenorrhea is an increase in prostaglandin F_{2a} production by the endometrium, leading to myometrial contractions. Dysmenorrhea in a nonhuman primate can include the clinical signs of abdominal pain, anorexia, and prostration during menstruation (Ruch, 1959). Treatment with nonsteroidal anti-inflammatory agents, which block prostaglandin synthesis through inhibition of the enzyme cyclooxygenase, can be beneficial. Progesterone also offers a similar benefit by inhibiting endometrial prostaglandin synthesis. Endometriosis or other lesions within the uterine cavity, cervical stenosis or endocervical polyps, are other causes of dysmenorrhea, and treatment for these conditions is directed toward removing the lesion.

Painful menstruation has been suspected in many cases of cyclical anorexia, corresponding to the menstrual cycle of the animal, in nonhuman primate breeding colonies. In some instances it has been treated empirically with nonsteroidal anti-inflammatory agents with mixed results. Four cases of membranous dysmenorrhea, confirmed histologically, have been reported in the chimpanzee, *Pan troglodytes* (Solleveld and van Zwieten, 1978). The animals experienced abnormal menstrual bleeding for 3–5 days every 35 days. Pain was not obvious in these animals, although the possibility that the animals were masking pain was considered by the author. During menstruation, a hemorrhagic pear-shaped, hollow sac-like structure with a rough granular red/brown inner surface and gray/pink outer surface was shed in the form of a more or less complete cast. Hormone analysis of urine and histologic examination of the mass ruled out abortion.

VI. OBSTETRICAL PROBLEMS

A. Pregnancy Diagnosis

An excellent review on the detection and monitoring of pregnancy is presented in this series in "Nonhuman Primates in

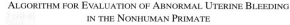

TABLE B.III

ALGORITHM FOR EVALUATION OF ABNORMAL UTERINE BLEEDING
IN THE NONHUMAN PRIMATE

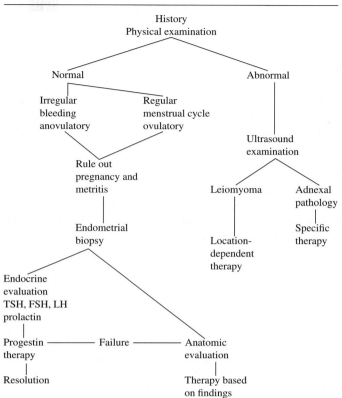

Biomedical Research: Biology and Management," Chapter 14 (Hendrickx and Dukelow, 1995b).

Amenorrhea and an enlarged abdomen are highly suggestive of pregnancy; however, several pathological lesions must also be considered. For example, leiomyomas can cause uterine enlargement. However, the uterus is more firm and irregular in contour than during pregnancy, and either amenorrhea or dysmenorrhea may be present. Alternatively, the soft consistency of an ovarian cyst can closely resemble that of the pregnant uterus, and amenorrhea is often associated. Hematometra as a result of vaginal or cervical stenosis may cause an enlarged, intermittently contractile uterus as well as amenorrhea. Ultrasonography is very useful in differentiating these disorders from pregnancy (Tarantal and Hendrickx, 1988; Conrad *et al.*, 1989).

B. Placental Disorders

1. Amniotic Band Syndrome

The fetal membranes normally line the uterine cavity and completely surround the fetus. These membranes are metabolically active in fetal development and play a critical role in protection throughout pregnancy. Clinical problems develop when the integrity of the membranes is compromised other than at the termination of pregnancy. The most striking placental malformation is commonly known as amniotic band syndrome. The amnion ruptures and a combination of mesoblastic proliferation and oligohydramnios form strands of different sizes that entangle and entrap the developing fetus. The mechanism of such ruptures is unknown and is not thought to recur in subsequent pregnancies of the same female. Amniotic band syndrome was diagnosed in a rhesus monkey by routine ultrasound examination at 110 gestational days, and the fetus was delivered by hysterotomy at 120 gestational days (Tarantal and Hendrickx, 1987). Resulting deformities of the cranial vault included incomplete ossification of the frontal and parietal regions of the skull; bilateral hydrocephalus with a communicating right occipital porencephalic cyst; a large midline facial cleft of the palate, maxilla, and nose; bulging orbits with unfused eyelids; and hydropic membranes. There is no treatment for this condition.

2. Extrachorial Placenta

Usually the membranous chorion inserts at the periphery of the villous chorion of the placental disc. If the membranes arise without bulky folding or thickening, the insertion is called circummarginate. If they arise from a cup-like fold that can be elevated at the insertion, they are called circumvallate. The circumvallate insertion has been associated with several clinical sequelae, including maternal bleeding in the second and third trimester, preterm labor, and abortion, but there are no precise correlations. A 15% incidence of circumvallate placenta has been reported in nonhuman primates, although the significance was unclear (Myers, 1972). Examination of 56 placentas from stump-tailed macaques (*Macaca arctoides*) identified two cases of placenta extracorialis (Johnson *et al.,* 1978). An annular ring of necrotic tissue and fibrin was apparent at the margin of the villous chorion. Furthermore, the placental tissue extended beyond the circumference of the chorionic plate, and the transition of the placenta from membranous chorion to villous chorion occupied an area smaller than the basal plate. The result was formation of a fibrous ring at the margin of the chorionic plate where fetal vessels appeared to terminate. In another review, 21 rhesus macaques had placental lesions but no recognizable instances of circumvallate placenta (Bunton, 1986).

3. Retained Placenta

Retained placentas are not uncommon in nonhuman primates. Many primates give birth unobserved during the evening, and many animals eat the placenta so it is difficult to know for certain if the placenta has been passed. If the placenta has not passed, the animal may present with a portion of the umbilical cord visible at the vulva or may hemorrhage excessively

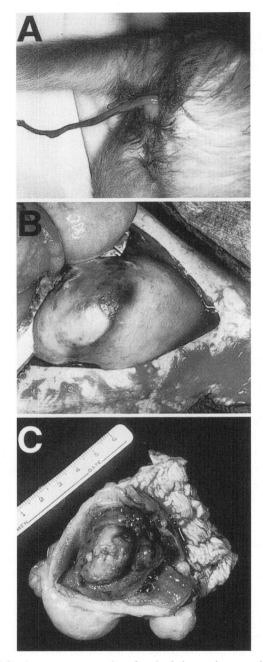

Fig. B.8. A common presentation of retained placenta is to note the umbilical cord protruding from the vulva (A). Alternatively, if the placenta is not removed expeditiously and the animal treated vigorously with appropriate antibiotics, the condition can rapidly progress to endometritis and necrosis of the uterus (B and C).

due to inadequate involution and contraction (Fig. B.8). Puerperal hemorrhage described in a pig-tailed macaque (*Macaca nemestrina*) (Ruch, 1959) resulted after the upper one-third of the placenta adhered firmly to the uterine wall, preventing uterine contraction. Clinical signs vary with the length of time postpartum and the degree of sepsis. The animal may be depressed with an enlarged uterus that is flaccid to spongy on palpation. Laboratory testing reveals anemia and indications of sepsis.

Placentas may be retained as a result of uterine inertia or abnormal adherence to the uterus. Placenta accreta and uterine inversion are unusual but serious problems. Placenta accreta denotes an abnormal placental adherence onto, into, or through the uterine wall, either partial or total, which leads to difficulty in delivery of the placenta. Additionally, postpartum bleeding may occur because the retained placenta fragments interfere with uterine involution. Treatment involves manually massaging the uterus to break down connections to the endometrium and to expel tissue and contents through the cervix. If this is not possible, surgical removal is required because pooling of blood and tissue debris make infection likely. Aggressive antibiotic therapy and, if the uterus is responsive, oxytocin (4–10 units IM every couple of hours) to facilitate uterine contraction help prevent endometritis. Hypofibrinogenemia resulting from disseminated intravascular coagulation is a possible complication.

C. Pregnancy Loss

Reproductive failure in nonhuman primates is a significant problem characterized by embryonic, fetal, and early neonatal death in addition to infertility of the mother (Andrews, 1971). Conservatively, prenatal mortality in nonhuman primates is thought to exceed 15% of all diagnosed pregnancies (Hendrickx and Nelson, 1971). In one report, 28% of all African green monkeys (*Cecopithecus aethiops*) underwent an abortion or stillbirth (Brady, 1983). The incidence in New World monkeys, *Saimiri* sp. and *Aotus* sp., is thought to be higher than in Old World monkeys (Rouse *et al.,* 1981; Taub, 1980). Moreover, the mean abortion rate of 156 owl monkeys (*Aotus trivirgatus*) was 48%. These spontaneous abortions usually occurred late in the second or third trimester, but handling, maternal anemia, season, or karyotype were not contributing causes, at least in this species (Rouse *et al.,* 1981). Factors that are known contributors to high rates of embryonic and fetal wastage include nonrepetitive, intrinsic chromosomal defects of the embryo and random, sporadic chromosomal aberrations of the parents. Infectious agents can also contribute to early or late term abortion and perinatal death directly or may complicate the case.

Most of the time there is no evidence, i.e., conceptus, that an animal has aborted. Bleeding can be the result of an abortion, a placental implantation sign in some species, or menstrual bleeding. Therefore, differentiating early abortion from infertility is difficult without circumstantial evidence that an abortion has occurred. A method has been developed to identify animals undergoing abortion and those already aborted. This method, which measures serum chorionic gonadotropin and estradiol at various time points, was then used with some success to manage a breeding colony of Bolivian squirrel monkeys (Diamond *et al.,* 1985). These animals, which had a history of poor repro-

ductive success, were identified as fertile with early abortion or infertile and appropriate therapy was initiated.

A variety of organisms can cause an infection that ascends through the maternal vagina and cervix to the fetal membranes, resulting in death of the fetus. Depending on the severity of the infection, the dam may show evidence of sepsis. In other instances, hematogenous spread from maternal circulation to the fetus can occur, which is usually associated with significant maternal morbidity and mortality preceding abortion.

Clinical signs vary with the etiologic agent. In general, dams with septic abortion present with fever and abdominal tenderness. In severe cases, the local infection may progress to septicemia, septic shock, and coagulation disorder. Complete blood counts reveal a high white blood cell count with a left shift, high total protein and fibrinogen levels. In cases of sepsis, a blood culture is valuable in identifying the etiologic agent. Optimal therapy includes complete evacuation of the contents of the uterus through gentle massage of the uterus or, if unsuccessful, hysterotomy and curettage of tissue debris. When the fetus has been dead for several days, careful palpation of the uterus may reveal overlapping fetal skull bones. Radiographs may demonstrate exaggerated curvature of the spine and possibly air in the cardiovascular system of the fetus. Prolonged *in utero* retention of a dead fetus may lead to sepsis and coagulation disorders. Aggressive antibiotic and supportive therapy, including administration of fluids, monitoring of renal function, and clotting panels, usually resolve the problem.

A number of organisms can cause early pregnancy loss. Some agents have a predilection for a specific gestational stage or mode of infection: ascending or hematogenous. The following is a review of case reports broken down by etiologic agent rather than by stage of pregnancy or mode of infection.

1. Bacterial Organisms

a. GRAM-POSITIVE BACTERIA. *Listeria monocytogenes* is a small gram-positive rod that causes significant infections primarily during late pregnancy. Intrauterine transfer of such infection from dam to fetus can lead to premature labor and delivery as well as fetal death. Placental involvement eventually causes fetal septicemia, typically involving several organ systems. A Gray's monkey (*Cercopithecus mona*) infected with *L. monocytogenes* aborted at term after about 150 gestational days, after which *Listeria* was isolated from the lung, liver, brain, and kidney of the fetus. The placenta contained gray-white spots of focal necrosis and fibrinous purulent inflammation (Vetesi *et al.,* 1972). In another case of listeriosis, a celebes black ape (*Macaca niger*) showed no clinical signs of infection before or after the infant was stillborn. In fact, diffuse fibrinopurulent placentitis was the only lesion (McClure and Strozier, 1975). Listeriosis in nonhuman primates with an emphasis on pathology has been reviewed by Anderson and McClure (1993).

Massive chorioamnionitis (inflammation of fetal membranes) was the apparent cause of abortion in an orangutan, *Pongo pygmaeus abeli* (Benirschke, 1983). These membranes contained gram-positive cocci, probably *Streptococcus viridans*. In another instance of chorioamnionitis, gram-positive cocci were cultured from an infant Duoc langur, *Pygathrix nemaeus* (Kaplan, 1979). A stillbirth in a Hanuman langur (*Presbytis entelles*) was reportedly caused by gram-positive rods, and a newborn spider monkey (*Ateles paniscus*) died from a mixed infection of gram-positive and gram-negative rods (Kaplan, 1979). In this group of bacterial disorders, parturient sepsis was described in a chimpanzee (*Pan troglodytes*) infected with staphylococci sp. and streptococci (Schmidt, 1978).

A midterm abortion in a rhesus macaque due to an ascending intrauterine infection was most likely caused by *Streptococcus* (Swindle *et al.*, 1982). Another female rhesus macaque developed severe streptococcal metritis and bacteremia, which led to placentitis, fetal septicemia, and fetal death. The dam also developed acute hemolytic uremic syndrome, which has been associated with complications of pregnancy and infectious septicemia in women (Wagner *et al.*, 1992).

b. GRAM-NEGATIVE BACTERIA.   An equally wide array of gram-negative organisms have been responsible for early pregnancy loss in nonhuman primates. Generally, disease from these agents follows a more acute course than provoked by gram-positive bacteria and often results in maternal morbidity and mortality as well.

Two septic abortions in Senegal bush babies (*Galago senegalensis*) were caused by an unknown gram-negative bacillus (Butler, 1970), after which both mothers were found dead. In one, blood was oozing from the vagina and, at necropsy, the uterus was enlarged and purple with a second fetus in the right uterine horn. The placenta and endometrium contained massive hemorrhages. The second female died while in the process of aborting.

After an abortion in an orangutan (*Pongo pygmaes*) caused by *E. coli* (Cambre *et al.*, 1980), the mother died within hours. *Escherichia coli* was isolated from many of her organs but was not found in the fetus. Evidently, the cause of this fetal death was the severity of maternal infection leading to distress rather than a shared maternal–fetal infection. Endotoxin is known to cause circulatory collapse and increased uterine activity in the pregnant dam. In related experimental studies with pregnant female baboons (*Papio cynocephalus*), the administration of endotoxin resulted in fetal death due to hypoxia and acidosis (Morishima *et al.*, 1978b).

Yersinia pseudotuberculosis has been associated both temporally and spatially with an epizootic in squirrel monkeys (Buhles *et al.*, 1981). Six animals died during this outbreak, including five pregnant females. In addition, two other animals aborted but did not die themselves. *Yersinia pseudotuberculosis* has also been reported to cause abortions in the owl monkey (*Aotus trivirgatus*) (Baggs *et al.*, 1976) and other nonhuman primates (McClure *et al.*, 1971).

Salmonella heidelberg, another gram-negative enteric organism, caused a septic abortion in a white-handed gibbon, *Hyalobates lar* (Thurman *et al.*, 1983). Although the gibbon was depressed and anorexic with marked vaginal hemorrhage, she responded well to subsequent antibiotic treatment.

Shigella has been implicated in abortions of rhesus monkeys (McClure *et al.*, 1976). *Shigella* was cultured from the cervix, rectum, and placenta of one such monkey who had aborted 1 day after the onset of severe diarrhea. Similarly a gorilla (*Gorilla gorilla*) infected with *Shigella flexneri* II aborted and later passed blood clots, probably due to the retained placenta and the inability of the uterus to contract and eliminate hemorrhage (Swenson and McClure, 1976). The umbilical cord of the fetus was present at the introitus, and the placenta was trapped by a constricted cervix. For treatment, the placenta was removed by massage and 10 units of oxytocin was administered to aid in uterine contraction. The fetal gorilla had congestion and petechiation over most of its body; subsequent culturing of its tissue revealed *S. flexneri* II and β-hemolytic *Streptococcus.*

c. MYCOPLASMA AND UREAPLASMS.   *Mycoplasma* has been suggested as a cause of reproductive failure in at least three species of monkeys (Kundsin *et al.*, 1975). Six of seven talapoins (*Miopithecus talapoin*) positive for *Mycoplasma* aborted. All patas monkeys (*Erythrocebus patas*) tested were positive for *Mycoplasma,* suggesting a possible contribution of this agent to the species' high incidence of abortion and stillbirth. Although *Mycoplasma* was also identified in cynomolgus macaques, the impact on reproduction was not investigated. Ureaplasms have been reported in marmosets and chimpanzees (Furr *et al.*, 1979; Brown *et al.*, 1976). These bacteria may be responsible for reproductive failure in chimpanzees (*Pan troglodytes*), as 8 of 23 females and 4 of 22 males were infected in one colony. When impregnated, only 3 of these 8 females succeeded in producing offspring, whereas in another group of 9 pregnant females that were negative for ureaplasm, 7 had successful pregnancies (Swenson and O'Leary, 1977).

2. Leptospirosis

An occurrence of severe icterohemorrhagic leptospirosis in a breeding colony of squirrel monkeys resulted in five abortions and peracute deaths of the females (Perolat *et al.*, 1992). *Leptospira interrogans* and *L. copenhageni* were identified as the etiologic agent at necropsy. Regions of the uterine wall were transmurally infarcted with rare intranuclear inclusions. Treatment with doxycycline appeared to be successful in preventing further abortion and death in the colony. In experimental studies, leptospirosis caused mild disease in patas, rhesus, vervets, and cebus monkeys, yet produced severe disease in the squirrel monkey (Palmer *et al.*, 1987).

3. Viral Disorders

The measles virus, a member of the paramyxovirus family, is highly contagious and spreads by infected respiratory droplets. After a 10- to 14-day incubation period, a prodrome of fever and malaise emerges followed by respiratory symptoms sometimes linked to a potentially serious complication of pneumonia. This infection is associated with spontaneous abortions either as a primary cause or through secondary immunosuppression resulting in other infections (McChesney *et al.*, 1989). Endometritis and cervicitis have also been observed in measles-infected rhesus monkeys (Renne *et al.*, 1973). Newly caught wild animals are stressed from capture and transport and have not been exposed to measles virus until they come in contact with humans. This combination of stress and naive immune status can result in severe morbidity and mortality for newly captured nonhuman primates. Eleven of 80 newly received monkeys developed a rash 6–15 days after arrival. One adult female aborted and then died 9 days later of giant cell pneumonia. She had previously been anorexic and had bilateral nasal discharge. Elsewhere, 9 of 21 (43%) newly captured, measles-infected animals aborted and 3 (14%) had stillborn offspring. Three of these adult females then died of measles virus-induced giant cell pneumonia. Another outbreak of abortions in wild-caught, measles-infected rhesus monkeys was described by Hertig *et al.* (1971), and an outbreak of measles at the California Primate Research Center at the University of California at Davis, resulted in significant fetal wastage (J. A. Roberts, personal communication, 1988). Measles virus in nonhuman primates with an emphasis on pathology has been reviewed (Lowenstine, 1993).

Other viruses have been implicated as causing abortions and stillbirths in nonhuman primates. Experimentally induced rubella in rhesus monkeys caused 60% of the infected females' pregnancies to end in abortion (Parkman *et al.*, 1965). Mumps-virus has also been described as causing abortions in this species (London *et al.*, 1971; St. Geme and Van Pelt, 1974). Experimentally inoculated SIV was responsible for two stillbirths. Three of the 13 infants, seronegative for SIV at birth, also seroconverted at 9–15 months of age, demonstrating mother–infant transmission through milk (McClure *et al.,* 1991). Lymphocytic choriomeningitis virus (LCMV) has been reported to cause abortion in early infections and anomalies in later infections in the baboon, *Papio cynocephalus* (Ackermann *et al.*, 1979).

4. Nutritional Deficiencies

Nutrition exerts important influences on the course and outcome of pregnancy. Although the consequences of severe nutritional deficiency for pregnant females are well understood, the impact of marginal nutrition imbalances is less apparent.

Restriction of protein to pregnant rhesus macaques to 3% of the total energy intake results in major fetal and perinatal problms. Control females given an adequate diet gained 1.3 kg during pregnancy, but protein-deprived animals gained only 0.02 kg. One of 15 infants born to the control group died shortly after birth; however, 8 of 16 infants whose dams were on the low protein diet were stillborn or died as newborns (Kohrs *et al.*, 1979). Surprisingly the birth weight of the protein-deprived group was only 15% lower than the control group. Heart rate, respiratory rate, and ability to maintain body temperature were evaluated in the newborns from the low protein group. These newborns had difficulty maintaining their own body temperature, which is a serious and potentially lethal side effect of severe protein calorie malnutrition (Kohrs *et al.*, 1979). Another study of rhesus monkeys established that severe protein deficiency resulted in 8 abortions, 5 stillbirths, and 30 live births (Roberts *et al.*, 1974). An additional effect of protein deprivation was that the group receiving 1 g of protein per kilogram of body weight had a shorter gestation period than those given 4 g per kilogram. Other factors that influence the length of gestation include season, size of mother, and sex of the infant (Riopelle and Hale, 1975). Like the rhesus monkeys, pregnant squirrel monkeys maintained on a diet containing only 8% calories from protein had a significantly higher incidence of stillbirths and abortions (61.5%) than their counterparts fed more protein. Particularly notable was that animals on the low protein diet ate the aborted fetus and products of conception within 20 min of delivery (Manocha, 1976).

Folate coenzymes function as donors of one carbon unit in the synthesis of cellular DNA, RNA, and proteins. These processes are intimately related to cell growth and proliferation. Unfortunately, folic acid deficiency occurs in many populations and is a particular problem during pregnancy. Folate deficiency in rhesus macaques led to an increase in the number of atresic and cystic ovarian follicles with degeneration of granulosa cells, a significant impairment of proliferation kinetics of granulosa cells, and a marked prolongation of pre-DNA synthesis time (Mohanty and Das, 1982). Deficiency of folate results in megaloblastic anemia, which is characterized by the presence of hypersegmented neutrophils and oval macrocytes in the blood with megaloblastic erythroid precursors and large myeloid cells in the bone marrow. Leukopenia and thrombocytopenia may also occur in severe cases. Signs of folic acid deficiency in nonhuman primates include loss of body weight, anorexia, gingivitis, diarrhea, dehydration, alopecia, scaly dermatitis, and petechial hemorrhages on various body parts (Wixson and Griffith, 1986). The requirement for this vitamin is markedly increased during pregnancy and lactation. High mean corpuscular volume (MCV) values have been observed during pregnancy in squirrel monkeys. Supplementation of squirrel monkeys with folic acid improved their hematologic and folate status, maternal weight gain during pregnancy, and infant birth weight. An estimated 109 μg/day of total folate during pregnancy is probably needed for optimal reproduction in this species (Rasmussen *et al.*, 1980).

Trace elements, usually mineral nutrients that are required in small amounts, serve essential roles as cofactors in metabolic processes. The trace mineral that has received the greatest attention, particularly with respect to reproduction, is zinc. Zinc deficiency during pregnancy can cause teratogenesis, growth retardation, prolonged parturition, and a variety of developmental disorders (Golub et al., 1984b). Accordingly, in pregnant rhesus macaques, abortions, stillbirths, and delivery complications were more common in zinc-deficient dams. In zinc-deficient bonnet macaques (Macaca radiata), none of the matings resulted in pregnancy, and after prolonged deficiency, menstrual cycles ceased altogether (Swenerton and Hurley, 1980). A marginal deficiency of dietary zinc can produce significant abnormalities of nutritional status and has the potential for producing serious immunohematological dysfunction during pregnancy (Golub et al., 1984a). Another deficiency, vitamin A, resulted in abortion in three of eight pregnant rhesus macaques, Macaca mulatta (O'Toole et al., 1974).

The overall effects of stress during pregnancy are largely unknown, but several studies suggest a relationship between stress or anxiety of the dam and fetal distress. In an experimental study, pregnant rhesus macaqus were deliberately stressed with bright lighting for various time periods. During the period of agitation, maternal arterial blood pressure and heart rate increased markedly, probably through an increase in sympathetic activity. Uterine activity also increased in most instances. Fetal bradycardia and decreased arterial oxygenation were noted. Maternal sedation improved these fetal conditions (Morishima et al., 1978a).

It has been suggested that housing might play an important role in determining reproductive success. When housing conditions were compared, female cynomolgus macaques individually housed in large cages were more likely to have reproductive success than animals pair housed in the same sized cages or females in smaller individual cages (Boot et al., 1985).

5. Environmental Factors

Experimental results have documented the reproductive dysfunction of rhesus macaques environmentally exposed to polychlorinated biphenyl (PCB), as well as the transplacental and mammary movement of PCB and its effect on infants (Barsotti et al., 1976; Allen and Barsotti, 1976). A spontaneous outbreak of PCB toxicity in rhesus macaques arose from PCB in the concrete sealant on the floor of a corn crib enclosure (Altman et al., 1979). Toxicity was characterized by weight loss, alopecia, acne, facial edema, and diarrhea. Breeding efficiency was impaired accompanied by a high incidence of abortions and stillbirths. Live offspring were small and unthrifty, contributing to a high perinatal mortality rate.

Transfer of lead across the placenta and its potential threat to the conceptus has been recognized. High doses of lead (5 mg/

kg/body weight/day) induced abortions and death in pregnant cynomolgus macaques. Lower doses produced lesions typical of lead toxicity in the newborn (Tachon et al., 1983).

Methylmercury exposure in Macaca fascicularis has been also associated with reproductive dysfunction (Burbacher et al., 1984). All control females conceived after exposure, but only four of the seven exposed females conceived. Moreover, no control animals aborted, although two of the four exposed pregnant females aborted.

D. Complications of Pregnancy

1. Ectopic Pregnancy

Ectopic pregnancy refers to implantation of the conceptus outside the uterine cavity. Many theories about the cause of ectopic pregnancies center on delayed transport of a fertilized ova due to aberrations of tubal architecture or of transport mechanisms that may depend on the hormonal milieu. The size and location of the pregnancy are critical in determining appropriate management. Locations can be tubal, abdominal, cervical, or ovarian. Amenorrhea and abdominal pain or irregular vaginal bleeding are the most common symptoms of ectopic pregnancy. Because the signs and symptoms are nonspecific, threatened or incomplete abortion, ruptured corpus luteum, dysfunctional bleeding, adnexal torsion, endometriosis, degenerating uterine leiomyomas, and salpingitis should be included in the differential diagnosis. Ultrasound and measurement of the serum hormones, chorionic gonadotropin (CG) and progesterone, are great assets in detecting and differentiating ectopic pregnancy from other conditions, including normal pregnancy. Despite the usefulness of serial CG measurements and ultrasound identification, direct visualization by laparoscopy or laparotomy is often necessary for definitive diagnosis. Treatment involves surgical evacuation or chemotherapy aimed at arresting trophoblastic cell growth. Ectopic pregnancy has been reported in the rhesus monkey (Jerome and Hendrickx, 1982) and the squirrel monkey (McClure and Chang, 1975). The rhesus monkey presented with anorexia, weight loss, and dried blood at the vulva. Blood was also present at the external cervical os. There was a firm area in the right cranial aspect of the uterus, and the ovaries were not palpable. Laparotomy revealed a tubal pregnancy. Although there was no evidence of tubal lesions that would predispose to tubal pregnancy, an ovariohysterectomy was performed. The squirrel monkey delivered a stillborn fetus and subsequently experienced severe postpartum hemorrhage and died. A mummified fetus, consisting principally of skeletal structures, was found in the mesentary, cranial to the uterus representing an ectopic pregnancy. Hemorrhage, due to an inability of the uterus to contract, was probably the cause of death of the dam.

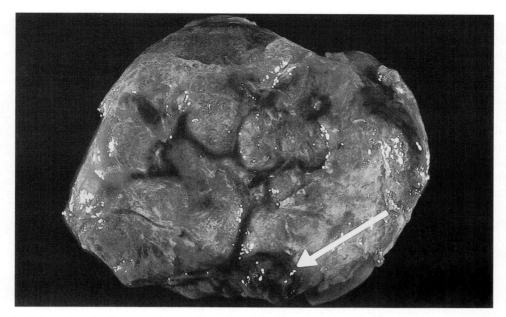

Fig. B.9. An example of placenta previa. The arrow identifies the portion of the placenta that was overlying the cervix. With each contraction, the placenta was forced into the canal. Subsequently, as the cervix dilates and the intrauterine pressure increases, the placenta becomes torn and hemorrhage ensues.

2. Mummified Fetus

A mummified fetus can be found in the abdomen or the uterus and is usually incidental to other findings. Prolonged *in utero* retention of a fetus may result from failure of fetal or maternal factors to initiate labor. An abdominal mummified fetus may result from an ovarian, tubal, or uterine pregnancy in which the fetus developed to near or full term, ruptured into the abdominal cavity, died, and became mummified and encapsulated. It may also result from a fertilized ovum that fails to transcend the uterine tubes, but instead enters the abdominal cavity, implants on the peritoneum, develops into a near- or full-term fetus, and dies. An owl monkey (*Aotus trivirgatus*) was found dead in the cage from *Klebsiella* infection that caused pneumonia. An incidental finding at necropsy was a full-term, encapsulated, abdominal mummified fetus (Bunte and Hildebrandt, 1975). Another abdominal mummified fetus was detected on routine physical examination in *Macaca assamensis*. The mass was closely attached by extensive fibrous adhesions to the ventral abdominal wall, the mesentery, the large intestine, and the left abdominal wall as well as the anterior border of the uterus by a fibrous peduncle. The probable cause was uterine rupture, subsequent fetal death, and mummification (Bosu and Barker, 1980). Two other intrauterine mummified fetuses were described in rhesus macaques (Mueller-Heubach and Batelli, 1981; Swindle *et al.,* 1981). In one, the only clinical sign was vaginal bleeding and, after removal of the fetus, the reproductive potential of the animal was considered good. In the other case, a fetus was maintained *in utero* for more than 700 days

without clinical signs before it was detected on routine examination.

3. Placenta Previa

Bleeding during the latter half of gestation can be inconsequential or signal a serious condition. Although lesions of the vagina and cervix are rarely the cause of significant bleeding late in pregnancy, polyps or invasive cervical carcinoma must be considered. The two most common causes of serious bleeding late in pregnancy, aside from abortion, are placenta previa and placental abruptio, which are potentially fatal to the mother and fetus (Pernoll, 1994).

Placenta previa is defined as implantation of the placenta in the lower uterine segment, with the placenta overlying or reaching the cervix (Fig. B.9). During late pregnancy, the lower uterine segment thins and the softening cervix begins to efface and dilate. If the placenta is implanted at the lower pole, the size and margins of the implantation site become altered by these uterine changes. Various degrees of detachment of the placenta result, and maternal bleeding occurs from the intervillous space. Blood loss may be slight or heavy and may discontinue, then recur with renewed intensity. Placenta previa can be total, partial, or marginal in position; however, all locations may be associated with life-threatening hemorrhage and do not necessarily predict different antepartum courses.

The specific etiology is usually unknown, but a number of factors may affect the location of placental implantation. These include abnormalities of endometrial vascularization, delayed ovulation, and prior trauma to the endometrium or myometrium.

The usual presentation is painless vaginal bleeding in the second half of pregnancy. Confirmation may be made with ultrasound, although placental migration confounds the traditional classification of placenta previa and may result in an inaccurate sonographic diagnosis. The earlier in pregnancy that sonography is performed, the more frequently the placenta appears to cover the cervix. Vaginal examination should be performed carefully as this may lead to profuse, even life-threatening, hemorrhage.

Once the diagnosis of placenta previa is confirmed by physical examination and sonography, management depends on the severity of the symptoms and the stage of gestation. Careful sonographic monitoring should continue. In the event the dam begins to hemorrhage, hemodynamic stability should be carefully assessed, lost blood replaced, and a cesarean section performed immediately.

Placenta previa has been reported in several species of non-human primates, including marmosets (*Callithrix jacchus*), tamarins (*Saguinus geoffroyi*) (Lunn, 1980), patas monkeys (*Erythrocebus patas*) (Wolf, 1971), orangutans (*Pongo pygmaes*) (Kingsley and Martin, 1979), and macaques (Ruch, 1959). The hallmark is variable amounts of vaginal bleeding without pain in the second to third trimesters. Vaginal examination, if possible, may reveal more blood clots and an effaced, patulous cervix. Rectal palpation may reveal a thick soft mass in the lower uterine segment. In some cases, as with the orangutan, vaginal bleeding may be intermittent for a fairly long time, but inconsequential to the animal. If placenta previa is not diagnosed and the pregnancy is allowed to proceed to term, the dam usually dies from massive hemorrhage during or after delivery.

4. Placenta Abruptio

Placenta abruptio refers to premature separation of the normally implanted placenta prior to the birth of the fetus. Etiological factors, such as short umbilical cord, uterine anomalies, trauma, and hypertension, may be responsible; however, the cause is obscure in most animals. The separation most often takes place in the third trimester, but can happen at any time. Frequently the placental separation is an acute process that increases in severity over a few hours. At other times, the episode varies from a self-limited one to one that becomes quiescent and then recurs. The placental separation may be complete, partial, or involve only the placental margin.

Separation of the placenta is initiated by bleeding into the decidua basalis. The bleeding splits the decidua and spreads beneath the placenta, shearing it off. As a hematoma forms, it causes additional separation of the placenta from the uterine wall with destruction and compression of adjacent placental tissue. Occasionally, blood extravasates into and through the myometrium to the peritoneal surface, giving the uterus a bluish color. The effects on the fetus depend mainly on the degree of disruption at the uteroplacental interface (Fig. B.10).

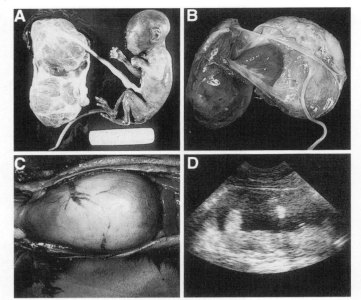

Fig. B.10. Placenta abruptio may present as acute, asymptomatic death of a pregnant female when the hemorrhage is concealed to profuse life-threatening hemorrhage. (A) and (B) Both resulted in maternal and fetal death. In both instances the blood loss occurred retroplacentally with no external hemorrhage (A) to a few drops (B). (C) Blood extravasated through the myometrium giving a blue color to the uterus. Bleeding was also concealed in this case. (D) Sonograph of a second trimester pregnant uterus indicating the marginal separation of the placenta. Careful monitoring of this animal resulted in no further evidence of separation and subsequent normal delivery of a healthy infant.

The diagnosis of placental abruption is based on clinical signs and ultrasound monitoring. Abdominal pain, pallor, uterine contractions, and uterine tenderness are primary clinical signs. Hemorrhage, however, may be visible, partially visible, or concealed. Hemorrhage may extravasate into the myometrium, into the amniotic fluid, or behind the placenta. A concealed abruption, which can be identified with ultrasound, must be differentiated from premature labor, uterine rupture, and severe preeclampsia. Visible hemorrhage during the second or third trimester must be differentiated from impending abortion, placenta previa, vaginal or cervical lacerations or polyps, cervical carcinoma, and ruptured uterus.

Placenta abrutio has been described in *Macaca mulatta* (Meyers, 1972), *M. fascicularis,* and *Saimiri scureus* (Cukierski *et al.,* 1985). Of the 21 cases in the latter review, 24% resulted in death of the dam and fetus and 52% in death of the fetus only. Approximately 75% had a history of abnormal vaginal bleeding during pregnancy and 19% had concealed hemorrage. Clinical signs were varied and included depression, pallor, little or no vaginal bleeding, and a painful abdomen. Fetal heart beats were slow and irregular, indicating distress. Of the predisposing factors, the most obvious were a thickened proliferative decidua (33%) and a history of abortions and/or abruptions (29%). Sequelae

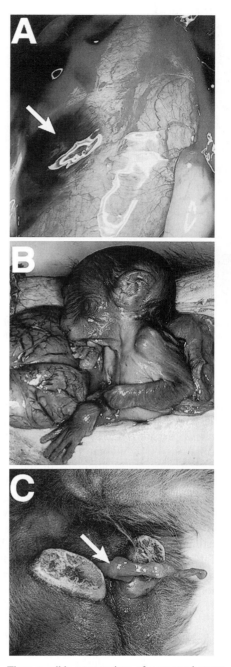

Fig. B.11. Three possible presentations of a ruptured uterus. (A) Strong evidence of a previously unrecognized uterine rupture resulting in a uterine wall defect. A common presentation is on examination of a postterm dam; there are no fetal heart sounds and the fetus is palpated free in the abdomen (B). An unusual presentation of ruptured uterus is the visualization of omentum protruding from the vulva (C).

included endometritis, hypovolemic shock, disseminated intravascular coagulation, and death (Cukierski *et al.,* 1985).

A 12-year-old multiparous lion-tailed macaque (*Macaca silensis*) suddenly became ataxic (Calle and Ensley, 1985). Phys-

ical examination revealed hypothermia, mucous membrane pallor, and a near-term fetus. The fetus was removed by hysterotomy after ultrasonic examination of the abdomen indicated its death. At the time of surgery, one-half to two-thirds of the placenta had separated from the uterus and the intervening space was occupied by a 10-cm fresh blood clot and approximately 75 ml of nonclotted blood.

Management depends on the stage of gestation and the condition of the dam and fetus. Marginal or mild degrees of premature separation can be monitored closely with frequent ultrasound examinations but no immediate intervention. Although external bleeding is typically moderate in amount, the total blood loss may be much greater. Additionally, the onset of symptoms may be gradual or abrupt with continuously progressing hemorrhage and contraction of the uterus. Greater degrees of abruption or progression require a more aggressive approach, involving stabilization of the dam and immediate surgical delivery of the fetus and placenta. Fetal distress is common. Placenta abruptio may also cause fetal brain damage secondary to hypoxia (Myers and Brann, 1976). Maternal hypotension, tachycardia, hypothermia, and oliguria indicate shock and should be aggressively managed with fluid therapy and whole blood transfusion. Postsurgically, the dam should be monitored for uterine involution, coagulopathy, and hypovolemic shock.

5. Ruptured Uterus

Spontaneous rupture of the uterus may occur before or during labor. This serious hazard to the dam usually causes the fetus to die if it is extruded into the peritoneal cavity or if maternal hypovolemia is so profound that fetal oxygenation becomes inadequate. The major cause of uterine rupture is a weakness of the uterine wall from previous surgeries or neglected, obstructed labor. Pain often, but not always, precedes the tear. Pain and shock may follow, but the pain may lessen after the rupture. Hemorrhage may be inapparent, scant, or heavy depending on the location of the rupture.

The uterus may rupture during difficult delivery of the infant and be inapparent until days later when the animal is depressed, moving slow, and, if delivery occurred, not caring for the newborn (Fig. B-11). The hallmark is abdominal adhesions to the uterus that can be easily broken down by gentle external palpation, indicating that the adhesions are recently formed. Additionally the uterus is flacid and has not involuted. A complete blood count usually indicates anemia, a high white blood cell count with a left shift, and hyperfibrinogenemia compatible with sepsis.

Treatment consists of surgical repair and aggressive antibiotic therapy after testing for sensitivity to the drug of choice. Recovery can be quick and complete, generally followed by reproductive success. In our experience it is not necessary to schedule cesarean delivery for all future pregnancies.

Uterine rupture was discovered in a common marmoset (*Callithrix jacchus*) (Lunn, 1985) that behaved normally after delivery of a single infant. Examination and routine weighing just

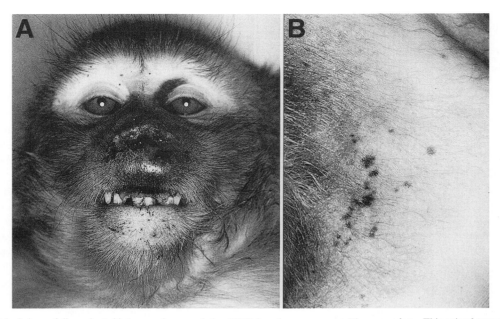

Fig. B.12. (A) Clinical signs of disseminated intravascular coagulation (DIC) in a rhesus macaque, *Macaca mulatta*. This animal presented with bruising and petechiation. Laboratory tests confirmed DIC. Note the discoloration, bruising, and thickened distorted facial features from extravasated blood. A closer look may reveal echymosis and petechiation (B).

after delivery revealed the presence of a large mass in the abdominal cavity in which a head and backbone could be identified, indicating a second infant. Subsequent surgery revealed the second infant free in the abdomen. The delivery had been effected through a circumferential tear in the posterior wall of the lower uterine segment close to the cervix. Consequently, multiple births or cephalopelvic disproportion may have been responsible for uterine rupture.

6. Coagulation Disorders

Disseminated intravascular coagulopathy (DIC) is not a distinct entity, it is a manifestation of various disease processes that have activation of intravascular clotting and fibrinolysis in common, resulting in an excess consumption of soluble coagulation components. Prolonged intrauterine fetal demise and placenta abruptio are the two leading causes of pregnancy-related DIC. Suspicious signals are excessive bleeding from surgical incision sites or from the postpartum uterus, bruising, or petechial hemorrhages (Fig. B.12). The prothrombin and partial thromboplastin times are relatively insensitive indicators of clotting status because these tests are not prolonged until 40–50% of the clotting factors have been consumed. Fibrinolytic split products and paracoagulation tests are more sensitive indicators of DIC. Treatment involves restoring circulating fluid volume, improvement in oxygen transport, and correction of coagulation disorders through transfusion of whole blood or components.

Consumption coagulopathy, associated with intrauterine fetal death, was described in the Duoc langur monkey, *Pygathrix nemaeus nemaeus* (Resnik *et al.,* 1978). Although the dam was clinically normal, the fetal skull bones overlapped, the amniotic fluid was green/brown, and radiographs of the dam demonstrated an exaggerated curvature of the spine and gas in the cardiovascular system, indicating that the fetus had been dead *in utero* for a prolonged period of time. Prothrombin and partial thromboplastin times were prolonged, and plasma protamine precipitate testing identified fibrin monomers in the blood from the mother. Table B.IV provides information on differential diagnosis for bleeding in late pregnancy (J. A. Roberts, personal communication, 1990).

7. Pregnancy-Induced Glucose Intolerance

Glucose metabolism changes during pregnancy. The major alteration is a lowering of fasting blood glucose levels, probably due to the constant drain of glucose to the uterus and developing fetus. Another major change during pregnancy is that β cells of the maternal pancreas hypertrophy and secrete two or three times as much insulin late in pregnancy as they do during the nonpregnant state. The insulin resistance of pregnancy is caused by a complex of metabolic functions carried on by the placenta, including its production of progesterone and estrogen, its alteration of cortisol dynamics, its degradation of insulin with insulinase, and its production of prolactin, placental lactogen, and growth hormone.

Clinical signs	Abortion	Moderate abruptio	Severe abruptio	Placenta previa	Uterine rupture
External hemorrhage	Mild	None to moderate	None to severe[a]	Mild to severe[b]	None to mild[c]
Pain	Slight	Moderate	Severe	None to slight	None to severe[d]
Uterine tone	Normal to increased	Increased	Hypertonic, "board like"	Normal	Normal
Fetal state	Dead	Alive but distressed	Dead or distressed	Alive	Dead or distressed
Shock	Uncommon	Frequent	Usual	Uncommon	Frequent
Coagulation disorder	Rare[e]	Occasional	Frequent	None	Rare

[a]Depends on whether the hemorrhage is concealed behind placenta, dissecting the myometrium, or breaking through to the amniotic fluid.
[b]Depends on how much the cervix is dilating and whether it is gradually or rapidly dilating.
[c]Depends on the location of the rupture; a rupture at the fundus bleeds intraabdominally whereas a lower uterine segment tear may ooze out the vagina.
[d]Pain may be severe during the buildup of pressure prior to rupture with some relief after the rupture.
[e]Coagulopathy may occur if the abortion is a result of maternal septicemia.

Gestational diabetes also affects nonhuman primates (Kessler *et al.,* 1985; Wagner *et al.,* 1992). The disease during pregnancy is usually mild and may be noted only retrospectively after delivery of a larger than normal infant or by an increase in fasting blood glucose. If this condition is suspected, intravenous glucose tolerance testing (IV-GGT) provides a definitive diagnosis. Either fasting normoglycemia or failure of the glucose levels to return to normal within 2 hr of oral glucose is indicative of gestational diabetes. In most cases of gestational diabetes, exogenous insulin is not required, and the animal reverts to normoglycemia postpartum. The hyperglycemic fetus releases large amounts of insulin, uses the glucose for energy to grow, and deposits calorie stores in glycogen and fat sites. Such a fetus becomes macrosomic. Periodic sonographic monitoring of the dam may be helpful in determining the need and timing for intervention by a cesarean section.

An aged rhesus macaque (*Macaca mulatta*) with gestational diabetes was diagnosed after a fasting blood glucose test of 151 mg/dl. One hour after the intravenous administration of glucose to assess glucose tolerance, the blood glucose was still above 200 mg/dl. The animal had a normal pregnancy, but delivered a 5-day postterm stillborn fetus weighing 840 g (normal weight range 300–600 g) (Kessler *et al.,* 1985). There was evidence of dystocia, most likely due to the size of the fetus.

8. Hypertensive Disorders

Hypertension preceding pregnancy is considered chronic hypertension whereas hypertension during pregnancy with resolution postpartum and recurrence with subsequent pregnancies is termed transient hypertension. Superimposed preeclampsia is defined as an exacerbation of hypertension, particularly when proteinuria or generalized edema develop that was not previously present (Fig. B.13).

Preeclampsia is a syndrome of pregnancy-induced hypertension accompanied by proteinuria, edema, and, frequently, disturbances in other organ systems. Abnormalities in blood pressure may range from minimal elevations to severe hypertension with multiorgan dysfunction. Hypertension in pregnancy jeopardizes the fetus because of compromised placental perfusion. Proteinuria is highly variable and usually a late sign of preeclampsia. Furthermore, the edema may be difficult to differentiate from normal physiological edema of pregnancy. Eclampsia is a more severe form of preeclampsia in which generalized seizures or coma ensue.

The etiology of preeclampsia is not known; however, the underlying abnormality involves general arteriolar constriction

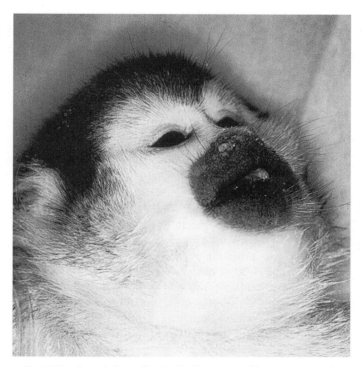

Fig. B.13. One of the earliest indications of possible preeclampsia in a breeding colony is facial edema, as depicted in this squirrel monkey, *Saimiri sciureus.* Edema may also be noted in the perineal area.

and increased vascular sensitivity to pressor hormones and ei-cosanoids, which affect many organ systems. Pregnancies complicated by preeclampsia show evidence of an inadequate maternal vascular response to placentation, including failure of normal trophoblastic invasion of the spiral arteries, which may lead to decreased placental function due to decreased blood flow, increasing the risk of placenta abruptio. Placental infarction was demonstrated as a result of preeclampsia in a patas monkey, *Erythrocebus patas* (Gille *et al.*, 1977). A gorilla diagnosed as having eclampsia had a placenta that was half the normal size and showed spotty calcifications, fibrotic areas, and infarcts (Baird, 1981).

In hypertensive animals whose malfunction is caused by a markedly increased peripheral resistance, cardiac output may decrease. The result can be pulmonary edema and congestive heart failure. Other indications include vasoconstriction and activation of the coagulation system. A selective reduction in platelet count is the most common coagulation abnormality, but hypofibrinogenemia may occur. These findings suggest that microangiopathy, not DIC, is involved in preeclampsia (Cunningham *et al.*, 1993a).

Central nervous system (CNS) changes in severe preeclampsia and eclampsia represent a form of hypertensive encephalopathy. Eclampsia, which is characterized by the onset of convulsions or other neurologic signs, appears to be restricted to the great apes. After a period of abnormal behavior and atypical postural changes, a 9-year-old multiparous gorilla (*Gorilla gorilla*) developed pedal edema and, several weeks prior to parturition, had a grand mal seizure. She was successfully treated with magnesium sulfate, delivered a healthy infant, and had no recurrence of seizure activity postpartum (Baird, 1981).

Changes in renal function include a reduced glomerular filtration rate and renal plasma flow that may progress to renal ischemia. Reduced blood flow through the kidneys is reflected in measurements of creatinine clearance. Hepatic dysfunction is evident by abnormal liver function tests and postmortem lesions.

The only definitive therapy is to deliver the fetus and the placenta. If the fetus is too immature, the alternative is palliative therapy directed primarily at reducing hypertension, which allows continuation of the pregnancy. There is little to suggest that therapy alters the underlying pathophysiology of preeclampsia. However, therapies in women that have been associated with a decrease in the progression of the disease include an intermittent administration of oral aspirin and calcium supplementation. The drug of choice to prevent seizures associated with eclampsia is magnesium sulfate. In the therapeutic range, magnesium slows neuromuscular conduction and depresses CNS irritability (Cunningham *et al.*, 1993a).

Preeclampsia, also called toxemia of pregnancy, has been reported both as a naturally occurring condition (Baird, 1981; Palmer *et al.*, 1979; Gille *et al.*, 1977; Swindle *et al.*, 1984) and as an experimentally induced model (Chez, 1976; Abitol *et al.*, 1977; Cavanagh *et al.*, 1985; Combs *et al.*, 1993) in New World

and Old World primates as well as in great apes. The condition in nonhuman primates covers the spectrum of disorders and is remarkably similar to preeclampsia in humans. Although most reports are isolated case studies, one group described 98 patas monkeys (*Erythrocebus patas*) with term pregnancies over a 1-year period; of these six developed a spontaneous disease characterized by edema, proteinuria, hypoproteinemia and hypertension (Palmer *et al.*, 1979). The highest incidence was manifested by primiparous animals, with 3 of 36 pregnancies affected. Five of the animals recovered spontaneously and were normal 14 days postpartum. Edema persisted for 30 days in one female that continued to be hypertensive and had persistent mild proteinuria and hypoproteinemia before progressing to severe renal disease. A method of monitoring fetal viability has been described and tested in a squirrel monkey with preeclampsia. The approach was to assemble a biophysical profile, including fetal heart rate and activity evaluated periodically by ultrasound, with the goal of identifying an appropriate point of intervention (J. Wimsatt, personal communication, 1987).

9. Hydronephrosis of Pregnancy

Upper ureteral dilation during pregnancy while the pelvic ureter remains normal is referred to as hydronephrosis of pregnancy. Hydronephrosis of pregnancy occurs so frequently in humans that it has been referred to as a physiologic state (Roberts and Wolf, 1971). The probable etiology is ureteral obstruction by the gravid uterus. The condition, which is not associated with decreased renal function, rapidly disappears after parturition and is assumed to be important only if it contributes to pyelonephritis of pregnancy. Bacteria entering the ureter under low pressure do not often cause pyelonephritis unless the ureter is obstructed. However, the presence of bacteria, even with partial ureteral obstruction, increases the chances of acute pyelonephritis.

Four species of nonhuman primates, *Macaca mulatta, M. arctoides, Erythrocebus patas,* and *Pan troglodytes,* were evaluated during pregnancy by means of excretory urograms and compared to those in a nonpregnant state. The roentgenograms show that, as in the human primate, significant upper ureteral dilation occurs during pregnancy (Roberts and Wolf, 1971; Roberts, 1976). As in humans, no clinical signs have been noted, and it is unknown whether there is an increased incidence of subacute pyelonephritis during pregnancy in these animals. Table B.V lists primary signs and complications of common obstetrical problems of nonhuman primates.

E. Maternal–Fetal Interactions

1. Antenatal Monitoring

Monitoring of growth and development of the conceptus is essential for the management of animals in captivity and for medical intervention, as described in Hendrickx and Dukelow

TABLE B.V
PRIMARY SIGNS AND COMPLICATIONS OF COMMON OBSTETRICAL PROBLEMS
OF NONHUMAN PRIMATES

Problem	Primary clinical signs	Complications
Ectopic pregnancy	Pain, depression, shock	Fetal death, maternal death
Placenta previa	Painless vaginal bleeding near term	Massive hemorrhage; fetal death, maternal death
Placenta abruptio	Depressed, pale; contracted uterus ± hemorrhage	Hypovolemic shock; coagulopathy; fetal death, maternal death
Ruptured uterus	Depressed, flacid uterus; recent adhesions ± hemorrhage	Septicemia, anemia; coagulopathy
Endometritis	Depressed, pyretic; poor uterine involution; leukocytosis, anemia	Peritonitis; pelvic abscess; septicemia; shock; coagulopathy; infertility
Pregnancy-induced glucose intolerance	Polyuria/polydipsia hyperglycemia; glucosuria	Macrosomic fetus; dystocia; placental insufficiency/fetal death
Preeclampsia eclampsia	Edema; hypertension; proteinuria	Placenta abruptio; coagulopathy; maternal death, fetal death

(1995b). Ultrasonic stethoscopy has been used extensively for the determination of fetal viability, distress, and placental localization. This procedure is an inexpensive, yet reliable, and convenient tool for antenatal monitoring (Mahoney and Eisele, 1976). Real time ultrasound is also invaluable for both pregnant and nonpregnant animals whenever diagnosis and interventive procedures are necessary. Readers are directed to the following references for related information (Logdberg, 1993; Pace *et al.,* 1991; Tarantal, 1990; Tarantal and Hendrickx, 1988; Brans *et al.,* 1990; Farine *et al.,* 1988; Shimizu, 1988; Nyland *et al.,* 1984).

2. Labor

Spontaneous parturition in nonhuman primates is discussed in Hendrickx and Dukelow (1995b). In a breeding colony, times of expected deliveries are usually determined through a combination of known time-mated dates, bimanual palpation of the uterus for confirmation of gestational day, and sonographic monitoring for fetal growth parameters. Intervention, either to induce labor or to perform a cesarean section, may be required if the animal does not deliver within a week of the day established for term pregnancy.

A scoring system adapted from the Bishop score in human medicine for quantitative evaluation of labor readiness in rhesus macaques has been published (Golub *et al.,* 1988). For a total

score of 10, the examiner rates cervical position, length or degree of effacement, softness, and dilation along with fetal head position. Cervical ripeness, particularly cervical dilation, is weighted in the labor-readiness index. Visual examination of the cervix with a speculum coupled with bimanual palpation provide the most information. The cervical score correlates closely with the onset of labor. However, one limitation of this technique in attempting to schedule precisely the date of induction is the variability among animals. For example, one animal progressed from a Bishop score of 3 to 7 in 2 days, whereas another animal progressed from 5 to only 7 over 24 days (Line *et al.,* 1986). Local application of prostaglandin E_2 gel leads to softening, effacement, and dilation of the cervix. Its effects were studied in pregnant Japanese macaques, *Macaca fuscata* (Shimizu *et al.,* 1994). Intracervical administration of prostaglandin E_2 gel caused cervical ripening and an increase in maternal plasma prostaglandin E_2 but no change in prostaglandin F_{2a}, demonstrating that its influence did not include induction of labor.

Induction and augmentation of labor are important tools in a breeding colony. When properly used for these purposes, oxytocin is a potent uterotonic agent that can be safe and effective. Oxytocin has two types of receptors in the uterus, and the total number of receptors increases with increasing gestational age. Because the preterm uterus is usually less sensitive to oxytocin than the term uterus, early induction of labor may require larger doses. Oxytocin affects the myometrium by increasing the strength, velocity, and frequency of contractions and by increasing intrauterine resting pressure. However, as a caution, after maximal efficiency is reached, an additional increase in oxytocin may result in excessive contraction, thereby decreasing the effectiveness of contractions and causing fetal distress.

Uterine contractions were monitored in nonhuman primates in order to detect a pattern that would predict delivery. Morgan *et al.* (1992) observed a switch of myometrial activity from low-amplitude, long-lasting, regular contractures of pregnancy to contractions. These switches, which always occurred around the onset of darkness, were repeated for several nights preceding spontaneous delivery, a pattern that clearly presaged birth.

To induce labor in an awake restrained animal (Line *et al.,* 1986), a dilute solution of oxytocin, 5 units per 100 ml in 5% dextrose solution, was administered intravenously by an infusion pump. The initial rate of oxytocin administration was 10 mU per hour and was later increased by 10 mU per hour increments at 10- to 20-min intervals to a maximum of 300 mU per hour. Once the uterine contractions are regular, oxytocin infusion is maintained at a constant rate until delivery of the infant. Maternal uterine contractions, pulse rate and blood pressure, and fetal heart rate should be monitored before and throughout oxytocin administration.

Hourly vaginal examinations are essential in monitoring the progress of birth during induced labor. Once the cervix is sufficiently dilated, rupturing the chorioamniotic membrane by grasping it with a pair of blunt forceps can hasten delivery.

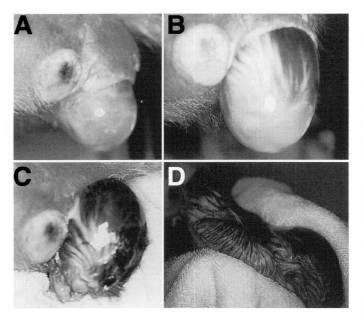

Fig. B.14. Sequence of events during normal induced labor in a rhesus macaque, *Macaca mulatta*. (A) The fetal membranes are bulging and visible at the vulva. (B) The fetal head is visible in the still intact membranes. (C) The membranes rupture and the fetal head is free. (D) The remainder of the animal is quickly delivered.

Delivery usually proceeds in approximately 1–3 hr from the time of membrane rupture (Fig. B.14). The placenta then usually passes within 15 min after delivery of the infant. At this time the infant should be monitored for respiration, heart rate, muscle tone, skin color, activity level, and temperature. If re-

quired for blood sampling, an umbilical arterial catheter can be placed at this time.

a. DYSFUNCTIONAL LABOR/DYSTOCIA.   Risks for dystocia include abnormal pelvic architecture, exceptionally large fetal size, unusual presentation or position, and dysfunctional uterine action or cervical resistance. Pelvic abnormalities may be due to traumatic fractures or metabolic bone diseases that alter the pelvic architecture, as well as soft tissue abnormalities, such as uterine masses. The size, presentation, and position of the fetus are important dystocic factors. Pelvic configuration and soft tissue masses influence fetal position and presentation. In a 35-year-old chimpanzee (*Pan troglodytes*), birth failure resulted from cervical blockage by a uterine fibroid tumor (Guilloud, 1969). New World nonhuman primates, *Saimiri* and *Callithrix,* in particular have very large offspring compared to the size of the mother (Hill, 1969). Newborn squirrel monkeys weigh an average 12% of the body weight of their mothers (Aksel and Abee, 1983). Other macrosomic fetuses, such as those resulting from gestational diabetes, hydrocephalus, fetal hydops (Cukierski *et al.,* 1986), and other disease processes, may also contribute to the incidence of dystocia. Multiple births can also predispose to position problems, resulting in dystocia (Fig. B.15)

Dystocia has been described in a De Brazza's monkey (*Cercopithecus neglectus*) (Pilkington, 1987) and in a marmoset (*Hapale jacchus*) (Hill, 1969). In the case of the marmoset, labor began in the evening but clearly was not progressing. Although a hysterotomy was attempted, the animal succumbed to shock. Two fetuses were found at postmortem. One, located in the vagina with a head presentation, had gross molding of the head that rendered the head completely misshapen. This case of dystocia resulted in a grossly distended bladder from marked

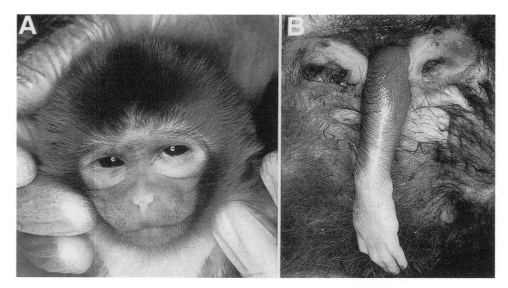

Fig. B.15.   Evidence of dystocia may be obvious (B) or circumstantial (A). The dam delivered this infant during the evening. In the morning, a bruised, swollen face indicates difficult but successful delivery.

urinary retention in the mother. The second fetus was positioned normally in the uterine cavity. Disproportion between the fetal head and the pelvic capacity or rickets from an earlier inadequate diet was assumed to be the predisposing condition. In another review, 21 of 32 monkeys with fetuses in the breech position on the day before delivery had stillbirths, but only 1 of 275 monkeys with normal cephalic presentation had a stillbirth (Cho *et al.*, 1985).

A breech birth described in a chimpanzee (*Pan troglodytes*) followed a difficult-to-detect labor whose onset was characterized only by restlessness. Subsequent labor was rapid and continuous, with the female shifting positions frequently. For delivery the female squatted as the neonate emerged legs first in tight flexion, but the full-term infant survived (Rushton and McGrew, 1980).

Pelvimetry has been developed to gain an impression of pelvic size and shape and to predict the outcome of labor in squirrel monkeys (Aksel and Abee, 1983) and cynomolgus macaques (Cho *et al.*, 1985). Comparison of pelvic outlets of the females with live born infants to those with stillbirths revealed a highly significant difference (Aksel and Abee, 1983).

Before parturition, the uterus must remain relatively quiet and the cervix firm. Within the last few weeks preceding parturition, the cervix undergoes a process of softening, effacement, and dilation. Uterine contractions increase in frequency, intensity, and coordination. In the abnormal counterpart of these events, functional uterine dystocia, one of two irregular contraction patterns occurs. A hypertonic pattern, consisting of an elevated resting pressure and contractions of increased frequency but decreased coordination, is often seen with fetal malpresentation and uterine overdistention. Hypotonic dysfunction, synchronous but weak or infrequent contractions, is more common and frequently responds to oxytocin. Alterations in myogenic control could be caused by inadequate depolarization with an impaired ionic milieu, hormonal deficiency, receptor deficiency, insufficient gap junction formation, inadequate muscle development, or lack of energy (Sokol *et al.*, 1994).

b. PRETERM LABOR.   Premature labor and delivery of a preterm, less than fully mature neonate is a clinical crisis. Labor begins when the mechanisms that produce labor override the maintenance of pregnancy. A variety of factors (maternal, placental, and fetal) may be responsible, although the specific etiology is not known. Hypertension, infection, antepartum hemorrhage, and cervical incompetence are all risk factors of preterm labor (Parsons and Spellacy, 1994).

The diagnosis of preterm labor is made when regular uterine contractions and cervical changes occur in an animal that has completed less than 85% of gestation. If there is doubt about the stage of gestation, ultrasound evaluation is effective at estimating the gestation day with a high degree of accuracy. The single most vital element for survival of the preterm infant is adequate pulmonary development. Although there are recognized differences in lung maturity and survival between male and female preterm infants of humans, this does not appear to be the case for nonhuman primates (Perelman *et al.*, 1986). When the fetus is thought to be mature but retarded in growth, amniocentesis and analysis of the lecithin–sphingomyelin ratio indicate the stage of fetal lung maturity. Additionally, glucocorticoids can be administered at specific time points during gestation to aid fetal lung development (Kotas and Kling, 1979).

Not all preterm labor is treated. If the fetus is dead or has major congenital anomalies or if the mother has medical problems such as severe preeclampsia, labor is allowed to progress. However, a tocolytic agent may be used to slow uterine contractions. The two most frequently used tocolytics are magnesium sulfate and β-mimetic drugs. High concentrations of magnesium sulfate have been shown to decrease uterine activity. Uterine relaxation caused by β-mimetic drugs increases the cyclic adenosine monophosphate concentration in the myometrial cell and causes calcium binding to the intracellular sarcoplasmic reticulum. This lowers the intracellular free calcium concentration, which in turn decreases the electrical potential of the myometrial cell. At present, several primate centers operate premature infant care centers. In these centers, evaluation techniques and treatment modes are being developed and much experience has been gained in the support of the preterm nonhuman primate.

3. Aspiration Distress

The transition from an intrauterine to an independent existence is hazardous. The vulnerability of the newborn exceeds that at any other point in life. Spontaneous gross and microscopic lesions were studied at autopsy in 82 perinatal and neonatal monkeys of various species. The site at greatest risk was the respiratory system. Differences in the type and distribution of lesions in the various systems were found between premature and mature infants (Anver *et al.*, 1973). Of these 82 neonatal deaths, 43 were caused by inflammatory diseases: mainly pneumonia, intrauterine distress, and trauma. Intrauterine distress and antepartum death with maceration were more common causes of death in premature infants; trauma and inflammatory disease occurred more often in mature infants (Price *et al.*, 1973). Aspiration of amniotic fluid and meconium causing and/or indicating fetal distress has been reported in newborn infants (Kosanke *et al.*, 1980; Block *et al.*, 1981).

Prematurity and perinatal mortality in the rhesus macaque were evaluated in relationship to birth weight and gestational age (Shaughnessy *et al.*, 1978). Results showed that gestational age was as important as birth weight in determining perinatal mortality. In another study, postnatal growth and skeletal maturation of experimental preterm macaques (*Macaca nemestrina*) were followed to assess the long-term sequelae of low birth weight and preterm birth. At cesarean section, the animals were of normal size and maturation for gestational age; however, skeletal maturation was delayed and required about 1 month to achieve the standard (Newell-Morris *et al.*, 1991).

4. Umbilical Cord Complications

Large variations in umbilical cord length are common. A short cord may cause complications in labor, such as interference with the descent of the fetus, premature separation of the placenta, inversion of the uterus, or cord rupture. A cord that is longer than average is likely to coil around fetal parts or prolapse through the birth canal, resulting in fetal asphyxia due to umbilical cord compression (Myers, 1971, 1975).

Loose umbilical cord knots are relatively common but a true knot, which is uncommon, may obstruct fetal circulation. The cord may differ in diameter and color on either side of a true knot, and thromboses within the adjacent umbilical cord and contiguous placental vessels are evidence of a true knot. A knotted umbilical cord of this kind was identified as the cause of death in an African green monkey (*Cercopithecus aethiops*) aborted during the third trimester (Brady, 1983). The maternal side of the cord was engorged, whereas the fetal side was devoid of blood. In such situations, unless the fetus is monitored throughout the labor, cord problems are difficult to detect. If fetal distress is detected for any reason, an immediate cesarean section is essential.

5. Erythroblastosis Fetalis

Erythroblastosis fetalis, which is a hemolytic disease of the newborn, is caused by an incompatibility between fetal and maternal blood. Maternal antibodies are formed against incompatible fetal blood, which often enters the maternal circulation during pregnancy and in the immediate postpartum period. Amniocentesis, placenta previa, placenta abruptio, trauma, multiple pregnancy, and cesarean section are factors that increase the risk of transplacental transfer of fetal red blood cells.

In the fetus, red blood cell destruction leads to anemia and ultimately erythroblastosis fetalis, which is characterized by heart failure, edema, ascites, pericardial effusion, and extramedullary hematopoiesis.

The severe anemia is associated with tissue hypoxia and acidosis. Extensive liver erythropoiesis replaces normal hepatic parenchyma and there is architectural distortion. Consequences include a decrease in protein production, portal hypertension, ascites, and generalized anasarca. Management depends on the severity of disease. Generally, a cesarean delivery is scheduled as early as possible, and support in the form of transfusions for the neonate is anticipated (Cunningham *et al.,* 1993b).

Naturally occurring transplacental immunization, caused by maternal–fetal blood group incompatibility in orangutans (*Pongo pygmaeus*), has been reported (van Foreest and Socha, 1981). Of the four pregnancies of one female orangutan, the first two resulted in normal births with subsequent normal development. The third offspring, although considered a normal term infant, died 10 days later. At necropsy, generalized anemia and jaundice constituted the principal findings. Microscopically, foci of extramedullary erythropoiesis were found in the liver, spleen, and lungs, suggesting immunologically mediated intravascular hemolysis. During the next pregnancy, when sera from the dam were tested to detect early symptoms of transplacental immunization, potent agglutinating antibodies directed against the red cells of the breeding mate of the female were present. Monitoring revealed a slow, steady rise in antibody titer. Immediately after a natural delivery, examination of the infant revealed severe anemia with marked jaundice, thrombocytopenia, normoblastosis, and quickly rising bilirubin levels. The infant was transfused with thoroughly washed maternal red cells, considered *a priori* to be compatible with the infant, and suspended in the serum from the father. The infant then recovered uneventfully.

A similar incident of erythroblastosis fetalis was reported in a tamarin, *Tamarinus nigricollis* (Gengozian *et al.,* 1966). Naturally occurring hemolytic disease of newborns in this species is of particular interest, as these primates frequently bear fraternal twins whose placental vascular anastomoses result in fetal hematopoietic chimerism (Gengozian, 1972, 1983). Both reports suggest that transplacental maternal–fetal incompatibility leading to perinatal death may constitute an important cause of fetal waste seen in New World monkey and Great Ape breeding colonies.

Although erythroblastosis fetalis represents a significant risk for successful management of pregnancy, species appear to differ in sensitivity to this condition. Great apes and marmosets appear to be more sensitive than rhesus and cynomolgus macaques and at least one species of baboon, *Papio hamadryas* (Wiener *et al.,* 1975, 1977). Socha (1993) has reviewed the literature, clinical presentation, and pathology of erythroblastosis fetalis in nonhuman primates.

VII. GENITAL SYSTEM: MALE

A. Introduction

An effective breeding program requires identification of those animals that are fertile and reproductively sound. Fertility is particularly important in males as most breeding colonies use fewer male breeders than female breeders. A ratio of 1 male to 10 females is not uncommon. Given these practices, 1 infertile male can have a tremendous impact on a breeding program. Lack of reproduction usually refers to inappropriate social interaction and copulatory behavior, whereas infertility implies a physiological problem. It is important to distinguish between the two because treatment is vastly different even if the mutual outcome is lack of offspring. Diagnosis and treatment of infertility in great apes have been reviewed (Gould, 1983).

B. Examination

A history of the clinical and behavioral background of the animal is important information in defining reproductive poten-

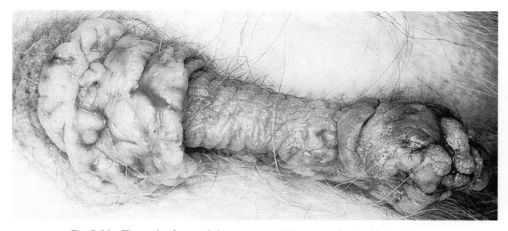

Fig. B.16.   The penis of an aged rhesus macaque (*Macaca mulatta*) with genital warts.

tial. As with females, knowing the background of reproductive and behavioral parameters, endocrine levels (Hendrickx and Dukelow, 1995ab), and possible environmental influences (Chik *et al.,* 1992) of males is essential.

If a male is behaving as expected, including copulation with intromission and ejaculation, yet no offspring are forthcoming, a complete physical examination, including all organ systems, is in order. Testicular atrophy was reported in a gorilla (*Gorilla gorilla*) associated with cardiopathy, neuropathy, and hemosiderosis, probably secondary to a nutritional disease (Steiner *et al.,* 1955). In another case, erectile failure in a cynomolgus monkey secondary to atherosclerosis of the penile artery was reported (Adams *et al.,* 1984). A thorough physical examination includes inspection of the male genital tract, including the penis, scrotum, testes, epididymis, and prostate. Particularly critical conditions to note include neoplastic or inflammatory lesions of the penis, prepuce or testicle, hematocele and varicocele, inguinal hernias, spermatic cord, and accessory gland abnormalities.

Seasonal variation in the reproductive cycle occurs in a number of species of prosimian, New and Old World primates. Although spermatogenesis may occur throughout the year, seasonal variations in sexual activity, believed to be controlled by accessory sex glands, are not unusual (Hendrickx and Dukelow, 1995a). The regressive phase of the normal, seasonal spermatogenic cycle of squirrel monkeys and rhesus monkeys must be differentiated from pathologic events that could lead to arrested spermatogenesis. Among the pathologic possibilities are cryptorchidism, hypopituitarism, estrogen-secreting neoplasms, malnutrition, obstruction of the vas deferens, and certain genetic disorders. Indirect therapy may involve eliminating stress, which affects the hypothalamic pituitary axis; improving nutrition; reaching and maintaining an ideal body weight; or identifying other nonspecific causes of arrested spermatogenesis. Hunt *et al.* (1993) have reviewed arrested spermatogenesis in *Aotus, Saimiri,* and *Macaca.*

An assessment of semen quality, including morphology, mobility, numbers of sperm, and volume of ejaculate, is important in assessing spermatogenesis and accessory gland function (Schaffer *et al.,* 1992; Valerio, 1970). Methods of obtaining samples vary from massage to electroejaculation (Bornman *et al.,* 1987; Gould and Mann, 1988). When these values 611072prove to be abnormal, a testicular biopsy described by Foster and Rowley (1982) may be helpful in identifying the stage of spermatogenesis interruption.

The measurement of gonadal and pituitary hormone levels may identify hypergonadotropic, normogonadoropic, or hypogonadism with implications for treatment. Finally, infertility may be associated with infectious agents. *Chlamydia trachomatis* caused epididymitis and urethritis in African green monkeys, *Cercopiethecus aethiops* (Moller and Mardh, 1980). Keeling (1982) reviewed agents potentially infectious for male great apes. Treatment with an appropriate antibiotic, based on culture and sensitivity, is important for primary bacterial infections and for preventing secondary infections. It is important to select an antibiotic that attains a high concentration in the prostate, seminal vesicles, testicles, or other target location.

C. Disorders and Diseases

1. Penis

The penis is affected by both bacterial and viral agents as well as by neoplasia and developmental or traumatic problems (Fig. B.16). An example is natural genital herpesvirus hominis type 2, isolated from pustulovesicular lesions on the external genitalia of two chimpanzees (McClure *et al.,* 1980). Typical herpetic changes that included necrosis, superficial ulceration, acute inflammatory cell infiltration, multinucleated syncytial giant cells, and intranuclear inclusions were noted. Another herpesvirus, simian agent 8, was identified in a colony of baboons, *Papio cynocephalus.* The lesions consisted of vesicles, ulcers,

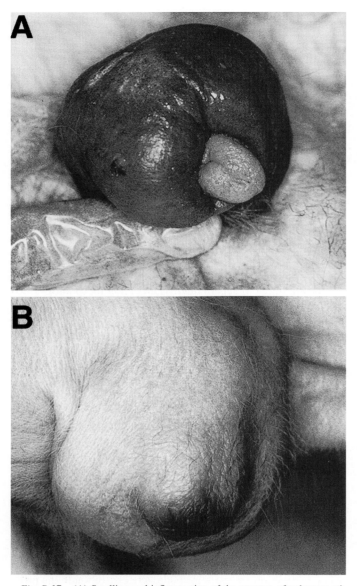

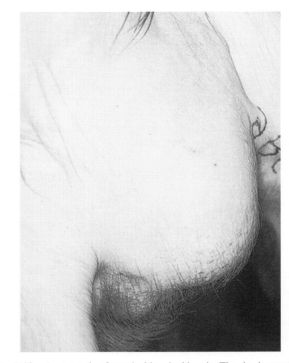

Fig. B.18. An example of a typical inguinal hernia. The size is noted in the health record of the animal, and the hernia is examined periodically for progression. The hernia will not be repaired unless it becomes progressively larger or there is evidence of a problem.

Fig. B.17. (A) Swelling and inflammation of the prepuce of unknown etiology. (B) Stricture in a weanling animal. The prepuce was noted to be swollen and erythematous. The stricture, which was corrected surgically, had contracted, causing difficulty in urination.

that the urethral meatus is located on the ventral surface of the penis, or perineum. A defect in embryonic development appears to be the cause. If the urethral meatus is located just proximal to the glans, it is referred to as glandular hypospadia; if it is on the penile shaft, it is termed penile hypospadia. A midshaft penile hypospadia was identified in an otherwise normal adult male rhesus macaque (Harrison, 1976).

2. Prepuce

The prepuce is a cutaneous fold over the glans penis. The fold or pocket, which can hold bacteria or viruses, is important in the transmission of venereal diseases. In addition, this tender skin can be torn or become inflamed (Fig. B.17A). Treatment is directed at removing the underlying cause while medicating the sites of inflammation and edema.

Phimosis is defined as tightness of the foreskin so that it cannot be drawn back over the glans. Phimosis has been observed in macaques, primarily young juveniles and occasionally infants, which usually resolves with age. In juveniles, it probably results from self-trauma either primary or secondary to an underlying infection. The prepuce is reddened, somewhat ulcerated, and contracted down through a combination of scar formation and adhesions (Fig. B.17B). If severe, it may result in incontinence and subsequent urine scald. Treatment involves

and pustules on the penis and prepuce. Transmission was consistent with the presence of a venereal disease (Levin *et al.,* 1988). Mycoplasmas and ureaplasms have also been isolated from chimpanzees and have been implicated in reproductive failure (Furr *et al.,* 1979; Swenson and O'Leary, 1977).

A squamous cell carcinoma with lymphatic metastasis was reported in a rhesus monkey (Hubbard *et al.,* 1983). Beniashvili (1989, 1995) has provided an extensive review of tumors of the male genital system.

Hypospadia is a congenital condition in which the urogenital sinus fails to complete its normal configuration. The result is surgically breaking down the adhesions and resecting the prepuce. Antibiotic therapy is helpful in preventing recurrence.

3. Testicles

Cryptorchidism refers to unilateral or bilateral undescended testes. Cryptorchidism may be associated with a decreased fertility rate in some species of nonhuman primates due to the temperature gradient; however, many species of nonhuman primates have retractable testes and carry them in the inguinal region much of the time. Cryptorchidism has been reported in a number of nonhuman primates, including three gibbons (*Hylobates lar*) and one proboscis monkey (*Nasalis larvatus*) (Ruch, 1959).

Like humans, these animals are subject to testicular tumors. An example is an adult male *Aotus nancymae* with a swollen left testicle that did not respond to antibiotic therapy. Subsequently, a mass that enlarged the testicle to about 2.5 times the normal size was removed surgically (Gozalo *et al.,* 1992). Although seminomas like this can be deadly in men, they apparently spread more slowly in the *Aotus*. Seminomas have also been reported in a howler monkey, *Alouatta caraya* (Maruffo and Malinow, 1966).

A testicular ademoma has been reported in the western lowland gorilla (*Gorilla gorilla*) (Jones *et al.,* 1980), and a malignant Leydig cell tumor was also described at this site (Brack, 1988).

4. Scrotum

Two relatively common conditions of older, overweight male macaques are inguinal hernia and scrotal edema. The inguinal hernia is usually of no consequence, but should be monitored. If it appears to be increasing in size, surgical reduction is required to prevent the necrosis of incarcerated omentum or prolapse and strangulation of the intestine (Fig. B.18). Although the cause of scrotal edema is not known, theoretically the normal posture of a macaque in a breeding cage coupled with the pressure of a large abdomen could result in venous congestion that eventually develops into dependent scrotal edema. The condition is usually intermittant, and the animals do not appear to be uncomfortable or to undergo any abnormality of hematological values.

5. Glands

The normal anatomy and selected pathological lesions of the prostate of nonhuman primates have been reported (Lewis *et al.,* 1981). In addition, experimental studies of prostatitis in nonhuman primates have provided information on bacterial adherence (Dilworth *et al.,* 1990) and ascending prostatitis (Neal *et al.,* 1990). Neoplastic and glandular growths of the prostate reported in the literature are a benign prostatic adenoma in *Lemur catta* and glandular hyperplasia in rhesus macaques and

squirrel monkeys (Roberts, 1972; Adams and Bond, 1979). Carcinoma of the prostate was reported in an aged rhesus macaque (Engle and Stout, 1940).

Although changes in male mammary glands are uncommon, a male was identified with gynecomastia, galactorrhea, and reddening of the sex skin. A spontaneous metastatic carcinoma was identified in this 6-year-old male rhesus macaque (Ringler and Abrams, 1972). The animal exhibited these signs for 6–8 weeks preceding other clinical signs. At necropsy, the origin of the tumor could not be identified. The histologic character of the neoplastic masses and nodules in the adrenal cortex, kidney, and liver of this animal suggested that any one could have been primary and could have contributed to abnormal hormone production resulting in mammary gland changes. Hormone production by neoplastic tissue is often the first indication of an occult carcinoma.

REFERENCES

Abee, C. R., and Aksel, S. (1983). Hysterosalpinography: A technique to aid in assessment of reproductive fitness of female squirrel monkeys (*Saimiri sciureus*). *Lab. Anim. Sci.* **33,** 593–596.

Abitbol, M. M., Ober, W. B., Gallo, G. R., Driscoll, S. G., and Pirani, C. L. (1977). Experimental toxemia of pregnancy in the monkey, with a preliminary report on renin and aldosterone. *Am. J. Pathol.* **86,** 573–590.

Ackermann, R., Kalter, S. S., Heberling, R. L., McCullough, B., Eichberg, J., and Rodriguez, A. R. (1979). Fetal infection of the baboon (*Papio cynocephalus*) with lymphocytic choriomeningitis virus. *Arch. Virol.* **60,** 311–323.

Adams, M. R., and Bond, M. G. (1979). Benign prostatic hyperplasia in a squirrel monkey *Saimiri sciureus. Lab. Anim. Sci.* **29,** 674–676.

Adams, M. R., Kaplan, J. R., Koritnik, D. R., Weaver, D. S., and Bond, M. G. (1984). Erectile failure in cynomolgus monkeys with atherosclerosis of the arteries supplying the penis. *J. Urol.* **131,** 571–573.

Adams, R. J., Rock, J. A., Swindle, M. M., Garnett, N. L., and Porter, W. P. (1985). Surgical correction of genital prolapse in three rhesus monkeys. *Lab. Anim. Sci.* **35,** 405–408.

Aksel, S., and Abee, C. R. (1983). A pelvimetry method for predicting perinatal mortality in pregnant squirrel monkeys (*Saimiri sciureus*). *Lab. Anim. Sci.* **33,** 165–167.

Allen, J. R., and Barsotti, D. A. (1976). The effects of transplacental and mammary movement of PCBs on infant rhesus monkeys. *Toxicology* **6,** 331–340.

Altman, N. H., New, A. E., McConnell, E. E., and Ferrell, T. L. (1979). A spontaneous outbreak of polychlorinated biphenyl (PCB) toxicity in rhesus monkeys (*Macaca mulatta*): Clinical observations. *Lab. Anim. Sci.* **29,** 661–665.

Ami, Y., Suzaki, Y., and Goto, N. (1993). Endometriosis in cynomolgus monkeys retired from breeding. *J. Vet. Med. Sci.* **55,** 7–11.

Anderson, D. C., and McClure, H. M. (1993). Listeriosis. *In* "Monographs of the Pathology of Laboratory Animals: Nonhuman Primates" (T. C. Jones, U. Mohr, and R. D. Hunt, eds.), Vol. 1, pp. 135–141. Springer-Verlag, Berlin and New York.

Andrews, E. J. (1971). Spontaneous abortions in *Macaca mulatta.* (Letter). *Lab. Anim. Sci.* **21,** 964.

Anver, M. R., Hunt, R. D., and Price, R. A. (1973). Simian neonatology. II. Neonatal pathology. *Vet. Pathol.* **10,** 16–36.

Baggs, R. B., Hunt, R. D., Garcia, F. G., Hajema, E. M., Blake, B. J., and Fraser, C. E. O. (1976). Pseudotuberculosis (*Yersinia enterocolitica*) in the owl monkey (*Aotus trivirgatus*). *Lab. Anim. Sci.* **26,** 1079–1083.

Baird, J. N. (1981). Eclampsia in a lowland gorilla. *Am. J. Obstet. Gynecol.* **141**, 345–346.

Barsotti, D. A., Marlar, R. J., and Allen, J. R. (1976). Reproductive dysfunction in rhesus monkeys exposed to low levels of polychlorinated biphenyls (Aroclor 1248). *Food Cosmet. Toxicol.* **14**, 99–103.

Baskin, G. B., Soike, K., Jirge, S. K., and Wolf, R. W. (1980). Ovarian teratoma in an African green monkey (*Cercopithecus aethiops*). *Vet. Pathol.* **19**(2), 219–221.

Beniashvili, D. Sh. (1989). An overview of the world literature on spontaneous tumors in nonhuman primates. *J. Med. Primatol.* **18**, 423–437.

Beniashvili, D. Sh. (1995). Tumors of the genitorurinary system. *In* "Experimental Tumors in Monkeys," pp. 87–113. CRC Press, Boca Raton, FL.

Benirschke, K. (1983). Chorioamnionitis as cause of abortion in orang-utan (*Pongo pygmaeus abeli*). *J. Zoo Anim. Med.* **14**, 56–60.

Bertens, A. P. M. G., Helmond, F. A., and Hein, P. R. (1982). Endometriosis in rhesus monkeys. *Lab. Anim.* **16**, 281–284.

Binhazim, A. A., Chapman, W. L., and Isaac, W. (1989). Multiple spontaneous lesions in an aged spider monkey. *Lab. Anim. Sci.* **39**, 355–357.

Block, M. F., Kallenberger, D. A., Kert, J. D., and Nerveux, R. D. (1981). *In utero* meconium aspiration by the baboon fetus. *Obstet. Gynecol.* **57**, 37–40.

Boot, R., Leussink, A. B., and Vlug, R. F. (1985). Influence of housing conditions on pregnancy outcome in cynomolgus monkeys (*Macaca fascicularis*). *Lab. Anim.* **19**, 42–47.

Bornman, M. S., van Vuuren, M., Meltzer, D. G. A., van der Merwe, C. A., and Rensburg, S. J. (1987). Quality of semen obtained by electroejaculation from chacma baboons (*Papio ursinus*). *J. Med. Primatol.* **17**, 57–61.

Bosu, W. T. K., and Barker, I. K. (1980). An abdominal mummified fetus in a *Macaca assamensis*. *J. Med. Primatol.* **9**, 71–75.

Brack, M. (1988). Malignant Leydig cell tumour in a *Tupaia belangeri*: Case report and literature review of male genital tumours in nonhuman primates. *Lab. Anim.* **22**(2), 131–134.

Brady, A. G. (1983). Knotted umbilical cord as a cause of death in a *Cercopithecus aethiops* fetus. *Lab. Anim. Sci.* **33**, 375–376.

Brans, Y. W., Kuehl, T. J., Hayashi, R. H., and Reyes, P. (1990). Maternal blood pressure and fetal ultrasonography in normal baboon pregnancies. *J. Med. Primatol.* **19**, 641–649.

Brown, R. J., and Kupper, J. L. (1972). Parovarian cysts (hydatid cyst of Morgagni) in a squirrel monkey (*Saimiri sciureus*). *Lab. Anim. Sci.* **22**, 741–742.

Brown, W. J., Jacobs, N. F., Arum, E. S., and Arko, R. J. (1976). T-strain mycoplasma in the chimpanzee. *Lab. Anim. Sci.* **26**, 81–83.

Brumsted, J. R., and Riddick, D. H. (1994). Menstruation and disorders of menstrual function *In* "Danforth's Obstetrics and Gynecology" (J. R. Scott, P. J. DiSaia, C. B. Hammond, and W. N. Spellacy, eds.), 7th ed., pp. 665–680. Lippincott, Philadelphia.

Buhles, W. C., Vanderlip, J. E., Russell, S. W., and Alexander, N. L. (1981). *Yersinia pseudotuberculosis* infection: Study of an epizootic in squirrel monkeys. *J. Clin. Microbiol.* **13**, 519–525.

Bunte, R. M., and Hildebrandt, P. K. (1975). Abdominal mummified fetus in an owl monkey. *J. Am. Vet. Med. Assoc.* **167**, 667–668.

Bunton, T. E. (1986). Incidental lesions in nonhuman primate placentae. *Vet. Pathol.* **23**, 431–438.

Bunton, T. E., and Lollini, L. (1983). Ovarian adenocarcinoma in a bonnet monkey: Histologic and ultrastructural features. *J. Med. Primatol.* **12**, 106–111.

Burbacher, T. M., Monnett, C., Grant, K. S., and Mottet, N. K. (1984). Methylmercury exposure and reproductive dysfunction in the nonhuman primate. *Toxicol. Appl. Pharmacol.* **75**, 18–24.

Butler, H. (1970). Septic abortion in the Senegal bush baby (*Galago senegalensis senegalensis*). *Folia Primatol.* **13**, 207–212.

Calle, P. P., and Ensley, P. K. (1985). Abruptio placentae in a lion-tailed macaque. *J. Am. Vet. Med. Assoc.* **187**, 1275–1276.

Cambre, R. C., Wilson, H. L., Spraker, T. R., and Favara, B. E. (1980). Fatal airsacculitis and pneumonia, with abortion, in an orangutan. *J. Am. Vet. Med. Assoc.* **177**, 822–824.

Cappuccio, A. L., Patton, D. L., Kuo, C.-c., and Campbell, L. A. (1994). Detection of *Chlamydia trachomatis* deoxyribonucleic acid in monkey models (*Macaca nemestrina*) of salpingitis by in situ hybridization: Implications for pathogenesis. *Am. J. Obstet. Gynecol.* **171**, 102–110.

Cavanagh, D., Rao, P. S., Knuppel, R. A., Desai, U., and Balis, J. U. (1985). Pregnancy-induced hypertension: Development of a model in the pregnant primate (*Papio anubis*). *Am. J. Obstet. Gynecol.* **151**, 987–999.

Chalifoux, L. V. (1993a). Ovarian teratoma, *Macaca mulatta*. *In* "Monographs on the Pathology of Laboratory Animals: Nonhuman Primates" (T. C. Jones, U. Mohr, and R. D. Hunt, eds.), Vol. 2, pp. 151–154. Springer-Verlag, Berlin and New York.

Chalifoux, L. V. (1993b). Endometrial adenocarcinoma, squirrel monkey. *In* "Monographs on the Pathology of Laboratory Animals: Nonhuman Primates" (T. C. Jones, U. Mohr, and R. D. Hunt, eds.), Vol. 2, pp. 161–164. Springer-Verlag, Berlin and New York.

Chez, R. A. (1976). Nonhuman primate models of toxemia of pregnancy. *Prospect Nephrol. Hypertens.* **5**, 421–424.

Chik, C. L., Almeida, O. F. X., Libre, E. A., Booth, J. D., Renquist, D., and Merriam, G. R. (1992). Photoperiod driven changes in reproductive function in male rhesus monkeys. *J. Clin. Endocrinol. Metab.* **74**, 1068–1074.

Cho, F., Hanari, K., Suzuki, M. T., and Honjo, S. (1985). Relationship between fetal position and stillbirth in the cynomolgus monkeys (*Macaca fascicularis*): Retrospective analysis. *J. Med. Primatol.* **14**, 169–174.

Combs, C. A., Katz, M. A., Kitzmiller, J. L., and Brescia, R. J. (1993). Experimental preeclampsia produced by chronic constriction of the lower aorta: Validation with longitudinal blood pressure measurements in conscious rhesus monkeys. *Am. J. Obstet. Gynecol.* **169**, 215–223.

Conrad, S. H., Sackett, G. P., and Burbacher, T. M. (1989). Diagnosis of early pregnancy by ultrasound in *Macaca fascicularis*. *J. Med. Primatol.* **18**, 143–154.

Cukierski, M. A., Anderson, J. H., and Ford, E. W. (1985). Premature separation of the normally implanted placenta (abruptio placentae) in nonhuman primates. *Abstr., In. Anat. Cong., 12th,* London.

Cukierski, M. A., Tarantal, A. F., and Hendrickx, A. G. (1986). A case of nonimmune hydrops fetalis with a rare cardiac anomaly in the rhesus monkey. *J. Med. Primatol.* **15**, 227–234.

Cunningham, F. G., MacDonald, P. C., Grant, N. F., Levino, K. J., and Gilstrap, L. C. (1993a). Hypertensive disorders of pregnancy. *In* "Williams Obstetrics," 19th ed., pp. 763–817. Appleton & Lange, Norwalk, CT.

Cunningham, F. G., MacDonald, P. C., Grant, N. F., Levino, K. J., and Gilstrap, L. C. (1993b). Disease and injuries of the fetus and newborn infant. *In* "Williams Obstetrics," 19th ed., pp. 1010–1029. Appleton & Lange, Norwalk, CT.

DaRif, C. A., Parker, R. F., and Schoeb, T. R. (1984). Endometriosis with bacterial peritonitis in a baboon. *Lab. Anim. Sci.* **34**, 491–493.

Davis, R. H., and Schneider, H. P. (1975). Cast of the Z shaped cervical canal of the uterus of the rhesus monkey. *Lab. Anim. Sci.* **25**, 506.

Diamond, E. J., Aksel, S., Hazelton, J. M., Barnet, S. B., Williams, L. E., and Abee, C. R. (1985). Serum hormone patterns during abortion in the Bolivian squirrel monkey. *Lab. Anim. Sci.* **35**, 619–623.

DiGiacomo, R. F. (1977). Gynecologic pathology in the rhesus monkey (*Macaca mulatta*). II. Findings in laboratory and free-ranging monkeys. *Vet. Pathol.* **14**, 539–546.

DiGiacomo, R. F., Hooks, J. J., Sulima, M. P., Gibbs, C. J., and Gajdusek, D. C. (1977). Pelvic endometriosis and simian foamy virus infection in pig-tailed macaque. *J. Am. Vet. Med. Assoc.* **171**, 859–861.

Dilworth, J. P., Neal, D. E., Fussell, E. N., and Roberts, J. A. (1990). I. Experimental prostatitis in nonhuman primates: Bacterial adherence in the urethra. *Prostate* **17**, 227–231.

Doyle, L., Young, C. L., Jang, S. S., and Hillier, S. L. (1991). Normal vaginal aerobic and anaerobic bacterial flora of the rhesus macaque (*Macaca mulatta*). *J. Med. Primatol.* **20**, 409–413.

Engle, E. T., and Stout, A. P. (1940). Spontaneous primary carcinoma of the prostate in a monkey (*Macaca mulatta*). *Am. J. Cancer* **39**, 334–337.

Eydelloth, R. S., and Swindle, M. M. (1983). Intraductal mammary carcinoma and benign ovarian teratoma in a rhesus monkey. *J. Med. Primatol.* **12**, 101–105.

Fanton, J. W., and Golden, J. G. (1991). Radiation-induced endometriosis in *Macaca mulatta*. *Radiat. Res.* **126**, 141–146.

Fanton, J. W., and Hubbard, G. B. (1983). Spontaneous endometriosis in a cynomolgus monkey (*Macaca fascicularis*). *Lab. Anim. Sci.* **33**, 597–599.

Fanton, J. W., Hubbard, G. B., and Wood, D. H. (1986a). Endometriosis: Clinical and pathologic findings in 70 rhesus monkeys. *Am. J. Vet. Res.* **47**, 1537–1541.

Fanton, J. W., Yochmowitz, M. G., Wood, D. H., and Salmon, Y. L. (1986b). Surgical treatment of endometriosis in 50 rhesus monkeys. *Am. J. Vet. Res.* **47**, 1602–1604.

Farine, D., MacCarter, G. D., Timor-Tritch, I. E., Yeh, M.-N., and Stark, R. I. (1988). Real-time ultrasonic evaluation of the baboon pregnancy: Biometric measurements. *J. Med. Primatol.* **17**, 215–221.

Felsburg, P. J., Heberling, R. L., Brack, M., and Kalter, S. S. (1973). Experimental genital herpes infection of the marmoset. *J. Med. Primatol.* **2**, 50–60.

Folse, D. S., and Stout, L. C. (1978). Endometriosis in a baboon (*Papio doguera*). *Lab. Anim. Sci.* **28**, 217–219.

Foster, J. W., and Rowley, M. J. (1982). Testicular biopsy in the study of gorilla infertility. *Am. J. Primatol, Suppl.* **1**, 121–125.

Foster, W. G., Stals, S. I., and McMahon, A. (1992). A prospective analysis of endometrial cycle changes by ultrasound in the female cynomolgus monkey. *J. Med. Primatol.* **21**, 30–34.

Fox, J. G., and Frost, W. W. (1974). *Corynebacterium ulcerans* mastitis in a bonnet macaque (*Macaca radiata*). *Lab. Anim. Sci.* **24**, 820–822.

Furr, P. M., Hetherington, C. M., and Taylor-Robinson, D. (1979). Ureaplasmas in the marmoset (*Callithrix jacchus*): Transmission and elimination. *J. Med. Primatol.* **8**, 321–326.

Gengozian, N. (1972). A blood factor in marmosets, *Sanguinus fuscicollis*. Its detection, mode of inheritance and species specificity. *J. Med. Primatol.* **1**, 272–286.

Gengozian, N. (1983). The marmoset as a model for clinical and basic immunology. *In* "Monographs in Primatology" (S. S. Kalter, ed.), Vol. 2, pp. 173–187. Liss, New York.

Gengozian, N., Lushbaugh, C. C., Humason, G. L., and Kniseley, R. M. (1966). 'Erythroblastosis foetalis' in the primate, *Tamarinus nigricollis*. *Nature (London)* **209**, 731–732.

Gille, J. H., Moore, D. G., and Sedgwick, C. J. (1977). Placental infarction: A sign of preeclampsia in a patas monkey (*Erythrocebus patas*). *Lab. Anim. Sci.* **27**, 119–121.

Golub, M. S., Gershwin, M. E., Hurley, L. S., Baly, D. L., and Hendrickx, A. G. (1984a). Studies of marginal zinc deprivation in rhesus monkeys. I. Influence on pregnant dams. *Am. J. Clin. Nutr.* **39**, 265–280.

Golub, M. S., Gershwin, M. E., Hurley, L. S., Baly, D. L., and Hendrickx, A. G. (1984b). Studies of marginal zinc deprivation in rhesus monkeys. II. Pregnancy outcome. *Am. J. Clin. Nutr.* **39**, 879–887.

Golub, M. S., Donald, J. M., Anderson, J. H., and Ford, E. W. (1988). A labor readiness index (Bishop score) for rhesus monkeys. *Lab. Anim. Sci.* **38**, 435–438.

Goodeaux, L. L., Anzalone, C. A., Webre, M. K., Graves, K. H., and Voelkel, S. A. (1990). Nonsurgical technique for flushing the *Macaca mulatta* uterus. *J. Med. Primatol.* **19**, 59–67.

Gould, K. G. (1983). Diagnosis and treatment of infertility in male great apes. *Zoo Biol.* **2**, 281–293.

Gould, K. G., and Mann, D. R. (1988). Comparison of electrostimulation methods for semen recovery in the rhesus monkey (*Macaca mulatta*). *J. Med. Primatol.* **17**, 95–103.

Gozalo, A., Nolan, T., and Montoya, E. (1992). Spontaneous seminoma in an owl monkey in captivity. *J. Med. Primatol.* **21**, 39–41.

Graham, C. E., and McClure, H. M. (1976). Sertoli-Leydig cell tumor in a chimpanzee. *Lab. Anim. Sci.* **26**, 948–950.

Graham, C. E., and McClure, H. M. (1977). Ovarian tumors and related lesions in aged chimpanzees. *Vet. Pathol.* **14**(4), 380–386.

Guilloud, N. B. (1969). The breeding of apes: Experience at the Yerkes Regional Primate Research Center and a brief review of the literature. *Ann. N. Y. Acad. Sci.* **162**, 297–300.

Harrison, R. M. (1976). Hypospadias in a male rhesus monkey. *J. Med. Primatol.* **5**, 60–63.

Hartman, C. G. (1932). Studies in the reproduction of the monkey Macacas (Pithecus) rhesus with special reference to menstruation and pregnancy. *Contrib. Embryol.* **23**(134), 1–161; *Carnegie Inst. Washington Publ.* **433**.

Hendrickx, A. G., and Dukelow, W. R. (1995a). Reproductive biology. *In* "Nonhuman Primates in Biomedical Research. Biology and Management" (B. T. Bennet, C. R. Abee, and R. V. Henrickson, eds.), pp. 147–191. Academic Press, San Diego, CA.

Hendrickx, A. G., and Dukelow, W. R. (1995b). Breeding. *In* "Nonhuman Primates in Biomedical Research. Biology and Management" (B. T. Bennet, C. R. Abee, and R. V. Henrickson, eds.), pp. 335–375. Academic Press, San Diego, CA.

Hendrickx, A. G., and Nelson, V. G. (1971). Reproductive failure. *In* "Comparative Reproduction of Nonhuman Primates" (E. S. Hafez, ed.), pp. 403–425. Thomas, Springfield, IL.

Herthelius, M., Gorbach, S. L., Mollby, R., Nord, C. E., Pettersson, L., and Winberg, J. (1989a). Elimination of vaginal colonization with *Escherichia coli* by administration of indigenous flora. *Infec. Immun.* **57**, 2447–2451.

Herthelius, M., Mollby, R., Nord, C. E., and Winberg, J. (1989b). Amoxicillin promotes vaginal colonization with adhering *Escherichia coli* present in faeces. *Pediatr./Nephrol.* **3**, 443–447.

Herthelius-Elman, M. Mollby, R., Nord, C. E., and Winberg, J. (1992). The effect of amoxycillin on vaginal colonization resistance and normal vaginal flora in monkeys. *J. Antimicrob. Chemother.* **29**, 329–340.

Hertig, A. T., King, N. W., and MacKey, J. (1971). Spontaneous abortion in wild-caught rhesus monkeys, *Macaca mulatta*. *Lab. Anim. Sci.* **21**, 510–519.

Hertig, A. T., MacKey, J. J., Feeley, G., and Kampschmidt, K. (1983). Dysplasia of the lower genital tract in the female monkey, *Macaca fascicularis,* the crab-eating macaque from Southeast Asia. *Am. J. Obstet Gynecol.* **145**, 968–980.

Hill, W. C. O. (1969). Obstetric mishaps in marmosets. *Acta Zool./Pathol. Antverp.* **48**, 149–154.

Holmberg, C. A., Sesline, D., and Osburn, B. (1978). Dysgerminoma in a rhesus monkey: Morphologic and biological features. *J. Med. Primatol.* **7**, 53–58.

Hubbard, G. B., Wood, D. H., and Fanton, J. W. (1983). Squamous cell carcinoma with metastasis in a rhesus monkey (*Macaca mulatta*). *Lab. Anim. Sci.* **33**, 469–472.

Hunt, R. D. (1993). Herpesviruses of primates: An introduction. *In* "Monographs on the Pathology of Laboratory Animals: Nonhuman Primates" (T. C. Jones, U. Mohr, and R. D. Hunt, eds.), Vol. 1, pp. 74–78. Springer-Verlag, Berlin and New York.

Hunt, R. D., Blake, B. J., and Chalifoux, L. V. (1993). Arrested spermatogenesis: *Aotus trivirgatus, Saimiri sciureus,* and *Macaca mulatta*. *In* "Monographs on the Pathology of Laboratory Animals: Nonhuman Primates" (T. C. Jones, U. Mohr, and R. D. Hunt, eds.), Vol. 2, pp. 164–168. Springer-Verlag, Berlin and New York.

James, A. E., Brayton, J. B., Novak, G., Wight, D., Shehan, T. K., Bush, R. M., and Sanders, R. C. (1976). The use of diagnostic ultrasound in evaluation of the abdomen in primates with emphasis on the rhesus monkey (*Macaca mulatta*). *J. Med. Primatol.* **5**, 160–175.

Jerome, C. P., and Hendrickx, A. G. (1982). A tubal pregnancy in a rhesus monkey (*Macaca mulatta*). *Vet. Pathol.* **19**, 239–245.

Johnson, A. P., Ison, C. A., Hetherington, C. M., Osborn, M. F., Southerton, G., London, W. T., Easmon, C. S. F., and Taykor-Robinson, D. (1985). Vaginal colonization of pig-tailed macaques by *Gardnerella vaginalis*. *Scand. J. Urol. Nephrol. Suppl.*, **86**, 207–210.

Johnson, L. D., Palmer, A. E., King, N. W., and Hertig, A. T. (1981). Vaginal adenosis in *Cebus apella* monkeys exposed to DES in utero. *Obstet. Gynecol.* **57**, 629–635.

Johnson, W. D., Hughes, H. C., Lang, C. M., and Stenger, V. G. (1978). Placenta extrachorialis in the stumptailed macaque (*Macaca arctoides*). *Lab. Anim. Sci.* **28**, 81–84.

Jones, D. M., Dixson, A. F., and Wadsworth, P. F. (1980). Interstitial cell tumour of the testis in a western lowland gorilla (*Gorilla gorilla gorilla*). *J. Med. Primatol.* **9**, 319–322.

Kaplan, C. G. (1979). Intrauterine infections in nonhuman primates. *J. Med. Primatol.* **8**, 233–243.

Keeling, M. E. (1982). Veterinary perspectives of infertility in male great apes. *Am. J. Primatol., Suppl.* **1**, 87–95.

Kessler, M. J., Howard, C. F., and London, W. T. (1985). Gestational diabetes mellitus and impaired glucose tolerance in an aged *Macaca mulatta*. *J. Med. Primatol.* **14**, 237–244.

Kingsley, S. R., and Martin, R. D. (1979). A case of placenta praevia in an orang-utan. *Vet. Rec.* **104**, 56–57.

Kohrs, M. B., Harper, A. E., and Kerr, G. R. (1976). Effects of a low protein diet during pregnancy of the rhesus monkey. I. Reproductive efficiency. *Am. J. Clin. Nutr.* **29**, 136–145.

Kohrs, M. B., Scheffler, G., and Kerr, G. (1979). Effects of a low protein diet during pregnancy of the rhesus monkey. II. Physiological adaptation of the infant. *Am. J. Clin. Nutr.* **32**, 1206–1213.

Kosanke, S. D., Campbell, G. A., Feeback, D. L., and White, G. L. (1980). Intrauterine aspiration of amniotic fluid in a chimpanzee. *VM/SAC, Vet. Med. Small Anim. Clin.*, **75**, 1743–1744.

Kotas, R. V., and Kling, O. R. (1979). Influence of glucocorticoid administration and inhibition on fetal baboon pulmonary maturity and the amniotic fluid L/S ratio. *J. Med. Primatol.* **8**, 88–94.

Kraemer, D. C., and Vera Cruz, N. C. (1972). The female reproductive system. *In* "Pathology of Simian Primates" (R. N. T.-W.-Fienes, ed.), Part 1, pp. 841–877. Karger, Basel.

Kundsin, R. B., Rowell, T., Shepard, M. C., Parreno, A., and Lunceford, C. D. (1975). T-strain mycoplasmas and reproductive failure in monkeys. *Lab. Anim. Sci.* **25**, 221–224.

Lang, C. M., and Benjamin, S. A. (1969). Acute pyometra in a rhesus monkey (*Macaca mulatta*). *J. Am. Vet. Med. Assoc.* **155**, 1156–1157.

Levin, J. L., Hilliard, J. K., Lipper, S. L., Butler, T. M., and Goodwin, W. J. (1988). A naturally occurring epizootic of Simian Agent 8 in the baboon. *Lab. Anim. Sci.* **38**, 394–397.

Lewis, R. W., Kim, J. C. S., Irani, D., and Roberts, J. A. (1981). The prostate of the nonhuman primate: Normal anatomy and pathology. *Prostate* **2**, 51–70.

Lindberg, B. S., and Busch, C. (1984). Endometriosis in rhesus monkeys. *Upsala J. Med. Sci.* **89**, 129–134.

Line, S. W., Golub, M. S., Mahoney, C. J., Ford, E. W., and Anderson, J. H. (1986). Parturition: Studies using the conscious rhesus monkey. *In* "Animal Models in Fetal Medicine (V). Parturition" (P. W. Nathanielsz, ed.), Monog. Fetal Physiol. Vol. 2, pp. 129–151. Perinatology Press, Ithaca, N.Y.

Logdberg, B. (1993). Methods for timing of pregnancy and monitoring of fetal body and brain growth in squirrel monkeys. *J. Med. Primatol.* **22**, 374–379.

London, W. T., Curfman, B., and Sever, J. L. (1971). Mumps infection of the rhesus monkey fetus. *Teratology* **4**, 234–235 (abstr.).

London, W. T., Nahmias, A. J., Naib, Z. M., Fuccillo, D. A., Ellenberg, J. H., and Sever, J. L. (1974). A nonhuman primate model for the study of the cervical oncogenic potential of herpes simplex virus type 2. *Cancer Res.* **34**, 1118–1121.

Lowenstine, L. J. (1993). Measles virus infection: Nonhuman primates. *In* "Monographs on Pathology of Laboratory Animals: Nonhuman Primates" (T. C. Jones, U. Mohr, and R. D. Hunt, eds.), Vol. 1, pp. 108–118. Springer-Verlag, Berlin and New York.

Lunn, S. F. (1980). A case of placenta praevia in a common marmoset (*Callithrix jacchus*). *Vet. Rec.* **106**, 414.

Lunn, S. F. (1985). Uterine rupture during labour in a common marmoset (*Callithrix jacchus*). *Vet. Rec.* **116**, 266–267.

MacKenzie, W. F., and Casey, H. W. (1975). Animal model of human disease. Endometriosis. Animal model: Endometriosis in rhesus monkeys. *Am. J. Pathol.* **80**, 341–344.

Mahoney, C. J. (1975). The accuracy of bimanual rectal palpation for determining the time of ovulation and conception in the rhesus monkey (*Macaca mulatta*). *In* "Breeding Simians for Developmental Biology," Lab. Anim. Handb. No. 6, pp. 127–140.

Mahoney, C. J., and Eisele, S. (1976). Use of an ultrasonic blood flow monitor for determining fetal viability in the rhesus monkey (*Macaca mulatta*). A preliminary study. *J. Med. Primatol.* **5**, 284–295.

Manocha, S. L. (1976). Abortion and cannibalism in squirrel monkeys (*Saimiri sciureus*) associated with experimental protein deficiency during gestation. *Lab. Anim. Sci.* **26**, 649–650.

Martin, C. B., Misenhimer, H. R., and Ramsey, E. M. (1970). Ovarian tumors in rhesus monkeys (*Macaca mulatta*). Report of three cases. *Lab. Anim. Care* **20**, 686–692.

Maruffo, C. A., and Malinow, M. R. (1966). Seminoma in a howler monkey (*Aloutta caraya*). *J. Pathol. Bacteriol.* **91**, 280–282.

McCann, T. O., and Myers, R. E. (1970). Endometriosis in rhesus monkeys. *Am. J. Obstet. Gynecol.* **106**, 516–523.

McCarthy, T. J., Beluhan, F. Z., Bardawil, W. A., and Bennett, B. T. (1989). Pyometra in a rhesus monkey secondary to prolonged therapy with medroxyprogesterone acetate. *Lab. Anim. Sci.* **39**, 71–72.

McChesney, M. B., Fujinami, R. S., Lerche, N. W., Marx, P. A., and Oldstone, M. B. A. (1989). Virus-induced immunosuppression: Infection of peripheral blood mononuclear cells and suppression of immunoglobulin synthesis during natural measles virus infection of rhesus monkeys. *J. Infect. Dis.* **159**, 757–760.

McClure, H. M. (1980). Neoplastic diseases of nonhuman primates: Literature review and observations in an autopsy series of 2176 animals. *In* "The Comparative Pathology of Zoo Animals" (R. J. Montali and G. Migaki, eds.), pp. 549–565. Smithsonian Institution Press, Washington, DC.

McClure, H. M., and Chang, J. (1975). Ectopic pregnancy in a squirrel monkey. *J. Am. Vet. Med. Assoc.* **167**, 654–655.

McClure, H. M., and Graham, C. E. (1973). Malignant uterine mesotheliomas in squirrel monkeys following diethylstilbestrol administration. *Lab. Anim. Sci.* **23**, 493–498.

McClure, H. M., and Strozier, L. M. (1975). Perinatal listeric septicemia in a Celebese black ape. *J. Am. Vet. Med. Assoc.* **167**, 637–638.

McClure, H. M., Weaver, R. E., and Kaufmann, A. F. (1971). Pseudotuberculosis in nonhuman primates: infection with organisms of the *Yersinia enterocolitica* group. *Lab. Anim. Sci.* **21**, 376–382.

McClure, H. M., Alford, P., and Swenson, R. B. (1976). Nonenteric shigella infections in nonhuman primates. *J. Am. Vet. Med. Assoc.* **169**, 938–939.

McClure, H. M., Swenson, R. B., Kalter, S. S., and Lester, T. L. (1980). Natural genital *Herpesvirus hominis* infection in chimpanzees (*Pan troglodytes* and *Pan paniscus*). *Lab. Anim. Sci.* **30**, 895–901.

McClure, H. M., Anderson, D. C., Fultz, P. N., Ansari, A. A., Jehuda-Cohen, T., Villinger, F., Klumpp, S. A., Switzer, W., Lockwood, E., Brodie, A., and Keyserling, H. (1991). Maternal transmission of SIV$_{smm}$ in rhesus macaques. *J. Med. Primatol.* **20**, 182–187.

Miller, C. J., Alexander, N. J., Vogel, P., Anderson, J., and Marx, P. A. (1992a). Mechanism of genital transmission of SIV: A hypothesis based on transmission studies and the location of SIV in the genital tract of chronically infected female rhesus macaques. *J. Med. Primatol.* **21**, 64–68.

Miller, C. J., Vogel, P., Alexander, N. J., Sutjipto, S., Hendrickx, A. G., and Marx, P. A. (1992b). Localization of SIV in the genital tract of chronically infected female rhesus macaques. *Am. J. Pathol.* **141,** 655–660.

Mohanty, D., and Das, K. C. (1982). Effect of folate deficiency on the reproductive organs of female rhesus monkeys: A cytomorphological and cytokinetic study. *J. Nutr.* **112,** 1565–1576.

Moller, B. R., and Freundt, E. A. (1983). Monkey animal model for study of mycoplasmal infections of the urogenital tract. *Sex. Transm. Dis.* **10,** Suppl., 359–362.

Moller, B. R., and Mardh, P.-A. (1980). Experimental epididymitis and urethritis in grivet monkeys provoked by *Chlamydia trachomatis. Fertil. Steril.* **34,** 275–279.

Moody, K. D., Percy, D. H., Papero, M. A., and Morgenstern, S. E. (1991). Use of leuprolide to treat endometriosis in a rhesus macaque. *Lab. Anim. Sci.* **41,** 427–431.

Morgan, M. A., Silavin, S. L., Wentworth, R. A., Figueroa, J. P., Honnebier, B. O. M., Fishburne, J. I., and Nathanielsz, P. W. (1992). Different patterns of myometrial activity and 24-H rhythms in myometrial contractility in the gravid baboon during the second half of pregnancy. *Biol. Reprod.* **46,** 1158–1164.

Morin, M. L., Renquist, D. M., and Allen, A. M. (1980). Squamous cell carcinoma with metastasis in a cynomolgus monkey (*Macaca fascicularis*). *Lab. Anim. Sci.* **30**(1), 110–112.

Morishima, H. O., Pedersen, H., and Finster, M. (1978a). The influence of maternal psychological stress on the fetus. *Am. J. Obstet. Gynecol.* **131,** 286–290.

Morishima, H. O., Niemann, W. H., and James, L. S. (1978b). Effects of endotoxin on the pregnant baboon and fetus. *Am. J. Obstet. Gynecol.* **131,** 899–902.

Mueller-Heubach, E., and Batelli, A. (1981). Prolonged in-utero retention and mummification of a *Macaca mulatta* fetus. *J. Med. Primatol.* **10,** 265–268.

Myers, R. E. (1971). Brain damage induced by umbilical cord compression at different gestational ages in monkeys. *Med. Primatol., Sel. Pap. Conf. Exp. Med. Surg. Primates, 2nd,* New York, 1969, pp. 394–425.

Myers, R. E. (1972). The gross pathology of the rhesus monkey placenta. *J. Reprod. Med.* **9,** 171–198.

Myers, R. E. (1975). Fetal asphyxia due to umbilical cord compression. Medibolic and brain pathologic consequences. *Biol. Neonate* **26,** 21–43.

Myers, R. E., and Brann, A. W. (1976). Abruptio placentae in rhesus monkey causing brain damage to the fetus. *Am. J. Obstet. Gynecol.* **126,** 1048–1049.

Neal, D. E., Dilworth, J. P., Kaack, M. B., Didier, P., and Roberts, J. A. (1990). Experimental prostatitis in nonhuman primates: II. Ascending acute prostatitis. *Prostate* **17,** 233–239.

Newell-Morris, L., Carrol, B., Covey, A., Medley, S., and Sackett, G. P. (1991). Postnatal growth and skeletal maturation of experimental preterm macaques (*Macaca nemestrina*). *J. Med. Primatol.* **20,** 17–22.

Nyland, T. G., Hill, D. E., Hendrickx, A. G., Farver, T. B., McGahan, J. P., Henrickson, R., Anderson, J., and Phillips, H. E. (1984). Ultrasonic assessment of fetal growth in the nonhuman primate (*Macaca mulatta*). *J. Clin. Ultrasound* **13,** 387–395.

O'Banion, M. K., Sundberg, J. P., Shima, A. L., and Reichmann, M. E. (1987). Venereal papilloma and papillomavirus in a colobus monkey, *Colobus guereza. Intervirology* **28,** 232–237.

Olson, L. C., and Sternfeld, M. D. (1987). A percutaneous method for obtaining uterine biopsies. *Lab. Anim. Sci.* **37,** 663–664.

O'Toole, B. A., Fradkin, R., Warkany, J., Wilson, J. G., and Mann, G. V. (1974). Vitamin A deficiency and reproduction in rhesus monkeys. *J. Nutr.* **104,** 1513–1524.

Pace, M., La Torre, R., Giulietti, M., Patella, A., and Turillazzi, P. G. (1991). Fetal death in a long-tailed macaque (*Macaca fascicularis*). Clinical and sonographic approaches. *Folia Primatol.* **57,** 216–220.

Palmer, A. E., London, W. T., Sly, D. L., and Rice, J. M. (1979). Spontaneous preeclamptic toxemia of pregnancy in the patas monkey (*Erythrocebus patas*). *Lab. Anim. Sci.* **29,** 102–106.

Palmer, M. F., Waitkins, S. A., Fitzgeorge, R. B., and Baskerville, A. (1987). Experimental infection of monkeys with *Leptospira interrogans* serovar *hardjo. Epidemiol. Infect.* **98,** 191–197.

Parkman, P. D., Phillips, P. E., and Meyer, H. M. (1965). Experimental rubella virus infection in pregnant monkeys. *Am. J. Dis. Child.* **110,** 390–394.

Parmley, T. H., Dubin, N. H., Blake, D. A., and King, T. M. (1983). Hysterosalpingography in cynomolgus monkeys. *J. Med. Primatol.* **12,** 41–48.

Parsons, M. T., and Spellacy, W. N. (1994). Causes and management of preterm labor. *In* "Danforth's Obstetrics and Gynecology" (J. R. Scott, P. J. DiSaia, C. B. Hammond, and W. N. Spellacy, eds.), 7th ed., pp. 289–304. Lippincott, Philadelphia.

Perelman, R. H., Engle, M. J., Palta, M., Kemnitz, J. W., and Farrell, P. M. (1986). Fetal lung development in male and female nonhuman primates. *Pediatr. Res.* **20,** 987–991.

Pernoll, M. L. (1994). Late pregnancy complication; 3rd trimester hemorrhage. *In* "Handbook of Obstetrics and Gynecology" (R. C. Benson and M. L. Pernoll, eds.), 9th ed., pp. 314–345. McGraw-Hill, New York.

Perolat, P., Poingt, J.-P., Vie, J.-C., Jouaneau, C., Baranton, G., and Gysin, J. (1992). Occurrence of severe leptospirosis in a breeding colony of squirrel monkeys. *Am. J. Trop. Med. Hyg.* **46,** 538–545.

Phillips-Conroy, J. E., Jolly, C. J., Petros, B., Allan, J. S., and Desrosiers, R. C. (1994). Sexual transmission of SIV$_{agm}$ in wild grivet monkeys. *J. Med. Primatol.* **23,** 1–7.

Pilkington, M. D. (1987). Dystocia in a De Brazza's monkey (letter). *Vet. Rec.* **120,** 603.

Price, R. A., Anver, M. R., and Hunt, R. D. (1973). Simian neonatology. III. The causes of neonatal mortality. *Vet. Pathol.* **10,** 37–44.

Rasmussen, K. M., Thenen, S. W., and Hayes, K. C. (1980). Effect of folic acid supplementation on pregnancy in the squirrel monkey (*Saimiri sciureus*). *J. Med. Primatol.* **9,** 169–184.

Reeves, W. C., Di Giacomo, R., and Alexander, E. R. (1981). A primate model for age and host response to genital herpetic infection: Determinants of latency. *J. Infect. Dis.* **143,** 554–557.

Renne, R. A., McLaughlin, R., and Jenson, A. B. (1973). Measles virus-associated endometritis, cervicitis, and abortion in a rhesus monkey. *J. Am. Vet. Med. Assoc.* **163,** 639–641.

Resnik, R., Robinson, P. T., Lasley, B., and Benirschke, K. (1978). Intrauterine fetal demise associated with consumption coagulopathy in a Douc langur monkey (*Pygathrix nemaeus nemaeus*). *J. Med. Primatol.* **7,** 249–253.

Ringler, D. H., and Abrams, G. D. (1972). Gynecomastia and galactorrhea in a male rhesus monkey (*Macaca mulatta*) with spontaneous metastatic carcinoma. *J. Med. Primatol.* **1,** 309–317.

Riopelle, A. J., and Hale, P. A. (1975). Nutritional and environmental factors affecting gestation length in rhesus monkeys. *Am. J. Clin. Nutr.* **28,** 1170–1176.

Roberts, J. A. (1972). The urinary system. In "Pathology of Simian Primates" (R.N.T.-W.-Fienes, ed.) Part 1, pp. 821–840. Karger, Basel.

Roberts, J. A. (1976). Hydronephrosis of pregnancy. *Urology* **8,** 1–4.

Roberts, J. A., and Wolf, R. H. (1971). Hydronephrosis of pregnancy: A naturally occurring disorder in non-human primates closely resembling that in man. *Folia Primatol.* **15,** 143–147.

Roberts, J. A., Hill, C. W., and Riopelle, A. J. (1974). Maternal protein deprivation and toxemia of pregnancy: Studies in the rhesus monkey (*Macaca mulatta*). *Am. J. Obstet. Gynecol.* **118,** 14–17.

Rohovsky, M. W., Fox, J. G., and Ghalifoux, L. V. (1977). Benign ovarian teratomas in two rhesus monkeys (*Macaca mulatta*). *Lab. Anim. Sci.* **27,** 280–281.

Rouse, R., Bronson, R. T., and Sehgal, P. K. (1981). A retrospective study of etiological factors of abortion in the owl monkey, *Aotus trivirgatus. J. Med. Primatol.* **10,** 199–204.

Ruch, T. C. (1959). Diseases of the endocrine, reproductive, and urinary systems. *In* "Diseases of Laboratory Primates" (T. C. Ruch, ed.), pp. 443–471. Saunders, Philadelphia.

Rushton, E., and McGrew, W. C. (1980). Breech birth of a chimpanzee (*Pan troglodytes*). A case report and literature review. *J. Med. Primatol.* **9**, 189–193.

Schaerdel, A. D. (1986). Pelvic endometriosis associated with infarctions of the colon in a rhesus monkey. *Lab. Anim. Sci.* **36**, 533–536.

Schaffer, N. E., McCarthy, T. J., Fazleabas, A. T., and Jeyendran, R. S. (1992). Assessment of semen quality in a baboon (*Papio anubis*) breeding colony. *J. Med. Primatol.* **21**, 47–48.

Schenken, R. S., Asch, R. H., Williams, R. F., and Hodgen, G. D. (1984a). Etiology of infertility in monkeys with endometriosis: Measurement of peritoneal fluid prostaglandins. *Am. J. Obstet. Gynecol.* **150**, 349–353.

Schenken, R. S., Asch, R. H., Williams, R. F., and Hodgen, G. D. (1984b). Etiology of infertility in monkeys with endometriosis: Leteinized unruptured follicles, luteal phase defects, pelvic adhesions, and spontaneous abortions. *Fertil. Steril.* **41**, 122–129.

Schenken, R. S., Williams, R. F., and Hodgen, G. D. (1987). Effect of pregnancy on surgically induced endometriosis in cynomolgus monkeys. *Am. J. Obstet. Gynecol.* **157**, 1392–1396.

Schiffer, S. P., Cary, C. J., Peter, G. K., and Cohen, B. J. (1984). Hemoperitoneum associated with endometriosis in a rhesus monkey. *J. Am. Vet. Med. Assoc.* **185**, 1375–1377.

Schmidt, R. E. (1978). Systemic pathology of chimpanzees. *J. Med. Primatol.* **7**, 274–318.

Scott, W. J., Fradkin, R., and Wilson, J. G. (1975). Ovarian teratoma in a rhesus monkey. *J. Med. Primatol.* **4**, 204–206.

Sesline, D. H., Simpson, J., and Henrickson, R. V. (1983). Neonatal deaths in bonnet monkeys born to dams with rudimentary papillae mammae. *Lab. Anim. Sci.* **33**, 467–468.

Severino, M. F. (1995). Dysfunctional uterine bleeding. *In* "Gynecology and Obstetrics" (J. J. Sciarra, ed.), Vol. 5, No. 20, pp. 1–6. Lippincott-Raven, Philadelphia and New York.

Shalev, M., Ciurea, D., and Deligdisch, L. (1992). Endometriosis and stromal tumor in a baboon (*Papio hamadryas*). *Lab. Anim. Sci.* **42**, 204–208.

Shaughnessy, P. W., DiGiacomo, R. F., Martin, D. P., and Valerio, D. A. (1978). Prematurity and perinatal morality in the rhesus (*Macaca mulatta*): Relationship to birth weight and gestational age. *Biol. Neonate* **34**, 129–145.

Shimizu, K. (1988). Ultrasonic assessment of pregnancy and fetal development in three species of macaque monkeys. *J. Med. Primatol.* **17**, 247–256.

Shimizu, K., Nozaki, M., and Oshima, K. (1994). Cervical ripening and uterine contraction induced by prostaglandin E2-gel in pregnant Japanese monkeys (*Macaca fuscata fuscata*). *J. Med. Primatol.* **23**, 23–31.

Simon, M. A., Daniel, M. D., Lee-Parritz, D., King, N. W., and Ringler, D. J. (1993). Disseminated B virus infection in a cynomolgus monkey. *Lab. Anim. Sci.* **43**, 545–550.

Singleton, W. L., Smikle, C. B., Hankins, G. D. V., Hubbard, G. B., Ehler, W. J., and Brasky, K. B. (1995). Surgical correction of severe vaginal introital stenosis in female baboons (*Papio* sp.) infected with simian agent 8. *Lab. Anim. Sci.* **45**(6), 628–630.

Skangalis, M., Swenson, C. E., Mahoney, C. J., and O'Leary, W. M. (1979). The normal microbial flora of the baboon vagina. *J. Med. Primatol.* **8**, 289–297.

Socha, W. W. (1993). Erythroblastosis fetalis. *In* "Monographs on the Pathology of Laboratory Animals: Nonhuman Primates" (T. C. Jones, U. Mohr, and R. D. Hunt, eds.), Vol. 2, pp. 215–220. Springer-Verlag, Berlin and New York.

Sokol, R. J., Brindley, B. A., and Dombrowski, M. P. (1994). Practical diagnosis and management of abnormal labor. *In* "Danforth's Obstetrics and Gynecology" (J. R. Scott, P. J. DiSaia, C. B. Hammond, and W. N. Spellacy, eds.), 7th ed., pp. 521–561. Lippincott, Philadelphia.

Solleveld, H. A., and van Zwieten, M. J. (1978). Membranous dysmenorrhea in the chimpanzee (*Pan troglodytes*). A report of four cases. *J. Med. Primatol.* **7**, 19–25.

Steiner, P. E., Rasmussen, T. B., and Fisher, L. E. (1955). Neuropathy, cardiopathy, hemosiderosis, and testicular atrophy in *Gorilla gorilla*. *AMA Arch. Pathol.* **59**, 5–25.

St. Geme, J. W., and Van Pelt, L. F. (1974). Fetal and postnatal growth retardation associated with gestational mumps virus infection of the rhesus monkey. *Lab. Anim. Sci.* **24**, 895–899.

Strozier, L. M., McClure, H. M., Keeling, M. E., and Cummins, L. B. (1972). Endometrial adenocarcinoma, endometriosis, and pyometra in a rhesus monkey. *J. Am. Vet. Med. Assoc.* **161**, 704–706.

Swenerton, H., and Hurley, L. S. (1980). Zinc deficiency in rhesus and bonnet monkeys, including effects on reproduction. *J. Nutr.* **110**, 575–583.

Swenson, C. E., and O'Leary, W. M. (1977). Genital *Ureaplasmas* in nonhuman primates. *J. Med. Primatol.* **6**, 344–348.

Swenson, R. B., and McClure, H. M. (1976). Septic abortion in a gorilla due to *Shigella flexneri*. *Proc. Annu. Meet., Am. Assoc./Zoo Vet., 1976*, pp. 195–196.

Swindle, M. M., Adams, R. J., and Craft, C. F. (1981). Intrauterine mummified fetus in a rhesus monkey (*Macaca mulatta*). *J. Med. Primatol.* **10**, 269–273.

Swindle, M. M., Craft, C. F., Marriott, B. M., Strandberg, J. D., and Luzarraga, M. (1982). Ascending intrauterine infections in rhesus monkeys. *J. Am. Vet. Med. Assoc.* **181**, 1367–1370.

Swindle, M. M., Marriott, B. M., and Frank, A. A. (1984). Incomplete abortion and hydrometrosis in a squirrel monkey (*Saimiri sciureus*). *Lab. Anim. Sci.* **34**, 290–292.

Tachon, P., Laschi, A., Briffaux, J. P., Brain, G., and Chambon, P. (1983). Lead poisoning in monkeys during pregnancy and lactation. *Sci. Total Environ.* **30**, 221–229.

Tarantal, A. F. (1990). Interventional ultrasound in pregnant macaques: Embryonic/fetal applications. *J. Med. Primatol.* **19**, 47–58.

Tarantal, A. F. (1992). Sonographic assessment of nongravid female macaques (*Macaca mulatta* and *Macaca fascicularis*). *J. Med. Primatol.* **21**, 308–315.

Tarantal, A. F., and Hendrickx, A. G. (1987). Amniotic band syndrome in a rhesus monkey: A case report. *J. Med. Primatol.* **16**, 291–299.

Tarantal, A. F., and Hendrickx, A. G. (1988). Use of ultrasound for early pregnancy detection in the rhesus and cynomolgus macaque (*Macaca mulatta* and *Macaca fascicularis*). *J. Med. Primatol.* **17**, 105–112.

Taub, D. M. (1980). Age at first pregnancy and reproductive outcome among colony-born squirrel monkeys (*Saimiri sciureus*, Brazilian). *Folia Primatol.* **33**, 262–272.

Thurman, J. D., Morton, R. J., and Stair, E. L. (1983). Septic abortion caused by *Salmonella heidelberg* in a white-handed gibbon. *J. Am. Vet. Med. Assoc.* **183**, 1325–1326.

Valerio, D. A., Leverage, W. E., and Munster, J. H. (1970). Semen evaluation in Macaques. *Lab. Anim. Care.* **20**, 734–740.

van Foreest, A. W., and Socha, W. W. (1981). Transplacental immunization in the course of incompatible pregnancy. *Proc. Annu. Meet., Am. Assoc./Zoo Vet., 1981.*

Van Pelt, L. F. (1974). Clinical assessment of reproductive function in female rhesus monkeys: Individual physical examination. *Lab. Anim.* **8**, 199–212.

Vetesi, F., Balsai, A., and Kemenes, F. (1972). Proceedings: Abortion in Gray's Monkey (*Cercopithecus mona*) associated with *Listeria monocytogenes*. *Acta Microbiol. Acad. Sci. Hung.* **19**, 441–443.

Wagner, J. D., Jayo, M. J., Bullock, B. C., and Washburn, S. A. (1992). Gestational diabetes mellitus in a cynomolgus monkey with group A streptococcal metritis and hemolytic uremic syndrome. *J. Med. Primatol.* **21**, 371–374.

Wagner, J. E., and Carey, K. D. (1976). Ovarian carcinoma with transcelomic metastasis in a Barbary ape. *J. Am. Vet. Med. Assoc.* **169**, 968–970.

Waterton, J. C., Breen, S. A., Dukes, M., Horrocks, M., and Wadsworth, P. F. (1993). A case of adenomyosis in a pigtailed monkey diagnosed by magnetic resonance imaging and treated with the novel pure antiestrogen, ICI 182,780. *Lab. Anim. Sci.* **43**, 247–251.

Wiener, A. S., Socha, W. W., Niemann, W., and Moor-Jankowski, J. (1975). Erythroblastosis models. A review and new experimental data in monkeys. *J. Med. Primatol.* **4,** 179–187.

Wiener, A. S., Socha, W. W., and Moor-Jankowski, J. (1977). Erythroblastosis models. II. Maternofetal incompatability in chimpanzee. *Folia Primatol.* **27,** 68–74.

Wixson, S. K., and Griffith, J. W. (1986). Nutritional deficiency anemias in nonhuman primates. *Lab. Anim. Sci.* **36,** 231–236.

Wolf, R. H. (1971). Placenta previa in a patas monkey (*Erythrocebus patas*). *Folia Primatol.* **14,** 80–83.

Chapter 9

Integumentary System

Joseph T. Bielitzki

I. INTRODUCTION

The skin is the largest organ of the body. It appears to be a homogeneous covering of the body, but regional differences exist both in function and in structure. Skin is accessible for inspection, evaluation, and diagnostic testing. The clinical findings associated with diseases of the skin are frequently subtle, and its response can be misleading. Both primary and secondary diseases are manifest by changes in the skin.

Primary dermatologic disease in the captive nonhuman primate is infrequent and the literature is scant. Case reports serve as the predominant source of information. Several factors contribute to the infrequent appearance of spontaneous skin disorders: (1) Natural selection in the wild is likely highly effective in removing those mutations or developmental anomalies that result in decreased camouflage, reduced ability to cope with the external environment, or provide increased susceptibility to parasitic or other infectious processes. (2) Most captive nonhuman primates are only a few generations removed from feral stock. (3) Animals with naturally occurring skin problems in a captive colony are removed from the breeding pool unless a specific genetic model is being developed or sought. (4) Importation of feral animals has decreased, reducing the prevalence of infectious and parasitic diseases that affect the skin. (5) Exporters have improved preventive health programs and screening in countries of origin.

II. STRUCTURE AND FUNCTION OF THE SKIN

Skin is composed of two distinct layers: the epidermis and the dermis. It varies in thickness over the body, and males tend to show greater thickness than females. Variations in color and pelage are common among the nonhuman primates, but the underlying structure remains fairly constant. Functionally, it serves as the barrier between the internal aqueous environment of the body and the dry and gaseous external environment.

A. Structure

The skin is composed of two distinct regions, the outer avascular epidermis and deeper vascular dermis. The epidermis lacks a vascular component and is dependent on diffusion from the underlying vascular dermis for nutrients.

There are four defined layers of cells, originating embryologically from ectoderm, that make up the epidermis: the basal cell layer, the stratum spinosum, the stratum granulosum, and the stratum corneum. The deepest is the basal or germinal layer, seen as a single row of mitotically active columnar cells. Functionally, this layer produces the cells that mature into the keratinocytes. Melanocytes are located among the cells of this layer, but derive from neural crest. Pigment produced by the melanocytes is incorporated into the surrounding epidermal cells. The next cellular layer is the stratum spinosum, which is involved in the production of keratin precursors. These cells are polyhedral or cuboidal with spinous processes between adjacent cells. In a number of primate species, this layer may be poorly defined. The next layer, the stratum granulosum, consists of squamous cells containing keratohyaline granules. The stratum corneum is the outermost layer of the epidermis. It is composed of dead keratinized cells arranged in a lamellar pattern. This surface layer sloughs continuously, and these aggregates of sloughed keratinized cells are seen as dander. Cells produced in the basal layer mature through each layer and are ultimately shed as dander. Hair follicles with associated apocrine and sebaceous glands are part of the dermis but pass through the epidermis. The epidermis and dermis interface at the noncellular basal lamina.

Skin structures characteristic of Old World monkeys are the ischial callosities. Callosities are greatly thickened areas of waxy keratin on which the animal may sit for extended periods of time without damage to the underlying soft tissue. In males, a crescent callosity originates at the ischial tuberosities and merges ventral to the anal orifice. In the female, separate callosities are present over each ischium and separated by the vaginal orifice. Corresponding structures are missing in New World species.

The dermis provides much of the support for the skin. It contains the vasculature, nerve endings associated with sensory input, and cellular components associated with the hair, nail, and glandular structures of the skin. Fibroblasts in the dermis produce collagen, elastin, and ground substance, which provides the flexibility and pliability needed for tissue movement and stretching during motion.

The dermis is richly vascular and contains a significant capillary bed. This vascular bed is capable of rapid dilation or constriction to accommodate to changes in ambient temperature for the purpose of maintaining homeothermy. The vascular supply is active in response to both primary and secondary disease. Changes in vascular permeability occur in response to a variety of systemic or local stimuli.

Skin is richly innervated and acts as the tactile organ of the body. Numerous sensory nerve endings are present in the skin; the greater the functional need of the area, the greater the number of nerve endings. These sensory nerve endings appear to decrease in number as the animal ages (Short et al., 1987). Prehensile areas on the tail of New World species contain numerous sensory nerve endings capable of enhanced input. Dermatoglyphs, the fine ridges of the skin, are obvious on both palmar and plantar surfaces of the hands and feet (Newell-Morris, 1979). Prehensile areas of the tail have skin ridges similar to those seen on hands and feet.

The Langerhans cell or dendritic macrophage originates in bone marrow and migrates through the epidermis. Monocytes, neutrophils, lymphocytes, basophils, and eosinophils migrate into and through the dermis. When disruptions in the integrity of the epidermis occur, these cell types may be seen near and in the defect. The Langerhans cells of the epidermis and the lymphocytes of the dermis act as an immunologic barrier. The Langerhans cells present antigens to the lymphocytes. The lymphoid cells of the skin make up the skin-associated lymphoid tissue (SALT), which is thought to function in a manner similar to the dedicated lymphoid tissue of the gut, gut-associated lymphoid tissue (GALT), acting as a first line source for immune recognition.

Hair provides significant protection to nonhuman primates. It acts as insulation to both heat and cold and provides a barrier between the skin and the environment. The color and distribution pattern of the pelage is important in species recognition and, in some cases, in gender identification. Hair may play a role for some species during aggressive interactions and territorial defense. Mediated by the sympathetic nervous system, the erector pilae muscles cause hair to extend away from the body, making an individual appear larger and more threatening.

Great variation in the color of pelage occurs among the various species of nonhuman primates. Within some species, pelage differs between sexes. An example of this is observed in forest baboons of the genus *Mandrillus*. The neonates of many New World and Old World species have coat coloration distinct from the adult. For example, the Colobus monkey infant, *Colobus* sp., is white at birth. The infant stump-tail macaque, *Macaca arctoides,* is white to buff; and the silver leaf langur infant, *Presbytis cristatus,* is brilliant gold. New World species, especially infant callithricids, lack adult coat color and pattern.

Alopecia is common in nonhuman primates. Total alopecia, where hair follicles failed to develop, has been reported in a rhesus macaque (*Macaca mulatta*) (Ratteree and Baskin, 1992) and in a common chimpanzee (*Pan troglodytes*) (Eichberg and De Villez, 1984). Pattern baldness is common and genetically inherited in the stump-tail macaque (*M. arctoides*). The stump tail shows an onset of the balding pattern with sexual maturity and both males and females may be affected (Uno, 1980, 1987). Seasonal thinning of the hair coat has been noted for rhesus macaques under both captive conditions and in the wild (Malley, 1968). Focal areas of alopecia may be associated with infectious conditions, burns, scarring, or behavioral abnormalities, such as overgrooming or barbering.

Defects in pigment deposition occur in nonhuman primates. Infrequently, true albinism has been reported, which is characterized by a total lack of pigment in the skin, the hair, and the eye (Sabater Pi, 1967). Dilute coat color, dirty white or yellow, is seen in amelanistic individuals (Hill *et al.*, 1970). Pigment, although reduced, is present, and eye color is less intense than in wild-type individuals.

B. Function

The skin forms a selectively permeable barrier between the body and the outside environment (Lehman *et al.*, 1988). The skin acts as the primary barrier for maintaining the internal aqueous environment necessary for continued cellular function. Electrolytes and fluid are prevented from escaping the body through evaporation by the physical barrier of skin. Hair provides an additional physical barrier against traumatic injury. The epidermis, which is constantly regenerating its keratinized layers, serves as a replaceable physical covering for the entire body. Skin heals rapidly following puncture, penetration, or exposure of the underlying dermis, assuring continued stability of the internal aqueous environment of the body. The absorption of compounds through the skin is variable, and the amount absorbed is determined by the location on the body and the pathological condition of the skin (Bronaugh *et al.*, 1986).

The epidermal barrier is richly innervated for maximal tactile sensory input. Receptors for temperature, pressure, and pain are present. In some species, vibrissae are present on the muzzle and around the eyes for enhanced sensory input during motion or nocturnal activity.

The rich vasculature of the skin helps maintain stable body temperatures through vasoconstriction and vasodilation. Perspiration is not a usual mechanism for temperature regulation in the nonhuman primate, although eccrine sweat glands are present. Pelage acts to insulate the body from thermal extremes, resulting in minimal heat loss during cool periods and protection from high ambient temperatures. Subcutaneous fat acts to insulate against environmental variations in temperature and serves as a caloric reservoir.

A number of species use glandular skin secretions to scent mark their environment (Epple, *et al.*, 1986; Tattersall, 1993). Several species have strong and characteristic odors. Of the laboratory species, the stump-tail macaque, *M. arctoides,* the owl monkey, *Aotus* sp., and the callithricids best define this

trait. Scent glands, which may be focal or diffuse, are located at the carpus, the perianal region, and along the sternum, depending on the species (Chapman *et al.,* 1985; Geissmann, 1987; Zeller *et al.,* 1988).

Several species of nonhuman primates commonly used in biomedical research exhibit sexual swelling associated with the estrous cycle. This sex skin peaks in size at or near ovulation. Sexual swellings vary from a slight enlargement of the labia minora to a turgid edematous enlargement of the skin of the perineum, labia, and base of the tail. In species that demonstrate enlargement or tumescence, the skin appears sclerotic at peak swelling. The degree and extent of the swelling vary by species. The extent of swelling may increase or decrease following puberty, depending on the species. The orangutan, *Pongo pygmaus,* demonstrates a swelling during early pregnancy.

The color of the sex skin may change slightly in the pregnant savanna baboon: from a gray pink to red (Strum and Western, 1982). Following the pregnancy, the facial pigment in patas monkeys, *Erythrocebus patas,* will change from black to white in subsequent pregnancies.

III. DEFINITIONS AND DESCRIPTIONS OF CHANGES TO THE SKIN

Standard nomenclature is used for describing the morphological lesions of the skin. The lesions can be defined as changes of color, the presence of lumps, and the type of material composing the core of these lumps; a thickening or thinning of the layers of the skin; and by defects in surface integrity of the skin.

Changes in color that are flat to the skin surface and circumscribed are called macules if under 1 cm in diameter and patches if greater than 1 cm. Color changes may be due to an increase in pigment deposition or hyperpigmentation; a reduction of pigment or hypopigmentation; or changes in vascularity. Hyperpigmentation can be observed in the presence or absence of an inflammatory response. Hypopigmentation can be associated with trauma, thermal or chemical burns, or exposure to ionizing radiation or laser. Vascular changes may be associated with normal physiological processes, such as ovarian cycles, or associated with pathologic changes, such as ecchymotic or petechial hemorrhage.

Lumps may vary in size and in the nature of the material within their core. Vesicles are small, less than 0.5 cm in diameter, liquid-filled elevations resulting from the infiltration of fluid between the epidermis and the dermis. Vesicles may form larger structures called bulla. Pustules contain purulent exudate within the core and may have originated as a vesicle or bulla that has become secondarily infected. Folliculitis is the accumulation of purulent material within an infected hair follicle. Infections of hair follicles may be called furuncles, and several coalesced furuncles make up the larger structures called carbuncles. Abscesses are the accumulation of exudate and the associated inflammatory response within the subcutaneous region. Cysts occur as a result of the obstruction of an orifice or duct, and the material within consists of glandular secretions.

Papules are small solid masses elevated above the surface of the skin. Their center is composed of metabolic deposits, mineral deposits, areas of cellular hyperplasia, or cellular infiltrates. As papules increase in size they are called nodules. When slow growing, nodules are often the result of a granulomatous reaction. Ulceration may occur as the blood supply is reduced as a result of trauma to the elevated skin mass. Neoplastic growths, or tumors, may originate in the skin or subcutis. Localized and circumscribed edema of the dermis is called a wheal and is generally elevated and flat. Reddened areas that extend beyond the circumscribed margins of a wheal are referred to as a flare. A delayed-type hypersensitivity, in response to the intradermal injection of tuberculin, is frequently described as a wheal-and-flare reaction.

Thickening of the skin that involves the epidermis is called hyperkeratosis. Thickening involving both the dermis and the epidermis is called lichenification and is characterized by both hardening and thickening. Both are generalized responses to chronic inflammation. Dried areas of the epidermis may slough at a greater than normal rate, and such areas appear gray or white and are referred to as scale. If edema, cellular infiltrates, or collagen proliferation occurs in the subcutaneous area, the pressure placed on the dermis may cause the epidermis to thin and harden. This process of sclerosis may be local or diffuse, and the affected area is characterized by having a transparent or translucent appearance. Affected areas are friable and lack elasticity.

Defects in the skin are defined in terms of size and cause. Ulcers refer to a loss of the epidermis and damage to the dermis and are caused by a rupture of vesicles, bullae, or pustules or the result of infarction or trauma. Erosions are similar in appearance, but are caused by trauma or abrasion. They appear as a depression in the epidermis. Excoriations are the loss of the epidermis and often the dermis caused by rubbing, scratching, or biting. This lesion is usually associated with pruritis. Fissures are cracks extending through the epidermis and dermis. During the healing process of any of these lesions a crust of dried serum, exudate, and blood covers the defect. Healing occurs beneath this crust (referred to as an eschar in thermal injury), and the defect is filled by fibrous tissue and is called a scar.

IV. EXAMINATION OF THE SKIN

The skin is the most easily visualized organ of the body. Changes in the condition of the skin often provide an early indication that clinical disease is present.

A. Physical Examination

An examination of the skin should occur with every routine physical examination. The distribution pattern of cutaneous lesions may provide clues as to whether the clinical problem is systemic or localized. Reddened macular areas, when diffuse, are characteristic of systemic disease. Vesicles and papules are often seen early with infectious conditions. Pustules and crateriform ulcers may represent a progression of a vesicular condition and are the result of secondary bacterial infection of the original vesicle. Pustules appearing in the absence of a previous vesicle may be associated with folliculitis. Such pustules are usually smaller than those following vesicles. Papules and nodules may be indicative of an early cellular response. Chronic granulomatous reactions occur when a poor immune response is mounted against the infectious agents. Diffuse ulcerated nodules are characteristic of an infectious process, whereas single ulcerated areas are more typical of neoplasia. Areas of alopecia should be noted and correlated to behavioral problems, such as self-directed behaviors. Lesions should be characterized as pruritic or nonpruritic. Defects in the skin should be described using standardized terminology and evaluated to determine the age or maturity of the lesion. Chronicity of skin lesions may be linked to the history. The amount of subcutaneous fat is an indicator of nutritional status (Altmann et al., 1993). Skin turgor, normally a good indicator of hydration in other species, is less reliable in the nonhuman primate.

B. Laboratory and Microscopic Examination

Clinical laboratory results can provide significant diagnostic information when evaluating skin lesions. Routine evaluation of blood parameters should initiate the diagnostic workup. Complete blood counts and serum chemistries are beneficial in determining if systemic disease is present. Serology is confirmatory for specific viral etiologies. Blood cultures may be beneficial when septicemia is suspected. Skin scrapings and skin cultures are beneficial in identifying problems associated with parasitic, mycotic, and bacterial agents. Bacterial culture and antibiotic sensitivity should be used when identifying and treating skin infections. Gram stains and acid-fast stains, along with the morphological characteristics of exudate or vesicle contents, can be diagnostic. The aspirated contents of vesicles and pustules may be submitted for cytological diagnostic evaluation. Zoonotic disease transmission should be considered when aspirating vesicles or when working with any material thought to be of an infectious nature. Laboratory personnel must be notified of the potential zoonotic risk, especially when dealing with suspected viral etiologies.

In the nonhuman primate, skin biopsies are especially beneficial. Microscopic examination of skin lesions can rapidly confirm an etiologic agent or indicate diagnostic direction. Special stains are available to assist in the diagnosis of a number of etiologic agents and pathologic conditions. The type of infiltrate and distribution of cells can further aid in diagnosis. Many viral etiologies have characteristic inclusion bodies.

V. DISEASES OF THE SKIN

A. Infectious Diseases

A number of infectious etiologies affect the skin either as primary pathogens or by causing systemic disease with cutaneous signs. The number of new etiologies being reported and the frequency of clinical problems have decreased in part because fewer animals originate from feral stock. In addition, preconditioning animals in countries of origin prior to exportation has contributed to this decrease.

Pox-like disease in nonhuman primates is caused by viral agents of two subgroups. Yaba monkey tumor poxvirus and Tana poxvirus are classified in the Yaba poxvirus subgroup (Espana, 1971; Whittaker and Glanister, 1985; Fenner, 1990). Yaba monkey tumor virus causes dermal histicytomas. The extent of the tumor is self-limiting (Ambrus *et al.,* 1969; Spencer, 1985). Biting insects may be associated with transmission of the agent between animals (Ambrus *et al.,* 1969). Tana poxvirus causes typical pox-like lesions. Monkeypox is an orthopoxvirus. This family also includes smallpox and vaccinia. Although infrequent, infections with monkeypox are more common than those of the Yaba poxviruses. Lesions associated with this subgroup are elevated or flat ulcerated areas (McNulty, 1972; Lane *et al.,* 1981), and both New World and Old World species may be affected. The natural reservoir of infection of monkeypox appears to be several African species of upper canopy squirrels (Khodakovich *et al.,* 1987). The occurrence of these agents in research colonies is rare. Most cases were reported in newly imported animals. The possibility for zoonotic transmission exists for all listed agents. Intracellular inclusion bodies are commonly observed on histological examination of the epidermis (McConnell, 1970; Fenner, 1990).

Papillomatous growths have been reported on several occasions in nonhuman primates: *Cebus, Colobus polykomos* (Boever and Kern, 1976), *C. guereza* (Rangan *et al.,* 1980), *Macaca mulatta* (Kloster *et al.,* 1988), and *M. nemestrina.* The lesions ranged from pedunculated cutaneous masses to flat or slightly elevated cauliflower-like growths. The size of the lesions varied from 1 to 20 mm in diameter and most showed multiple growths. Viral particles consistent with the morphology of the papillomavirus were identified in the nuclei of the stratum granulosum of affected tissue. Papillomaviruses in other animal species have been linked to certain cutaneous and genital tumors, and some serotypes are capable of malignant transformation (Sundberg and O'Banion, 1989; Sundberg and Reichmann, 1993). Papillomaviruses have not been reported with any frequency in the nonhuman primate, making a strong correlation with tumorogenesis difficult.

Nonhuman primates have a resident skin flora. *Staphylococcus* and *Streptococcus* are frequently found on the skin during nondisease states and appear important in maintaining skin pH and for inhibiting nonresident pathogens from becoming established. Resident bacteria are genetically monomorphic for the host (Zimmerman, 1977), and resident organisms evolve to adapt to the host (Kloos and Wolfshohl, 1979, 1983).

Increased numbers of nonresident pathogens are typical of cutaneous disease. Immunodeficiency disease may allow normal flora to produce clinical lesions. Such infections respond poorly to conventional therapy.

An impetigo-like condition characterized by moist pyoderma on the abdomen and dark discoloration of the adjacent skin is commonly seen in nursery-reared macaques in which incubator substrates are wet, thus keeping the skin moist. Streptococcal organisms are usually isolated, and the condition responds readily to antibiotics and improved sanitary conditions.

A broad spectrum of bacterial agents may be associated with cutaneous and subcutaneous infections. Enteric pathogens are frequently isolated from injuries. *Pseudomonas aeruginosa* and *Proteus mirabilis* are often isolated and difficult to treat; the associated cellutitis is extensive and necrotizing (Line *et al.,* 1984). Unexpected organisms, such as *Haemophilus influenzae,* have been isolated from subcutaneous abscesses (Burr and Kulshrestha, 1982). *Corynebacterium ulcerans* has been reported (May, 1972). *Clostridium* sp. may also be isolated from traumatic injuries (Boncyk and Kalter, 1980). Penetrating wounds of the skin with a subsequent infection with *Clostridium tetani* may result in paralytic disease (Kessler and Brown, 1979). This is especially a potential problem in nonhuman primates maintained outdoors. Infections associated with *Pseudomonas pseudomallei,* an organism endemic to southeast Asia, have been reported in animals imported from this region. The typical presentation is a nonhealing or recurrent fistula with a purulent discharge. The infection is generally related to an underlying infection in the bony structure. The organism is highly resistant to most antibiotics. Affected animals should be removed from the colony and care taken to prevent zoonotic transmission (Douglas *et al.,* 1971).

A variety of mycotic infections are reported in the nonhuman primate. Most are commonly reported in other species of vertebrate animals. Mycotic infections are more ubiquitous in the host range than are other pathogens.

Nonhuman primates may be infected with a variety of common dermatomycoses. In colonies, the most frequent sources of infection are from infected human contacts. Dermatophytes common to humans and domestic pets have been reported in nonhuman primates maintained in laboratories and zoological gardens. *Trichophyton mentagrophytes* (Bagnall and Gruenberg, 1972), *T. rumbrum, T. violacea, Microsporum canis* (Kaplan *et al.,* 1958; Klokke and de Vries, 1963), and *M. gypseum* are associated with humans or contact with domestic pets. *Microsporum distortum* (Kaplan *et al.,* 1957), *M. audouini* (Fisher and Lederer, 1960), *M. cookei,* and *T. gallinae* are reported less frequently and were seen in newly imported animals (Migaki, 1986).

The clinical signs associated with dermatomycoses are dry scaly lesions with circumscribed areas of alopecia. Alopecia is not uniformly present. The infection may spread rapidly within a colony when animals are group housed. Treatment with topicals is difficult because of the need for frequent application. Griseofulvin continues to be a simple and effective treatment. Ketoconizole is effective but has more significant side effects.

Periodic reports identify *Dermatophilus congolensis* as a cause of necrotic dermatitis, characterized by parakeratosis, hyperkeratosis, and acanthosis with or without abscess formation. Predisposing factors are trauma and a moist environment (Migaki and Seibold, 1976; Klumpp and McClure, 1993).

Actinomyces has been reported from a granulomatous abscess. Diagnostic confirmation is made by the presence of sulfur granules in the exudate (Weidman, 1935).

Candida albicans has been reported in a rhesus monkey associated with preputial inflammation and discharge and lytic lesions of the fingernails and nail beds (Kerber *et al.,* 1968). Yeast infections of the skin may also be seen in the folds of the sex skin of periovulatory nonhuman primates.

African histoplasmosis or large form histoplasmosis, *Histoplasma capsulatum* var. *duboisii,* has been reported in baboons from central Africa. The agent differs from the related organism, *H. capsulatum,* in both appearance and disease pathogenesis. Infections are often seen in newly imported animals. The typical lesions are ulcerated cutaneous nodules located on the buttocks, hands, feet, and face. Underlying bony structures may be involved. The lesions become elevated and granulomatous if the infection persists for long periods. Surgical excision of affected areas involving the cutaneum has proven to be a successful treatment modality (Butler *et al.,* 1988).

Sporothrix schenkii is infrequently reported as a cause of cutaneous nodules and ulcerations. Regional lymphnodes may be enlarged. The infection is often associated with a penetrating injury (Saliba *et al.,* 1968).

Animals housed in the southwest region of the United States may develop infections with *Coccidioides immitis.* Bony involvement may result in cutaneous fistulas from the affected region. Culling of these animals is appropriate due to the poor response of the organism to treatment.

A number of rickettsial agents have been reported as causing disease in nonhuman primates, with accompanying skin lesions. The agent of scrub typhus, *Rickettsia tsutsugamushi* (*R. orientalis*), is transmitted by the southeast Asian trombiculid mites of the genus *Leptotrombidium* from a reservoir rodent host. The characteristic lesion is an eschar at the site of inoculation. Generalized skin reactions are not seen in the nonhuman primate (Philip, 1980; Kitaoka, 1972). *Rickettsia rickettsii,* the etiologic agent of Rocky Mountain spotted fever, can be transmitted to nonhuman primates through ticks of the genera *Dermacentor* or *Rhipicephalus.* Lesions are characterized as a macular rash on the limbs, perineum, head, and lower back (Saslaw and Carlisle, 1966). Appropriate control of the arthropod vector or the reservoir host in endemic areas prevents infections in primate colonies housed in outdoor corrals. Although not reported as a naturally occurring infection, north Asian tick typhur caused by *R. sibirica*

can experimentally cause cutaneous and subcutaneous hemorrhages in the primate host (Burgdorfer, 1980).

Ectoparasites are frequently reported in nonhuman primates. Three types of mite infestations are of concern: demodectic, psoregatic, and sarcoptic. *Demodex* sp. lesions were nonpruritic (Loebel and Nutting, 1973; Hickey *et al.,* 1983). *Psoregates* sp. produced rough, scaly, elevated, circumscribed, nonpruritic papules (Lee *et al.,* 1981; Baskin *et al.,* 1984). Lesions in the periorbital area caused by psoregates may result in a yellow discoloration of the skin (Raulston, 1972). Sarcoptic lesions are papular, erythematous, and frequently pruritic. Zoonotic transmission of scabies has been reported (Goldman and Feldman, 1949).

The nematode *Anatrichosoma cutaneum* has been reported as causing subcutaneous migration tracts, which are most evident in the palmar and plantar surfaces. The affected skin is dry, white, and scaly (Breznock and Pulley, 1975; Harwell and Dalgard, 1979; Anonymous, 1980; Kessler, 1982).

B. Noninfectious Diseases

Enteric disease is the leading cause of morbidity and mortality in colonies of nonhuman primates. Morbidity and mortality as a result of trauma rank second. Pair or group housing of animals increases the likelihood of traumatic injury. Following injury, healing of the skin occurs across most species in a similar manner. The type and severity of the injury determine the rate of healing. Large defects and infected wounds heal more slowly. Following injury, growth factors are released locally, stimulating reepithelialization across the defect. Initial coverage of the defect by epithelial cells occurs deep to the crust of serum, which forms an initial barrier over the wound. Following the initial coverage of the defect by serum, the deeper layers of the epidermis and dermis begin to regenerate.

Trauma frequently involves injury to tissues deep to the skin. Systemic responses to injury may accompany severe trauma and associated tissue damage necessitating treatment for shock, sepsis, and multiple organ failure.

Lacerations may be deep or superficial and respond readily to suturing. The area may require covering or protection if self-directed behaviors become increased during wound repair. Lacerations of the sex skin in species that show tumescence are difficult to suture because the epidermis is friable. The fully tumesced skin lacks tensile strength and repair is best accomplished after the swelling is reduced. Even when detumesced, wound repair is difficult and healing by secondary intention is often necessary.

Crush injuries to the skin are commonly associated with animal bites. In many cases the skin is not penetrated, but several days after the bite has occured, injured areas demonstrate ischemic necrosis, characterized by black discoloration of dry devitalized skin. Secondary infections of the areas are common and abscessation may occur. Tissue under the skin may also be devitalized and require debridement. Large defects can be repaired following the control of secondary bacterial infection and generation of a healthy bed of granulation tissue. The application of wet to dry dressings has proven beneficial in the management of these cases. Surgical intervention, such as debridement, plasty, or skin flaps, serves to reduce the size of the defect and reduces the opportunity for bacterial growth, which results in a more rapid healing process (Rosenberg *et al.,* 1981; Fanton, 1985; Line and Morykwas, 1993). Large untreated defects will develop into large areas of sclerosis, resulting in an area of increased friability, reduced elasticity, and a high probability of reinjury.

Penetrating bite wounds may result in abscess formation. Mixed populations of bacteria are often cultured from such wounds. Appropriate antibiotic therapy is essential to hasten the healing process. Drains may be beneficial but are difficult to keep in place due to the dexterity of the patient.

Occasionally, calcinosis circumscripta is reported in nonhuman primates. The lesions appear as firm subcutaneous nodules without inflammation. Biopsy reveals metastatic calcium deposition. The lesion is felt to be a consequence of an earlier traumatic injury.

Thermal injury to the skin is often associated with exposure to supplemental heat. Thermal injury may occur during extended surgical procedures or recovery periods, when water blankets or heat sources are used. Contact with water heating pads for greater than 30 min at temperatures as low as 106°F may cause injury. Contact points at bony protuberances are the most frequent site of injury. Tissue damage can be avoided by periodically changing the position of the patient or by reducing the temperature of the heating pad to below 102°F. The use of heat lamps may result in local burns or hyperthermia. Serious problems may be avoided if the distance between the lamp and the cage front is maintained at a distance of at least 4 feet (1.3 m). Treatment involves prevention of secondary bacterial infection to the traumatized skin. Severe injury may result in the need for surgical debridement and the application of wet to dry dressings. Large defects may require grafting or other appropriate techniques.

A number of species show poor adaptation to cold environmental temperatures (Laber-Laird *et al.,* 1988). Nonacclimated animals may develop injuries associated with localized vasoconstriction, even at temperatures above freezing. Frostbite and vasoconstrictive injuries result in ischemic necrosis to the affected body parts, most often the distal tail and digits. Surgical amputation of injured tissue is the treatment of choice. Secondary infection is common during the early stages of frostbite.

Contact dermatitis associated with the use of chemical disinfectants and cleaning agents may occur. Tissue damage ranges from mild inflammation to loss of epidermal integrity. Most frequently injury is located on the hands and feet, where sloughing of keratinized layers may occur. More serious injuries involve exposure of the underlying dermis with the opportunity for secondary infection. Areas of frequent surface contact are affected; the lateral aspects of the arms, legs, pelvis, and shoulder girdle are most often involved. The ischial callosities may be affected at the junction of the keratinized callosity and the surrounding skin. If the injury is severe the callosity may slough or become deeply infected; the prognosis under these circumstances is guarded.

Ionizing and electron radiation cause skin injury under experimental conditions. Lesions range from erythema with mild exposure to wet designation and skin ulceration with secondary infection with greater exposures. Injuries may resemble thermal or chemical injuries. Most exposure to radiation at high levels is experimental and lesions should be anticipated based on the dose and duration of exposure (Lippincott *et al.,* 1973). Glomangiomas have been reported following experimental irradiation in macaques (Hubbard and Wood, 1984). Disruption of the skin integrity may cause long-term localized alteration in skin pigment and color following healing (Jelinek, 1985).

C. Neoplasia

There are numerous reports of skin neoplasia. Malignant and benign tumor types are reported with equal frequency (Lowenstine, 1986). From cells of epidermal origin, basal cell carcinomas (Fisher and Robinson, 1976; Yanai *et al.,* 1995) and squamous cell carcinomas (Richter and Buyukmichi, 1979; Migaki *et al.,* 1971) have been reported. Dermal tumors derive from a variety of sources. Leiomyosarcoma (Brunnert *et al.,* 1990), liposarcomas, fibrosarcomas, hemangiomas, papillary carcinoma associated with apocrine sweat glands (Cameron and Conroy, 1976), and mammary adenocarcinomas have been reported. Malignant melanomas are rare, even though most primate skin is highly pigmented. A benign melanocytoma has been reported in the rhesus macaque (Frazier *et al.,* 1993).

Skin can be the source of metastases or act as the final destination of metastatic tumors. Lymphomas associated with STLV-1 infection (Yakovleva *et al.,* 1993) and simian immunodeficiency virus (SIV) infection are commonly found in subcutaneous areas. Malignant lymphoma is frequently seen in multiple locations in the skin.

Clinical treatment of neoplasia of the skin is possible, however, often the tumor is identified late in the course of the disease, making intervention difficult. Both surgical intervention and chemotherapy are possible and, when employed, should be aggressive.

D. Manifestations of Systemic Disease

A number of agents and conditions have clinical manifestations of disease that affect the skin even though the skin is not the primary site for the agent. Systemic manifestations of disease are generally diffuse in distribution.

The herpesviruses frequently present clinically with cutaneous involvement (Kalter, 1988). The neurotrophic alphaherpes viruses, herpes simiae (herpes B virus), simian agent 8 (SA 8), and herpes simplex (herpes hominis) (McClure *et al.,* 1980; Heldstab *et al.,* 1981; Hunt, 1993a,b), may cause vesicle, pustule, or ulcer formation in skin and at the mucocutaneous junction. These viruses are persistent and latent, localizing in specific neural locations during latency (Brack, 1977; Hunt and Blake, 1993a,b).

Herpes simiae virus resides within the neurons of the trigeminal ganglion and the lumbosacral plexus. During periods of viral reactivation, skin lesions are noted at the nerve endings of the distribution of the ganglion or plexus. Characteristic vesicle formation occurs on the mucous membranes and mucocutaneous border of the nose and oral cavity, on the skin of the nose and the eyelids, and conjunctiva. When genital involvement occurs due to reactivation of a lumbosacral plexus infection, lesions are present on the skin of the prepuce and the vulva (Zwartouw *et al.,* 1984). Venereal transmission may occur in infected colonies (Weigler *et al.,* 1994). Primary infections have been noted in macaque infants less than 30 days of age (Anderson *et al.,* 1994). Herpes simiae virus has significant zoonotic potential with a number of fatalities being reported.

A number of herpes agents related to the varicella-zoster viruses of humans have been reported (Padovan and Cantrelli, 1986; Roberts, 1993). Isolates include the Liverpool vervet monkey virus (Clarkson *et al.,* 1967), the patas monkey herpesvirus (McCarthy *et al.,* 1968; Schmidt *et al.,* 1983), delta herpesvirus (Ayres, 1971; Gard and London, 1983), and the Medical Lake macaque virus (Lourie *et al.,* 1971; Blakely *et al.,* 1973). The cutaneous lesions are similar for each virus; they comprise a diffuse maculopapular rash with crusts. Vesicles may occur prior to ulceration and crust formation. Ulcerated lesions occur and are most often seen at mucocutaneous junctions and may extend into the oral cavity. Secondary bacterial infection of ulcerated areas is common. Subcutaneous hemorrhage may occur. The disease is accompanied by fever, anorexia, lymphadenopathy, and respiratory signs.

A variety of organ systems are affected. High morbidity is common during the initial outbreak with a variable mortality. Diagnosis can be made serologically. Cross-protection may be possible using human varicella virus (Felsenfeld and Schmidt, 1979) or the human varicella vaccine. Human varicella has been reported in a captive gorilla (Myers *et al.,* 1987). Exacerbation of latent infections has been seen following the stress of colony reorganization.

Hemorrhagic fevers are often fatally acute in the nonhuman primate. Primary focal hemorrhage is more likely to affect internal organs. Skin lesions are typically macular and associated with hemorrhage from capillary fragility or a rapidly developing thrombocytopenia. Hemorrhage in the form of bruising may develop at pressure points. Simian hemorrhagic fever (SHF) requires exposure to an inapparent carrier species, the patas monkey or baboon.

A number of New World and Old World species are susceptible to measles. Cutaneous lesions are described as viral exanthems, the hematogenous dissemination of virus to the skin.

Generalized eruption of a macular or papular rash follows fever and respiratory signs (Renne *et al.,* 1973; Remfrey, 1976; Montroy *et al.,* 1980; Roberts *et al.,* 1988). Diagnosis can be made by serology and history. Measles is decreasing in prevalence in the human population, and because humans are the primary source of infection for nonhuman primates, this reduces the potential of colony outbreaks. Potentially infected or exposed humans should be excluded from contact with nonhuman primates. Another source of infection is research utilizing live virus for molecular or vaccine stidies (Lowenstine, 1993).

Juvenile and adult macaques infected with SRV type 2 have developed noma, which is a necrotizing skin lesion affecting the skin over the maxillary dental arcade. It is seen as a rapidly developing ischemic area on the midline of the face involving the tissues of the nose and lips. The mucous membranes and bony structures of the upper dental arcade may also be affected. Involved tissues become reddened, edematous, ischemic, necrotic, and slough over a course of 3–4 days. Soft tissue lesions respond to supportive care and wound debridement; the resulting cutaneous defect persists for life. When bone necrosis and an accompanying osteomyelitis are present, the response to therapy is poor and mortality is high. Specific etiologic agents have not been identified from the lesions. Mixed bacterial flora are identified in necrotic areas. The mandible is less often affected. Lesions are generally restricted to a single portion of the dental arcade. Noma has also been reported in the cotton-top marmoset (*Saguinus oedipus*) (Brack, 1982). In this case, the condition was not associated with an identified retroviral infection.

Subcutaneous lesions similar to the lesions of Kaposi's sarcoma have been reported in *Macaca nemestrina* infected with SRV type 2 (Tsai *et al.,* 1985; Tsai, 1993). The more common presentation of this type of fibroid lesion is as retroperitoneal fibromatosis (Giddens *et al.,* 1979).

A maculopapular rash in the axillary and inguinal area is reported in both SIV- and HIV-infected macaques. Although not uniformly present, it is reported consistently under experimental conditions. Similar skin lesions are not reported in endemically infected African species. The appearance of the rash appears to correlate to Langerhans cell density in the area (Ringler *et al.,* 1987). This lesion precedes the appearance of clinical signs of acquired immunodeficiency syndrome (AIDS) in the animal and is often the first indication of infection. Secondary skin infection caused by bacterial and fungal agents can be observed following immunosuppression. Granulomatous skin lesions have been reported for SIV-infected rhesus macaques (Horvarth *et al.,* 1993).

Borrelia burgdorferi has been reported in nonhuman primates. The disease requires exposure to infected ticks of the genus *Dermacentor* or *Rhipicephalus*. Lesions are reported as concentric red rings radiating from the central area of the bite. The lesion, erythema migrans, develops several days to weeks following the tick bite (Philipp *et al.,* 1993). Exposure to the infected arthropod vector is essential for transmission. A history of outdoor housing with access to grassy areas may be indicative of Lyme disease without the presence of the characteristic skin lesion. Postexposure findings are fever and lameness due to chronic arthralgia (Roberts *et al.,* 1995). Serological tests for antibody are beneficial in the diagnosis.

Spontaneous *Mycobacterium leprae* infection has been reported in the sooty mangabey, *Cercocebus atys* (Meyers *et al.,* 1985), and the common chimpanzee, *Pan troglodytes* (Leininger *et al.,* 1978, 1980; Baskin, 1993). The initial case of leprosy in the mangabey was felt to have been transmitted from humans. The possibility for animal-to-human transmission exists but has not been verified (Hagstad, 1983a,b). Tuberculoid leprosy is characterized by cutaneous granuloma formation, which frequently ulcerates. In lepromatous leprosy, a weaker host immune response occurs, resulting in more numerous lesions. The cutaneous lesions of leprosy are seen most often on areas of the body with slightly lower skin temperatures, such as the ears, hands, feet, tail, and brow ridges. Lepromin intradermal testing may be beneficial; serological tests for antibody are more consistent in reaching a diagnosis. Acid-fast staining of impression smears of ulcerated areas does not always demonstrate organisms.

Mycobacterium sp. have been isolated from subcutaneous fistulas, tracts, and abscesses (Rush, 1977; Hines *et al.,* 1995) and with generalized infections (Chandrasekharan and Krishnamurthi, 1951; Lindsey and Melby, 1966). Regional lymph nodes may fistulate and act as a nidus for recurrence. The lesion is poorly responsive to therapy (Wolf *et al.,* 1988). Generally the etiologic agent is an atypical *Mycobacterium. Mycobacterium kansasii* was reported in a rhesus colony (Valerio *et al.,* 1978). Concurrent infection with an immunosuppressive retrovirus may predispose nonhuman primates to mycobacterial infection.

Disseminated intravascular coagulopathy is an acute, life-threatening condition and indicative of generalized sepsis (White *et al.,* 1980). The cutaneous response may be variable; however, diffuse thrombus formation is characteristic. When affecting the vascular beds of the skin, thrombi cause stellate-shaped areas of hemorrhage. If the animal stabilizes, these lesions may become necrotic due to ischemia. The associated thrombocytopenia results in ecchymotic or diffuse hemorrhage as platelets are consumed during the clotting cascade. Skin lesions have a generalized distribution, with hemorrhage being more common at contact points.

Atopic dermatitis is seen in nonhuman primates housed on wood-based contact bedding or over pans containing chips. Atopy has been associated with exposure to tree pollens in the Japanese macaque (*Macaca fuscata*) (Yokota *et al.,* 1987). The route of exposure to the allergen is respiratory. The affected animal presents with pruritis, regional alopecia, and scaly, hyperkeratotic areas with lichenification. Thickening is most prominent over the shoulders and in the flank. Hyperpigmentation (acanthosis) may occur in more chronic cases. Moist pyoderma may be a secondary feature and excoriations are common. Diagnostic testing includes intradermal allergen testing. Canine preparations can be used and should include regional plant ma-

terials and, when possible, allergens contained within the bedding. Anaphylaxis is possible during the following testing due to the high allergen load present in the test materials. Skin biopsies of the affected areas are confirmatory.

Reports indicate that dermatitis with autologous bone marrow transplantation (Feldman *et al.,* 1995) or toxic epidermal necrolysis with heterologous bone marrow transplantation may occur. Debate exists as to an association with graft-versus-host response (Krueger, 1973).

Psoriasiform dermatosis has been reported in *Macaca mulatta* (Lowe *et al.,* 1982; Lowe, 1985; Rubel, 1993) and in a single *Macaca fascicularis* (Jayo *et al.,* 1988) with lesions similar to those of humans. The characteristic epidermal lesions were parakeratosis, microabscesses, suprapapillary epidermal thinning, inflammatory cells within the epidermis, and reduction of the stratum granulosum. The vasculature of the dermis was tortuous with infiltration of neutrophils, lymphocytes, and monocytes.

Seborrheic dermatitis has been observed in a rhesus macaque (Newcomer *et al.,* 1984), characterized by an increase in sebaceous gland activity. Affected areas demonstrated fine scale without erythema. Lesions are often symmetrical in humans and are associated with the yeast *Pityosporum. Pemphigus vulgaris* has been reported in a baboon (Rosenberg *et al.,* 1987) and a pig-tailed macaque (Wolff *et al.,* 1986) with characteristic lesions of parakeratosis, acanthosis, secondary skin infection, increased sebaceous secretions, and antinuclear antibodies. Spontaneous hypercholesterolemia with cutaneous deposition of cholesterol resembling xanthoma plana, yellow orange fatty plaques, has been reported in the titi monkey (*Callicebus moloch*) (Roberts *et al.,* 1986).

In most mammalian species, endocrine imbalances result in alterations to skin and hair. In the nonhuman primate, few documented cases exist to verify endocrine abnormalities as a cause of skin pathology. Hypothyroidism with typical skin lesions has been reported in a single chimpanzee (Miller *et al.,* 1983). In three congenitally hypothyroid baboons, the gross and histopathologic appearance of the skin failed to demonstrate classic signs. Myxedema was evident in two of the three animals shortly after birth; both became obese and one demonstrated retarded skeletal growth. It is likely that additional endocrine cases exist and remain to be reported.

Congenital defects in the skin occur, but the frequency of these occurrences makes detailed evaluations of the conditions difficult. A review of developmental abnormalities included skin problems (Hendrickx and Binkerd, 1993).

REFERENCES

Altmann, J., Schoeller, D., Altmann, S. A., Muruthi, P., and Sapolsky, R. M. (1993). Body size and fatness of free-living baboons reflect food availability and activity levels. *Am. J. Primatol.* **30**(2), 149–161.

Ambrus, J. L., Strandstrom, H. V., and Kawinski, W. (1969). "Spontaneous" occurrence of Yaba tumor in a monkey colony. *Experientia* **25,** 64.

Anderson, D. C., Swenson, R. B., Orkin, J. L., Kalter, S. S., and McClure, H. M. (1994). Primary Herpesvirus simiae (B-virus) infection in infant macaques. *Lab. Anim. Sci.* **44**(5), 526–530.

Anonymous. (1980). Note on *Anatrichosoma* in primates and request for information. *Lab. Primate Newsl.* **19**(1), 7.

Ayres, J. P. (1971). Studies of the Delta herpesvirus isolated from the patas monkey (*Erythrocebus patas*). *Laboratory Animal Science* **21**, 685–695.

Bagnall, B. G., and Gruenberg, W. (1972). Generalized *Trichophyton mentagrophytes* ringworm in capuchin monkeys (*Cebus nigrivitatus*). *Br. J. Dermatol.* **87**, 565–570.

Baskin, G. B. (1993). Leprosy. *In* "Nonhuman Primates II" (T. C. Jones, U. Mohr, and R. D. Hunt, eds.), pp. 8–14. Springer-Verlag, Berlin.

Baskin, G. B., Eberhard, M. L., Watson, E., and Fish, R. (1984). Diagnostic exercise. [Cutaneous acariasis of sooty mangabeys.] *Lab. Anim. Sci.* **34**(6), 602–603.

Bellinger, D. A., and Bullock, B. C. (1988). Cutaneous *Mycobacterium avium* infection in a cynomolgus monkey. *Lab. Anim. Sci.* **38**(1), 85–86.

Beniashvili, D. S. (1989). An overview of the world literature on spontaneous tumors in nonhuman Primates. *J. Med. Primatol.* **18**(6), 423–437.

Biberstein, E. L., Jang, S. S., and Hirsh, D. C. (1984). Species distribution of coagulase-positive *Staphylococci* in animals. *J. Clin. Microbiol.* **19**(5), 610–615.

Blakely, G. A., Lourie, B., Morton, W. G., Evans, H. H., and Kaufmann, A. F. (1973). A varicella-like disease in macaque monkeys. *J. Infect. Dis.* **127**, 617–625.

Boever, W. J., and Kern, T. (1976). Papillomas in black and white colobus monkeys (*Colobus polykomus*). *J. Wildl. Dis.* **12**, 180–181.

Boncyk, L. H., and Kalter, S. S. (1980). Bacteriological findings in a nonhuman primate colony. *Dev. Biol. Stand.* **45**, 23–28.

Brack, M. (1977). Morphological and epidemiological aspects of simian herpesvirus infections, *SCRIFTENREIHE VERSUCHSTIERKUNDE* **5**, 1–63.

Brack, M. (1982). Noma in *Saguinus oedipus*: A report of 2 cases. *Lab. Anim.* **16**(4), 361–363 (Ger. summ.).

Brack, M., and Martin, D. P. (1984). Trichoepithelioma in a Barbary ape (*Macaca sylvanus*): Review of cutaneous tumors in nonhuman primates and case report. *J. Med. Primatol.* **13**(3), 159–164.

Breznock, A. W., and Pulley, L. T. (1975). *Anatrichosoma* infection in two white-handed gibbons. *J. Am. Vet. Med. Assoc.* **167**, 631–633.

Bronaugh, R. L., Weingarten, D. P., and Lowe, N. J. (1986). Differential rates of percutaneous absorption through the eczematous and normal skin of a monkey. *J. Invest. Dermatol.* **87**(4), 451–453.

Brunnert, S. R., Herron, A. J., and Altman, N. H. (1990). Subcutaneous leiomyosarcoma in a Peruvian squirrel monkey (*Saimiri*). *Vet. Pathol.* **27**(2), 126–128.

Burgdorfer, W. (1980). The spotted fever-group diseases. *In* "CRC Handbook Series in Zoonoses" (H. Stoenner, W. Kaplan, and M. Torten, eds.), Sect. A, Vol. 2, pp. 279–301. CRC Press, Boca Raton, FL.

Burr, E. W., and Kulshrestha, S. B. (1982). *Hemophilus influenza* recorded from a subcutaneous abscess of a rhesus monkey in Uttar Pradesh, India. *Indian Vet. J.* **59**, 10–11.

Butler, T. M., Gleiser, C. A., Bernal, J. C., and Ajello, L. (1988). Case of disseminated African histoplasmosis in a baboon. *J. Med. Primatol.* **17**(3), 153–161.

Cameron, A. M., and Conroy, J. D. (1976). Papillary carcinoma of apocrine sweat glands in a capuchin monkey (*Cebus albifrons*). *J. Med. Primatol.* **5**, 56–59.

Chandrasekharan, K. P., and Krishnamurthi, D. (1951). A case of generalized tuberculosis in a monkey (*Macaca* sp.). *Indian Vet. J.* **27**, 381–385.

Chapman, W. L., Jr., Hanson, W. L., Hayre, H. D., and Harrison, D. P. (1985). An enlarged aggregate of apocrine glands on the chest of karyotype I owl monkeys. *Lab. Anim. Sci.* **35**(5), 491–492.

Clarkson, M. J., Thorpe, E., and McCarthy, K. (1967). A virus disease of captive vervet monkeys (*Cercopithecus aethiops*) caused by a new herpesvirus. *Archiv. für die gesamte Virusforschung* **22**, 219–233.

Donham, K. J., and Leininger, J. R. (1977). Spontaneous leprosy-like disease in a chimpanzee. *J. Infect. Dis.* **136**, 132–136.

Douglas, J. D., Cronin, R. J., and Kaufmann, A. F. (1971). Spontaneous melioidosis in recently imported monkeys. *In* "Medical Primatology 1970" (E. I. Goldsmith and J. Moor-Jankowski, eds.), pp. 742–747. Karger, Basel.

Eichberg, J. W., and De Villez, R. L. (1984). Alopecia totalis in a chimpanzee. *J. Med. Primatol.* **8**, 81–88.

Epple, G., Belcher, A. M., and Smith, A. B., III (1986). Chemical signals in callitrichid monkeys: A comparative review. *In* "Chemical Signals in Vertebrates 4: Ecology, Evolution, and Comparative Biology" (D. Duvall, D. Mueller-Schwarze, and R. M. Silverstein, eds.), pp. 653–672. Plenum, New York.

Espana, C. (1971). A pox disease of monkeys transmissible to man. *In* "Medical Primatology 1970" (E. I. Goldsmith and J. Moor-Jankowski, eds.), pp. 694–708. Karger, Basel.

Espana, C. (1973). Herpesvirus simiae infection in *Macaca radiata*. *Am. J. Phys. Anthropol.* **38**, 447–454.

Fanton, J. W. (1985). Cosmetic repair of chronic head restraint defects. *J. Med. Primatol.* **14**(1), 29–34.

Feldman, S. H., Metzger, M., and Hoyt, F. R., Jr. (1995). Dermatitis in a rhesus macaque after autologous bone marrow transplantation. *Lab. Anim.* **24**(3), 17–19.

Felsenfeld, L., and Schmidt, N. J. (1979). Varicella-zoster virus immunizes patas monkeys against simian varicella-like disease. *J. Gen. Virol.* **42**, 171–178.

Fenner, F. (1990). Poxviruses of laboratory animals. *Lab. Anim. Sci.* **40**(5), 469–480.

Fisher, L. E., and Lederer, H. A. (1960). Ringworm infection of zoo animals *VM/SAC, Vet. Med. Small Anim. Clin.* **55**(4), 52–53.

Fisher, L. F., and Robinson, F. R. (1976). Basal cell tumor in a DeBrazza monkey. *Vet. Pathol.* **13**, 449–450.

Fleischman, R. W., and McCracken, D. (1977). Paecilomycosis in a nonhuman primate (*Macaca mulatta*). *Vet. Pathol.* **14**, 387–391.

Fleming, M. P. (1979). Laboratory diagnosis of dermatomycosis (ringworm) in animals. *Primate Supply* **4**(1), 13–14.

Fox, J. G., Campbell, L. H., Reed, C., Snyder, S. B., and Soave, O. A. (1973). Dermatophilosis (cutaneous stretothricosis) in owl monkeys. *J. Am. Vet. Med. Assoc.* **163**, 642–644.

Frazier, K. S., Herron, A. J., Hines, M. E., II, and Altman, N. H. (1993). Immunohistochemical and morphologic features of an nevocellular nevus (benign intradermal junctional melanocytoma) in a rhesus monkey (*Macaca mulatta*). *Vet. Pathol.* **30**(3), 306–308.

Gard, E. A., and London, W. T. (1983). Clinical history and viral characterization of Delta herpesvirus infection in a patas monkey colony. *In* "Viral and Immunological Diseases In Nonhuman Primates" (S. S. Kalter, ed.), pp. 211–212. Liss, New York.

Geissmann, T. (1987). A sternal gland in the siamang gibbon (*Hylobates syndactylus*). *Int. J. Primatol.* **8**(1), 1–15.

Georg, L. K. (1954). The diagnosis of ringworm in animals. *VM/SAC, Vet. Med. Small Anim. Clin.* **49**, 157–166.

Giddens, W. E., Jr., Bielitzki, J. T., Morton, W. R., Ochs, H. D., Myers, M. S., Blakely, G. A., and Boyce, J. T. (1979). Idiopathic retroperitoneal fibrosis: An enzootic disease in the pigtail monkey (*Macaca nemestrina*). *Lab. Investi.* **40**, 294 (abstr.).

Goldman, L., and Feldman, M. D. (1949). Human infestation with scabies of monkeys. *Arch. Dermatol. Syphilol.* **59**, 175–178.

Gough, A. W., Barsoum, N. J., Gracon, S. I., Mitchell, L., and Sturgess, J. M. (1982). Poxvirus infection in a colony of common marmosets (*Callithrix jacchus*). *Lab. Anim. Sci.* **32**, 87–90.

Hagstad, H. V. (1983a). Leprosy in sub-human primates: Potential risk for transfer of *Mycobacterium leprae* to humans. *Lepr. Rev.* **54**(4), 353–356 (letter).

Hagstad, H. V. (1983b). Leprosy in sub-human primates: Potential risk for transfer of *M. leprae* to humans. *Int. J. Zoonoses* **10**(2), 127–131.

Harwell, G. L., and Dalgard, D. (1979). *Anatrichosoma cutaneum* dermatitis in non-human primates. *Proc. Annu. Meet., Am. Assoc. Zoo Vet.*, pp. 83–86a.

Heldstab, A., Ruedi, D., Sonnabend, W., and Deinhardt, F. (1981). Spontaneous generalized Herpesvirus hominis infection of a lowland gorilla (*Gorilla gorilla gorilla*). *J. Med. Primatol.* **10**, 129–135.

Hendrickx, A. G., and Binkerd, P. E. (1993). Congenital malformations in nonhuman primates. *In* "Nonhuman Primates I" (T. C. Jones, U. Mohr, and R. D. Hunt, eds.), pp. 170–180. Springer-Verlag, Berlin.

Hickey, T. E., Kelly, W. A., and Sitzman, J. E. (1983). Demodectic mange in a tamarin (*Saguinus geoffroy*). *Lab. Anim. Sci.* 33(2), 192–193.

Hill, WCO, Sabater, Pi, J. (1970). Notes on two anomalies in mandrills (*Mandrillus spinx Linn.*). *Folia Primatologica,* 12, 290–295.

Hines, M. E. II, Kreeger, J. M., Herron, A. J. (1995). Mycobacterial infections of animals: Pathology and pathogenesis. *Laboratory Animal Science* 45(4), 334–351.

Hubbard, G. B., and Wood, D. H. (1984). Glomangiomas in four irradiated *Macaca mulatta. Vet. Pathol.* 21(6), 609–610.

Hunt, R. D. (1993a). Herpesviruses of Primates: An introduction. *In* "Nonhuman Primates I" (T. C. Jones, U. Mohr, and R. D. Hunt, eds.), pp. 74–78. Springer-Verlag, Berlin.

Hunt, R. D. (1993b). Herpesvirus simplex infection. *In* "Nonhuman Primates I" (T. C. Jones, U. Mohr, and R. D. Hunt, eds.), pp. 82–86. Springer-Verlag, Berlin.

Hunt, R. D., and Blake, B. J. (1993a). Herpesvirus B infection. *In* "Nonhuman Primates I" (T. C. Jones, U. Mohr, and R. D. Hunt, eds.), pp. 78–81. Springer-Verlag, Berlin.

Hunt, R. D., and Blake, B. J. (1993b). Herpesvirus Platyrhinae infection. *In* "Nonhuman Primates I" (T. C. Jones, U. Mohr, and R. D. Hunt, eds.), pp. 100–103. Springer-Verlag, Berlin.

Hunt, R. D., Garcia, F. G., Barahona, H. H., King, N. W., Fraser, C. E. O., and Melendez, L. V. (1973). Spontaneous herpesvirus *Saimiri* lymphoma in an owl monkey. *J. Infect. Dis.* 127, 723–725.

Jayo, M. J., Zanolli, M. D., and Jayo, J. M. (1988). Psoriatic plaques in *Macaca fascicularis. Vet. Pathol.* 25(4), 282–285.

Jelinek, F. (1985). Local dermatitis with subsequent pigmentation in green monkeys (*Cercopithecus aethiops*). *Z. Versuchstierkd.* 27(3-4), 121–124 (Ger. summ.).

Kalter, S. S. (1988). Herpesvirus infection in Old and New World monkeys. *Dev. Vet. Virol.* 6, 101–133.

Kaplan, W., George, L. K., Hendricks, S. L., Leeper, R. A. (1957). Isolation of Microsporum distortum from animals in the United States. *Journal of Infectious Diseases,* 28, 449–453.

Kessler, M. J. (1982). Nasal and cutaneous anatrichosomiasis in the free-ranging rhesus monkeys (*Macaca mulatta*) of Cayo Santiago. *Am. J. Primatol.* 3(1-4), 55–60.

Kessler, M. J., and Brown, R. J. (1979). Clinical description of tetanus in squirrel monkeys (*Saimiri sciureus*). *Lab. Anim. Sci.* 29, 240–242.

Kohdakovich, L., Szczeniowski, M., Manbu-ma-Disu, Jezek, Z., Marennikova, S., Nakano, J., and Messinger, D. (1987). The role of squirrels in maintaining monkeypox transmission. *Trop. Geogr. Med.* 39(2), 115–122.

Kitaoka, M. (1972). Serological survey of scrub typhus on monkeys imported from the Southeast Pacific area. *J. Hyg. Epidemiol. Microbiol. Immunol.* 16, 257–260.

Klokke, A. H., and de Vries, G. A. (1963). Tinea capitis in chimpanzees caused by *Microsporum canis,* Bodin 1902, resembling *M. obesum,* Conant 1937. *Sabouraudia* 2, 268–270.

Kloos, W. E., and Wolfshohl, J. F. (1979). Evidence for deoxyribonucleotide sequence divergence between *Staphylococci* living on human and other primate skin. *Curr. Microbiol.* 3, 167–172.

Kloos, W. E., and Wolfshohl, J. F. (1983). Deoxyribonucleotide sequence divergence between *Staphylococcus cohnii* subspecies populations living on primate skin. *Curr. Microbiol.* 8(2), 115–121.

Kloster, B. E., Manias, D. A., Ostrow, R. S., Shaver, M. K., McPherson, S. W., Rangen, S. R. S., Uno, H., and Faras, A. J. (1988). Molecular cloning and characterization of the DNA of two papilloviruses from monkeys. *Virology* 166(1), 30–40.

Klumpp, S. A., and McClure, H. M. (1993). Dermatophilosis, skin. *In* "Nonhuman Primates II" (T. C. Jones, U. Mohr, and R. D. Hunt, eds.), pp. 14–18. Springer-Verlag, Berlin.

Krueger, G. R. F. (1973). Graft-versus-host disease and toxic epidermal necrolysis. *Lancet* 1, 268–269 (letter).

Laber-Laird, K., McDole, G., and Jerome, C. (1988). Unexpected frostbite in cynomolgus macaques after a short exposure to snow. *Lab. Anim. Sci.* 38(3), 325–326.

Lane, J. M., Steele, J. H., and Beran, G. W. (1981). Pox and parapox virus infections. *In* "CRC Handbook Series in Zoonoses" (G. W. Beran, ed), Sect. B, Vol. 2, pp. 365–385. CRC Press, Boca Raton, FL.

Lebel, R. R., and Nutting, W. B. (1973). Demodectic mites of subhuman primates. I. Demodex sarnini sp., N. (Acari: Demodicidae) from the squirrel monkey; Saimiri sciureus. *Journal of Parasitology.* 59, 719–722.

Lee, K. J., Lang, C. M., Hughes, H. C., and Hartshorn, R. D. (1981). Psorergatic mange (Acari: *Psotergatidae*) of the stumptail macaque (*Macaca arctoides*). *Lab. Anim. Sci.* 31, 77–79.

Lehman, P. A., Slattery, J. T., and Franz, T. J. (1988). Percutaneous absorption of retinoids: Influence of vehicle, light exposure, and dose. *J. Invest. Dermatol.* 91(1), 56–61.

Leininger, J. R., Donham, K. J., and Rubino, M. J. (1978). Leprosy in a chimpanzee: Morphology of the skin lesions and characterization of the organism. *Vet. Pathol.* 15, 339–346.

Leininger, J. R., Donham, K. J., and Meyers, W. M. (1980). Leprosy in a chimpanzee: Postmortem lesions. *Int. J. Lepr.* 48, 414–421,

Lindsey, J. R., and Melby, E. C., Jr. (1966). Naturally occurring primary cutaneous tuberculosis in the rhesus monkey. *Lab. Anim. Care* 16, 369–385.

Line, A. S., and Morykwas, M. J. (1993). Use of cultured human epidermal xenografts for treatment of large wounds in nonhuman primates. *Am. J. Primatol.* 30(4), 328 (abstr.).

Line, S., Dorr, T., Roberts, J., and Ihrke, P. (1984). Necrotizing cellulitis in a squirrel monkey. *J. Am. Vet. Med. Assoc.* 185(11), 1378–1379.

Lippincott, S. W., Montour, J. L., and Wilson, J. D. (1973). Electron irradiation of monkey skin. *Acta Radiol.: Thera. Phys. Biol.* 12, 347–352 (Ger. and Fr. summ.).

Loebel, R. R., and Nutting, W. B. (1973). Demodectic mites of sub-human primates. I. *Demodex samiri* sp., N. (*Acari: Demodicidae*) from the squirrel monkey, *Samiri sciureus. J. Parasitol.* 59, 719–722.

Lourie, B., Morton, W. G., Blakely, G. A., and Kaufman, A. F. (1971). Epizootic vesicular disease in macaque monkeys. *Lab. Anim. Sci.* 21, 1079–1080.

Lowe, N. J. (1985). Psoriasiform dermatosis in a nonhuman primate. *In* "Models in Dermatology" (H. I. Maiback and N. J. Lowe, eds.), Vol. 1, pp. 181–186. Karger, Basel.

Lowe, N. J., Breeding, J., Chalet, M., and Russell, D. H. (1982). Psoriasiform process in a rhesus monkey: Epidermal measurements. *Psoriasis, Proc. Int. Symp., 3rd, 1981,* pp. 349–350.

Lowenstine, L. J. (1986). Neoplasms and proliferative disorders in nonhuman primates. *In* "Primates: The Road to Self-Sustaining Populations" (K. Benirschke, ed.), pp. 781–814. Springer-Verlag, New York.

Lowenstine, L. J. (1993). Measles virus infection, nonhuman primates. *In* "Nonhuman Primates I" (T. C. Jones, U. Mohr, and R. D. Hunt, eds.), pp. 108–118. Springer-Verlag, Berlin.

Malley, A. (1968). Skin manifestations of drug toxicity as revealed in nonhuman primates. *In* "Conference on Nonhuman Primate Toxicology" (C. O. Miller, ed.), pp. 141–144. U.S. Printing Office, Washington, DC.

May, B. D. (1972). *Corynebacterium ulcerans* infections in monkeys. *Lab. Anim. Sci.* 22, 609–513.

McClure, H. M., Swenson, R. B., Kalter, S. S., and Lester, T. L. (1980). Natural genital Herpesvirus hominis infection in chimpanzees (*Pan troglodytes* and *Pan paniscus*). *Lab. Anim. Sci.* 30, 895–901.

McConnell, S. (1970). Simian pox viruses. *In* "Infections and Immunosuppression in Sub-human Primates" (H. Balner and W. I. B. Beveridge, eds.), pp. 83–86. Williams & Wilkins, Baltimore.

McNulty, W. P. (1972). Pox diseases in primates. *In* "Pathology of Simian Primates" (R. N. T.-W.-Fiennes, T. Orihel, and J. Ayers, eds.), Part 2, pp. 612–645. Karger, Basel.

Meyers, W. M., Walsh, G. P., Brown, H. L., Binford, C. H., Imes, G. D., Jr., Hadfield, T. L., Schlagel, C. J., Fukunishi, Y., Gerone, P. J., Wolf, R. H., Gormus, B. J., Martin, L. N., Harboe, M., and Imaeda, T. (1985). Leprosy in a mangabey monkey: Naturally acquired infection. *Int. J. Lepr.* 53(1), 1–14.

Migaki, G. (1986). Mycotic infections in nonhuman primates. *In* "Primates: The Road to Self-Sustaining Populations" (K. Benirschke, ed.), pp. 557–570. Springer-Verlag, New York.

Migaki, G., and Seibold, H. R. (1976). Dermatophilosis in a titi monkey (*Callicebus moloch*). *Am. J. Vet. Res.* **37**, 1225–1226.

Migaki, G., DiGiacomo, R., and Garner, F. M. (1971). Squamous cell carcinoma of skin in a rhesus monkey (*Macaca mulatta*): Report of a case. *Lab. Anim. Sci.* **21**, 410–411.

Miller, R. E., Albert, S. G., and Boever, W. J. (1983). Hypothyroidism in a chimpanzee. *J. Am. Vet. Med. Assoc.* **183**(11), 1326–1328.

Montroy, R. D., Huxsoll, D. L., Hildebrandt, P. K., Booth, B. W., and Arimbalam, S. (1980). An epizootic of measles in captive silvered leaf-monkeys (*Presbytis cristatus*) in Malaysia. *Lab. Anim. Sci.* **30**, 694–697.

Myers, M. G., Kramer, L. W., and Stanberry, L. R. (1987). Varicella in a gorilla. *J. Med. Virol.* **23**(4), 317–322.

Newcomer, C. E., Fox, J. G., Taylor, R. M., and Smith, D. E. (1984). Seborrheic dermatitis in a rhesus monkey (*Macaca mulatta*). *Lab. Anim. Sci.* **34**(2), 185–187.

Newell-Morris, L. (1979). Midlo and Cummins updated: Primate dermatoglyphics today and tomorrow. *Birth Defects, Orig. Artic. Ser.* **15**, 739–764.

Padovan, D. (1982). The pathology of Delta herpesvirus. *Proc. Annu. Meet., Am. Assoc. Zoo Vet.*, p. 41.

Padovan, D., and Cantrell, C. A. (1986). Varicella-like herpesvirus infections of nonhuman primates. *Lab. Anim. Sci.* **36**(1), 7–13.

Philip, R. N. (1980). Scrub typhus. *In* "CRC Handbook Series in Zoonoses" (H. Stoenner, W. Kaplan, and M. Torten, eds.), Sect. A, Vol. 2, pp. 303–315. CRC Press, Boca Raton, FL.

Philipp, M. T., Aydintug, M. K., Bohm, R. P., Cogswell, F. B., Dennis, V. A., and Lanners, H. N. (1993). Early and early disseminated phases of Lyme disease in the rhesus monkey: A model for infection in humans. *Infec. Immunol.* **61**, 3047–3059.

Rangan, S. R. S., Gutter, A., Baskin, G. B., and Anderson, D. (1980). Virus associated papillomas in colobus monkeys (*Colobus guereza*). *Lab. Anim. Sci.* **30**, 885–889.

Ratteree, M. S., and Baskin, G. B. (1992). Congenital hypotrichosis in a rhesus monkey. *Lab. Anim. Sci.* **2**(4), 410–412.

Raulston, G. L. (1972). Psorergatic mites in patas monkeys. *Lab. Anim. Sci.* **22**, 107–108.

Remfrey, J. (1976). A measles epizootic with five deaths in newly imported rhesus monkeys (*Macaca mulatta*). *Lab. Anim.* **10**, 49–57.

Renne, R. A., McLaughlin, R., and Jenson, A. B. (1973). Measles virus-associated endometritis, cervicitis, and abortion in a rhesus monkey. *J. Am. Vet. Med. Assoc.* **163**, 639–641.

Richter, C. B., and Buyukmihci, N. (1979). Squamous cell of the epidermis in an aged white-lipped tamarin (*Saguinus fuscicollis leucogenys*, Gray). *Vet. Pathol.* **16**, 263–265.

Ringler, D. J., Hancock, W. W., King, N. W., and Murphy, G. F. (1987). Langerhans cells: Population dynamics, morphologic changes and immunophenotypic evidence suggesting their role as target cells in the rash of SIV-infected rhesus monkeys. *Lab. Invest.* **56**(1), 64a (abstr. only).

Roberts, E. D. (1993). *Simian varicella. In* "Nonhuman Primates I" (T. C. Jones, U. Mohr, and R. D. Hunt, eds.), pp. 93–100. Springer-Verlag, Berlin.

Roberts, E. D., Bohm, R. P., Jr., Cogswell, F. B., Lanners, H. N., Lowrie, R. C., Jr., Povinellie, L., Piesman, J., and Philipp, M. T. (1995). Chronic Lyme disease in a rhesus monkey. *Lab. Invest.* **72**(2), 146–160.

Roberts, J., Line, S., and Blanchard, P. (1986). Spontaneous hypercholesterolemia and atherosclerosis in a titi monkey. *J. Med. Primatol.* **15**(2), 131–138.

Roberts, J. A., Lerche, N. W., Anderson, J. H., Markovits, J. E., *et al.* (1988). Epizootic measles at the California Primate Research Center. *Lab. Anim. Sci.* **38**(4), 492 (abstr. only).

Rosenberg, D. P., Anderson, J. H., Silberg, B., and Henrickson, R. V. (1981). Advances in wound care for non-human primates. *Proc. Annu. Meet., Am. Assoc. Zoo Vet.*, pp. 65–57.

Rosenberg, D. P., De Villez, R. L., and Gleiser, C. A. (1987). Pemphigus vulgaris in a baboon. *Lab. Anim. Sci.* **37**(4), 489–491.

Rubel, G. R. (1993). Psoriasiform dermatosis, in a captive-born rhesus monkey. *Contemp. Top. Anim. Sci.* **32**(4), 13 (abstr.).

Rush, H. G. (1977). What's your diagnosis? [Cutaneous tuberculosis.] *Lab. Anim.* **6**(6), 16–18.

Sabater Pi, J. (1967). An albino gorilla from Rio Muni, West Africa, and notes on its adaptation to captivity. *Folia Primatologica*, **7**, 155–160.

Saliba, A. M., Matero, E. A., Moreno, G. (1968). Sporotrichosis in a chimpanzee. *Mod. Vet. Pract.* **49**, 74.

Saslaw, S. and Carlisle, H. N. (1966). Aerosol infection of monkeys with Rickettsia rickettsii. *Bacteriol. Rev.* **30**, 636.

Schmidt, N. J., Arvin, A. M., Martin, D. P., and Gard, E. A. (1983). Serological investigation of an outbreak of Simian varicella in *Erythrocebus patas* monkeys. *J. Clin. Microbiol.* **18**(4), 901–904.

Short, R., Williams, D. D., and Bowden, D. M. (1987). Cross-sectional evaluation of potential biological markers of aging in pigtailed macaques: Effects of age, sex and diet. *J. Gerontol.* **42**(6), 644–664.

Singleton, W. L., Smikle, C. B., Hankins, G. D., Hubbard, G. B., Ehler, W. J., and Brasky, K. B. (1994). Reconstructive vaginal surgery in the female baboon (*Papio* sp.) with Simian Agent 8. *Contemp. Top. Lab. Anim. Sci.* **33**(4), A-11 (abstr.).

Spencer, A. J., Anness, S. H., Fine, B. S. (1984). Spontaneous degenerative maculopathy in the monkey. *Opthomology.* **81**(5), 513–521.

Strum, S. C., and Western, J. D. (1982). Variations in fecundity with age and environment in olive baboons (*Papio anubis*). *Am. J. Primatol.* **3**(1-4), 61–76.

Sundberg, J. P., and O'Banion, M. K. (1989). Animal papillomaviruses associated with malignant tumors. *Adv. Viral Oncol.* **8**, 55–71.

Sundberg, J. P., and Reichmann, M. E. (1993). Papillomavirus infections. *In* "Nonhuman Primates II" (T. C. Jones, U. Mohr, and R. D. Hunt, eds.), pp. 1–8. Springer-Verlag, Berlin.

Tattersall, L. (1993). Madagascar's lemurs. *Sci. Am.* **268**(1), 110–117.

Tsai, C.-C. (1993). Fibromatosis in macaques infected with type D retroviruses. *In* "Nonhuman Primates I" (T. C. Jones, U. Mohr, and R. D. Hunt, eds.), pp. 48–57. Springer-Verlag, Berlin.

Tsai, C.-C., Warner, T. F. C. S., Uno, H., Giddens, W. E., Jr., and Ochs, H. D. (1985). Subcutaneous fibromatosis associated with an acquired immune deficiency syndrome in pig-tailed macaques. *Am. J. Pathol.* **120**(1), 30–37.

Uno, H. (1980). Baldness. *Comp. Pathol. Bull.* **12**(3), 2, 4.

Uno, H. (1987). Stumptailed macaques as a model of male-pattern baldness. *In* "Models in Dermatology" (H. I. Maiback and N. J. Lowe, eds.), pp. 159–169. Karger, Basel.

Valerio, D. A., Dalgard, D. W., Voelker, R. W., McCarrol, N. E., and Good, R. C. (1978). *Mycobacterium kansasii* infection in rhesus monkeys. *In* "Mycobacterial Infections of Zoo Animals" (R. J. Montalli, ed.), pp. 145–150. Smithsonian Institution Press, Washington, DC.

Weidman, F. D. (1935). Dermatoses of monkeys and apes. 9th Int. Congress of Dermatology, **1**, 600–606.

Weigler, B. J., Scinicariello, F., and Hilliard, J. K. (1994). Risk of veneral B Virus transmission in rhesus monkeys (*Macaca mulatta*) through use of molecular epidemiology. *Contemp. Top. Lab. Anim. Sci.* **33**(4), A-12 (abstr.).

White, G. L., Kosanke, S. D., Feeback, D. L., Reid, M. C., and Koehn, G. S. (1980). A clinically suspected case of disseminated intravascular coagulopathy in a female chimpanzee (a case report). *VM/SAC, Vet. Med. Small Anim. Clin.* **75**, 685–689.

Whittaker, D., and Glanister, J. R. (1985). A Yaba-like condition in a young baboon (*Papio anubis*). *Lab. Anim.* **19**(3), 177–179 (Ger. summ.).

Wolf, R. H., Gibson, S. V., Watson, E. A., and Baskin, G. B. (1988). Multidrug chemotherapy of tuberculosis in rhesus monkeys. *Lab. Anim. Sci.* **38**(1), 25–33.

Wolff, P. L., Garden, J. M., Marder, R., Rosenberg, D. P., and Sundberg, J. P. (1986). Pemphigus vulgaris in a pigtail macaque. *J. Am. Vet. Med. Assoc.* **189**(9), 1220–1221.

Yakavleva, L. A., Lennert, K., Chikobava, M. G., Indizhiya, L. V., Klotz, I. N., Lapin, B. A. (1993). Morphological characteristics of malignant T-cell lymphomas in baboons. *Pathological Anatomy and Histopathology.* **422**(2), 109–120.

Yanai, T., Wakabayashi, S., Masegi, T., Iwasaki, T., Yamazoe, K., Iskikawa, K., and Ueda, K. (1995). Basal cell tumor in a Japanese macaque (*Macaca fuscata*). *Vet. Pathol.* **32**(3), 318–320.

Yokota, A., Minezawa, M., Nakamura, S., Kanaizuk, T., Gotoh, S., and Baba, S. (1987). Naturally occurring Japanese cedar (*Cryptomeria japonia*) pollen-sosis in Japanese monkeys (*Macaca fuscata*) inhabiting Miyajima Island. *Reichorui Kenkyu/Primate Res.* **3**(2), 112–118.

Zeller, U., Epple, G., Kuederling, I., and Kuhn, H.-J. (1988). The anatomy of the circumgenital scent gland of *Saguinus fuscicollis* (Callitrichidae, Primates). *J. Zool.* **214**(1), 141–156.

Zimmerman, R. J. (1977). The population structure and electrophoretic analysis of *Staphylococcus* species isolated from mammalian skin. *Diss. Abstr. Int. B* **37**, 3773.

Zwartouw, H. T., MacArthur, J. A., Boulter, E. A., Seamer, J. H., Marston, J. H., and Chamove, A. S. (1984). Transmission of virus infection between monkeys especially in relation to breeding colonies. *Lab. Anim.* **18**(2), 125–130. (Ger. summ).

Chapter 10

Digestive System

Alan G. Brady and Daniel G. Morton

NONHUMAN PRIMATES IN BIOMEDICAL RESEARCH: DISEASES

TABLE I
DENTAL FORMULAS FOR PERMANENT TEETH

Source and location[a]	Incisors	Canines	Premolars	Molars[b]	Total
Old World primates					
U	2	1	2	3	32
L	2	1	2	3	
Cebidae					
U	2	1	3	3	36
L	2	1	3	3	
Callitrichidae					
U	2	1	3	2	32
L	2	1	3	2	
Prosimians					
U	2	1	3	3	36
L	2	1	3	3	

[a] U, upper; L, lower.
[b] Substantial variation in molar number exists between and within species; for a detailed discussion, see Napier and Napier (1967).

I. INTRODUCTION: DIAGNOSIS AND TREATMENT OF GASTROINTESTINAL DISEASE

Signs of gastrointestinal disease are among the most common problems seen in nonhuman primates (Holmberg *et al.*, 1982b). Some diseases producing gastrointestinal (GI) signs are limited to the gastrointestinal tract, whereas others may be multisystemic. This chapter focuses on the diagnosis and treatment of diseases of the gastrointestinal system. The reader is referred to other chapters in which diseases are discussed by etiology for more detailed descriptions of most of the diseases mentioned in this chapter.

The most common clinical sign that alerts the clinician to gastrointestinal disease in nonhuman primates is diarrhea (Hird *et al.*, 1984; Paul-Murphy, 1993). Vomiting and constipation are less commonly observed. Other, less specific, clinical signs observed in some cases of gastrointestinal disease include cachexia, abnormal stool, abdominal pain, distended abdomen, and straining to defecate. Diseases that primarily affect other organ systems may first present as gastrointestinal problems. For example, renal failure, hepatic failure, and pancreatitis can present with vomiting; hepatic diseases and right heart failure can be accompanied by diarrhea; and neoplastic or inflammatory masses in the abdomen may cause vomiting, diarrhea, or constipation. Vomiting most frequently is associated with diseases of the stomach or diseases within other organ systems.

II. ORAL CAVITY

A. Teeth

The teeth and dental pathology of nonhuman primates and humans are sufficiently similar to make nonhuman primates an appropriate and common model for dental research (Friskopp and Blomlof, 1988; Steinberg *et al.*, 1986; Page and Schroeder, 1982). Such common human dental conditions as caries, plaque, periodontal disease, dental abscesses, and fractures all occur spontaneously in primate species. Examination of the eruption pattern of the teeth of feral primates also has important husbandry implications; dental eruption and osseus development are the most useful indicators of general bodily maturity (Watts, 1977). A good program of dental preventive medicine is an important part of a comprehensive program of preventive medicine for any primate colony, as dental disease can lead to other more serious problems such as weight loss, imbalanced food selection, bacteremia (which can, among other things, complicate studies of catheterized animals and implants), and mandibular fractures.

1. Dental Eruption

Dental formulas for primates are shown in Table 1. Dental eruption tables for age determination in common laboratory primate species are shown in Tables II and III, with references for further reading provided in Table IV. It should be noted that studies examining teeth radiographically showed earlier eruption times than those using visual oral examination, but this difference is probably not substantial (Thorington and Vorek, 1976). Deciduous teeth erupt in three groups, incisors first, then canines and first molars, and finally second molars. The greatest variability occurs in eruption of the canine tooth. Comparative studies have been done on dental development in captive versus feral apes. Although they indicate that captivity has no effect, these studies are questionable because of lack of documentation regarding age and history of many of the animals included (Thoden Van Hozen, 1967). In the rhesus, eruption of permanent teeth is similar in males and females, except for the canines, which erupt later in males than in females (Cheverud, 1981). No sex differences exist in dental eruption patterns between male and female common marmosets (*Callithrix jacchus*) (Goss, 1984). In a radiographic study of the mandibular cheek teeth of *Cebus albifrons*, eruption occurred earlier in males (Fleagle and Schaffler, 1982).

2. Dental Abscesses

Dental abscesses are a recognized clinical entity in most common species of laboratory primates. Abscessed canine teeth are very common in squirrel monkeys (Abee, 1985; Olfert, 1974). In a breeding colony of approximately 400 *Saimiri* sp. (with a variety of ages represented) over a 3-year period, 51 animals had dental abscesses, with a majority being abscessed canine teeth. Other abscesses were usually associated with molars (S. D. Dillard-Palughi, personal communication, 1992).

Dental abscessation in nonhuman primates is not due to any one etiologic agent, rather to opportunistic infection as a result

TABLE II

OLD WORLD PRIMATE DENTAL ERUPTION

Species and type[a]	Incisors	Canines	Premolar	Molars	Reference
Gorilla gorilla					
D					
P	64–90	77–124	71–103	36–157	Smith *et al.* (1994)
Pan troglodytes					
D	60–200	256–565		84–431	Mooney *et al.* (1991)
P	59–92	96–121	73–100	36–163	Smith *et al.* (1994)
Macaca mulatta					
D	7–26	44–77		47–179	Gavan (1967)
P	22–37	47–73	37–49	14–74	Cheverud (1981)
M. fascicularis					
D	0–2	1–3	2–4		
P	23–37	36–51	37–49	14–49	Bowen and Koch (1970)
Cercopithecus aethiops					
D	6–34	35–45	45–75		
P	12–24	36–40	20–36	8–48	Ockerse (1959)
Papio sp.					
D					Smith *et al.* (1994)
P	35–41.5	48.5–56	49–56	21.5–72	Hummer (1967)

[a] D, deciduous (days); P, permanent (months).

of other dental problems (Kilgore, 1989; Lovell, 1990), some of which have not yet been identified. Any condition that causes exposure of the pulp cavity and/or tooth root can result in abscessation. Such conditions include excessive dental wear, caries, dental trauma resulting in loose or fractured teeth, periodontal disease, and endodontic procedures (see the section on cutting of canine teeth).

Animals having abscessed teeth usually present with facial swelling or a draining tract on the face. Maxillary canine tooth abscesses characteristically first appear as a swelling or draining tract below the eye. There may also be periorbital swelling and discharge associated with conjunctivitis on the affected side. Occasionally, a decrease in appetite, reluctance to use one side of the mouth, or other signs may be noted. Molar abscesses or other abscesses that have been present for an extended period may result in sepsis with associated systemic signs. In cases where the swelling is generalized (which often happens with

TABLE III

NEW WORLD PRIMATE DENTAL ERUPTION

Species and type[b]	Incisors	Canines	Premolars	Molars	Reference
Saimiri sp.					
D	0–21	14–28	28–63		
P	8–14	19–22	12–16	11–22	Long and Cooper (1968)
Callithrix iacchus					
D	1–13	7–32	14–53		Smith *et al.* (1994)
P					
Saguinus nigricollis					
D	At birth	At birth	0–28		
P	4–6	9–9.5	6–9	3–7	Smith *et al.* (1994)
Cebus albifrons[a]					
D					
P					Smith *et al.* (1994)
Aotus sp.					
D					
P					Smith *et al.* (1994)

[a] Only premolar data provided.

[b] D, deciduous (days); P, permanent (months).

TABLE IV
DENTAL ERUPTION IN SELECTED PRIMATES[a]

Species	References
Gorilla gorilla	Smith *et al.* (1994); Keiter (1981); Wiloughby (1978)
Pan troglodytes	Smith *et al.* (1994); Kuykendall *et al.* (1992); Nissen and Riesen (1945, 1964); Kraemer *et al.* (1982); Mooney *et al.* (1991)
Macaca fascicularis	Honjo *et al.* (1966) in Iwamoto *et al.* (1984); Spiegel (1929, 1934); Berkson (1968); Bowen and Koch (1970); Smith *et al.* (1994)
M. mulatta	Cheverud (1981); Hurme and van Wagenen (1953, 1961); Kuksova (1958); Gavan (1967); McNamara *et al.* (1977); Smith *et al.* (1994); Turnquist and Kessler (1990)
M. nemestrina	Sirianni and Swindler (1985); Smith *et al.* (1994)
Cercopithecus aethiops	Ockerse (1959); Smith *et al.* (1994)
Papio cynocephalus	Siegal and Sciulli (1973); Smith *et al.* (1994); Reed (1973); Lawrence *et al.* (1982)
P. hamadryas	Kuksova (1958); Smith *et al.* (1994); Hummer (1967)
Saimiri sciureus	Long and Cooper (1968); Smith *et al.* (1994); Galliari and Colillas (1985); Tappen and Severson (1971)
Callithrix jacchus	Kuster (1983); Smith *et al.* (1994); Tappen and Severson (1971); Johnston *et al.* (1970); Goss (1984)
Saguinus nigricollis	Chase *et al.* (1969); Smith *et al.* (1994)
Cebus albifrons	Fleagle and Schaffler (1982); Smith *et al.* (1994); Tappen and Severson (1971)
Aotus sp.	Hall *et al.* (1979); Smith *et al.* (1994); English (1934); Thorington and Vorek (1976)

[a] Adapted from Smith *et al.* (1994).

molar abscesses), close examination for loose and/or devitalized teeth (characterized by their dark appearance) or drainage around the tooth or teeth (more than one may be affected) may be useful in identifying the affected tooth. As in human dentistry, dental radiographs can provide definitive information regarding this condition. Dental abscesses must be differentiated from other conditions that result in facial swelling and/or drainage, such as trauma, hypoproteinemia, and renal disease.

Treatment for dental abscesses consists of extraction of the affected tooth or teeth and establishing drainage of purulent material. In animals showing signs of sepsis, systemic antibiotics and supportive treatment may be required (parenteral fluids, special diet, etc.). Failure to treat abscesses aggressively may result in loss of an eye due to retroorbital abscess or fatal extension of infection to the brain, respiratory tract, or other body systems.

3. Dental Fractures

Although little has been written regarding the management of broken teeth in primates, the approach to treatment should be considered similar to that in other animals. Extraction is the treatment of choice unless (as may be the case with well-developed canine teeth) this treatment could result in infection of a large open alveolus, malocclusion with associated pain, or inability to eat. In such cases, a root canal procedure may be considered if the fracture is fresh and the remaining tooth and root are in good condition. The use of this procedure for dental fractures has been described in other species (Ross and Myers, 1970).

4. Canine Tooth Extraction/Cutting/Blunting to Disarm Primates

The practice of cutting or extracting canine teeth in primates is one method used to reduce fight-related injuries associated with housing primates in groups and to reduce the potential of serious trauma among personnel handling these animals. Early techniques directed toward complete extraction of the canine teeth (Gibson and Hall, 1970) were invasive, substantial surgical procedures that had the potential for infection of the alveolus and malocclusion due to large gaps in the dental arcades left by the missing canines. Subsequent techniques were pulpectomies (removal of pulp from the dental pulp chamber and root canal) or pulpotomies (surgical excision of the coronal portion of the dental pulp) in which the tooth is excised at the desired level, the pulp cavity prepared, and then capped using amalgam or dental composite material. Most published procedures are abbreviated versions of human endodontic procedures (Reynolds and Hall, 1979; Thomson *et al.,* 1979). Although these avoid some of the more readily apparent problems associated with extraction, one study (Curtis *et al.,* 1986) of skulls from 47 *Macaca fascicularis* euthanatized 2 years after the procedure of Reynolds and Hall (1979) demonstrated osseous evidence of abscess formation in 79% of canines where the pulp chamber was exposed and 17% of cut canines with the pulp chamber not exposed. Pulpotomies and pulpectomies have a number of distinct advantages over extraction if a disarming procedure is required; however, the technique requires adherence to the same principles of human endodontic therapy: meticulous removal of pulp material from the root canal, careful preparation of all surfaces, and complete filling of the space with materials designed for the purpose. A procedure has been described (Schofield *et al.,* 1991). in which the tooth is amputated below the alveolar bone crest and the exposed pulp is covered by a mucoperiosteal gingival flap. This procedure may circumvent many of the problems associated with amputating the tooth. Blunting of canines is another alternative technique (Carter and Houghton, 1987).

5. Caries, Plaque, and Malocclusion

Dental caries have been described in many species of nonhuman primates. Evidence shows that these are not exclusively due to diets found in captivity, as has sometimes been assumed. One South African study of teeth from 50 newly captured vervets showed that 38% had carious lesions. The caries were primarily molar occlusal and in the interproximal areas of the anterior teeth (Gardy *et al.,* 1982). Other studies have confirmed the predisposition of the molars to caries in primates, with more caries occurring in the maxillary than mandibular molars (Cohen and Goldman, 1960). Housing arrangement may also play a role in carie formation; one study of *Saimiri* indicates that *Streptococcus* sp., which are more or less cariogenic depending on the serotype, tend to be the same among cagemates, but different between different cages of animals, even when animals with a different serotype are housed in the same room (Beighton and Hayday, 1982). There is evidence (also in *Saimiri*) that soft diets used in some research protocols affect dental occlusion; the lack of forceful chewing required for natural diets inhibits jaw growth, resulting in dental crowding and malocclusion (Corrucini and Beecher, 1982). In the past, these conditions have been largely ignored until a tooth abscesses or other acute condition arose. The anticipated holding of animals for extended periods makes a program of early intervention and more sophisticated preventive dentistry worthwhile. Such a program might include fluoride supplementation, dietary adjustment to reduce processed sugars and increase fibrous, hard-to-chew items (unless an animal has a preexisting condition that would make consumption of such items difficult), periodic dental exams, cleaning, and early treatment of caries, malocclusive conditions, and other nonacute dental conditions that have serious sequelae.

B. Periodontal Tissues

Periodontal Disease and Gingivitis

Gingivitis and periodontal disease strongly resemble these conditions in humans, both in etiology and in pathogenesis. Gingivitis and periodontal disease have several predisposing factors that promote both direct damage to gingival and periodontal tissue and colonization by opportunist pathogenic bacteria that cause additional invasion and damage. Bacterial flora associated with diseased periodontal tissue include *Actinomyces, Veilonella, Bacteroides,* and *Vibrio* bacteria (Page and Schroeder, 1982). Studies have demonstrated the presence of *Bacteroides gingivalis* in squirrel monkey gingiva, with infection associated with gingival disease in this species. *Bacteroides gingivalis* is one of the major etiologic agents for periodontitis in humans (Clark *et al.,* 1988). The enteric pathogen *Shigella flexneri* has also been implicated as a cause of periodontal disease (Armitage *et al.,* 1982, 1983).

Clinical signs for gingivitis consist primarily of mild inflammation of the soft tissues surrounding the teeth, often associated with plaque and/or calculus on the tooth enamel in the coronal region. As the condition progresses to periodontal disease, there is generalized inflammation of the periodontal tissue, receding of the gingival tissue, bone erosion, and foul breath. Tissues bleed easily when probed. Erosion of soft tissue and bone may cause loosening or loss of teeth and dental abscesses. In small primates, bone erosion may be sufficient to cause pathologic fractures of the mandible. Animals in advanced stages may be reluctant to eat or eat only soft foods and lose weight. At necropsy, the bone erosion, bone cratering due to abscesses, and increased vascular channels are visible on defleshed specimens.

Histologically, inflammatory infiltrates are visible in gingival and periodontal tissue. Gingivitis and periodontal disease must be differentiated from other inflammatory-erosive conditions of the mouth such as noma and viral ulcers. Localization of lesions to the area surrounding the teeth is characteristic of this condition.

Treatment of gingivitis and periodontal disease consists of removal of the inciting dental plaque and calculus from the teeth. Minimum safety precautions for the procedure include adequate chemical restraint and a properly fitted speculum for the animal and a face shield, high efficiency particulate air (HEPA) filtered respirator, and gloves for the person performing the procedure. Thorough cleaning within the periodontal pocket surrounding each tooth is especially important. Cleaning may be done either mechanically, using a sharp dental curette, or with an ultrasonic dental scaler. Ultrasonic scaling should only be done in a biohazard cabinet capable of protecting the operator and others from the substantial aerosol that results from this technique. Removal of plaque and calculus should be followed by polishing of the teeth using a rotating rubber cup ("prophy cup") and a mild abrasive cleaner designed for the purpose; this helps prevent adhesion of further material to the dental enamel. As with humans, routine cleaning of this type on a semiannual or annual basis as a preventive medicine procedure is superior to attempting to treat the advanced disease.

The feed additive sodium hexametaphosphate shows promise in decreasing the rate of calculus formation in primates (Willis *et al.,* 1996).

An important complication to primate research caused by periodontal disease and gingivitis is the ability of these conditions to provide a route for bacterial agents entering the general circulation. This represents a known hazard where artificial joints, heart valves, and other implantable devices are used and could also compromise studies of infection and immunity, efficacy of antibacterial agents, and so on. A preventive dental health program like the one just described is a necessary part of any study when there is concern about bacterial seeding on this type.

C. Bacterial and Fungal Diseases of the Oral Cavity

1. Necrotic Stomatitis/Noma

Noma (derived from the Greek word "to devour") is an acute gangrenous condition of the oral cavity that can spread to the maxilla, mandible, and surrounding soft tissue. Noma in primates is considered to be similar to the condition of the same name seen in humans. As in human noma, there is believed to be no specific etiologic agent; the condition is secondary to immunosuppressive conditions, poor nutrition, and/or poor dental hygiene (Adams and Bishops, 1980). Noma has been reported in macaques and tamarins (Lackner *et al.,* 1994; Buchanan *et al.,* 1981; Brack, 1982). Clinically, noma is characterized by rapidly progressive necrosis of oral soft tissue, exposing and ultimately destroying underlying bone, often resulting in sequestrum formation. Death due to noma and its

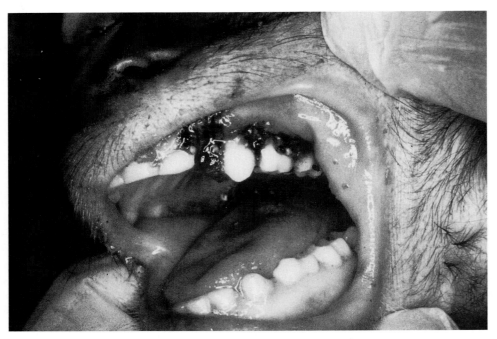

Fig. 1. Noma in a rhesus monkey infected with simian retrovirus. Photograph provided by Dr. Linda Lowenstine, University of California at Davis.

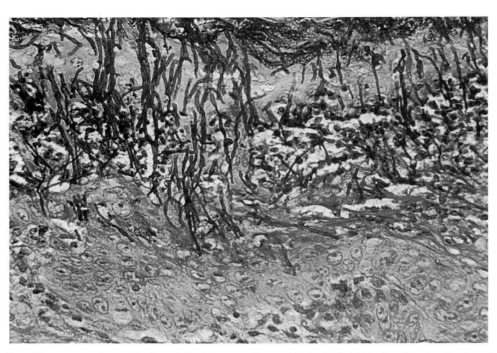

Fig. 2. Candidiasis. Branching, segmented pseudohyphae of *Candida* sp. can be seen histologically within the affected oral and esophageal epithelium using PAS or silver fungal stains. PAS stain. Photograph provided by Dr. Gary Baskin, Tulane Primate Center.

sequelae is common. Differential diagnosis in early stages includes acute ulcerative gingivitis. Severe, ruptured dental abscesses may also have a facial lesion similar to early stages of noma. Neither of these conditions demonstrate the rapid, invasive progression that is characteristic of this disease.

Grossly, noma may start as a small mucosal ulcer and then progress, with gangrenous destruction of tissue in the oral cavity and on the face (Fig. 1). Gingiva, lips, and cheeks are most often and most severely affected. Microscopically, circumscribed areas of necrosis are surrounded by well-demarcated margins of inflammatory cells and bacteria. Tissue beyond the margin may be edematous and be more diffusely infiltrated with inflammatory cells (Lackner and Wilson, 1993; Adams and Bishop, 1980). Treatment of noma through the use of standard therapies such as antibiotics, lesion debridement, and supportive care has met with little success. In cases where noma is secondary to systemic disease, treatment of the primary disease may be of some use. One report described the successful use of 2-ethoxy-6,9-diaminoacridine lactate (Rivanol; Chinosolfabrik der Riedal de Haen AG, Seelze, Germany) in a single *Saguinus oedipus*. This topical agent stimulates wound granulation and epithelization; it was used without systemic antibiotics (Brack, 1982).

To prevent noma, animals that are nutritionally deficient, have immunosuppressive diseases, or are being treated with immunosuppressive drugs should be identified as being at high risk. These animals should receive more frequent oral examinations and close attention should be paid to oral hygiene.

2. Oral Candidiasis

As in other species, fungal diseases of the primate gastrointestinal tract usually occur as a manifestation of systemic disease.

"Thrush" (the oral form of the disease) or moniliasis of the gastrointestinal tract occurs primarily in immunosuppressed animals and animals being treated with broad-spectrum antibiotics. Etiologic agents are the opportunist organisms of the genus *Candida,* most commonly *Candida albicans.*

Grossly, lesions of moniliasis usually appear as irregular, yellow-white pseudomembranous, or plaque-like, formations on the mucosa. On microscopic examination (Fig. 2), *Candida* organisms can be seen on superficial layers of the mucosae, with numerous pseudohyphae visible (Migaki, 1986). Moniliasis can be most effectively treated in the early stages. Treatment consists of nystatin suspension given orally at a dose of approximately 22,000 units per kilogram per day in doses divided three or four times daily, to be continued 2 days past full recovery (Hawk and Leary, 1995). For those animals known to be at risk for the disease (e.g., those with immunosuppressive conditions or those being treated with broad-spectrum antibiotics, consideration should be given to a routine daily oral check for thrush. Moniliasis of other parts of the gastrointestinal tract should be included in the differential diagnosis whenever animals at risk show signs of inflammatory GI disease: loss of appetite, vomiting, and diarrhea.

D. Viral Diseases and Oral Ulcers

Oral ulcers are a clinical sign for several important systemic viral infections of primates, including the herpes viruses and measles. Immunosuppressive viruses in the retrovirus group can also cause oral lesions indirectly by making primates susceptible to a variety of opportunistic pathogens. Table V lists viral agents and the lesions they cause. Readers are referred to the chapter on viral diseases elsewhere in this volume for more detailed information on these viruses.

E. Nutritional Diseases of the Oral Cavity

1. Scurvy: Vitamin C Deficiency

Oral lesions associated with vitamin C deficiency are known to occur in Old World primates. Deficiency of vitamin C results in the inability of animals to produce hydroxyproline and intracellular cement, which are required for maintaining the integrity of blood vessels, bone, and a variety of other tissues. Lesions include gingival hemorrhage and lossening of teeth. Oral lesions have not been seen in squirrel monkeys; cephalohematomas are the predominant lesion in this species (Ratteree *et al.,* 1990; Roberts, 1993b). Treatment for vitamin C deficiency consists of ascorbic acid injections; 25 mg/kg given intramuscularly twice daily for 5 days. The diet deficiency should also be corrected, and additional items containing vitamin C may be supplemented (Ratterree *et al.,* 1990). Vitamin C deficiency can usually be avoided by feeding an appropriate diet and by paying close attention to feed storage time and conditions of storage and shipment. Diets containing vitamin C have a shelf life of only 3 months without refrigeration. The use of stabilized vitamin C can extend the shelf life of feed (National Research Council, 1996).

2. Cheilosis: Folic Acid Deficiency

Cheilosis (fissuring, scaling of the lips, and labial commissures) has been experimentally induced in marmosets fed diets deficient in folic acid. The condition begins with mottling and mild inflammation at the commissures and can progress to severe inflammation, necrosis, and sloughing of labial tissue. Differential diagnosis should include other conditions that cause erosive/inflammatory lesions of the lips, including thrush, noma, and herpes virus infections (see Table V). Histologically, the condition begins with a leukocytic infiltrate of epithelium at the mucocutaneous junction and enlargement of nuclei in the stratum spinosum and stratum germinativum. As the condition progresses, the epithelium becomes edematous, necrotic, and then sloughs entirely. In advanced cases, there are deep fissures containing necrotic material that extends into the connective tissue and muscle of the labial commissure. Folic acid is also necessary for the maturation of erythrocytes and has been associated with gestational anemia in squirrel monkeys (Rasmussen *et al.,* 1980). Folic acid-associated cheilosis is rapidly

TABLE V

VIRAL CAUSES OF ORAL LESIONS

Agent	Known susceptable species	Lesion description	Comment	Reference
Herpes B (monkey B virus, herpes simiae, Cercopthecine herpesvirus)	*Macaca* sp.	Vesicles and ulcers of oral mucous membranes, usually self-limiting in primate reservoir hosts; rarely may cause severe oral–esophageal lesions and/or fatal systemic disease in these animals	Macaques are reservoir host; most show no lesions	Hunt and Blake (1993a); Cole *et al.* (1968)
Simian Varicella Delta herpes Medical Lake macaque virus Patas herpesvirus	*E. patas* *C. aethiops* *Macaca* sp. *Pan* sp. *Gorilla* sp.	Mucosal ulcers, white plaques, and hemorrhage throughout GI tract	Virus is similar to, but antigenically distinct from, varicella-zoster virus (cause of chicken pox and shingles in humans)	Roberts (1993a); Padovan and Cantrell (1986) Wolf *et al.,* (1974)
Herpes simplex (herpes hominis)	All primate species are probably susceptible; severe systemic disease in *Aotus, Saguinus, Callithrix, Hylobates*	Plaques and ulcers of the oral cavity; extension into esophagus and systemic disease in severe cases		Hunt (1993b)
Herpes tamarinus	*Aotus, Saguinus, Callthrix, Saimiri* (*Saimiri* is the reservoir host)	Resembles herpes simplex infection in *Aotus, Saguinus,* and *Callithrix*; causes oral ulcers in *Saimiri*		Abee (1985); Hunt (1993b)
Simian AIDS retrovirus 1 (SRV-1), simian immuno-suppressive virus (SIV)	*Macaca* sp.	See descriptions for thrush, acute necrotizing ulcerative gingivitis (ANUG), and noma	Oral lesions are result of opportunistic agents rather than primary viral infection	Shiodt *et al.* (1988); Lowenstine (1993a)
Measles virus (Paramyxovirus)	All primate species apparently are susceptible	1-mm-diameter raised white oral lesions with red margin and bluish center; usually associated with skin lesions, pneumonia, and diarrhea	Oral lesions are known as Koplick spots	Lowenstine (1993b); Hall *et al.* (1971)

reversible with administration of dietary or supplemental folic acid (Dreizen and Levy, 1969). Consideration of folic acid content should be a part of any evaluation of a primate diet.

F. Developmental Anomalies

1. Cleft Palate

Cleft palate and harelip are congenital abnormalities that have been reported in primates (Swindler and Merrill, 1971; Schultz, 1972). Cleft palate (Fig. 3) results from the failure of the lateral palatine processes to fuse during the first trimester of pregnancy. Studies in mice suggest that both genetic and environmental factors may play a role in cleft palate (Patten and Carlson, 1974). The prevalence of this defect in primates is unknown; it is most frequently reported in squirrel monkeys. One colony reported 2.4% of the 169 squirrel monkeys born in the colony to be affected (Baker *et al.,* 1977). In humans, cleft palate occurs in approximately 1 out of every 800 births (Berman, 1991). Clinical signs of cleft palate in the neonate include milk coming from the nares during feeding, chronic upper respiratory infection, weight loss, and difficulty with nursing. Animals with cleft palate may also have other congenital anomalies; they should receive a full physical examination to check for such anomalies. At necropsy, infants may show pharyngitis, inflammation, and infection of the nasopharynx and aspiration pneumonia, in addition to the defect itself.

Repair of cleft palate is routinely performed in humans and has been described in domestic animals (Howard, 1983). If repair is to be attempted, an orogastric tube feeding should be started when the problem is diagnosed to reduce the chance of aspiration pneumonia before the defect can be repaired. If repair is not performed, the animal should be euthanized for humane reasons. The reproductive history of the dam and sire should be examined for other offspring with congenital anomalies. If anomalies have occured previously, consideration should be given to culling the parent(s) with which the anomalies are associated from the breeding colony. Examination for cleft palate and other abnormalities should be a part of any evaluation of the primate neonate.

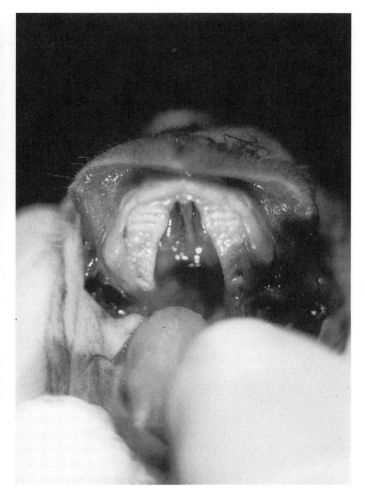

Fig. 3. Cleft palate in an aborted squirrel monkey fetus. Photograph provided by Dr. Susan Gibson, University of South Alabama.

G. Oral Hyperplasia and Neoplasia

HYPERPLASIA

1. Gingival Hyperplasia

Gingival hyperplasia is a chronic inflammatory condition seen with gingivitis. In humans, it has also been associated with pregnancy, diabetes mellitus, and the use of diphenylhydantoin (T. Kaufman, personal communication, 1993). In primates, it has been associated with the use of diphenylhydantoin (Fagan and Ooosterhuis, 1979) and has occurred without any known etiology (Sheldon, 1967). Teeth may become obscured with gingival hyperplasia. Gingiva also bleed easily and animals may eat with difficulty or be reluctant to eat. Grossly, this tissue has the bright red/pink granular surface of classic granulation tissue; it bleeds with even slight manipulation. Microscopically, mature fibrous tissue is seen with extended rete peges of the musocal epithelium. Inflammatory cells are seen in submucosal areas, but few of these cells are present in fibrous tissue.

Gingival hyperplasia is best treated by surgical excision of hyperplastic tissue (gingivectomy) and treatment of any underlying gingivitis (Sheldon, 1967). A good dental prophylaxis program, with periodic dental scaling and cleaning, may be helpful in the prevention of gingival hyperplasia.

NEOPLASIA

Oral–pharyngeal tumors are relatively common in primates. One report states that nearly one-half of all reported primate neoplasms are in the mouth, pharynx, and esophagus. Oral–pharyngeal tumors reported in primates include squamous cell carcinoma, lymphoma, odontoma, adamantinoma, papilloma, and fibroma (De Paoli and McClure, 1982; Squire *et al.,* 1978). Squamous cell carcinoma and lymphoma are among the most frequently reported of these tumors.

1. Squamous Cell Carcinoma

Squamous cell carcinoma (SCC) has been reported in both Old World and New World primates (Betton, 1983; Montesdeoca *et al.,* 1993; Grana *et al.,* 1992; Morris, 1994; Sasaki *et al.,* 1961; Fincham *et al.,* 1982; Cran, 1969; S. V. Gibson, personal communication, 1991). Clinical signs include facial swelling/asymmetry, weight loss and/or reluctance to eat, loosened teeth, foul breath, and purulent oral discharge. Differential diagnosis includes dental abscess, sialocoele, and lymphadenopathy. Serum chemistry may reveal greatly elevated serum alkaline phosphatase (believed to be due to the local invasion of bone). Gross appearance of SCC is usually of a firm, locally invasive mass that may invade into the hard palate, maxilla, or mandible. The mass may ulcerate as it grows. Teeth in the area of the tumor may be loosened or absent. Metastasis into the lymph nodes and lungs has been reported (Betton, 1983). Microscopically, there are nests and sheets of epithelial cells of variable size with nuclei also varying in size. Keratin "pearls" (condensed keratin in the center of concentric layers of epithelial cells) may also be visible. A search of the literature revealed no published reports of successful treatment of SCC in nonhuman primates. Presumably, excision of the mass using techniques similar to those references later for odontoma would be of some use in slowing the growth of this tumor.

2. Lymphoma

Oral–pharyngeal lymphoma has been reported in macaques (Jaax *et al.,* 1988; Cohen and Goldman, 1960) and in one lowland gorilla (Prowten *et al.,* 1985). Because lymphoma has been described in a variety of Old World and New World species and in prosimians, it is probably safe to assume that this tumor may occur in the GI tract of any primate. Lymphoma is associated with infection with herpes saimiri virus in *Aotus,* tamarins, marmosets, spider monkeys, and howler monkeys and with infection with simian immunodeficiency virus (SIV) or type D retrovirus (the latter two probably due to immunosuppression, making the animal more susceptible to another carcinogenic agent) (Hunt, 1993a). Clinical signs include loss of appetite, weight loss, reluctance to swallow, nasal discharge, and generalized weakness. Clinical pathology results may include leukopenia, anemia, hyproteinemia/hypoalbuminemia, and increased alkaline phosphatase (ALP). Grossly, lymphoma may appear as a mass or masses anywhere in the GI tract. Diagnosis may be tentatively made by observing characteristic abnormal lymphocytes on impression smears. Definitive diagnosis may be made by microscopic examination of a biopsy. Microscopically, sheets of large round cells are observed with enlarged nuclei and prominent nucleoli. Ultrastructurally, lymphocytic cells were observed with convoluted nuclei and abundant ribosomes. Cells with small nuclei had an abundant well-developed Golgi complex and endoplasmic reticulum (Jaax *et al.,* 1988). Radiation and chemotherapy were attempted in the gorilla with little affect on the progression of tumor growth and metastasis.

3. Ameloblastic Odontoma

An ameloblastic odontoma has been described in a 15-year-old *Macaca fascicularis* (Davis, 1988). The animal presented with unilateral swelling of the maxilla. Radiographically, the mass was well delineated, irregular in density, and surrounded by a maxillary canine, obscuring the tooth itself. Histologically, the mass contained a mixture of dental tissue types with nests and cords of cuboidal and columnar cells predominating. Mitotic figures were rare. Treatment consisted of excision of the mass and curettage of the surrounding area (Banks *et al.,* 1988). Odontomas have also been reported in chimpanzees (Cohen and Goldman, 1960). Other oral tumors described include osteogenic sarcoma of the mandible in a rhesus (Cohen and Goldman, 1960).

H. Foreign Bodies of the Oral Cavity and Gastrointestinal Tract

The natural curiosity of primates and their tendency to put objects in their mouths puts them at risk for foreign body obstruction and/or damage to the gastrointestinal tract. Ingestion of foreign bodies is especially common in recently captured feral animals. Trichobezoars (hairballs) are foreign bodies that may be found in the primate stomach or intestine, particularly in animals that have a history of pulling hair from their own coat or that of other animals, or where animals have access to fibrous materials.

Clinical signs of foreign bodies may include loss of appetite, weight loss, drooling, draining tracts of the neck (especially in macaques and *Cercopithecus* sp. that have cheek pouches), abdominal pain or tenderness, hunched posture, diarrhea, and an abnormal mass or masses palpated in the abdomen. Radiographs and contrast radiography are often useful in making a definitive diagnosis. If perforation of the GI tract occurs, animals (especially small primates) can be expected to deteriorate rapidly. In these cases, contrast procedures using barium sulfate or other irritating agents should be avoided and surgical repair should be undertaken as an emergency procedure. Differential diagnosis for foreign body obstruction/damage includes stomach torsion, intestinal intussusception, acute gastroenteritis, and gastrointestinal neoplasia.

Most oral and cheek pouch foreign bodies may be removed under anesthesia with forceps. Esophageal and stomach foreign bodies may be removed with a flexible endoscope and appropriate forceps. In more distal areas of the tract, smaller foreign bodies may be removed using mineral oil or emetics, provided the size and the shape of the object permit easy passage (as with barium sulfate, avoid the use of oral agents if perforation is suspected). Surgery for the removal of foreign bodies and the repair of resulting damage to the tract have been discussed elsewhere (Dulisch, 1983; Krahwinkel and Richardson, 1983).

Prevention of foreign body ingestion requires that animal housing and all items placed in or on primate cages be designed in such a way that small parts cannot be ingested. Such housing and related items must be inspected regularly for damage that may loosen small parts and make them susceptible to ingestion. Shade cloth used for outdoor enclosures, steel fiber from tires used in environmental enrichment, and even fibrous plant material from supplemental foods such as coconut husks are potential foreign bodies. Personnel should not enter animal housing with small, unsecured items that are easily dropped (e.g., hypodermic needles, wire twist ties) and they should be aware that leaving items within reach on tables, carts, or on the floor outside of a cage is an invitation to ingestion. Animal care staff should check housing areas following the entry of maintenance personnel for hardware (nails, nuts, bolts, wire, wire insulation, broken glass, etc.) that may have been left behind. For animals housed outdoors, care should be taken to prevent the growth of grasses, such as foxtail, that can be ingested and result in penetration of the gastrointestinal tract.

III. PHARYNX, ESOPHAGUS, AND STOMACH

A. Approach to Vomiting Diagnosis and Treatment

Nonhuman primates differ from several commonly used laboratory animals in their ability to vomit (Davis, 1980). This can be an important protective mechanism for these animals and (as described later) can be a highly visible, important clinical sign in diagnosing serious health problems. Chronic nausea and vomiting can also result in serious discomfort for primates. Human patients and nurses identify nausea and vomiting as the most distressing side effect of cancer chemotherapy (Jenns, 1994). Chronic vomiting also disrupts fluid, electrolyte, and acid/base homeostasis.

TABLE VI

ANTIMETICS IN HUMAN AND VETERINARY MEDICINE

Drug or drug class	Primate dose[a]	Indication	Comment
Antihistamines (diphenhydramine, dimenhydrinate, meclozine, doxylamine promethazine, L-hyoscine)	None established	Nausea associated with vestibular stimulation (motion sickness)	Considered to be specific for motion sickness in veterinary literature; doxylamine and meclozine have been used to treat morning sickness in humans; terratogenic potential of these drugs is controversial. Other side effects for antihistamines are sedation and xerostomia
Phenothiazines (chlorpromazine, prochlorperazine, trifluoperazine, perphenazine, pipamazine, mepazine)	Chlorpromazine 1–3 mg/kg IM, 3–5 mg/kg PO[a,b]	All causes of nausea with exception of vestibular stimulation	Sedation is common side effect
Butyrophenones (droperidol)	None established	Used in human cancer chemotherapy	Marked sedation is side effect
Benzodiazepines (diazepam, lorazepam, midazolam)	Diazepam 1.0 mg/kg IM, IV[a,b]	Used in human cancer chemotherapy	Commonly used in combination with other antiemetic agents; only short-acting benzodiazepines appear to be effective antiemetics; sedation is side effect
Steroids (dexamethasone)	0.25–1.0 mg/kg IM[a,b]	Used in human cancer chemotherapy	Moderate antimemetic action when given as a single high dose; only side effect noted is transient rectal pain in humans if administered too rapidly[d]
Pyridoxine (vitamin B_6)	None established	Has been recommended for use in human patients with pregnancy-associated nausea (morning sickness)[c]	Efficacy has not been well demonstrated. Endogenous status and lack of side effects may make it worthy of trial in controlled primate studies where other drugs would cause unacceptable variables
5HT3 receptor antagonists (ondansetron and others)	None established	Broad spectrum	Highly effective in human chemotherapy and postoperative patients. Efficacy of oral form may be less than injectable[e]

[a] Dose not established for antiemetic use in primates. Doses shown is that used for other indications.
[b] From Hawk *et al.* (1995).
[c] From Mitchelson (1992).
[d] From Krosnow (1991)
[e] From Cooke (1994)

Thus, the control of nausea and vomiting in nonhuman primates is important for both humane and medical reasons.

For a detailed discussion of the diagnostic approach to vomiting, readers are referred to several excellent general reviews on the subject (Tams, 1989; Mitchelson, 1992). Briefly, it is diagnostically important to differentiate among retching, vomiting, and regurgitation. Retching is a nonproductive spasmodic series of contractions that occur prior to vomiting; vomiting is a forceful ejection of gastrointestinal contents through the mouth; and regurgitation is a passive, retrograde movement of ingested material. Vomiting is associated with a wide variety of etiologies: dietary, toxins/drug agents, metabolic disorders, mechanical gastrointestinal obstruction (foreign body, tumor, torsion, etc.), or neurogenic causes (vestibular stimulation). Regurgitation is usually associated with some type of esophageal disorder: primary or secondary megaesophagus, esophageal foreign bodies, strictures (including vascular ring anomalies, scar tissue, extraluminal masses pressing on the esophagus),

diverticula and esophageal masses (granuloma, abscess, tumor), or segmental motility disorders of the esophagus. Other clinical observations that are important include time elapsed since feeding, the contents of emesis, and results of physical, radiographic, and endoscopic examinations.

Treatment priorities in vomiting are (1) resolution of the primary problem causing vomiting, (2) controlling vomiting, and (3) treating resulting hydration, electrolyte, and acid/base abnormalities. Table VI lists the types of drugs in common use for the control of vomiting in human and veterinary medicine. Established doses for primates are shown for some drugs; dose and treatment regimens must be extrapolated for other agents.

B. Parasitic Diseases

The increasing sophistication of conditioning programs for feral primates (especially the routine use of broad-spectrum parasiticides and quarantine for newly arrived animals) and the use of animals that are raised in domestic colonies have greatly decreased the prevalence of esophageal and gastric parasites. As a result, most clinical descriptions are from older reports. Reports of protozoal gastric infections are rare; two cases of gastric infection with *Entamoeba histolytica* in primates have been reported, one in colobus monkeys (*Colobus guereza*) (Loomis *et al.*, 1983) and the other in a silver leaf monkey (*Presbytis cristatus*) (Palmierei *et al.*, 1984). Primate gastric/esophageal parasites include *Nochtia nochti*, *Physaloptera dilatata* and *P. tumefaciens*, *Protospirura muricola*, and *Spirura guainensis*. A more complete discussion of parasites may be found elsewhere in this volume.

1. *Nochtia nochti*

Nochtia nochti is a trichostrongyle nematode that inhabits the gastric mucosae of macaques. Adult males and females are 5.7–6.5 and 7.6–10 mm in length, respectively, with both being bright red; eggs are ellipsoid, thin shelled, and 35–42 μm × 60–80 μm in size. Their life cycle is direct with infection by ingestion. *Nochtia* usually produces no clinical disease; ova are contained in gastric lesions along with adults; when eggs are seen in primate feces they are usually embryonated, which differentiates them from the eggs of *Strongyloides*. Gastric lesions resemble adenomas and are most frequently located between the pylorus and the fundus of the stomach. As mentioned earlier, both adults and ova are contained in the lesions. Histologically, lesions contain hyperplastic fronds of gastric mucosae and inflammatory tissue (Shadduck and Pakes, 1978; Toft, 1986). Because infection is usually diagnosed postmortem as an incidental finding, no treatment has been described for *Nochtia* (presumably, broad-spectrum nematicides such as ivermectin would be effective against this parasite).

2. *Physaloptera*

Physaloptera sp. adults resemble ascarids and are found in the stomach and small intestine of nonhuman primates. *Physaloptera tumefaciens* is found in macaques, whereas *P. dilatata* is found in capuchins, marmosets, and woolly monkeys. Their life cycle is indirect, with cockroaches, beetles, crickets, and other arthropods acting as intermediate hosts. Heavily infected animals may lose weight, be anemic, and show signs of gastritis and enteritis, including melena. Diagnosis may be made from fecal parasite examination or by identification of adult worms in the stomach and duodenum at necropsy. At necropsy, adult *Physaloptera* may be differentiated from *Ascaris* by their firm attachment to the mucosae of the stomach and duodenum.

A consistent finding of *Physaloptera* within a primate colony would suggest the need for insect control within the facility. The ability of *Physaloptera* to cause clinical signs would make it a consideration in many areas of primate research. No effective treatment protocol has been published for this parasite, pre-sumably because of the low incidence of infection with improved husbandry and the use of broad-spectrum nematicides, such as ivermectin.

3. *Protospirura muricola*

Protospirura muricola is found in the stomach and esophagus of owl monkeys, marmosets, and other New World primates. Primates are an aberrant host with rodents believed to be the definitive host; primates are infected by ingesting the intermediate host (cockroaches). Male and female *Protospirura* are 2.5–4.0 and 4.0–7 cm in length, respectively. Although infection in the rat is restricted to a relatively benign infection of the stomach, in primates the parasite proliferates in the esophagus, stomach, and peritoneal cavity, resulting in mechanical obstruction and lesions. The terminal esophagus is most severely affected; burrowing worms and mechanical pressure from parasites in the lumen can result in destruction of the mucosae and bacterial invasion of the submucosae (Foster and Johnson, 1939). As with other nematodes in this section, no treatment protocol has been published (see note earlier regarding *Nochtia*).

4. *Spirura guainensis*

Spirura guainensis is found in the esophagus of tamarins. Clinical disease is rare with infestation; lesions are usually limited to mild inflammatory changes in the esophagus. Little is known regarding the life cycle of this parasite and no treatment has been described.

C. Bacterial Diseases

1. Gastric Bloat/Torsion

Gastric bloat continues to be an important cause of death in nonhuman primates despite improved understanding of the pathogenesis and etiology of the disease since it was first described by Chapman in 1967. The immediate cause of bloat is the rapid production of gas by clostridial organisms, with *Clostridium perfringens* the organism most frequently isolated. Prepared diets ("monkey biscuits") have been proposed as a source for *C. perfringens* in these cases (Bennet *et al.*, 1980). A number of predisposing factors have been implicated in the disease, most are related to diet and food intake. These include a sudden change in diet, antibiotic therapy, anesthesia, shipping, and fasting followed by *ad libitum* feeding. The disease has been reported in both Old World and New World primates, and all primate species are believed to be susceptible. Primates with gastric dilatation are most frequently found dead without any premonitory clinical signs (Pond *et al.*, 1982). Animals found alive with this condition are usually in shock with gross distension of the abdomen, dyspnea, and other symptoms related to shock. Death usually occurs within a matter of hours. Cases are usually sporadic; however, the death of 29 marmosets due to bloat over a 5-week period following antibiotic therapy has been described (Stein *et al.,* 1981). At necropsy, the stomach is distended by gas and fermented food material. Stomach rupture may occur in some cases. Subcutaneous hemorrhage, edema, and emphysema may be present, especially in the abdominal area. The intestine and other abdominal viscera may be congested as a result of vascular changes. *Clostridium perfringens* may be isolated from stomach contents, blood cultures, liver, and other tissues. This condition must be differentiated from normal postmortem gas accumulation in the gastrointestinal tract. If gas accumulation is postmortem, animals are unlikely to have changes in other tissues, such as subcutaneous hemorrhage, edema, and congestion of viscera.

Treatment for bloat has consisted of emptying and lavage of the stomach, fluid therapy, antibiotics to combat bacteremia, and corticosteroids for shock. Careful observation and early treatment may improve an animal's chance for survival. Treatment is often unrewarding and recurrence is common.

Husbandry and clinical procedures that are potentially useful in preventing bloat include limiting feed intake after fasting and anesthesia, gradual changes in diet, judicious use of broad-spectrum antibiotics that affect gut flora, measures that equalize feed distribution in social groups where dominant animals may monopolize feed, and limiting the use of treats that encourage animals to engorge themselves.

2. *Helicobacter* sp.

Helicobacter sp. have been widely studied for the effects of stomach colonization on animals and human health (Bronsdon *et al.,* 1991). Preliminary studies indicate that the organism causes a mild, asymptomatic gastritis in primates. A urea breath test has been developed for noninvasive diagnosis of *Helicobacter* infection in primates (Stadtlander and Stutzenberger, 1995).

IV. SMALL AND LARGE INTESTINE

A. Approach to Diarrhea Diagnosis and Treatment

Diarrhea in captive nonhuman primates affects up to 10–15% of animals in some colonies each year and accounts for approximately one-third of deaths not related to research (Hird *et al.,* 1984; Holmberg *et al.,* 1982b; Paul-Murphy, 1993; Russel *et al.,* 1987). Some species, such as *Erthyrocebus patas,* have relatively high incidence and mortality rates associated with diarrhea, whereas genera such as *Saimiri* and *Papio* have a lower incidence. In nursery-reared *Macaca nemestrina,* the incidence of diarrhea was highest during the first months of life and multiple episodes were common. Diarrhea in macaques raised with their mothers in large breeding colonies was less common than in hand-reared macaques. The peak incidence in those reared

by their dams occurred between 6 and 12 months of age, following weaning (Russell *et al.,* 1987). Diarrhea is defined as stool with increased water content. Increased fecal water results in increased stool volume, which is often accompanied by an increased frequency of defecation. Ninety-five percent of the water delivered to the digestive tract by ingestion and secretions normally is absorbed by the intestinal tract. In humans, about 85–90% of the total fluid normally is absorbed in the small intestine (Bayliss *et al.,* 1988). The remainder of the fluid must be absorbed from the cecum and colon. The cecum and colon have a considerable reserve absorptive capacity. Mechanisms of diarrhea have been reviewed (Ammon, 1995; Banwell, 1990; Drazner, 1983; Krejs, 1988; Jergens, 1995; Walker *et al.,* 1986). In small intestinal disease, the reserve absorptive capacity of the large bowel must be exceeded before diarrhea is observed. The cause of diarrhea may be decreased fluid absorption, increased fluid secretion, or a combination of decreased absorption and increased secretion. Some bacterial toxins, such as cholera toxin, cause increased fluid secretion in the small intestine. Damage to intestinal epithelium mediated by infectious agents or chemicals, inhibition of normal gastrointestinal motility, impairment of venous or lymphatic drainage, or increased vascular permeability with leakage of excess fluid into the bowel lumen are several possible mechanisms associated with increased fecal fluid loss.

The clinical history and the nature of the stool may provide the clinician with valuable diagnostic clues (Jergens, 1995). Environmental factors, such as housing, feed, and social interactions, should be assessed. Recent stress related to shipment, environmental changes, or research protocols may be associated with the onset of diarrhea. Loose, watery stools containing undigested food or digested blood suggest stomach or small bowel dysfunction. Mucus and/or fresh blood in stools ranging from liquid to normal consistency suggests disease of the large bowel. Straining to defecate and painful defecation indicate involvement of the colon, rectum, or anus. It should be noted that some primate species, such as those in the genus *Saimiri,* may normally have a stool with a relatively high water content without showing any evidence of the electrolyte loss, weight loss, and dehydration that are associated with true diarrhea (Abee, 1997).

The intensity of the recommended diagnostic effort and therapy usually is based on the duration and severity of the diarrhea (Ammon, 1995; Bayliss *et al.,* 1988; Donowitz *et al.,* 1995). The intervention required depends on a variatey of factors, including age and size of the animal and past history. Chronic or recurrent diarrhea often has different pathophysiologic mechanisms compared to acute diarrhea and merits different diagnostic procedures and therapies. Mild diarrhea lasting only a few days and resulting in no other clinical signs may be treated by observation and perhaps isolation. Psychogenic stress is an important cause of diarrhea in many species, and it is likely that stress contributes to some cases of mild diarrhea in nonhuman primates (Bayliss *et al.,* 1988). Examination of fresh direct fecal smears for neutrophils or pathogenic protozoa and fecal flotation for intestinal parasites are inexpensive and rapid diagnostic procedures appropriate for cases of mild acute diarrhea. Fecal samples for smears should be collected in a dry container or directly into fixative, as water and urine destroy amebic parasites (Donowitz *et al.*, 1995). Formalin adequately preserves protozoan cysts, helminth ova, and larvae, whereas polyvinyl alcohol is preferable for identifying protozoa in the trophozoite stage. Polyvinyl alcohol also preserves cysts (Matherne *et al.*, 1992; Swenson, 1993). A Merthiolate (thimerosal)–iodine–formaldehyde fixative containing Lugols iodine also preserves trophozoites and cysts (Owne, 1992). Dimethyl sulfoxide (DMSO)-modified acid fast stains may be used to identify *Cryptosporidium* spp. (Bronsdon, 1984). Diagnostic kits with appropriate fixatives and sample containers are available from laboratory supply vendors. Smears may be examined fresh or stained with Wright's stain, new methylene blue, or other stains to assist in the identification of leukocytes and erythrocytes (Paul-Murphy, 1993). Fecal cultures for bacterial pathogens such as *Shigella, Campylobacter, Salmonella,* enteropathogenic *Escherichia coli, Yersinia,* and *Mycobacterium* may indicate specific therapy.

Mild diarrhea that persists for more than a few days without evidence of dehydration or debilitation warrants more aggressive action. A thorough physical examination should be performed. Repeated examinations of stool for protozoal and helminth parasites should be performed if initial tests are negative. Repeated bacterial cultures may be necessary to isolate *Shigella, Salmonella,* and *Campylobacter* species. A successful *Campylobacter* sp. culture requires the use of special isolation medium and culture techniques (see Chapter 2). Isolation of *Yersina* spp. is enhanced by culturing at 24–28°C (Carniel and Mollaret, 1990). The proper selection of specimens should be verified with laboratory personnel before the samples are collected. Radiographs, hematology and clinical chemistry panels, and other diagnostic tests may assist in making a diagnosis and providing appropriate treatment. Examination of the stool using electron microscopy may demonstrate enteric viruses as the etiology in some cases of diarrhea in young or immunosuppressed animals. Often the cause of mild diarrhea cannot be determined, and a therapeutic trial using antibiotics, antiparasitic drugs, and/or dietary modification may result in the remission of diarrhea.

Acute severe diarrhea results in dehydration, loss of body condition, and loss of normal behavioral patterns. In some cases, dehydration and death may occur rapidly before diarrhea is first observed. Diagnostic procedures for acute, severe diarrhea must occur concurrently with aggressive therapy. Diagnostic tests should include a physical examination, direct microscopic fecal examination, fecal flotation, fecal cultures including cultures for *Campylobacter* spp., and hematology and clinical chemistry profiles. Large numbers of leukocytes and blood in the stool suggest infections with invasive organisms such as *Shigella* spp. but may also be seen with some severe *Campylobacter* spp. infections or in other conditions (Paul-Murphy, 1993). In one study, examination of the stool for leukocytes and erythrocytes was not useful

in diagnosing *Shigella* infections (Hirsh *et al.*, 1980). Fever and fibrinogen levels in excess of 400 mg/dl are suggestive of *Shigella* infection. Additional diagnostic procedures, such as acid fast stains of fecal smears for *Mycobacterium,* must be selected using professional judgment.

The cause of chronic gastrointestinal disease in nonhuman primates often remains undetermined. Even in animals that were submitted for necropsy, one study found that complete postmortem examination and diagnostic testing identified the etiology in less than 50% of the animals with diarrhea (Holmberg *et al.*, 1982b).

Repeated examinations for enteric bacterial pathogens, pathogenic protozoa, and helminths may be necessary to identify an infectious agent. Bacterial culture and examination for protozoal parasites should be performed on at least three separate occasions, preferably at intervals of at least 24 hr, unless a cause is identified. Concurrent treatment and certain diagnostic procedures can produce negative results. For example, radiologic studies using barium interfere with the identification of amebae in stool samples (Donowitz *et al.*, 1995). Additional studies, including radiographs, hematology and clinical chemistry profiles, tests of digestive function, and serology for specific agents, may identify the cause(s) of persistent diarrhea. In one study, endoscopic colonic biopsies of rhesus monkeys with chronic diarrhea demonstrated nonspecific chronic inflammation, but were not helpful in determining a cause or effective therapy (Gullett *et al.*, 1996).

Diarrhea causes losses of water, sodium, chloride, bicarbonate, and potassium. In one retrospective study of rhesus monkeys, hyponatremia and hypochloremia were present in most animals with diarrhea (George and Lerche, 1990). Metabolic acidosis related to a loss of bicarbonate and dehydration, as indicated by decreased total serum carbon dioxide and increased anion gap, was present in 59% of these animals. Serum potassium levels were variable and unpredictable, with equal numbers of hypokalemic, normokalemic, and hyperkalemic animals. Vomiting combined with diarrhea is uncommon in nonhuman primates, but if vomiting and diarrhea occur together, metabolic alkalosis (increased total carbon dioxide), mixed metabolic acidosis and alkalosis (normal total carbon dioxide and increased anion gap), and/or severe potassium deficits are possible (George and Lerche, 1990; Paul-Murphy, 1993). Fluid and electrolyte replacement therapy is essential for diarrheic, dehydrated animals.

Fluid replacement therapy for the treatment of fluid and electrolyte losses associated with diarrhea has been reviewed (Ammon, 1995; DiBartola, 1992; Johnson, 1992; Muir and DiBartola, 1983; Paul-Murphy, 1993). Oral fluids are preferred when patients will consume adequate quantities to replace intestinal losses and meet maintenance requirements. Oral fluids should not be given to animals that are vomiting. Commercially available or homemade oral glucose–electrolyte solutions may be used (Ammon, 1995; Johnson, 1992; Paul-Murphy, 1993; Schiller, 1995). Glucose promotes the absorption of fluids and electrolytes. Solutions containing rice syrup solids may be more effective than solutions made with pure glucose for reducing stool volume and for promoting the retention of fluid and electrolytes (Pizzarro *et al.,* 1991). Several oral rehydration solutions for humans are useful for the treatment of nonhuman primates with diarrhea, e.g., WHO oral rehydration salts (Gains Brothers Packaging, Kansas City, MO), Ricelyte (Mead-Johnson, Evansville, IN), and Rehydralyte (Ross Laboratories, Columbus, OH). Some oral solutions available commercially (e.g., Lytren, Pedialyte, and Gatorade) are low in sodium and are not adequate for fluid replacement therapy in severely dehydrated animals (Ammon, 1995; Guerrant and Bobak, 1991; Paul-Murphy, 1993). A satisfactory homemade oral fluid and electrolyte solution for the treatment of fluid/electrolyte loss accompanying diarrhea can be made by mixing ½ teaspoon potassium chloride, ½ teaspoon sodium bicarbonate, ½ teaspoon sodium chloride, and 2 tablespoons glucose or 4 tablespoons sucrose in 1 liter of water (Ammon, 1995). This mixture can be stored indefinitely in the dry state and keeps for approximately 24 hr once water is added. The palatability of oral fluid/electrolyte replacement solutions may be improved by adding a small amount of powdered, sweetened orange drink to the solution. The addition of large amounts can alter solution osmolality and should be avoided (Paul-Murphy, 1993).

Oral rehydration fluids should be given at a minimum rate of 60 ml/kg within the first 2 hr. Approximately 30–40 ml/kg can be given safely by gavage to most animals as a single dose. Neonates should be given smaller volumes. Once dehydration is corrected, maintenance solutions such as Pedialyte (Abbott Laboratories, Columbus, OH) should be continued at volumes of approximately 100–150 ml/kg/day (Paul-Murphy, 1993).

Intravenous fluids should be administered to all animals with dehydration exeeding 12% and to animals that are weak, debilitated, or depressed (Paul-Murphy, 1993). Intravenous fluid replacement should be considered in animals with diarrhea that weigh less than 2 kg and whenever infants, aged, or debilitated animals present with diarrhea. A blood sample for hematology and serum chemistry should be obtained prior to fluid therapy. When diarrhea is not accompanied by vomiting, lactated Ringer's solution is recommended for intravenous therapy (DiBartola, 1992). Isotonic sodium chloride may be used when vomiting and diarrhea occur concurrently, especially if the acid–base status of the patient is unknown. Serum potassium levels may be decreased, normal, or elevated in nonhuman primates with diarrhea. Potassium supplementation should be implemented with caution if the serum potassium concentration is not known (Paul-Murphy, 1993). Fluids may be supplemented with 15 mEq/liter potassium when a potassium deficit is determined (DiBartola, 1992). Intravenous potassium should not be given at a rate exceeding 1.0 mEq/kg/hr. Administration of diluted potassium gluconate elixir orally can be used to replace depleted potassium. Metabolic acidosis often resolves in response to rehydration without specific corrective therapy. A bolus dose of 1 mEq/kg of sodium bicarbonate is indicted if serum pH is below 7.1 or pH and total carbon dioxide are both low after the first hour of rehydration therapy (Paul-Murphy, 1993). In dehydrated animals, fluids may be replaced intavenously for up to 1 hr at a maximal rate of 60–90 ml/kg/hr (about one blood volume per hour). When intravenous infusions are performed at rapid rates, patients should be monitored for signs of fluid overload. Evidence of overhydration may include serous nasal discharge, chemosis, restlessness, shivering, tachycardia, cough, tachypnea, dyspnea, pulmonary crackles and edema, ascites, polyuria, exophthalmos, diarrhea, and vomiting (Cornelius *et al.,* 1978). Fluid and electrolyte replacement therapy and supportive care may be the only appropriate treatment in cases of viral diarrhea for which specific treatment is not available (Miller *et al.,* 1990b).

Specific therapies that eliminate infectious agents or correct the underlying problem are always desirable, and therapeutic considerations for many specific diseases involving the gastrointestinal tract are covered in other chapters of this text. An accurate diagnosis and specific therapy usually are required to successfully treat cases of chronic diarrhea. In many cases the etiology of diarrhea is never determined. Many cases of acute diarrhea are self-limiting, and the patients recover if proper supportive care is provided. However, in cases of acute diarrhea, antibiotic therapy may be indicated before bacterial cultures and other diagnostic tests can be completed. Indications for antibiotic use in acute cases of diarrhea include fever or the presence of blood, leukocytes, or necrotic debris in the stool. These findings indicate that the mucosal barrier has been damaged and that the intestinal wall is susceptible to bacterial invasion. In these cases, a broad-spectrum antibiotic that is effective against *Shigella* sp. and other gram-negative aerobes should be selected. Drugs that do not destroy normal anaerobic flora are preferred. Trimethoprim/sulfonamide combinations, chloramphenicol, and fluoroquinolone antibiotics such as enrofloxacin (Baytril, Mobay Corporation, Shawnee, KS) and ciprofloxacin (Cipro, Bayer Corp., West Haven, CT) have been efficacious in nonhuman primats with severe acute diarrhea (Line *et al.,* 1992; Salam and Bennish, 1991; Paul-Murphy, 1993). Concurrent administration of parenteral trimethoprim–sulfamethoxazole and oral erythromycin or a fluoroquinolone antibiotic given as the sole agent have been recommended as initial therapies prior to receiving culture results. Trimethoprim–sulfamethoxazole is a treatment of choice for *Shigella* and *Salmonella,* whereas erythromycin is effective against most *Campylobacter* isolates (Paul-Murphy, 1993). Ampicillin is one of the drugs of choice for shigellosis in humans and may be considered for use in nonhuman primates. *Salmonella* and *Campylobacter* are often resistant to ampicillin (Salam and Bennish, 1991; Paul-Murphy, 1993). Strains of these two genera that are resistant to tetracycline are also relatively common (Paul-Murphy, 1993). Susceptible strains of all three major bacterial enteric pathogens generally are eliminated from the body after 2–5 days of treatment, with the exception of *Salmonella* infection involving multiple organs. Animals not treated with antibiotics often shed

Campylobacter organisms for up to 10 days, so treatment may be of value in controlling the spread of the pathogen within a colony. Five days of antibiotic therapy may be adequate for some infections; treatment regimens of 10–14 days have been recommended by some authors (Bryant *et al.,* 1983; Line *et al.,* 1992; Paul-Murphy, 1993, Pucak *et al.,* 1977). Once antibiotic sensitivity testing has been performed on pathogenic isolates, antibiotic therapy should be changed if appropriate.

Fasting may be indicated in larger species when vomiting and diarrhea occur concurrently, but is not indicated in cases of diarrhea without vomiting (Ammon, 1995). In small, debilitated, or infant animals, caloric needs must be supplied orally or parenterally, preferably by providing multiple small meals (Paul-Murphy, 1993). Intestinal motility is decreased in most cases of diarrhea, and anticholinergic agents generally are contraindicated (Burrows, 1988; Bywater and Newsome, 1982; Paul-Murphy, 1993). Other symptomatic and adjunctive nonspecific therapies for diarrhea are reviewed elsewhere (Ammon, 1995; Bywater and Newsome, 1982; Krejs, 1988; Paul-Murphy, 1993; Schiller, 1995).

When fatalities occur or animals with diarrhea are euthanatized, complete necropsies should be performed and appropriate samples should be submitted for the identification of viral, bacterial, and parasitic agents. If tuberculin tests are suspicious or positive, or gross lesions are compatible with tuberculosis, fixed and fresh samples of bronchial lymph node, lung, liver, and spleen should be collected for histologic examination, acid fast stains, and mycobacterial identification [Centers for Disease Control (CDC), 1993]. In a survey of necropsy findings in macaques, most fatalities associated with diarrhea had lesions in the large intestine (Holmberg *et al.,* 1982b). In this survey, complete necropsy procedures and postmortem diagnostic testing identified the etiology in less than 50% of cases with diarrhea.

B. Bacterial and Fungal Diseases

1. *Shigella* sp.

Gastrointestinal diseases caused by *Shigella* sp. traditionally represent some of the greatest threats to primate health in terms of prevalence and seriousness. This genus is characterized as a nonmotile, nonencapsulated, non-spore-forming gram-negative rod in the family Enterobacteriaceae. Species of *Shigella* most often implicated are *Shigella flexneri* and *S. sonnei* (McClure *et al.,* 1986). Transmission of *Shigella* is fecal–oral; efforts to control infection spread are greatly complicated by the existence of a nonclinical carrier state in from 5 to 67% of the animals in some colonies and the inability to consistently culture this organism from infected animals. A high prevalence of *Shigella* in primate colonies within a zoological park has also been described (Banish *et al.,* 1993a). Flies may mechanically transmit the organism (Russell and Detolly, 1993). It is interesting to note that *Shigella* infection is apparently only acquired in captivity; the organism has not been isolated from primates cultured in the wild (Cooper, 1976).

Periodontal disease associated with *Shigella* has been discussed previously under oral diseases. In *Shigella* enteritis, animals may initially be quiet and inactive. This is rapidly followed by the passage of liquid stools, which may contain blood and/or mucous. The animal may become prostrate, develop edema of the face and neck, rectal prolapse, or symptoms associated with intestinal intussusception. Some animals that survive the acute phase of the disease slowly deteriorate over the next 2–3 weeks and die. Differential diagnosis should include yersiniosis and salmonellosis. *Campylobacter*-associated enteritis may show some of the same clinical signs, but is usually less severe. Definitive diagnosis requires culture of the organism from a rectal swab or fresh stool specimen; a 1- to 2-g fresh, uncontaminated stool specimen is preferred. The sample should be rapidly transported to the laboratory for immediate culture to optimize conditions for isolation (Dow *et al.,* 1989). Banish *et al.* (1993a) have described a detailed procedure for the isolation of *Shigella* from primates in a zoological park collection. Repeated cultures may be required to isolate *Shigella*. Laboratory evaluation of animals with shigellosis should also include the assessment of hydration, electrolyte, and acid–base status and hematocrit.

Lesions of shigellosis are primarily in the cecum and colon. The colon and cecal walls are often thickened with edema. Associated mesenteric lymph nodes may be enlarged, congested, and edematous (Russell and Detolly, 1993; Cooper, 1976). Opening the lumen reveals a catarrhal or diphtheritic colitis/typhlitis with variable amounts of hemorrhage and necrosis. Some animals may have ulcers that penetrate through the mucosa and reach almost to the serosa. The spleen may be enlarged and have subcapsular, petechial hemorrhages (Mulder, 1971). Histologically, there are early changes of epithelial cells from columnar to cuboidal. Subsequent death of the epithelial cells leaves eroded areas that progress to deep ulcers. The lamina propria becomes infiltrated with neutrophils and mononuclear cells. Diphtheritic colitis is characterized by the presence of a pseudomembrane containing fibrin, erythrocytes, inflammatory cells, bacteria, and dead epithelial cells that overlie eroded and ulcerated areas of the intestinal wall. Immunohistology studies have demonstrated the presence of *Shigella* in epithelial cells of the mucosa (Ogawa *et al.,* 1966). When the colitis is diphtheritic, they may be seen in the diphtheritic membrane. In ulcerative colitis, *Shigella* may be seen in the lamina propria and Peyer's patches (Ogawa *et al.,* 1964; Mulder, 1971). Gastritis associated with *Shigella* infection has been described (Kent *et al.,* 1967), but lesions are usually absent in the small intestine. Animals that survive the acute disease may show connective tissue formation and some epithelial regeneration. In ultrastructural studies, there are low numbers of intracellular *Shigella* contained in vacuoles of epithelial cells early in the disease. As the disease progresses, the epithelial cells die and are replaced by fibrinous exudate (Russell and Detolly, 1993).

Treatment for shigellosis should include antibiotic therapy based on sensitivity testing and aggressive correction of deficits in hydration, acid–base balance, and electrolytes. Some clinicians claim better results giving oral antibiotics than giving parenteral, even to the point of giving preparations designed for parenteral use orally (This works best with drugs such as gentamicin and metronidazole that remain unabsorbed and unchanged in the gastrointestinal tract.) Fluid therapy should follow established principles for this type of treatment (Short, 1980; Paul-Murphy, 1993). A discussion of fluid therapy may be found in Section IV,A.

Important research and management benefits can be derived from treating *Shigella* as a colony preventive medicine problem as opposed to treating individuals animals. Antibiotic treatment of individual animals as they become ill is often unsuccessful and has led to the development of multiply-resistant strains of *Shigella* (Lindsey *et al.*, 1971). Elimination of the *Shigella* carrier state has been reported in research and commercial macaque colonies (Pucak *et al.*, 1977; Olson *et al.*, 1986) and in a zoologic park collection of primates (Banish *et al.*, 1993b). A successful program to eliminate *Shigella* from a colony should include:

1. Identification and isolation of carrier animals through repeated culturing using a meticulous culture technique.
2. Antibiotic treatment of carrier animals using adequate doses of an antibiotic to which the organism has been found to be susceptible through sensitivity testing.
3. Repeated culturing of carrier animals posttreatment using the same meticulous culture technique with retreatment or culling of animals that continue to carry *Shigella*.
4. Careful attention to hygiene. A program has its best chance of success if a complete change in housing can be timed to coincide with treatment. Schedules for cage washing, cage-washing temperatures, appropriate use of disinfectants, and other factors can influence the success of such a program.

One study has shown a predisposition of animals with hypovitaminosis C to shigellosis (Honjo *et al.*, 1969). Colonies where this disease is endemic should be checked to ensure that dietary levels of vitamin C provide for the needs of all animals. It is possible that animals with clinical infection may benefit from parenteral supplementation of this and other vitamins.

2. *Salmonella* sp.

Salmonella is grouped with *Shigella* in the Enterobacteriaceae family and shares some of the same characteristics. It is a gram-negative, non-spore-forming, motile, rod-shaped bacteria. There are over 2000 closely related serovars. Infected animals frequently do not demonstrate clinical illness, which complicates efforts at control in infected colonies.

Clinical signs for *Salmonella* include stools that vary from soft to watery, with occasionally mucus or a small amount of blood (Klumpp *et al.*, 1986). In experimental infections, most animals have diarrhea within 24 hr of inoculation (Kent *et al.*, 1966). Animals that become septicemic may show a variety of clinical signs.

Salmonellosis in nonhuman primates is less common than shigellosis or *Campylobacter*-associated diarrhea. Studies published in the 1960s and 1970s showed that from 1 to 12% of newly arrived or recently captured animals were infected with *Salmonella*. Of 632 cases of diarrhea at one importer facility, 2.7% cultured positive for *Salmonella* as opposed to 8.7% positive for *Shigella* (Tribe and Fleming, 1983; Kourany *et al.*, 1969; Arya *et al.*, 1973; Agarwal and Chakravarti, 1969; Deinhardt *et al.*, 1967). With the increase in captive-breeding programs, improved husbandry and monitoring, and more stringent requirements for imported animals, the number of cases appears to have declined. *Salmonella* should still be considered along with *Shigella* and *Campylobacter* in the differential diagnosis of nonhuman primates with diarrheal disease.

Diagnosis of salmonellosis requires isolation of the organism from a rectal swab or stool culture. The same principles described for *Shigella* isolation also apply to *Salmonella*: a recently passed, uncontaminated stool sample of 1–2 g that is rapidly placed on appropriate growth media and incubated provides the best chance for isolation. The large number of *Salmonella* serovars makes serotyping useful for epidemiologic investigators.

Lesions of salmonellosis are primarily in the ileum and colon. Grossly, both become edematous, reddened, and dilated. The colonic mucosae becomes smooth, with ulcers and diphtheritic lesions. The mesenteric lymph nodes may be enlarged. Microscopically, there is hyperplasia and erosion of the mucosal epithelium in the colon with necrotic debris in the lumen and inflammatory infiltrate in the lamina propria. Microabscessation of colon lymphoid tissue is occasionally seen. In cases where the animal becomes septicemic, areas of focal necrosis may be seen in the liver and spleen (Kent *et al.*, 1966; Potkay, 1992).

Treatment for salmonellosis is similar to that used for *Shigella*: use of an antibiotic to which the organism is known to be sensitive and supportive care to compensate for the loss of fluids, electrolytes, and acid–base imbalance resulting from the diarrhea.

The zoonotic potential of *Salmonella* and the difficulty in eliminating the carrier state may make it necessary to cull carrier animals. As with humans, *Salmonella* has been isolated from the gallbladder of apparently healthy nonhuman primates (Bokkenheuser, 1962). Rodents, opossums, raccoons, and birds (along with most other animals) are potential reservoirs for *Salmonella,* and flies and other insects can mechanically transmit the organism. Control of these animals and insects in primate housing can be important in the prevention of infection.

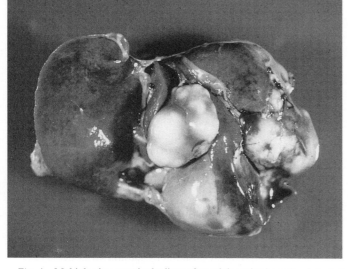

Fig. 4. Multiple abscesses in the liver of an adult squirrel monkey infected with *Yersinia enterocolitica*. Photograph provided by Dr. Susan Gibson, University of South Alabama.

3. *Campylobacter* sp.

Formerly designated as the genus *Vibrio*, *Campylobacter* bacteria are characterized as slender, curved, or comma-shaped gram-negative bacteria with a single polar flagellum (Fox, 1982). *Campylobacter* has been described as the most common bacterial cause of acute enterocolitis in humans. As with *Shigella*, some evidence suggests that primate infection is nonexistent in the wild (Morton *et al.*, 1983). In captive primate colonies, the incidence of infection can range from 0 to 100%, with a higher incidence in primate nurseries and other groupings of younger animals (Russell *et al.*, 1988). Transmission is fecal–oral. Some primates can be nonclinical carriers of the organism (Bryant *et al.*, 1983), *Campylobacter jejeuni* and *C. coli* are the isolates most frequently reported.

Enteritis due to *Campylobacter* tends to be less severe and more chronic than *Shigella* enteritis. In experimental infections, diarrhea begins 36–48 hr postinoculation and lasts for 7–11 days, with most severe clinical signs lasting for 2–5 days. Shedding of the organism continues for an average of 3 weeks (Russell *et al.*, 1989). Most animals have inappetence, straining, and mild diarrhea. Severe signs such as rectal prolapse and intestinal intussusception are rare and mortality from *Campylobacter* enteritis is low. Although diarrhea tends to be less severe than *Shigella*, cases of severe dysentery with large amounts of blood in watery stools have been reported.

The special conditions required to isolate and grow this organism prevented clinicians from becoming aware of its significance in primate colonies prior to 1980. *Campylobacter* is macroaerophilic, requires a 5–10% carbon dioxide environ-

ment, and is easily overgrown by other enteric bacteria without selective media and growing conditions. Gram stains of fecal smears may be useful in making an early diagnosis (McClure *et al.*, 1986). As with all diarrheal diseases, laboratory evaluation should also include an assessment of hydration, electrolyte, and acid–base status. Hematocrit, mean corpuscular volume, and hemoglobin have been found to be reduced, and leukocyte and blood urea nitrogen (BUN) levels are increased in primates with *Campylobacter* enteritis (Goodwin *et al.*, 1983).

Gross lesions of *Campylobacter* enteritis include a thickened, turgid distal ileum, cecum, and colon. Mesenteric and celiac lymph nodes can be enlarged. Intestinal contents may be liquid to semisolid from the jejunum through the colon, and the mucosal surface of the ileum, cecum, and colon is coated with mucus or blood. On microscopic examination, villi of the jejunum and ileum may be shortened and lacteals dilated (Bryant *et al.*, 1983). The epithelium of the colon may be replaced by squamous cells in severe cases. There is a loss of goblet cells, and inflammatory infiltrates may be present between crypt epithelial cells, in the crypts and lymphatics, and in the lamina propria. Ultrastructure examination reveals loss of microvilli in the epithelium and degenerated erythrocytes and epithelial cells in the colon lumen (Russell *et al.*, 1989; Russell and Detolly, 1993). *Campylobacter* has also been found to cause gastritis in primates (Newell *et al.*, 1987; Bronsdon and Schoenknecht, 1988; Baskerville and Newell, 1988; Newell *et al.*, 1988).

Unlike *Shigella* colitis, *Campylobacter* enteritis has generally responded well to appropriate antibiotic therapy, with few problems associated with resistant strains of the bacteria. This, of course, will probably change if antibiotic use continues to be widespread and indiscriminate. Erythromycin is given orally at a dose of 15–25 mg/kg twice daily for 10 days. Oral and parenteral fluids and electrolytes should be provided as needed to correct imbalances in hydration, electrolytes, and acid–base homeostasis.

Birds are a potential reservoir for primates housed outdoors and the organism has also been isolated from flies (Pazzaglia *et al.*, 1994), suggesting that control of these may be of use in limiting infections. The infection rate in primate nurseries is high (Russell *et al.*, 1988); strict hygiene in these areas is especially important. An ELISA test has been developed for *Campylobacter* that should be useful for epidemiology studies (Kohno *et al.*, 1988).

4. *Yersinia enterocolitica* and *Y. pseudotuberculosis*

Yersinia enterocolitica and *Y. pseudotuberculosis* both cause a disease known as pseudotuberculosis in nonhuman primates. Both are gram-negative coccobacilli in the family Enterobacteriaceae.

It is difficult to identify any marked differences in the clinical syndromes associated with these two agents in nonhuman primates. Both cause diarrhea (sometimes with blood), dehydration, depression, anorexia, and weight loss. Hepatomegaly, splenomegaly, and lymphadenopathy may also be seen (Skavlen *et al.,* 1985; Baggs *et al.,* 1976; Bronson *et al.,* 1972). Illness can also follow a peracute course, where animals appear to be healthy, then are either found dead or rapidly deteriorate and die a short time after discovery. Abortion and stillbirth have been reported with *Y. pseudotuberculosis* infection; they have not been reported with *Y. enterocolitica.* The highly invasive nature of *Y. enterocolitica,* however, suggests that even this distinction between the two is questionable. Although sustained enzootics of pseudotuberculosis have been reported (Rosenberg *et al.,* 1980; Baggs *et al.,* 1976), cases are often sporadic. Such sporadic infection may coincide with visits to a primate enclosure by birds or rodents that act as reservoir hosts for these agents (Bronson *et al.,* 1972).

Differential diagnosis for pseudotuberculosis should include other causes of bacterial enteritis and systemic disease. *Shigella* and *Salmonella* may cause somewhat similar clinical signs. *Mycobacterium tuberculosis* may cause liver and spleen enlargement (granulomas), but lesions (especially those in the intestine) differ from those of *Y. entercolitica* and *Y. pseudotuberculosis* and tuberculosis tends to have a more chronic course. *Campylobacter* infection generally causes a milder disease than pseudotuberculosis and is not known to cause septicemia.

Yersinia enterocolitica and *Y. pseudotuberculosis* may be isolated from rectal swabs or blood from septicemic animals. Isolates may also be obtained from liver, spleen, lymph nodes, kidney, or other organs that have lesions. As with *Campylobacter,* special conditions are required for the culture of *Y. enterocolitica* and *Y. pseudotuberculosis.* Failure to provide these conditionis may lead to an inability to correctly diagnose this infection (see elsewhere in this volume). Animals with pseudotuberculosis may have pronounced leukopenia or leukocytosis (Skavlen *et al.,* 1985; McClure *et al.,* 1971; Rosenberg *et al.,* 1980).

Pseudotuberculosis causes ulcerative gastroenteritis and septicemia in nonhuman primates. Grossly, there is mucosal ulceration of the gastrointestinal tract that may occur in any part or throughout; lesions can be diphtheritic. The intestine may also be congested and/or hemorrhagic. There can be hepatomegaly and splenomegaly and yellow/white foci in the liver (Fig. 4), spleen, lymph nodes, and adrenal cortex. The organism has also been isolated from the uterus in infected animals that have abortion/stillbirth (Rosenberg *et al.,* 1980). In chronic disease, large abscesses of the liver and spleen may be seen. Microscopically, there is ulcerative enteritis and multifocal necrosis of the spleen and liver, with coccobacilli visible in affected areas (McClure *et al.,* 1971; Baggs *et al.,* 1976; Skavlen *et al.,* 1985; Bronson *et al.,* 1972).

Pseudotuberculosis in nonhuman primates is a disease that is frequently not identified until it is far advanced; as such, treatment is often unrewarding. Aggressive treatment with a systemic antibiotic to which the organism is sensitive may be therapeutic in the early stages of the disease. This should be combined with fluid therapy to correct resulting deficits. In chronic cases, there may be some benefit derived from splenectomy and/or hepatic lobectomy where isolated abscesses are present.

Birds and rodents are known carriers of *Y. enterocolitica* and *Y. pseudotuberculosis,* and control of these carriers in and around primate housing can greatly assist in reducing the number of cases. Cockroaches were suspected as carriers in one outbreak (S. V. Gibson, personal communication, 1995). Primates can also be carriers (Skavlen *et al.,* 1985). Rectal swabs may be used to screen for carrier animals, followed by a course of antibiotic therapy for carriers and those with whom they are housed.

Some evidence suggests that pseudotuberculosis is a zoonotic disease (Wilson *et al.,* 1976). Personnel should follow appropriate precautions when working with infected animals, tissues, or body fluids.

5. *Mycobacterium avium–intracellulare* Complex

Atypical tuberculosis (synonyms include avian tuberculosis and Runyon's type III tuberculosis) is a disease caused by bacteria in the *Mycobacterium avium–intracellulare* complex (*M. avium* and *M. intracellulare* were once considered to be separate organisms and are seen as such in older literature, but these are now grouped together as the "*Mycobacterium avium–intracellulare* complex"). These bacteria are common inhabitants of soil, water, and plants and are considered to be opportunistic pathogens.

Clinical signs for atypical tuberculosis include chronic diarrhea and weight loss, dehydration, splenomegaly, hepatomegaly, and lymphadenopathy (Sesline *et al.,* 1975). The disease usually has an extended course, with death occurring after a year or more (Sesline, 1975). Cutaneous granuloma formation has also been described with *M. avium* infection (Bellinger and Bullock, 1988). Animals with atypical tuberculosis may react positively to a tuberculin skin test using mammalian old tuberculin (Sedgwick *et al.,* 1970). Tuberculosis caused by *Mycobacterium tuberculosis* or *M. bovis* should be considered in the differential diagnosis. Although clinical signs and lesions of atypical tuberculosis are primarily in the gastrointestinal system and those of tuberculosis are in the respiratory system, clinical signs and lesions for these mycobacteria can be quite similar (Goodwin *et al.,* 1988). Definitive diagnosis may be made by culture and demonstration of characteristic lesions in necropsy or biopsy specimens (Sesline, 1975).

Laboratory findings in animals with atypical tuberculosis include normocytic, normochromic anemia, lymphopenia, and neutrophilic leukocytosis. Increases in serum aspartate aminotransferase (AST, formerly known as SGOT) and globulin and a decrease in albumin may also be seen.

Animals with atypical tuberculosis may have no gross lesions early in the disease. In more advanced cases, the primary lesions are usually in the intestine. There is thickening of the intestinal

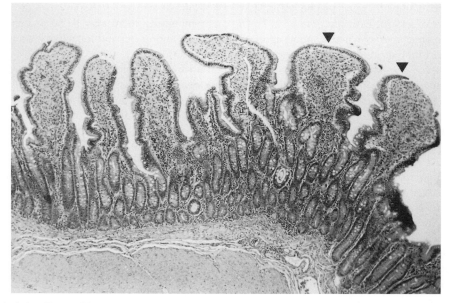

Fig. 5. Atypical tuberculosis in a 7-year-old *Macaca nemestrina.* The lamina propria of the small intestinal villi are mildly to moderately distended with a sheet of epithelioid-type macrophages that are characteristic of an atypical mycobacterial infection. Magnification: ×75. Photograph provided by Yerkes Primate Center.

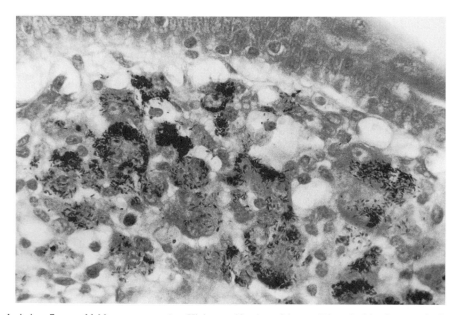

Fig. 6. Atypical tuberculosis in a 7-year-old *Macaca nemestrina.* High magnification of the small intestinal lamina propria shows variable numbers of acid fast bacilli within the cytoplasm of epithelioid macrophages. Kinyouns acid fast stain. Magnification: ×740. Photograph provided by Yerkes Primate Center

wall and the serosa may have a roughened, granular appearance or have yellow-white nodules on the surface. The lymph nodes (espcially mesenteric nodes), liver, and spleen may be enlarged, and the liver and spleen have areas of tan or yellow discoloration. Colonic contents are often fluid, and the mucosal wall can be thickened into sometimes yellowish folds (Smith *et al.,* 1972; Fleischman *et al.,* 1982; Holmberg *et al.,* 1982a; King, 1993b). Microscopically, there is diffuse infiltration of large numbers of macrophages in the lamina propria of the intestine (Fig. 5). Acid fast staining reveals many mycobacteria contained within these cells (Fig. 6). In disseminated cases, similar cells may be seen in the liver, spleen, lymph nodes, and other locations. In rare cases, animals with atypical tuberculosis may exhibit granuloma formation similar to that seen in tuberculosis (Goodwin *et al.,* 1988; Bellinger and Bullock, 1988).

As with tuberculosis, the treatment of animals with atypical tuberculosis is often unrewarding. In most cases, the disease is far advanced by the time it is diagnosed. Affected animals should be evaluated for immunocompromising disease or conditions (Holmberg *et al.,* 1985). In cases where the cause of immunosuppression can be corrected (e.g., chronic use of steroids or radiation exposure), removal of the immunosuppressive agent combined with the use of an antimicrobial agent to which the organism has been proven sensitive may be of benefit. Bacteria in the *M. avium–intracellulare* complex are often resistant to many of the antimicrobial agents commonly used against the mycobacteria. Atypical tuberculosis is considered to be a zoonotic disease (Hugh-Jones *et al.,* 1995), but the opportunistic nature of these bacteria makes primate-to-human transmission unlikely if proper procedures are in effect for screening of exposed personnel, hygiene, protective clothing, and animal monitoring.

6. *Mycobacterium paratuberculosis*

Mycobacterium paratuberculosis has been identified as the agent causing a wasting disease in a colony of *Macaca arctoides.* This organism causes Johne's disease in a variety of species. In primates, infection resulted in granulomatous lesions of the intestine, liver, and mesenteric lymph nodes. In the *M. arctoides* outbreak, investigators reported successful treatment of some animals with the drug Rifabutine (Farmitalia Carlo Erba, Milan, Italy). The low number of reported cases of Johne's disease in primates may, at least in part, be the result of problems associated with culturing the agent (McClure *et al.,* 1987; Anderson and McClure, 1993).

7. Pseudomembranous enterocolitis

Fatal pseudomembranous enterocolitis has been associated with antibiotic therapy in callitrichids, a howler monkey, and an owl monkey (Torgerson *et al.,* 1992). Most of these animals had histories of chronic diarrhea and all were on antibiotic therapy at the time of death. Toxins of *Clostridium difficile* were identified in the majority of these cases, and the pathogenesis is believed to be similar to that of pseudomembranous entercolitis associated with the use of certain antibiotics in humans.

C. Viral Diseases

Many viral infections that involve the gastrointestinal tract are disseminated infections involving multiple organs. The following examples of viral diseases have diarrhea or other intestinal signs. The reader is referred to the chapter on viral diseases elsewhere in this volume for more information.

1. Simian Hemorrhagic Fever

Simian hemorrhagic fever is an acute, highly fatal, togavirus infection of macaques that causes disseminated vascular damage, disseminated intravascular coagulation, and hemorrhage from most body orifices and in many internal organs (Allen *et al.,* 1968; Gravell *et al.,* 1980; London, 1977). A dark tarry stool indicative of intestinal hemorrhage is a common clinical sign. Severe mucosal hemorrhage of the proximal duodenum, beginning at the pylorus and extending distally 5–10 cm, occurs in many infected animals and is considered highly suggestive of this disease. Widespread necrosis of lymphoid tissue is characteristic. Patas monkeys, African green monkeys, and baboons can carry the virus asymptomatically for long periods of time, and asymptomatic African primates have been implicated as the sources of several outbreaks in macaques.

2. *Paramyxovirus saguinus*

Paramyxovirus infections in nonhuman primates may present initially or primarily with diarrhea. A paramyxovirus, tentatively named *Paramyxovirus saguinus,* has been reported to cause severe gastroenteritis, leading to diarrhea, dehydration, and death in tamarins and marmosets (Fraser *et al.,* 1978; Hunt and Blake, 1993c). Foci of mucosal hemorrhage and necrosis are grossly visible in the stomach, cecum, and colon of acutely infected animals and may extend deeply into the lamina propria. Microscopic intestinal epithelial necrosis is most severe in the small intestine, but also occurs in the cecum and colon. Multinucleated syncytial giant cells formed from intestinal and colonic epithelial cells, blunted intestinal villi, and hyperplastic intestinal and colonic crypt epithelium accompany lesions of intestinal necrosis. Indistinct eosinophilic intranuclear inclusion bodies that generally fill the nuclei of epithelial cells and syncytial cells are present, and eosinophilic intracytoplasmic inclusions are observed less frequently. Syncytial cells with intranuclear or intracytoplasmic inclusion bodies may be seen in the epithelium of bile ducts, pancreatic ducts, and the urinary bladder and in hepatocytes and renal tubules, but necrosis is not present at these sites.

3. Measles

Measles also causes severe clinical signs in marmosets and tamarins as well as in other Old World and New World primates (Levy and Mirkovic, 1971; Lowenstine, 1993b). In marmosets, measles commonly causes necrosis, syncytial cells, and intranuclear and intracytoplasmic viral inclusions in the gastrointestinal epithelium and may be accompanied by severe diarrhea and dehydration. Syncytia and inclusion bodies also occur in the lamina propria and gut-associated lymphoid tissue anywhere in the small and large intestine, but may no longer be detectable when New World primates die of measles infection. Measles in all susceptible primates usually is accompanied by clinical signs and lesions of respiratory disease and cutaneous rash with syncytial cells and inclusion bodies in the lungs, airways, and other organ systems (Albrecht *et al.,* 1980). Macaques with clinical measles infection may have gastrointestinal lesions and diarrhea, but these are less common than respiratory signs, conjunctivitis, and cutaneous rash (Hall *et al.,* 1971). Oral and esophageal foci of necrosis (Koplick's spots) are seen occasionally in macaques. Measles in marmosets and macaques can be prevented by vaccination. One facility (J. Roberts, personal communication, 1996) uses a live virus vaccine (Attenuvax, Merck) at 6 months of age or during quarantine for newly arrived animals; 0.5 cc of the vaccine is administered subcutaneously. A canine distemper vaccine (Vanguard, Norden) that contains measles virus has been suggested as a less expensive alternative to human measles vaccine (Staley *et al.,* 1995). The efficacy and safety of this vaccine in nonhuman primates have not been thoroughly tested.

4. Cytomegalovirus: Other Herpes Viruses

Disseminated cytomegalovirus and varicella-like herpesvirus infections in macaques can cause lesions and perhaps diarrhea in macaques, particularly in immunosuppressed animals. Cytomegalic cells with intranuclear and intracytoplasmic inclusions have been described in the lamina propria of the small and large intestine of macaques with disseminated cytomegalovirus infections (Baskin, 1993). Cytomegalovirus rarely infects surface epithelial cells. Intense infiltration of neutrophils into the lamina propria is a common intestinal lesion of cytomegalovirus infection in macaques. Diarrhea and other intestinal signs of cytomegalovirus infection usually are less common and less severe than signs associated with other organs. Foci of intestinal epithelial necrosis and ulceration with intranuclear inclusion bodies also have been reported in macaques with disseminated varicella-like herpesvirus infections (Baskin, 1987; Padovan and Cantrell, 1986; Roberts, 1993a). Disseminated herpesvirus infections in owl monkeys infected with *Herpesvirus tamarinus* (*H. platyrrhinae* or *Herpes i*) may be accompanied by necrosis and hemorrhage in the gastrointestinal tract and eosinophilic intranuclear inclusion bodies (Hunt and Blake, 1993b).

5. Rotavirus

Antibodies to group A rotavirus have been documented in a high proportion of captive and feral cynomolgus monkeys monkeys, and the prevalence of antibodies was similar in adults and juveniles (Awang and Yap, 1990). This report suggests that cynomolgus monkeys are probably infected at a very young age. Experimental infections with simian and/or human rotaviruses have been produced in newborn cynomolgus monkeys, rhesus monkeys, and baboons (Leong and Awang, 1990). Formula-fed

cynomolgus inoculated orally within 24 hr of birth with either simian or human group A rotavirus consistently shed virus for 1–6 days. All monkeys inoculated with the simian virus and most inoculated with the human rotavirus within the first day of life developed diarrhea lasting 1–6 days. Most monkeys inoculated with the simian rotavirus at 2–10 days of age also developed diarrhea and shed virus in the stool. Animals inoculated at 2 weeks to 3 months of age did not develop diarrhea, although some shed low levels of virus for several days. No vomiting was observed in any monkeys infected with the rotavirus. The presence of maternal antibodies to group A rotavirus in formula-fed infants did not prevent viral shedding or diarrhea in infected newborn cynomolgus monkeys. Less than one-half of the inoculated animals developed antibodies to group A rotavirus following experimental infection (Leong and Awang, 1990). These studies suggest that the rotavirus should be considered as a possible cause of diarrhea in newborn nonhuman primates.

6. Immunodeficiency Viruses

Chronic diarrhea is a typical feature of simian acquired immunodeficiency syndrome in macaques associated with either simian immunodeficiency virus 1 (SIV-1) or type D simian retroviruses (SRV). Diarrhea often is the cause of death in animals that develop immunodeficiency. In most cases, secondary infections can be implicated as the cause(s) of diarrhea in severely immunosuppressed animals. Enteric pathogens reported in animals with simian immunodeficiency syndrome include *Shigella* spp., *Campylobacter* spp., *Mycobacterium avium–intracellulare, Rhodococcus equi, Cryptosporidium, Giardia, Yersinia* spp., *Balantidium coli,* trichomonads, and cytomegalovirus (Baskin *et al.,* 1988; Henrickson *et al.,* 1984; King, 1993a; Lackner *et al.,* 1990; Lowenstine, 1993a; Osborn *et al.,* 1984). However, in a significant number of cases, secondary infections could not be identified, and diarrhea was attributed to the primary lentivirus or type D retrovirus infection. Rhesus monkeys infected experimentally with SIV_{mac} developed severe intestinal villous blunting with variable crypt hyperplasia; however, SIV was not detectable in enterocyte (King, 1993a). Type D simian retrovirus can infect enterocyte, lymphoid cells, and macrophages, and SRV infection of rhesus monkeys has been associated with villous blunting and mucosal lymphoplasmacytic infiltrates (Lackner *et al.,* 1990; Lowenstine, 1993a).

Fibroblastic neoplasms of the lymph nodes and mesentery at the ileocecocolic junction are associated with infections with certain strains of type D simian retroviruses in *Macaca nemestrina, M. mulatta, M. fascicularis,* and *M. fuscata* (Giddens *et al.,* 1985; Tsai, 1993). This syndrome, known as retroperitoneal fibromatosis, may be localized to the ileocecocolic area or may spread throughout the abdominal viscera and occasionally to the pleural cavity. Neoplastic tissue may completely surround the bowel and migrate distally and proximally along the intestinal tract, almost always remaining beneath the peritoneal surface. Occasionally the neoplastic tissue invades the tunica muscularis and submucosa of the intestinal tract. Some masses consist primarily of large fibroblasts, whereas others contain more collagen and fewer, smaller cells. The pattern of fibrosis is irregular and disorganized. Retroperitoneal fibromatosis lacks the high cellularity and anaplasia of typical fibrosarcomas. Variable numbers of retroperitoneal fibromatosis cells stain positively for factor VIII-related antigen (Giddens *et al.,* 1985). Lymphoid infiltrates are seen commonly within neoplastic masses. Affected animals usually present with either diarrhea or evidence of intestinal obstruction, although complete obstruction of the bowel is rarely evident at necropsy. Masses are detectable by abdominal palpation. Affected animals usually develop other signs of immunodeficiency syndrome, including secondary infections.

D. Intestinal Parasites

Intestinal parasitism may be associated with no clinical signs, diarrhea, general poor body condition, intestinal obstruction, and, in some cases, peritonitis and intestinal adhesions. Any animal with clinical signs suggesting gastrointestinal disease should be examined for internal parasites and treated appropriately. Because a complete discussion of intestinal protozoal and helminth parasites is beyond the scope of this chapter, the reader is referred to the chapter on parasitic diseases elsewhere in this volume for information regarding enteric parasites.

E. Toxic and Metabolic Diseases

1. Polychlorinated Biphenyl Intoxication

Ingestion of toxic substances can result in diarrhea, e.g., polychlorinated biphenyl compounds in concrete sealer were reported to cause diarrhea, weight loss, alopecia, photophobia, acne, and facial edema in rhesus monkeys (Altman *et al.,* 1979).

2. Amyloidosis

The small intestine is the most common site of amyloid deposition in rhesus monkeys and pig-tailed macaques with generalized amyloidosis, but the colon, cecum, liver, spleen, and other organs may also contain amyloid deposits (Blanchard, 1993; Blanchard *et al.,* 1986; Slattum *et al.,* 1989a,b). Although systemic amyloidosis is best described in rhesus monkeys and pig-tailed macaques, the syndrome probably occurs in many other species. In most cases of amyloidosis in nonhuman primates, amyloid deposition is a sequela to chronic inflammation. In rhesus monkeys and pig-tailed macaques, amyloid deposition commonly is a sequela of chronic diarrhea and inflammatory lesions of the intestine, cecum, and colon. Pig-tailed macaques with retroperitoneal fibromatosis and simian retrovirus type D infection are more likely to have amyloidosis than normal animals (Slattum *et al.,* 1989a). Intestinal amyloid in

macaques is of the AA type. An AA amyloid is formed from an acute-phase protein (serum amyloid A protein) released by the liver in response to inflammation. Amyloidosis is discussed in further detail in the section on liver diseases elsewhere in this volume.

3. Protein-Losing Enteropathy

Protein-losing enteropathy with associated chronic weight loss, hypoalbuminemia, and diarrhea has been described in *Macaca mulatta* and one *M. arctoides* (Rodger *et al.,* 1980). These cases were associated with one or more of the following: intestinal lymphangiectasia, intestinal mast cell proliferation, intestinal infection with *Pseudomonas* spp., intestinal goblet cell hyperplasia with excessive mucin production, and intestinal amyloidosis.

4. Colitis/Adenocarcinoma of Marmosets and Tamarins

A syndrome of severe chronic weight loss, anorexia, diarrhea, wasting, and death in tamarins has been associated with a variety of gastrointestinal lesions (Chalifoux *et al.,* 1982). The most common of these is acute to chronic colitis that can occur in 50–100% of cotton-top tamarins (*Saguinus oedipus oedipus*) and less frequently in *Callithrix jacchus* and *Saguinus fuscicollis illigeri* (Chalifoux *et al.,* 1985, 1993a; Lushbaugh *et al.,* 1985a,b). Diarrhea is first apparent in juvenile callitrichids and continues persistently or intermittently if not treated. The clinical course may last for years; however, tamarins less than 1 year of age frequently die from secondary septicemia. The early lesions of tamarin colitis include diffuse or widespread infiltrates of neutrophils in the lamina propria and epithelium of the colon, cecum, and rectum. Reddening or petechial hemorrhages may be observed grossly, but often the colon and cecum have no visible gross lesions. Crypt abscesses form in the mucosal glands, with attenuation and destruction of epithelium. Crypt epithelium frequently extends into the submucosa, especially in areas of submucosal lymphoid aggregates, and inflammation extends laterally from these herniated crypts, resulting in ulceration that occasionally can be observed grossly. Lymphocytes, plasma cells, and macrophages become numerous as the inflammatory process progresses whereas neutrophils persist in active inflammatory lesions. Glands become more tortuous and goblet cells are decreased. Atrophy or hyperplasia of epithelium may occur. Extensive hyperplasia may result in papillary proliferation of the colonic or cecal mucosa. Cellular atypia in hyperplastic crypts can exhibit pseudostratification, a high mitotic index, cellular pleomorphism, and loss of cellular polarity. In cases that have subsided, inflammation may be absent, goblet cells are present, and the irregular appearance of the mucosa may persist, The cause of this syndrome is not known. Differences in intestinal mucins have been observed in clinically normal tamarins and tamarins with colitis (Chalifoux *et al.,* 1993a; Podolsky, 1985). Oral treatment with 10–50 mg/kg/day sulfasalazine has been reported to cause significant clinical improvement in many affected cotton-top tamarins (Chalifoux *et al.,* 1985; Madara, 1985). Sulfasalazine is a combination of sulfapyridine and salicylic acid. Bacteria convert salicylic acid to 5-aminosalicylate, which is believed to act by inhibiting prostaglandin and leukotriene production in the colon, cecum, and anus (Bayliss *et al.,* 1988). Colitis in cotton-top tamarins has been studied as a model for human chronic ulcerative colitis, which also responds to sulfasalazine.

In some cotton-top tamarins with chronic colitis, foci of cellular proliferation and atypia can progress to colonic adenocarcinoma (Chalifoux *et al.,* 1993b; Lushbaugh *et al.,* 1978, 1985b). Colonic adenocarcinoma arising from chronic colitis has not been reported in species other than cotton-top tamarins (*Saguinus oedipus oedipus*). Colonic adenocarcinomas usually occur in cotton-top tamarins 5–7 years of age (ranging from 21 months to 12 years) (Chalifoux *et al.,* 1993b). Up to 20% of tamarins in a colony may be affected. Colonic adenocarcinomas arise deep within the colonic mucosal glands. Early neoplastic lesions may be confined to white plaques in the ileal, cecal, colonic, or rectal mucosa. Neoplastic cells often aggressively invade the intestinal wall, but do not form polypoid or papillary masses. Poorly organized cords, sheets, and glandular structures of cells exhibit cellular pleomorphism, lack of orientation to basement membranes, and signet ring cells containing periodic acid–Schiff (PAS)-positive mucin or diffuse cytoplasmic PAS staining. Periodic acid–Schiff staining assists in the identification of neoplastic cells beneath the mucosa and at metastatic sites such as lymph nodes. In some neoplasms, argentaffin-positive neuroendocrine cells may accompany mucus-secreting cells (Swartzendruber and Richter, 1980). Mucin may be seen in small lakes surrounding neoplastic foci. Adenocarcinomas commonly metastasize to abdominal lymph nodes and spread less frequently to lung, liver, and spleen. Metastases in lymph nodes and other organs usually are firm and white. Inflammatory reactions similar to those seen in chronic colitis may be present, and reactive fibrous tissue often surrounds neoplastic cells. Dilatation of the bowel may be seen proximal to areas of fibrosis and stricture.

Additional differential diagnoses for diarrhea in young tamarins include focal ulcerative ileocolitis of unknown etiology, Tyzzer's disease, pseudomembranous enterocolitis associated with *Clostridium difficile,* and the more common bacterial and parasitic infections seen in other species of nonhuman primates (Snook, 1993; Snook *et al.,* 1989). Focal ulcerative ileocolitis has been reported in cotton-top tamarins under 1 year of age from a single colony. These animals presented with inappetence, diarrhea, nonregenerative hemolytic anemia, severe thrombocytopenia, and widespread hemorrhages in the intestinal tract and elsewhere. Septicemia was a common complication. The disease usually progressed rapidly to death. At necropsy, these tamarins had focal ulceration at the ileocolic junction, with or without reactive fibroplasia and inflammation. Lesions usually were limited to a zone within a few centimeters

of the ulcer. Tyzzer's disease typically had hepatic or cardiac necrosis and inflammation, and intracytoplasmic bacteria could be visualized in lesions using Steiner's silver stain (Snook, 1993). Pseudomembranous enterocolitis associated with *Clostridium difficile* usually had an acute clinical course and lesions of acute mucosal necrosis and fibrin exudation.

5. Idiopathic Colitis of Young Macaques

Chronic colitis of unknown etiology occurs in macaques and is associated with diarrhea and emaciation (Adler *et al.,* 1993). The published report concerned macaques less than 3 years of age. These animals typically have chronic or intermittent diarrhea that has not responded well to antibiotic therapy. The cecum and colon are distended with fluid. The mucosa of the large bowel appears diffusely thickened and granular, and there may be erosions or small uclers visible grossly. In the lamina propria of the large bowel, there are diffuse microscopic infiltrates of lymphocytes and plasma cells, with scattered foci of macrophages and neutrophils. Mucosal glands in the cecum and proximal colon become filled with neutrophils, form crypt abscesses, and ulcerate. Mucosal epithelial hyperplasia may be accompanied by glandular tortuosity, karyomegaly, epithelial pseudostratification, goblet cell depletion, and damage to superficial epithelium. Herniation of mucosal glands into the submucosal lymphoid patches is common, and these lesions can lead to larger ulcers. About one-half of the cases of chronic colitis have similar lesions in the terminal ileum. Enlarged, hyperplastic mesenteric lymph nodes, thymic atrophy, and chronic inflammation of stomach, gallbladder, and liver accompany colonic lesions in some cases. Chronic colitis with a similar appearance may occur in adult macaques and in other nonhuman primate species.

F. Constipation

Constipation may include increased stool firmness and decreased moisture, decreased stool volume, motility disorders associated with intestinal transit and defecation, painful or difficult defecation, and reduced frequency of defecation (Bayliss *et al.,* 1988; Koch, 1995). In some cases of impaired motility, the stool may be soft or may even be classified as diarrhea. When evaluating a nonhuman primate with constipation, the clinical and experimental history should be reviewed. Adhesions or other sequelae of prior abdominal surgery may impair gastrointestinal motility or transit. Opiate analgesics, anticholinergic agents, calcium channel blockers, and other drugs may produce signs of constipation in otherwise normal animals (Koch, 1995).

Constipation usually is not a clinical emergency and often may have no medical significance. Nonspecific treatment of constipation may include increasing dietary fiber and the use of laxatives. Popcorn and peanuts are high in dietary fiber and may be used in moderation to add fiber to diets of constipated non-human primates. The pathophysiology, clinical evaluation, and treatment of constipation in humans has been reviewed, and many of the principles apply equally well to nonhuman primates (Koch, 1995). Nonhuman primates presented with constipation should be examined to determine if an underlying disease is causing the clinical signs. Specific treatment of underlying diseases usually is preferable to symptomatic therapy.

Cases of constipation involving impaired intestinal motility are more likely to respond to specific therapy than other types of constipation if the primary cause can be identified. Blockage of flow of ingesta through the intestinal tract may be caused by intestinal foreign bodies, trichobezoars, intussusception or volvulus, or heavy burdens of intestinal parasites. Ileus related to intestinal obstruction, trauma, surgery, or intestinal inflammation may reduce the movement of ingesta through the bowel, leading to either diarrhea or constipation. Endometriosis and enteric neoplasms (such as the colonic adenocarcinoma of *Saguinus oedipus,* lymphosarcoma involving the bowel, and retroperitoneal fibromatosis) may surround and constrict the bowel lumen, preventing the normal passage of ingesta. These cases may present as constipation or diarrhea.

G. Intestinal Neoplasia

Neoplasms of the small and large intestines are included in this section because they usually impair motility and result in abnormal stool. Nonhuman primates with primary intestinal neoplasms often present with weight loss, a palpable abdominal mass, and diarrhea (DePaoli and McClure, 1982). Some of the intestinal neoplasms reported in nonhuman primates include small intestinal adenocarcinoma in *Callicebus moloch, Cebus apella, Macaca mulatta, M. radiata,* and *Saguinus fuscicollis*; small intestinal polyposis associated with oxyurid parasites in *Pan troglodytes*; colonic carcinoma in *M. mulatta*; duodenal carcinoid in *M. fascicularis*; colonic leiomyosarcoma in *M. mulatta*; and rectal adenocarcinoma in *M. sinica* (DePaoli and McClure, 1982; Klumpp and McClure, 1993; Lowenstine, 1986; Toft *et al.,* 1976). Colorectal cancer has been reported to be relatively common in *M. mulatta* older than 20 years of age. Authors of one study (Kemnitz *et al.,* 1996) found colon cancer in 21 of 175 (12%) *M. mulatta* aged 21–36 years.

H. Idiopathic Megacolon

An idiopathic acquired megacolon syndrome has been reported in adult female *M. fascicularis* (Eisele *et al.,* 1991). Clinical signs included diarrhea, abdominal distention, increased mucus in the stool, anorexia, and failure to defecate. The colons of all affected animals were greatly distended with gas and ingesta. Four of five affected animals had histories of prior abdominal surgeries. Five animals were cured following partial surgical resection of the dilated bowel. At surgery, all monkeys had abdominal adhesions and three had volvulus of the colon. Histologically, there was degeneration and fibrosis of the colonic wall, primarily in the outer longitudinal muscle layer.

V. LIVER

A. Diagnosis of Liver Disease

1. Metabolism

The functional anatomy of the liver has been reviewed (McCuskey, 1993; Miyai, 1991; Sasse *et al.,* 1992; Herlong, 1988; Ockner, 1988a). The physiologic roles of the liver in human and nonhuman primates are similar. The liver plays a critical role in energy metabolism. Following a meal, the liver creates cytoplasmic reserves of glycogen and processes carbohydrates into fat. During fasting, the liver metabolizes stored and circulating lipids, generates glucose from glycogen stores, and converts amino acids into simple sugars. The liver stores enough glycogen to maintain blood glucose levels for approximately 1 day of fasting. During a long fast, the body mobilizes fat reserves and the liver oxidizes fatty acids as its primary source of energy. Carbohydrate substrates required during fasting are made by deamination of amino acids within hepatocytes. Excessive storage of fat in the liver may occur in a variety of conditions, including obesity, prolonged fasting or malnutrition, endocrine disorders such as diabetes mellitus or with corticosteroid therapy, and some forms of hepatotoxicity. Hepatic lipidosis results in liver enlargement, but by itself is not believed to cause significant hepatic dysfunction (Ockner, 1988a).

The liver produces large quantities of plasma proteins, including albumin, clotting factors, complement, and specialized carrier proteins. Generally, liver disease must be advanced and severe for primary liver failure to result in functionally significant reductions in protein synthesis. Failure to maintain sufficient protein levels in the blood can produce edema, and failure to produce coagulation proteins may result in coagulopathy and hemorrhage (see Section V,A,3). In addition to protein synthesis, the liver is important in the metabolism of amino acids. The liver converts ammonia, which is produced naturally during the deamination of amino acids to carbohydrates, to urea by the Kreb–Henseleit urea cycle. Chronic liver disease can result in increased plasma levels of ammonia, aromatic amino acids, and other nitrogenous compounds and in decreased levels of branched chain amino acids, contributing to the neurologic syndrome of hepatic encephalopathy (Maddison, 1992).

The production and metabolism of lipids are important functions of the liver. Free fatty acids are converted to triglycerides, and most cholesterol produced endogenously is produced in the liver. The enzyme lecithin–cholesterol acyltransferase (LCAT) is produced in heaptocytes and is responsible for the esterification of cholesterol. The liver synthesizes bile salts, conjugates them, and excretes them in the bile. Bile salts emulsify digested fats and facilitate absorption of lipids by the intestine. The liver also synthesizes carrier proteins, including lipoproteins, permitting the release of complex lipids into the bloodstream.

Hepatic metabolism of xenobiotics and endogenous substrates such as hormones usually involves one of two key pathways. The cytochrome P450 system within the smooth endoplasmic reticulum of the hepatocytes oxidizes a wide variety of xenobiotics in the presence of NADPH. These reactions detoxify certain chemicals and increase the reactivity and toxicity of other molecules. There are multiple classes of P450 enzymes, and the distribution of these enzymes within the liver is not uniform. Very reactive, toxic metabolites tend to cause damage to the cells in which the toxic metabolites are formed, resulting in predilections of specific toxins for certain portions of the hepatic lobule. The second metabolic system involves covalent bonding (conjugation) of substrates to glucuronic acid or sulfate. Both reactions increase the water solubility of the metabolites and facilitate direct biliary excretion or reabsorption into the blood and subsequent renal excretion.

2. Clinical Signs

Clinical signs of liver disease often are nonspecific and may initially seem unrelated to the liver (Ockner, 1988a). Because the liver has a great functional reserve and regenerative capacity, striking lesions may be present in animals that appear clinically normal. The broad spectrum of hepatic functions may also complicate the diagnosis of primary liver disease, and the liver may be involved secondarily in a wide range of diseases involving other organs. Most clinical signs that suggest liver disease can also be caused by diseases in other systems, so a careful evalaution of history, clinical examination, selected laboratory test results, and special procedures is required to reach an accurate diagnosis. One of the most obvious signs suggesting liver disease is icterus; however, icterus may also be caused by hemolysis or extrahepatic biliary obstruction. Patients with hepatic disease may present with hemorrhage, neurologic signs, diarrhea, steatorrhea, ascites, prostration, weight loss, or unexpected reactions to drugs or chemicals that are metabolized in the liver. When liver disease is suspected, laboratory tests including hematology and serum biochemical profiles containing markers for hepatic disease generally provide the clinician with sufficient information to diagnose, or at least suspect, liver disease (Herlong, 1988).

3. Clinical Pathologic Diagnosis

Much of what is known about the clinical pathologic features of human liver disease can be applied directly to the understanding of liver disease in nonhuman primates. The literature regarding human disease is extensive and should be used when necessary to supplement the veterinary literature. Liver function tests should be included in any standard, complete clinical chemistry profile. The most commonly used tests of liver dysfunction include serum concentrations of hepatic intracellular enzymes and actively secreted enzymes, bilirubin, cholesterol, and albumin. Hypoglycemia, low BUN concentrations, elevated serum bile acid concentrations, abnormal coagulation parameters, and other clinicopathologic findings also may occur in some cases of liver disease. It is particularly important to examine more than one test for liver dysfunction because many of the tests are not specific for liver disease when performed alone, and not all parameters will be abnormal in all cases of liver disease (Herlong, 1988). Reviews of clinical chemistry considerations and normal values in nonhuman primates are available (Cornelius, 1991; Loeb, 1989). It is helpful, when possible, to compare test values from animals that may have disease to values obtained from healthy animals of the same species using the same laboratory and testing procedures.

Alanine transaminase (ALT, previously known as serum glutamic pyruvic transaminase, SGPT) and aspartate transaminase (AST, previously known as serum pyruvic oxaloacetic transaminase, SGOT) are cytoplasmic enzymes abundant within hepatocytes. Aspartate transaminase also exists within mitochondria. These enzymes are elevated in serum when cellular damage causes these enzymes to leak from the cytoplasm (Benjamin, 1978; Herlong, 1988; Ockner, 1988b). Liver injury sufficient to produce large elevations in these enzymes may not be fatal to hepatocytes, and rapid recovery is possible. Alanine transaminase is considered relatively specific for hepatic disease. However, ALT is not always elevated when the liver is damaged, and large quantities of ALT are produced in the hearts of some nonhuman primates (reviewed by Hoffman et al., 1989). Aspartate transaminase resides in liver, myocardium, and skeletal muscle and may be elevated when muscle is injured. Elevations of both ALT and AST usually are diagnostic of hepatic or biliary disease; however, myocardial disease may occasionally produce similar enzyme elevations. The degree of transaminase elevations generally can be used to estimate the severity and/or extent of liver damage (Benjamin, 1978; Herlong, 1988). Alanine transaminase and AST often are elevated in cases of biliary obstruction, but elevations tend to be highest in cases of viral hepatitis and toxic liver damage (Herlong, 1988). Because these enzymes have a relatively short half-life in the blood (hours to a few days), ALT and AST levels in serum or plasma can be used to monitor the course of liver disease once a diagnosis has been made. Normal values for ALT and AST have been published for several species of clinically healthy nonhuman primates (Cornelius, 1991; Loeb, 1989; Malaga et al., 1991).

Serum alkaline phosphatase (SAP), γ-glutamyl transpeptidase (GGT), and serum bilirubin levels are frequently used to diagnose hepatobiliary disease. Alkaline phosphatase is found in liver, bone, kidney, placenta, intestine, and leukocytes, but most serum alkaline phosphatase originates in liver and bone (Herlong, 1988). Serum alkaline phosphatase is secreted in greater quantities during hepatobiliary diseases, but does not passively leak through damaged membranes as do ALT and

AST. Very large elevations in serum alkaline phosphatase are seen with the obstruction of extrahepatic or intrahepatic bile ducts or with hepatic masses (Herlong, 1988). High SAP with normal bilirubin levels may be found in humans with granulomatous lesions of the liver, such as tuberculosis, and in cases of amyloidosis. Findings in some nonhuman primates may be similar. Because elevated SAP levels may be found in growing animals and in animals with bone diseases, other tests must be used to confirm the presence of biliary or hepatic disease. Interpretation of elevated alkaline phosphatase should be made in conjunction with serum bilirubin levels and with other tests indicative of cholestasis, such as GGT, 5'-nucleotidase, or leucine aminopeptidase. Of these, GGT is most commonly used in veterinary medicine. γ-Glutamyl transpeptidase is helpful in identifying the source of elevated alkaline phosphatase, but GGT is present in many organs and its elevation indicates liver disease only when combined with other tests.

Bilirubin is the primary degradation product of heme. Most bilirubin in the normal animal is produced during the destruction of aging erythrocytes, and the most common cause of increased bilirubin production is the increased destruction of erythrocytes (hemolysis) (Scharschmidt, 1988). Hepatocytes conjugate bilirubin to glucoronic acid, which greatly increases the water solubility of bilirubin and facilitates its excretion. The ability of the liver to conjugate bilirubin normally exceeds the capacity of the liver to excrete conjugated bilirubin into the bile. Van den Bergh's test distinguishes the conjugated (direct) form of bilirubin from the unconjugated (indirect) form (Benjamin, 1978). Elevated conjugated bilirubin usually indicates biliary obstruction or an impairment of biliary secretion with loss of bilirubin from hepatocytes into the bloodstream. Elevated unconjugated bilirubin suggests a hemolytic crisis that temporarily exceeds the conjugation capacity of the liver and usually is not related to primary hepatic disease (Kruckenberg and Kidd, 1989). Inter- and intraspecies variations occur. For example, Bolivian squirrel monkeys (*Saimiri sciureus boliviensis*) have total bilirubin levels of less than 0.5 mg/dl when animals are sampled without fasting, but fasting mean bilirubin levels rise to 2.0 mg/dl because bilirubin production is high in this species and the activity of UDP-glucuronosyltransferase is low (Cornelius and Freedland, 1992). In normal Brazilian squirrel monkeys (*S. sciureus sciureus*), fasting total bilirubin levels are less than 0.5 mg/dl.

Determination of the serum bile acid concentrations is a very sensitive test for hepatic disease that is being used increasingly in veterinary medicine. Bile acids are produced in hepatocytes, secreted in the bile, absorbed from the ileum into the blood, and taken up again in the hepatocytes (Herlong, 1988). Bile acids may be elevated when hepatocellular damage results in a decreased secretion of bile acids into bile or when intestinal venous drainage bypasses the liver, such as in protocaval shunts.

When liver disease is suspected or confirmed biochemically, but the cause is unknown, it often is helpful to perform a liver biopsy. Wedge biopsies allow greater histologic evaluation of

hepatic architecture and permit better surgical evaluation of the liver and other abdominal viscera than do needle biopsies. However, needle biopsies may provide a less invasive method of diagnosis in some cases. The development of laparoscopic techniques and their increased use in veterinary medicine offer the clinician the opportunity to thoroughly examine the abdomen and select appropriate biopsy specimens without creating a large surgical incision. Laparoscopic techniques may be particularly useful for critically ill patients when the cause of illness has not been determined using less invasive techniques and for research in which major surgery is unacceptable or multiple samples must be taken at different times.

B. Parasitic Diseases

Readers are referred to the chapter on parasitic diseases for more information on liver parasites of nonhuman primates.

C. Viral Diseases

Only viral diseases that have the liver as a primary target organ are included in this chapter. More complete information on viral diseases of nonhuman primates can be found elsewhere in this volume.

1. Yellow Fever Virus

Nonhuman primates are the primary host for the arbovirus that causes yellow fever (Stokes *et al.,* 1928; Monath, 1982). The etiologic agent is an RNA virus, genus *Flavivirus* in the family Togaviridae (Rice *et al.,* 1985). Two cycles of transmission are recognized. In the sylvatic cycle, the virus is transmitted between primates by mosquitoes (primarily of the genus *Aedes*). In the urban cycle, the virus is transmitted between humans by *Aedes*.

Yellow fever is one of the hemorrhagic fevers. The severity of the disease in primates varies, with neotropical primates more seriously affected than African species. Yellow fever is not seen in Asia, but Asian primate species are highly susceptible to experimental infection and are considered to be a good model for the human disease (Hugh-Jones *et al.,* 1995b). Among neotropical primates, those of genus *Allouatta* and *Ateles* are more seriously affected than other genera. The initial clinical signs in susceptible primates are similar to those seen in humans: fever, nausea, and vomiting. As the disease progresses, animals develop kidney and liver disease (the name "yellow fever" derives from the jaundice associated with liver disease) and bleeding from body orifices. Mortality is high in animals that develop hemorrhage and kidney and liver disease. Differential diagnosis includes other hemorrhagic fever viruses and depends on the exposure of the animal to the mosquito vector. Diagnosis can be confirmed through virus isolation (note that handling of this agent requires biosafety level 3 conditions). Serologic testing is available, but some cross-reactivity exists between this and other flaviviruses. Gross lesions in animals with yellow fever include hemorrhage and fatty degeneration of the liver. Microscopically, Councilman bodies (acidophilic round bodies in hepatic cells), intranuclear inclusions, and midzonal hepatic necrosis are characteristics of the disease (Felsenfeld, 1972).

Treatment for yellow fever is supportive. A vaccine is available for human use that is effective experimentally in primates (Hahn *et al.*, 1987).

2. Callitrichid Hepatitis

Callitrichid hepatitis (CH) is caused by the same virus that causes lymphocytic choriomeningitis in rodents, an RNA virus in the Arenaviridae family (Stephenson *et al.*, 1995). All reported outbreaks have been in neotropical primates from the family Callitrichidae.

Animals with CH may be found dead or die shortly after illness is discovered. In experimentally infected marmosets, illness began 7 days postinoculation and animals were either severely ill or dead by day 9 (Montali *et al.*, 1989). Clinical signs can include rapidly progressive weakness and anorexia. Treatment of CH is often unrewarding and mortality is high. Laboratory findings in animals with CH include elevated serum aspartate aminotransferase (AST, formerly known as SGOT), elevated total bilirubin, and serum alkaline phosphatase and lymphocytosis. Differential diagnosis for animals with CH includes yellow fever. *Herpes tamarinus* infection (see the chapter on viral diseases) resembles CH, but gross lesions differ and animals have characteristic intranuclear inclusions in the liver and other tissues.

At necropsy, animals with CH have discoloration of the liver, which may range from mottled to uniformly tan. The liver may also be enlarged. Microscopically, the liver has multifocal areas of necrosis, fatty degeneration, and periportal infiltrates of lymphocytes and macraophages (Fig. 7). Less consistently, necrosis in lymphoid tissues and the adrenal glands has been reported (Lucke and Bennett, 1982; Ramsay *et al.*, 1989). Electron microscopy studies have demonstrated 85- to 105-nm-diameter, enveloped, virus particles within hepatocyte vesicles (Montali *et al.*, 1989; Montali, 1993).

All published reports of callitrichid hepatitis outbreaks have been from zoos and animals parks, indicating that husbandry practices or housing used exclusively in these institutions may play a role in infection. It has been suggested that feral rodents in or near exhibits, rodents on exhibit, and/or the practice of feeding mouse neonates as a food supplement for callitrichids may play a role in infection. Lymphocytic choriomeningitis virus (LCMV) is a known zoonotic agent, and two people who cared for LCMV-infected callitrichids seroconverted to LCMV following outbreaks of CH (Stephenson *et al.*, 1991; Montali, 1993). Biosafety level 2 precautions should be taken when handling infected animals, animal tissues, and body fluids. Biosafety level 3 precautions are required for procedures involving

concentrated virus (Centers for Disease Control and Prevention *et al.*, 1993).

3. Ebola Reston (Ebola-like) Virus

Readers are referred to the chapter on viral diseases elsewhere in this volume for complete information on Ebola virus infection.

4. Other Hepatitis Viruses

The agent for hepatitis A (infectious heaptitis) is an enterovirus for which humans and nonhuman primates are reservoirs. Several species of primates have been experimentally infected, including owl monkeys, African green monkeys, cynomolgus macaques, rhesus macaques, and chimpanzees (Eichberg and Kalter, 1980). Infection in humans and chimpanzees is frequently inapparent. Transmission is fecal–oral and the disease in primates has low morbidity and mortality. Numerous cases of hepatitis A transmission from primates to humans have been reported. Many cases involved transmission during the importation process. Cases of disease transmission from experimentally infected animals also occurred.

The agent for hepatitis B (serum hepatitis) is a hepadnavirus that rarely causes clinical disease in monkeys. Apes are susceptible but are often asymptomatic. Spontaneous infection and disease have been reported in other primate species (Kornegay *et al.*, 1985). Approximately 10% of infected humans and chimpanzees become chronic carriers (Kornegay *et al.*, 1985). Many hepatitis B carriers develop hepatocellular carcinoma or cirrhosis. Transmission is usually by the exposure of mucous membranes or broken skin to infected body fluids (Zuckerman *et al.*, 1975).

The agent for hepatitis C has now been classified as a member of a new genus within the Flaviviridae family. The hepatitis C virus is primarily transmitted via infected blood. There is growing evidence for sexual transmission. Although chimpanzees have been experimentally infected with the hepatitis C virus, spontaneous infections of nonhuman primates have not been reported (Hugh-Jones *et al.*, 1995a).

The hepatitis E virus is the major etiology of non-A, non-B epidemic, or enteric hepatitis (Lee, personal communication, 1997). The hepatitis E virus is currently unclassified (Koonin *et al.*, 1992). Owl monkeys, cynomolgus monkeys, and tamarins have been experimentally infected with the virus (Krawczynski and Bradley, 1989; Ticehurst *et al.*, 1992; Tabar and Gerety, 1983; Tabar, 1989; Uchida *et al.*, 1990). Transmission is fecal–oral. In humans, the clinical features are similar to hepatitis A, although hepatitis E more often results in fulminant hepatitis and has up to 20% mortality in pregnant women.

Evidence suggests that the hepatitis G virus is distantly related to the hepatitis C virus (20–26% homology) and thus is provisionally included in the flavivirus family. Hepatitis G virus infections usually results in no overt clinical symptoms and controversy exists concerning designation as a hepatitis virus. Two closely related viruses termed GBV-A and GBV-B have been isolated from tamarins (Lee, personal communication, 1997).

Experimental infection of nonhuman primates with any of these agents has only caused illness in tamarins (Leary *et al.,* 1996).

For more information on hepatitis virus infections, readers are referred to the chapter on viral diseases elsewhere in this volume.

D. Metabolic Disorders

1. Fatal Fatty Liver Syndrome

Fatal fatty liver syndrome (FFLS also known as fatal fasting syndrome or fat macaque syndrome) is an acute metabolic syndrome of high mortality. At present, the pathogenesis of this condition is poorly understood, but predisposing factors include

1. Obesity.
2. Species. Macaques, especially cynomolgus and rhesus, are predisposed. The syndrome has been reported less commonly in other species.
3. Sex. Females are predisposed, although the syndrome has been reported in males.
4. Stress or other causes of sudden fasting.
5. Age. In one retrospective study where the ages of animals were known, the mean age was 9 years (Laber-Laird *et al.,* 1987).

This syndrome is similar in many ways to diseases seen in cats, guinea pigs, sheep, cattle, and horses (Gliatto and Bronson, 1993).

Clinical signs include anorexia, depression, and substantial weight loss. Animals with the syndrome may lose up to 30% of their normal weight. Laboratory results may include elevated BUN and creatinine and anemia. The presence of ketones, glucose, and protein in the urine of affected animals has also occasionally been reported. Other causes of fatty change in the liver that need to be considered in the differential diagnosis of FFLS should include diabetes mellitus, hypothyroidism, and a variety of toxic agents (Laber-Laird *et al.,* 1987). The history and presence or absence of predisposing factors in the animal described earlier should be used in making a final diagnosis.

The lesion found most consistently at necropsy of FFLS animals is an enlarged, yellow or tan liver. The fatty change in the liver may be so severe that thinly cut slices float in formalin. Fatal fatty liver syndrome animals also have abundant adipose tissue and may lack intestinal contents. Fat necrosis (manifested by discoloration or granular appearance) may also be apparent. Microscopically, there is a severe, diffuse, fatty change in the liver. Fat vacuoles in the cytoplasm of hepatocytes may be demonstrated with Sudan IV or Oil Red O stain. Fat vacuoles may also be seen in the proximal tubular epithelium of the kidneys, along with evidence of tubular necrosis. Many animals have dilated pancreatic acini and focal areas of pancreatic necrosis (Bronson *et al.,* 1982b; Gliatto and Bronson, 1993).

There is no well-established treatment available for FFLS. In an unpublished report, the syndrome has been treated success-

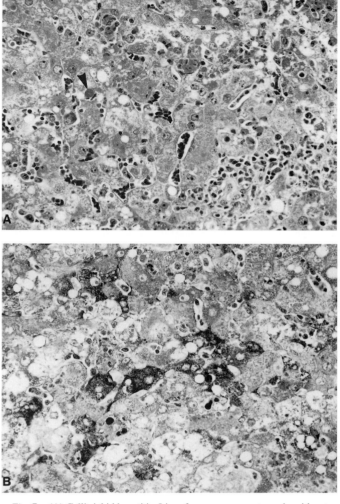

Fig. 7. (A) Callitrichid hepatitis. Liver from an emperor tamarin with naturally occurring callitrichid hepatitis (LCMV$_{CH}$ infection). Hepatic plates are disrupted and contain necrotic hepatocytes, degenerating hepatocytes, infiltrates of lymphocytes, and a few neutrophils. Note acidophilic body (arrow) typical of those seen in LCMV$_{CH}$-infected livers. Hematopylin and eosin (H&E) stain. Magnification: ×300. (B) Immunoperoxidase labeling shows LCMV$_{CH}$ viral antigen (dark granular material) mostly in misshapen, abnormal-appearing hepatocytes from the same tamarin liver in (A). Magnification: ×300. Reprinted by permission from Montali *et al.* (1995).

fully with nutritional support by enteral feeding (C. R. Valverde, personal communication, 1997) by implantation of a percutaneous endoscopic gastrostomy (PEG) tube (Armstrong and Hardie, 1989) and use of a liquid diet (Ensure, Ross) at less than 30 ml/kg given two to three times daily. The exact volume and frequency are based on the calculation of metabolic requirements (DeBiasse and Wilmore, 1994). This feeding regimen may need to be continued for as long as 4–8 weeks. Pre- and postprandial bile acid studies, weight monitoring, and liver biopsies can be used to monitor therapeutic progress. A regular diet should always be available to animals during treatment and a record kept of the number of biscuits eaten. Animals should be weaned off the liquid diet slowly by mixing the liquid diet with increasing amounts of solid food. A potential complication of the PEG tube procedure includes the leakage of gastric contents into the abdominal cavity. This can be prevented by a careful technique during introduction of the PEG tube. Wound care of the ostomy site is important in ensuring successful maintenance of the tube.

Weight control and careful management of situations that might result in stress or fasting may be useful in preventing FFLS in animals that are predisposed.

2. Amyloidosis

Amyloidosis is characterized by the extracellular accumulation of amyloid protein fibrils in many organs. Amyloid is commonly classified as primary (AL) and secondary (AA), which differ in both molecular structure and origin. Primary amyloid is associated with plasma cell dyscrasias, myeloma, and reticulum cell sarcomas. Secondary amyloid is associated with chronic inflammatory processes. The most commonly reported amyloid of nonhuman primates is the AA type (Blanchard, 1993).

Although amyloid is a secondary condition, deposition of amyloid in organ systems can interfere with vital organ system functions to cause illness or death above and beyond damage caused by the primary illness.

Clinical signs of amyloidosis include hepatomegaly, splenomegaly, chronic weight loss, and diarrhea. Animals with amyloidosis often have a history of chronic inflammatory disease: colitis, osteoarthritis, lung mite infestation, etc. (Chapman et al., 1977; Slattum et al., 1989a,b). Differential diagnosis for amyloidosis should include other causes of chronic weight loss and diarrhea, including malabsorption, mycobacterial infection (tuberculosis or pseudotuberculosis), and neoplasia. It should be noted that a mycobacterial infection can cause amyloidosis because of the chronic inflammation that is characteristic of these infections. Thus, animals may have a mycobacterial infection and amyloidosis simultaneously. Intestinal and/or liver biopsy is useful in the diagnosis of amyloidosis, as clinical pathology studies are usually unrevealing (Blanchard et al., 1986).

At necropsy, there may be no gross lesions in mild cases. In more advanced amyloidosis, animals have enlarged, firm livers with focal or diffuse areas of tan or yellow discoloration. Cut surfaces may have a waxy texture. The spleen may be enlarged and firm and the intestinal wall may be thickened, with fibrous strictures of the colon. The mucosal surface of the large intestine may be ulcerated. Microscopically, amyloid is identified as an amorphous hyaline substance that stains light pink to purple with hematoxylin and eosin. When stained with Congo red, amyloid exhibits characteristic green birefringence when illuminated by polarized light. When stained sections are treated with potassium permanganate, AA amyloid is no longer stained by Congo red, a characteristic that differentiates it from AL amyloid (Kisilevsky, 1983). In the liver, amyloid deposits are seen lining the hepatic cords and extending into the sinusoid. Moderate to severe amyloidosis may result in the atrophy of hepatocytes (Slattum et al., 1989a,b). Deposits in the spleen are primarily in and around the lymphoid follicles. In the intestine there are deposits in both the small and the large intestine, with the deposits more commonly found in the small intestine. Inflammatory changes and ulceration are more apparent in the large intestine (Slattum et al., 1989b; Blanchard et al., 1986). Amyloid deposits may also be seen in the heart, kidney, stomach, lungs, brain, and gallbladder (Blanchard, 1993). On electron microscopic examination, amyloid appears as parallel arrays of protein fibrils 70 to 100 Å in diameter.

Oral DMSO has been used successfully to treat intestinal amyloidosis in a rhesus monkey. The dose used to treat the animal was 80 mg/kg SID. Marked improvement in stools was noted after 10 days. Treatment was continued for 6 months and response was confirmed by intestinal biopsy (Jayo et al., 1990).

E. Nutritional Diseases

1. Cholelithiasis

Spontaneous cholelithiasis has been reported in several species of nonhuman primates, including owl monkeys, marmosets, baboons, orangutans, and rhesus macaques (McSherry et al., 1971; Anver et al., 1972; Chalifoux et al., 1993a). Most choleliths in nonhuman primates are composed of cholesterol, but other composition has been reported (Kessler, 1982; Pissinatti et al., 1987). Cholesterol gallstones result from the precipitation of excess cholesterol in bile. Cholelithiasis can be induced in some primate species by feeding an atherogenic diet. Virtually 100% of some Saimiri species fed an atherogenic diet develop gallstones. Cercopithecus aethiops are moderately susceptible, and macaques and Bolivian squirrel monkeys are relatively resistant (Kessler, 1982; Portman et al., 1980; Osuga and Portman, 1971). As in humans, females appear to be predisposed to cholelithiasis. Animals are often asymptomatic, with choleliths simply found at necropsy. Some animals may have weight loss, vomiting, and abdominal pain. Diagnosis is best done by ultrasonographic or radiographic examination. Spontaneous cholelithiasis in owl monkeys has been proposed as a model for the human disease (Baer et al., 1990).

VI. EXOCRINE PANCREAS

Pancreatic exocrine insufficiency and primary pancreatic diseases are uncommon in nonhuman primates. As in other species, pancreatic exocrine insufficiency in nonhuman primates would be expected to result in a maldigestion/malabsorption syndrome as it does in other species. Elevated serum amylase levels in nonhuman primates suggest pancreatitis, but are not specific and can occur in other disease syndromes; therefore, other tests should be used to confirm a diagnosis of pancreatitis (Gatesman, 1992).

A. Pancreatic Disease

1. Adenoviral Pancreatitis

Adenoviral pancreatitis has been reported in rhesus monkeys infected with simian immunodeficiency virus (SIV/Delta) and in a juvenile rhesus monkey that developed diarrhea and died (Baskin *et al.*, 1988; Chandler *et al.*, 1974). Necrosis of pancreatic acini, infiltrates of mononuclear cells, and interstitial fibrosis were accompanied by basophilic, smudgy inclusions that usually filled the nuclei of pancreatic acinar cells. Intranuclear inclusion bodies also were seen in pancreatic ductular cells, submucosal duodenal glands, intestinal and gastric epithelial cells, and renal tubules, but necrotic and inflammatory lesions were seen only in pancreatic acini.

B. Parasitic Disease

The spirurid nematode *Trichospirura leptostoma* has been proposed as a cause of wasting disease in marmosets (Beglinger *et al.*, 1988). *Trichospirura leptostoma* inhabits the pancreatic ducts of marmosets, squirrel monkeys, owl monkeys, and perhaps other New World primates.

Clinical signs in marmosets include weight loss, debilitation, anemia, and osteomalacia (a sequella to malabsorption). Differential diagnosis should include other causes of weight loss and debilitation, including other parasitic infections.

Fecal examination of animals with *T. leptostoma* infection may reveal that characteristic ova. Repeated fecal examinations are recommended because the presence of ova in the stool is sporadic. Other abnormal clinical pathology results in marmosets with *T. leptostoma* associated wasting include elevated ALT, AST, and SAP and kentonuria (Beglinger *et al.*, 1988; Wolff, 1993).

At necropsy, affected animals have adult *T. leptostoma* in the pancreatic ducts and may have enlarged adrenal glands and cardiomegaly with pericardial effusion. Lesions found on histologic examination include mild to severe chronic pancreatitis with periductal inflammation and fibrosis (Beglinger *et al.*, 1988; Potkay, 1992), with adult *T. leptostoma* visible in the ducts and ova visible in the ductules.

Broad-spectrum nematicides like ivermectin and the benzimidoles have been proposed for treatment of *T. leptostoma* infection. One study (Hawkins *et al.*, 1997) found that fenbendazole given daily at a dosage of 50 mg/kg body weight by gavage tube for 14 days was a more effective treatment than ivermectin.

The cockroach is an intermediate host for *T. leptostoma*. Control of cockroaches in primate housing areas may be useful in preventing the wasting disease (Beglinger *et al.*, 1988; Potkay, 1992).

C. Pancreatic Neoplasia

Neoplastic processes may involve the pancreas. Pancreatic adenocarcinomas have been reported in *Cercopithecus aethiops* and *Papio cynocephalus* (Lowenstine, 1986). Tumors that spread through the peritoneal cavity may secondarily affect the pancreas or the pancreatic ducts.

D. Other Pancreatic Diseases

Pancreatic lesions may be seen secondary to other disease states. In the fatal fasting syndrome of obese macaques, rapid weight loss, hepatic lipidosis, and fat necrosis may be accompanied by a pale or red, firm pancreas (Gliatto and Bronson, 1993). Histologically, there may be small foci of pancreatic necrosis, dilatation of pancreatic acini with acinar cell atrophy and zymogen depletion, and interstitial fat necrosis. Similar histologic lesions have been seen in uremic *Macaca mulatta* and *M. fascicularis* (Bronson *et al.*, 1982b).

ACKNOWLEDGMENTS

The assistance of Dr. Susan Gibson, University of South Alabama, Dr. Sherry Klumpp, Yerkes Primate Center, Dr. D. Rick Lee, University of Texas/M.D. Anderson Cancer Center, Dr. Melissa Stoller, University of Chicago, and Dr. James Curtis, Medical College of Georgia is gratefully acknowledged. We thank Sheila Morse, Marilyn Holladay, and Jeanie Fincher for assistance in the preparation of the manuscript.

REFERENCES

Abee, C. R. (1985). Medical care and management of the squirrel monkey. *In* "Handbook of Squirrel Monkey Research" (L. A. Rosenblum and C. L. Coe, eds.), pp. 447–488. Plenum, New York.

Adams, R. J., and Bishop, J. L. (1980). An oral disease resembling noma in six rhesus monkeys (*Macaca mulatta*). *Lab. Anim. Sci.* **30**, 85–91.

Adler, R. R., Moore, P. F., Schmucker, D. L., and Lowenstine, L. J. (1993). Chronic colitis, juvenile *Macaca mulatta*. *In* "Monographs on the Pathology of Laboratory Animals: Nonhuman Primates" (T. C. Jones, U. Mohr, and R. D. Hunt, eds.), Vol. 2, pp. 81–87. Springer-Verlag, Berlin and New York.

Agarwal, K. C., and Chakravarti, R. N. (1969). Preliminary observations on the intestinal bacterial flora of wild rhesus monkeys with special reference to shigellosis, salmonellosis and vibriosis. *J. Assoc. Physicians India* **17**, 409–412.

Albrecht, P., Lorenz, D., Klutch, M. J., Vickers, J. H., and Ennis, F. A. (1980). Fatal measles infection in marmosets, pathogenesis and prophylaxis. *Infect. Immun.* **27**, 969–978.

Allen, A. M., Palmer, A. E., Tauraso, N. M., and Shelokov, A. 1968). Simian hemorrhagic fever. II. Studies in pathology. *Am. J. Trop. Med. Hyg.* **17**, 413–421.

Altman, N. H., New, A. E., McConnell, E. E., and Ferrell, T. L. (1979). A spontaneous outbreak of polychlorinated biphenyl (PCB) toxicity in rhesus monkeys (*Macaca mulatta*): Clinical observations. *Lab. Anim. Sci.* **29**, 661–665.

Ammon, H. V. (1995). Diarrhea. *In* "Bockus Gastroenterology" (W. S. Haurbrich, F. Schaffner, and J. E. Berk, eds.), Vol. 1, pp. 87–101. Saunders, Philadelphia.

Anderson, D. C., and McClure, H. M. (1993). Paratuberculosis, nonhuman primates. *In* "Monographs on the Pathology of Laboratory Animals: Nonhuman Primates" (T. C. Jones, U. Mohr, and R. D. Hunt, eds.), Vol. 1, pp. 148–154. Springer-Verlag, Berlin and New York.

Anver, M. R., Hunt, R. D., and Chalifoux, L. V. (1972). Cholesterol gallstones in *Aotus trivirgatus*. *J. Med. Primatol.* **1**, 241–246.

Armitage, G. C., Newburn, E., Hoover, C. I., and Anderson, J. H. (1982). Periodontal disease associated with *Shigella flexneri* in rhesus monkeys. *J. Periodont. Res.* **17**, 131–144.

Armitage, G. C., Banks, T. A., Newburn, E., Greenspan, J. S., Hoover, C. I., and Anderson, J. H. (1983). Immunologic observations in macaques with *Shigella*-associated periodontal disease. *J. Periodont. Res.* **18**, 139–148.

Armstrong, P. J., and Hardie, E. M. (1989). Percutaneous endoscopic gastrostomy. *Vet. Med. Rep.* **1**, 404–411.

Arya, S. C., Agarwal, D. S., Verghese, A., and Pal, S. C. (1973). Shigellosis in rhesus monkeys in quarantine. *Lab. Anim.* **7**, 101–109.

Awang, A., and Yap, K. L. (1990). Group A rotavirus infection in animals from an animal house and in wild-caught monkeys. *J. Diarrheal. Dis. Res.* **8**, 82–86.

Baer, J. F., Weller, R. E., Dagle, G. E., Malaga, C. A., and Lee, S. P. (1990). Cholelithiasis in owl monkeys: Seven cases. *Lab. Anim. Sci.* **40**, 629–633.

Baggs, R. B., Hunt, R. D., Garcia, F. G., Hajema, E. M., Blake, B. J., and Fraser, E. O. (1976). Pseudotuberculosis (*Yersinia enterocolitica*) in the owl monkey (*Aotus trivirgatus*). *Lab. Anim. Sci.* **26**, 1079–1083.

Baker, C. A., Hendrick, A. G., and Cooper, R. W. (1977). Spontaneous malformations in squirrel monkey (*Saimiri sciureus*) fetuses with emphasis on cleft lip and palate. *J. Med. Primatol.* **6**, 13–22.

Banish, L. D., Sims, R., Sack, D., Montali, R. J., Phillips, L., and Bush, M. (1993a). Prevalence of shigellosis and other enteric pathogens in a zoologic collection of primates. *J. Am. Vet. Med. Assoc.* **203**, 126–132.

Banish, L. D., Sims, R., Bush, M., Sack, D., and Montali, R. (1993b). Clearance of Shigella flexneri carriers in a zoologic collection of primates. *JAVMA, J. Am. Vet. Med. Assoc.* **203**, 133–136.

Banks, R. E., Davis, J. A., Bach, D. E., and Beattie, R. J. (1968). Surgical excision of an ameloblastic odontoma in a cynomolgus monkey (*Macaca fascicularis*). *Lab. Anim. Sci.* **38**, 316–319.

Banwell, J. G. (1990). Pathophysiology of diarrheal disorders. *Rev. Infect. Dis.* **112**, Suppl. 1, S30–S35.

Baskerville, A., and Newell, D. G. (1988). Naturally occurring chronic gastritis and *C. pylori* infection in the rhesus monkey: A potential model for gastritis in man. *Gut* **29**, 465–472.

Baskin, G. B. (1987). Disseminated cytomegalovirus infection in immunodeficient rhesus monkeys. *Am. J. Pathol.* **129**, 345–352.

Baskin, G. B. (1993). Cytomegalovirus in nonhuman primates. *In* "Monographs on the Pathology of Laboratory Animals: Nonhuman Primates" (T. C. Jones, U. Mohr, and R. D. Hunt, eds.), Vol. I, pp. 32–37. Springer-Verlag, Berlin and New York.

Baskin, G. B., Murphey-Corb, M., Watson, E. A., and Martin, L. N. (1988). Necropsy findings in rhesus monkeys experimentally infected with cultured simian immunodeficiency virus (SIV)/Delta. *Vet. Pathol.* **25**, 456–467.

Bayliss, T. M., Schuster, M. M., and Hendrix, T. R. (1988). Diarrhea and constipation. *In* "The Principles and Practice of Medicine" (A. N. Harvey, R. J. Johns, V. A. McKusick, A. J. Owens, Jr., and R. S. Ross, eds.), pp. 812–822. Appleton & Lange, Norwalk, CT.

Beglinger, R., Illgen, B., and Heider, P. K. (1988). The parasite trichospirura leptostoma associated with wasting disease in a colony of common marmosets. *Callithrix jacchus. Folia Primatol.* **51**, 45–51.

Beighton, D., and Hayday, H. (1982). The effect of communal caging on the streptococcal flora of the dental plaque of monkeys (*Macaca fascicularis*). *Lab. Anim.* **16**, 68–70.

Bellinger, D. A., and Bullock, B. C. (1988). Cutaneous *Mycobacterium avium* infection in a cynomolgus monkey. *Lab. Anim. Sci.* **38**, 85–86.

Benjamin, M. M. (1978). Liver function tests. *In* "Outline of Veterinary Clinical Pathology," pp. 233–264. Iowa State University Press, Ames.

Bennett, T. B., Cuasay, L., Welsh, T. J., Beluhan, F. Z., and Schofield, L. (1980). Acute gastric dilatation in monkeys: A microbiologic study of gastric contents, blood and feed. *Lab. Anim. Sci.* **30**, 241–244.

Berkson, G. (1968). Weight and tooth development during the first year in *Macaca irus. Lab. Anim. Care* **18**, 352–355.

Berman, S. (1991). Ear, nose and throat. *In* "Handbook of Pediatrics" (G. Merenstein, D. Kaplan, and A. Rosenberg, eds.), 16th ed., p. 647. Appleton & Lange, Norwalk, CT.

Betton, G. R. (1983). Spontaneous neoplasms of the marmoset (*Callithrix jacchus*). Oral and nasopharyngeal squamous cell carcinomas. *Vet. Pathol.* **21**, 193–197.

Blanchard, J. L. (1993). Generalized amyloidosis. *In* "Monographs on the Pathology of Laboratory Animals: Nonhuman Primates" (T. C. Jones, U. Mohr, and R. D. Hunt, eds.), Vol. I, pp. 194–197. Springer-Verlag, Berlin and New York.

Blanchard, J. L., Baskin, G. B., and Watson, E. A. (1986). Generalized amyloidosis in rhesus monkeys. *Vet. Pathol.* **23**, 425–430.

Bokkenheuser, V. (1962). *Salmonella* and *Shigella* in gall-bladders from man and monkey. *S. Afr. J. Med. Sci.* **27**, 60–64.

Bowen, W. H., and Koch, G. (1970). Determination of age in monkeys (*Macaca irus*) on the basis of dental development. *Lab. Anim.* **4**, 113–123.

Brack, M. (1982). Noma in *Saguinus oedipus:* A report of 2 cases. *Lab. Anim.* **16**, 361–363.

Bronsdon, M. A. (1984). Rapid dimethyl sulfoxide-modified acid fast stain of *Cryptospordium* oocysts in stool specimens. *J. Clin. Microbiol.* **19**, 952–953.

Bronsdon, M. A., and Schoenknecht, F. D. (1988). *Campylobacter pylori* isolated from the stomach of the monkey, *Macaca nemestrina*. *J. Clin. Microbiol.* **26**, 1725–1728.

Bronsdon, M. A., Goodwin, C. S., Sly, L. I., Chilvers, T., and Schoenknecht, F. D. (1991). *Helicobacter nemestrinae* sp. nov., a spiral bacterium found in the stomach of a pigtailed macaque (*Macaca nemestrina*). *Int. J. Syst. Bacteriol.* **41**, 148–153.

Bronson, R. T., May, B. D., and Ruebner, B. H. (1972). An outbreak of infection by *Yersinia pseudotuberculosis* in nonhuman primates. *Am. J. Pathol.* **69**, 289–303.

Bronson, R. T., O'Connell, M., Klepper-Kilgore, N., Chalifoux, L. V., and Sehgal, P. (1982a). Fatal fasting syndrome of obese macaques. *Lab. Anim. Sci.* **32**, 187–192.

Bronson, R. T., Strauss, W., and Wheeler, W. (1982b). Pancreatic ectasia in uremic macaques. *Am. J. Pathol.* **106**, 342–347.

Bryant, J. L., Stills, H. F., Lentsch, R. H., and Middleton, C. C. (1983). *Campylobacter jejuni* isolated from patas monkeys with diarrhea. *Lab. Anim. Sci.* **33**, 303–305.

Buchanan, W., Sehgal, P., Bronson, R. T., Rodger, R. F., and Horton, J. E. (1981). Noma in nonhuman primate. *Oral Surg.* **52**, 19–22.

Burrows, C. F. (1988). The treatment of diarrhea. *Curr. Vet. Ther.* **8**, 784–790.

Bywater, R. J., and Newsome, P. M. (1982). Diarrhea. *J. Am. Vet. Med. Assoc.* **181**, 718–720.

Carniel, E., and Mollaret, H. H. (1990). Yersiniosis. *Comp. Immunol. Microbiol. Infect. Dis.* **13**, 51–58.

Carter, K. K. D.V.M., and Houghton, P. (1987). Blunting canine teeth in Macaques: A possible alternative to extraction or endodontics. *Lab. Anim.* **16**, 27–33.

Centers for Disease Control (CDC) (1993). Tuberculosis in imported nonhuman primates—United States, June 1990–May 1993. *Morbid. Mortal. Wkly. Rep.* **42**, 972–576.

Centers for Disease Control and Prevention, U.S. Department of Health and Human Services, and National Institutes of Health (1993). Agent: Lymphocytic choriomeningitis virus. *In* "Biosafety in Microbiological and Biomedical Laboratories," pp. 112–113. CDC/USDHHS/NIH, Washington, DC.

Chalifoux, L. V., and Anver, M. R. (1993). Cholesterol gallstones, owl monkeys. *In* "Monographs on the Pathology of Laboratory Animals: Nonhuman Primates" (T. C. Jones, U. Mohr, and R. D. Hunt, eds.), Vol. 2, pp. 63–64. Springer-Verlag, Berlin and New York.

Chalifoux, L. V., Bronson, R. T., Escajadillo, A., and McKenna, S. (1982). An analysis of the association of gastrointestinal lesions with chronic wasting syndrome of marmosets. *Vet. Pathol.* **19**, Suppl. 7, 141–162.

Chalifoux, L. V., Brieland, J. K., and King, N. W., Jr. (1985). Evolution and natural history of colonic disease in cotton-topped tamarins (*Saguinus oedipus*). *Dig. Dis. Sci.* **30**, Suppl., 54S–58S.

Chalifoux, L. V., King, N. W., Jr., and Johnson, L. D. (1993a). Acute and chronic colitis, cotton-top tamarins. *In* "Monographs on the Pathology of Laboratory Animals: Nonhuman Primates" (T. C. Jones, U. Mohr, and R. D. Hunt, eds.), Vol. 2, pp. 75–80. Springer-Verlag, Berlin and New York.

Chalifoux, L. V., King, N. W., Jr., and Johnson, L. D. (1993b). Adenocarcinoma, colon, cotton top tamarin. *In* "Monographs on the Pathology of Laboratory Animals: Nonhuman Primates" (T. C. Jones, U. Mohr, and R. D. Hunt, eds.), Vol. 2, pp. 87–94. Springer-Verlag, Berlin and New York.

Chandler, F. W., Callaway, C. S., and Adams, S. R. (1974). Pancreatitis associated with an adenovirus in a rhesus monkey. *Vet. Pathol.* **11**, 165–171.

Chapman, W. L. (1967). Acute gastric dilatation in *Macaca mulatta* and *Macaca speciosa* monkeys. *Lab. Anim. Care* **17**, 130–136.

Chapman, W. L., and Crowell, W. A. (1977). Amyloidosis in rhesus monkeys with rheumatoid arthritis and enterocolitis. *J. Am. Vet. Med. Assoc.* **171**, 855–858.

Chase, J. E., and Cooper, R. W. (1969). *Saguinus nigricollis*—physical growth and dental eruption in a small population of captive-born individuals. *Am. J. Phys. Anthropol* **30**, 111–116.

Cheverud, J. M. (1981). Epiphyseal union and dental eruption in *Macaca mulatta*. *Am. J. Phys. Anthropol.* **56**, 157–167.

Clark, W. B., Magnusson, I., Abee, C. R., Collins, B., Beem, J. E., and McArthur, W. P. (1988). Natural occurrence of black-pigmented *Bacteroides* species in the gingival crevice of the squirrel monkey. *Infect. Immun.* **56**, 2392–2399.

Cohen, D. W., and Goldman, H. M. (1960). Oral disease in primates. *Ann. N. Y. Acad. Sci.* **85**, 889–909.

Cole, W. C., Bostrom, R. E., and Whitney, R. A., Jr. (1968). Diagnosis and handling of B virus in a rhesus monkey (*Macaca mulatta*). *J. Am. Vet. Med. Assoc.* **153**, 894–898.

Cooke, C. E. (1994). Oral ondansetron for preventing nausea and vomiting. *Am. J. Hosp. Pharm.* **51**, 762–771.

Cooper, J. E., Needham, J. R. (1976). An outbreak of shigellosis in laboratory marmosets and tamarins (Family: Callithricidae). *J. Hyg. Camb.* **76**, 415–425.

Cornelius, C. E. (1991). Liver function tests in the differential diagnosis of hepatotoxicity. *In* "Hepatotoxicology" (R. G. Meeks, S. D. Harrison, and R. J. Bull, eds.), pp. 181–213. CRC Press, Boca Raton, FL.

Cornelius, C. E., and Freedland, R. A. (1992). Fasting hyperbilirubinemia in normal fasting squirrel monkeys. *Lab. Anim. Sci.* **42**, 35–37.

Cornelius, L. M., Finco, D. R., and Culver, D. H. (1978). Physiologic effects of rapid infusion of lactated Ringer s solution into dogs. *Am. J. Vet. Res.* **39**, 1185–1190.

Corruccini, R. S., and Beecher, R. M. (1982). Occlusal variation related to soft diet in squirrel monkeys. *Science* **218**, 74–76.

Cran, J. A. (1969). An epithelial tumour occurring in the jaws of a black faced spider monkey. *Oral Surg., Oral Med. Oral Pathol.* **27**, 494–498.

Curtis, J. W., Jr., Brodish, D. L., Weaver, D. S., and Brady, A. G. (1986). Periapical abscesses of cut canine teeth in cynomolgus macaques. *Lab. Anim.* **20**, 277–280.

Davis, L. E. (1980). Pharmacologic control of vomiting. *J. Am. Vet. Med. Assoc.* **176**, 241–242.

Davis, J. A. (1988). Ameloblastic odontoma in a cynomolgus monkey (*Macaca fascicularis*). *Lab. Anim. Sci.* **38**, 312–315.

DeBiasse, M. A., and Wilmore, D. W. (1994). What is optimal nutritional support? *New Horizons* **2**, 122–130.

Deinhardt, F., Holmes, A. W., Devine, J., Deinhardt, J. (1967). *Lab. Anim. Care* **17**, 48–70.

De Paoli, A., and McClure, H. M. (1982). Gastrointestinal neoplasms in nonhuman primates. *Vet. Pathol.* **19**, Suppl. 7, 104–125.

DiBartola, S. P. (1992). Introduction to fluid therapy. *In* "Fluid Therapy in Small Animal Practice" (S. P. DiBartola, ed.), pp. 321–340. Saunders, Philadelphia.

Donowitz, M., Kokke, F. T., and Saidi, R. (1995). Evaluation of patients with chronic diarrhea. *N. Engl. J. Med.* **332**, 725–729.

Dow, S. W., Jones, R. L., and Rosychuk, R. A. (1989). Bacteriologic specimens: Selection, collection, and transport for optimum results. *Compend. Contin. Educ. Prac. Vet.* **11**, 686–702.

Drazner, F. H. (1983). Mechanisms of diarrheal disease. *Curr. Vet. Ther.* **8**, 773–783.

Dreizen, S., and Levy, B. M. (1969). Histopathology of experimentally induced nutritional deficiency cheilosis in the marmoset (*Callithrix jacchus*). *Arch. Oral Biol.* **14**, 577–582.

Dulisch, M. L. (1983). Gastrotomy. *In* "Current Techniques in Small Animal Surgery" (M. J. Bojrab, S. W. Crane, and S. P. Arnoczky, eds.), 2nd ed., p. 157. Lea & Febiger, Philadelphia.

Eichberg, J. W., and Kalter, S. S. (1980). Hepatitis A and B: Serologic survey of human and non-human primate sera. *Lab. Anim. Sci.* **30**, 541–543.

Eisele, P. H., Markovits, J. E., and Paul-Murphy, J. R. (1991). Partial colectomy for treating acquired megacolon in long-tailed macaques. *Lab. Anim. Sci.* **41**, 436–441.

English, W. L. (1934). Notes on the breeding of a douroucouli (*Aotus trivirgatus*) in captivity. *Proc. Zool. Soc. London*, pp. 143–144.

Fagan, D., and Oosterhuis, J. (1979). Gingival hyperplasia induced by diphenylhydantoin in a gorilla. *J. Am. Vet. Med. Assoc.* **175**, 960–961.

Felsenfeld, A. D. (1972). The yellow fever. *In* "Pathology of Simian Primates" (R. N. T.-W.-Fiennes, T. Orihel, and J. Ayers, eds.), Vol. 2, pp. 523–536. Karger, Basel.

Fincham, J. E., Van Rensburg, S. J., and Kriek, N. P. J. (1982). A Squamous cell carcinoma in an african green monkey. *Vet. Pathol.* **19**, 450–453.

Fleagle, J. G., and Schaffler, M. B. (1982). Development and eruption of mandibular cheek teeth in *Cebus albifrons*. *Folia Primatol.* **38**, 158–169.

Fleischman, R. W., du Moulin, G. C., Esber, H. J., Ilievski, V., and Bogden, A. E. (1982). Nontuberculous mycobacterial infection attributable to *Mycobacterium intracellulare* serotype 10 in two rhesus monkeys. *J. Am. Vet. Med. Assoc.* **181**, 1358–1362.

Foster, A. O., and Johnson, C. M. (1939). A preliminary note on the identity life-cycle and pathogenicity of an important nematode parasite of captive monkeys. *Am. J. Trop. Med. Hyg.* **19**, 265–277.

Fox, J. G. (1982). Campylobacteriosis—a "new" disease in laboratory animals. *Lab. Anim. Sci.* **32**, 626–637.

Fraser, C. E. O., Chalifoux, L., Sehgal, P., Hunt, R. D., and King, N. W., Jr. (1978). A paramyxovirus causing fatal gastroenterocolitis in marmoset monkeys. *Primates Med.* **10**, 261–270.

Friskopp, J., and Blomlof, L. (1988). Spontaneous periodontitis in a sample group of the monkey *Macaca fascicularis*. *J. Periodont. Res.* **23**, 265–267.

Galliari, C. A., and Colillas, O. J. (1985). Sequences and timing of dental eruption in Bolivian captive-born squirrel monkeys (*Saimiri sciureus*). *Am. J. Primatol.* **8**, 195–204.

Gardy, A. G., Hatchuel, D. A., and Sher, J. (1982). The oral pathological conditions of the hard tissues of the vervet monkey in their natural environment. *Diastema*, 20th Anniversary Issue, pp. 43–49.

Gatesman, T. J. (1992). Serum amylase values in callitrichids. *Lab. Anim. Sci.* **42**, 46–50.

Gavan, J. A. (1967). Eruption of primate deciduous dentition: A comparative study. *J. Dent. Res.* **46**, 984–988.

George, J. W., and Lerche, N. W. (1990). Electrolyte abnormalities associated with diarrhea in rhesus monkeys: 100 cases (1986–1987) *J. Am. Vet. Med. Assoc.* **196**, 1654–1658.

Gibson, W. E., and Hall, A. S. (1970). Surgical removal of the maxillary canine tooth in the rhesus monkey (*Macaca mulatta*). *J. Am. Vet. Med. Assoc.* **157**, 717–722.

Giddens, W. E., Jr., Tsai, C.-C., Morton, W. R., Ochs, H. D., Knitter, G. H., and Blakeley, G. A. (1985). Retroperitoneal fibromatosis and acquired immunodeficiency syndrome in macaques. *Am. J. Pathol.* **119**, 253–263.

Gliatto, J. M., and Bronson, R. T. (1993). Fatal fasting syndrome of obese macaques. *In* "Monographs on the Pathology of Laboratory Animals: Nonhuman Primates" (T. C. Jones, U. Mohr, and R. D. Hunt, eds.), Vol. 2, pp. 198–202. Springer-Verlag, Berlin and New York.

Goodwin, B. T., Jerome, C. P., and Bullock, B. C. (1988). Unusual lesion morphology and skin test reaction for *Mycobacterium avium* complex in macaques. *Lab. Anim. Sci.* **38**, 20–24.

Goodwin, T., Adams, M. R., Lehner, N. D., and Jerome, C. P. (1983). *Yersinia enterocolitica* septicemia in *Erythrocebus patas*. *Lab. Anim. Sci.* **33**, 481.

Goss, A. N. (1984). A comparison of tooth eruption patterns between two colonies of young marmosets (*Callithrix jacchus*). *J. Dent. Res.* **63**, 44–46.

Grana, D., Mareso, E., and Gomez, E. (1992). Oral squamous cell carcinoma in capuchin monkeys (*Cebus apella*). Report of two cases. *J. Med. Primatol.* **21**, 384–386.

Gravell, M., Palmer, A. E., Rodriguez, M., London, W. T., and Hamilton, R. S. (1980). Method to detect asymptomatic carriers of simian hemorrhagic fever virus. *Lab. Anim. Sci.* **30**, 988–991.

Guerrant, R. L., and Bobak, D. A. (1991). Bacterial and protozoal gastroenteritis. *N. Engl. J. Med.* **325**, 327–340.

Gullett, P. A., Tarara, R., and Markovits, J. E. (1996). Colon biopsy in the management of chronic diarrhea in rhesus monkeys. *Contemp. Top. Lab. Anim. Sci.* **35**, 74–75.

Hahn, C. S., Dalrymple, J. M., Strauss, J. H., and Rice, C. M. (1987). Comparison of the virulent Asibi strain of yellow fever virus with the 17D vaccine strain derived from it. *Proc. Natl. Acad. Sci. U.S.A.* **84**, 2019–2023.

Hall, R. D., Beattie, R. J., Wyckoff, G. H. (1979). Weight gains and sequence of dental eruptions in infant owl monkeys (*Aotus trivirgatus*). *In* "Nursery Care of Nonhuman Primates" (G. C. Ruppenthal, ed.) Plenum, New York, pp. 321–328.

Hall, W. C., Kovatch, R. M., Herman, P. H., and Fox, J. G. (1971). Pathology of measles in rhesus monkeys. *Vet. Pathol.* **8**, 307–319.

Hawk, C. T., Leary, S. L. (1995). Formulary for laboratory animals. Iowa State University Press, Ames, Iowa.

Hawkins, J. V., Clapp, N. K., Carson, R. L., Henke, M. A., McCracken, M. D., Faulkner, C. T., and Patton, S. (1997). Diagnosis and treatment of Trichospirura leptostoma infection in common marmosets (*Callithrix jacchus*). *Contemp. Top.* **36**(1), 52–53.

Henrickson, R. V., Maul, D. H., Lerche, N. W., Osborn, K. G., Lowenstine, L. J., Prahalada, S., Sever, J. L., Madden, D. L., and Gardner, M. B. (1984). Clinical features of simian acquired immunodeficiency syndrome (SAIDS) in rhesus monkeys. *Lab. Anim. Sci.* **34**, 140–145.

Herlong, H. F. (1988). Normal and abnormal hepatic physiology: Biochemical and radiologic assessment of the liver and classification of diseases of the liver. *In* "The Principles and Practice of Medicine" (A. N. Harvey, R. J. Johns, V. A. McKusick, A. J. Owens, Jr., and R. S. Ross, eds.), pp. 831–836. Appleton & Lange, Norwalk, CT.

Hird, D. W., Anderson, J. H., and Bielitzki, J. T. (1984). Diarrhea in non-human primates: A survey of primate colonies for incidence rates and clinical opinion. *Lab. Anim. Sci.* **34**, 465–470.

Hirsh, D. C., Davidson, J. N., Beards, L. R., Anderson, J. H., Budd, C. P., and Henrickson, R. V. (1980). Microscopic examination of stools from non-

human primates as a way of predicting the presence of *Shigella*. *J. Clin. Microbiol.* **11**, 65–67.

Hoffman, W. E., Kramer, J., Main, A. R., and Torres, J. L. (1989). Clinical enzymology. *In* "The Clinical Chemistry of Laboratory Animals" (W. F. Loeb and F. W. Quimby, eds.), pp. 237–278. Pergamon, New York.

Holmberg, C. A., Henrickson, R. V., Malaga, C., Schneider, R., and Gribble, D. (1982a). Nontuberculous mycobacterial disease in rhesus monkeys. *Vet. Pathol.* **19**, Suppl. 7, 9–16.

Holmberg, C. A., Leininger, R., Wheeldon, E., Slater, D., Henrickson, R., and Anderson, J. (1982b). Clinicopathological studies of gastrointestinal disease in macaques. *Vet. Pathol.* **19**, Suppl. 7, 163–170.

Holmberg, C. A., Henrickson, R., Lenniger, R., Anderson, J., Hayashi, L., and Ellingsworth, L. (1985). Immunologic abnormality in a group of *Macaca arctoides* with high mortality due to atypical mycobacterial and other disease processes. *Am. J. Vet. Res.* **46**, 1192–1196.

Honjo, S., Takasaka, M., Fujiwara, T., and Imaizumi, K. (1966). Shigellosis in cynomolgus monkeys (*Macaca irus*). IV. Bacteriological and histopathological observations on the earlier stage of experimental infection with *Shigella flexneri* 2A. *Jpn. J. Med. Sci. Biol.* **19**, 23–32.

Honjo, S., Takasaka, M., Fujiwara, T., Imaizumi, K., and Ogawa, I. (1969). Shigellosis in cynomolgus monkeys (*Macaca irus*). VII. Experimental production of dystentery with a relatively small dose of *Shigella flexneri* 2A in ascorbic acid deficiency monkeys. *Jpn. J. Med. Sci. Biol.* **22**, 149–162.

Howard, D. R. (1983). Repair and reconstruction of cleft palate and other oronasal fistulas. *In* "Current Techniques in Small Animal Surgery" (M. J. Bojrab, S. W. Crane, and S. P. Arnoczky, eds.), 2nd ed., pp. 109–113. Lea & Febiger, Philadelphia.

Hugh-Jones, M. E., Hubbert, W. T., and Hagstad, H. V. (1995a). Bacterial zoonoses. *Zoonoses Recognition Control Prev.* **8**, 285–286.

Hugh-Jones, M. E., Hubbert, W. T., and Hagstad, H. V. (1995b). Yellow fever. *Zoonoses Recognition Control Prev.* **8**, 352–353.

Hummer, R. L. (1967). Preventive medicine practices in baboon colony management. *In* "The Baboon in Medical Research" (H. Vagtbarg, ed.), Vol. 2, pp. 51–52. University of Texas Press, Austin.

Hunt, R. D. (1993a). Herpesviruses of primates: An introduction. *In* "Monographs on the Pathology of Laboratory Animals: Nonhuman Primates" (T. C. Jones, U. Mohr, and R. D. Hunt, eds.), Vol. 1, pp. 74–77. Springer-Verlag, Berlin and New York.

Hunt, R. D. (1993b). Herpesvirus simplex infection. *In* "Monographs on the Pathology of Laboratory Animals: Nonhuman Primates" (T. C. Jones, U. Mohr, and R. D. Hunt, eds.), Vol. 1, pp. 82–86. Springer-Verlag, Berlin and New York.

Hunt, R. D., and Blake, B. J. (1993a). Herpesvirus B Infection. *In* "Monographs on the Pathology of Laboratory Animals: Nonhuman Primates" (T. C. Jones, U. Mohr, and R. D. Hunt, eds.), Vol. I, pp. 78–81. Springer-Verlag, Berlin and New York.

Hunt, R. D., and Blake, B. J. (1993b). *Herpesvirus platyrrhinae* infection. *In* "Monographs on the Pathology of Laboratory Animals: Nonhuman Primates" (T. C. Jones, U. Mohr, and R. D. Hunt, eds.), Vol. I, pp. 100–103. Springer-Verlag, Berlin and New York.

Hunt, R. D., and Blake, B. J. (1993c). Gastroenteritis due to paramyxovirus. *In* "Monographs on the Pathology of Laboratory Animals: Nonhuman Primates" (T. C. Jones, U. Mohr, and R. D. Hunt, eds.), Vol. 2, pp. 32–37. Springer-Verlag, Berlin and New York.

Hurme, V. O., and van Wagenen, G. (1953). Basic data on the emergence of deciduous teeth in the monkey (*Macaca mulatta*). *Proc. Am. Philos Soc.* **97**, 291–315.

Hurme, V. O., and van Wagenen, G. (1961). Basic data on the emergence of permanent teeth in the rhesus monkey (*Macaca mulatta*). *Proc. Am. Philos. Soc.* **105**, 105–140.

Iwamoto, M., Hamada, Y., and Watanabe, T. (1984). Eruption of deciduous teeth in Japanese monkeys (*Macaca fuscata*). *J. Anthropol. Soc. Nippon* **92**, 273–279.

Jaax, N. K., Petrali, J. P., and Jaax, J. P. (1988). Lymphoma of the pharynx and abdominal wall in two cynomolgus monkeys. *Lab. Anim. Sci.* **38**, 198–200.

Jayo, J. M., Sajuthi, D., Wagner, J. D., Bullock, B. C., and McDole, G. K. (1990). Intestinal amyloidosis in a rhesus monkey responsive to treatment with dimethyl sulfoxide. *Lab. Anim. Sci.* **40**, 548.

Jenns, K. (1994). Importance of nausea (Review). *Cancer Nurs.* **17**, 488–493.

Jergens, A. E. (1995). Diarrhea. *In* "Textbook of Veterinary Internal Medicine: Diseases of the Dog and Cat" (S. J. Ettinger and E. C. Feldman, eds.), Vol. 1, pp. 111–114. Saunders, Philadelphia.

Johnson, S. E. (1992). Fluid therapy for gastrointestinal, pancreatic, and hepatic disease. *In* "Fluid Therapy in Small Animal Practice" (S. P. DiBartola, ed.), pp. 507–528. Saunders, Philadelphia.

Johnston, G. W., Dreizen, S., and Levy, B. M. (1970). Dental development in the cotton ear marmoset (*Callithrix jacchus*). *Am. J. Phys. Anthropol.* **33**, 41–48.

Jones, T. C., Mohr, V., Hunt, R. D., Russell, R. G., and DeTolla, L. J. (1993). Shigellosis. *In* "Monographs on the Pathology of Laboratory Animals: Nonhuman Primates" (T. C. Jones, U. Mohr, and R. D. Hunt, eds.), Vol. 2, pp. 45–63. Springer-Verlag, Berlin and New York.

Keiter, M. D. (1981). Hand-rearing and development of a lowland gorilla at Woodland Park Zoo, Seattle. *Int. Zoo Yearb.* **21**, 229–253.

Kemnitz, J. W. (1996). Rhesus monkeys and other primate models. *In* "The Encyclopedia of Aging, 2nd Edition" (G. Maddox, ed.). Springer Publishing, Inc., New York, pp. 829–830.

Kent, T. H., Formal, S. B., and Labrec, E. H. (1966). Salmonella gastroenteritis in rhesus monkeys. *Arch. Pathol.* **82**, 272–279.

Kent, T. H., Formal, S. B., LaBrec, E. H., Sprinz, H., Maenza, R. M. (1967). Gastric shigellosis in rhesus monkeys. *Am. J. Path.* **51**, 259–267.

Kessler, M. J. (1982). Clinical note, Calcium bilirubinate gallstones in an aged rhesus monkey (*Macaca mulatta*). *Am. J. Primatol.* **2**, 291–294.

Kilgore, L. (1989). Dental pathologies in ten free-ranging chimpanzees from Gombe National Park, Tanzania. *Am. J. Phys. Anthropol.* **80**, 219–227.

King, N. W., Jr. (1993a). Simian immunodeficiency virus infections. *In* "Monographs on the Pathology of Laboratory Animals: Nonhuman Primates" (T. C. Jones, U. Mohr, and R. D. Hunt, eds.), Vol. I, pp. 5–20. Springer-Verlag, Berlin and New York.

King, N. W., Jr. (1993b). *Mycobacterium avium-intracellulare* infection. *In* "Monographs on the Pathology of Laboratory Animals: Nonhuman Primates" (T. C. Jones, U. Mohr, and R. D. Hunt, eds.), Vol. I, pp. 57–63. Springer-Verlag, Berlin and New York.

King, N. W., Jr. (1993c). Tuberculosis. *In* "Monographs on the Pathology of Laboratory Animals: Nonhuman Primates" (T. C. Jones, U. Mohr, and R. D. Hunt, eds.), Vol. I, pp. 141–148. Springer-Verlag, Berlin and New York.

Kisilevsky, R. (1983). Biology of disease: Amyloidosis: A familiar problem in the light of current pathogenetic developments. *Lab. Invest.* **49**, 381–389.

Klumpp, S. A., and McClure, H. M. (1993). Carcinomas, gastrointestinal tract. *In* "Monographs on the Pathology of Laboratory Animals: Nonhuman Primates" (T. C. Jones, U. Mohr, and R. D. Hunt, eds.), Vol. 2, pp. 53–60. Springer-Verlag, Berlin and New York.

Klumpp, S. A., Weaver, D. S., Jerome, C. P., and Jokinen, M. P. (1986). Salmonella osteomyelitis in a rhesus monkey. *Vet. Pathol.* **23**, 190–197.

Koch, T. R. (1995). Constipation. *In* "Bockus Gastroenterology" (W. S. Haurbrich, F. Schaffner, and J. E. Berk, eds.), Vol. 1, pp. 102–112. Saunders, Philadelphia.

Kohno, A., Terao, K., Takasaka, M., and Honjo, S. (1988). The serodiagnosis of *Campylobacter* infection in infant cynomolgus monkeys (*Macaca fascicularis*) 2 to 18 weeks old by enzyme-linked immunosorbent assay. *Lab. Anim. Sci.* **38**, 715–721.

Koonin, E. V., Borbalenya, A. E., Purdy, M. A., Rozanov, M. N., Reyes, G. R., and Bradley, D. W. (1992). Computer-assisted assignment of functional domains in the nonstructural polyprotein of hepatitis E virus: Delineation of an additional group of positive-strand RNA plant and animal viruses. *Proc. Natl. Acad. Sci. U.S.A.* **89**, 8259–8263.

Kornegay, R. W., Giddens, E. W. Jr., Van Hoosier, G. L., Martan, B. L. (1985). Subacute nonsuppurative hepatitis associated with hepatitis B virus infection in two cynomolgus monkeys. *Lab. Anim. Sci.* **35**, 400–404.

Kourany, M., Porter, J. A. (1969). A survey for enteropathogenic bacteria in Panamanian primates. *Lab. Anim. Care* **19**, 336–341.

Kraemer, H. C., Horvat, J. R., Doering, C., and McGinnis, P. R. (1982). Male chimpanzee development focusing on adolescence: Integration of behavioral with physiological changes. *Primates* **23**, 393–405.

Krahwinkel, D. J., and Richardson, D. C. (1983). Surgery of the small intestine. *In* "Current Techniques in Small Animal Surgery" (M. J. Bojrab, S. W. Crane, and S. P. Arnoczky, eds.), 2nd ed., pp. 162–174. Lea & Febiger, Philadelphia.

Krawczynski, K., and Bradley, D. W. (1989). Enterically transmitted non-A, non-B hepatitis: Identification of virus-associated antigen in experimentally infected cynomolgus macaques. *J. Infect. Dis.* **159**, 1042–1049.

Krejs, G. J. (1988). Diarrhea. *In* "Cecil's Textbook of Medicine" (J. B. Wyngaarden and L. H. Smith, eds.), pp. 725–732. Saunders, Philadelphia.

Krosnow, S. H. (1991). New directions in managing chemotherapy-related emesis. *Medline* **5**, 19–24.

Kruckenberg, S., and Kidd, R. (1989). Liver function tests; bilirubin, exogenous dyes, and urobilinogen. *In* "The Clinical Chemistry of Laboratory Animals" (W. F. Loeb and F. W. Quimby, eds.), pp. 309–319. Pergamon, New York.

Kuksova, M. I. (1958). The eruption of milk teeth in the hamadryas baboon. *Sov. Antropol.* **2**, 17–21.

Kuster, J. (1983). Longitudinal study of the physical development of hand-reared common marmosets (*Callithrix jacchus*). *In* "Perspectives in Primate Biology. New Delhi: Today and Tomorrow" (P. K. Seth, ed.), pp. 147–159.

Kuykendall, K. L., Mahoney, C. J., and Conroy, G. C. (1992). Probit and survival analysis of tooth emergence ages in a mixed-longitudinal sample of chimpanzees. (*Pan troglodytes*). *Am. J. Phys. Anthropol.* **89**, 379–399.

Laber-Laird, K. E., Jokinen, M. D., and Lehner, N. D. M. (1987). Fatal fatty liver-kidney syndrome in obese monkeys. *Lab. Anim. Sci.* **37**, 205–209.

Lackner, A. A., and Wilson, D. W. (1993). Cyptosporidiosis, intestines, pancreatic duct, bile duct, gall bladder, *Macaca mulatta*. *In* "Monographs on the Pathology of Laboratory Animals: Nonhuman Primates" (T. C. Jones, U. Mohr, and R. D. Hunt, eds.), Vol. 2, pp. 41–46. Springer-Verlag, Berlin and New York.

Lackner, A. A., Armitage, G. C., Schiodt, M. (1993). Noma, *Macaca mulatta*. *In* "Monographs on the Pathology of Laboratory Animals: Nonhuman Primates" (T. C. Jones, U. Mohr, and R. D. Hunt, eds.), Vol. 2, pp. 70–73.

Lackner, A. A., Moore, P. F., Marx, P. A., Munn, R. J., Gardner, M. B., and Lowenstine, L. J. (1990). Immunohistochemical localization of type D retrovirus serotype 1 in the digestive tract of rhesus monkeys with simian AIDS. *J. Med. Primatol.* **19**, 339–349.

Lawrence, W. A., Coelho, A. M., and Relethford, J. H. (1982). Sequence and age of eruption of deciduous dentition in the baboon (*Papio* sp.) *Am. J. Primatol.* **2**, 295–300.

Leary, T. P., Desai, S. M., Yamaguchi, J., Chalmers, M. L., Schlauder, G. G., Dawson, G. J., and Mushahwar, I. K. (1996). Species-specific variants of GB virus A in captive monkeys. *J. Virol.* **70**(12), 9028–9030.

Leong, Y. K., and Awang, A. (1990). Experimental group A rotaviral infection in cynomolgus monkeys raised on formula diet. *Microbiol. Immunol.* **34**, 153–162.

Levy, B. M., and Mirkovic, R. R. (1971). An epizootic of measles in a marmoset colony. *Lab. Anim. Sci.* **21**, 33–39.

Lindsey, J. R., Hardy, P. H., Jr., Baker, H. J., and Melby, E. C., Jr. (1971). Observations on shigellosis and development of multiply resistant shigellas in *Macaca mulatta*. *Lab. Anim. Sci.* **21**, 832–844.

Line, A. S., Paul-Murphy, J., Aucoin, D. P., and Hirsh, D. C. (1992). Enrofloxacin treatment of long-tailed macaques with acute bacillary dysentery due to multiresistant *Shigella flexneri* IV. *Lab. Anim. Sci.* **42**, 240–244.

Loeb, W. F. (1989). The nonhuman primate. *In* "The Clinical Chemistry of Laboratory Animals" (W. F. Loeb and F. W. Quimby, eds.), pp. 59–69. Pergamon, New York.

London, W. T. (1977). Epizootiology, transmission and approach to prevention of fatal simian haemorrhagic fever in rhesus monkeys. *Nature (London)* **268**, 344–345.

Long, J. O., and Cooper, R. W. (1968). Physical growth and dental eruption in captive-bred squirrel monkeys. In "The Squirrel Monkey" (L. A. Rosenblum and R. W. Cooper, eds.), pp. 193–205. Academic Press, New York.

Loomis, M. R., Britt, J. O., Jr., Gendron, A. P., Holshuh, H. J., and Howard, E. B. (1983). Hepatic and gastric amebiasis. J. Am. Vet. Med. Assoc. 183, 1188–1191.

Lovell, N. (1990). Skeletal and dental pathologies of free ranging lowland gorillas. Am. J. Phys. Anthropol. 81, 399–412.

Lowenstine, L. J. (1986). Neoplasms and proliferative disorders in nonhuman primates. In "Primates: The Road to Self-Sustaining Populations" (K. Benirschke, ed.), pp. 781–814. Springer-Verlag, Berlin and New York.

Lowenstine, L. J. (1993a). Type D retrovirus infection, Macaques. In "Monographs of the Pathology of Laboratory Animals: Nonhuman Primates" (T. C. Jones, U. Mohr, and R. D. Hunt, eds.), Vol. I, pp. 20–32. Springer-Verlag, Berlin and New York.

Lowenstine, L. J. (1993b). Measles virus infection nonhuman primates. In "Monographs on the Pathology of Laboratory Animals: Nonhuman Primates" (T. C. Jones, U. Mohr, and R. D. Hunt, eds.), Vol. I, pp. 108–118. Springer-Verlag, Berlin and New York.

Lucke, V. M., and Bennett, A. M. (1982). An outbreak of hepatitis in marmosets in a zoological collection. Lab. Anim. 16, 73–77.

Lushbaugh, C. C., Humason, G. L., Swartzendruber, D. C., Richter, C. B., and Gengozian, N. (1978). Spontaneous colonic adenocarcinoma in marmosets. Primates Med. 10, 119–134.

Lushbaugh, C., Humanson, G., and Clapp, N. (1985a). Histology of colitis: Saguinus oedipus oedipus and other marmosets. Dig. Dis. Sci. 30, Suppl., 45S–51S.

Lushbaugh, C., Humanson, G., and Clapp, N. (1985b). Histology of colon cancer in Saguinus oedipus oedipus. Dig. Dis. Sci. 30, Suppl., 1195–1255.

Madara, J. L. (1985). Structural characterization of spontaneous colitis in cotton-top tamarins (Saguinus oedipus). Dig. Dis. Sci. 30, Suppl., 52S–53S.

Maddison, J. E. (1992). Hepatic encephalopathy: Current concepts of the pathogenesis. J. Vet. Intern. Med. 6, 341–353.

Matherne, C. M., Herring, D. L., Hill, M. J., and Keeling, M. E. (1992). Idenfification of intestinal parasites in laboratory animals using formalin-ethyl acetate concentrations and permanent trichrome stains. Lab. Anim. Sci. 42, 422.

Malaga, C. A., Weller, R. E., Buschbom, R. L., and Ragan, H. A. (1991). Serum chemistry of the wild caught karyotype I night monkey (Aotus nancymai). Lab. Anim. Sci. 41, 143–145.

McClure, H. M., Weaver, R. E., and Kaufman, A. F. (1971). Pseudotuberculosis in nonhuman primates: Infection with organisms of the Yersinia enterocolitica group. Lab. Anim. Sci. 21, 376–382.

McClure, H. M., Brodie, A. R., Anderson, D. C., and Swenson, R. B. (1986). Bacterial infections of nonhuman primates. In "Primates: The Road to Self-Sustaining Populations" (K. Benirschke, ed.), pp. 43, 531–556. Springer-Verlag, Berlin and New York.

McClure, H. M., Chiodini, R. J., Anderson, D. C., Swenson, R. B., Thayer, W. R., and Coutu, J. A. (1987). Mycobacterium paratuberculosis infection in a colony of stumptail macaques (Macaca arctoides). J. Infect. Dis. 155, 1011–1019.

McCuskey, R. S. (1993). Functional morphology of the liver with emphasis on microvasculature. In "Hepatic Transport and Bile Secretion: Physiology and Pathophysiology" (N. Tavolonic and P. D. Berk, eds.), pp. 1–10. Raven Press, New York.

McNamara, J. A., Foster, D. L., and Rosenstein, B. D. (1977). Eruption of the deciduous dentition in the rhesus monkey. J. Dent. Res. 56, 701.

McSherry, C. K., Javitt, N. B., De Carvalho, J. M., and Glenn, F. (1971). Cholesterol gallstones and the chemical composition of bile in baboons. Ann. Surg. 173, 569–577.

Migaki, G. (1986). Mycotic Infections in nonhuman primates. In "Primates: The Road to Self-Sustaining Populations" (K. Benirschke, ed.), pp. 557–570. Springer-Verlag, Berlin and New York.

Miller, R. A., Bronsdon, M. A., and Morton, W. R. (1990a). Experimental crytosporidiosis in a primate model. J. Infect. Dis. 161, 312–315.

Mitchelson, F. (1992). Pharmacological agents affecting emesis. Drugs 43, 443–463.

Miyai, K. (1991). Structural organization of the liver. In "Hepatotoxicology" (R. G. Meeks, S. D. Harrison, and R. J. Bull, eds.), pp. 1–65. CRC Press, Boca Raton, FL.

Monath, T. P. (1982). Yellow fever. In "Cecil's Textbook of Medicine" (J. B. Wyngaarden and L. H. Smith, eds.), 16th edition, pp. 1686–1691. Saunders, Philadelphia.

Montali, R. (1993). Callitrichid hepatitis. In "Monographs on the Pathology of Laboratory Animals: Nonhuman Primates" (T. C. Jones, U. Mohr, and R. D. Hunt, eds.) Vol. 2, pp. 61–62. Springer-Verlag, Berlin and New York.

Montali, R. J., Ramsay, E. C., Stephensen, C. B., Worley, M., Davis, J. A., and Holmes, K. V. (1989). A new transmissible viral hepatitis of marmosets and tamarins. J. Infect. Dis. 160, 759–765.

Montali, R. J., Connolly, B. M., Armstrong, D. L., Scanga, C. A., and Holmes, K. V. (1995). Pathology and immunohistochemistry of Callitrichid hepatitis, an emerging disease of captive new world primates caused by lymphocytic choriomeningitis virus. Am. J. Pathol. 148, 1441–1449.

Montesdeoca, D., Roberts, J., and Donnelly, T. M. (1993). Asymmetry of the face of a squirrel monkey. Lab. Anim. Sci. 21, 18–21.

Mooney, M. P., Seigal, M. I., Eichberg, J. W., Lee, R. D., and Swan, J. (1991). Deciduous dentition eruption sequence of the laboratory-reared chimpanzee (Pan troglodytes). J. Med. Primatol. 20, 138–139.

Morris, T. H. (1994). A further case of squamous cell carcinoma in the oral cavity of a squirrel monkey. J. Med. Primatol. 23, 317–318.

Morton, W. R., Bronsdon, M., Mickelsen, G., Knitter, G., Rosenkranz, S., Kuller, L., and Sajuthi, D. (1983). Identification of Campylobacter jejeuni in Macaca fascicularis imported from Indonesia. Lab. Anim. Sci. 33, 187–188.

Muir, W. W., and DiBartola, S. P. (1983). Fluid therapy. Curr. Vet. Ther. 8, 28–40.

Mulder, J. B. (1971). Shigellosis in nonhuman primates: A review. Lab. Anim. Sci. 21, 734–738.

Napier, J. R., and Napier, P. H. (1967). The teeth, digestion and diet. In "A Handbook of Living Primates," pp. 21–27. Academic Press, London.

National Research Council (1996). Animal Environment, Housing and Management. In "Guide to the Care and Use of Laboratory Animals" pp. 21–55. National Academy Press, Washington, D.C.

Newell, D. G., Hudson, M. J., and Baskerville, A. (1987). Naturally occurring gastritis associated with Campylobacter pylori infection in the rhesus monkey. Lancet 1338.

Newell, D. G., Hudson, M. J., and Baskerville, A. (1988). Isolation of a gastric Campylobacter-like organism from the stomach of four rhesus monkeys, and identification as Campylobacter pylori. J. Med. Microbiol. 27, 41–44.

Nissen, H. W., and Riesen, A. H. (1945). The deciduous dentition of chimpanzee. Growth 9, 265–274.

Nissen, H. W., and Riesen, A. H. (1964). The eruption of the permanent dentition of chimpanzee. Am. J. Phys. Anthropol. 22, 285–294.

Ockerse, (1959). Eruption sequence and eruption times of the teeth of the vervet monkey. J. Dent. Assoc. S. Afr. 14, 422–424.

Ockner, R. K. (1988a). Diseases of the liver, gallbladder, and bile ducts. In "Cecil's Textbook of Medicine" (J. B. Wyngaarden and L. H. Smith, eds.), Vol. 1, pp. 808–811. Saunders, Philadelphia.

Ockner, R. K. (1988b). Laboratory tests in liver disease. In "Cecil's Textbook of Medicine" (J. B. Wyngaarden and L. H. Smith, eds.), Vol. I, pp. 814–817. Saunders, Philadelphia.

Ogawa, H., Takahashi, R. (1964). Shigellosis in cynomolgus monkeys (Macaca inus) III. Histopathological studies on natural and experimental shigellosis. Jap J. M. Sc. and Biol 17, 321–332.

Olfert, E. D. (1974). Tooth root abscess and fistula in the squirrel monkey. Can. Vet. J. 15, 171–172.

Olson, L. C., Bergquist, D. Y., and Fitzgerald, D. L. (1986). Control of Shigella flexneri in Celebes black macaques Macaca nigra). Lab. Anim. Sci. 36, 240–242.

Osborn, K. G., Prahalada, S., Lowenstine, L. J., Gardner, M. B., Maul, D. H., and Hendrickson, R. V. (1984). The pathology of an epizootic of acquired immunodeficiency in rhesus monkeys. Am. J. Pathol. 114, 94–103.

Osuga, T., and Portman, O. W. (1971). Experimental formation of gallstones in the squirrel monkey. *Proc. Soc. Exp. Biol. Med.* **136,** 722–726.

Owen, D. G. (1992). "Laboratory Animal Handbook," No. 12, p. 9. Royal Society of Medicine Services Limited, London.

Padovan, D., and Cantrell, C. A. (1986). Varicella-like herpesvirus infections of nonhuman primates. *Lab. Anim. Sci.* **36,** 7–13.

Page, R. C., and Schroeder, H. E. (1982). Periodontitis in man and other animals. *In* "Periodontitis in other Mammalian Animals," pp. 187–212. Karger, Basel.

Palmieri, J. R., Dalgard, D. W., and Connor, D. H. (1984). Gastric amebiasis in a silvered leaf monkey. *J. Am. Vet. Med. Assoc.* **185,** 1374–1375.

Patten, B. M., and Carlson, B. M. (1974). "Foundations of Embryology," 3rd ed., pp. 442–445. McGraw-Hill, New York.

Paul-Murphy, J. (1993). Bacterial enterocolitis in non-human primates. *In* "Zoo and Wildlife Medicine" (M. E. Fowler, ed.), Curr. Vol. 3, pp. 344–351. Saunders, Philadelphia.

Pazzaglia, G., Widjaja, S., Soebekti, D., Tjaniadi, P., Simanjuntak, L., Lesmana, M., and Jennings, G. (1994). Persistent recurring diarrhea in a colony of orangutans (*Pongo pygmaeus*) caused by multiple strains of *Campylobacter spp. Acta Trop.* **57,** 1–10.

Pissinatti, A., da Cruz, J. B., Massinegto, D., and Silva, R. B. (1987). Spontaneous cholelithiasis species of callitrichidae. *Int. J. Primatol.* **8,** 514.

Pizarro, D., Posada, G., Sandi, L., and Moran, J. R. (1991). Rice-based oral electrolyte solutions for the management of infantile diarrhea. *N. Engl. J. Med.* **324,** 517–521.

Podolsky, D. K. (1985). Colonic glycoproteins in cotton-top tamarin, relationship to chronic colitis. *Dig. Dis. Sci.* **30,** Suppl., 36S–37S.

Pond, C. L., Newcomer, C. E., and Anver, M. R. (1982). Acute gastric dilation in primates; review and case studies. *Vet. Pathol.* **19,** Suppl. 7, 126–133.

Portman, O. W., Alexander, M., Tanaka, N., and Osuga, T. (1980). Relationships between cholesterol gallstones, biliary function, and plasma lipoproteins in squirrel monkeys. *J. Lab. Clin. Med.* **96,** 90–101.

Potkay, S. (1992). Diseases of the callitrichidae: A review. *J. Med. Primatol.* **21,** 189–236.

Prowten, A. W., Lee, R. V., Krishnamsetty, R. M., Satchidanand, S. K., and Srivastave, B. I. S. (1985). T cell lymphoma associated with immunologic evidence of retrovirus infection in a lowland gorilla. *J. Am. Vet. Med. Assoc.* **187,** 1280–1282.

Pucak, G. J., Orcutt, R. P., Judge, R. J., and Rendon, F. (1977). Elimination of the *Shigella* carrier state in rhesus monkeys (*Macaca mulatta*) by trimethoprim sulfamethoxazole. *J. Med. Primatol.* **6,** 127–132.

Ramsay, E. C., Montali, R. J., Vorley, M., Stephensen, C. B., and Holmes, K. V. (1989). Callitrichid hepatitis: Epizootiology of a fatal hepatitis in zoo tamarins and marmosets, *J. Zoo Wild. Med.* **20,** 178–183.

Rasmussen, K. M., Thenen, S. W., and Hayes, K. C. (1980). Effect of folic acid supplementation on pregnancy in the squirrel monkey (*Saimiri sciureus*). *J. Med. Primatol.* **9,** 169–184.

Ratterree, M. S., Didier, P. J., Blanchard, J. L., Clarke, M. R., and Schaffer, D. (1990). Vitamin C deficiency in captive nonhuman primates fed commercial primate diet. *Lab. Anim. Sci.* **40,** 165–168.

Reed, O. M. (1973). *Papio cynocephalus* age determination. *Am. J. Phys. Anthropol.* **38,** 309–314.

Reynolds, J. A., and Hall, A. S. (1979). A rapid procedure for shortening teeth of nonhuman primates. *Lab. Anim. Sci.* **29,** 521–524.

Rice, C. M., Lenches, E. M., Eddy, S. R., Shin, S. J., Sheets, R. L., and Strauss, J. H. (1985). Nucleotide sequence of yellow fever virus: Implications for flovirus gene expression and evolution. *Science* **229,** 726–733.

Roberts, D. E. (1993a). Simian varicella. *In* "Monographs on the Pathology of Laboratory Animals: Nonhuman Primates" (T. C. Jones, U. Mohr, and R. D. Hunt, eds.), Vol. I, pp. 93–100. Springer-Verlag, Berlin and New York.

Roberts, D. E. (1993b). Vitamin C deficiency, old and new world monkeys. *In* "Monographs on the Pathology of Laboratory Animals: Nonhuman Primates" (T. C. Jones, U. Mohr, and R. D. Hunt, eds.), Vol. I, pp. 202–206. Springer-Verlag, Berlin and New York.

Rodger, R. R., Bronson, R. T., McIntyre, K. W., and Nicolosi, R. J. (1980). Protein-losing enteropathy in six macaques. *J. Am. Vet. Med. Assoc.* **177,** 863–866.

Rosenberg, D. P., Lerche, N. W., and Henrickson, R. V. (1980). *Yersinia pseudotuberculosis* infection in a group of *Macaca fascicularis. J. Am. Vet. Med. Assoc.* **177,** 818–819.

Ross, D. L., and Myers, J. W. (1970). Endodontic therapy for canine teeth in dogs. *J. Am. Vet. Med. Assoc.* **157,** 1713–1718.

Russell, R. G., and Detolly, L. J. (1993). Shigellosis. *In* "Monographs on the Pathology of Laboratory Animals: Nonhuman Primates" (T. C. Jones, U. Mohr, and R. D. Hunt, eds.), Vol. 2, pp. 45–53. Springer-Verlag, Berlin and New York.

Russell, R. G., Rosenkranz, S. L., Lee, L. A., Howard, H., DiGiacomo, R. F., Bronsdon, M. A., Blakley, G. A., Tsai, C-C., and Morton, W. R. (1987). Epidemiology and etiology of diarrhea in colony-born *Macaca nemestrnia. Lab. Anim. Sci.* **37,** 309–316.

Russell, R. G., Krugner, L., Tsai, C.-C., and Ekström, R. (1988(. Prevalence of *Campylobacter* in infant, juvenile and adult laboratory primates. *Lab. Anim. Sci.* **38,** 711–714.

Russell, R. G., Blaser, M. J., Sarmiento, J. I., and Fox, J. (1989). Experimental *Campylobacter jejeuni* infection in *Macaca nemestrina. Infect. Immun.* **57,** 1438–1444.

Salam, M. A., and Bennish, M. L. (1991). Antimicrobial therapy for shigellosis. *Rev. Infect. Dis.* **13,** Suppl. 4, S332–S341.

Sasaki, T., Hirokawa, M., and Usizima, H. (1961). A spontaneous squamous cell carcinoma of the lower jaw in *Macaca mulatta. Primates* **3,** 82–87.

Sasse, D., Spornitz, U. M., and Maly, I. P. (1992). Liver architecture. *Enzyme* **46,** 8–32.

Scharschmidt, B. F. (1988). Bilirubin metabolism and hyperbilirubinemia. *In* "Cecil's Textbook of Medicine" (J. B. Wyngaarden and L. H. Smith, eds.), Vol. 1, pp. 811–814. Saunders, Philadelphia.

Schiller, L. R. (1995). Review article: Antidiarrhoeal pharmacology and therapeutics. *Aliment. Pharmacol. Ther.* **9,** 87–106.

Schiodt, M., Lackner, A., Armitage, G., Lerche, N., Greenspan, J. S., and Lowenstein, L. (1988). Oral lesions in rhesus monkeys associates with infection by simian AIDS retrovirus, serotype-I (SRV-1). *Oral Surg. Oral Med. Oral Pathol.* **65,** 50–55.

Schofield, J. C., Alves, M. E. A. F., Hughes, K. W., and Bennett, B. T. (1991). Disarming canine teeth of nonhuman primates using the submucossal vital root retention technique *Lab. Anim. Sci.* **41,** 128–133.

Schultz, A. H. (1972). Developmental abnormalities. *In* "Pathology of Simian Primates" (R. N. T.-W.-Fiennes, ed.), Part I, pp. 161–166. Karger, Basel.

Sedgwick, C., Parcher, J., and Durham, R. (1970). Atypical mycobacterial infection in the pig-tailed macaque (*Macaca nemestrina*). *J. Am. Vet. Med. Assoc.* **157,** 724–725.

Sesline, H., Schwartz, L. W., Osburn, B. I., Thoen, C. O., Holmberg, C., Anderson, J. H., and Henrickson, R. V. (1975). *Mycobacterium avium* infection in three rhesus monkeys. *J. Am. Vet. Med. Assoc.* **167,** 639–645.

Shadduck, J. A., and Pakes, S. P. (1978). Protozoal and metazoal diseases. *In* "Pathology of Laboratory Animals" (K. Benirschke, F. M. Garner, and T. C. Jones, eds.), Vol. 2, pp. 1652–1654. Springer-Verlag, Berlin and New York.

Sheldon, W. G. (1967). Fibrous gingival hyperplasia of a mustache guenon monkey (*Cercopithecus cephus*). *Lab. Anim. Care* **17,** 140–143.

Short, C. E. (1980). Fluid and electrolyte therapy. *Curr. Vet. Ther.* **7,** 49–53.

Siegal, M. I., and Sciulli, P. W. (1973). Eruption sequence of the deciduous dentition of *Papio cynocephalus. J. Med. Primatol.* **2,** 247–248.

Sirianni, J. E., and Swindler, D. R. (1985). "Growth and Development of the Pigtailed Macaque." CRC Press, Boca Raton, FL.

Skavlen, P. A., Stills, H. F., Steffan, E. K., and Middleton, C. C. (1985). Naturally occurring *Yersinia enterocolitica* septicemia in patas monkeys, (*Erythrocebus patas*). *Lab. Anim. Sci.* **35,** 488–490.

Slattum, M. M., Rosenkranz, S. L., DiGiacomo, R. F., Tsai, C.-C., and Giddens, W. E., Jr. (1989a). Amyloidosis in pigtailed macaques (*Macaca nemestrina*): Epidemiologic aspects. *Lab. Anim. Sci.* **39,** 560–566.

Slattum, M. M., Tsai, C.-C., DiGiacomo, R. F., and Giddens, W. E., Jr. (1989b). Amyloidosis in pigtailed macaques (*Macaca nemestrina*): Pathologic aspects. *Lab. Anim. Sci.* **39,** 567–570.

Smith, B. H., Crummett, T. L., and Brandt, K. L. (1994). Ages of eruption of primate teeth: A compendium for aging individuals and comparing life histories. *Yearb. Phy. Anthropol.* **37**, 177–231.

Smith, H. A., Jones, T. C., and Duncan, R. D. (1972). "Vet Pathology," 4th ed. Lea & Febinger, Philadelphia.

Snook, S. S. (1993). Focal ulcerative ileocolitis, cotton-top tamarin. *In* "Monographs on the Pathology of Laboratory Animals: Nonhuman Primates" (T. C. Jones, U. Mohr, and R. D. Hunt, eds.), Vol. 2, pp. 94–98. Springer-Verlag, Berlin and New York.

Snook, S. S., Canfield, D. R., Sehgal, P. K., and King, N. W., Jr. (1989). Focal ulcerative ileocolitis with terminal thrombocytopenic purpura in juvenile cotton top tamarins (*Saguinus oedipus*). *Lab. Anim. Sci.* **39**, 109–114.

Spiegel, A. (1929). Biologische Beobachtungen an Javamakaken *Macacus irus* F. Cuv. (*Cynomolgus L.*) *Zool. Anz.* **81**, 45–46.

Spiegel, A. (1934). Der zeitliche Ablauf der Bezahnung und des Zahnwechsels bei Javamakaken (*Macaca irus mordax Th. and Wr.*). *Z. Wiss. Zool.* **145**, 711–732.

Squire, R. A., Goodman, D. G., Valerio, M. G., Federickson, T. N., Strandberg, J. D., Levitt, M. H., Lingeman, C. H., Harshbarger, J. C., and Dawe, C. J. (1978). Digestive system and pancreas. *In* "Pathology of Laboratory Animals" (K. Benirschke, F. M. Garner, and T. C. Jones, eds.), Vol. 2, pp. 1125–1130. Springer-Verlag, Berlin and New York.

Stadtlander, C., and Stutzenberger, F. J. (1995). Adaptation of the (^{13}C) urea breath test as a noninvasive method for detection of *Helicobacter pylori* infection in squirrel monkeys (*Saimiri* spp.). *Lab. Anim. Sci.* **45**, 239–243.

Staley, E. C., Southers, J. L., Thoen, C. O., and Easley, S. P. (1995). Evaluation of tuberculin testing and measles prophylaxis procedures used in rhesus macaque quarantine/conditioning protocols. *Lab. Anim. Sci.* **45**, 125–130.

Stein, F. J., Lewis, D. H., and Sis, R. F. (1981). Acute gastric dilatation in common marmosets. *Lab. Anim. Sci.* **31**, 522–523.

Steinberg, L. M., Strom, J. L., Harbo, J. N., and Mandel, I. D. (1986). The squirrel monkey as a model in gingivitis studies. *Quintessence Int.* **17**, 113–118.

Stephenson, C. B., Jacob, J. R., Montali, R. J., Holmes, K. V., Muchmore, E., Compans, R. W., Arms, E. D., Buchmeier, M. J., and Lanford, R. E. (1991). Isolation of an arenavirus from a marmoset with callitrichid hepatitis and its serological association with disease. *J. Virol.* **65**, 3995–4000.

Stephenson, C. B., Park, J. Y., Blount, S. R. (1995). cDNA sequence analysis confirms that the etiologic agent of callitrichid hepatitis is lymphocytic chariomeningitis virus. *J. Virology* **69**, 1349–1352.

Stokes, A., Bauer, J. H., and Hudson, N. P. (1928). Experimental transmission of yellow fever to laboratory animals. *Am. J. Trop. Med.* **2**, 103–164.

Swartzendruber, D. C., and Richter, C. B. (1980). Mucous and argentaffin cells in colonic adenocarcinomas of tamarins and rats. *Lab. Invest.* **43**, 523–529.

Swenson, B. R. (1993). Protozol parasites of great apes. *In* "Zoo and Wildlife Medicine" (M. E. Fowler, ed.), Curr. Ther., Vol. 3, pp. 352–355. Saunders, Philadelphia.

Swindler, D. R., and Merrill, O. M. (1971). Spontaneous cleft lip and palate in a living non human primate *Macaca mulatta*. *Am. J. Phys. Anthropol.* **34**, 435–440.

Tabor, E. (1989). Nonhuman primate models for Non-A, Non-B Hepatitis. *Cancer Detec. Prev.* **14**(2), 221–225.

Tabor, E., Purcell, R. H., and Gerety, R. J. (1983). Primate animal models and titered inocula for the study of human Hepatitis A, Hepatitis B, and Non-A, Non-B. *J. Med. Primatol.* **12**, 305–318.

Tams, T. R. (1989). Vomiting, regurgitation and dysphagia. *In* "Textbook of Veterinary Internal Medicine" (S. Ettinger, ed.), pp. 27–32. Saunders, Philadelphia.

Tappen, N. C., and Severson, A. (1971). Sequence of eruption of permanent teeth and epiphyseal union in new world monkeys. *Folia Primatol.* **15**, 293–312.

Thoden Van Hozen, S. K. (1967). Does captivity influence the morphogenesis of animal the skull and teeth? *Ned. T????? T????.* **74**, Suppl., 17–42.

Thomson, F. N., Schulte, J. M., and Bertsch, M. L. (1979). Root canal procedure for disarming nonhuman primates. *Lab. Anim. Sci.* **29**, 382–386.

Thorington, R. W., Jr., and Vorek, R. E. (1976). Observations on the geographic variation and skeletal development of *A?????Sci.* **26**, 1006–1021.

Ticehurst, J., Rhodes, J. L. L., Krawczynski, K., Asher, L. V. S., Engler, W. F., Mensing, T. L., Caudill, J. D., Sjögren, M. H., Hoke, C. H., LeDuc, J. W., Bradley, D. W., and Binn, L. N. (1992). Infection of owl monkeys (*Aotus tivirgatus*) and cynomolgus monkeys (*Macaca fascicularis*) with Hepatitis 5 virus from Mexico. *J. Infect. Dis.* **165**, 835–845.

Toft, J. D. (1982). The pathoparasitology ??????? entary tract and pancreas of nonhuman primates: A review. *Vet. Pathol.* **1**, ?????, pp. 44–92.

Toft, J. D., Schmidt, R. E., and DePaoli, A. (1976). Intestinal polyposis associated with oxyurid parasites in a chimpanzee (*Pan troglodytes*). *J. Med. Primatol.* **5**, 360–364.

Torgerson, R., Chalifoux, L., King, N., Ringler, D., and Snook, S. (1992). Antibiotic associated pseudomembranous entercolitis in new world primates. *Vet. Pathol.* **29**, 454.

Tribe, G. W., and Fleming, M. P. (1983). Biphasic enteritis in imported cynomolgus (*Macaca fascicularis*) monkeys infected with *Shigella, Salmonella* and *Campylobacter* species. *Lab. Anim.* **17**, 65–69.

Tsai, C.-C. (1993). Fibromatosis in macaques infected with type D retroviruses. *In* "Monographs on the Pathology of Laboratory Animals: Nonhuman Primates" (T. C. Jones, U. Mohr, and R. D. Hunt, eds.), Vol. I, pp. 48–57. Springer-Verlag, Berlin and New York.

Turnquist, J. E., and Kessler, M. J. (1990). Dental eruption in free-ranging *Macaca mulatta* on Cayo Santiago. *Am. J. Phys. Anthropol.* **81**, 309 (abstr.).

Uchida, T., Win, K. M., Suzuki, K., Komatsu, K., Iida, F., Shikata, T., Rikihisa, T., Mizuno, K., Soe, S., Myint, H., Tin, K. M., and Nakane, K. (1990). Serial transmission of a putative causative virus of enterically transmitted Non-A, Non-B Hepatitis to *Macaca fascicularis* and *Macaca mulatta*. *Jpn. J. Exp. Med.* **60**, 13–21.

Walker, R. J., Caldwell, M. B., Lee, E. C., Guerry, P., Trust, T. J., and Ruiz-Palacios, G. M. (1986). Pathophysiology of *Campylobacter* enteritis. *Microbiol. Rev.* **50**, 81–94.

Watts, E. S. (1977). Some guidelines for collection and reporting of nonhuman primate growth data. *Lab. Anim. Sci.* **27**, 85–89.

Willis, G. P., Kapustin, N. K., Warrick, J. M., and Hopkins, D. T. (1996). Reducing dental calculus formation in lemurs. *Proc. Annu. Meet., Am. Assoc. Zoo Vet. 1996*, pp. 586–586.

Willoughby, D. P. (1978). "All About Gorillas." A. S. Barnes & Noble, South Brunswick, NJ.

Wilson, H. D., McCormick, J. B., and Feely, J. C. (1976). *Yersinia enterocolitica* infection in a 4 month old infant associated with infection in household dogs. *J. Pediatr.* **89**, 767–769.

Wolf, R. H., Smetana, H. F., Allen, W. P., and Felsenfeld, A. D. (1974). Pathology and clinical history of delta herpesvirus infection in patas monkeys. *Lab. Anim. Sci.* **24**, 218–221.

Wolff, P. L. (1993). Parasites of new world primates. *Zoo Wild Anim. Med.* **3**, 378–389.

Zuckerman, A. J., Scalise, G., Mazaheri, M. R., Kremastinou, J., Howard, C. R., and Sorenson, K. (1975). Transmission of hepatitis B to the rhesus monkey. *Dev. Biol. Stand.* **30**, 236–239.

Chapter 11

Diseases of the Musculoskeletal System

Kenneth P. H. Pritzker and Matt J. Kessler

I. INTRODUCTION

Among primate species, there is widespread variation in body mass, body proportion, and locomotive biomechanics (Preuschoft, 1989; Demes and Gunther, 1989; Ruff, 1989). Notwithstanding the major differences in functional morphology and scale, growth, maturation, composition, metabolism, and biomechanical properties of nonhuman primate musculoskeletal tissues closely resemble those of humans. Further, these similarities exist despite profound differences in habitat, diet, and locomotor behavior (Rawlins and Kessler, 1986; R. G. Rawlins, 1976). Thus, it is not surprising that nonhuman primates are subject to natural musculoskeletal diseases similar to humans. Further, experimentally induced musculoskeletal diseases in nonhuman primates resemble natural diseases of humans exposed to similar pathogenic agents. Most diseases described in this chapter are spontaneous and sporadic. Their principal values for medical research include

1. Generalization of musculoskeletal diseases found in humans to other species in the primate order as well as exclusion of disease restriction to human primates.
2. Exclusion of factors present in human environments but absent in nonhuman primates as obligate etiologic or pathogenic factors in musculoskeletal disease.
3. Recognition of common pathogenic factors for musculoskeletal disease present in both human and nonhuman primate environments.
4. For some disorders, recognition that the nonhuman primate may be used as models for human musculoskeletal diseases (Cornelius and Rosenberg, 1983).

Criteria for animal models of musculoskeletal disease have been discussed extensively for osteoarthritis (Pritzker, 1994b), but similar considerations prevail for other musculoskeletal disorders. At present, only a few spontaneous nonhuman primate musculoskeletal diseases such as osteoarthritis and periodontitis are suitable for comparative research purposes. For a few other diseases, most notably nutritional deficiencies (vitamins C and D), type II collagen-induced arthritis, and osteoporosis, the nonhuman primate has proved useful for research in experimentally induced model diseases. For both spontaneous and experimentally induced musculoskeletal diseases, the resemblance to human disease is limited by temporal differences in factors such as the response to pain, wound healing rate, hormonal status (e.g., menopause), and aging. Nonetheless, comparison between human and nonhuman musculoskeletal diseases can provide insight into musculoskeletal evolutionary adaptations among primate species. As a practical matter, this knowledge can be useful in preventing musculoskeletal disease in captive primate populations.

II. ARTHRITIS

Arthritis can be broadly classified into degenerative and inflammatory disorders. Degenerative arthritis represents a broad class of chronic joint diseases in which the primary target tissue is articular cartilage and/or subchondral bone. The classification "degenerative joint disease" is complicated because some types of arthritis, most notably crystal-associated arthritis such as gout and calcium pyrophosphate dihydrate (CPPD) crystal deposition disease arthropathy, have both inflammatory and degenerative components. Further, secondary degenerative arthritis can supervene on joints initially damaged by inflammatory processes. Inflammatory arthritis represents joint diseases that affect vascularized articular tissues primarily. Although joint capsules, ligaments, and tendons can be affected, the most prominent lesions are seen in the synovium and the synovial space. Inflammatory arthritis is usually classified on the basis of the infectious etiologic agent where known, e.g., mycoplasma, or by the clinical pattern of joint involvement, e.g., rheumatoid arthritis. For each arthritic disease, the reaction of each tissue within the joint, articular cartilage, subchondral bone, synovium, synovial fluid, ligament, and capsule varies in character, intensity, and specificity, depending on the type, activity, and stage of arthritis. This section discusses the characteristics of each type of arthritis affecting nonhuman primates in the previously mentioned context.

A. Joint Biology

The relatively few studies of normal nonhuman primate joints indicate that while nonhuman primate articular tissues may differ in some gross morphologic features (Renxian et al., 1987; Le Minor, 1990), there is remarkable similarity to humans in microscopic structural features (Pidd and Gardner, 1987; Chateauvert et al., 1990; Luder and Schroeder, 1992), tissue composition (Stanescu et al., 1980; Stanescu and Pham, 1986; Chateauvert et al., 1989; Grynpas et al., 1994), biomechanical properties (Bourdella et al., 1931; Athanasiou et al., 1991, 1995), and reaction to injury (Gibson et al., 1976; Zeman et al., 1989, 1991; Malinin et al., 1994). Of particular interest for arthritis models, the knee joint articular contact surfaces of the Cercopithecidae, which includes rhesus macaques, closely resembles that of humans (Renxian et al., 1987). Scanning electron microscopy of baboon (*Papio anubis*) knee joint cartilage demonstrated that these primates share with humans the general structural features of cartilage matrix, namely collagen fiber architecturally arranged in a proteoglycan gel (Pidd and Gardner, 1987). This similarity extends to the organization of chondrocytes within articular cartilage (Chateauvert et al., 1990), the mineralization pattern of the deep cartilage matrix (Luder and Schroeder, 1992), and the response to cartilage transplantation (Kandel et al., 1983; Malinin et al., 1994). Biochemically, nonhuman primate articular cartilage contains type II collagen (Grynpas et al., 1994), noncollagenous proteins (Chaminade et al., 1982), and proteoglycans (Stanescu et al., 1980; Stanescu and Pham, 1986) in a distribution similar to humans. Estrogen receptors have been found in baboon chondrocytes (Sheridan et al., 1985).

Cartilage lesions induced by intraarticular injection of specific agents provide an example of how nonhuman primate cartilage reacts to injury similar to humans but differently from other species such as the rabbit (Tenenbaum *et al.,* 1981b; Ohira and Ishikawa, 1986). Unlike rabbits, repeated intraarticular corticosteroid injections into the knee joint of the cynomolgus macaque (*Macaca fascicularis*) resulted in only superficial fibrillation and degeneration of cartilage without any increase in calcification (Gibson *et al.,* 1976). In other studies, Zeman *et al.* (1989, 1991) induced hemarthrosis in rhesus macaque knee joints by intraarticular injection of autologous blood. This injury elicited a reaction consisting predominantly of synovial cell proliferation and synoviocyte erythrophagocytosis with only transient and mild changes in the articular cartilage morphology. This reaction was similar in time (7–14 days) and extent to that found in human spontaneous hemarthrosis.

B. Arthritis: Natural Prevalence

Interest in nonhuman primate arthritis is relatively recent. For example, Ruch's (1959c) comprehensive monograph devotes only one page to arthritis noting osteologic findings and sporadic cases, but failing to classify or otherwise describe these disorders. These early studies demonstrated the presence of arthritis in skeletons from a variety of primates, including the gorilla, orangutan, baboon, and mandrill (Rollet, 1891; Fox, 1939; Schultz, 1939; Randall, 1942; Ruch, 1959c). Fox failed to find arthritis in 36 macaque skeletons examined, but made passing mention of a macaque with arthritis at the London zoo (Fox, 1939; Ruch, 1959c). In the same institution, arthritis was noted in living primates as early as 1939 (Hamerton, 1939; Ruch, 1959c). The arthritis found in skeletons of large primates was attributed to the size and relative weight of these animals. The relative paucity of arthritis in laboratory primates was attributed to the use of small and juvenile animals for biomedical research. From these early observations, the implicit conclusion was that arthritis was a disorder of aging, accelerated by the body mass bearing on joints.

Although the relative prevalence may differ, it is now recognized that nonhuman primates appear to be subject to the entire spectrum of arthritic diseases (Rothschild and Woods, 1993). As with other species, these diseases are seldom documented in wild or feral animals, partly because the diseases generally occur in the aged and partly because field observers do not concentrate on disease recognition. A prominent example is the degenerative osteoarthritis in rhesus macaques at the Caribbean Primate Research Center in Puerto Rico. Despite a clinical prevalence of >25%, this disease was not widely recognized until DeRousseau (1978) conducted her doctoral dissertation research at Cayo Santiago in the 1970s and a complex degenerative joint disease was discovered in a nonhuman primate by Kandel *et al.* (1983; Pritzker *et al.,* 1989) in 1981. A second example is alkaptonuria, which has been observed in the cynomolgus macaque (Walker *et al.,* 1988). Although this condition is associated with arthritis in humans, this has not yet been described in nonhuman primates.

Joint disease in nonhuman primates can be extensive without obvious clinical physical signs. An example is the case of Legg-Calvé-Perthes disease described in a lowland gorilla (Douglass, 1981). This disorder, in which the capitular femoral epiphysis becomes necrotic with secondary deformation of femoral head, was discovered only because the lesions were observed on routine radiography.

C. Degenerative Arthritis

Particularly in the North American literature, degenerative joint disease and osteoarthritis are often used as synonymous terms encompassing a wide spectrum of arthritic disorders (Mankin *et al.,* 1986; Watt and Dieppe, 1990; Cushnaghan and Dieppe, 1991; Schumacher, 1992). This classification tends to confuse our understanding as it groups together specific forms of degenerative arthritis such as posttraumatic arthropathy, acromegalic arthropathy, crystal-associated arthropathy, and ochronotic arthropathy, that have diverse etiologic factors and pathogenic mechanisms. Further, this broad disease classification confuses our approach to understanding the pathogenic mechanisms of "primary" osteoarthritis, a set of conditions considered separately later in which the etiologic factors are less well understood.

As in humans, nonhuman primates are subject to degenerative arthritic diseases in specific joints. The spontaneous temporomandibular joint arthropathy that occurrs in baboons is illustrative (Haskin *et al.,* 1993; Haskin and Cameron, 1994). This disorder, which progresses with age, is characterized by pigmentation and perforation of the fibrocartilagenous meniscal discs with cartilage erosion in the adjacent joint surfaces. This condition has been replicated by perforating the temporomandibular meniscal disc of adult cynomolgus macaques (*Macaca fascicularis*) using surgical electrocautery (Helmy *et al.,* 1988). This surgical procedure led to synovial hyperplasia and synovial chondrometaplasia (Helmy *et al.,* 1989). Surgical repair using a synovial flap over the perforation restored the integrity of the temporomandibular disc and prevented degeneration of the cartilaginous joint surfaces (Sharawy *et al.,* 1994).

A model of one form of degenerative arthritis, pigmented villonodular synovitis, has been developed in rhesus macaques (Singh *et al.,* 1969). The animals were subjected to weekly intraarticular injections into the knee and ankle joints of autologous blood, plasma from autologous blood, or 4% gum acacia solution. Both the iron/dextrin and the autologous blood-injected groups developed pain and limitation of movement. Histologically, the synovium showed villous fronds with synovial lining cell hyperplasia, hemosiderin deposition, extensive macrophage infiltration, and collagen fiber formation. The histologic changes were greater in the iron/dextrin group than in animals receiving autologous blood. The plasma-injected group showed minimal inflammation whereas the gum acacia group showed synovial edema with infiltration of chronic inflammatory cells.

This study demonstrated that pigmented villonodular arthritis can be modeled by iron or blood intraarticular injection and that gum acacia injection was capable of including a local chronic inflammatory arthritis with minimal synovial lining cell hyperplasia.

D. Osteoarthritis

Osteoarthritis, or osteoarthrosis as it is known in the European literature, is a group of degenerative joint diseases of unknown etiology that share many clinical features, morphologic appearances, and histologic processes. Within the group, the disorders differ in the progression of articular structural changes. For example, in some forms of osteoarthritis, the disease primarily affects articular cartilage, in others, subchondral bone; and still others, articular cartilage and bone simultaneously.

Osteoarthritis has been defined as a group of arthritic disorders usually involving multiple joints characterized at the tissue level by degenerative, regenerative, and reparative structural changes in cartilage, synovium, and bone (Pritzker, 1992, 1997; Gahunia et al., 1995a,b). Osteoarthritis has been present since ancient times (Dieppe and Rogers, 1993; Rothschild, 1993b; Rothschild and Martin, 1993; Jurmain and Kilgore, 1995); it is geographically widespread and affects many species besides humans (Sokoloff, 1960; Jurmain, 1989; Pritzker, 1994b). Because it is a leading cause of chronic disability in Western human populations, osteoarthritis is a major public health problem (Badley et al., 1994; Felson et al., 1995).

Based on osteologic criteria, osteoarthritis affects many Old World nonhuman primate species (Taylor et al., 1955; Sokoloff, 1956; Stecher, 1958a,b; DeRousseau, 1978, 1988; Rothschild and Woods, 1992a; Jurmain and Kilgore, 1995), including the gorilla (Gorilla gorilla), chimpanzee (Pan), gibbon (Hylobates), baboon (Papio), and rhesus and cynomolgus monkeys (Macaca mulatta, M. fascicularis). Although there are differences in joint involvement between wild and captive species, the knee joint is commonly affected in arthritic animals in both environments (Lovell, 1990a,b, 1991; Rothschild and Woods, 1992a).

The etiologic factors that contribute to osteoarthritis are poorly understood. Former simplistic ideas that osteoarthritis was caused only by mechanical wear and tear or that osteoarthritis is primarily a disease of aging have been disproved by formal critical studies, some involving nonhuman primates (Pritzker et al., 1989, 1990; Chateauvert et al., 1989, 1990; Carlson et al., 1994; Gahunia et al., 1995a,b). Although joint injury and secondary degenerative arthritis can be induced naturally and experimentally by excessive trauma, this is an insufficient explanation for the symmetrical polyarthritis affecting large joints commonly seen in osteoarthritis (Pritzker, 1994b). Further, study populations of free-ranging nonhuman primates in which osteoarthritis is prevalent do not appear subject to

excessive locomotor trauma (Kessler et al., 1985). Similarly, it is now recognized in both human (Hogan and Pritzker, 1985) and nonhuman primates (Macaca mulatta) (Chateauvert et al., 1989, 1990) that osteoarthritis begins shortly after skeletal maturation but may persist and progress with age. Many constitutional, environmental, and biochemical factors have been studied in an effort to elucidate the pathogenesis of osteoarthritis (Howell et al., 1992). Among the constitutional factors, osteoarthritis appears as a polygenetic disease. In both human and nonhuman primates, this disease is more common in females than in males and, in at least a subset, may be associated with obesity (Carlson et al., 1996). The resemblance of the joint lesions to acromegalic arthropathy (Bluestone et al., 1971; Layton et al., 1988) suggests that increased circulating growth factors (including the hormone insulin) or an increased tissue response to growth factors may be implicated in osteoarthritis pathogenesis. An intriguing observation seen in the Cayo Santiago macaque population is the frequency of obesity (7–10%) (Schwartz et al., 1993) and the association of obesity with type II diabetes mellitus (Howard et al., 1986; Schwartz, 1989; Howard and Yasuda, 1990). As yet, no study has attempted to correlate these observations with the prevalence of spontaneous osteoarthritis in this population. Nonhuman primate studies have demonstrated that osteoarthritis occurs independently of dietary and habitat differences between humans and rhesus macaques (Chateauvert et al., 1989; Pritzker et al., 1989; Chateauvert et al., 1990).

Based on comparative primate studies, Alexander (1994) has advanced the idea suggested by Harrison et al. (1953) that synovial joints require frequent motion over the full range of the articular surfaces to maintain anatomical integrity and function. This hypothesis is supported by the osteologic studies of Rothschild and Woods (1993) who found that osteoarthritis was very uncommon in free-ranging arboreal New World primates. From a human evolutionary perspective, it has been suggested that the reduction of full joint excursion formerly required for arboreal movement contributes to the development of osteoarthritis (Alexander, 1994). Like humans, adult rhesus macaques are terrestrial animals that utilize only a portion of their joint excursion capability (R. G. Rawlins, 1976). In these animals, passive joint excursion decreased with age (DeRousseau et al., 1983; Turnquist and Kessler, 1989). However, free-ranging animals were subject both to more restricted passive joint extension and to more osteoarthritis than caged animals. These findings indicate that at least a portion of the documented restriction in joint motion may be secondary to osteoarthritis (Kessler et al., 1986).

Clinically, osteoarthritis in nonhuman primates can present with a reduction of active joint movement, often resulting in a gait disorder (Bayne, 1985; DeRousseau et al., 1986). Limitation of joint movement related to joint contracture is common in many forms of arthritis and in nonarticular diseases such as amyloidosis associated with severe debilitation (Blanchard et al., 1986). In contrast, osteoarthritis is usually observed in other-

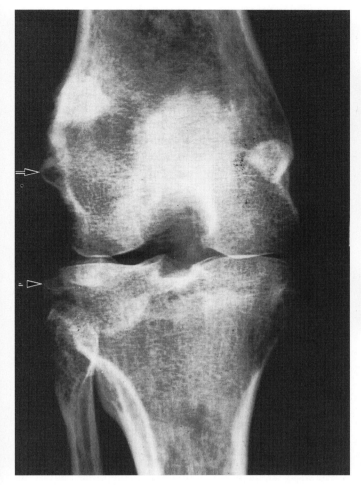

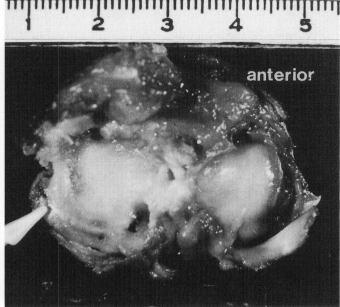

Fig. 2. A right tibial plateau from a rhesus macaque with moderate osteo-arthritis. Note the irregular surface indicative of cartilage fibrillation. The medial surface (⇑) is more severely affected.

Fig. 1. Anterior posterior specimen X-ray of knee joint of a rhesus macaque with severe osteoarthritis. Note the loss of joint space, periarticular bone sclerosis, and osteophyte formation (↑).

wise healthy animals. In advanced disease, visible hypertrophic deformation of the joints can be seen (Chateauvert *et al.,* 1989; Pritzker *et al.,* 1989). In osteoarthritic rhesus macaques, hypertrophic deformation of the proximal and distal interphalangeal joints of the hands has also been observed (Lim *et al.,* 1995, 1996). Unlike humans, joints at the thumb base were spared, a consequence of major differences in functional anatomy. Unlike humans, synovial effusion is rarely observed. It has been suggested that limitation of joint movement may affect adversely the social rank of nonhuman primates, but this has not been well documented. Osteoarthritis can affect the spine, producing visible dorsal kyphotic deformity. However, as described later, fixed deformity of the spine is more often the result of spondyloarthropathy, a disease with a different pathogenesis and clinical course (Rothschild, 1993a; Rothschild and Martin, 1993; Rothschild and Woods, 1989, 1993; Rothschild *et al.,* 1997).

Conventional radiography of the affected joints is the clinical technique used to confirm the diagnosis of osteoarthritis. Radiologic features include narrowing of the joint space, increased radiodensity (sclerosis of the subchondral bone), remodeling (deformation of the articular plate), subchondral bone cysts, and the demonstration of marginal osteophytes (Kessler *et al.,* 1986; Pritzker *et al.,* 1989; Gahunia *et al.,* 1995a) (Fig. 1). Although research has been extensive, no serological biomarker has been found that is acceptable for diagnosis or assessment of osteoarthritis (Carlson *et al.,* 1995; Lohmander *et al.,* 1995).

The gross and microscopic lesions of nonhuman primate osteoarthritis, well studied in rhesus and cynomolgus macaques (Chateauvert *et al.,* 1990; Pritzker, 1992; Carlson *et al.,* 1994; Gahunia *et al.,* 1995a,b), appear identical to the human disease. On gross examination, early disease is characterized by the softening of cartilage and superficial fibrillation (Fig. 2). As the disease progresses, these changes are accompanied by erosion of the articular cartilage, leaving articular surfaces consisting of eburnated bone. With advanced disease, the articular surface deforms and osteophytes develop at the articular surface margins. Microscopically, cartilage matrix fibrillation, condensation of collagen, proteoglycan depletion in the cartilage superficial layers, chondrocyte necrosis, and chondrocyte proliferation are features (Fig. 3). The subchondral bone is thicker than normal (Carlson *et al.,* 1996) and shows increased osteoblasts and osteoclasts on the bone surfaces. There is a slight

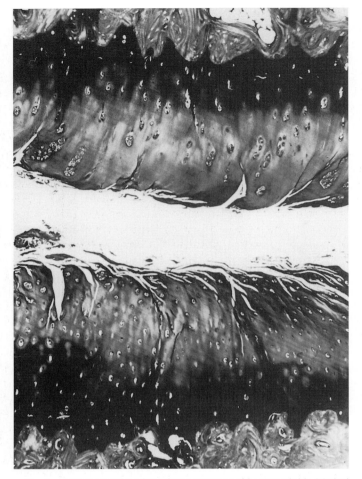

Fig. 3. Articular cartilage from rhesus macaque with osteoarthritis. Marked fibrillation and hypercellularity of the cartilage are shown. Toluidine blue stain. Magnification: ×25.

Most experimental models of osteoarthritis, including experimentally induced nonhuman primate osteoarthritis (Lufti, 1975; Helmy *et al.,* 1988), are essentially models of a single episode of joint injury and repair rather than generalized disease. In contrast, spontaneous osteoarthritis in the nonhuman primate, particularly rhesus (Pritzker *et al.,* 1989, 1990; Pritzker, 1994b) and cynomolgus (Carlson *et al.,* 1994, 1995) macaques, is now well accepted as an excellent model for human osteoarthritis with many research advantages over most other experimentally induced models or even the human disease itself (Sokoloff, 1990; Pritzker, 1994b). Comparative biology has demonstrated similarities (female preponderance, obesity association, pattern of joint involvement) and differences (diet, habitat) between human and nonhuman primates with the disease. The model has been used to explore and define the natural history (Chateauvert *et al.,* 1989), histopathology (Chateauvert *et al.,* 1990; Pritzker, 1992), cartilage biochemistry (Chateauvert *et al.,* 1989, Grynpas *et al.,* 1990, 1994; Carlson *et al.,* 1995), and bone mineral abnormalities (Grynpas *et al.,* 1993b) associated with osteoarthritis. Further, because the natural disease can be studied in cross-sectional age sequences through the technique of advanced magnetic resonance imaging, the model has been instrumental in defining disease progression (Gahunia *et al.,* 1993, 1995a,b). High-resolution magnetic resonance imaging has demonstrated a layered pattern in normal articular cartilage and its progressive disruption with osteoarthritis (Fig. 4). This in turn has led to the clarification of early osteoarthritic lesions and to concepts related to the heterogenous sequence of matrix degeneration and regeneration that characterizes osteoarthritis progression in articular cartilage (Gahunia *et al.,* 1995a). Indeed, the utility of this nonhuman primate as a spontaneous osteoarthritis model appears limited only by the availability of sufficient mature and aged animals in appropriate study environments.

E. Spontaneous Osteonecrosis of the Knee

Spontaneous osteonecrosis of the knee is a disorder presenting in humans with sudden pain in the knee (Houpt *et al.,* 1983). The usual underlying lesion is a microfracture through the articular plate of the femoral condyle. The condition is usually self-limited, persisting either as a central defect of the articular surface or as healing by elaboration of fibrocartilage. The lesion is often associated with a "loose body" containing necrotic bone covered by fibrocartilage. By the tissue within the "loose body," this lesion can be distinguished from osteochondritis dissecans, a disorder of aberrant growth plate within articular cartilage. Spontaneous osteonecrosis of the knee has been observed in two rhesus macaques from the Caribbean Primate Research Center (Pritzker *et al.,* 1997). Fibrocartilage healing in the defect was demonstrated on histopathological examination. Although this lesion has been associated with osteoporosis in humans, osteoporosis was not eviden in primate cases.

proliferation of synovial lining cells with a modest lymphocytic, inflammatory infiltrate in the synovium. In advanced osteoarthritis, the synovium shows fibrosis arranged parallel to the synovial surface as well as circumferential to synovial capillary blood vessels. Biochemically, osteoarthritic cartilage is characterized in early disease by edema, increased glycosaminoglycans, and increased concentrations of calcium and phosphorus (Chateauvert *et al.,* 1989; Grynpas *et al.,* 1990), features that are similar to the human disease (Pritzker *et al.,* 1987). Like humans with advanced disease, nonhuman primate osteoarthritic hyaline articular cartilage shows proteoglycan depletion and expresses reparative type I collagen (Grynpas *et al.,* 1994). Although there is no specific therapy for osteoarthritis, provision of an environment that allows adequate exercise and control of obesity may delay the onset and reduce the rate of progression of the disease.

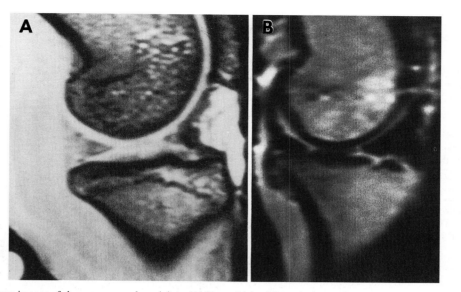

Fig. 4. Magnetic resonance images of rhesus macaque knee joints. (A) Normal joint. The articular cartilage demonstrates higher signal intensity, a smooth contour, and uniform thickness. (B) Osteoarthritis. Narrowing of the joint space is seen. The articular cartilage shows focal loss and focal increase of signal intensity, thinning, and focal disruption of the articular surface.

F. Crystal-Associated Arthritis

Of the common crystal-associated arthritic disorders that affect humans, gout (monosodium urate) remains undescribed in nonhuman primates, and calcific periarthritis (calcium apatite arthropathy) is the subject of only a few case reports (Thompson *et al.,* 1959; Line *et al.,* 1984; Van Linthoudt *et al.,* 1992). Of note, calcium pyrophosphate dihydrate crystal arthropathy has been found in several primate species and is useful as an aging indicator as well as a model disease (Kandel *et al.,* 1983; Roberts *et al.,* 1984a,b; Pritzker *et al.,* 1985, 1989; Renlund *et al.,* 1985, 1986, 1989). In contrast, CPPD crystal arthropathy has been documented only rarely in other mammals, principally in the dog [two cases (Gibson and Roenigk, 1972; Heimann *et al.,* 1990)].

Common to these diseases is that the pathogenic agents, crystals, can be detected easily in affected tissues. Further, the structure of the pathogenic agent, the crystal, is specific and can be identified with great precision. As the crystal deposition is usually the result of known metabolic processes, the pathogenic mechanisms of articular crystal deposition can be relatively well understood.

1. Calcium Pyrophosphate Dihydrate Crystal Arthropathy

Calcium pyrophosphate dihydrate crystal arthropathy is a very common degenerative arthritis in humans. In humans and nonhuman primates, this disease is most frequently associated with advanced age (Kandel *et al.,* 1983; Roberts *et al.,* 1984a,b; Renlund *et al.,* 1986; Pritzker *et al.,* 1988, 1989; Ryan and

McCarty, 1993; Pritzker, 1994a). More rarely, CPPD crystal arthropathy has been reported in certain human families or in such conditions as hypercalcemia, e.g., hyperparathyroidism, hypomagnesium, hypophosphatasia (familial deficiency in alkaline phosphatase), or iron excess (hemochromatosis) (Ryan and McCarty, 1993; Pritzker, 1994a). Unlike urate crystals in gout, CPPD crystal deposition appears restricted to articular tissues. Investigations of pathogenesis have been centered on the special characteristics of these tissues that facilitate crystal formation. As tissue ionic calcium concentrations are constant within a very narrow range, studies have focused on pyrophosphate ion formation and matrix characteristics that promote or inhibit crystal nucleation (Pritzker *et al.,* 1985). It is known that the source of extracellular pyrophosphate generation is at the chondrocyte cell membrane and that soluble pyrophosphate accumulates in cartilage matrix prior to crystallization (Ryan and McCarty, 1995). Although osteoarthritis can coexist with CPPD crystal arthropathy, cartilage lesions associated with crystals are usually distinct and related to the differences in tissue compliance between the crystal-bearing and the non-crystal-bearing cartilage matrix. Superficial to the crystal deposits, the cartilage matrix becomes edematous, permitting the crystals to migrate to and shed from the articular surface. Once the crystals reach the synovial fluid space, the crystals can incite the acute inflammation characteristic of pseudogout (Ryan and McCarty, 1993). There is no specific therapy for this disease.

The specific mechanisms of how pyrophosphate is formed and whether pyrophosphate is generated in excess or degraded too slowly and which enzymes (NTP pyrophosphohydrolase or alkaline phosphatase) may be involved are the subjects of much current study (Tenenbaum *et al.,* 1981a; Xu *et al.,* 1991, 1994; Derfus *et al.,* 1995; Ryan and McCarty, 1995; Shinozaki *et al.,* 1995; Shinozaki and Pritzker, 1995, 1996). Among nonhuman primates, CPPD arthropathy has been found in rhesus macaque (*Macaca mulatta*), Barbary ape (*M. sylvanus*), and mandrill (*Mandrillus leukophaeus*) (Renlund *et al.,* 1989). Although acute arthritis with synovial effusion has been reported, most cases have been associated with fixed joint deformities or have been asymptomatic. Radiographic examination of large joints such as the knee can demonstrate cartilage mineralization, as linear radiodensities corresponding to meniscal calcification. Occasionally, more extensive chondrocalcinosis in which the articular cartilage is also involved can be seen (Rubenstein and Pritzker, 1989). However, in macaques, it has been difficult to visualize chondrocalcinosis by radiography (Kessler *et al.,* 1986) (Fig. 5).

Calcium pyrophosphate dihydrate crystal arthropathy preferentially affects large joints and intervertebral discs. Gross examination demonstrates the crystals as punctate white deposits *wthin* the articular tissues (Fig. 6). This contrasts with gout in which the crystals aggregate as a white paste *on* the articular surfaces. Calcium pyrophosphate dihydrate crystals are commonly seen within meniscal fibrocartilage, but in advanced cases they can also be found in hyaline articular cartilage, tendon insertions, and synovium.

With polarized light microscopy using a λ compensator, CPPD crystals can be detected with considerable precision in synovial fluids as blue intracellular and extracellular positively birefringent rhomboid paralleliped crystals 1–20 μm in length. The microscopic detection of these crystals in tissues is dependent on the examination of undecalcified sections preferably unstained under compensated polarized light (Fig. 7). The identification of CPPD crystals is a more elaborate task involving X-ray or electron powder diffraction analysis (Cheng *et al.,* 1983).

The definitive accepted criteria for the diagnosis of CPPD crystal arthropathy is the detection of CPPD crystals in synovial fluid or articular tissue by compensated polarized light microscopy (McCarty, 1992). To date, CPPD crystals have been found only in soft articular tissues. Although putative CPPD crystals have been observed in bone (Keen *et al.,* 1991), these crystals were later discovered not to be CPPD but rather calcium hydrogen phosphate dihydrate ($CaHPO_4.2H_2O$) (brushite). Brushite is a calcium phosphate crystal with similar compensated polarized light microscopy morphology and a Ca:P elemental ratio of 1:1 identical to CPPD (Keen *et al.,* 1995).

Based on naked eye observations of skeletal osseous articular surface concretions and indentations, Rothschild attempted to extend the definition of CPPD crystal arthropathy in human (Rothschild *et al.,* 1992) and nonhuman primates to broader criteria (Rothschild and Woods, 1992a, 1993; Rothschild, 1996). To date, CPPD crystals have not been detected in osseous material. It is likely that Rothschild's "CPPD arthropathy" are osseous changes from a non-crystal-related arthropathy. However, the possibility remains, at least in some cases, that his

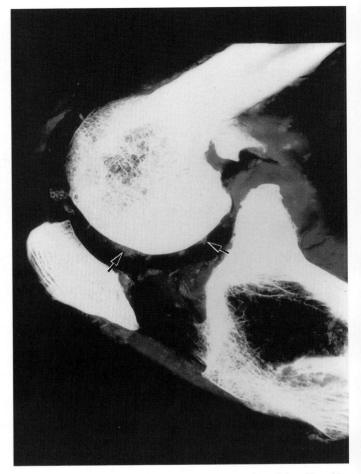

Fig. 5. Lateral specimen X-ray of rhesus macaque knee joint affected by calcium pyrophosphate dihydrate (CPPD) crystal arthropathy. Radiodensities representing cartilage and meniscal calcifications are seen (↑).

findings may represent the osseous substrate of CPPD crystal deposition disease. To resolve this controversy, additional studies that correlate the presence of CPPD crystals in cartilage with macroscopic changes in bone are needed.

Ultrastructurally, CPPD crystals form as aggregates in articular cartilage at the junction of the territorial and interterritorial matrix, predominantly in the midzone. In most studies, the crystals appear unrelated to either matrix vesicles or collagen fibers (Boivin and Lagier, 1983; Pritzker *et al.,* 1988). Formation of CPPD crystals without a specific relationship to collagen fibers has been observed in model hydrogels (Pritzker *et al.,* 1978; Hunter *et al.,* 1987). Nonetheless, Beutler *et al.* (1993) found CPPD crystals aligned to collagen fibers in synovium. In these studies, however, the crystals formed in a matrix with dense parallel collagen fibers. Therefore, it was not surprising to see the crystals in this tissue aligned parallel to the collagen fiber direction.

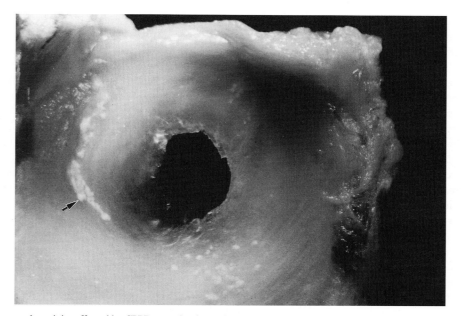

Fig. 6. Rhesus macaque knee joint affected by CPPD crystal arthropathy. Extensive punctate calcifications within the meniscus are observed (↑).

To date, it has not been possible to induce CPPD crystal formation experimentally in articular tissues of any animals. The association of CPPD crystal arthropathy in nonhuman primates with traumatic hemarthrosis has been suggested. However, following experimentally induced hemarthrosis, no CPPD crystals were found in joints (Roberts *et al.,* 1984b; Zeman *et al.,* 1989). As expected, intraarticular CPPD crystal injection does reproduce the pathological features of acute CPPD crystal arthritis (Fam *et al.,* 1995).

As a disease model, naturally occurring CPPD crystal arthropathy in aged macaque primates has been of great utility and offers much promise for future research. Prior to its description in the barbary ape (*Macaca sylvanus*), CPPD arthropathy was unknown in primates other than humans. At that time, al-

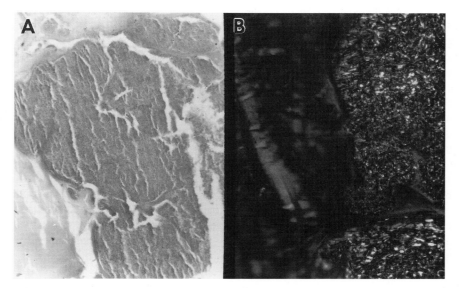

Fig. 7. Rhesus macaque articular cartilage with CPPD crystal deposition. (A) With conventional sections, the crystals appear as granular aggregates forming "geodes" with cartilage. Hematoxylin and eosin section. Magnification: ×250. (B) Positively birefringent crystals are most easily seen in unstained sections viewed under compensated polarized light. Unstained section. Magnification: ×250.

though there had been a case reported in a dog (Gibson and Roenigk, 1972), the common articular calcification in other species was calcium apatite (Yosipovitch and Glimcher, 1972; Woodard et al., 1982). The discovery of CPPD crystal deposition disease in nonhuman primate joints demonstrated that primate articular tissues share similar aging processes with humans. In rhesus macaques, there appears to be significant differences in the two populations found to have the disease. In the Cayo Santiago population at the Caribbean Primate Research Center, the animals were generally healthy, free-ranging, and old (Renlund et al., 1986). At the Tulane (formerly Delta) Regional Primate Research Center, five of six animals were debilitated from chronic diarrhea or other infectious diseases (Roberts, 1993b; Roberts et al., 1984b). This suggests that an electrolyte disorder may have contributed to the disease pathogenesis in this group. When sufficient animals become available, the presence of CPPD crystal arthropathy in nonhuman primates will present an opportunity to study the comparative natural history of this important disease of aging humans.

2. Calcium Apatite Crystal Deposition Disease

Calcium apatite crystal deposition disease is a heterogenous group of disorders in which calcium phosphate [$Ca_{10}(PO_4)_5OH$] crystals form in articular or periarticular tissues (Schumacher et al., 1997, 1981; Fam et al., 1981; McCarty et al., 1981; Kandel et al., 1986; Fam and Rubenstein, 1989; Halverson, 1992; Fam and Pritzker, 1992; Slavin et al., 1993). In humans, apatite crystal deposition disease can present an acute arthritis stimulating gout (Fam and Rubenstein, 1989), as bursitis (Fam et al., 1981; McCarty et al., 1981), as a periarticular mass (Fam et al., 1981; Kandel et al., 1986; Slavin et al., 1993), or as an asymptomatic radiologic finding (Halverson, 1992). In calcium apatite arthropathy associated with scleroderma, apatite crystals appearing in the sinus tract to the skin can simulate the pus of septic fasciitis or arthritis (Fam and Pritzker, 1992). Apatite crystal deposition in either a periarthritic tumoral nodule or an apatite crystal deposition within bursas is a common association with chronic renal failure (LeGeros et al., 1973; Irby et al., 1975; Rubin et al., 1984; Goldstein et al., 1985).

In the few cases of nonhuman primate apatite arthritis described, the disease presents as a radiodense periarticular mass (Thompson et al., 1959; Line et al., 1984; Van Linthoudt et al., 1992). In each of the four cases reported, lesions occurred in the hand or foot, suggesting trauma as a contributory factor. In the older literature, this mass was termed calcinosis circumscripta. More recently, the terms "calcific periarthritis" and "tumoral calcinosis" are frequently used (Schumacher et al., 1977; Kindblom and Gunterberg, 1988). Calcium apatite crystal arthropathy is found in many species, including the turtle (Frye and Dutra, 1976), dog (Woodard et al., 1982), horse (Dodd and Raker, 1970), buffalo (Ikede, 1979), and rabbit (Yosipovitch and Glimcher, 1972). The differential diagnosis of the tumoral form of apatite arthropathy is the tumoral presentation of CPPD

crystal deposition disease (Pritzker et al., 1976; Sissons et al., 1989).

In the two cases of local soft tissue apatite deposition in rhesus macaques, the clinical presentation was a nonpainful mass on the right foot (Line et al., 1984). There was no history of trauma or systemic disease in these cases.

Van Linthoudt et al. (1992) described tumoral apatite crystal deposition in a Diana monkey (Cercopithecus diana diana) with chronic renal insufficiency. The disease presented with a subcutaneous mass on the left carpus. Radiologic examination demonstrated a multilobulated radiodensity on the palmar surface of the carpus. Aspiration of the mass revealed typical nonbirefringent particulate matter that stained positive with Alizarin red (Van Linthoudt et al., 1992).

As Alizarin red will stain many phases in which calcium is present, the diagnosis of calcium apatite deposition is established by more precise crystal identification (Pritzker and Luk, 1976; Schumacher et al., 1977; Halverson et al., 1984). Individual apatite crystals are submicroscopic, having dimensions typically $40 \times 10 \times 10$ nm. Material seen on light microscopy of synovial fluid consists of crystal agglomerates. When arranged in spheroidal collections, the appearances are that of "coin bodies" of varied size. This material is not birefringent and may be mistaken for dust contaminant on the microscopic slide. Calcium apatite crystals are identified by transmission electron microscopy by demonstrating aggregates of needle-shaped crystals with a Ca:P ratio by X-ray spectroscopy of 1.67:1 and by the characteristic electron powder diffraction pattern.

The therapy for this disease consists of addressing underlying causes of the calcium imbalance such as renal failure. In some cases without renal failure, spontaneous resolution of the periarticular apatite mass has been reported (Fam et al., 1981; Fam and Pritzker, 1992).

G. Diffuse Idiopathic Skeletal Hyperostosis

Diffuse idiopathic skeletal hyperostosis (DISH) is a term coined by Resnick et al. (1978) encompassing hyperostotic spondylosis (spinal hyperostosis) (Forestier and Rotes-Querol, 1950, 1971) as well as disproportionate osteophytosis affecting bones adjacent to peripheral joints (Resnick et al., 1978; Utsinger, 1985). Diffuse idiopathic skeletal hyperostosis appears to be a condition distinct from spinal osteoarthritis or spondylosis deformans and the chronic inflammatory seronegative spondyloarthropathies. Known etiologic factors for DISH include diabetes mellitus and hypervitaminosis A. In humans, DISH is associated with diabetes mellitus complicated by hyperuricemia and/or dyslipidemia (Boulet and Mirouse, 1954; Julkunen and Heinonen, 1971; Vezyroglou et al., 1996). It has been suggested that the osteophyte production is related to excessive growth factor stimuli or response on bone (Fornasier et al., 1983; Littlejohn, 1985). Diffuse idiopathic skeletal hyperostosis is also recognized in humans as a complication of long-term therapy with vitamin A analogs (retinoids) for skin disorders such as psoriasis (Wilson *et al.*, 1988). Cervical thoracic spinal hyperostosis accompanied by exostoses of peripheral bones is a feature of natural hypervitaminosis A in the cat (Seawright and English, 1964). These lesions can be induced by experimental hypervitaminosis A in both the cat and the rat (Seawright and English, 1967; Clark, 1971; Ishizawa, 1992). Hypervitaminosis A-induced spinal hyperostosis leading to spinal ankylosis has been observed in Callitrichidae (*Callithrix jacchus, Saguinus nigricollis,* and *Saguinis geoffroyi*) housed in a zoo setting (Demontoy *et al.*, 1979). The animals presented with musculoskeletal lameness, paresis, as well as debilitation, alopecia, and cachexia. X-rays demonstrated dense new bone formation on the entire vertebral column, lesions that were confirmed at necropsy. Common to spinal hyperostosis associated with hyperinsulinemia and hypercalcemia is hyperlipemia (Clark, 1971; Vezyroglou *et al.*, 1996). It remains unknown whether hyperlipemia is a coincident biomarker for DISH or whether it is involved in DISH pathogenesis.

In humans, DISH is common in elderly males and may be accompanied by osteoporosis (Utsinger, 1985). The early phases of the disease are asymptomatic, but DISH may present as stiffness and mild pain in the thoracic area. The diagnosis is made by the radiologic appearance of anterolateral spinal osteophytosis particularly affecting the thoracic vertebrae (Jones *et al.*, 1988) and by the observation of peripheral osteophytosis with intact articular architecture (Resnick *et al.*, 1978; Utsinger, 1985). In advanced disease, extension of the spinal osteophytes produces a fixed dorsal kyphosis. The differential diagnosis of DISH includes two conditions producing spinal osteophytosis that are commonly found in nonhuman primates: osteoarthritis and inflammatory spondyloarthropathy. The differential diagnosis of DISH should also include ossification of the posterior longitudinal spinous ligament, a condition commonly recognized in Japan (Ono *et al.*, 1977; Tsuyama, 1984; Jones *et al.*, 1988). The diseases can be distinguished radiologically and on gross examination from DISH by the pattern and distribution of osteophytes (Jones *et al.*, 1988).

Spinal hyperostosis is widespread, but uncommon, among mammalian species irrespective of their posture or locomotion (du Boulay and Crawford, 1968; du Boulay *et al.*, 1972; Woodard *et al.*, 1985; Lagier, 1989). Although the different types of spondylosis have not always been distinguished clearly in osteologic studies, DISH has been found in a variety of nonhuman primates, including the gorilla (Lovell, 1990b) and the rhesus macaque (Sokoloff *et al.*, 1968). Kandel *et al.* (1983) found DISH associated with CPPD crystal deposition disease in an aged barbary ape (*Macaca sylvanus*). It has been speculated that DISH in nonhuman primates represents a nutritional osteodystrophy (du Boulay *et al.*, 1972). However, no specific evidence has been offered to support this hypothesis.

In the spine, the gross pathology consists of osteophytes extending from the articular margins along the articular ligaments. This appears to be a metaplastic process unassociated with inflammation. Within the osteophyte, the marrow is hematopoietic marrow and is contiguous to the marrow in the vertebral body (Fornasier *et al.*, 1983). When ankylosis supervenes, atrophy and collapse of the intervertebral disc space follow (Resnick and Niwayama, 1976; Resnick *et al.*, 1978; Revell and Pirie, 1981; Lagier, 1989). The rearrangement of biomechanical forces may induce secondary degenerative arthritis in the adjacent spinal facet joints. Presently, the major biomedical research implication of DISH in nonhuman primates is its distinction from inflammatory spondyloarthropathy, a condition associated with peripheral joint erosive arthritis.

H. Miscellaneous Degenerative Spinal Disorders

The anatomy and histomorphology of the nonhuman primate spinal column bear close resemblance to humans, despite differences in posture (Tominaga *et al.*, 1995). Therefore, it is expected that nonhuman primates would be suitable models for experimental spinal diseases.

Degenerative disc disease, perhaps the most common spinal disease in humans, has been observed with increasing age among baboons (*Papio cynocephalus anubis*), a nonhuman primate that commonly sits in an upright posture (Cheung *et al.*, 1984). Experimental degenerative disc disease has been induced in nonhuman primates by surgical incision of the intervertebral disc (Cheung *et al.*, 1984) and by intervertebral injection of collagenase (Stern and Coulson, 1976). Spinal osteoarthritis or spondylosis deformans differs from DISH in several morphologic characteristics. In spondylosis deformans, the osteophytes are circumferential extensions of the vertebral articular plate, the subchondral bone is normal or thickened, and ankylosis is uncommon. Vitamin A toxicity, another noninflammatory ankylosing arthropathy, has not been described in nonhuman primates.

Nonhuman primates appear subject to idiopathic kyphotic scoliosis. This disease has been found in the pig-tailed macaque (*Macaca nemestrina*). In this case, investigations failed to demonstrate any arthritis or intraosseous disease that predisposed to the kyphosis (Srikanth *et al.*, 1995).

Nonhuman primates are also subject to spontaneous malformations of the vertebral column. Cerroni *et al.* (1991), studying skeletons from the patas monkey (*Erythrocebus patas*), demonstrated five spontaneous malformations of the neural arch among 194 skeletons. These defects ranged from spinal bifida occulta to lack of the development of the vertebral lamina (Cerroni *et al.*, 1991).

I. Inflammatory Arthritis

Spontaneous and experimentally induced inflammatory arthritis has been extensively studied in nonhuman primates principally to better our understanding of pathogenic mechanisms of rheumatoid and articular seronegative polyarthritis. Common to these forms of arthritis is persistent, and therefore, dysregulated joint inflammation and pain.

The role of the nervous system in mediating the acute arthritis induced by intraarticular carageenan and kaolin injection has been investigated in depth by Dougherty and colleagues (Dougherty *et al.*, 1992; Westlund *et al.*, 1992; Sluka *et al.*, 1992; Sorkin *et al.*, 1992). Their findings, which may be applicable to all types of arthritis, indicate a broad increase in neurotransmitters and neuromodulators along the peripheral nerves and spinal tracts from the affected joint but differential increases in mediators with joint movement and with time after induction of arthritis. These studies are illuminating the relative roles of various endogenous chemicals in the regulation of peripheral inflammation and nocioceptive afferent transmission.

1. Septic Arthritis

Septic arthritis, arthritis secondary to microorganisms, has been described infrequently in nonhuman primates. Septic arthritis in multiple joints secondary to *Streptococcus aureus* has been reported in a neonatal male orangutan *Pongo pygmaeus*) (Hoopes *et al.*, 1978). This animal, given penicillin prophylactically at birth, developed septicemia and septic arthritis from pencillin-resistant staphylococci and streptococci. Septic arthritis has also been described in association with hematogenous osteomyelitis in the rhesus macaque (Klumpp *et al.*, 1986).

2. Rheumatoid Arthritis and Chronic Polyarthritis

The syndrome of bilateral symmetrical chronic polyarthritis is a common presentation for many different types of arthritis, the most common of which is rheumatoid arthritis (Hoffman, 1978). In addition to rheumatoid arthritis, arthritis associated with inflammatory bowel disease, postinfectious reactive arthritis, arthritis associated with mixed connective tissue diseases, and ankylosing spondylitis appear particularly relevant to nonhuman primates. The key feature common to many forms of chronic inflammatory arthritis is that the diseases behave in a similar manner to arthritis associated with systemic infections, but the disease cannot be transmitted from animal to animal, nor can microorganisms be found in the affected joint tissues. Chronic inflammatory arthritis has been noted with an annual prevalence of 0.5% in one colony of rhesus macaques (Ford *et al.*, 1986). Given the prevalence of chronic inflammatory arthritis in humans of about 3%, it is peculiar that relatively few cases have been described in nonhuman primates. This is probably a consequence of underreporting.

Rheumatoid arthritis is a chronic systemic inflammatory disease that affects the connective tissues of many organs but primarily assaults the joints. Within an affected joint, the principal lesion is a nonsuppurative proliferative synovitis that can progressively erode and cover the articular surfaces (pannus), leading to joint destruction and fibrous ankylosis (Silman, 1994;

Zvaifler, 1995). Despite intense investigation, the etiologic agent of rheumatoid arthritis is not known (Silman, 1994). Genetic studies have identified a shared epitope in the HLA-DRB1 gene as a predisposing factor. The disease is more common in females, particularly in premenopausal females. Rheumatoid arthritis patients appear to have abnormal responses to endocrine stimulation of the hypothalamic–pituitary–adrenal glucocorticoid axis (Masi and Chrousos, 1996).

Oral contraceptives appear to be a protective factor. Gonadal androgens also have protective effects in rheumatoid arthritis (Cutolo *et al.*, 1995). This effect is thought to be related to downregulation by androgens of cytokine production by macrophages and T cells (Cutolo *et al.*, 1995). Rheumatoid arthritis is associated with rheumatoid factor autoantibodies to IgG. Not only are rheumatoid factors serologic biomarkers found in approximately 80% of patients with rheumatoid arthritis but, when present in immune complexes, can participate in the pathogenesis of lesions, particularly vasculitis. Because of the autoimmune phenomena in rheumatoid arthritis, immunologic imbalance or deficiency has been implicated in its pathogenesis. Again, the cause of this abnormality is not known, but both viruses and mycoplasma organisms have been suspected as pathogenic agents (Cole and Cassell, 1979; Wilder, 1994).

Bywaters (1981) has reviewed the early literature on nonhuman primate chronic polyarthritis. It is interesting that amyloidosis was a prominent feature in most of the cases described (Gillman and Gilbert, 1954; Benditt and Eriksen, 1972; Casey *et al.*, 1972; Obeck *et al.*, 1976; Chapman and Crowell, 1977). The amyloid AA protein is produced by macrophagic inflammatory cells and is deposited in tissues in many types of chronic inflammation (Tan and Pepys, 1994). By its accumulation in connective tissue within blood vessels and vascular sinusoids, amyloid can depress immunologic and inflammatory responses, thereby perpetuating chronic inflammation (Tan and Pepys, 1994). Bywaters (1981) found symmetrical polyarthritis in only 1 of 152 rhesus macaques studied in a colony used to make polio vaccine. Radiologically, erosive lesions were seen in the metacarpal phalangeal and interphalangeal joints. Microscopically, synovial cell hyperplasia with prominent lymphocyte infiltration was seen. Vasculitis and rheumatoid nodules were not observed.

Brown and colleagues (1970, 1974) described polyarthritis associated with systemic disease and a positive rheumatoid factor in lowland gorillas housed in zoo environments. In these animals, mycoplasma was isolated from the synovial membrane. Further, these animals responded to prolonged therapy with tetracycline. In total, six gorillas (three males and three females) from five different zoos were described with the disease. The disease presented with migratory polyarthritis and failure to grow. The synovial biopsy from the first animal showed very mild synovial lining cell proliferation with edema and focal nodular lymphocytic infiltrate around some synovial capillary blood vessels. It is interesting that these inflammatory changes were not as exuberant as that often seen in human disease.

Chronic polyarthritis was described in 6 of 16 gorillas in the colony at the Cincinnati zoo (Hess *et al.,* 1983). The arthritis was characterized by pain and swelling of peripheral joints. No serologic, microbiologic, or articular radiologic abnormalities were detected. The animals responded to tetracycline. Of note, one of the animals caretakers had HLA-B27 associated Reiter's syndrome at the same time as the arthritis outbreak among the gorillas.

Mycoplasma has been isolated from the joints of monkeys with polyarthritis (Valerio *et al.,* 1971). In contrast, in the case of polyarthritis in a female rhesus macaque, the synovium showed inflammatory and proliferative changes similar to that seen in humans (Obeck *et al.,* 1976). Although the mycoplasma complement fixation titer rose fourfold over the first 3 months of the illness, microorganisms could not be recovered from joints or other tissues. As Obeck *et al.* (1976) noted, the association of polyarthritis and mycoplasma in humans and non-human primates is controversial. Mycoplasma can induce polyarthritis in mice, rats, and swine (Alspaugh and Van Hoosier, 1973; Harwick *et al.,* 1973; Sokoloff, 1973; Cole and Cassell, 1979). Mycoplasma has been recovered frequently from the oral cavity of nonhuman primates that do not have arthritis (Obeck *et al.,* 1976). Chimpanzees (*Pan troglodytes*) inoculated intraarticularly with mycoplasma cultured from synovial aspirates of immunosuppressed patients with septic arthritis developed a local and self-limiting septic arthritis (Barile *et al.,* 1994). Animals previously inoculated systemically with mycoplasma were protected from the arthritis, suggesting that the experimental arthritis was mediated by an immune reaction.

A case of polyarthritis seronegative for rheumatoid factor in a male lion-tailed macaque (*Macaca silenus*) has been described (Anderson and Schiller, 1991). A similar isolated case was described in male juvenile rhesus macaque by Lipman *et al.* (1991). Their pathologic findings were typical of seronegative polyarthritis. The relationship of all of these cases to human rheumatoid arthritis should be interpreted with caution. Rheumatoid factor was positive only in the gorilla cases. However, rheumatoid factor can be positive in other forms of inflammatory arthritis that do not meet the criteria for rheumatoid arthritis. Similarly, while the culture of mycoplasma organisms and the response to tetracycline is very provocative, mycoplasma in humans has not been found in joints of patients with rheumatoid arthritis and the response to trials of tetracycline has been equivocal (Greenwald *et al.,* 1987, 1988; Cole *et al.,* 1994). Tetracycline has actions other than its antimicrobial activity, principally as an inhibitor of synovial and cartilage collagenase. In contrast to the female preponderance in human disease, there is no gender predilection for chronic polyarthritis in nonhuman primates in zoo collections.

3. Reactive Arthritis

Reactive arthritis secondary to bacterial enteritis (*Shigella flexneri*) has been described in gorillas (Raphael *et al.,* 1995).

Polyarthritis developed 4 weeks to 6 months after the onset of chronic intermittent diarrhea. Aspiration of joint fluid failed to demonstrate bacterial organisms. One of the animals had a major histocompatibility antigen similar to HLA-B26. Typical HLA-B27 ankylosing spondylitis has also been documented in the gorilla (R. F. Adams *et al.,* 1987). This animal had both spinal and peripheral arthritis and presented with rigid gait, joint contractures, and general debilitation.

4. Inflammatory Spondyloarthropathy

Spondyloarthropathy is a term used for a group of inflammatory arthritic disorders in which involvement of the spinal entheses (ligament insertions) is prominent (Thomson and Inman, 1990). In humans, these disorders include ankylosing spondylitis, postinfectious reactive arthritis, Reiter's syndrome (postreactive urethritis, conjunctivitis and arthritis), psoriatic arthritis, and arthritis associated with inflammatory bowel disease (Thomson and Inman, 1990; Mielants *et al.,* 1991; El-Khoury *et al.,* 1996). Although the spine is commonly affected, these disorders are often associated with arthritis affecting synovial joints, particularly the sacroiliac joints (Thomson and Inman, 1990). From skeletal studies, spondyloarthropathy appears widespread among mammalian species (Rothschild and Woods, 1992b; Rothschild and Rothschild, 1994; Rothschild *et al.,* 1993, 1994, 1997). Many species, including bears, hyenas, and elephants, are susceptible to this disorder. Both Old World primates such as the gorilla (Rothschild and Woods, 1989), gibbon, chimpanzee, baboon, Diana monkey, and rhesus macaque (Sokoloff *et al.,* 1968; Nall and Bartels, 1973; Rothschild and Woods, 1991, 1992b,c; Swezey *et al.,* 1991; Rothschild *et al.,* 1997) and New World primates such as marmosets (*Callithrix jacchus*) (Rothschild, 1993a) can be affected. Spondyloarthropathy appears particularly prevalent among wild and captive contemporary baboon populations (Rothschild and Rothschild, 1996), suggesting the presence of a new pathogenic factor in the environment.

In humans, the histocompatibility marker HLA-B27 is associated but not exclusively associated with predisposition to ankylosing spondylitis. Common to patients with spondyloarthropathy is enhanced reactivity to bacterial (Repo *et al.,* 1990) and chlamydial antigens (Rahman *et al.,* 1992). This exaggerated reaction to injury preferentially affects neutrophil inflammatory responses and T lymphocyte activity (Repo *et al.,* 1990; Toussirot *et al.,* 1994). It is likely that multiple etiologic agents induce this abnormal inflammatory activity. Beyond genetic factors, chronic viral infection, including immunodeficiency virus, must be considered (Mijiyawa, 1993). Of particular interest for nonhuman primate spondyloarthropathy is the association of human spondyloarthropathy and reactive arthritis following gram-negative bacterial entercolitis. Bacterial enterocolitis is a common enzootic disorder among nonhuman primates in both captive and wild populations (Paul-Murphy, 1993; Raphael *et al.,* 1995). As with humans,

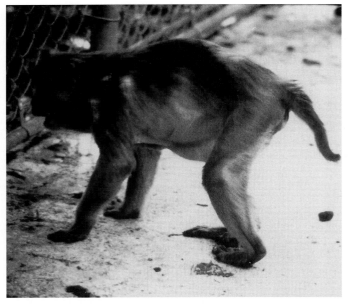

Fig. 8. Rhesus macaque with spondyloarthropathy. Note the fixed dorsal kyphosis.

it is reasonable to suggest that a portion of the nonhuman primate population has exaggerated inflammatory reactivity to bacterial antigens. The preferential spinal and sacroiliac distribution of this disease is thought to be related to the tracking of bacterial or chlamydial antigens from the sites of bowel or urethral inflammation to ligament insertions on vertebrae. However, the proximity of the inflammation to the spine may not be an obligate requirement. Polyarthritis and ossifying enthesopathy can be induced in rats using type II collagen injection into the foot pad as a pathogenic agent (Gillet *et al.,* 1989). The principal characteristics of spondyloarthritic inflammation are its persistence at low intensity and induction of new bone formation. The erosive lesions and the joint lesions appear related to synovial cell hyperplasia and the release of cytokines, whereas the growth of osteophytes and the ultimate process of ankylosis must be considered as an exaggerated repair process to chronic inflammation.

Smith *et al.* (1973) attempted to experimentally induce reactive arthritis in rhesus macaques by intraarticular injection of Bedsonia organisms isolated from the joint of a patient with Reiter's syndrome. However, only a limited and local arthritis in the injected joint was observed (Smith *et al.,* 1973).

Chronic spondyloarthropathy produces a visible fixed deformity of the dorsal spine (Fig. 8). On gross examination, the most typical finding in spondyloarthropathy is osteophytosis, which develops on the lateral aspects of the vertebral bodies. Extension and coalescence of osteophytes result in ankylosis. Ankylosis can affect other joints, particularly the sacroiliac joints. In both the spine and the peripheral joints, an erosive arthritis consisting of disruption of the bone and articular surface of the

joint margins can be seen. Microscopically, in areas of active disease, a mixed acute and chronic inflammatory reaction consisting of neutrophils, lymphocytes and plasma cells can be observed (Sokoloff *et al.,* 1968; Cawley *et al.,* 1972; Agarwal *et al.,* 1990). These cells are present in a loose fibrous connective tissue with prominent capillary blood vessels. Where synovial joints are affected, synovial lining cell hyperplasia is seen. Similar to rheumatoid arthritis, synovium can be seen at the leading edge of the erosions invading the articular margin.

The susceptibility of nonhuman primates to both spondyloarthropathy and chronic enterocolitis suggests that these animals are particularly suited for the development of a model disease. Such a model could lead to better understanding of spondyloarthropathy in humans. Experimental attempts to develop such models with bacterial or chlamydial antigens overlap proposed models for rheumatoid arthritis. These models will be discussed later in this chapter.

J. Experimental Inflammatory Arthritis

1. Experimental Rheumatoid Arthritis

Rheumatoid arthritis is a systemic disease characterized by persistent chronic inflammation in multiple joints and other connective tissues and by serological autoimmune phenomena such as the production of rheumatoid factor type antibodies. Because of these features, an infectious etiology has been postulated often for this disease but never proven. Nonhuman primates have been studied both as candidate species to attempt to transmit the disease (Jurmain and Kilgore, 1995) and as an animal model to emulate the major pathologic features (Lucherini *et al.,* 1964a,b, 1965a,b, 1966; Lucherini and Porzio, 1996a,b, 1967).

In an effort to transmit rheumatoid arthritis, synovial fluid cells and synovial membrane-cultured cells from patients with rheumatoid arthritis were inoculated intravenously and intraarticularly into the right knee joints of female baboons *(Papio cynocephalus)* (Hunneyball *et al.,* 1979; Mackay *et al.,* 1983). The animals were followed clinically for up to 36 months. No serological abnormality or arthritis was found in these animals. Explanations offered for the lack of disease transmission included (1) no transmisssible agent was present in the cell inoculates, (2) baboons were not susceptible to the infectious agent, or (3) the incubation period for rheumatoid arthritis was longer than the observation time, implying that rheumatoid arthritis was caused by a slow virus.

Of course, the negative results also provide support that rheumatoid arthritis may not be a specific infection but rather a nonspecific aberrant and persistent inflammatory response to different exogenous stimuli.

Following these experiments, the capacity of the baboon to respond to exogenous antigen was tested by an intramuscular injection of ovalbumin in Freund's complete adjuvant followed by challenge with an intraarticular injection of ovalbumin

(Alexander *et al.,* 1983). As expected, the procedure induced a local inflammatory arthritis that persisted until the experiment was concluded 20 days later. Histologically, the affected joints showed chronic inflammatory synovitis with the presence of plasma cells in the synovium. Immunoglobulin G (IgG) was found by immunofluorescence in the synovial blood vessels of the affected joints, indicating that immune complexes contributed to the arthritis. Similar experiments were performed on marmosets (*Callithrix jacchus*) with similar limited results (Hunneyball, 1983). Polyarthritis was induced successfully in baboons by a daily subcutaneous injection of muramyl dyspeptide, a synthetic analog to a bacterial cell wall component (Gardner *et al.,* 1991). This inflammatory arthritis was characterized by synovial lining cell hyperplasia but only slight synovial lymphocyte infiltration.

Lucherini and colleagues investigated extensively a model for rheumatoid arthritis induced by experimental autoimmunity to human fibrin (Lucherini *et al.,* 1964a,b, 1965a,b,c 1966; Lucherini and Porzio, 1996a, 1967). Yearling macaques were inoculated subcutaneously in the interscapular region with 10 mg of fibrin in Freund's complete adjuvant. This was followed 21 days later by injection of 10 mg fibrin intramuscularly into the right lateral deltoid muscle. These animals developed acute and later chronic erosive polyarthritis characterized pathologically by synovial proliferation and pannus formation. These animals also demonstrated a mildly positive rheumatoid factor. In an attempt to replicate this study in marmosets (*Callithrix jacchus*), only local arthritis was found 16 days following the intraarticular injection of fibrin into sensitized animals (Hunneyball, 1983). Although this is a shorter time interval than the studies of Lucherini, it does suggest that the marmoset is less sensitive to human fibrin than the rhesus macaque. The variability of these studies also suggests that nonhuman primates are relatively resistant to the induction of autoimmune arthritis by conventional antigens. As discussed later, this may relate to genetic differences in major histocompatibility complex alleles.

2. Experimental Lyme Disease Arthritis

A systemic disease with features similar to juvenile rheumatoid arthritis was first described in Lyme, Connecticut, in 1977 (Steere *et al.,* 1977; Steere, 1989; Roberts *et al.,* 1995). The causative agent was identified in 1983 as the spirochete *Borrelia burgdorferi* (Burgdorfer, 1984). The disease is transmitted primarily by hard ticks of the genus *Ixodes* for which many species of mammals and birds act as hosts. However, the main reservoir for the organism is the white-footed mouse (*Peromyscus*), which serves as a host for the tiny deer tick, *Ixodes dammini*. White-tailed deer, field dogs, and wild birds serve as transport hosts for infected ticks (Nielsen, 1989).

In human beings, Lyme disease has three stages, which include an expanding skin rash at the site of the tick bite (erythema migrans) and a flu-like syndrome but without respiratory signs. The second stage occurs several weeks later and consists

of cardiac or neurological signs such as myocarditis and transient arrhythmias or meningitis and cranial nerve neuropathies. The final stage occurs several months later and is characterized by polyarthritis of the major joints with pain and swelling.

Although Lyme disease has been reported in dogs, cattle, and horses causing arthritis and lameness, there is yet to be any case report of spontaneous Lyme disease affecting nonhuman primates. However, male rhesus monkeys experimentally inoculated with *Borrelia burgdorferi* developed an infection that mimics both the early and the later stages of the human Lyme disease, including skin rash, neurological signs, and arthritis (Philipp *et al.,* 1993; Philipp and Johnson, 1994; Roberts *et al.,* 1995). Six months after spirochetal inoculation by tick bites, male rhesus macaques developed chronic polyarthritis with proliferative synovitis, pannus formation, and cartilage erosion (Roberts *et al.,* 1995). With immunohistochemistry, *B. burgdorferi* spirochetes could be demonstrated intracellularly in the synovial macrophages, which was accompanied by peripheral nerve infection, inflammation, and fibrosis. In both humans and nonhuman primates, the peripheral nerve involvement tends to be subclinical. Nonetheless, this suggests that a neuropathic component may contribute to the development of the polyarthritis.

The diagnosis of Lyme disease is based on clinical signs and recovery of the organism. The development of an enzyme-linked immunosorbent assay (ELISA) test for Lyme disease has greatly facilitated its diagnosis and therapy. Prompt diagnosis is extremely important because the infection can be treated successfully with tetracyclines in the early stages of the disease.

The rhesus macaque appears to be a very good model in which to study Lyme disease infection. The presence of this experimental disease also suggests that nonhuman primates in endemic areas could be susceptible to the spontaneous disease.

3. Experimental Simian Immunodeficiency Virus Arthritis

Arthralgia and nonerosive polyarthritis are recognized features of acquired immunodeficiency syndrome (AIDS) (Berman *et al.,* 1988). The underlying pathology appears to be a mild and nonspecific synovitis. Acquired immunodeficiency syndrome-associated arthritis is likely a heterogenous group of disorders mediated by impaired immunologic reactions to opportunistic microorganisms (Espinoza *et al.,* 1992; Hughes *et al.,* 1992). African green monkeys (*Cercopithecus aethiops*) and sooty mangabey monkeys (*Cercocebus atys*) are the asymptomatic natural carriers of simian immunodeficiency virus (SIV) (Fultz *et al.,* 1986; Hendry *et al.,* 1986), a virus with similar biologic characteristics to human immunodeficiency viruses (Lowenstine *et al.,* 1986; Franchini *et al.,* 1987; Payne *et al.,* 1987).

Rhesus macaques infected with SIV are widely used as a model for AIDS (Letvin *et al.,* 1985; Baskin *et al.,* 1986). Roberts and Martin (1991) studied the joints of 36 animals inoculated with SIV 8 months to 3 years previously. Although clinical signs of arthritis prior to death were minimal, 40% of the animals had morphologic findings of synovitis at autopsy. These findings consisted of synovial lining cell proliferation and nodular infiltrates composed of lymphocytes and macrophages in the synovial connective tissue. Occasional multinucleated macrophages present in advanced lesions stained positively for immunohistochemical markers for SIV. The synovitis was much less severe than that reported by the same group of investigators in experimental Lyme arthritis (Roberts *et al.*, 1995) and much milder than that seen in human rheumatoid arthritis. The identification of viral epitopes within synovial macrophages suggests that SIV synovitis is a primary viral reaction. Retroviruses have been proposed as pathologic agents for human arthritis such as chronic rheumatoid arthritis (Rodahl, 1989). Nonetheless, the possibility remains that the polyarthritis in SAIDS reflects the T-lymphocyte immunodeficiency in these animals and is secondary to other viral etiologic agents (Beilke *et al.*, 1996).

4. Experimental Type II Collagen Polyarthritis

The hypothesis that rheumatoid arthritis is an autoimmune disease, that at least a portion of the autoimmune reaction is directed toward an endogenous articular component, and that collagen is antigenic (Steffen and Timpl, 1963) led to the development of experimental polyarthritis in rodents induced by sensitization to the major protein of articular cartilage, type II collagen (Trentham *et al.*, 1978; Trentham, 1982; Holmdahl *et al.*, 1989, 1990). This arthritis does have some species specificity, as guinea pigs and rabbits appear not to be susceptible (Yoo *et al.*, 1988). Because this experimental arthritis has many genetic immunologic and pathologic features similar to human rheumatoid arthritis and because the spontaneous rheumatoid-like polyarthritis is recognized in gorillas (Hess *et al.*, 1983), several investigators have extended this model to nonhuman primates (Kang *et al.*, 1984; Cathcart *et al.*, 1986; Rubin *et al.*, 1987; T. C. Yoo *et al.*, 1986; T. D. Yoo *et al.*, 1988; Terato *et al.*, 1989; Bakker *et al.*, 1990; Roberts, 1993a). Collectively, these studies have shown that type II collagen arthritis can be induced in both New World primates, squirrel monkeys (*Saimiri sciureus*) (Cathcart *et al.*, 1986), and Old World primates, rhesus and cynomolgus macaques (Kang *et al.*, 1984; Rubin *et al.*, 1987; Terato *et al.*, 1989; Yoo *et al.*, 1988; Bakker *et al.*, 1990). The experimental disease has interesting species gender and genetic susceptibilities. Under similar immunization conditions, squirrel monkeys (*S. sciureus*) develop acute and fulminant polyarthritis whereas Cebus monkeys (*Cebus albifrons*) appear completely resistant (Cathcart *et al.*, 1986). Although the disease can be induced in males, females appear more susceptible and have more severe arthritis (Terato *et al.*, 1989; Bakker *et al.*, 1990). Further, the disease can be induced by type II collagen derived from either chick (Terato *et al.*, 1989) or bovine (Rubin *et al.*, 1987; Yoo *et al.*, 1988; Bakker *et al.*, 1990) collagen. Most studies employed Freund's complete adjuvant in the sensitization procedure, but the disease can be induced by the intraperitoneal implantation of type II collagen adsorbed onto nitrocellulose filters (Healy *et al.*, 1989). As the filter is inert, this method permits induction of the arthritis by immunization with type II collagen antigens alone. Clinically, 5–8 weeks or more following immunization, the animals present with persistent chronic polyarthritis characterized by joint swelling, tenderness, and restricted movement, primarily affecting the small joints of the hands and feet. The restriction of the tissue response to peripheral joints may be species specific. Type II collagen-induced arthritis in Wistar rats induces a polyarthritis involving not only small joints but also the spine. The axial ossifying enthesiopathy in these animals resembles the spondyloarthropathy of ankylosing spondylitis or reactive spondyloarthropathy (Gillet *et al.*, 1987, 1989).

The severity of the inflammation appears to vary with the method and dose of immunization as well as with gender and age. For example, in studies done by Bakker *et al.* (1990), the arthritis was often acute and fulminant. In contrast, other investigators induced acute inflammation that progressed to chronic polyarthritis (Rubin *et al.*, 1987; Yoo *et al.*, 1988; Healy *et al.*, 1989; Terato *et al.*, 1989). Affected animals experienced weight loss, appetite loss, and decreased mobility, features characteristic of systemic illness. On radiologic examination, joint space narrowing, marginal erosions, juxtaarticular radiolucencies, and eventually joint subluxation and destruction were observed predominantly in the synovial joints of the hands and feet. At necropsy, both small and large diarthoidal joints were affected, demonstrating synovial hyperplasia and synovial fluid exudate. The synovitis extended as pannus eroding the articular cartilage. The microscopic findings of synovial inflammation, cartilage erosion, subchondral bone porosis, and eventual fibrous ankylosis emulated closely the pathologic features of human rheumatoid arthritis. With the onset of arthritis, the standard serological indicators of inflammation, including the erythrocyte sedimentation rate and the C reactive protein, increased. Leukocytosis was invariably observed. A normocytic anemia was seen in some animals.

Immunologically, all animals had serum antibodies to the inducer collagen (bovine or chick). Only animals susceptible to the arthritis had elevated antibody levels to monkey type II collagen (Terato *et al.*, 1989; Bakker *et al.*, 1991b). In susceptible animals, the predominant antibody response was IgM, whereas IgG was predominant in resistant animals (Bakker *et al.*, 1991b). Susceptible animals showed enhanced B- and T-cell reactivity to bovine type II antigen, whereas resistant animals did not (Bakker *et al.*, 1991a,b; 't Hart *et al.*, 1991).

The genetic association of major histocompatibility complex (MHC) genes with rheumatoid arthritis (Silman, 1994) and homology of MHC complex class I alleles between humans and pongidae nonhuman primates (orangutan, chimpanzee, gorilla) (Lawlor *et al.*, 1990) stimulated investigations on the genetic susceptibility of the rhesus macaque to type II collagen arthritis. Bakker *et al.* 1992; 't Hart *et al.*, 1993) found that juvenile macaques possessing the MHC class I allele (Mamu-A26) were resistant to disease whereas the allele was absent in all young animals with type II collagen arthritis. This resistance appears confined to reactivity to type II collagen by T lymphocytes and does not extend to antigens associated with other experimental autoimmune diseases. With age, the expression of the Mamu-A26 allele decreases. Older animals with this allele become susceptible to type II collagen arthritis, although less severely than animals genetically deficient in this allele (Bakker *et al.,* 1992).

In rhesus macaques, type II collagen arthritis can be abrogated completely by the immunosuppressant cyclosporin administered between immunization and the time of onset of clinical symptoms (Bakker *et al.,* 1993). This resistance persists even after booster immunization with type II collagen. Suppression of the disease is accompanied by a serological decrease in type II collagen antibodies (Bakker *et al.,* 1993).

The pathologic role of collagen antibodies in chronic inflammatory arthritis has yet to be determined. Typically, these antibodies follow the onset of the human disease. Collagen type II antibody titers are inconstantly related to disease severity (Pereira *et al.,* 1985; Jasin, 1985; Charriere *et al.,* 1988; Mottonen *et al.,* 1988; Morgan *et al.,* 1989; Morgan, 1990; Jonker *et al.,* 1991). These antibodies are secreted by immunocompetent cells present in rheumatoid synovium (Tarkowski *et al.,* 1989). Antibody secretion can persist in synovial explant culture (Londei *et al.,* 1989).

When collagen type II antibodies bind to chondrocytes at the cell membrane, the secretion of collagenase increases (Takagi and Jasin, 1992). This effect is not seen with antibodies to other collagens. This phenomenon suggests a direct pathologic link between collagen type II antibodies and cartilage matrix destruction, provided that the effector cells such as chondrocytes are exposed to the antibody.

Experimentally induced collagen type II arthritis has proved to be a superb model for illuminating the pathogenic mechanisms associated with human rheumatoid arthritis. The nonhuman primate model has been especially useful for defining genetic-, species-, and tissue-specific responses to autoimmune inflammation affecting joints.

5. Experimental Interleukin-3 Polyarthritis

Interleukin-3 (IL-3) is a cytokine that simulates hematopoiesis along multiple lineages. Interleukin-3 receptors are present on macrophages, basophils, and eosinophils. Juvenile rhesus macaques given daily subcutaneous injections of IL-3 for 1 week developed acute polyarthritis that affected the proximal interphalangeal joints of the hands and feet (van Gils *et al.,* 1993). This arthritis was characterized by synovial edema with mononuclear inflammatory cell infiltration and neovascularization. A fibrinous exudate was present in the synovial space. In contrast to experimental collagen type II arthritis, which has association with MHC allele A[26], affected monkeys had a higher frequency of MHC alleles B9 and DR5 than controls.

III. CONNECTIVE TISSUE DISORDERS

A. Systemic Lupus Erythematosus

Systemic lupus erythematosus (SLE) has been described occurring as a spontaneous disease in the rhesus macaque (Anderson and Klein, 1993) and as a disease induced by an alfalfa sprout-enriched diet in cynomolgus macaques (Bardana *et al.,* 1982; Malinow *et al.,* 1982).

In the spontaneous case, a mature male macaque on a normal diet developed fever with leukocytosis, autoimmune hemolytic anemia, and splenomegaly as well as an elevated serum antinuclear antibody titer. At necropsy, in addition to membranoproliferative glomerulonephritis, and Libman–Sacks-type endocarditis, nonerosive arthritis characterized by synovitis was seen in the small joints of the hands (Anderson and Klein, 1993). These features are in keeping with the current diagnostic criteria for SLE. This animal was from the same colony as the solitary case of spontaneous eosinophilic fasciitis, which is described in the next section (Anderson and Klein, 1992).

In studies of alfalfa meal used as an oral agent to reduce plasma cholesterol and control atherosclerosis, autoimmune pancytopenia with raised antinuclear antibody titers developed in both a human volunteer and in female cynomolgus macaques (Malinow *et al.,* 1981). Three of five animals fed a 45% alfalfa seed-enriched diet for 6 months or more developed a systemic illness characterized by autoimmune hemolytic anemia, facial rash, chronic dermal inflammation with the presence of granular IgG at the dermal–epidermal junction, an immune complex type of glomerulonephritis, and raised antinuclear antibody titers (Bardana *et al.,* 1982). This disease remitted with withdrawal of alfalfa from the diet and, in some cases, by corticosteroid therapy. Dietary administration of L-canavanine sulfate, an amino acid found in alfalfa sprouts, reactivated the disease in three animals within 2 months and induced the disease *de novo* in two animals after 10 months (Malinow *et al.,* 1982).

These studies show that nonhuman primates can acquire SLE. The selective susceptibility suggests that genetic factors are implicated. The induction of this disease by a purified dietary substance, L-canavanine, suggests that nonhuman primates may be a very suitable model to study the pathogenesis of this disease.

B. Eosinophilic Fasciitis

Eosinophilic fasciitis has been reported in a female rhesus macaque from the same colony as a spontaneous case of systemic lupus erythematosus (Anderson and Klein, 1993). This animal presented with contractures and taut skin symmetrically arranged on the hind limbs. Laboratory examination showed a peripheral eosinophilia. A biopsy showed chronic inflammation at the muscle fascia junction. This inflammation persisted and was observed at necropsy 6 months later. Isolated sarcosporidial cysts were also seen in the muscle. The surrounding areas were devoid of inflammation. The authors discounted the known association of this muscle parasite with peripheral fasciitis and eosinophilia (Terrell and Stookey, 1972). There was no description of the diet.

Eosinophilic fasciitis, a variant of scleroderma, was first described in North America by Shulman (1975). It is likely that the case described in the macaque was observed because of the outbreak of eosinophilia myalgia syndrome in 1989 (Centers for Disease Control, 1989; Serratrice *et al.,* 1990; Lin *et al.,* 1992). This syndrome, in which peripheral eosinophila and fasciitis are prominent, was associated with over-the-counter preparations of L-tryptophan used as dietary supplements. There has been no attempt to induce this disease in nonhuman primates using this agent.

C. Retroperitoneal Fibromatosis

A peculiar form of retroperitoneal fibromatosis frequently associated with simian acquired immunodeficiency syndrome has been described in a mixed colony of macaques (*Macaca nemestrina, M. mulatta, M. fascicularis, M. fuscata*) at the Washington Regional Primate Research Center (Giddens *et al.,* 1985; Tsai *et al.,* 1985a,b). This disease can present in a localized modular or more diffuse form. Retroperitoneal fibromatosis is characterized histologically by extensive fibrovascular proliferation starting at the root of the mesentery. Nuclear activity may be observed in both fibroblast and endothelial cells. This disease can be transmitted by the intraperitoneal injection of affected retroperitoneal fibromatosis tissue into allogenic nonhuman primates but not into xenogenic rodents or marmosets (*Saguinus labiatus*). Type D retrovirus gene sequences have been isolated for lymphoid and retroperitoneal fibromatosis tissue of affected macaques (Bryant *et al.,* 1986). Retroperitoneal fibromatosis in SAIDS-affected macaques appears analogous to the development of Kaposi's sarcoma in humans with AIDS (Giddens *et al.,* 1985).

IV. SKELETAL MUSCLE DISEASES

The histologic architecture of skeletal muscles is well conserved in primates. The distribution of type I and type II fibers in humans is also present in both prosimian (Brooke and Kasier, 1970; Sickles and Pinkstaff, 1981) and simian (Beatty *et al.,* 1966; McIntosh *et al.,* 1985; Acosta and Roy, 1987; Suzuki and Hayama, 1991) nonhuman primates. The effects of aging on muscle fiber size and the accumulation of the lipid oxidation product, lipofuscin, have been studied in rhesus macaques (Beatty *et al.,* 1982). With increasing age, the average muscle fiber diameter decreased. As with humans (Jennekens *et al.,* 1971; Beatty *et al.,* 1982), focal neuropathic lesions were observed. Again, similar to humans, the number of lipofuscin granules within muscle fibers increased with age. Lipofuscin accumulations were greater in muscles in which oxidative fibers predominated.

Despite the similarity of the muscle fiber composition to humans, very little is known about spontaneous skeletal muscle diseases in nonhuman primates. With the exception of viral myositis, there has been little experimental investigation directed toward muscle disorders in nonhuman primates.

A. Polymyositis

Spontaneous myositis has been reported in primates housed in zoo environments, but this condition has not been well studied (Schmidt *et al.,* 1986). Muscle weakness secondary to polymositis is a prominent clinical feature in about 50% of rhesus macaques affected with SAIDS. Simian acquired immunodeficiency syndrome is associated with chronic infection by type D retroviruses (Dalakas *et al.,* 1986, 1987). Although the pathologic findings are similar, the incidence of myositis is much higher in nonhuman primates than that found in humans with AIDS. The histopathology resembles human inclusion body myositis (Carpenter *et al.,* 1978). Perivascular lymphocytic infiltrates of the OKT4 and OKT8 types and perimysial infiltrates consisting of lymphocytes and macrophages are observed. Focal single fiber myonecrosis is seen. Vacuoles containing basophilic granules are occasionally seen within the muscle fibers. As the disease advances, type II fiber atrophy and extensive perimysial fibrosis are seen. In tissue culture, muscle fibers can be infected with the retrovirus without cytopathic changes. It is presumed that muscle fibers in infected animals are similarly affected. Like the synovitis observed in SAIDS, the virus can be detected by immunofluorescence in macrophages associated with the inflammation. The mechanisms of polymyositis associated with SAIDS or AIDS are not clear. Although it is possible that the polymyositis represents a response to a primary viral infection of muscle, it is also conceivable that the viral-infected macrophages are part of the inflammatory response to another pathogenic agent in these immunodeficient animals. One such agent is human lymphotropic T virus type I (HLTV-1), a virus frequently concomitant with the AIDS virus. HLTV-I induced polymyositis and arthritis after intravenous injection into young rhesus macaques (Beilke *et al.,* 1996). The resistance of at least 50% of nonhuman primates to polymyositis suggests that genetic factors may modulate the muscle-specific inflammatory response. As with experimental inflammatory arthritis, experimental nonhuman primate viral myositis may be the most useful in understanding determinants of resistance or susceptibility to chronic inflammation that may also be operative in humans.

B. Wasting Marmoset Syndrome

Wasting marmoset syndrome is a term used for a syndrome of profound weight loss, muscle atrophy, progressive "cage paralysis," and hair loss associated with chronic diarrhea, colitis, and hemolytic anemia. This syndrome was prevalent in captive colonies of marmosets and tamarins (Callitrichidae) (King, 1976; Morin, 1983; Potkay, 1992). The etiology for this disease is unknown, but primary nutritional deficiencies of vitamin E (Hayes, 1974; Chadwick *et al.,* 1979; Baskin *et al.,* 1983) and protein deficiency secondary to chronic diarrhea (Shimwell *et al.,* 1979; Brack and Rothe, 1981; Chalifoux *et al.,* 1982; Murgatroyd, 1985) have been postulated.

In this disorder, the skeletal muscle shows extensive type II fiber atrophy, rounding up of fiber cross-sectional profiles, focal necrosis, and fibrosis (Murgatroyd, 1985). A diet deficient in vitamin E can induce all the features of the wasting syndrome without gastrointestinal involvement (Dinning and Day, 1957; Nelson *et al.,* 1981; Baskin *et al.,* 1983). Marmosets demonstrated hemolytic anemia, fat necrosis, and panniculitis as well as extensive muscle necrosis. Although vitamin E administration could not reverse the disease, vitamin E and selenium provided to animals newly arrived within the colony could prevent the syndrome (Baskin *et al.,* 1983). Currently, wasting marmoset syndrome is prevented by the dietary administration of supplements containing vitamin E, selenium, zinc, and copper.

C. Cage Paralysis

Cage paralysis is a general term referring to reluctance to move exhibited by any animal in a cage or confined environment (Ruch, 1959b). This condition, which was first recognized in zoo monkeys in 1904 (Brooks and Blair, 1904), occurs sporadically in captive animals housed under a variety of conditions (Campbell and Cleland, 1919). The disorder can develop in individual caged or corralled monkeys but has not been reported in free-ranging primates. Cage paralysis presents as progressive reluctance to move, motor weakness, and ultimately with joint contractures that affect the hind limbs predominantly. Cage paralysis appears to encompass a wide group of diseases, including peripheral, neural (Kark *et al.,* 1974; Agamanolis *et al.,* 1976), muscular (Dalakas *et al.,* 1986), arthritic (Sokoloff *et al.,* 1968), and general debilitative nutritional disorders (Ruch, 1959b; Brack and Rothe, 1981; Blanchard *et al.,* 1986).

Because the disorder is sporadic, restricted to animals in captivity, and begins in the lower limbs, a common nutritional factor has been sought. Experimental studies using rhesus monkeys have led to the speculation that chronic vitamin B_{12} deficiency might be involved with the syndrome. Rhesus macaques on vitamin B_{12}-deficient diets developed visual impairment. As the disease progresses, gradual spastic paralysis of the hind limbs ensues (Kark *et al.,* 1974; Agamanolis *et al.,* 1976). Physical examination of affected monkeys revealed a reduced range of motion in the knee joints, but radiologically the joints appear normal, at least initially. Following limitation of movement, there is joint swelling and pain, muscle wasting, and tendon contraction. The condition appears irreversible. Many of

these animals compensated for the hind limb deficit by learning to "walk" on their hands with their torso and hind limbs extended above their head. In B_{12}-deficient animals, the involvement of optic nerve and dorsal spinal cord similar to B_{12} deficiency in humans was observed. In rhesus macaques, the major difference is that the central nervous system appears more vulnerable to B_{12} deficiency and the hematopoietic system.

Although the studies of B_{12} deficiency are illuminating, it must be stressed that cage paralysis does not appear to be restricted to animals with vitamin B_{12} deficiency. Indeed, cage paralysis appears to be a late common syndrome for numerous chronic peripheral neural, arthritic, nutritional, and infectious debilitative disorders affecting nonhuman primates.

V. BONE DISEASES

A. Bone Biology

The growth, metabolism, architecture, composition, and biomechanical properties of bone in nonhuman primates resemble humans more closely than other species commonly used in biomedical research. Like humans, but unlike rodents, the epiphyses of nonhuman primates close toward the end of adolescence (Bowden *et al.,* 1979; Cheverud, 1981). One consequence of this biological similarity is that nonhuman primate bones undergo bone remodeling with a formation of osteons (Haversian systems) in the cortical bones. Cortical bone osteons do not usually form in rodents, making them poor models for most types of comparative osteological studies. Among primates, the fraction of cortical bone that is composed of osteons increases progressively from arboreal through terrestrial quadrupeds to humans (Schaffler and Burr, 1984). The rate of osteoid remodeling varies with anatomical site. In the macaque, rib osteons remodel comparably to humans whereas femoral cortical remodeling is slower (Schock *et al.,* 1972; Przybeck, 1985; Burr, 1992). Using tetracycline labeling, it has been demonstrated that juvenile macaques have a cortical mineral apposition rate greater than juvenile humans (Schock *et al.,* 1972). When synthetic progesten was administered to rhesus macaques, the bone apposition rate and activation frequency decreased compared to controls (Duncan *et al.,* 1977). In studies of selective thyroid ablation in neonatal rhesus macaques using I^{131}, thyroid deficiency resulted in a profound reduction in bone growth, an increase in radiologic bone density, and a delay in appearance in secondary ossification centers (Lusted *et al.,* 1953; Crane *et al.,* 1954).

The early studies of bone disease in nonhuman primates were stimulated by the presence of bone deformities observed in captive animals (Ruch, 1959c). The recognition that these deformities had a nutritional basis led to the study of nonhuman primates as models for nutritional, vitamin C, vitamin D, protein, and caloric deficiencies and as models for the toxic effects of environmental substances on bone. More recently, natural diseases such as periodontitis have been studied in nonhuman primates. Experimental model diseases such as osteonocrosis and osteoporosis have also been induced in nonhuman primates.

B. Bone Induction and Bone Grafts

Following trauma or surgical procedures, bone grafts from various sources have been used to facilitate or accelerate bone repair. There is considerable interest in the biologic capacity to accelerate bone differentiation and to induce new bone formation using natural or biomimetic materials. A major test system for bone induction is heterotopic bone formation following intramuscular implantation of bone material. Bone induction using allogeneic demineralized bone powder can be achieved in rodents (Urist et al., 1969; Reddi, 1981; Sampath and Reddi, 1983). However, early attempts using demineralized bone powder to induce bone in rhesus macaques (Hosny and Sharawy, 1985) and squirrel monkeys (Aspenberg et al., 1988, 1991; Hayes 1974) were less successful. Initially, the lack of bioavailability of bone morphogenic proteins or the inflammatory response to the transplanted bone material was considered a critical factor. Subsequently, supplementation of demineralized bone with human bone morphogenetic protein-2 induced new bone formation (Asperberg et al., 1992). Substitution of collagen I for allogeneic demineralized bone did not increase bone induction, implicating inflammation as the principal inhibitory process in bone formation (Aspenberg and Turek, 1996).

Ripamonti et al., (1991) implanted antigen-extracted allogenic (AAA) bone removed from adult male Chacma baboons (Papio ursinus) intermuscularly into other adult male baboons. The animals were followed for up to 9 months. Histologically, bone resorption occurred, which was followed by exuberant bone formation. These studies demonstrated that nonhuman primates retain bone-inducible proteins in the bone matrix.

In further studies, osteogenin, a bone morphogenic protein isolated from demineralized baboon bone matrix, was an effective osteoinductive agent when implanted intramuscularly with porous hydroxyapatite into nonhealing calvarial bone defects surgically prepared in adult male baboons (Ripamonti et al., 1991, 1992a–d; Ripamonti, 1992).

Porous hydroxyapatite itself has been found to induce heterotropic bone formation in baboons, but not in rabbits or dogs, thus demonstrating the importance of the nonhuman primate for this model system (Ripamonti et al., 1992a, 1993a,b; Ripamonti, 1995).

Recombinant human osteogenic protein-1 (bone morphogenetic protein-7) was implanted in large segmental ulnar and tibial defects surgically induced in green monkeys (Cercopithecus aethiops) (Cook et al., 1995). Osseous repair was stimulated with substantial restoration of mechanical integrity within 20 weeks following surgery. As nonhuman primates are less responsive to fracture healing than rodents or canines, success-

ful healing in this model has more direct application to therapy for human conditions than other species.

C. Nutritional Disorders

1. "Simian Bone Disease" and Hyperparathyroidism

The history of "simian bone disease" has been extensively reviewed (Ruch, 1959c; Krook and Barrett, 1962; Barker and Herbert, 1972). These descriptions are of immense interest as they reveal the development of our understanding of nutritional bone disease affecting nonhuman primates over the first 60 years of the 20th century. Initially, "simian bone disease" was thought to resemble goundou, a human disorder found in Central Africa that resulted in the formation of symmetrical painless swellings and exostoses on the side of the nose. Similar findings were observed in monekys in 1908 (Roques and Bouffard, 1908). With further studies, the controversy arose as to whether these changes represented Paget's disease or von Recklinghausen's disease of bone (osteitis fibrosa of hyperparathyroidism) (Corson-White, 1922). Krook and Barrett (1962) pointed out that "simian bone disease" was described before it was recognized that von Recklinghausen's disease was related to hyperparathyroidism. They described two such cases and demonstrated that the disease, in fact, was related to hyperparathyroidism secondary to an inadequate dietary calcium intake. A similar disorder was found in a group of captive lemurs (Lemur catta and L. varegatus) (Tomson et al., 1980). These animals presented with impaired mobility. On radiologic examination, long bone deformities and cystic endocortical erosions were seen. Blood chemistry demonstrated decreased serum calcium and elevated phosphate and alkaline phosphatase. This clinical picture is characteristic of secondary hyperparathyroidism. When the dietary calcium was raised, the lesions remitted.

It is important to note that the effects of excess parathyroid hormone secretion are manifest in bone tissue long before tertiary hyperparathyroidism, i.e., hypercalcemia, ensues. This state of severe secondary hyperparathyroidism with nonsuppressible parathyroid hormone secretion is termed refractory secondary parathyroidism. Histologically, the findings of the early phase of Paget's disease and the osteitis fibrosa of hyperparathyroidism are extremely similar. These findings include extensive bone resorption with osteoclasts and fibrosis in the marrow. With extensive disease, radiologic bone "cysts," which correspond to histologic "brown tumors," form typically in the mandible, maxilla, or long bones. Brown tumors received their name from the brown color of the old blood and hemosiderin present in the lesional tissue. Brown tumors arise from expansion of the cortical bone secondary to endocortical bone resorption and the increased intraosseous pressure from vascular congestion. The histologic appearance includes the presence of numerous osteoclasts, capillary blood vessels, macrophages, and fibroblasts, the latter cells often containing hemosiderin. In "simian bone disease," brown tumors likely underlie the facial masses originally described in pseudogoundou. Brown tumors in "simian bone disease" likely represent the bone effects of refractory secondary hyperparathyroidism, i.e., autonomous hyperparathyroid activity developing in parathyroid glands previously stimulated by calcium deficiency to secondary reactive hyperplasia (Galbraith and Quarles, 1993). The case of a brown tumor arising in a woolly monkey (*Lagothrix lagotrichia*) is instructive as the lesion, an expansile tumor of the humerus, was thought clinically to be a malignant bone tumor (Smith *et al.*, 1978).

Clinically, animals with "simian bone disease" presented with decreased locomotion, kyphosis, propensity to bend or fracture long bones, and marked thickening of the maxillary and mandibular bones accompanied by dental displacement. This was particularly true in young animals with adequate nutrition. "Simian bone disease" has virtually disappeared from laboratory primates, primate centers, and zoological parks. The disorder remains a sporadic problem in pet monkeys maintained on unbalanced or inadequate diets (Smith, *et al.*, 1978).

2. Periarticular Periosteal Hyperostosis

Periarticular periosteal hyperostosis affecting the distal femur and proximal tibia as well as other long bones has been described in lemurs (Tomson *et al.*, 1980; Junge *et al.*, 1994; Weber *et al.*, 1995). Although the etiologic factors may vary from nutritional calcium deficiency (Tomson *et al.*, 1980) to chronic renal disease (Junge *et al.*, 1994), the clinical presentation and histologic features are those of secondary hyperparathyroidism. X-ray examination shows exuberant subperiosteal new bone formation at the distal ends of bones. The irregular and often radiate pattern distinguishes the lesion from hypertrophic osteoarthropathy often associated with intrathoracic lesions. Histologically, irregular bone resorption and new bone formation with marrow fibrosis, features characteristic of parathyroid hormone activity on bone, were observed. In one report, indices for parathyroid hormone activity were normal, further suggesting that the hyperparathyroidism was secondary (Weber *et al.*, 1995). The differences in these lesions from those in rickets affecting Old World monkeys such as rhesus macaques appear more related to the anatomical distribution than to pathogenesis (Simon and Garman, 1970).

3. Protein Deficiency

Kwashiorkor, a syndrome of growth failure, anemia, hypoproteinemia, and edema, is common in severely undernourished children and can be replicated in young nonhuman primates (Follis, 1957; Ramalingaswami *et al.*, 1961; Deo *et al.*, 1965; Jha *et al.*, 1968; Kerr *et al.*, 1973). Follis (1957) induced kwashiorkor by feeding juvenile green monkeys (*Cercopithecus aethiops*) a diet of cornmeal supplemented by vitamin C. Even though epiphyseal growth was orderly, maturation failure of cortical bone, i.e., failure to develop osteons (Haversian sys-

tems), was observed. Jha and colleagues (Ramalingaswami *et al.*, 1961; Deo *et al.*, 1965; Sood *et al.*, 1965; Jha *et al.*, 1968) studied a synthetic protein-deficient diet administered to rhesus macaques and compared the results to animals receiving a diet containing 20% protein. Animals on the protein-deficient diet had a selective decrease in serum calcium while maintaining serum calcium, phosphorous, and alkaline phosphatase. Using tetracycline labeling, a decrease in appositional new bone formation was seen that was progressive with the duration of the protein deficiency. The epiphyseal zones were decreased in thickness, but no deformity or mineralization disorder was observed. In similar studies in infant rhesus macaques, a decrease in growth of all organs, incuding muscle and bone, was seen. However, temporary protein deprivation reduced bone mineralization but not bone width; the effect was reversible on restoration of a normal diet (Leutenegger *et al.*, 1973; Riopelle *et al.*, 1976; Riopelle and Favret, 1977; Murchison *et al.*, 1984).

These studies suggest that adequate dietary protein is required to maintain bone growth, bone mass, and bone remodeling. Apart from kwashiorkor, these studies have important implications for osteoporosis. First, protein deficiency during growth can lead to osteoporosis. This situation, which occurred in children of young women during World War II in China and Japan, may be a major factor in the prevalence of osteoporosis in these areas at the present time. Second, osteoporosis therapy to restore bone is not effective unless the dietary protein intake is sufficient in quantity and quality. With regard to mechanisms, dietary protein is required not only for collagenous and noncollagenous bone structures, but also for the peptide hormones that stimulate bone growth.

4. Caloric Restriction

Caloric restriction with adequate protein, vitamins, and other nutrients has been shown to retard aging and increase the mean and maximum life span in rodents (Weindruch and Walford, 1988). Presentation of a calorie-restricted diet to nonhuman primates results in decreased crown–rump lengths and decreased serum alkaline phosphatase, both indirect indicators of decreased bone growth (Lane *et al.*, 1992; Weindruch *et al.*, 1995). In further studies, juvenile, adult, and old rhesus macaques were investigated longitudinally (Lane *et al.*, 1995). The animals were pair housed in standard rhesus monkey cages, an environment that limits physical activity and social interaction. In this study, which extended over 6 years, food-deprived animals demonstrated a decline in alkaline phosphatase as well as retarded bone maturation. Food restriction decreased the total bone mineral content but not bone densities. This reflects the observation that these animals had smaller bones but the bone was normally mineralized. Of note, the serum calcium concentration in food-restricted animals was substantially lower than controls. Interleukin-6 (IL-6) is a cytokine that stimulates bone resorption by accelerating osteoclast formation (Ershler, 1993). Recombinant human IL-6 administered in pharmacologic doses to rhesus monkeys also decreased bone formation (Binkley *et al.*, 1994). Food-deprived animals did not show the expected increase in IL-6 levels with age (Ershler *et al.*, 1993). Hormonal aspects of food deprivation have been studied predominantly from the viewpoint of carbohydrate metabolism and insulin sensitivity in animals predisposed to obesity (Cutler *et al.*, 1992; Bodkin *et al.*, 1993a, b, 1995; Hansen and Bodkin, 1993; Ortmeyer *et al.*, 1993; Kemnitz *et al.*, 1994; Hansen *et al.*, 1995). Similarly, serum insulin-like growth factor 1 levels of growing rhesus macaques correlate with body weight (Styne, 1991). Food restriction in rhesus macaques restores insulin sensitivity and reduces serum insulin levels. This downregulation of insulin and perhaps other growth factors may have direct effects on the skeletal system by decreasing the rate of bone growth and retarding bone maturation.

5. Scurvy

L-Ascorbic acid (vitamin C) is an essential cofactor for many enzyme oxidation processes, including EC 1-5-3 proline oxidase, EC 1-4-3-13 lysyl oxidase (collagen formation and maturation), and dopamine β-oxidase (conversion of dopamine to the neurotransmitter noradrenaline), for folate metabolism, and for iron absorption (Levine, 1986; Hallberg *et al.*, 1987; Padh, 1990). Ascorbate serves as an important tissue antioxidant (Gershoff, 1993; Rose and Bode, 1993). Ascorbate is also required for the expression of alkaline phosphatase by cells (Leboy *et al.*, 1989).

Because of the lack of cellular L-gulono-γ-lactone oxidase, humans and nonhuman primates, with the possible exception of some prosimians, require dietary L-ascorbic acid (Nishikimi and Udenfriend, 1976). Scurvy, a dietary deficiency of the vitamin C, is manifested in the musculoskeletal system by joint pain and tenderness, reluctance to move, lameness or abnormal locomotion, muscle wasting, subperiosteal hemorrhages, and epiphyseal fractures (Shaw *et al.*, 1945; Machlin *et al*, 1979). Juvenile animals are most susceptible, with clinical manifestations varying among species. In juvenile rhesus macaques, acute ascorbate deprivation presents clinically with weight loss and joint tenderness. Chronic ascorbate deficiency is characterized by gingival swelling, hyperemia, injury, and hemorrhage as well as by periodontal bone resorption, epiphyseal injury, and fractures of long bones (Shaw *et al.*, 1945). In juvenile squirrel monkeys, large acute cephalohematomas are a common pathognomic presentation (Blackwell *et al.*, 1974; Demaray *et al.*, 1978; Kessler, 1980; Ratterree *et al.*, 1990). In young rhesus monkeys the earliest sign may be subtle lameness (Eisele *et al.*, 1992). Other signs include generalized weakness, weight loss, scruffy hair coat, gingival and subcutaneous petechial hemorrhages, a propensity for easily bruising, and anemia. Vitamin C is required to mediate some effects of other vitamins (Hayes, 1974), and biotin is required to modulate vitamin C levels (Furukawa *et al.*, 1992). Therefore, the differential diagnosis of weakness and peripheral neuropathy includes mixed vitamin deficiencies, including those secondary to parasites. Scurvy may be associated with a macrocytic anemia related to the re-

quirement of ascorbate for folate metabolism. Failure to form collagen adequately results in major connective tissue lesions attributed to scurvy, including subcutaneous and gingival petechial hemorrhages, a propensity to bruising, and, in bones, subperiosteal hematomas and epiphyseal disruption (Sabin, 1939). Periosteal elevation in long bones is a characteristic radiological finding in scurvy. In newborn squirrel monkeys, periosteal elevation can be seen in the skull. These observations are secondary to hemorrhage from the fragile capillaries in the inner (cambium) layer of the periosteum. Epiphyseal disruption occurs secondary to hemorrhage from capillaries present within the bone marrow and from failure of collagen maturation during the repair process. Epiphyseal/metaphyseal sites in growing bones are sites where collagen turnover and capillary blood vessel formation are most rapid and therefore most vulnerable to ascorbate deficiency. These lesions are reversible with administration of vitamin C. Following treatment, X-rays show subperiosteal radiodensities representing ossification followed by remodeling toward normal structure. With administration of vitamin C, the epiphyseal lesions also return toward normal morphology. Deficiency of L-ascorbic acid can potentiate the abnormal bone formation in experimental fluorosis in rhesus macaques. Again, these effects are reversed with adequate ascorbate supplementation (Reddy and Rao, 1971; Reddy and Srikantia, 1971). Historically, ascorbate deficiency was a contributing factor to "simian bone disease." Experimental vitamin C deficiency in rhesus macaques can produce scorbutic lesions within bones as early as 4 weeks following the initiation of ascorbic acid-deficient diets (Baskin *et al.*, 1983). While all commercial nonhuman primate diets contain vitamin C in concentrations sufficient to prevent scurvy, a manufacturing error in the production of monkey diet led to outbreaks of scurvy in the course of 2–3 months in rhesus and squirrel monkeys at several primate facilities (Ratterree *et al.*, 1990; Eisele *et al.*, 1992). Additionally, prolonged storage or heat can destroy vitamin C in diets.

The diagnosis of vitamin C deficiency is based on clinical signs, radiologic lesions, and ascorbic acid levels in the serum. The treatment for vitamin C deficiency in nonhuman primates must include the parenteral injection of ascorbic acid, as well as dietary supplementation with citrus fruit and other ascorbic acid dietary sources. Dietary supplementation alone appears insufficient to reverse scurvy in nonhuman primates. Squirrel monkeys respond to a single intramuscular injection of 50 mg of ascorbic acid (Kessler, 1980) and dietary supplementation. Others have used two doses of 250 mg ascorbic acid intramuscularly plus oral supplementation (Eisele *et al.*, 1992) or 25 mg per kilogram ascorbic acid intramuscularly given twice daily for 5 days (Ratterree *et al.*, 1990).

6. Rickets and Osteomalacia

Rickets is a disorder of growing bones manifest by epiphyseal deformities and failure of bone mineralization. Osteomalacia is a similar disorder in the mature skeleton characterized by failure to mineralize osteoid, the connective tissue matrix of bone. Both disorders can result from diseases of diverse etiology and pathogenesis. Rickets has been recognized in nonhuman primates since ancient times (von den Driesch and Boessneck, 1985, 1993). Signs, symptoms, and pathology of advanced rickets and osteomalacia have been reviewed extensively by Ruch (1959c) as well as by Krook and Barrett (1962). These diseases share common dietary deficiencies and/or metabolic defects in vitamin D, calcium, or phosphate metabolism (Mankin, 1974b). An extensive discussion of the metabolic pathways contributing to rickets is beyond the scope of this review. Briefly, vitamin D_3 (cholecalciferol, vitamin D_3) can be synthesized endogenously in the epidermis from 7-dehydrocholesterol by the activity of ultraviolet radiation from sunlight. Dietary vitamin D is required under conditions of decreased sun exposure, pregnancy, and lactation (Holick, 1995). Vitamin D is a family of compounds that includes vitamin D_2 (ergocalciferol) derived from the plant sterol and vitamin D_3 (cholecalciferol) derived from animal sources. This distinction has important consequences for the prevention of rickets in nonhuman primates. Vitamin D_3 is hydroxylated in the liver to 25-$(OH)D_3$ and is further hydroxylated in the kidney to the active hormone 1,25-$(OH)_2D_3$ (Vieth and Cole, 1996). Dietary deficiency, malabsorption, and liver and kidney diseases as well as end organ hormone resistance can each give rise to rickets or osteomalacia. 1,25-Dihydroxyvitamin D_3 has many activities that promote bone development and bone mineralization (Vieth and Cole, 1996). These include terminal differentiation of cell lines such as epiphyseal chondrocytes and the modulation of hormonal biorhythms (Stumpf, 1988; Stumpf and Privette, 1991; Walters, 1992). As dietary vitamin D requirement is partial and variable among species and even among members of the same species between sun-exposed and sun-deprived environments, the relative contribution of vitamin D, calcium, and phosphate deficiencies to the pathogenesis of nutritional rickets and osteomalacia is controversial (Simon and Garman, 1970).

The requirement for vitamin D in nonhuman primates has been demonstrated by dietary experiments. Rhesus macaques fed vitamin D-deficient diets with calcium/phosphorus ratios varying from 1:2 to 1.3:1 developed clinical rickets reversible by the administration of cod liver oil or exposure to ultraviolet light (Gerstenberger, 1938). Juvenile animals that are rapidly growing and are deprived of sunlight are most susceptible to rickets (Gerstenberger, 1938; Simon and Garman, 1970; Morrisey et al., 1994, 1995).

New World monkeys such as marmosets (*Callithrix jacchus*) have much higher circulating levels of the active hormone 1,25-$(OH)_2$ D_3 and require higher vitamin D in diets compared to Old World primates such as rhesus monkeys (Shinki et al., 1983). New World monkeys are subject to osteomalacia, which has clinical biochemical features in common with vitamin D-dependent rickets type II (end organ resistance rickets) in humans (Brooks et al., 1978; Yamaguchi et al., 1986; Vieth and Cole, 1996). The mechanism of the 1,25-$(OH)_2D_3$ resistance has not been determined. In these animals, it has been suggested

that 1,25-$(OH)_2D_3$ is more tightly bound to serum proteins (Yamaguchi et al., 1986). However, osteomalacic animals did show a decrease in serum 25-$(OH)D_3$ compared to normal animals, suggesting a relative lack of dietary vitamin D_3. Comparative species differences in vitamin D metabolism among nonhuman primates and humans have been subject to considerable investigation (Gray et al., 1982; Shinki et al., 1983; Liberman et al., 1985; J. S. Adams et al., 1985a, b, 1987; Takahashi et al., 1985; Vieth et al., 1987, 1990; Zucker et al., 1988; Adams and Gacad, 1988; Gacad and Adams, 1989, 1991, 1992, 1993; Padh, 1990, 1993; Cleve et al., 1991; Gacad et al., 1992). New World monkeys have circulating 1,25-$(OH)_2D_3$ levels up to 10 times that of Old World primates (Shinki et al., 1983; Adams et al., 1985a). Old World primates (rhesus macaques) also have higher 1,25-$(OH)_2D_3$ levels than humans (Vieth et al., 1987), suggesting that nonhuman primates have 1,25-$(OH)_2D_3$ end organ resistance or, alternatively, that humans have 1,25-$(OH)_2D_3$ end organ sensitivity compared to other primates. Humans have a larger fraction of free 25-$(OH)D_3$ than nonhuman primates (Vieth et al., 1990). Perhaps adaption of terrestrial environment, to higher latitudes, and to clothing has induced 1,25$(OH)_2D_3$ end organ sensitivity in humans.

In contast to vitamin D metabolism, the serum parathyroid hormone concentration (J. S. Adams et al., 1987) and parathyroid hormone responses to hypocalcemic stimuli nonhuman primates resemble those of humans (Fincham et al., 1993).

Experimental vitamin D deficiency rickets in baboons (*Papio ursinus*) is manifested clinically by failure to grow, enlargement of wrists and knees, and bowing of long bones. Radiologically, enlargement and deformity (cupping) of the epiphyses and decreased bone density are seen. Histologically, there is epiphyseal plate hypertrophy with chondrocyte hyperplasia and failure to mineralize and resorb the hypertrophic epiphyseal cartilage matrix. Pure nutritional vitamin D deficiency is accompanied by increased serum alkaline phosphatase but little change in other biochemical parameters. Cereals such as maize exacerbate the disease as well as serum biochemical abnormalities. Under maize-replete, vitamin D_3-deplete conditions, serum phosphorous and magnesium levels are low and serum calcium declines late in the disease (Sly et al., 1984).

Osteomalacia in a group of free-ranging Japanese macaques (*Macaca fuscata*) has been extensively studied (Snyder et al., 1980). These animals were translocated to a habitat with abundant sunlight but very different from their natural environment. On a diet consisting of foraged natural vegetation, which included dried corn and cattle cubes, they developed lameness followed by bowing of the extremities. Radiologically, a general decrease in bone density with multiple fractures of long bones was demonstrated. Blood chemistry revealed elevated serum alkaline phosphatase, hypophosphatemia, and normal serum calcium. Bone biopsy showed an increased osteoid width (30 μm) on the bone surfaces, a feature characteristic of osteomalacia.

Daily supplements of commercial monkey ration reversed the disease. In these animals, the available diet had a low calcium/phosphorous ratio, suggesting that calcium deficiency was a prime etiologic factor. Similarly, osteopenia has been demonstrated in capuchin monkeys (*Cebus albifrons*) on diets with a low Ca:P ratio (Anderson *et al.*, 1977). Juvenile baboons on low Ca:P diets also developed rickets and, after 16 months, secondary hyperparathyroidism (Pettifor *et al.*, 1984).

Gross examination of bones with rickets demonstrated enlargement and deformity of the epiphyseal growth plate cartilage. In both rickets and osteomalacia, the bone is soft. Histologically, in rickets the epiphyseal plate is elongated with persistence of the chondrocytes giving rise to an appearance of hyperplasia (Lapin and Yakovleva, 1960; Mankin, 1974a). Mechanical forces on the soft epiphyseal cartilage result in transverse "pseudofractures," which, when calcified, provide the radiologic sign of Looser's lines (Mankin, 1974a). Chondrocyte persistence, with an excess accumulation of nonmineralized matrix together with transverse pseudofractures, gives rise to epiphyseal deformities seen radiologically as cupping. At the cartilage bone junction, there is decreased mineralization of the cartilage matrix.

With osteomalacia in the adult skeleton, principal lesions are seen on trabecular bone surfaces and within cortical osteons at sites of remodeling. At these sites, there is an increase in the osteoid width and an increase in the percentage of bone surface covered by osteoid. Other histologic features are variable. In nutritional deficiencies where osteoid is mineralizable, osteoblasts are present on osteoid surfaces. When previously administered systemically, tetracycline uptake can be seen at the mineralization front beneath these surfaces. When osteoid is not mineralizable, such as in some types of renal osteodystrophy, bone surfaces are hypocellular and refractory to tetracycline uptake. When secondary hyperparathyroidism is present, increased osteoclasts and fibrosis at sites of resorption of the residual mineralized bone are observed (Simon and Garman, 1970; Mankin, 1974a).

Therapy for rickets and osteomalacia is dependent on accurate diagnosis of the underlying cause and on an adequate appreciation of the vitamin D resistance, particularly in nonhuman primate species. Dietary therapy with vitamin D_2 derived from ultraviolet irradiation of plant ergosterol appears adequate for Old World primates (Morrisey *et al.*, 1995). However, squirrel monkeys given vitamin D_2 developed rickets (Lehner *et al.*, 1967), possibly because of more rapid metabolism of $1,25\text{-}(OH)_2$ vitamin D_2. It is now recognized that vitamin D_3 from animal sources is required to prevent rickets in New World monkeys (Hunt *et al.*, 1967a, b). In addition to providing adequate vitamin D_3 supplementation, therapy should be directed toward correcting underlying systemic disease if present, e.g., malabsorption.

7. Zinc Deficiency

Zinc is an essential trace metal for skeletal growth and development (Berg and Shi, 1996). Zinc has many biologic functions on skeletal tissue, not least as a component of the active site of metalloenzymes such as alkaline phosphatase (Wuthier and Register, 1984). Zinc is taken up by bone with only slight preference to soft tissues (Jowsey and Orvis, 1967). Spontaneous zinc deficiency in marmosets (*Saguinas mystax*) presented with

alopecia and thickened skin, particulary involving the tail (Chadwick *et al.*, 1979). Experimental marginal zinc deficiency in pregnant rhesus primates resulted in retarded skeletal growth and a rickets-like syndrome in the newborn offspring that persisted over the clinical follow-up of 3 years (Golub *et al.*, 1984; Leek *et al.*, 1984, 1988). Based on radiologic observations, zinc deficiency retarded periosteal and trabecular bone formation but permitted endosteal bone resorption. Similar lesions induced by the alkaline phosphatase inhibitor cadmium can be reversed by administrating zinc (Bonner *et al.*, 1980). These observations provide evidence that the skeletal manifestations of zinc deficiency are mediated by the negative effect of zinc deficiency on alkaline phosphatase. Moderate dietary zinc deprivation in adolescent female rhesus macaques resulted in slower skeletal growth, motivation, and mineralization than controls, particularly in the postmenorrheal rapid growth period (Golub *et al.*, 1996).

D. Bone Mineralization Toxic Disorders

1. Lead

More than 90% of lead found in the body is stored in the skeleton. In adults, lead is found distributed preferentially in cancellous bone reflecting the higher fraction of active bone surfaces found on bone trabeculae (Wittmers *et al.*, 1988). Lead within bone is relatively inert as it is surrounded by the bone mineral calcium apatite (Eisenstein and Kawanoue, 1975).

Isolated cases of lead poisoning in nonhuman primates associated with the use of lead base paints for cages have been recognized since 1938 (van Bogaert and Scherer, 1938; Fisher, 1954; de Bisschop, 1956; McIntosh, 1956; Cordy, 1957; Ruch, 1959b; Hausman *et al.*, 1961). However, the skeletal manifestations have been noted in only a few reports (Fisher, 1954; de Bisschop, 1956; Cordy, 1957). Calcium deficiency in rhesus macaques facilitated lead ingestion possibly by inhibition of the adverse taste effects of lead (Jacobson and Snowdon, 1976). Perhaps, the most significant outbreak of lead poisoning occurred in juvenile Cercopithecinae at the National Zoological Park in Washington, D.C. (Zook and Paasch, 1980). The source of the lead was traced to the pica of infant and juvenile primates gnawing at cage bars covered by lead-based paints (Zook *et al.*, 1973). These animals presented with amaurotic epilepsy that was later recognized as a manifestation of lead encephalopathy.

In studies of experimental lead encephalopathy in juvenile rhesus macaques, lead could be demonstrated radiologically as a metaphyseal-radiodense transverse zone. These "lead lines" corresponded to zones of pathologically mineralized cartilage matrix surrounded by a thin layer of bone. These mineralized nodules were surrounded by osteoclasts or chondroclasts that contained intracellular crystals (Eisenstein and Kawanoue, 1975). Electron microscopy of these crystals demonstrated membrane limited crystal and amorphous electron-dense inclusions. Because the extracellular lead deposition is amorphous, it is assumed that the lead crystal formation was a result of solubilization and recrystallization of the lead. These findings were accompanied by decreased bone formation on the normally mineralized epiphyseal cartilage trabeculae. Environmental lead toxicity associated with nonhuman primates is now mostly of historical interest as lead-based paints, lead water pipes, and devices containing lead solder are no longer used in zoo environments.

2 Cadmium

Itai Itai disease, a disorder found in Japan, is characterized by renal insufficiency and painful bones secondary to osteomalacia. Chronic cadmium toxicity combined with malnutrition were thought to be etiologic factors. To study the relative roles of cadmium, protein, and vitamin D deficiency, extensive long-term dietary experiments were performed on rhesus macaques (Kimura, 1986). In the presence of a low protein diet, cadmium ingestion appears to inhibit mineralization on osteoid, an effect that may be related directly to the effects of cadmium on bone cells. Cadmium nephrotoxicity at the doses employed did not interfere with vitamin D hydroxylation in the kidney.

3. Fluoride

Fluoride is a substance with special affinity for bone as it is preferentially incorporated into the bone mineral apatite (Grynpas, 1990). Administered in drinking water at low concentrations (1 ppm), fluoride protects against dental caries (Murray et al., 1990). The effect of fluoride on bone has been investigated extensively as a therapy for osteoporosis and as a toxic agent in fluorosis. There have been relatively few studies of fluoride in nonhuman primates (Wadhwani, 1955; Griffiths et al., 1975). These studies demonstrate that the presence of fluoride can protect against osteoporosis and that with dietary calcium deficiency, fluoride administrations can lead to osteomalacia (Griffiths, et al., 1975).

4. Tetracycline

Rhesus macaques have been used to study the toxic effects of excessive tetracycline administration on bone (Yen et al., 1972; Simmons et al., 1983). In young macaques, oral tetracycline has been shown to retard endochondral ossification and linear growth of bone (Yen and Shaw, 1957, 1974; Yen et al., 1972). The rate of membranous bone growth can be retarded for up to 2 weeks by the adminstration of a single intraperitoneal dose of tetracycline at 80 mg/kg (Yen et al., 1972). In a long-term study, mature female rhesus macaques were given 50 mg of tetracycline intramuscularly daily for 1 year, a dose known to affect bone structure adversely (Simmons et al., 1983). Tetracycline decreased bone remodeling and decreased the density of bone mineralization. The calcium:phosphorous ratio in newly formed bone mineral was increased.

E. Bone Inflammation

Nonhuman primates appear susceptible to the same range of bone inflammation and bone infections as humans. These diseases include local and hematogenous osteomyelitis, aggressive orofacial granulomatous inflammation (noma), and chronic periodontitis. In most instances, the microorganisms and the reactions to injury are similar to the human diseases.

1. Osteomyelitis

Osteologic studies on more than 1400 primate skeletons from a large variety of collections demonstrated osteomyelitis in about 1% of cases. In most instances, only one bone was involved, suggesting local osteomyelitis (Rothschild and Woods, 1992a). A case of cranial osteomyelitis was found on examination of 31 mountain gorilla skeletons (Lovell, 1990b). Local osteomyelitis in nonhuman primate colonies may be less reported than rare as the disease secondary to fracture or fight wounds is well recognized (Klumpp et al., 1986). Of interest, nonhuman primates can survive in the wild with chronic local osteomyelitis (Fox, 1937).

Hematogenous osteomyelitis was found in a rhesus macaque 42 days after the onset of salmonella enteritis (Klumpp et al., 1986). This infection presented with fever and a fluctuant mass at the medial aspect of the left knee. Subsequently, bones of both legs became involved. On postmortem examination, an extensive sequestrum and involucrum was seen involving the left femur. The distal right femur and the proximal tibia and fibula were involved with bone erosions. There was some evidence that this animal was immunosuppressed compared to other animals in his group (Klumpp et al., 1986).

Local osteomyelitis secondary to an overlying skin wound was observed in the femur of a stump-tailed macaque (Macaca arctoides) (Battles et al., 1985). This animal demonstrated many typical features of osteomyelitis: fistual arts, sequestrum, and circumferential periosteal new bone formation (involucrum).

Considering the importance and the extensive study of tuberculosis in nonhuman primates, tuberculosis involving bone has been described infrequently (Martin et al., 1968; Kennard, 1941; Southard, 1906). Many older descriptions may represent other diseases such as spondyloarthropathy (Nail and Ray, 1955; Ruch, 1959c). Tuberculous osteomyelitis presents with paresis and eventual paralysis of the hind limbs accompanied by kyphosis. Radiologic examination shows circumscribed radiolucencies typically involving a thoracic vertebral body eventual collapse. The histological reaction is characterized by caseous necrosis and granulomas with macrophages and giant cells of the Langhans type. The bone adjacent to the granulomatous inflammation shows resorption. In nonhuman primates, subperiosteal new bone formation can be observed (Martin et al., 1968). Traditionally, microorganisms were identified by special histologic stains, but molecular techniques are now available for tuberculosis. Experimentally, tuberculosis spondylitis was induced in juvenile cynomolgus monkeys (Macaca fascicularis) by intratracheal installation of tubercle bacilli. In this model, high doses of bacilli produced fulminant pneumonia, whereas lower doses resulted in chronic granulomatous spondylitis (Gordon et al., 1986).

Granulomatous osteomyelitis secondary to coccidioidomycosis has been reported involving the T_{11} dorsal spinous process in a rhesus macaque (Castleman *et al.,* 1980) and in the T_{12}–L_2 vertebra bony segments in a baboon (Rosenberg *et al.,* 1984). In these cases, the bone involvement was presumed to be secondary to hematogenous spread from a lund infection. Vertebral and rib involvement by coccidioidomycosis has been demonstrated in macerated oseologic material from chimpanzees (Long and Merbs, 1981). In these cases, the osseous involvement was predominantly axial.

Granulomatous osteomyelitis secondary to *Histoplasmosis duboisii* was found in 2 of 21 affected animals in an epizootic outbreak in Texas at the Southwest Foundation for Biomedical Research's colony of 3400 baboons. While the source of the organism was considered to be respiratory inhalation from soil, the bone infections represented direct invasion from adjacent soft tissue lesions.

2. Noma (Cancrum Oris)

Noma is an old clinical term for a spreading sore that begins on the mucosal membrane at the alveolar margin of the mouth. Noma (cancrum oris or Vincent's disease) is now used to describe a severe, aggressive gangrenous infection of the orofacial tissues, including bone. Lesions in the bone include osteonecrosis and osteomyelitis with sequestration.

The disease usually affects malnourished, debilitated young children living in underdeveloped tropical countries following systemic infections such as malaria, measles, primary herpes simplex, or enteritis (Loesche, 1976). Noma, and a milder form of the disease called acute ulcerative necrotizing gingivitis (ANUG) or simply ulcerative necrotizing gingivitis, has been associated with at least three species of the spirochete *Treponema* and *Bacillus fusiformis,* which normally inhabit the oral cavity of humans. There is also an association between noma and nonhemolytic streptococci, *Staphylococcus aureus* and *Bacteriodes melaninogenicus* (Adams and Bishop, 1980). Prior to the advent of antibiotics, death often resulted from the complications of noma such as osteomyelitis, bronchopneumonia, pulmonary necrosis, and cachexia. An underlying immunological defect or compromise has been suspected to play a role in the pathogenesis of noma (Enwonwu, 1972; Buchanan *et al.,* 1981). Recent cases in monkeys immunosuppressed with retrovirus infections have added credence to this hypothesis.

Although the organisms that are associated with noma can be found in the oral cavity of normal and, to a greater extent, in malnourished monkeys (Ruch, 1959a), only a few noma cases have been reported in nonhuman primates. In 1931, two spontaneously occurring cases of noma were reported in chimpanzees (Bourdella *et al.,* 1931). In 1933, two cases of noma were reported in macaques experimentally infected with *Leishmania donovani* (Krishnan, 1933; Smith, 1933) and 10 years later rhesus monkeys on a folic acid-deficient diet developed gingivitis and orofacial lesions consistent with noma (Weisman *et*

al., 1943). Several other nutritional deficiency studies using rhesus monkeys also resulted in gingivitis and lesions similar to noma. Noma in nonhuman primates was not reported again until the 1980s when Adams and Bishop (1980) and Buchanan *et al.,* (1981) described spontaneously occurring lesions in six rhesus monkeys and one *Macaca cyclopis,* respectively. Another two cases were reported in cotton-topped marmosets (Brack, 1982), the first and only report of noma to date in New World primates. A high sugar diet was considered the predisposing cause of infection and disease in the marmosets. The most recently reported cases of noma in nonhuman primates have occurred in *M. cyclopis* with an acquired immunodeficiency syndrome from infection with a retrovirus (King *et al.,* 1983; Letvin *et al.,* 1983; Letvin and King, 1984). These monkeys exhibited immunosuppression and a variety of opportunistic infections, including *Pneumocystis carnii,* cytomegalovirus, simian virus 40 (SV40) with noma lesions, and lymphomas. In all of the cases reported in nonhuman primates, the acute onset, course of infection, and lesions were similar or identical to those of the human disease. Histologically, the disease is characterized by necrotizing and often granulomatous inflammation with extensive bone destruction and development of bone and tooth sequestra (Adams and Bishop, 1980). In most cases, there was a predisposing factor involved such as malnutrition, enteritis, debility, and/or immunosuppression from infection with retroviruses. These findings in nonhuman primates support the hypothesis that noma is a disease from opportunistic infection and disease. Treatment, if successful, must include systemic antibiotics and, if possible, correction of the underlying cause(s) of infection.

3. Periodontal Disease

Chronic periodontitis is characterized by acute and chronic gingival inflammation associated with bone resorption and bone periodontal ligament resorption surrounding the teeth. Chronic periodontitis is common in aged human and nonhuman primates (Page *et al.,* 1975). Cohen and Goldman (1960) reviewed the early literature on nonhuman primate periodontal disease and described the periodontal lesions in animals dying of debilitation secondary to enteritis. The etiologic agent of spontaneous periodontis is unknown. In osteological studies, periodontal bone resorption was observed in orangutan and chimpanzee skulls, but gibbons and simiangs were spared (Cohen and Goldman, 1960). Periodontal disease resulting in tooth loss has been reported in captive *Callithrix jacchus* (Lucas *et al.,* 1937; Shaw and Auskaps, 1954).

Periodontal bone resorption has been induced in cotton-topped marmosets (*Saguinus oedipus*) by a repeated intramuscular injection of cortisone (Dreizen *et al.,* 1971). Cortisone-treated animals showed much less gingival inflammation than controls but much more extensive bone resorption. This protocol is a problematic model for periodontal disease as extensive osteoporosis in other bones of the treated animals was reported.

A more controlled model is local periodontal disease induced by ligature-induced attachment loss (Giannobile *et al.,* 1994). In this model, in cynomolgus monkeys (Kornman *et al.,* 1981; Kiel *et al.,* 1983; Brecx *et al.,* 1985, 1986; Holt *et al.,* 1988) or squirrel monkeys (Heijl *et al.,* 1976; Adams *et al.,* 1979), a notch is placed surgically into the tooth root at the crest of the alveolar bone and a ligature is placed around the tooth separating the tooth from the periodontal ligament. Periodontitis commences within 7 days but requires up to 4 months to demonstrate bone loss. Application of platelet-derived growth factor (PDGF) and insulin-like growth factor (IGF-1) into the defect can accelerate healing in this model (Schou *et al.,* 1993). Systemic bisphosphonate, administered at the onset of the surgical procedure, also reduces bone resorption without reducing gingival inflammation (Kornman *et al.,* 1990; Brunsvold *et al.,* 1992; Weinreb *et al.,* 1994).

F. Dysbaric Osteonecrosis

In an attempt to induce dysbaric osteonecrosis, squirrel monkeys (*Saimiri sciureus*) were subjected to pressures of 2.4 kg/cm^2 (25 m seawater equivalent) for 3 hr weekly for 26 weeks followed by 13 months of observation (Kupper, 1976). No clinical, radiologic, or histologic evidence of dysbaric osteonecrosis was discovered under these conditions.

G. Infantile Cortical Hyperostosis

Symmetrical diaphyseal enlargement secondary to subperiosteal new bone formation accompanied by incomplete epiphyseal ossification are the hallmarks of infantile cortical hyperostosis. This syndrome has been seen in both sporadic and familial presentations in rhesus macaques (Cicmanec *et al.,* 1972; Chesney *et al.,* 1973; Snook and King, 1989; Snook, 1993). In the familial case, a female rhesus macaque had congenital cortical hyperostosis. Eleven years later, she gave birth to a stillborn with the disease. Five other infants were unaffected.

Although radiologic photographs and descriptions are similar, other case reports have classified this disease as polyostotic osteophytosis (Cicmanec *et al.,* 1972) or as a variant of progressive diaphyseal dysplasia (Chesney *et al.,* 1973). In the case examined histologically, the subperiosteal bone appears to demonstrate new bone formation with progressive maturation. The radiologic and histologic appearances of this syndrome resemble infantile cortical hyperostosis (Caffey's disease) in humans (Caffey, 1968; Staheli *et al.,* 1968). The etiology of this disease is unknown.

H. Hypertrophic Osteoarthropathy and Hypertrophic Pulmonary Osteoarthropathy

Hypertrophic osteoarthropathy is a disorder characterized by bilateral symmetrical subperiosteal new bone formation at the ends of long bones. Most commonly, but not exclusively, the condition is associated with destructive chronic lung disease or lung tumors. The mechanism of hypertrophic osteoarthropathy associated with intrathoracic lesions is not known, but it is thought to be mediated by neural reflexes (Holling *et al.,* 1961; Epstein *et al.,* 1979). There have been case reports of hypertrophic osteoarthropathy in a chimpanzee (Marzke and Merbs, 1984), an orangutan (Hime *et al.,* 1972), and a gibbon (Ryder-Davies and Hime, 1972). These lesions must be distinguished from the periarticular periosteal new bone formation associated with secondary hyperparathyroidism (Krook and Barrett, 1962; Tomson *et al.,* 1980; Junge *et al.,* 1994).

I. Fractures

Healed fractures are frequently found in skeletons from wild nonhuman primates (Duckworth, 1902, 1911; Schultz, 1939; Ruch, 1959c; Bramblett, 1967; Lovell, 1990b). In a systematic study, skeletal material from free-ranging Cayo Santiago rhesus macaques, including 126 animals of various ages from the same social group, were examined for the presence of healed fractures in long bones (Buikstra, 1975). In this group, fracture incidence increased with age. Fracture prevalence was similar for males and females, but fractures in females tended to occur at a younger age. The craniocaudal increase in fractures in rhesus macaques, the distribution of fractures to both proximal and distal limb (compared to gibbons), and the preponderance of clavicle fractures in males are indicators of specialized locomotor activity (Buikstra, 1975). Although spontaneous fractures in nonhuman primates are a common occurrence, little study of normal or pathological fracture healing in living nonhuman primates has been done. Fractures associated with osteoporosis have not been reported in nonhuman primates.

J. Osteoporosis

Osteoporosis is a systemic skeletal disorder of diverse etiology characterized by decreased bone mass and microarchitectural deterioration of bone tissue with a consequent increase in bone fragility and fracture susceptibility. Dual photon absorptiometry and radiologic morphometry are the noninvasive techniques currently used to assess bone mass in human and nonhuman primates (Wiers, 1971; Jayo *et al.,* 1990b, 1994; Shively *et al.,* 1991; Grynpas *et al.,* 1993b; Yoshida, 1993; Kammerer *et al.,* 1995; Champ *et al.,* 1996). More precise measurements of bone architecture are available using histomorphometry on iliac crest bone biopsies (Goodwin and Jerome, 1987; Lipkin, 1996). Many blood and urine biochemical markers have been studied as surrogate markers for bone turnover (Sin *et al.,* 1984). Among the available markers, bone collagen cross-links, deoxypyridinoline and pyridinoline, are useful as indices of bone resorption. Measurement of the markers in 24 rhesus macaques ranging in age from 3 to 25 years showed that the pyrodinoline:deoxypyrodinoline ratio was inversely related to bone density, an observation that parallels changes seen in humans (Hearn and Russell, 1980). Natural bone loss in nonhuman primates has been studied with aging and in model diseases induced by disuse related to restricted movement or more extensive immobilization and after experimental cessation of ovarian function.

1. Age-Associated Osteoporosis

Osteopenia with preferential disposition to trabecular bone of the axial skeleton is characteristic of human aging (Mazess, 1982). Osteoporosis in the aged has been attributed in part to subclinical vitamin D deficiency inducing secondary hyperparathyroidism and, in part, to decreased storage of IGF-1 and transforming growth factor β (TGF-β) within bone. These deficiencies result in decreased coupling between bone resorption and bone formation (Boonen et al., 1995).

Radiologic studies of free-ranging rhesus macaques (DeRousseau, 1985) and osteologic studies of skeletons from free-ranging chimpanzees (Sumner et al., 1989) have demonstrated similar findings regarding loss of cortical bone. Using conventional radiographic techniques, cortical bone thickness decreases with age in rhesus macaques. In females, recent pregnancy was a risk factor for osteopenia. In both sexes, coexistent osteoarthritis was protective (DeRousseau, 1985). These studies have been extended by measuring bone density on spinal vertebrae from rhesus macaque skeletons collected at the Caribbean Primate Research Center (Cerroni et al., 1997). With this technique, generalized osteoporosis identified with aging was observed selectively in both male and female rhesus macaques (Fig. 9). Similar studies by Bowden in caged pigtailed macaques (Macaca nemestrina) and long-tailed macaques (M. fascicularis) demonstrated that cortical bone decreased in both males and females with age (Bowden et al., 1979; Williams and Bowden, 1984). Examination of osteons from the right sixth rib of rhesus macaques showed decreased osteon formation with age accompanied by erosion of the endosteal surfaces (Przybeck, 1985). Bone density studies on skeletal material from free-ranging Gombe chimpanzees confirmed the age-related osteopenia with endosteal bone loss (Sumner et al., 1989). In all these studies, and in contrast to humans, cortical bone loss was greater than cancellous bone. A contributing factor to this difference is the younger relative age of the nonhuman primates compared to elderly humans. Skeletal study of a male Japanese macaque (M. fuscata) with an estimate age of 40 years demonstrated extensive vertebral osteoporosis (Tasumi, 1969).

Investigations in male green monkeys (Cerpithecus aethiops) confirmed the decrease in bone density at ages greater than 10 years (Yoshida, 1993). Mature female cynomolgus macaques demonstrated decreased bone density with age (Jayo et al., 1994). Subordinate female cynomolgus macaques have been

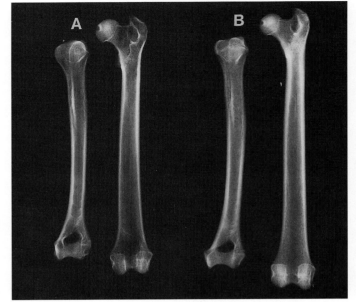

Fig. 9. Humerus and femoral bones from age-associated osteoporotic (A) and normal (B) rhesus macaques. Photograph courtesy of Antonietta Cerroni and Jean Turnquist, Caribbean Primate Research Center, Puerto Rico.

observed to have decreased ovarian function with an increased ratio of anovulatory cycles (Fleisch et al., 1966; Bisaz et al., 1976). Radiologic morphometry indicators for bone mass have been studied in the baboon (Papio hamadryas) colony at the Southwest Foundation for Biomedical Research (Aufdemorte et al., 1993; Hughes et al., 1994; Kammerer et al., 1994, 1995). Cortical bone width and cortical bone width/total bone diameter ratios decreased with age in both males and females. These studies and others indicate that peak bone mass is achieved by age 10 years and declines beyond age 12 to 15 years (Pope et al., 1989; Jayo et al., 1994; Champ et al., 1996). Prior studies using single photon densitometry in rhesus macaques showed similar results (Aguilo and Cabrera, 1989). In females, social subordination was linked both to lower bone densities and to fewer ovulatory cycles (Shively et al., 1991). Statistical analysis of bone mass indicators in a baboon colony demonstrated hereditability of bone mass. This finding, together with the suggested hereditable component for human bone mass (Pocock et al., 1987; Morrison et al., 1994), indicates that nonhuman primates may be useful to model the genetic factors associated with age-associated osteoporosis.

In addition to quantitative measurements of bone mass, the evaluation of bone material composition, particularly bone mineral, is an important determinant of bone quality (Grynpas, 1993). With age in human and nonhuman primates, there is a shift to higher bone mineral densities reflecting denser packing of the bone mineral, calcium apatite (Grynpas et al., 1989, 1993b;

Grynpas, 1993). The calcium content of trabecular bone in rhesus macaques has also been shown to decline with age (Lei and Young, 1979; Grynpas *et al.,* 1993a). These effects appear independent of dietary protein content (Grynpas *et al.,* 1993a).

2. Osteoporosis Models

a. DISUSE OSTEOPOROSIS. Mechanical forces from weight bearing (gravity) and muscle content (movement) are required to maintain bone integrity (Kazarian and von Gierke, 1969; Panin *et al.,* 1971). In early experiments under microgravity conditions of space flight, a decrease in bone density in humans occurs within 14 days (Whedon *et al.,* 1967; Kazarian and von Gierke, 1969). Similar changes were observed in a pig-tailed macaque (*Macaca nemestrina*) after an orbital spaceflight of 8.8 days (Mack, 1971). Stimulated by problems of spaceflight, disuse osteoporosis has been studied extensively in rhesus macaques under conditions ranging from chair restraint (Schock *et al.,* 1975; Cann *et al.,* 1980; Young and Schneider, 1981; Young *et al.,* 1983, 1986; Zerath *et al.,* 1994) to immobilization in a full body plastic cast (Kazarian and von Gierke, 1969, 1971; Kazarian *et al.,* 1981; Wronski and Morey, 1983; Simmons *et al.,* 1984, 1986; Grynpas *et al.,* 1986). With immobilization, there is loss of both cortical and trabecular bone. In cortical bone, resorption increases by the increased activity of existing osteoclast units, which results in increased cortical porosity (Young *et al.,* 1983, 1986). Immobilization results in an increased average density of cortical bone (Grynpas *et al.,* 1986) and an increased mineralized bone fraction (Mechanic *et al.,* 1986). These findings are reconciled by the observation that mineral from the less mineralized newly formed bone is preferentially resorbed. During immobilization, reducible bone collagen cross-links increase whereas nonreducible cross-links remained unchanged (Yamauchi *et al.,* 1988). This reflects high collagen tumor in the mineralized bone. This is compatible with resorption during immobilization of less dense bone mineral that is usually located closer to the bone surfaces. In trabecular bone, inhibition of new bone formation is prominent (Wronski and Morey, 1983). These differential findings have activation of existing osteoclasts and diminished coupling of osteoblasts in common. Reambulation tends to reverse cellular changes (Young *et al.,* 1983, 1986) and mineralization changes (Grynpas *et al.,* 1986). However, it is unclear whether the repair process is capable of restoring fully resorbed trabecular plates. Although many of these experiments were set up to simulate microgravity conditions, they are representative only of disuse osteoporosis under normal gravity. Microgravity induces additional changes in body fluid distribution, hormone, and immune responses as well as neural reflexes, all of which may be expected to interact in special ways on bone resorption and formation (Grindeland *et al.,* 1992).

Examination of skeletons from chimpanzees affected with poliomyelitis show focal hypoplasia and a decrease in mineral

density in bones of paralyzed limbs compared to the control opposite limb (Morbeck *et al.,* 1991). This study demonstrates the roles of muscle in maintaining bone quality.

b. POSTMENOPAUSAL OSTEOPOROSIS. Animal models for postmenopausal osteoporosis in species other than primates have been limited by fundamental differences in hormone cycles, bone growth dynamics, and bone biomechanics (Rodgers *et al.,* 1993). Female nonhuman primates such as rhesus macaques undergo menopause between age 24 and 26 (Walker, 1995). As there are insufficient animals of this age available for research, surgical ovariectomy is commonly used to induce the cessation of ovarian function (Adams *et al.,* 1985a; Bowles *et al.,* 1985; Jerome *et al.,* 1986, 1994, 1995a; Miller *et al.,* 1986; Mazess *et al.,* 1987; Longcope *et al.,* 1989; Jayo *et al.,* 1990a; Lundon and Grynpas, 1993; Carlson *et al.,* 1993; Kasra and Grynpas, 1994). Surgical ovariectomy simulates many but not all menopausal conditions. In contrast to menopause, which produces a slow progressive decline in hormones, surgical ovariectomy results in an abrupt hormone decrease with rapid compensating effects in other components of the endocrine system. Nonetheless, mature animals developed osteopenia (Miller *et al.,* 1986; Mazess *et al.,* 1987; Jerome *et al.,* 1995a). Ovariectomized cynomolgus macaques (*Macaca fascicularis*) showed decreased cortical bone density (Lundon and Grynpas, 1993). Increased eroded surfaces and increased basic multicellular units of bone were seen on the trabeculae (Jerome *et al.,* 1994; Lundon *et al.,* 1994). In cynomolgus monkeys, ovariectomy decreased the biomechanical competence of cortical bone as reflected by a decrease in the elastic modulus, shear modulus, failure shear stress, and failure torque in the tibia (Kasra and Grynpas, 1994). These studies demonstrated no difference in the trabecular bone biomechanics between ovariectomized and control animals. Intact female cynomolgus macaques given weak (androsteinedione) or strong (testosterone) androgen supplements showed increased mechanical properties in both cortical and trabecular bones. More substantive bone mechanical and histomorphometric restorative effects were observed after administration of the strong androgen (Kasra and Grynpas, 1995; Lundon *et al.,* 1997).

The surgical ovariectomy nonhuman primate model for osteoporosis has been sufficiently well established to be used in pharmaceutical studies of bone antiresorptive agents such as bisphosphonates and parathyroid hormone. These studies in the baboon (*Papio anubis*) have demonstrated that bisphosphonates can prevent bone resorption and the loss of mechanical properties that are induced by the surgical ovariectomy osteoporosis model (Geusens *et al.,* 1992; Thompson *et al.,* 1992; Balena *et al.,* 1993). Administration of parathyroid hormone 1–34 peptide over 3 months restored cancellous but not cortical bone (Jerome *et al.,* 1995b).

Osteoporosis has been induced in macaques following pharmacologic oophorectomy by infusion of the gonadotropin-releasing hormone (GnRH) agonist (Mann *et al.,* 1990). The GnRH agonist, when administered by intravenous infusion, stimulates excessive luteinizing hormone and follicle-stimulating hormone secretion, interrupts the cyclic responses of these hormones, and decreases estrogen and progesterone secretion. Nine months of GnRH agonist treatment is required to induce 11–14% bone loss. Termination of treatment restores menstrual cycles within 4 weeks with eventual restoration of bone mass. Under GnRH agonist treatment conditions, bone mass can be preserved by the administration of human growth hormone (Mann *et al.,* 1992).

VI. MUSCULOSKELETAL NEOPLASIA

Spontaneous tumors affecting soft connective tissue in bone have been described infrequently in nonhuman primates (O'Gara and Adamson, 1978; Lowenstine, 1986; Beniashvili, 1989). Studies of specific primate populations have confirmed the rarity of these lesions (Seibold and Wolf, 1973; McClure, 1980). Like humans, soft tissue and bone tumors in nonhuman primates have varied histological appearances (Jacobson, 1971; Sembrat and Fritz, 1979; Beniashvili, 1989; Chalifoux, 1993). The facial bones appear susceptible to neoplasia (Chalifoux, 1993), which are often lymphomas (Jayo *et al.,* 1988; Beniashvili, 1989).

Extraosseous osteosarcoma has been reported in a rhesus macaque (Takagi and Jasin, 1992). O'Gara and Adamson (1978) have reviewed the literature on bone tumors induced in nonhuman primates either by direct implantation of chemical carcinogens or by internal or external ionizing radiation. The induction of tumors by these means and the range of tumor histology appear similar to tumors induced in other experimental animals. As with humans, it is important to recognize that metabolic diseases such as hyperparathyroidism can simulate skeletal neoplasia (Smith *et al.,* 1978). Neoplasia in nonhuman primates is more extensively discussed elsewhere in this volume.

ACKNOWLEDGMENTS

We thank Dr. Marc Grynpas, Dr. Rita Kandel, Dr. Richard Rawlins, Dr. Richard Renlund, Dr. Bruce Rothschild, and Dr. Jean Turnquist for helpful discussions. This chapter is based in part on a bibliography of primate musculoskeletal disease from 1940 through 1996 compiled by Ms. Debra Paros of the Primate Information Center, Regional Primate Research Center, University of Washington, Seattle, Washington, for bibliographic assistance. We are indebted to Ms. Paros for her assistance and to Ms. Anna Vaccaro for assembling of the manuscript. The collaborative comparative primate musculoskeletal research program between the Caribbean Primate Research Center, University of Puerto Rico, Medical Sciences Campus, and the Connective Tissue Research Group, Mount Sinai Hospital, University of Toronto, Toronto, Canada, has been sponsored by USPHS Grant RR03640 from the National Institutes of Health, National Center for Research Resources, Comparative Medicine Program, the University of Puerto Rico, and the Arthritis Society of Canada.

REFERENCES

Acosta, L., Jr., and Roy, R. R. (1987). Fiber-type composition of selected hindlimb muscles of a primate (cynomolgus monkey). *Anat. Rec.* **218,** 136–141.

Adams, J. S., and Gacad, M. A. (1988). Phenotypic diversity of the cellular 1,25-dihydroxyvitamin D_3-receptor interaction among different genera of New World primates. *J. Clin. Endocrinol. Metab.* **66,** 224–229.

Adams, J. S., Gacad, M. A., Baker, A. J., Gonzales, B., and Rude, R. K. (1985a). Serum concentrations of 1,25-dihydroxyvitamin D_3 in platyrrhini and catarrhini: A phylogenetic appraisal. *Am. J. Primatol.* **9,** 219–224.

Adams, J. S., Gacad, M. A., Baker, A. J., Keuhn, G., and Rude, R. K. (1985b). Diminished internalization and action of 1,25-dihydroxyvitamin D_3 in dermal fibroblasts cultured from New World primates. *Endocrinology (Baltimore)* **116,** 2523–2527.

Adams, J. S., Gacad, M. A., Rude, R. K., Deseran, M., Endres, D. B., and Mallette, L. E. (1987). Immunoreactive parathyroid hormone levels in platyrrhini and catarrhini: A comparative analysis with three different assays. *Am. J. Primatol.* **13,** 425–433.

Adams, R. A., Zander, H. A., and Polson, A. M. (1979). Cell populations in the transseptal fiber region before, during and after experimental periodontitis in squirrel monkeys. *J. Periodontol.* **50,** 7–12.

Adams, R. F., Flinn, G. S., and Douglas, M. (1987). Ankylosing spondylitis in a nonhuman primate: A monkey tale. *Arthritis Rheum.* **30,** 956–957.

Adams, R. J., and Bishop, J. L. (1980). An oral disease resembling Noma in six rhesus monkeys (*Macaca mulatta*). *Lab. Anim. Sci.* **30,** 85–91.

Agamanolis, D. P., Chester, E. M., Victor, M., Kark, J. A., Hines, J. D., and Harris, J. W. (1976). Neuropathology of experimental vitamin B_{12} deficiency in monkeys. *Neurology* **26,** 906–914.

Agarwal, A. K., Reidbord, H. E., Kraus, D. R., and Eisenbeis, C. H., Jr. (1990). Variable histopathology of discovertebral lesion (spondylodiscitis) of ankylosing spondylitis. *Clin. Exp. Rheumatol.* **8,** 67–69.

Aguilo, F., and Cabrera, R. (1989). Validation of single photon absorptiometry in estimating bone mineral mass in rhesus monkey skeletons. *P. R. Health Sci. J.* **8,** 205–209.

Alexander, C. J. (1994). Utilization of joint movement range in arboreal primates compared with human subjects: An evolutionary frame for primary osteoarthritis. *Ann. Rheum. Dis.* **53,** 720–725.

Alexander, I. S., Gardner, D. L., and Skelton-Stroud, P. N. (1983). Synovial response of *Papio cynocephalus* to exogenous antigen: Histological and immunoperoxidase observations. *Ann. Rheum. Dis.* **42,** 448–451.

Alspaugh, M. A., and Van Hoosier, G. L., Jr. (1973). Naturally-occurring and experimentally-induced arthritides in rodents: A review of the literature. *Lab. Anim. Sci.* **23,** 724–742.

Anderson, M. P., Hunt, R. D., Griffiths, H. J., McIntyre, K. W., and Zimmerman, R. E. (1977). Long-term effect of low dietary calcium: Phosphate ratio on the skeleton of Cebus albifrons monkeys. *J. Nutr.* **107,** 834–839.

Anderson, S. T., and Klein, E. C. (1992). Eosinophilic fasciitis in a rhesus macaque. *Arthritis Rheum.* **35,** 714–716.

Anderson, S. T., and Klein, E. C. (1993). Systemic lupus erythematosus in a rhesus macaque. *Arthritis Rheum.* **36,** 1739–1742.

Anderson, S. T., and Schiller, C. A. (1991). Rheumatoid-like arthritis in a lion tailed macaque. *J. Rheumatol.* **18,** 1247–1250.

Aspenberg, P., and Turek, T. (1996). BMP-2 for intramuscular bone induction. *Acta Orthop. Scand.* **67,** 3–6.

Aspenberg, P., Lohmander, L. S., and Thorngren, K.-G. (1988). Failure of bone induction by bone matrix in adult monkeys. *J. Bone and Jt. Surg., Br. Vol.* **70B,** 625–627.

Aspenberg, P., Lohmander, L. S., and Thorngren, K.-G. (1991). Monkey bone matrix induces bone formation in the athymic rat, but not in adult monkeys. *J. Orthop. Res.* **9,** 20–25.

Aspenberg, P., Wang, E., and Thorngren, K.-G. (1992). Bone morphogenetic protein induces bone in the squirrel monkey, but bone matrix does not. *Acta Orthop. Scand.* **63,** 619–622.

Athanasiou, K. A., Rosenwasser, M. P., Buckwalter, J. A., Malinin, T. I., and Mow, V. C. (1991). Interspecies comparisons of in situ intrinsic mechanical properties of knee joint cartilage. *J. Orthop. Res.* **9,** 330–340.

Athanasiou, K. A., Agarwal, A., Muffoletto, A., Dzida, F. J., Constantinides, G., and Clem, M. (1995). Biomechanical properties of hip cartilage in experimental animal models. *Clin. Orthop. Relat. Res.* **316,** 254–266.

Aufdemorte, T. B., Fox, W. C., Miller, D., Buffum, K., Holt, G. R., and Carey, K. D. (1993). A non-human primate model for the study of osteoporosis and oral bone loss. *Bone* **14,** 581–586.

Badley, E. M., Rasooly, I., and Webster, G. K. (1994). Relative importance of musculoskeletal disorders as a cause of chronic health problems, disability, and health care utilization: Findings from the 1990 Ontario Health Survey. *J. Rheumatol.* **21,** 505–514.

Bakker, N. P. M., van Erck, M. G., Zurcher, C., Faaber, P., Lemmens, A., Hazenberg, M., Bontrop, R. E., and Jonker, M. (1990). Experimental immune mediated arthritis in rhesus monkeys. A model for human rheumatoid arthritis? *Rheumatol. Int.* **10,** 21–29.

Bakker, N. P. M., van Erck, M. G. M., 't Hart, B. A., and Jonker, M. (1991a). Acquired resistance to type II collagen-induced arthritis in rhesus monkeys is reflected by a T cell low-responsiveness to the antigen. *Clin. Exp. Immunol.* **86,** 219–223.

Bakker, N. P. M., van Erck, M. G. M., Botman, C. A. D., Jonker, M., and 't Hart, B. A. (1991b). Collagen-induced arthritis in an outbred group of rhesus monkeys comprising responder and nonresponder animals—relationship between the course of arthritis and collagen-specific immunity. *Arthritis Rheum.* **34,** 616–624.

Bakker, N. P. M., van Erck, M. G. M., Otting, N., Lardy, N. M., Noort, R. C., 't Hart, B. A., Jonker, M., and Bontrop, R. E. (1992). Resistance to collagen-induced arthritis in a nonhuman primate species maps to the major histocompatibility complex Class I region. *J. Exp. Med.* **175,** 933–937.

Bakker, N. P. M., van Besouw, N., Groenestein, R., Jonker, M., and 't Hart, B. A. (1993). The anti-arthritic and immunosuppressive effects of cyclosporin A on collagen-induced arthritis in the rhesus monkey. *Clin. Exp. Immunol.* **93,** 318–322.

Balena, R., Toolan, B. C., Shea, M., Markatos, A., Myers, E. R., Lee, S. C., Opas, E. E., Seedor, J. G., Klein, H., Frankenfield, D., Quartuccio, H., Floravanti, C., Clair, J., Brown, E., Hayes, W. C., and Rodan, G. A. (1993). The effects of 2-year treatment with the aminobisphosphonate alendronate on bone metabolism, bone histomorphometry, and bone strength in ovariectomized nonhuman primates. *J. Clin. Invest.* **92,** 2577–2586.

Bardana, E. J., Malinow, M. R., Houghton, D. C., McNulty, W. P., Wuepper, K. D., Parker, F., and Pirofsky, B. (1982). Diet-induced systemic lupus erythematosus (SLE) in primates. *Am. J. Kidney Dis.* **1,** 345–352.

Barile, M. F., Kapatais-Zoumbos, K., Snoy, P., Grabowski, M. W., Sneller, M., Miller, L., and Chandler, D. K. F. (1994). Experimentally induced septic arthritis in chimpanzees infected with mycoplasma hominis, mycoplasma pneumoniae, and ureaplasma urealyticum. *Clin. Infect. Dis.* **18,** 694–703.

Barker, M. J. M., and Herbert, R. T. (1972). Diseases of the skeleton. *In* "Pathology of Simian Primates" (R. Fiennes, T. Orihel, and J. Ayers, eds.), Vol. 2, p. 433. Karger, Basel.

Baskin, G. B., Wolf, R. H., Worth, C. L., Soike, K., Gibson, S. V., and Bieri, J. G. (1983). Anemia, steatitis, and muscle necrosis in marmosets *(Saguinus labiatus) Lab. Anim. Sci.* **33,** 74–80.

Baskin, G. B., Martin, L. N., Rangan, S. R. S., Gormus, B. J., Murphey-Corb, M., Wolf, R. H., and Soike, K. F. (1986). Transmissible lymphoma and simian acquired immunodeficiency syndrome in rhesus monkeys. *J. Natl. Cancer Inst.* **77,** 127.

Battles, A. H., Parker, R. B., and Collins, B. R. (1985). Periosteal reaction consistent with osteomyelitis in a stump-tailed macaque. *J. Am. Vet. Med. Assoc.* **187,** 1276–1277.

Bayne, K. A. L. (1985), Qualitative observations of idiosyncratic behavior in old monkeys. *In* "Behavior and Pathology of Aging in Rhesus Monkeys" (R. T. Davis and C. W. Leathers, eds.), p. 201. Liss, New York.

Beatty, C. H., Basinger, G. M., Dully, C. C., and Bocek, R. M. (1966). Comparison of red and white voluntary skeletal muscles of several species. *J. Histochem.* **14,** 590–600.

Beatty, C. H., Bocek, R. M., Herrington, P. T., Lamy, C., and Hoskins, M. K. (1982). Aged rhesus skeletal muscle: Histochemistry and lipofuscin content. *Age* **5,** 1–9.

Beilke, M. A., Traina-Dorge, V., England, J. D., and Blanchard, J. L. (1996). Polymyositis, arthritis, and uveitis in a macaque experimentally infected with human T lymphotropic virus type I. *Arthritis Rheum.* **39,** 610–615.

Benditt, E. P., and Eriksen, N. (1972). Chemical characteristics of the substance of typical amyloidosis in monkeys. *Acta Pathol. Microbiol. Scand.* 233, 103–108.

Beniashvili, D. S. (1989). An overview of the world literature spontaneous tumors in nonhuman primates. *J. Med. Primatol.* **18,** 423–437.

Berg, J. M., and Shi, Y. (1996). The galvanization of biology: A growing appreciation for the roles of zinc. *Science* **271,** 1081–1085.

Berman, A., Espinosza, L. R., Diaz, J. D., Aguilar, J. L., Rolando, T., Vasey, F. B., Germain, B. F., and Lockey, R. I. (1988). Rheumatic manifestations of human immunodeficiency virus infection. *Am. J. Med.* **85,** 59.

Beutler, A., Rothfuss, S., Clayburne, G., Sieck, M., and Schumacher, H. R., Jr. (1993). Calcium pyrophosphate dihydrate crystal deposition in synovium. *Arthritis Rheum.* **36**(5), 704–715.

Binkley, N. C., Sun, W. H., Checovich, M. M., Roecker, E. B., Kimmel, D. B., and Ershler, W. B. (1994). Effects of recombinant human interleukin-6 administration on bone in rhesus monkeys. *Lymphokine Cytokine Res.* **13,** 221–226.

Bisaz, S., Felix, R., Hansen, N. M., and Fleisch, H. (1976). Disaggregation of hydroxyapatite crystals. *Biochim. Biophys. Acta* **451,** 560–566.

Blackwell, C. A., Manning, P. J., and Fisk, S. K. (1974). Cranial hyperostosis of squirrel monkeys *(Saimiri sciureus). Lab. Anim. Sci.* **24,** 541–544.

Blanchard, J. L., Baskin, G. B., and Watson, E. A. (1986). Generalized amyloidosis in rhesus monkeys. *Vet. Pathol.* **23,** 425–430.

Bluestone, R., Bywaters, E., Haratog, M., Holt, P. J. L., and Hyde, S. (1971). Acromegalic arthropathy. *Ann. Rheum. Dis.* **30,** 243–258.

Bodkin, N. L., Hannah, J. S., Ortmeyer, H. K., and Hansen, B. C. (1993a). Central obesity in rhesus monkeys: Association with hyperinsulinemia, insulin resistance, and hypertriglyceridemia? *Int. J. Obes.* **17,** 53–61.

Bodkin, N. L., Ortmeyer, H. K., and Hansen, B. C. (1993b). Diversity of insulin resistance in monkeys with normal glucose tolerance. *Obes. Res.* **1,** 364–370.

Bodkin, N. L., Ortmeyer, H. K., and Hansen, B. C. (1995). Long-term dietary restriction in older-aged rhesus monkeys: Effects on insulin resistance. *J. Gerontol.* **50**(3), B142–B147.

Boivin, G., and Lagier, R. (1983). An ultrastructural study of articular chondrocalcinosis in cases of knee osteoarthritis. *Virchows Arch. A: Pathol. Anat. Histopathol.* **400,** 13–29.

Bonner, F. W., King, I. J., and Parke, D. V. (1980). Cadmium-induced reduction of bone alkaline phosphatase and its prevention by zinc. *Chem.-Biol. Interact.* **29,** 369–372.

Boonen, S., Aerssens, J., Broos, P., Pelemans, W., and Dequeker, J. (1995). Age-related bone loss and senile osteoporosis: Evidence of both secondary hyperparathyroidism and skeletal growth factor deficiency in the elderly. *Aging Clin. Exp. Res.* **7,** 414–422.

Boulet, P., and Mirouse, J. (1954). Les ostéoses diabétiques (ostéoporose et hyperostose). *Ann. Med. (Paris)* **55,** 674–721.

Bourdella, P. E., Urbain, A., and Davosne, J. (1931). Deux cas de gingivostomatite gangreneuse (noma) due a *B. perfringens* chez le chimpanze. *Bull. Soc. Pathol. Exot.* **24,** 787–789.

Bowden, D. M., Teets, C., Witkin, J., and Young, D. M. (1979). Long bone calcification and morphology. In "Aging in Nonhuman Primates" (D. M. Bowden, ed.), p. 335. Van Nostrand-Reinhold, New York.

Bowles, E. A., Weaver, D. S., Telewski, F. W., Wakefield, A. H., Jaffe, M. J., and Miller, L. C. (1985). Bone measurement by enhanced contrast image analysis: Ovariectomized and intact *Macaca fascicularis* as a model for human postmenopausal osteoporosis. *Am. J. Phys. Anthropol.* **67,** 99–103.

Brack, M. (1982). Noma in *Saguinus oedipus*: A report of 2 cases. *Lab. Anim.* **16**, 361–363.

Brack, M., and Rothe, H. (1981). Chronic tubulointerstitial nephritis and wasting disease in marmosets *(Callithrix jacchus). Vet. Pathol.* **18**, 45–54.

Bramblett, C. A. (1967). Pathology in the Darajani baboon. *Am. J. Phys. Anthropol.* **26**, 331–340.

Brecx, M. C., Nalbandian, J., Ooya, K., Kornman, K. S., and Robertson, P. B. (1985). Morphological studies on periodontal disease in the cynomolgus monkey. II. Light microscopic observations on ligature-induced periodontitis. *J. Periodont. Res.* **20**, 165–175.

Brecx, M. C., Nalbandian, J., Kornman, K. S., and Robertson, P. B. (1986). Morphological studies on periodontal disease in the cynomolgus monkey. III. Electron microscopic observations. *J. Periodont. Res.* **21**, 137–153.

Brooke, M. H., and Kasier, K. K. (1970). Muscle fiber types: How many and what kinds? *Arch. Neurol. (Chicago)* **23**, 369–379.

Brooks, H., and Blair, W. R. (1904). Osteomalacia of primates in captivity. A clinical and pathological study of "cage paralysis." *Rep. N. Y. Zool. Soc.* **9**, 135–175.

Brooks, M. H., Bell, N. H., Love, L., Stern, P. H., Orfei, E., Queener, S. F., Hamstra, A. J., and DeLuca, H. F. (1978). Vitamin D-dependent rickets type II: Resistance of target organs to 1,25-dehydroxy-vitamin D. *N. Engl. J. Med.* **298**, 996–999.

Brown, T. M., Clark, H. W., Bailey, J. S., and Gray, C. W. (1970). A mechanistic approach to treatment of rheumatoid type arthritis naturally occurring in a gorilla. *Trans. Am. Clin. Climatol. Assoc.* **82**, 227–247.

Brown, T. M., Clark, H. W., and Bailey, J. S. (1974). Natural occurrence of rheumatoid arthritis in great apes—a new animal model. *Proc. Zool. Soc. Philos. Centen. Symp.,* pp. 43–79.

Brunsvold, M. A., Chaves, E. S., Kornman, K. S., Aufdemorte, T. B., and Wood, R. (1992). Effects of a bisphosphonate on experimental periodontitis in monkeys. *J. Periodontol.* **63**, 825–830.

Bryant, M. L., Marx, P. A., Shiigi, S. M., Wilson, B. J., McNulty, W. P., and Gardner, M. B. (1986). Distribution of Type D retrovirus sequences in tissues of macaques with simian acquired immune deficiency and retroperitoneal fibromatosis. *Virology* **150**, 149–160.

Buchanan, W., Sehgal, P., Bronson, R. T., Rodger, R. F., and Horton, J. E. (1981). Noma in a nonhuman primate. *Oral Surg., Oral Med. Oral Pathol.* **52**, 19–22.

Buikstra, J. E. (1975). Healed fractures in *Macaca mulatta*: Age, sex, and symmetry. *Folia Primatol.* **23**, 140–148.

Burgdorfer, W. (1984). The New Zealand white rabbit: An experimental host for infecting ticks with Lyme disease spirochetes. *Yale J. Biol. Med.* **57**, 609–612.

Burr, D. B. (1992). Estimated intracortical bone turnover in the femur of growing macaques: Implications for their use as models in skeletal pathology. *Anat. Rec.* **232**, 180–189.

Bywaters, E. G. L. (1981). Observations on chronic polyarthritis in monkeys. *J. R. Soc. Med.* **74**, 794–799.

Caffey, J. P. (1968). "Pediatric X-Ray Diagnosis," pp. 961–987. Chicago Year Book Medical Publishers, Chicago.

Campbell, A. W., and Cleland, J. B. (1919). Cage paralysis in monkeys. *J. Comp. Pathol.* **32**, 95–104.

Cann, C. E., Genant, H. K., and Young, D. R. (1980). Comparison of vertebral and peripheral mineral losses in disuse osteoporosis in monkeys. *Radiology* **134**, 525–529.

Carlson, C. S., Tulli, H. M., Jayo, M. J., Loeser, R. F., Tracy, R. P., Mann, K. G., and Adams, M. R. (1993). Immunolocalization of noncollagenous bone matrix proteins in lumbar vertebrae from intact and surgically menopausal cynomolgus monkeys. *J. Bone Min. Res.* **8**, 71–81.

Carlson, C. S., Loeser, R. F., Jayo, M. J., Weaver, D. S., Adams, M. R., and Jerome, C. P. (1994). Osteoarthritis in cynomolgus macaques: A primate model of naturally occurring disease. *J. Orthop. Res.* **12**, 331–339.

Carlson, C. S., Loeser, R. F., Johnstone, B., Tulli, H. M., Dobson, D. B., and Caterson, B. (1995). Osteoarthritis in cynomolgus macaques. II. Detection of modulated proteoglycan epitopes in cartilage and synovial fluid. *J. Orthop. Res.* **13**, 399–409.

Carlson, C. S., Loeser, R. F., Purser, C. B., Gardin, J. F., and Jerome, C. P. (1996). Osteoarthritis in cynomolgus macaques. III. Effects of age, gender and subchondral bone thickness on the severity of disease. *J. Bone Miner. Res.* **11**, 1209–1217.

Carpenter, S., Karpati, G., Heller, I., and Eisen, A. (1978). Inclusion body myositis: A distinct variety of idiopathic inflammatory myopathy. *Neurology* **28**, 8–17.

Casey, H. W., Kirk, J. H., and Splitter, G. A. (1972). Generalized amyloidosis in a rhesus monkey. *Lab. Anim. Sci.* **22**, 587–593.

Castleman, W. L., Anderson, J., and Holmberg, C. A. (1980). Posterior paralysis and spinal osteomyelitis in a rhesus monkey with coccidioidomycosis. *J. Am. Vet. Med. Assoc.* **177**, 933–934.

Cathcart, E. S., Hayes, K. C., Gonnerman, W. A., Lazzari, A. A., and Franzblau, C. (1986). Experimental arthritis in a nonhuman primate. I. Induction by bovine type II collagen. *Lab. Invest.* **54**, 26–31.

Cawley, M. I. D., Chalmers, T. M., Kellgren, J. H., and Ball, J. (1972). Destructive lesions of vertebral bodies in ankylosing spondylitis. *Ann. Rheum. Dis.* **31**, 345–358.

Centers for Disease Control (1989). Eosinophilia-myalgia syndrome and L-tryptophan-containing products—New Mexico, Minnesota, Oregon and New York. *Morbid. Mortal. Wkly. Rep.* **38**, 785–788.

Cerroni, A., Grynpas, M. D., Pritzker, K. P. H., Turnquist, J. E., Kessler, M. J., and Melbye, F. J. (1991). Spontaneous malformations of the vertebral column in patas monkeys. *Can. Assoc. Phys. Anthropol., 19th Ann. Meet.,* Abstract.

Cerroni, A. M., Grynpas, M. D., and Turnquist, J. E. (1997). Bone mineral density and osteoporosis in the rhesus monkeys of Cayo Santiago. *Am. J. Phys. Anthropol.,* pp. 89–90. Annual meeting issue, April 3, 1997, St-Louis.

Chadwick, D., May, J., and Lorenz, D. (1979). Spontaneous zinc deficiency in marmosets *(S. mystax). Lab. Anim. Sci.* **29**, 482–485.

Chalifoux, L. V. (1993). Chondrosarcoma, squirrel monkey. *In* "Monographs on the Pathology of Laboratory Animals: Nonhuman Primates (T. C. Jones, U. Mohr, and R. D. Hunt, eds.), Vol. 2, p. 128. Springer-Verlag, New York.

Chalifoux, L. V., Bronson, R. T., Escajadillo, A., and McKenna, S. (1982). An analysis of the association of gastroenteric lesions with chronic wasting syndrome of marmosets. *Vet. Pathol.* **19**, Suppl. 7, 141–162.

Chaminade, F., Stanescu, V., Stanescu, R., Maroteaux, P., and Peyron, J. G. (1982). Noncollagenous proteins in cartilage of normal subjects and patients with degenerative joint disease. *Arthritis Rheum.* **25**, 1078–1083.

Champ, J. E., Binkley, N., Havighurst, T., Colman, R. J., Kenmitz, J. W., and Roecker, E. B. (1996). The effect of advancing age on bone mineral content of female rhesus monkeys. *Bone* **19**, 485–492.

Chapman, W. L., Jr., and Crowell, W. A. (1977). Amyloidosis in rhesus monkeys with rheumatoid arthritis and enterocolitis. *J. Am. Vet. Med. Assoc.* **171**, 855–858.

Charriere, G., Hartmann, D. J., Vignon, E., Ronziere, M.-C., Herbage, D., and Ville, G. (1988). Antibodies to types I, II, IX and XI collagen in the serum of patients with rheumatic diseases. *Arthritis Rheum.* **31**, 325–331.

Chateuvert, J. M. D., Pritzker, K. P. H., Kessler, M. J., and Grynpas, M. D. (1989). Spontaneous osteoarthritis in rhesus macaques. I. Chemical and biochemical studies. *J. Rheumatol.* **16**, 1098–1104.

Chateauvert, J. M. D., Grynpas, M. D., Kessler, M. J., and Pritzker, K. P. H. (1990). Spontaneous osteoarthritis in rhesus macaques. II. Characterization of disease and morphometric studies. *J. Rheumatol.* **17**, 73–83.

Cheng, P.-T., Pritzker, K. P. H., Kandel, R. A., and Reid, A. (1983). Analytical scanning and transmission electron microscopy and x-ray microdiffractometry of calcium pyrophosphate dihydrate crystal deposits in tissues. *Scanning Electron Microsc.,* Volume 1, pp. 369–377.

Chesney, C. F., Hanlon, G. F., Scheffler, G., and Houser, W. D. (1973). Differential diagnosis of an obscure bone disease in an infant rhesus monkey. *Lab. Anim. Sci.* **23**, 414–422.

Cheung, H. S., Story, M. T., and McCarty, D. J. (1984). Mitogenic effects of hydroxyapatite and calcium pyrophosphate dihydrate crystals on cultured mammalian cells. *Arthritis Rheum.* **27**, 668–674.

Cheverud, J. M. (1981). Epiphyseal union and dental eruption in *Macaca mulatta. Am. J. Phys. Anthropol.* **56**, 157–167.

Cicmanec, J. L., Enlow, D. H., and Cohen, B. J. (1972). Polyostotic osteophytosis in a rhesus monkey. *Lab. Anim. Sci.* 22, 237–241.

Clark, L. (1971). Hypervitaminosis A: A review. *Aust. Vet. J.* 47, 568–570.

Cleve, H., Constans, J., and Scheffrahn, W. (1991). Vitamin-D-binding protein or group-specific component in chimpanzees *(Pan troglodytes* and *Pan paniscus). Folia Primatol.* 57, 232–236.

Cohen, D. W., and Goldman, H. M. (1960). Oral disease in primates. *Ann. N.Y. Acad. Sci.* 85, 889–909.

Cole, A. A., Chubinskaya, S., Luchene, L. J., Chlebek, K., Orth, M. W., Greenwald, R. A., Kuettner, K. E., and Schmid, T. M. (1994). Doxycycline disrupts chondrocyte differentiation and inhibits cartilage matrix degradation. *Arthritis Rheum.* 37, 1727–1734.

Cole, B. C., and Cassell, G. H. (1979). Mycoplasma infections as models of chronic joint inflammation. *Arthritis Rheum.* 22, 1375–1381.

Cook, S. D., Wolfe, M. W., Salkeld, S. L., and Rueger, D. C. (1995). Effect of recombinant human osteogenic protein-1 on healing of segmental defects in non-human primates. *J. Bone J. Surg., Am. Vol* 77-A, 734–750.

Cordy, D. R. (1957). Osteodystrophia fibrosa accompanied by visceral accumulations of lead. *Cornell Vet.* 47, 480.

Cornelius, C. E., and Rosenberg, D. P. (1983). Nonhuman primates with spontaneous diseases as animal models. *Am. J. Med.* 74, 169–171.

Corson-White, E. P. (1922). Osteitis deformans in monkeys. *Arch. Intern. Med.* 30, 790–796.

Crane, J. T., Pickering, D. E., van Wagenen, G., and Smyth, F. S. (1954). Growth and metabolism in normal and thyroid-ablated infant rhesus monkeys *(Macaca mulatta).* VII. Morphology of normal and thyroid-ablated infant rhesus monkeys *(Macaca mulatta). Am. J. Dis. Child.* 87, 708–723.

Cushnaghan, J., and Dieppe, P. (1991). Study of 500 patients with limb joint osteoarthritis. I. Analysis by age, sex, and distribution of symptomatic joint sites. *Ann. Rheum. Dis.* 50, 8–13.

Cutler, R. G., Davis, B. J., Ingram, D. K., and Roth, G. S. (1992). Plasma concentrations of glucose, insulin, and percent glycosylated hemoglobin are unaltered by food restriction in rhesus and squirrel monkeys. *J. Gerontol. Biol. Sci.* 47, B9–B12.

Cutolo, M., Sulli, A., Barone, A., Seriolo, B., and Accardo, S. (1995). The role of androgens in the pathophysiology of rheumatoid arthritis. *Fundam. Clin. Immunol.* 3, 9–18.

Dalakas, M. C., London, W. T., Gravell, M., and Sever, J. L. (1986). Polymyositis in an immunodeficiency disease in monkeys induced by a type D retrovirus. *Neurology* 36, 569–572.

Dalakas, M. C., Gravell, M., London, W. T., Cunningham, G., and Sever, J. L. (1987). Morphological changes of an inflammatory myopathy in rhesus monkeys with Simian Acquired Immunodeficiency Syndrome. *Proc. Soc. Exp. Biol. Med.* 185, 368–376.

de Bisschop, D. (1956). A case of lead poisoning in a gorilla. *Antwerp: Soc. R. Zoo. d'Anvers,* p. 5.

Demaray, S. Y., Altman, N. H., and Ferrell, T. L. (1978). Suspected ascorbic acid deficiency in a colony of squirrel monkeys *(Saimiri sciureus). Lab. Anim. Sci.* 28, 457–460.

Demes, B., and Gunther, M. M. (1989). Biomechanics and allometric scaling in primate locomotion and morphology. *Folia Primatol.* 53, 125–141.

Demontoy, M.-C., Berthier, J. L., and Letellier, F. (1979). Vitamine A et spondylose ankylosante chez des ouistitis. *Erkr. Zootiere Verhandlungsber. Int. Symp. 21st,* Berlin, Vol. 13, pp. 33–35.

Deo, M. G., Sood, S. K., and Ramalingaswami, V. (1965). Experimental protein deficiency; Pathological features in the rhesus monkey. *Arch. Pathol.* 80, 14–23.

Derfus, B., Steinberg, M., Mandel, N., Buday, M., Daft, L., and Ryan, L. (1995). Characterization of an additional articular cartilage vesicle fraction that generates calcium pyrophosphate dihydrate crystal in vitro. *J. Rheumatol.* 22, 1514–1519.

DeRousseau, C. J. (1978). Osteoarthritis in non human primates: A locomotion model of joint degeneration. Ph.D. Thesis, Northwestern University, Evanston, IL.

DeRousseau, C. J. (1985). Aging in the musculoskeletal system of rhesus monkeys: III. Bone loss. *Am. J. Phys. Anthropol.* 68, 157–167.

DeRousseau, C. J. (1988). "Osteoarthritis in Rhesus Monkeys and Gibbons: A Locomotor Model of Joint Degeneration." Karger, Basel.

DeRousseau, C. J., Rawlins, R. G., and Denlinger, J. L. (1983). Aging in the musculoskeletal system of rhesus monkeys: I. Passive joint excursion. *Am. J. Phys. Anthropol.* 61, 483–494.

DeRousseau, C. J., Bito, L. Z., and Kaufman, P. L. (1986). Age-dependent impairments of the rhesus monkey visual and musculoskeletal systems and apparent behavioral consequences. In "The Cayo Santiago Macaques. History, Behavior and Biology" (R. Rawlins and M. J. Kessler, eds.), p. 233. State University of New York Press, Albany.

Dieppe, P., and Rogers, J. M. (1993). Skeletal paleopathology of rheumatic disorders. In "Arthritis and Allied Conditions" (D. J. McCarty and W. J. Koopman, eds.), p. 9. Lea & Febiger, Philadelphia.

Dinning, J. S., and Day, P. L. (1957). Vitamin E deficiency in the monkey. I. Muscular dystrophy, hematologic changes, and the excretion of urinary nitrogenous constituents. *J. Exp. Med.* 105, 395–402.

Dodd, D. C., and Raker, C. W. (1970). Tumoral calcinosis (calcinosis circumscripta) in the horse. *J. Am. Vet. Med. Assoc.* 157, 968–972.

Dougherty, P. M., Sluka, K. A., Sorkin, L. S., Westlund, K. N., and Willis, W. D. (1992). Neural changes in acute arthritis in monkeys. I. Parallel enhancement of responses of spinothalamic tract neurons to mechanical stimulation and excitatory amino acids. *Brain Res. Rev.* 17, 1–13.

Douglass, E. M. (1981). Legg-Calve-Perthes disease in a lowland gorilla. *Vet. Med.,* 76(1), 101–103.

Dreizen, S., Levy, B. M., and Bernick, S. (1971). Studies on the biology of the periodontium of Marmosets: X. Cortisone induced periodontal and skeletal changes in adult cotton top Marmosets. *J. Periodontol.* 42, 217–224.

du Boulay, G. H., and Crawford, M. A. (1968). Nutritional bone disease in captive primates. *Symp. Zool. Soc. London* 21, 223–236.

du Boulay, G. H., Hime, J. M., and Verity, P. M. (1972). Spondylosis in captive wild animals. A possible relationship with nutritional osteodystrophy. *Br. J. Radiol.* 45, 841–847.

Duckworth, W. L. H. (1902). Les fractures de os des orangs-outangs et la lésion femorale du *Pithecanthropus erectus. Anthropologie, Paris* 13, 204–206.

Duckworth, W. L. H. (1911). On the natural repair of fractures, as seen in the skeletons of anthropoid apes. *J. Anat.* 46, 81–85.

Duncan, H., Parfitt, A. M., Villanueva, A. R., Crouch, M. M., Mathews, C. H. E., Kayan, S., and Weikel, J. H. (1977). Effect of melengestrol acetate on bone dynamics of monkey ribs. *Calcif. Tissue Res.* 22, 542–544.

Eisele, P. H., Morgan, J. P., Line, A. S., and Anderson, J. H. (1992). Skeletal lesions and anemia associated with ascorbic acid deficiency in juvenile rhesus macaques. *Lab. Anim. Sci.* 42, 245–249.

Eisenstein, R., and Kawanoue, S. (1975). The lead line in bone—A lesion apparently due to chondroclastic indigestion. *Am. J. Pathol.* 80, 309–316.

El-Khoury, G. Y., Kathol, M. H., and Brandser, E. A. (1996). Seronegative spondyloarthropathies. *Radiol. Clin. North Am.* 34, 343–357.

Enwonwu, C. O. (1972). Epidemiological and biochemical studies of necrotizing ulcerative gingivitis and noma (cancrum oris) in Nigerian children. *Arch. Oral Biol.* 17, 1357–1371.

Epstein, O., Adjukiewicz, A. B., Dick, R., and Sherlock, S. (1979). Hypertrophic hepatic osteoarthropathy. Clinical, roentgenologic, biochemical, hormonal and cardiorespiratory studies, and review of the literature. *Am. J. Med.* 67, 88–97.

Ershler, W. B. (1993). Interleukin-6: A cytokine for gerontologists. *J. Am. Geriatr. Soc.* 41, 176–181.

Ershler, W. B., Sun, W. H., Binkley, N., Gravenstein, S., Volk, M. J., Kamoske, G., Klopp, R. G., Roecker, E. B., Daynes, R. A., and Weindruch, R. (1993). Interleukin-6 and aging: Blood levels and mononuclear cell production increase with advancing age and in vitro production is modifiable by dietary restriction. *Lymphokine Cytokine Res.* 12, 225–230.

Espinoza, L. R., Jara, L. J., Espinoza, C. G., Silveira, L. H., Martinez-Osuna, P., and Seleznick, M. (1992). There is an association between human immunodeficiency virus infection and spondyloarthropathies. *Rheum. Dis. Clin. North Am.* 18, 257–266.

Fam, A. G., and Pritzker, K. P. H. (1992). Acute calcific periarthritis in scleroderma. *J. Rheumatol.* 19, 1580–1585.

Fam, A. G., Rubenstein, J. (1989). Hydroxyapatite pseudopodagra. A syndrome of young women. *Arthritis and Rheum.* **32**, 741–747.

Fam, A. G., Pritzker, K. P. H., Stein, J. L., Houpt, J. B., and Little, A. H. (1981). Apatite-associated arthropathy: A clinical study of 14 cases and of 2 patients with calcific bursitis. *Arthritis Rheum.* **24**, 461–471.

Fam, A. G., Morava-Protzner, I., Purcell, C., Young, B. D., Bunting, P. S., and Lewis, A. J. (1995). Acceleration of experimental lapine osteoarthritis by calcium pyrophosphate microcrystalline synovitis. *Arthritis Rheum.* **38**, 201–210.

Felson, D. T., Zhang, Y., Hannan, M. T., Naimark, A., Weissman, B. N., Aliabadi, P., and Levy, D. (1995). The incidence and natural history of knee osteoarthritis in the elderly. *Arthritis Rheum.* **38**, 1500–1505.

Fincham, J. E., Wilson, G. R., Belonje, P. C., Seier, J. V., Taljaard, J. J. F., McIntosh, M., Gruger, M., and Voget, M. (1993). Parathyroid hormone, ionized calcium, and potentially interacting variables in plasma of an Old World primate. *J. Med. Primatol.* **22**, 246–252.

Fisher, L. E. (1954). Lead poisoning in a gorilla. *J. Am. Vet. Med. Assoc.* **125**, 478–479.

Fleisch, H., Russell, R. G. G., and Straumann, F. (1966). Effect of pyrophosphate on hydroxyapatite and its implications in calcium homeostasis. *Nature (London)* **212**, 901–903.

Follis, R. H., Jr. (1957). A kwashiorkor-like syndrome observed in monkeys fed maize. *Proc. Soc. Exp. Biol. Med.* **96**, 523–528.

Ford, E., Hird, D., Franti, C., and Lerche, N. (1986). Analysis of factors associated with sixty cases of chronic arthritis in rhesus monkeys at the California Primate Research Center. *Lab. Anim. Sci.* **36**, 561 (abstr).

Forestier, J., and Rotes-Querol, J. (1950). Senile ankylosing hyperostosis of the spine. *Ann. Rheum. Dis.* **9**, 321–330.

Forestier, J., and Rotes-Querol, J. (1971). Ankylosing hyperstosis of the spine. *Clin. Orthop. Relat. Res.* **74**, 65–83.

Fornasier, V. L., Littlejohn, G., Urowitz, M. B., Keystone, E. C., and Smythe, H. A. (1983). Spinal entheseal new bone formation: The early changes of spinal diffuse idiopathic skeletal hyperostosis. *J. Rheumatol.* **10**, 939–947.

Fox, H. (1937). Notes on the skeleton of a chimpanzee found in the wild, with serious chronic inflammation of one posterior extremity. *Rep. Penrose Res. Lab.,* pp. 18–26.

Fox, H. (1939). Chronic arthritis in wild mammals. *Trans. Am. Philos. Soc.* **[N.S.] 31**, 73–148.

Franchini, G., Gurgo, C., Guo, H. G., Gallo, R. C., Collatin, E., Fargnoli, K. A., Hall, L. F., Wong-Stoal, E., and Reitz, M. S., Jr. (1987). Sequence of simian immunodeficiency virus and its relationship to the human immunodeficiency viruses. *Nature (London)* **328**, 539.

Frye, F. L., and Dutra, F. R. (1976). Articular pseudogout in a turtle *(Chrysemys s. elegans). VM/SAC, Vet. Med. Small Anim. Clin.,* **71**(5), 655–659.

Fultz, P. N., McClure, H. M., Anderson, D. S., Swenson, R. B., Arnand, R., and Srinivasan, A. (1986). Isolation of a T-lymphotropic retrovirus from naturally infected sooty mangabey monkeys *(Cercocebus atys). Proc. Natl. Acad. Sci. U.S.A.* **83**, 5286.

Furukawa, Y., Kinoshita, A., Satoh, H., Kikuchi, H., Ohkoshi, S., Maebashi, M., Makino, Y., Sato, T., Ito, M., and Kimura, S. (1992). Bone disorder and reduction of ascorbic acid concentration induced by biotin deficiency in osteogenic disorder rats unable to synthesize ascorbic acid. *J. Clin. Biochem. Nutr.* **12**, 171–182.

Gacad, M. A., and Adams, J. S. (1989). Immunoblot analysis of the 1,25-dihydroxyvitamin D receptor in cultured primate cells. *J. Bone Miner. Res.* **4**, 5225 (abstr.).

Gacad, M. A., and Adams, J. S. (1991). Endogenous blockade of 1,25-dihydroxyvitamin D-receptor binding in New World primate cells. *J. Clin. Invest.* **87**, 996–1001.

Gacad, M. A., and Adams, J. S. (1992). Specificity of steroid binding in New World primate cells with a vitamin D-resistant phenotype. Endocrinology **31**(6), 2581–2587.

Gacad, M. A., and Adams, J. S. (1993). Identification of a competitite binding component in vitamin D-resistant New World primate cells with a low affinity but high capacity for 1,25-dihydroxyvitamin D_3. *J. Bone Miner. Res.* **8**, 27–35.

Gacad, M. A., Deseran, M. W., and Adams, J. S. (1992). Influence of ultraviolet B radiation on vitamin D_3 metabolism in vitamin D_3-resistant New World primates. *Am. J. Primatol.* **28**, 263–270.

Gahunia, H. K., Lemaire, C., Cross, A. R., Kessler, M. J., and Pritzker, K. P. H. (1993). Osteoarthritis in rhesus macaques: Assessment of cartilage matrix quality by quantitative magnetic resonance imaging. *In* "Joint Destruction in Arthritis and Osteoarthritis" (W. B. van den Berg and P. L. E. M. van Lent, eds.), p. 255. Birkhaeuser, Basel.

Gahunia, H. K., Babyn, P., Lemaire, C., Kessler, M. J., and Pritzker, K. P. H. (1995a). Osteoarthritis staging: Comparison between magnetic resonance imaging, gross pathology and histopathology in the rhesus macaque. *Osteoarthritis Cartilage* **3**, 169–180.

Gahunia, H. K., Lemaire, C., Babyn, P. S., Cross, A. R., Kessler, M. J., and Pritzker, K. P. H. (1995b). Osteoarthritis in rhesus macaque knee joint: Quantitative magnetic resonance imaging tissue characterization of articular cartilage. *J. Rheumatol.* **22**, 1747–1756.

Galbraith, S. C., and Quarles, L. D. (1993). Tertiary hyperparathyroidism and refractory secondary hyperparathyroidism. *In* "Primer on the Metabolic Bone Diseases and Disorders of Mineral Metabolism" (M. J. Favus, ed.), p. 159. Raven Press, New York.

Gardner, D. L., Skelton-Stroud, P. N., and Fitzmaurice, R. J. (1991). Akute Muramyl-Dipeptid-induzierte arthritis beim Pavian *Papio cynocephalus. Z. Rheumatol.* **50**, 86–92.

Gershoff, S. N. (1993). Vitamin C (ascorbic acid): New roles, new requirements? *Nutr. Rev.* **51**, 313–326.

Gerstenberger, H. J. (1938). Rickets in monkeys *(Macacus rhesus). Am. J. Dis. Child.* **56**, 694.

Geusens, P., Nijs, J., Van der Perre, G., Van Audekercke, R., Lowet, G., Goovaerts, S., Barbier, A., Lacheretz, F., Remandet, B., Jiang, Y., and Dequeker, J. (1992). Longitudinal effect of tiludronate on bone mineral density, resonant frequency, and strength in monkeys. *J. Bone Miner. Res.* **7**, 599–609.

Giannobile, W. V., Finkelman, R. D., and Lynch, S. E. (1994). Comparison of canine and nonhuman primate animal models for periodontal regenerative therapy. *J. Periodontol.* **65**, 1158–1168.

Gibson, J. P., and Roenigk, W. J. (1972). Pseudogout in a dog. *J. Am. Vet. Med. Assoc.* **161**, 912–915.

Gibson, T., Burry, H. C., Poswillo, D., and Glass, J. (1976). Effect of intraarticular corticosteroid injections on primate cartilage. *Ann. Rheum. Dis.* **36**, 74–79.

Giddens, W. E., Tsai, C.-C., Morton, W. R., Ochs, H. D., Knitter, G. H., and Blakley, G. A. (1985). Retroperitoneal fibromatosis and acquired immunodeficiency syndrome in macaques. Pathologic observations and transmission studies. *Am. J. Pathol.* **119**, 253–263.

Gillet, P., Bannwarth, B., Netter, P., Morel, O., Pere, P., and Gaucher, A. (1987). Experimental autoimmune spondylodiscitis associated with type II collagen arthritis. *J. Rheumatol.* **14**, 856–857.

Gillet, P., Bannwarth, B., Charriere, G., Leroux, P., Fener, P., Netter, P., Hartmann, D. J., Pere, P., and Gaucher, A. (1989). Studies of Type II collagen induced arthritis in rats: An experimental model of peripheral and axial ossifying enthesopathy. *J. Rheumatol.* **16**, 721–728.

Gillman, J., and Gilbert, C. (1954). Some connective tissue diseases (amyloidosis, arthritis, reticulosarcoma) in the baboon *(Papio ursinus). S. Afr. J. Med. Sci.* **18**, 112–113.

Goldstein, S., Winston, E., Chung, T. J., Chopra, S., and Pariser, K. (1985). Chronic arthropathy in long-term hemodialysis. *Am. J. Med.* **78**, 82–86.

Golub, M. S., Gershwin, M. E., Hurley, L. S., Saito, W., and Hendrickx, A. G. (1984). Studies of marginal zinc deprivation in rhesus monkeys. IV. Growth of infants in the first year. *Am. J. Clinic. Nutr.* **40**, 1192–1202.

Golub, M. S., Keen, C. L., Gershwin, M. E., Styne, D. M., Takeuchi, P. T., Ontell, F., Walter, R. M., and Hendrickx, A. G. (1996). Adolescent growth and maturation in zinc-deprived rhesus monkeys. *Am. J. Clinic. Nutr.* **64**, 274–282.

Goodwin, B. T., and Jerome, C. P. (1987). Iliac biopsy for histomorphometric analysis of trabecular bone in cynomolgus monkeys and baboons. *Lab. Anim. Sci.* **37**, 213–216.

Gordon, T. P., Reid, C., Rozenbilds, M. A. M., and Ahern, M. (1986). Crystal shedding in septic arthritis: Case reports and in vivo evidence in an animal model. *Aust. N.Z. J. Med.* **16**, 336–340.

Gray, T. K., Lester, G. E., Moore, G., Crews, D., Simons, E. L., and Stuart, M. (1982) Serum concentrations of calcium and vitamin D metabolites in Prosimians. *J. Med. Primatol.* **11**, 85–90.

Greenwald, R. A., Golub, L. M., Lavietes, B., Ramamurthy, N. S., Gruber, B., Laskin, R. S., and McNamara, T. F. (1987). Tetracyclines inhibit human synovial collagenase in vivo and in vitro. *J. Rheumatol.* **14**, 28–32.

Greenwald, R. A., Simonson, B. G., Moak, S. A., Rush, S. W., Ramamurthy, N. S., Laskin, R. S., and Golub, L. M. (1988). Inhibition of epiphyseal cartilage collagenase by tetracyclines in low phosphate rickets in rats. *J. Orthop. Res.* **6**, 695–703.

Griffiths, H. J., Hunt, R. D., Zimmerman, R. E., Finberg, H., and Cuttino, J. (1975). The role of calcium and fluoride in osteoporosis in rhesus monkeys. *Investig. Radiol.* **10**, 263–268.

Grindeland, R. E., Ballard, R. W., Connolly, J. P., and Vasques, M. F. (1992). Cosmos 2044 mission. *J. Appl. Physiol.* **73**, 1S–3S.

Grynpas, M. D. (1990). Fluoride effects on bone crystals. *J. Bone Miner. Res.* **5**, S169–S175.

Grynpas, M. D. (1993). Age and disease-related changes in the mineral of bone. *Calcif. Tissue Inter.* **53**, Suppl. 1, S57–S64.

Grynpas, M. D., Patterson-Allen, P., and Simmons, D. J. (1986). The changes in quality of mandibular bone mineral in otherwise totally immobilized rhesus monkeys. *Calcif. Tissue Inter.* **39**, 57–62.

Grynpas, M. D., Huckell, B., Pritzker, K. P. H., Hancock, R. G. V., and Kessler, M. J. (1989). Bone mineral and osteoporosis in aging rhesus monkeys. *P. R. Health Sci. J.* **8**, 197–204.

Grynpas, M. D., Chateauvert, J. M. D., and Pritzker, K. P. H. (1990). Determining the elemental composition of articular cartilage: A comparison between human and non-human primates. *Methods Cartilage Res.* **49**, 194–196.

Grynpas, M. D., Hancock, R. G. V., Greenwood, C., Turnquist, J., and Kessler, M. J. (1993a). The effects of diet, age, and sex on the mineral content of primate bones. *Calcif. Tissue Int.* **52**, 399–405.

Grynpas, M. D., Huckell, C. B., Reichs, K. J., DeRousseau, C. J., Greenwood, C., and Kessler, M. J. (1993b). Effect of age and osteoarthritis on bone mineral in rhesus monkey vertebrae. *J. Bone Miner. Res.* **8**, 909–917.

Grynpas, M. D., Gahunia, H. K., Yuan, J., Pritzker, K. P. H., Hartmann, D., and Tupy, J. H. (1994). Analysis of collagens solubilized from cartilage of normal and spontaneously osteoarthritis rhesus monkeys. *Osteoarthritis Cartilage* **2**, 227–234.

Hallberg, L., Brune, M., and Rossander-Hulthen, L. (1987). Is there a physiological role of vitamin C in iron absorption? *Ann. N. Y. Acad. Sci.* **498**, 324–332.

Halverson, P. B. (1992). Arthropathies associated with basic calcium phosphate crystals. *Scanning Microsc.* **6**, 791–797.

Halverson, P. B., Garancis, J. C., and McCarty, D. J. (1984). Histopathological and ultrastructural studies of synovium in Milwaukee shoulder syndrome—a basic calcium phosphate crystal arthropathy. *Ann. Rheum. Dis.* **43**, 734–741.

Hamerton, A. E. (1939). Review of mortality rates and report on the deaths occurring in the Society's gardens during the year 1938. *Proc. Zool. Soc. London* **B109**, 281–327.

Hansen, B. C., and Bodkin, N. L. (1993). Primary prevention of diabetes mellitus by prevention of obesity in monkeys. *Diabetes* **42**, 1809–1814.

Hansen, B. C., Ortmeyer, H. K., and Bodkin, N. L. (1995). Prevention of obesity in middle-aged monkeys: Food intake during body weight clamp. *Obes. Res.* **3**, 1995–2045.

Harrison, M. H. M., Schajowicz, F., and Trueta, J. (1953). Osteoarthritis of the hip; study of the nature and evolution of the disease. *J. Bone Jt. Surg., Br. Vol.* **35B**, 598–626.

Harwick, H. J., Kalmanson, G. M., Fox, M. A. and Guze, L. B. (1973). Arthritis in mice due to infection with mycoplasma pulmonis. I. Clinical and microbiological features. *J. Infect. Dis.* **128**, 533–540.

Haskin, C., and Cameron, I. (1994). Inflammatory changes occur independently of degenerative temporomandibular joint changes in baboons. *J. Dent. Res.* **73**, 304 (abstr.).

Haskin, C., Cameron, I., and Rice, K. (1993). Age dependent pathological changes in baboon temporomandibular disks and condyles. *J. Dent. Res.* **72**, 151 (abstr.).

Hausman, R., Sturtevant, R. A., and Wilson, W. J. (1961). Lead intoxication in primates. *J. Forensic Sci.* **6**, 180.

Hayes, K. C. (1974). Pathophysiology of vitamin E deficiency in monkeys. *Am. J. Clin. Nutr.* **26**, 1130–1140.

Healy, C. T., Martin, L. N., Roberts, E. D., and Rubin, A. S. (1989). Methods in laboratory investigation. Experimental arthropathy induced in rhesus monkeys and DBA/1 mice by a novel method: Intraperitoneal implantation of type II collagen adsorbed onto nitrocellulose filters. *Lab. Invest.* **60**, 462–470.

Hearn, P. R., and Russell, R. G. G. (1980). Formation of calcium pyrophosphate crystals in vitro: Implications for calcium pyrophosphate crystal deposition disease (pseudogout). *Ann. Rheum. Dis.* **39**, 222–227.

Heijl, L., Rifkin, B. R., and Zander, H. A. (1976). Conversion of chronic gingivitis to periodontitis in squirrel monkeys. *J. Periodontol.* **47**, 710–716.

Heimann, M., Carpenter, J. L., and Halverson, P. B. (1990). Calcium pyrophosphate deposition (chondrocalcinosis) in a dog. Case reports. *Vet. Pathol.* **27**, 122–124.

Helmy, E. S., Bays, R., and Sharawy, M. (1988). Osteoarthrosis of the temporomandibular joint following experimental disc perforation in *Macaca fascicularis. J. Oral Maxillofacial Surg.* **46**, 979–990.

Helmy, E. S., Bays, R. A., and Sharawy, M. M. (1989). Synovial chondromatosis associated with experimental osteoarthritis in adult monkeys. *J. Oral Maxillofacial Surg.* **47**, 823–827.

Hendry, R. M., Wells, M. A., Phelan, M. A., Schneider, A. L., Epstein, J. S., and Quinnan, G. V. (1986). Antibodies to simian immunodeficiency virus in African green monkeys in Africa in 1957–62. *Lancet* **2**, 455.

Hess, E. V., Kramer, L., Linnemann, C. C., Herzig, E., Adams, L. E., and Balz, G. (1983). Arthritis in gorillas. *Arthritis Rheum.* **26**, S56 (abstr.).

Hime, J. M., Keymer, I. F., and Appleby, E. C. (1972). Hypertrophic pulmonary osteoarthropathy in an orang-utan (*Pongo pygmaeus*). *Vet. Rec.* **91**, 334–337.

Hoffman, G. S. (1978). Polyarthritis: The differential diagnosis of rheumatoid arthritis. *Semin. Arthritis Rheum.* **8**, 115–141.

Hogan, D. B., and Pritzker, K. P. H. (1985). Synovial fluid analysis—another look at the mucin clot test. *J. Rheumatol.* **12**, 242–244.

Holick, M. F. (1995). Environmental factors that influence the cutaneous production of vitamin D1-3. *Am. J. Clin. Nutr.* **61**, 638S–645S.

Holling, H. E., Brody, R. S., and Boland, H. C. (1961). Pulmonary hypertrophic osteoarthropathy. *Lancet* **2**, 1269–1274.

Holmdahl, R., Andersson, M. E., Goldschmidt, T. J., Jansson, L., Karlsson, M., Malmstrom, V., and Mo, J. (1989). Collagen induced arthritis as an experimental model for rheumatoid arthritis: Immunogenetics, pathogenesis and autoimmunity. *APMIS* **97**, 575–584.

Holmdahl, R., Andersson, M., Goldschmidt, T. J., Gustafsson, K., Jansson, L., and Mo, J. A. (1990). Type II collagen autoimmunity in animals and provocations leading to arthritis. *Immunol. Rev.* **118**, 193.

Holt, S. C., Ebersole, J. L., Felton, J., Brunsvold, M., and Kornman, K. S. (1988). Implantation of Bacteroids gingivalis in non-human primates initiates progression of periodontis. *Science* **239**, 55–57.

Hoopes, P. J., McKay, D. W., Daisley, G. W., Jr., Kennedy, S., and Bush, M. (1978). Suppurative arthritis in an infant orangutan. *J. Am. Vet. Med. Assoc.* **173**, 1145–1147.

Hosny, M., and Sharawy, M. (1985). Osteoinduction in rhesus monkeys using demineralized bone powder allografts. *J. Oral Maxillofacial Surg.* **43**, 837–844.

Houpt, J. B., Pritzker, K. P. H., Alpert, B., Greyson, M. D., and Gross, A. E. (1983). Osteonecrosis of the knee—a review. *Semin. Arthritis Rheum.* **13**, 212–227.

Howard, C. F., Jr., and Yasuda, M. (1990). Diabetes mellitus in nonhuman primates: Recent research advances and current husbandry practices. *J. Med. Primatol.* **19**, 609–625.

Howard, C. F., Jr., Kessler, M. J., and Schwartz, S. (1986). Carbohydrate impairment and insulin secretory abnormalities among *Macaca mulatta* from Cayo Santiago. *Am. J. Primatol.* **11**, 147–162.

Howell, D. S., Treadwell, B. V., and Trippel, S. B. (1992). Etiopathogenesis of osteoarthritis. *In* "Osteoarthritis. Diagnosis and Medical/Surgical Management" (R. W. Moskowitz, D. S. Howell, V. M. Goldberg, and H. J. Mankin, eds.), p. 233. Saunders, Philadelphia.

Hughes, K. P., Kimmel, D. B., Kammerer, C. M., Davies, K. M., Rice, K. S., and Recker, R. R. (1994). Vertebral morphometry in adult female baboons. *J. Bone Miner. Res.* **9**, S209.

Hughes, R. A., Rowe, I. F., Shanson, D., and Keat, A. C. (1992). Septic bone, joint and muscle lesions associated with human immunodeficiency virus infection. *Br. J. Rheumatol.* **31**, 381–388.

Hunneyball, I. M. (1983). Investigations into the induction of chronic experimental arthritis in the common marmoset (*Callithrix jacchus*). *Rheumatol. Int.* **3**, 69–74.

Hunneyball, I. M., Harrison, G. B. L., and Stanworth, D. R. (1979). The production of experimental arthritis in baboons. *IRCS Med. Sci:Libr. Compend.* **7**, 517.

Hunt, R. D., Garcia, F. G., and Hegsted, D. M. (1967a). A comparison of vitamin D_2 and D_3 in New World primates. Part I. *Lab. Anim. Care* **17**, 222.

Hunt, R. D., Garcia, F. G., Hegsted, D. M., and Kaplinsky, N. (1967b). Vitamins D_2 and D_3 in New World primates: Influence on calcium absorption. *Science* **157**, 943.

Hunter, G. K., Grynpas, M. D., Cheng, P.-T., and Pritzker, K. P. H. (1987). Effect of glycosaminoglycans on calcium pyrophosphate crystal formation in collagen gels. *Calc. Tissue Int.* **41**, 164–170.

Ikede, B. O. (1979). Calcinosis circumscripta in the buffalo (*Bos bubalis*). *Vet. Pathol.* **16**, 260–262.

Irby, R., Edwards, W. M., and Gatter, R. (1975). Articular complications of homotransplantation and chronic renal hemodialysis. *J. Rheumatol.* **2**, 91–99.

Ishizawa, N. (1992). Experimental study of hyperostosis induced by hypervitaminosis A. *J. Jpn. Orthop. Assoc.* **66**, 919–930.

Jacobson, J. L., and Snowdon, C. T. (1976). Increased lead ingestion in calcium-deficient monkeys. *Nature (London)* **262**, 51–52.

Jacobson, S. A. (1971). "The Comparative Pathology of the Tumors of Bone." Thomas, Springfield, IL.

Jasin, H. E. (1985). Autoimmunity specificities of immune complexes requested in articular cartilage of patients with rheumatoid arthritis and osteoarthritis. *Arthritis Rheum.* **28**, 241–248.

Jayo, M. J., Jayo, J. M., Jerome, C. P., Krugner-Higby, L., and Reynolds, G. D. (1988). Maxillo-orbital lymphoma (Burkitt's-Type) in an infant *Macaca fascicularis*. *Lab. Anim. Sci.* **38**, 722–726.

Jayo, M. J., Weaver, D. S., Adams, M. R., and Rankin, S. E. (1990a). Effects on bone of surgical menopause and estrogen therapy with or without progesterone replacement in cynomolgus monkeys. *Am. J. Obstet. Gynecol.* **163**, 614–618.

Jayo, M. J., Weaver, D. S., Rankin, S. E., and Kaplan, J. R. (1990b). Accuracy and reproducibility of lumbar bone mineral status determined by dual photon absorptiometry in live male cynomolgus macaques (*Macaca fascicularis*). *Lab. Anim. Sci.* **40**, 266–269.

Jayo, M. J., Jerome, C. P., Lees, C. J., Rankin, S. E., and Weaver, D. S. (1994). Bone mass in female cynomolgus macaques: A cross-sectional and longitudinal study by age. *Calcif. Tissue Int.* **54**, 231–236.

Jennekens, F. G. I., Tomlinson, B. E., and Walton, J. N. (1971). Histochemical aspects of five limb muscles in old age. *J. Neurol. Sci.* **14**, 259–276.

Jerome, C. P., Kimmel, D. B., McAlister, J. A., and Weaver, D. S. (1986). Effects of ovariectomy on iliac trabecular bone in baboons (*Papio anubis*). *Calcif. Tissue Int.* **39**, 206–208.

Jerome, C. P., Carlson, C. S., Register, T. C., Bain, F. T., Jayo, M. J., Weaver, D. S., and Adams, M. R. (1994). Bone functional changes in intact, ovariectomized, and ovariectomized, hormone-supplemented adult cynomolgus monkeys (*Macaca fascicularis*) evaluated by serum markers and dynamic histomorphometry. *J. Bone Miner. Res.* **9**, 527–539.

Jerome, C. P., Lees, C. J., and Weaver, D. S. (1995a). Development of osteopenia in ovariectomized cynomolgus monkeys (*Macaca fascicularis*). *Bone* **17**, 403S–408S.

Jerome, C. P., Johnson, C. S., and Lees, C. J. (1995b). Effect of treatment for 3 months with human parathyroid hormone 1-34 peptide in ovariectomized cynomolgus monkeys (*Macaca fascicularis*). *Bone* **17**, 415S–420S.

Jha, G. J., Deo, M. G., and Ramalingaswami, V. (1968). Bone growth in protein deficiency. *Am. J. Pathol.* **53**, 1111–1123.

Jones, M. D., Pais, M. J., and Omiya, B. (1988). Bony overgrowths and abnormal calcifications about the spine. *Radiol. Clin. North Am.* **26**, 1213–1233.

Jonker, M., Bakker, K., Slierendregt, B., 't Hart, B., and Bontrop, R. (1991). Autoimmunity in non-human primates: The role of major histocompatibility complex and T cells, and implications for therapy. *Hum. Immunol.* **32**, 31–40.

Jowsey, J., and Orvis, A. L. (1967). Comparative deposition of 45Ca, 65Zn, and 91Y in bone. *Radiat. Res.* **31**, 693–698.

Julkunen, H., and Heinonen, O. P. (1971). Hyperostosis of the spine in an adult population, its relationship to hyperglycemia and obesity. *Ann. Rheum. Dis.* **30**, 605–612.

Junge, R. E., Mehren, K. G., Meehan, T. P., Crawshaw, G. J., Duncan, M. C., Gilula, L., Gannon, F., Finkel, G., and Whyte, M. P. (1994). Periarticular hyperostosis and renal disease in six black lemurs of two family groups. *J. Am. Vet. Med. Assoc.* **205**, 1024–1029.

Jurmain, R. (1989). Trauma, degenerative disease, and other pathologies among the Gombe chimpanzees. *Am. J. Phys. Anthropol.* **80**, 229–237.

Jurmain, R. D., and Kilgore, L. (1995). Skeletal evidence of osteoarthritis: A palaeopathological perspective. *Ann. Rheum. Dis.* **54**, 443–450.

Kammerer, C. M., Sparks, M., Whittam, N., and Rogers, J. (1994). Genetic and age effects on trabecular and compact bone mass variation in Papio baboons. *J. Bone Miner. Res.* **9**, S324.

Kammerer, C. M., Sparks, M. L., and Rogers, J. (1995). Effects of age, sex, and heredity on measures of bone mass in baboons (*Papio hamadryas*). *J. Med. Primatol.* **24**, 236–242.

Kandel, R. A., Renlund, R. C., Cheng, P.-T., Rapley, W. A., Mehren, K. G., and Pritzker, K. P. H. (1983). Calcium pyrophosphate dihydrate crystal deposition disease with concurrent vertebral hypertosis in a barbary ape. *Arthritis Rheum.* **26**, 682–687.

Kandel, R. A., Cheng, P.-T., and Pritzker, K. P. H. (1986). Localized apatite synovitis of the wrist. *J. Rheumatol.* **13**, 667–669.

Kang, A. H., Yoo, T. J., Yazawa, Y., Orchik, D., Floyd, R., Olson, G., Sudo, N., Ishibe, J. J., and Takeda, T. (1984). Induction of type II collagen autoimmune arthritis and ear disease in monkey. *Fed. Proc., Fed. Am. Soc. Exp. Biol.* **43**, 1994 (abstr.).

Kark, J. A., Victor, M., Hines, J. D. and Harris, J. W. (1974). Nutritional vitamin B_{12} deficiency in rhesus monkeys. *Am. J. Clin. Nutr.* **27**, 470–478.

Kasra, M., and Grynpas, M. D. (1994). Effect of long-term ovariectomy on bone mechanical properties in young female cynomolgus monkeys. *Bone* **15**, 557–561.

Kasra, M., and Grynpas, M. D. (1995). The effects of androgens on the mechanical properties of primate bone. *Bone* **17**, 265–270.

Kazarian, L., Cann, C., Parfitt, M., Simmons, D., and Morey-Holton, E. (1981). A 14-day ground-based hypokinesia study in nonhuman primates: A compilation of results. *NASA Tech. Memo.* **NASA TM-81268**, 62.

Kazarian, L. E., and von Gierke, H. E. (1969). Bone loss as a result of immobilization and chelation. *Clin. Orthop. Relat. Res.* **65**, 67–75.

Kazarian, L. E., and von Gierke, H. E. (1971). Disuse atrophy in *Macaca mulatta* and its implications for extended spaceflight. *NASA [Spec. Publ.] SP NASA SP-269*, 129–144.

Keen, C. E., Crocker, P. R., Brady, K., Hasan, N., and Levison, D. A. (1991). Calcium pyrophosphate dihydrate deposition disease: Morphological and microanalytical features. *Histopathology* 19, 529–536.

Keen, C. E., Crocker, P. R., Brady, K., Buk, S. J. A., and Levison, D. A. (1995). Intraosseous secondary calcium salt crystal deposition: An artifact of acid decalcification. *Histopathology* 27, 181–185.

Kemnitz, J. W., Roecker, E. B., Weindruch, R., Elson, D. F., Baum, S. T., and Bergman, R. T. (1994). Dietary restriction increases insulin sensitivity and lowers blood glucose in rhesus monkeys. *Am. J. Physiol.* 266, E540–E547.

Kennard, M. A. (1941). Abnormal findings in 246 consecutive autopsies on monkeys. *Yale J. Biol. Med.* 13, 701–712.

Kerr, G. R., Waisman, H. A., Allen, J. A., Wallace, J., and Scheffler, G. (1973). Malnutrition studies in *Macaca mulatta*. II. The effect on organ size and skeletal growth. *Am. J. Clin. Nutr.* 26, 620–630.

Kessler, M. J. (1980). Cephalhematomas due to suspected ascorbic acid deficiency in young squirrel monkeys (*Saimuri sciureus*). *J. Med. Primatol.* 9, 314–318.

Kessler, M. J., London, W. T., Rawlins, R. G., Gonzalez, J., Martinez, H. S., and Sanchez, J. (1985). Management of a harem breeding colony of rhesus monkeys to reduce trauma-related morbidity and mortality. *J. Med. Primatol.* 14, 91–98.

Kessler, M. J., Turnquist, J. E., Pritzker, K. P. H., and London, W. T. (1986). Reduction of passive extension and radiographic evidence of degenerative knee joint diseases in cage-raised and free-ranging aged rhesus monkeys (*Macaca mulatta*). *J. Med. Primatol.* 15, 1–9.

Kiel, R. A., Kornman, K. S., and Robertson, P. B. (1983). Clinical and microbiology effects of localized ligature-induced periodontitis of a non-ligated sites in the cynomolgus monkey. *J. Periodont. Res.* 18, 200–211.

Kimura, M. (1986). Summary of seven years observations on cadmium-fed monkeys under various nutritional conditions. *Ed. Proc.—Int. Cadmium conf., 5th, 1986*, pp. 105–107.

Kindblom, L.-G., and Gunterberg, B. (1988). Tumoral calcinosis. An ultrastructural analysis and consideration of pathogenesis. *APMIS* 96, 368–376.

King, G. (1976). An investigation into ''Wasting Marmoset Syndrome'' at Jersey Zoo. *Annu. Rep., Jersey Wildl. Preserv. Trust*, pp. 97–107.

King, N. W., Hunt, R. D., and Letvin, N. L. (1983). Histopathologic changes in macaques with an acquired immunodeficiency syndrome (AIDS). *Am. J. Pathol.* 113, 382–388.

Klumpp, S. A., Weaver, D. S., Jerome, C. P., and Jokinen, M. P. (1986). Salmonella osteomyelitis in a rhesus monkey. *Vet. Pathol.* 23, 190–197.

Kornman, K. S., Holt, S. C., and Robertson, P. B. (1981). The microbiology of ligature-induced periodontitis in the cynomolgus monkey. *J. Periodont. Res.* 16, 363–371.

Kornman, K. S., Blodgett, R. F., Brunsvold, M., and Holt, S. C. (1990). Effects of topical application of meclofenamic acid and ibuprofen on bone loss, subgingival microbiota and gingival PMN response in the primate *Macaca fascicularis*. *J. Periodont. Res.* 25, 300–307.

Krishnan, K. V. (1933). Vincent's disease in a *Macaca irus* monkey. *Indian Med. Gaz.* 68, 455–456.

Krook, L., and Barrett, R. B. (1962). Simian bone disease—A secondary hyperparathyroidism. *Cornell Vet.* 52, 459–492.

Kupper, J. L. (1976). Evaluation of the squirrel monkey (*Saimiri sciureus*) as an experimental animal model for dysbaric osteonecrosis. *Nav. Aerosp. Med. Res. Lab. Rep.* 1221, 1–7.

Lagier, R. (1989). Spinal hyperostosis in comparative pathology. A useful approach to the concept. *Skeletal Radiol.* 18, 99–107.

Lane, M. A., Ingram, D. K., Cutler, R. G., Knapka, J. J., Barnard, D. E., and Roth, G. S. (1992). Dietary restriction in nonhuman primates: Progress report on the NIA study. *In* ''Physiopathological Processes of Aging: Towards a Multicausal Interpretation'' (N. Fabris, D. Harman, D. L. Knook, E. Steinhagen-Thiessen,

and I. Zs-nagy, eds.), Ann. N. Y. Acad. Sci., vol. 673, pp. 36–45. New York Acad. Sci., New York.

Lane, M. A., Reznick, A. Z., Tilmont, E. M., Lanir, A., Ball, S. S., Read, V., Ingram, D. K., Cutler, R. G., and Roth, G. S. (1995). Aging and food restriction alter some indices of bone metabolism in male rhesus monkeys (*Macaca mulatta*). *J. Nutr.* 125, 1600–1610.

Lapin, B. A., and Yakovleva, L. A. (1960). Noninfectious diseases. *In* ''Comparative Pathology in Monkeys'' (Anonymous), p. 239. Thomas, Springfield, IL.

Lawlor, D. A., Warren, E., Ward, F. E., and Parham, P. (1990). Comparison of class I MHC alleles in humans and apes. *Immunol. Rev.* 113, 147–185.

Layton, M. W., Fudman, E. J., Barkan, A., Braunstein, E. M., and Fox, I. H. (1988). Acromegalic arthropathy. Characteristics and response to therapy. *Arthritis Rheum.* 31, 1022–1027.

Leboy, P. S., Vaias, L., Uschmann, B., Golub, E., and Adams, S. L. (1989). Ascorbic acid induces alkaline phosphatase, type X collagen, and calcium deposition in cutured chick chondrocytes. *J. Biol. Chem.* 264, 17281–17286.

Leek, J. C., Vogler, J. B., Gershwin, M. E., Golub, M. S., Hurley, L. S., and Hendrickx, A. G. (1984). Studies of marginal zinc deprivation in rhesus monkeys. V. Fetal and infant skeletal effects. *Am. J. Clin. Nutr.* 40, 1203–1212.

Leek, J. C., Keen, C. L., Vogler, J. B., Golub, M. S., Hurley, L. S., Hendrickx, A. G., and Gershwin, M. E. (1988). Long-term marginal zinc deprivation in rhesus monkeys. IV. Effects on skeletal growth and mineralization. *Am. J. Clin. Nutr.* 47, 889–895.

LeGeros, R. Z., Contiguglia, S. R., and Alfrey, A. C. (1973). Pathological calcifications associated with uremia. Two types of calcium phosphate deposits. *Calcif. Tissue Res.* 13, 173–185.

Lehner, N. D. M., Bullock, B. C., Clarkson, T. B., and Lofland, H. B. (1967). Biological activities of vitamins D_2 and D_3 for growing squirrel monkeys. *Lab. Anim. Care* 17, 483–493.

Lei, K. Y., and Young, L. C. (1979). Mineral content of bone and other tissues. *In* ''Aging in Nonhuman Primates'' (D. M. Bowden, ed.), p. 348. Van Nostrand-Reinhold, New York.

Le Minor, J. M. (1990). Comparative morphology of the lateral meniscus of the knee in primates. *J. Anat.* 170, 161–171.

Letvin, N. L., and King, N. W. (1984). Clinical and pathologic features of an acquired immune deficiency syndrome (AIDS) in macaque monkeys. *Adv. Vet. Sci. Comp. Med.* 28, 237–265.

Letvin, N. L., Eaton, K. A., Aldrich, W. R., Sehgal, P. K., Blake, B. J., Schlossman, S. F., King, N. W., and Hunt, R. D. (1983). Acquired immunodeficiency syndrome in a colony of macaque monkeys. *Proc. Natl. Acad. Sci. U.S.A.* 80, 2718–2722.

Letvin, N. L., Daniel, M. D., Sehgal, P. K., Desrosiers, R. C., Hunt, R. D., Waldron, L. M., MacKey, J. J., Schmidt, D. K., Chalifoux, L. V., and King, N. W. (1985). Induction of AIDS-like disease in macaque monkeys with T-cell tropic retrovirus STLV-III. *Science* 230, 71.

Leutenegger, W., Larsen, R. M., and Bravo, S. (1973). The effects of temporary protein deprivation on bone width and bone mineral content in rhesus macaques. *Growth* 37, 369–372.

Levine, M. (1986). New concepts in the biology and biochemistry of ascorbic acid. *Semin. Med. Beth Isr. Hosp., Boston* 314, 892–902.

Liberman, U. A., deGrange, D., and Marx, S. J. (1985). Low affinity of the receptor for 1,25-dihydroxyvitamin D_3 in the marmoset, a New World monkey. *FEBS Lett.* 182, 385–389.

Lim, K. K. T., Rogers, J., Shepstone, L., and Dieppe, P. A. (1995). The evolutionary origins of osteoarthritis: A comparative skeletal study of hand disease in 2 primates. *J. Rheumatol.* 22, 2132–2134.

Lim, K. K. T., Kessler, M. J., Pritzker, K. P. H., Turnquist, J., and Dieppe, P. A. (1996). Osteoarthritis of the hand in a non-human primate: A clinical, radiographic and skeletal survey of the Cayo Santiago macaques. *J. Med. Primatol.* 25, 301–308.

Lin, J. D., Phelps, R. G., Gordon, M. L., Hilfer, J. B., Wolfe, D. E., Venkataseshan, V. S., and Fleischmajer, R. (1992). Pathologic manifestations of the eosinophilia myalgia syndrome: Analysis of 11 cases. *Hum. Pathol.* **23,** 429–437.

Line, S. W., Ihrke, P. J., and Prahalada, S. (1984). Calcinosis circumscripta in two rhesus monkeys. *Lab. Anim. Sci.* **54,** 616–618.

Lipkin, E. W. (1996). Regional histomorphology of cancellous bone in *Macaca fascicularis. Am. J. Primatol.* **39,** 179–187.

Lipman, N. S., Schelling, S. H., Otto, G., and Murphy, J. C. (1991). Juvenile rheumatoid arthritis in a rhesus monkey (*Macaca mulatta*). *J. Med. Primatol.* **20,** 82–88.

Littlejohn, G. O. (1985). Insulin and new bone formation in diffuse idiopathic skeletal hyperostosis. *Clin. Rheumatol.* **4,** 294–300.

Loesche, W. J. (1976). Periodontal disease and the treponemes. *In* "The Biology of Parasitic Spirochetes" (R. C. Johnson, ed.), p. 261. Academic Press, New York.

Lohmander, S., Saxne, T., and Heinegard, D. (1995). Molecular markers for joint and skeletal diseases. Acta Orthopaedica Scandinavia, Suppl. 266, Vol. 66, October 1995. An Eric K. Fernström Symposium, Scandinavian University Press, Oslo-Copenhagen-Stockholm.

Londei, M., Savill, C. M., Verhoef, A., Brennan, F., Leech, Z. A., Duance, V., Maini, R. N., and Feldmann, M. (1989). Persistance of collagen type II-specific T cell clones in the synovial membrane of a patient with rheumatoid arthritis. *Proc. Natl. Acad. Sci. U.S.A.* **86,** 636–640.

Long, J. C., and Merbs, C. F. (1981). Coccidioidomycosis: A primate model. *In* "Buikstra, Prehistoric Tubercolis in the Americas" (Anonymous). Northwestern University Archeological Program, Evanston, IL.

Longcope, C., Hoberg, L., Steuterman, S., and Baran, D. (1989). The effect of ovariectomy on spine bone mineral density in rhesus monkeys. *Bone* **10,** 341–344.

Lovell, N. C. (1990a). "Patterns of Injury and Illness in Great Apes: A Skeletal Analysis." Smithsonian Institution Press, Washington, DC.

Lovell, N. C. (1990b). Skeletal and dental pathology of free-ranging mountain gorillas. *Am. J. Phys. Anthropol.* **81,** 399–412.

Lovell, N. C. (1991). An evolutionary framework for assessing illness and injury in nonhuman primates. *Yearb. Phys. Anthropol.* **34,** 117–155.

Lowenstine, L. J. (1986). Neoplasms and proliferative disorders in nonhuman primates. *In* "Primates: The Road to Self-Sustaining Populations" (K. Benirschke, ed.), p. 781. Springer-Verlag, Berlin and New York.

Lowenstine, L. J., Pedersen, N. C., Higgins, J., Pallis, K. C., Uyeda, A., Marx, P., Lerche, N. W., Munn, R. J., and Gardner, M. B. (1986). Serologic-epidemiologic survey of captive Old-World primates for antibodies to human and simian retroviruses, and isolation of a lentivirus from sooty mangabeys (*Cercocebus atys*). *Int. J. Cancer* **38,** 563.

Lucas, N. S., Hume, E. M., and Smith, H. H. (1937). On the breeding of the common marmoset (*Hapale jacchus, Linn*) in captivity when irradiated with ultraviolet rays. II. A ten years' family history. *Proc. Zool. Soc. London* **107,** 205–211.

Lucherini, T., and Porzio, F. (1966a). Study of the provocation of experimental arthritis in the rhesus monkey: V. Conclusions. *Minerva Med.* **57,** 1851–1856.

Lucherini, T., and Porzio, F. (1966b). Studi sulla provocazione di un'artrite sperimentale nel rhesus. *Minerva Med.* **57,** 1851–1856.

Lucherini, T., and Porzio, F. (1967). The provocation of experimental arthritis in the rhesus monkey. *Rass. Clin.-Sci. Ist. Biochimi. Ital.* **43,** 1–7.

Lucherini, T., Cecchi, E., Porzio, F., and D'Amore, A. (1964a). The experimental provocation of rheumatoid-like nodules. *Minerva Med.* **55,** 2377–2380.

Lucherini, T., Cecchi, E., Porzio, F., and D'Amore, D. (1964b). Study of the provocation of experimental arthritis in rhesus monkey: I. Results obtained with the use of mycobacterial adjuvant. *Minerva Med.* **55,** 4059–4065.

Lucherini, T., Cecchi, E., Porzio, F., and D'Amore, A. (1965a). Study of the provocation of experimental arthritis in the rhesus monkey: II. Results obtained with the use of fibrin. *Minerva Med.* **56,** 323–328.

Lucherini, T., Cecchi, E., Porzio, F., and D'Amore, A. (1965b). Study of the provocation of experimental arthritis in the rhesus monkey: III: Further results using fibrin. *Minerva Med.* **56,,** 1509–1512.

Lucherini, T., Cecchi, E., Porzio, F., and D'Amore, A. (1965c). Study of the provocation of experimental arthritis in the rhesus monkey: IV. Effects of protein deficiency of fibrin induced arthritis. *Minerva Med.* **56,** 1549–1554.

Lucherini, T., Cecchi, E., and Porzio, F. (1966). Induction of an experimental arthritis in the rhesus. *Reumatismo* **18,** 189–219.

Luder, H. U., and Schroeder, H. E. (1992). Light and electron microscopic morphology of the temporomandibular joint in growing and mature crab-eating monkeys (*Macaca fascicularis):* The condylar calcified cartilage. *Anat. Embryol.* **185,** 189–199.

Lufti, A. M. (1975). Morphological changes in the articular cartilage after meniscectomy: An experimental study in the monkey. *J. Bone Jnt. Surg., Br. Vol.* **57B,** 525–528.

Lundon, K., and Grynpas, M. D. (1993). The longterm effect of ovariectomy on the quality and quantity of cortical bone in the young cynomolgus monkey: A comparison of density fractionation and histomorphometric techniques. *Bone* **14,** 389–395.

Lundon, K., Dumitriu, M., and Grynpas, M. D. (1994). The long-term effect of ovariectomy on the quality and quantity of cancellous bone in young macaques. *Bone Miner.* **24,** 135–149.

Lundon, K., Dumitriu, M., and Grynpas, M. D. (1997). Supraphysiologic levels of testosterone affect cancellous and cortical bone in the young female cynomolgus monkey. *Calcif. Tissue Int.* **60,** 54–62.

Lusted, L. B., Pickering, D. E., Fisher, D. E., and Smyth, F. S. (1953). Growth and metabolism in normal and thyroid-ablated infant monkeys (*Macaca mulatta*). V. Roentgenographic features of skeletal development in normal and thyroid-ablated infant rhesus monkeys (*Macaca mulatta*). *Am. J. Dis. Child.* **86,** 426–435.

Machlin, L. J., Garcia, F., Kuenzig, W., and Brin, M. (1979). Antiscorbutic activity of ascorbic acid phosphate in the rhesus monkey and the guinea pig. *Am. J. Clin. Nutr.* **32,** 325–331.

Mack, P. B. (1971). Bone density changes in a *Macaca nemestrina* monkey during the Biosatellite III Project. *Aerosp. Med.* **42,** 828–833.

Mackay, J. M. K., Sim, A. K., McCormick, J. N., Marmion, B. P., McCraw, A. P., Duthie, J. J. R., and Gardner, D. L. (1983). Aetiology of rheumatoid arthritis: An attempt to transmit an infective agent from patients with rheumatoid arthritis to baboons. *Ann. Rheum. Dis.* **42,** 443–447.

Malinin, T. I., Mnaymneh, W., Lo, H. K., and Hinkle, D. K. (1994). Cryopreservation of articular cartilage. Ultrastructural observations and long-term results of experimental distal femoral transplantation. *Clin. Orthop. Relat. Res.* **303,** 18–32.

Malinow, M. R., Bardana, E. J., and Goodnight, S. H. (1981). Pancytopenia during ingestion of alfalfa seeds. *Lancet* **8220,** 615.

Malinow, M. R., Bardana, E. J., Pirofsky, B., Craig, S., and McLaughlin, P. (1982). Systemic lupus erythematosus-like syndrome in monkeys fed alfalfa sprouts: Role of a nonprotein amino acid. *Science* **216,** 415–417.

Mankin, H. J. (1974a). Rickets, osteomalacia, and renal osteodystrophy. Part I. *J. Bone Jt. Surg., Am. Vol.* **56-A,** 101–128.

Mankin, H. J. (1974b). Rickets, osteomalacia, and renal osteodystrophy. Part II. *J. Bone Jt. Surg., Am. Vol.* **56-A,** 352–386.

Mankin, H. J., Brandt, K. D., and Shulman, L. E. (1986). Workshop on etiopathogenesis of osteoarthritis. Proceedings and recommendations. *J. Rheumatol.* **13,** 1130–1160.

Mann, D. R., Gould, K. G., and Collins, D. C. (1990). A potential primate model for bone loss resulting from medical oophorectomy or menopause. *J. Clin. Endocrinol. Metab.* **71,** 105–110.

Mann, D. R., Rudman, C. G., Akinbami, M. A., and Gould, K. G. (1992). Preservation of bone mass in hypogonadal female monkeys with recombinant human growth hormone administration. *J. Clin. Endocrinol. Metab.* **74,** 1263–1269.

Martin, J. E., Cole, W. C., and Whitney, R. A., Jr. (1968). Tuberculosis of the spine (Pott's Disease) in a rhesus monkey (*Macaca mulatta*). *J. Am. Vet. Med. Assoc.* **153,** 914–917.

Marzke, M. W., and Merbs, C. F. (1984). Evidence of hypertrophic pulmonary osteoarthropathy in a chimpanzee, *Pan troglodytes. J. Med. Primatol.* **13,** 135–145.

Masi, A. T., and Chrousos, G. P. (1996). Hypothalamic-pituitary-adrenal-glucocorticoid axis function in rheumatoid arthritis. *J. Rheumatol.* **23,** 577–581.

Mazess, B., Vetter, J., and Weaver, D. S. (1987). Bone changes in oophorectomized monkeys: CT findings. *J. Comput. Assist. Tomogr.* **11,** 302–305.

Mazess, R. B. (1982). On aging bone loss. *Clin. Orthop. Relat. Res.* **165,** 239–252.

McCarty, D. J. (1992). Identification of calcium pyrophosphate dihydrate crystals. *Clin. Exp. Rheumatol.* **10,** 555–556.

McCarty, D. J., Halverson, P. B., Carrera, G. F., Brewer, B. J., and Kozin, F. (1981). "Milwaukee Shoulder"—Association of microspheroids containing hydroxyapatite crystals, active collagenase, and neutral protease with rotator cuff defects. *Arthritis Rheum.* **24,** 464–473.

McClure, H. M. (1980). Neoplastic diseases in nonhuman primates: Literature review and observations in an autopsy series of 2,176 animals. *In* "The Comparative Pathology of Zoo Animals" (R. J. Montali and G. Migaki, eds.), p. 549. Smithsonian Institution Press, Washington, DC.

McIntosh, I. G. (1956). Lead poisoning in animals. *Vet. Rev. Anat.* **2,** 57.

McIntosh, J. S., Ringqvist, M., and Schmidt, E. M. (1985). Fiber type composition of monkey forearm muscle. *Anat. Rec.* **211,** 403–409.

Mechanic, G. L., Young, D. R., Banes, A. J., and Yamauchi, M. (1986). Nonmineralized and mineralized bone collagen in bone of immobilized monkeys. *Calcif. Tissue Int.* **39,** 63–68.

Mielants, H., Veys, E. M., Goemaere, S., Goethals, K., Cuvelier, C., and De Vos, M. (1991). Gut inflammation in the spondyloarthropathies: Clinical, radiologic, biologic and genetic features in relation to the type of histology. A prospective study. *J. Rheumatol.* **18,** 1542–1551.

Mijiyawa, M. (1993). Spondyloarthropathies in patients attending the rheumatology unit of Lome Hospital. *J. Rheumatol.* **20,** 1167–1169.

Miller, L. C., Weaver, D. S., McAlister, J. A., and Koritnik, D. R. (1986). Effects of ovariectomy on vertebral trabecular bone in the cynomolgus monkey (*Macaca fascicularis*). *Calcif. Tissue Int.* **38,** 62–65.

Morbeck, M. E., Zihlman, A. L., Richman Sumner, D., Jr., and Galloway, A. (1991). Poliomyelitis and skeletal asymmetry in Gombe chimpanzees. *Primates* **32,** 77–91.

Morgan, K. (1990). What do anti-collagen antibodies mean? *Ann. Rheum. Dis.* **49,** 62–65.

Morgan, K., Clague, R. B., Collins, I., Ayad, S., Phinn, S. D., and Holt, P. J. L. (1989). A longitudinal study of anticollagen antibodies in patients with rheumatoid arthritis. *Arthritis Rheum.* **32,** 139–145.

Morin, M. L. (1983). A different approach in examining a wasting syndrome. *Lab. Anim.* **12,** 36–41.

Morrisey, J. K., Reichard, T., Janssen, D. D., Lloyd, M., and Bernard, J. B. (1994). Vitamin D deficiency rickets in colobinae monkeys. *Proc. Annu. Meet., Am. Assoc. Zoo Vet., 1994,* pp. 381–383.

Morrisey, J. K., Reichard, T., Lloyd, M., and Bernard, J. (1995). Vitamin-D-deficiency rickets in three colobus monkeys (*Colobus guereza kikuyuensis*) at the Toledo Zoo. *J. Zoo Wildl. Med.* **26,** 564–568.

Morrison, N. A., Qi, J. C., Tokita, A., Kelly, P. J., Crofts, L., Nguyen, T. V., Sambrook, P. N., and Eisman, J. A. (1994). Prediction of bone density from vitamin D receptor alleles. *Nature (London)* **367,** 284–287.

Mottonen, T., Hannonen, P., Oka, M., Rautiainen, J., Jokinen, I., Arvilommi, H., Palosuo, T., and Aho, K. (1988). Antibodies against native type II collagen do not precede the clinical onset of rheumatoid arthritis. *Arthritis Rheum.* **31,** 776–779.

Murchison, M. A., Owsley, D. W., and Riopelle, A. J. (1984). Transverse line formation in protein-deprived rhesus monkeys. *Hum. Biol.* **56,** 173–182.

Murgatroyd, L. B. (1985). "Symposium on Marmoset Pathology." ICI Pharmaceuticals Division, Macclesfield, Cheshire.

Murray, T. M., Harrison, J. E., Bayley, T. A., Josse, R. G., Sturtridge, W. C., Chow, R., Budden, F., Laurier, L., Pritzker, K. P. H., Kandel, R., Vieth, R., Strauss, A., and Goodwin, S. (1990). Fluoride treatment of postmenopausal osteoporosis: Age, renal function, and other clinical factors in the osteogenic response. *J. Bone Miner. Res.* **5,** S27–S35.

Nair, C. P., and Ray, A. P. (1955). Observations on the incidence and types of tuberculosis in rhesus monkeys on autopsy studies. *Indian J. Malariol.* **9,** 185–189.

Nall, J. D., and Bartels, J. E. (1973). Spondylitis in Diana Guenon monkey. *J. Zoo Anim. Med.* **4,** 22–23.

Nelson, J. S., Fitch, C. D., Fischer, V. W., Brown, G. O. Jr., and Chou, A. C. (1981). Progressive neuropathologic lesions in vitamin E deficient rhesus monkeys. *J. Neuropathol. Exp. Neurol.* **40,** 166–186.

Nielsen, S. W. (1989). Lyme borreliosis. *Comp. Pathol. Bull.* **21,** 1–4.

Nishikimi, M., and Udenfriend, S. (1976). Immunologic evidence that the gene for L-gulono-gamma-lactone oxidase is not expressed in animals subject to scurvy. *Proc. Natl. Acad. Sci. U.S.A.* **73,** 2066–2068.

Obeck, D. K., Toft, J. D. I., and Dupuy, H. J. (1976). Severe polyarthritis in a rhesus monkey: Suggested mycoplasma etiology. *Lab. Anim. Sci.* **26,** 613–618.

O'Gara, R. W., and Adamson, R. H. (1978). Spontaneous and induced neoplasms in nonhuman primates. *Proc. Sympo.,* National Zoological Park, Smithsonian Institution, Part I, pp. 190–238.

Ohira, T., and Ishikawa, K. (1986). Hydroxyapatite deposition in articular cartilage by intra-articular injections of methylprednisolone. A histological, ultrastructural, and x-ray microprobe analysis in rabbits. *J. Bone Jt. Surg., Amer. Vol.* **68-A,** 509–520.

Ono, K., Ota, H., Tada, K., Hamada, H., and Takaoka, K. (1977). Ossified posterior longitudinal ligament: A clinicopathologic study. *Spine* **2,** 126–138.

Ortmeyer, H. K., Bodkin, N. L., and Hansen, B. C. (1993). Insulin-mediated glycogen synthase activity in muscle of spontaneously insulin-resistant and diabetic rhesus monkeys. *Am. J. Physiol.* **265,** R552–R558.

Padh, H. (1990). Cellular functions of ascorbic acid. *Biochem. Cell Biol.* **68,** 1166–1173.

Page, R. C., Simpson, D. M., and Ammons, W. F. (1975). Host tissue response in chronic inflammatory periodontal disease. IV. The periodontal and dental status of a group of aged great apes. *J. Periodontol.* **46,** 144–155.

Panin, N., Gorday, W. J., and Paul, B. J. (1971). Osteoporosis in hemiplegia. *Stroke* **2,** 41–47.

Paul-Murphy, J. (1993). Bacterial enterocolitis in non-human primates. *In* "Zoo and Wild Animal Medicine" (M. E. Fowler, ed.), p. 344. Curr. Ther., Vol. 3, Saunders, Philadelphia.

Payne, S. L., Fang, F. D., Liu, C. P., Dhruva, B. R., Rwanbo, P., Issel, C. J., and Montelaro, R. C. (1987). Antigenic variation and lentivirus persistence. Variations in envelope gene sequences during EIAV infection resemble changes reported for sequential isolates of HIV. *Virology* **61,** 321.

Pereira, R. S., Black, C. M., Duance, V. C., Jones, V. E., Jacoby, R. K., and Welsh, K. I. (1985). Disappearing collagen antibodies in rheumatoid arthritis. *Lancet* **2,** 501–502.

Pettifor, J. M., Marie, P. J., Sly, M. R., du Bruyn, D. B., Ross, F., Isdale, J. M., de Klerk, W. A., and van der Walt, W. H. (1984). The effect of differing dietary calcium and phosphorus contents on mineral metabolism and bone histomorphometry in young vitamin D-replete baboons. *Calcif. Tissue Int.* **36,** 668–676.

Philip, M. T., and Johnson, B. J. (1994). Animal models of Lyme disease: Pathogenesis and immunoprophylaxis. *Trends Microbiol.* **2,** 431–437.

Philipp, M. T., Aydintug, M. K., Bohm, R. P., Jr., Cogswell, F. B., Dennis, V. A., Lanners, H. N., Lowerie, R. C., Jr., Roberts, E. D., Conway, M. D., and Karacorlu, M. (1993). Early and early disseminated phases of Lyme disease in the rhesus monkey: A model for infection in humans. *Infect. Immun.* **61,** 3047–3059.

Pidd, J. G., and Gardner, D. L. (1987). Surface structure of baboon (*Papio anubis*) hydrated articular cartilage: Study of low temperature replicas by transmission electron microscopy. *J. Med. Primatol.* **16,** 301–309.

Pocock, N. A., Eisman, J. A., Hooper, J. L., Yeates, M. G., Sambrook, P. N., and Eberl, S. (1987). Genetic determinants of bone mass in adults. *J. Clin. Invest.* **80,** 706–710.

Pope, N. S., Gould, K. G., Anderson, D. C., and Mann, D. R. (1989). Effects of age and sex on bone density in the rhesus macaque. *Bone* **10,** 109–112.

Potkay, S. (1992). Diseases of the Callitrichidae: A review. *J. Med. Primatol.* **21,** 189–236.

Preuschoft, H. (1989). Quantitative approaches to primate morphology. *Folia Primatol.* **53**, 82–100.

Pritzker, K. P. H. (1992). Cartilage histopathology in human and rhesus macaque osteoarthritis. *In* "Articular Cartilage and Osteoarthritis" (K. E. Kuettner, R. Schleyerbach, V. C. Hascall, J. G. Reyron, eds.) p. 473. Raven Press, New York.

Pritzker, K. P. H. (1994a). Calcium pyrophosphate dihydrate crystal deposition and other crystal deposition diseases. *Curr. Opin. Rheumatol.* **6**, 442–447.

Pritzker, K. P. H. (1994b). Animal models for osteoarthritis: Processes, problems and prospects. *Ann. Rheum. Dis.* **53**, 406–420.

Pritzker, K. P. H. (1997). Pathology of osteoarthritis. *In* "Osteoarthritis" (K. D. Brandt, S. Lohmander, and M. Doherty, eds.) Oxford University Press, pp. 106–130. Oxford.

Pritzker, K. P. H., and Luk, S. C. (1976). Apatite associated arthropathies: Preliminary ultrastructural studies. *Scanning Electron Microsc.,* pp. 493–499.

Pritzker, K. P. H., Phillips, H., Luk, S. C., Koven, I. H., Kiss, A., and Houpt, J. B. (1976). Pseudotumor of temporomandibular joint: Destructive calcium pyrophosphate dihydrate arthropathy. *J. Rheumatol.* **3**, 70–81.

Pritzker, K. P. H., Cheng, P.-T., Adams, M. E., and Nyburg, S. C. (1978). Calcium pyrophosphate dihydrate crystal formation in model hydrogels. *J. Rheumatol.* **5**, 469–473.

Pritzker, K. P. H., Cheng, P.-T., Hunter, G. K., Grynpas, M. D., Kessler, M. J., and Renlund, R. C. (1985). In vitro and in vivo models of calcium pyrophosphate crystal formation. *In* "The Chemistry and Biology of Mineralized Tissues" (W. T. Butler, ed.), p. 381. Ebsco Media, Birmingham.

Pritzker, K. P. H., Chateauvert, J. M. D., and Grynpas, M. D. (1987). Osteoarthritic cartilage contains increased calcium, magnesium and phosphorus. *J. Rheumatol.* **14**, 806–810.

Pritzker, K. P. H., Cheng, P.-T., and Renlund, R. C. (1988). Calcium pyrophosphate crystal deposition in hyaline cartilage: Ultrastructural analysis and implications for pathogenesis. *J. Rheumatol.* **15**, 828–835.

Pritzker, K. P. H., Chateauvert, J., Grynpas, M. D., Renlund, R. C., Turnquist, J., and Kessler, M. J. (1989). Rhesus macaques as an experimental model for degenerative arthritis. *P. R. Health Sci. J.* **8**, 99–102.

Pritzker, K. P. H., Chateauvert, J. M. D., Grynpas, M. D., and Kessler, M. J. (1990). Studies of naturally degenerative arthritis in rhesus macaques as a model for degenerative arthritis in man. *In* "Methods in Cartilage Research" (A. Maroudas and K. E. Kuettner, eds.), p. 341. Academic Press, London.

Pritzker, K. P. H., Gahunia, H., and Kessler, M. J. (1997). *Spontaneous osteonecrosis of the knee in human primates.* (In preparation).

Przybeck, T. R. (1985). Histomorphology of the rib: Bone mass and cortical remodeling. *In* "Behavior and Pathology of Aging in Rhesus Monkeys" (R. T. Davis and C. W. Leathers, eds.), p. 303. Liss, New York.

Rahman, M. U., Cheema, M. A., Schumacher, H. R., and Hudson, A. P. (1992). Molecular evidence for the presence of chlamydia in the synovium of patients with Reiter's syndrome. *Arthritis Rheum.* **35**, 521–529.

Ramalingaswami, V., Deo, M. G., and Sood, S. K. (1961). Protein deficiency in rhesus monkeys. *Publi.* **843.,** National Academy of Sciences, National Research Council, Washington, D.C., pp. 365–375.

Randall, F. E. (1942). Osteological growth and variation in *Gorilla gorilla.* Ph.D. Thesis, Harvard University, Cambridge, MA.

Raphael, B. L., Calle, P. P., Haramati, N., Watkins, D. J., Stetter, M. D., and Cook, R. A. (1995). Reactive arthritis subsequent to Shigella Flexneri Enteritis in two juvenile lowland gorillas (*Gorilla gorilla gorilla*). *J. Zoo Wildl. Med.* **26**, 132–138.

Ratterree, M. S., Didier, P. J., Blanchard, J. L., Clarke, M. R., and Schaeffer, D. (1990). Vitamin C deficiency in captive nonhuman primates fed commercial primate diet. *Lab. Anim. Sci.* **40**, 165–168.

Rawlins, R. G. (1976). Locomotor ontogeny in Macaca mulatta I: Behavioral strategies and tactics. *Am. J. Phys. Anthropol.* **44**, 201.

Rawlins, R. G., and Kessler, M. J., eds. (1986). "The Cayo Santiago Macaques: History Behavior and Biology." State University of New York Press, Albany.

Reddi, A. H. (1981). Cell biology and biochemistry of endochondral bone development. *Collagen Relat. Res.: Clin. Exp.* **1**, 209.

Reddy, G. S., and Rao, B. S. N. (1971). Effect of dietary calcium, vitamin C and protein in development of experimental skeletal fluorosis. II. Calcium turnover with 45Ca; calcium and phosphorus balances. *Metab., Clin. Exp.* **20**, 650–656.

Reddy, G. S., and Srikantia, S. G. (1971). Effect of dietary calcium, vitamin C and protein in development of experimental skeletal fluorosis. I. Growth, serum chemistry, and changes in composition, and radiological appearance of bones. *Metab., Clin. Exp.* **20**, 642–649.

Renlund, R. C., Pritzker, K. P. H., and Kessler, M. J. (1985). Rhesus primates (*Macaca mulatta*) as a model for calcium pyrophosphate dihydrate crystal deposition disease. *Lab. Invest.* **52**, 55A (abstr.).

Renlund, R. C., Pritzker, K. P. H., and Kessler, M. J. (1986). Rhesus monkey (*Macaca mulatta*) as a model for calcium pyrophosphate dihydrate crystal deposition disease. *J. Med. Primatol.* **15**, 11–16.

Renlund, R. C., Pritzker, K. P. H., and Kessler, M. J. (1989). Calcium pyrophosphate dihydrate crystal deposition disease: A common disease of aging human and non-human primates. *Lab. Invest.* **60**, 78A (abstr.).

Renxian, Z., Zuyun, L., Wenji, Q., Hongzi, Z., and Ming, L. (1987). Comparative study of the femoral articular facies of knees of the primates. *Sci. Sinica, Ser. B (Engl. Ed.)* **30**, 960–966.

Repo, H., Ristola, M., and Leirisalo-Repo, M. (1990). Enhanced inflammatory reactivity in the pathogenesis of spondyloarthropathites. *Autoimmunity* **7**, 245–254.

Resnick, D., and Niwayama, G. (1976). Radiographic and pathologic features of spinal involvement in diffuse idiopathic skeletal hyperostosis. *Diagn. Radiol.* **119**, 559–568.

Resnick, D., Shapiro, R. F., Wiesner, K. B., Niwayama, G., Utsinger, P. D., and Shaul, S. R. (1978). Diffuse idiopathic skeletal hyperostosis (DISH). [Ankylosing hyperostosis of Forestier and Rotes-Querol.] *Semin. Arthritis Rheum.* **7**, 153–187.

Revell, P. A., and Pirie, O. J. (1981). The histopathology of ankylosing hyperostosis of the spine. *Rhumatologie (Paris)* **33**, 99–104.

Riopelle, A. J., and Favret, R. (1977). Protein deprivation in primates: XIII. Growth of infants born of deprived mothers. *Hum. Biol.* **49**, 321–333.

Riopelle, A. J., Hale, D. A., and Watts, E. S. (1976). Protein deprivation in primates: VII. Determinants of size and skeletal maturity at birth in rhesus monkeys. *Hum. Biol.* **48**, 203–222.

Ripamonti, U. (1991). Bone induction in nonhuman primates. An experimental study on the baboon. *Clin. Orthop. Relat. Res.* **269**, 284–294.

Ripamonti, U. (1992). Calvarial regeneration in primates with autolysed antigen-extracted allogeneic bone. *Clin. Orthop. Relat. Res.* **282**, 293–303.

Ripamonti, U. (1995). Osteoinduction in porous hydroxyapatite implanted in heterotopic sites of different animal models. *Biomaterials (Guildford, Engl.)* **17**, 31–35.

Ripamonti, U., Magan, A., Ma, S., van den Heever, B., Moehl, T., and Reddi, A. H. (1991). Xenogenic osteogenin, a bone morphogenetic protein, and demineralized bone matrices, including human, induce bone differentiation in athymic rats and baboons. *Matrix* **11**, 404–411.

Ripamonti, U., Ma, S., and Reddi, A. H. (1992a). The critical role of geometry of porous hydroxyapatite delivery system in induction of bone by osteogenin, a bone morphogenic protein. *Matrix* **12**, 202–212.

Ripamonti, U., Ma, S., Cunningham, N. S., Yeates, L., and Reddi, A. H. (1992b). Initiation of bone regeneration in adult baboons by osteogenin, a bone morphogenetic protein. *Matrix* **12**, 369–380.

Ripamonti, U., Ma, S. S., and Reddi, A. H. (1992c). Induction of bone in composites of osteogenin and porous hydroxyapatite in baboons. *Plast. Reconstr. Surg.* **89**, 731–739.

Ripamonti, U., Ma, S., van den Heever, B., and Reddi, A. H. (1992d). Osteogenin, a bone morphogenic protein, adsorbed on porous hydroxyapatite substrata induces rapid bone differentiation in calvarial defects of adult primates. *Plas. Reconstr. Surg.* **90**, 382–393.

Ripamonti, U., van den Heever, B., and van Wyk, J. (1993a). Expression of the osteogenic phenotype in porous hydroxyapatite implanted extraskeletally in baboons. *Matrix* **13**, 491–502.

Ripamonti, U., Yeates, L., and van den Heever, B. (1993b). Initiation of chromatographic adsorption of osteogenin, a bone morphogenetic protein, onto porous hydroxyapatite. *Biochem. Biophys. Res. Commun.* **193**, 509–517.

Roberts, E. D. (1993a). Type II collagen arthropathy. *In* "Nonhuman Primates. 2. Monographs on the Pathology of Laboratory Animals" (T. C. Jones, U. Mohr, and R. D. Hunt, eds.), p. 133. Springer-Verlag, Berlin.

Roberts, E. D. (1993b). Pyrophosphate arthropathy, *Macaca mulatta*. *In* "Nonhuman Primates. 2. Monographs on the Pathology of Laboratory Animals" (T. C. Jones, U. Mohr, and R. D. Hunt, eds.), p. 138. Springer-Verlag, Berlin.

Roberts, E. D., and Martin, L. N. (1991). Arthritis in rhesus monkeys experimentally infected with Simian immunodeficiency virus (SIV/DELTA). *Lab. Invest.* **65**, 637–643.

Roberts, E. D., Baskin, G. B., Watson, E., Henk, W. G., and Shelton, T. C. (1984a). Calcium pyrophosphate deposition disease (CPPD) in nonhuman primates. *Am. J. Pathol.* **116**, 359–361.

Roberts, E. D., Baskin, G. B., Watson, E., Henk, W. G., Shelton, T. C., and Bowen, M. S. (1984b). Calcium pyrophosphate deposition in non-human primates. *Vet. Pathol.* **21**, 592–596.

Roberts, E. D., Bohm, R. P. J., Cogswell, F. B., Lanners, H. N., Lowrie, R. C. J., Povinelli, L., Piesman, J., and Philipp, M. T. (1995). Chronic Lyme disease in the rhesus monkey. *Lab. Invest.* **72**, 146–160.

Rodahl, E. (1989). Retroviruses and chronic arthritis. Possible significance of some recent observations. *Scand. J. Rheumatol.* **18**, 335–339.

Rodgers, J. B., Monier-Faugere, M.-C., and Malluche, H. (1993). Animal models for the study of bone loss after cessation of ovarian function. *Boned* **14**, 369–377.

Rollet, E. (1891). Les maladies osseuses des grands singes. *Bull. Soc. Anthropol. Lyon* **10**, 84–103.

Roques, L., and Bouffard, G. (1908). Un cas de groundou chez le cynocéphale. *Bull. Soc. Pathol. Exot. Ses Fil.* **1**, 295–296.

Rose, R. C., and Bode, A. M. (1993). Biology of free radical scavengers: An evaluation of ascorbate. *FASEB J.* **7**, 1135–1142.

Rosenberg, D. P., Gleiser, C. A., and Carey, K. D. (1984). Spinal coccidioidomycosis in a baboon. *J. Am. Vet. Med. Asso.* **185**, 1379–1381.

Rothschild, B. M. (1993a). Arthritis of the spondyloarthropathy variety in *Callithrix jacchus*. *J. Med. Primatol.* **22**, 313–316.

Rothschild, B. M. (1993b). Skeletal paleopathology of rheumatic diseases: The sub-homo connection. *In* "Arthritis and Allied Conditions" (D. J. McCarty and W. J. Koopman, eds.), p. 3. Lea & Febiger, Philadelphia.

Rothschild, B. M. (1996). Paleopathology as a clinical science with implications for patient care, education, and research. *J. Rheumatol.* **23**, 1469–1475.

Rothschild, B. M., and Martin, L. D. (1993). "Paleopathology: Disease in the Fossil Record." CRC Press, Boca Raton, FL.

Rothschild, B. M., and Rothschild, C. (1994). No laughing matter: Spondyloarthropathy and osteoarthritis in hyaenidae. *J. Zoo Wildl. Med.* **25**, 259–263.

Rothschild, B. M., and Rothschild, C. (1996). Is there an epidemic/epizootic of spondyloarthropathy in baboons? *J. Med. Primatol.* **25**, 69–70.

Rothschild, B. M., and Woods, R. J. (1989). Spondyloarthropathy in gorillas. *Semin. Arthritis Rheum.* **18**, 267–276.

Rothschild, B. M., and Woods, R. J. (1991). Reactive erosive arthritis in chimpanzees. *Am. J. Primatol.* **25**, 49–56.

Rothschild, B. M., and Woods, R. J. (1992a). Osteoarthritis, calcium pyrophosphate deposition disease, and osseous infection in Old World primates. *Am. J. Phy. Anthropol.* **87**, 341–347.

Rothschild, B. M., and Woods, R. J. (1992b). Spondyloarthritis as an Old World phenomenon. *Semin. Arthritis Rheum.* **21**, 306–316.

Rothschild, B. M., and Woods, R. J. (1992c). Erosive arthritis and spondyloarthropathy in Old World primates. *Am. J. Phys. Anthropol.* **88**, 389–400.

Rothschild, B. M., and Woods, R. J. (1993). Arthritis in New World monkeys: Osteoarthritis, calcium pyrophosphate deposition disease, and spondyloarthropathy. *Int. J. Primatol.* **14**, 61–78.

Rothschild, B. M., Woods, R. J., and Rothschild, C. (1992). Calcium pyrophosphate deposition disease: Description in defleshed skeletons. *Clin. Exp. Rheumatol.* **10**, 557–564.

Rothschild, B. M., Wang, X., and Cifelli, R. (1993). Spondyloarthropathy in Ursidae: A sexually transmitted disease? *Na. Geogr. Res. Explor.* **9**, 381–383.

Rothschild, B. M., Wang, X., and Shoshani, J. (1994). Spondyloarthropathy in proboscideans. *J. Zoo Wildl. Med.* **25**, 360–366.

Rothschild, B. M., Hong, N., and Turnquist, J. E. (1997). Naturally occurring inflammatory arthritis of the spondyloarthropathy variety in Cayo Santiago rhesus macaques (*Macaca mulatta*). *Clin. Exp. Rheumatol.* **15**, 45–52.

Rubenstein, J., and Pritzker, K. P. H. (1989). Crystal-associated arthropathies. *Am. J. Radiol.* **152**, 685–695.

Rubin, A. S., Healy, C. T., Martin, L. N., Baskin, G. B., and Roberts, E. D. (1987). Experimental arthropathy induced in rhesus monkeys (*Macaca mulatta*) by intradermal immunization with native bovine Type II collagen. *Lab. Invest.* **57**, 524–534.

Rubin, L. A., Fam, A. G., Rubenstein, J., Campbell, J., and Saiphoo, C. (1984). Erosive azotemic osteoarthropathy. *Arthritis Rheum.* **27**, 1086–1094.

Ruch, T. C. (1959a). Diet and disease, including nutritional diseases. *In* "Diseases of Laboratory Primates" (T. C. Ruch, ed.), p. 4. Saunders, Philadelphia.

Ruch, T. C. (1959b). Diseases of the central nervous system and sense organisms. *In* "Diseases of Laboratory Primates" (T. C. Ruch, ed.), p. 380. Saunders, Philadelphia.

Ruch, T. C. (1959c). Bone diseases. *In* "Diseases of Laboratory Primates" (T. C. Ruch, ed.), p. 472. Saunders, Philadelphia.

Ruff, C. B. (1989). New approaches to structural evolution on limb bones in primates. *Folia Primatol.* **53**, 142–159.

Ryan, L. M., and McCarty, D. J. (1993). Calcium pyrophosphate crystal deposition disease; pseudogout; articular chondrocalcinosis. *In* "Arthritis and Allied Conditions" (D. J. McCarty and W. J. Koopman, eds.), p. 1835. Lea & Febiger, Philadelphia.

Ryan, L. M., and McCarty, D. J. (1995). Understanding inorganic pyrophosphate metabolism: Toward prevention of calcium pyrophosphate dihydrate crystal deposition. *Ann. Rheum. Dis.* **54**, 939–941.

Ryder-Davies, P., and Hime, J. M. (1972). Hypertrophic osteoarthropathy in a gibbon (*Hylobates lar*). *J. Small Anim. Pract.* **13**, 655–658.

Sabin, A. B. (1939). Vitamin C in relation to experimental poliomyelitis. With incidental observations on certain manifestations in *Macacus rhesus* monkeys on a scorbutic diet. *J. Exp. Med.* **69**, 507–516.

Sampath, T. K., and Reddi, A. H. (1983). Homology of bone-inductive proteins from human, monkey, bovine and rat extracellular matrix. *Proc. Natl. Acad. Sci. U.S.A.* **80**, 6591–6595.

Schaffler, M. B., and Burr, D. B. (1984). Primate cortical bone microstructure: Relationship to locomotion. *Am. J. Phys. Anthropol.* **65**, 191–197.

Schmidt, R. E., Hubbard, G. B., and Fletcher, K. C. (1986). Systemic survey of lesions from animals in a zoologic collection: VII. Musculo-skeletal system. *J. Zoo Anim. Med.* **17**, 37–42.

Schock, C. C., Noyes, F. R., and Villaneuva, A. R. (1972). Measurement of Haversian bone remodelling by means of tetracycline labelling in the rib of rhesus monkeys. *Henry Ford Hosp. Med. Bull.* **20**, 131–144.

Schock, C. C., Noyes, F. R., Crouch, M. M., and Mathews, C. H. E. (1975). The effects of immobility on long bone remodeling in the rhesus monkey. *Henry Ford Hosp. Med. Bull.* **23**, 107–116.

Schou, S., Holmstrup, P., and Kornman, K. S. (1993). Non-human primates used in studies of periodontal disease pathogenesis: A review. *J. Periodontol.* **64**, 497–508.

Schultz, A. H. (1939). Notes on diseases and healed fractures of wild apes, and their bearing on the antiquity of pathological conditions in man. *Bull. Hist. Med.* **7**, 571–582.

Schumacher, H. R., Somlyo, A. P., Tse, R. L., and Maurer, K. (1977). Arthritis associated with apatite crystals. *Ann. Intern. Med.* **87**, 411–416.

Schumacher, H. R., Miller, J. L., Ludivico, C., and Jessar, R. A. (1981). Erosive arthritis associated with apatite crystal deposition. *Arthritis Rheum.* **24**, 31–37.

Schumacher, H. R., Jr. (1992). Secondary osteoarthritis. *In* "Osteoarthritis. Diagnosis and Medical/Surgical Management" (R. W. Moskowitz, D. S. Howell, V. M. Goldberg, and H. J. Mankin, eds.), p. 367. Saunders, Philadelphia.

Schwartz, S. M. (1989). Characteristics of spontaneous obesity in the Cayo Santiago rhesus macaque: Preliminary report. *P. R. Health Sci. J.* **8,** 103–106.

Schwartz, S. M., Kemmitz, J. W., and Howard, C. F., Jr. (1993). Obesity in free-ranging rhesus macaques. *In. J. Obes.* **17,** 1–9.

Seawright, A. A., and English, P. B. (1964). Deforming cervical spondylosis in the cat. *J. Pathol. Bacteriol.* **88,** 503–509.

Seawright, A. A., and English, P. B. (1967). Hypervitaminosis A and deforming cervical spondylosis of the cat. *J. Comp. Pathol. Ther.* **77,** 29–39.

Seibold, H. R., and Wolf, R. H. (1973). Neoplasms and proliferative lesions in 1065 nonhuman primate necropsies. *Lab. Anim. Sci.* **23,** 533–539.

Sembrat, R. F., and Fritz, G. R. (1979). Long bone osteosarcoma in a rhesus monkey. *J. Am. Vet. Med. Assoc.* **175,** 971–974.

Serratrice, G., Pellissier, J. F., Roux, H., and Quilichini, P. (1990). Fasciitis, perimyositis, myositis, polymyositis, and eosinophilia. *Muscle & Nerve* **13,** 385–395.

Sharawy, M. M., Helmy, E. S., Bays, R. A., and Larke, V. B. (1994). Repair of temporomandibular joint disc perforation using a synovial membrane flap in *Macaca fascicularis* monkeys: Light and electron microscopy studies. *J. Oral Maxillofacial Surg.* **52,** 259–270.

Shaw, J. H., and Auskaps, A. M. (1954). Studies on the dentition of the marmoset. *Oral Surg. Oral Med. Oral Pathol.* **7,** 671–677.

Shaw, J. H., Phillips, P. H., and Elvehjem, C. A. (1945). Acute and chronic ascorbic acid deficiencies in the rhesus monkey. *J. Nutr.* **29,** 365–372.

Sheridan, P. J., Aufdemorte, T. B., Holt, G. R., and Gates, G. A. (1985). Cartilage of the baboon contains estrogen receptors. *Rheumatol. Int.* **5,** 279–281.

Shimwell, M., Warrington, B. F., and Fowler, J. S. L. (1979). Dietary habits relating to "wasting marmoset syndrome" (WMS). *Lab. Anim.* **13,** 139.

Shinki, T., Shiina, Y., Takahashi, N., Tanioka, Y., Koizumi, H., and Suda, T. (1983). Extremely high circulating levels of 1,25-dihydroxyvitamin D_3 in the marmoset, a New World monkey. *Biochem. Biophy. Res. Commun.* **114,** 452–457.

Shinozaki, T., and Pritzker, K. P. H. (1995). Polyamines enhance calcium pyrophoshate dihydrate crystal dissolution. *J. Rheumatol.* **22,** 1907–1912.

Shinozaki, T., and Pritzker, K. P. H. (1996). Regulation of alkaline phosphatase: Implications for calcium pyrophosphate dihydrate crystal dissolution and other alkaline phosphatase functions. *J. Rheumatol.* **23,** 677–683.

Shinozaki, T., Xu, Y., Cruz, T. F., and Pritzker, K. P. H. (1995). Calcium pyrophosphate dihydrate (CPPD) crystal dissolution by alkaline phosphatase: Interaction of alkaline phosphatase on CPPD crystals. *J. Rheumatol.* **22,** 117–123.

Shively, C. A., Jayo, M. J., Weaver, D. S., and Kaplan, J. R. (1991). Reduced vertebral bone mineral density in socially subordinate female cynomolgus macaques. *Am. J. Primatol.* **24,** 135 (abstr.).

Shulman, L. E. (1975). Diffuse fasciitis with eosinophilia: A new syndrome? *Trans. Assoc. Am. Physicians* **88,** 70–86.

Sickles, D. W., and Pinkstaff, C. A. (1981). Comparative histochemical study of prosimian primate hindlimb muscles. I. Muscle fiber types. *Am. J. Anat.* **160,** 175–186.

Silman, A. J. (1994). Epidemiology of rheumatoid arthritis. *APMIS* **102,** 721–728.

Simmons, D. J., Chang, S.-L., Russell, J. E., Grazman, B., Webster, D., and Oloff, C. (1983). The effect of protracted tetracycline treatment on bone growth and maturation. *Clin. Orthop. Relat. Res.* **180,** 253–259.

Simmons, D. J., Russell, J. E., Walker, W. V., Grazman, B., Oloff, C., and Kazarian, L. (1984). Growth and maturation of mandibular bone in otherwise totally immobilized rhesus monkeys. *Clin. Orthop. Relat. Res.* **182,** 220–230.

Simmons, D. J., Parvin, C., Smith, K. C., Frame, P., and Kazarian, L. (1986). Effect of rotopositioning on the growth and maturation of mandibular bone in immobilized rhesus monkeys. *Aviat. Space Environ. Med.* **57,** 157–161.

Simon, W. H., and Garman, R. A. (1970). Simian bone disease: Unrecognized rickets in rhesus monkeys. *Clin. Orthop. Rela. Res.* **73,** 232–240.

Sin, Y. M., Sedgwick, A. D., Moore, A., and Willoughby, D. A. (1984). Studies on the clearance of calcium pyrophosphate crystals from facsimile synovium. *Ann. Rheum. Dis.* **43,** 487–492.

Singh, R., Grewal, D. S., and Chakravarti, R. N. (1969). Experimental production of pigmented villo-nodular synovitis in the knee and ankle joints of rhesus monkeys. *J. Pathol.* **98,** 137–142.

Sissons, H. A., Steiner, G. C., Bonar, F., May, M., Rosenberg, Z. S., Samuels, H., and Present, D. (1989). Tumoral calcium pyrophosphate deposition disease. *Skeletal Radiol.* **18,** 79–87.

Slavin, R. E., Wen, J., Kumar, D., and Evans, E. B. (1993). Familial tumoral calcinosis. A clinical, histopathologic, and ultrastructural study with an analysis of its calcifying process and pathogenesis. *Am. J. Surg. Pathol.* **17,** 788–802.

Sluka, K. A., Dougherty, P. M., Sorkin, L. S., Willis, W. D., and Westlund, K. N. (1992). Neural changes in acute arthritis in monkeys. III. Changes in substance P, calcitonin gene-related peptide and glutamate in the dorsal horn of the spinal cord. *Brain Res. Rev.* **17,** 29–38.

Sly, M. R., van der Walt, W. H., du Bruyn, D. B., Pettifor, J. M., and Marie, P. J. (1984). Exacerbation of rickets and osteomalacia by Maize: A study of bone histomorphometry and composition in young baboons. *Calcif. Tissue Int.* **36,** 370–379.

Smith, D. E., James, P. G., Schachter, J., Engleman, E. P., and Meyer, K. F. (1973). Experimental bedsonial arthritis. *Arthritis Rheum.* **16,** 21–29.

Smith, K., Dillingham, L., and Giddens, W. E. J. (1978). Metabolic bone disease resembling osteosarcoma in a wooly monkey (*Lagothrix lagotricha*). *Lab. Anim. Sci.* **28,** 451–456.

Smith, R. O. A. (1933). Cancrum oris in a monkey infected with *Leishmania donovani*. *Indian Med. Gaz.* **68,** 455.

Snook, S. S. (1993). Infantile cortical hyperostosis, rhesus monkey. *In* "Nonhuman Primates. 2. Monographs on the Pathology of Laboratory Animals" (T. C. Jones, U. Mohr, and R. D. Hunt, eds.), p. 123. Springer-Verlag, Berlin.

Snook, S. S., and King, N. W. J. (1989). Familial infantile cortical hyperostosis (Caffey's Disease) in rhesus monkeys (*Macaca mulatta*). *Vet. Pathol.* **26,** 274–277.

Snyder, S. B., Omdahl, J. L., Law, D. H., and Froelich, J. W. (1980). Osteomalacia and nutritional secondary hyperparathyroidism in a semi-ranging troop of Japanese monkeys. *In* "The Comparative Pathology of Zoo Animals" (R. J. Montali and G. Migaki, eds.), p. 51. Smithsonian Institution Press, Washington, DC.

Sokoloff, L. (1956). Natural history of degenerative joint disease in small laboratory animals. 1. Pathologic anatomy of degenerative joint disease in mice. *Arch. Pathol.* **62,** 118–128.

Sokoloff, L. (1960). Comparative pathology of arthritis. *Adv. Vet. Sci. Comp. Med.* **6,** 193–250.

Sokoloff, L. (1973). Rheumatoid arthritis, animal model: Arthritis due to mycoplasma in rats and swine. *Am. J. Pathol.* **73,** 261–264.

Sokoloff, L. (1990). Animal models of osteoarthritis. *J. Rheumatol.* **17,** 5–6.

Sokoloff, L., Snell, K. C., and Stewart, H. L. (1968). Spinal ankylosis in old rhesus monkeys. *Clin. Orthop. Relat. Res.* **61,** 285–293.

Sood, S. K., Deo, M. G., and Ramalingaswami, V. (1965). Anemia in experimental protein deficiency in the rhesus monkey with special reference to iron metabolism. *Blood* **29,** 421.

Sorkin, L. S., Westlund, K. N., Sluka, K. A., Dougherty, P. M., and Willis, W. D. (1992). Neural changes in acute arthritis in monkeys. IV. Time-course of amino acid release into the lumbar dorsal horn. *Brain Res. Rev.* **17,** 39–50.

Southard, E. E. (1906). A case of Pott's Disease in the monkey. *J. Med. Res.* **14,** 393–398.

Srikanth, S., Devenny, M., and Coan, P. N. (1995). P65 idiopathic scoliosis and kyphosis in *Macaca nemestrina. Lab. Anim. Sci.* **45,** 470.

Staheli, L. T., Church, C. C., and Ward, B. H. (1968). Infantile cortical hyperostosis (Caffey's disease). Sixteen cases with a late follow-up of eight. *JAMA, J. Am. Med. Assoc.* **203,** 384–388.

Stanescu, V., and Pham, T. D. (1986). Gel electrophoresis of proteoglycan monomers of baboon articular cartilage separated by zonal rate centrifugation in sucrose gradients. *Connec. Tissue Res.* **14**, 169–177.

Stanescu, V., Maroteaux, P., and Sobczak, E. (1980). Proteoglycan populations of baboon (*Papio papio*) cartilages from different anatomical sites. Gel electrophoretic analysis of dissociated proteoglycans and of fractions obtained by density gradient centrifugation. *Biochim. Biophys. Acta* **629**, 371–381.

Stecher, R. M. (1958a). Osteoarthritis in the gorilla: Description of a skeleton with involvement of the knee and the spine. *Lab. Invest.* **7**, 445–457.

Stecher, R. M. (1958b). Osteoarthritis of the hip in a gorilla: Report of a third case. *Clin. Orthop.* **12**, 307–314.

Steere, A. C. (1989). Lyme disease. *N. Engl. J. Med.* **321**, 586–596.

Steere, A. C., Malawista, S. E., and Snydman, D. R. (1977). Lyme arthritis: An epidemic of oligo-articular arthritis in children and adults in three Connecticut communities. *Arthritis Rheum.* **20**, 7–17.

Steffen, C., and Timpl, R. (1963). Antigenicity of collagen and its application in the serologic investigation of rheumatoid arthritis sera. *Int. Arch. Allergy Appl. Immunol.* **22**, 333–349.

Stern, W. E., and Coulson, W. F. (1976). Effects of collagenase upon the intervertebral disc in monkeys. *J. Neurosurg.* **44**, 32–44.

Stumpf, W. E. (1988). Vitamin D-Soltriol. The heliogenic steroid hormone: Somatotrophic activator and modulator. *Histochemistry* **89**, 209–219.

Stumpf, W. E., and Privette, T. H. (1991). The steroid hormone of sunlight soltriol (vitamin D) as a seasonal regulator of biological activities and photoperiodic rhythms. *J. Steroid Biochem. Mol. Biol.* **39**, 283–289.

Styne, D. M. (1991). Serum insulin-like growth factor 1 concentrations in the developing rhesus monkey. *J. Med. Primatol.* **20**, 334–337.

Sumner, D. R., Morbeck, M. E., and Lobick, J. J. (1989). Apparent age-related bone loss among adult female gombe chimpanzees. *Am. J. Phys. Anthropol.* **79**, 225–234.

Suzuki, A., and Hayama, S. (1991). Histochemical classification of myofiber types in the triceps surae and flexor digitorum superficialis muscle of Japanese macaques. *Acta Histochem. Cytochem.* **24**, 323–328.

Swezey, R. L., Cox, C., and Gonzales, B. (1991). Ankylosing spondylitis in nonhuman primates: The drill and the siamang. *Semin. Arthritis Rheum.* **21**, 170–174.

Takagi, T., and Jasin, H. E. (1992). Interactions between anticollagen antibodies and chondrocytes. *Arthritis Rheum.* **35**, 224–230.

Takahashi, N., Suda, S., Shinki, T., Horiuchi, N., Shiina, Y., Tanoika, Y., Koizumi, H., and Suda, T. (1985). The mechanism of end-organ resistance to 1,25-hydroxycholecalciferol in the common marmoset. *Biochem. J.* **227**, 555–563.

Tan, S. Y., and Pepys, M. B. (1994). Amyloidosis. *Histopathology* **25**, 403–414.

Tarkowski, A., Klareskog, L., Carlsten, H., Herberts, P., and Koopman, W. J. (1989). Secretion of antibodies to types I and II collagen by synovial tissue cells in patients with rheumatoid arthritis. *Arthritis Rheum.* **32**, 1087–1092.

Tasumi, M. (1969). Senile features in the skeleton of an aged Japanese monkey. *Primates* **10**, 263–272.

Taylor, H. W. Y., King, J. B., and Stecher, R. M. (1955). Osteoarthritis of the hip on gorillas: Report of two cases. *Clin. Orthop.* **6**, 149–157.

Tenenbaum, J., Muniz, O., Schumacher, R., Good, A. E., and Howell, D. S. (1981a). Comparison of phosphohydrolase activities from articular cartilage in calcium pyrophosphate deposition disease and primary osteoarthritis. *Arthritis Rheum.* **24**, 492–500.

Tenenbaum, J., Pritzker, K. P. H., Gross, A. E., Cheng, P.-T., Renlund, R. C., and Tenenbaum, H. (1981b). The effects of intraarticular corticosteroids on articular cartilage. *Semin. Arthritis Rheum.* **11**, Suppl. 1, 140–141.

Terato, K., Arai, H., Shimozuru, Y., Fukuda, T., Tanaka, H., Watanabe, H., Nagai, Y., Fujimoto, K., Okubo, F., Cho, F., Honjo, S., and Cremer, M. A. (1989). Sex-linked differences in susceptibility of cynomolgus monkeys to Type II collagen-induced arthritis. Evidence that epitope-specific immune suppression is involved in the regulation of Type II collagen autoantibody formation. *Arthritis Rheum.* **32**, 748–758.

Terrell, T. G., and Stookey, J. L. (1972). Chronic eosinophilic myositis in a rhesus monkey infected with sarcosporidiosis. *Vet. Pathol.* **9**, 266–271.

't Hart, B. A., Botman, C. A. D., and Bakker, N. P. M. (1991). Induction of type II collagen-specific antibody production in blood lymphocyte cultures of rhesus monkeys (*Macaca mulatta*) with collagen-induced arthritis using the immobilized native antigen. *Clin. Exp. Immunol.* **83**, 375–378.

't Hart, B. A., Baaker, N. P. M., Jonker, M., and Bontrop, R. E. (1993). Resistance to collagen-induced arthritis in rats and rhesus monkeys after immunization with attenuated type II collagen. *Eur. J. Immunol.* **23**, 1588–1594.

Thompson, D. D., Seedor, J. G., Quartuccio, H., Solomon, H., Fioravanti, C., Davidson, J., Klein, H., Jackson, R., Clair, J., Frankenfield, D., Brown, E., Simmons, H. A., and Rodan, G. A. (1992). The bisphosphonate, aledronate, prevents bone loss in ovariectomized baboons. *J. Bone Miner. Res.* **7**, 951–960.

Thompson, S. W., II, Sullivan, D. J., and Pedersen, R. A. (1959). Calcinosis circumscripta. A histochemical study of the lesions in man, dogs, and a monkey. *Cornell Vet.* **49**, 265–285.

Thomson, G. T. D., and Inman, R. D. (1990). Diagnostic conundra in the spondyloarthropathies: Towards a base for revised nosology. *J. Rheumatol.* **17**, 426–429.

Tominaga, T., Dickman, C. A., Sonntag, V. K. H., and Coons, S. (1995). Comparative anatomy of the baboon and the human cervical spine. *Spine* **20**, 131–137.

Tomson, F. N., Keller, G. L., and Knapke, F. B. (1980). Nutritional secondary hyperparathyroidism in a group of lemurs. *In* "The Comparative Pathology of Zoo Animals" (R. J. Montali and G. Migaki, eds.), p. 59. Smithsonian Institution Press, Washington, DC.

Toussirot, E., Lafforgue, P., Boucraut, J., Despieds, P., Schiano, A., Bernard, D., and Acquaviva, P. C. (1994). Serum levels of interleukin 1-B, tumor necrosis factor-x, soluble interleukin 2 receptor and soluble DC8 in seronegative spondyloarthropathies. *Rheumatol. Int.* **13**, 175–180.

Trentham, D. E. (1982). Collagen arthritis as a relevant model for rheumatoid arthritis. *Arthritis Rheum.* **25**, 911–916.

Trentham, D. E., Townes, A. S., Kang, A. H., and David, J. R. (1978). Humoral and cellular sensitivity to collagen in type II collagen-induced arthritis in rats. *J. Clin. Invest.* **61**, 89–96.

Tsai, C. C., Giddens, W. E., Jr., Morton, W. R., Rosenkranz, S. L., Ochs, H. D., and Benveniste, R. E. (1985a). Retroperitoneal fibromatosis and acquired immunodeficiency in macaques: Epidemiologic studies. *Lab. Anim. Sci.* **35**, 460–464.

Tsai, C. C., Warner, T. F., Uno, H., Giddens, W. E., Jr., and Ochs, H. D. (1985b). Subcutaneous fibromatosis associated with an acquired immune deficiency syndrome in pig-tailed macaques. *Am. J. Pathol.* **120**, 30–37.

Tsuyama, N. (1984). Ossification of the posterior longitudinal ligament of the spine. *Clin. Orthop. Relat. Res.* **184**, 71–84.

Turnquist, J. E., and Kessler, M. J. (1989). Free-ranging Cayo Santiago rhesus monkeys (*Macaca mulatta*): II. Passive joint mobility. *Am. J. Primatol.* **19**, 15–23.

Urist, M. R., Hay, P. H., Dubuc, F., and Buring, K. (1969). Osteogenic competence. *Clin. Orthop. Relat. Res.* **64**, 194.

Utsinger, P. D. (1985). Diffuse idiopathic skeletal hyperostosis. *Clin. Rheum. Dis.* **11**, 325–351.

Valerio, D. A., Valerio, M. G., Ulland, B. M., and Innes, J. R. M. (1971). Clinical conditions and diseases encountered in a large simian colony. *Proc. Int. Cong. Primatol. 3rd*, Zurich, 1970, Vol. 2, 205–212.

van Bogaert, L., and Scherer, H. J. (1938). Acute amaurotic epilepsy in *Macacus rhesus*. *Arch. Neurol. Psychiatry* **40**, 521.

van Gils, F. C. J. M., Mulder, A. H., van den Bos, C., Burger, H., van Leen, R. W., and Wagemaker, G. (1993). Acute side effects of homologous interleukin-3 in rhesus monkeys. *Am. J. Pathol.* **143**, 1621–1633.

Van Linthoudt, D., Schumacher, H. R. J., Burus, R. B., Hinshaw, K. C., and Pierce, V. (1992). Apatite crystal deposition disease in a Diana monkey (*Cercopithecus diana diana*). *J. Zoo Wildl. Med.* **23**, 346–352.

Vezyroglou, G., Mitropoulos, A., Kyriazis, N., and Antoniadis, C. (1996). A metabolic syndrome in diffuse idiopathic skeletal hyperostosis. A controlled study. *J. Rheumatol.* **23**, 672–676.

Vieth, R., and Cole, E. C. (1996). The vitamin D endocrine system. *In* "Handbook of Endocrinology" (Anonymous), p. 33. CRC Press, Boca Raton, FL.

Vieth, R., Kessler, M. J., and Pritzker, K. P. H. (1987). Serum concentrations of vitamin D metabolites in Cayo Santiago rhesus macaques. *J. Med. Primatol.* **16**, 349–357.

Vieth, R., Kessler, M. J., and Pritzker, K. P. H. (1990). Species differences in the binding kinetics of 25-hydroxyvitamin D₃ to vitamin D binding protein. *Can. J. Physiol. Pharmacol.* **68**, 1368–1371.

von den Driesch, A., and Boessneck, J. (1985). Pathologically altered skeletal remains of baboons from ancient Egyptian time. *Tieraerztl. Praxis* **13**, 367–372.

von den Driesch, A., and Boessneck, J. (1993). The raising and worship of monkeys in the late period of ancient Egypt. *Tieracrztl. Praxis* **21**, 95–101.

Wadhwani, T. K. (1955). Effect of fluorine on the composition of bones: Changes in the composition of bones of monkeys (*Macaca radiata*). *Indian J. Med. Res.* **43**, 321–330.

Walker, M. D., Krugner-Higby, L., Baker, H. J., and Wood, P. A. (1988). Alkaptonuria in a cynomolgus macaque (*Macaca fascicularis*). *Lab. Anim. Sci.* **38**, 494 (abstr.).

Walker, M. L. (1995). Menopause in female rhesus monkeys. *Am. J. Primatol.* **35**, 59–71.

Walters, M. R. (1992). Newly identified actions of the vitamin D endocrine system. *Endoc. Rev.* **13**, 719–764.

Watt, I., and Dieppe, P. (1990). Osteoarthritis revisited. *Skeletal Radiol.* **19**, 1–3.

Weber, M., Lamberski, N., and Heriot, K. (1995). An idiopathic proliferative disease of bone in two subspecies of ruffed lemur (*Varecia variegata variegata* and *Varecia variegata rubra*). *Proc. J. Conf. AAZV/WDA/AAWVP.*, 268 (abstr.).

Weindruch, R., and Walford, R. L. (1988). "The Retardation of Aging and Disease by Dietary Restriction." Thomas, Springfield, IL.

Weindruch, R., Marriott, B. M., Conway, J., Knapka, J. J., Lane, M. A., Cutler, R. G., Roth, G. S., and Ingram, D. K. (1995). Measures of body size and growth in rhesus and squirrel monkeys subjected to long-term dietary restriction. *Am. J. Primatol.* **35**, 207–288.

Weinreb, M., Quartuccio, H., Seedor, J. G., Aufdemorte, T. B., Brunsvold, M., Chaves, E., Kornman, K. S., and Rodan, G. A. (1994). Histomorphometrical analysis of the effects of the bisphosphonate alendronate on bone loss caused by experimental periodontitis in monkeys. *J. Periodont. Res.* **29**, 35–40.

Weisman, H. A., Rasmussen, A. F., Jr., Elvehjem, C. A., and Clark, P. F. (1943). Studies on the nutritional requirements of the rhesus monkeys. *J. Nutr.* **26**, 205–218.

Westlund, K. N., Sun, Y. C., Sluka, K. A., Dougherty, P. M., Sorkin, L. S., and Willis, W. D. (1992). Neural changes in acute arthritis in monkeys. II. Increased glutamate immunoreactivity in the medial articular nerve. *Brain Res. Rev.* **17**, 15–27.

Whedon, G. D., Lutwak, L., and Neuman, W. (1967). Calcium and nitrogen balance. *NASA* [*Spec. Publ.*] *SP* NASA SP-121, 127.

Wiers, B. H. (1971). Precipitation boundaries in calcium-pyrophosphate and calcium-ethane-1-hydroxy-1, 1-diphosphonate systems. *Inorg. Chem.* **10**, 2581–1584.

Wilder, R. L. (1994). Hypothesis for retroviral causation of rheumatoid arthritis. *Curr. Opin. Rheumatol.* **6**, 295–299.

Williams, D. D., and Bowden, D. M. (1984). A nonhuman primate model for the osteopenia of aging. *In* "Comparative Pathobiology of Major Age-related Diseases: Current Status and Research Frontiers (D. G. Scarpelli, G. Migaki, eds.), p. 207. Liss, New York.

Wilson, D. J., Kay, V., Charig, M., Hughes, D. G., and Creasy, T. S. (1988). Skeletal hyperostosis and extraosseous calcification in patients receiving long-term etretinate (Tigason). *Br. J. Dermatol.* **119**, 597–607.

Wittmers, L. E., Wallgren, J., Alich, A., Aufderheide, A. C., and Rapp, G. (1988). Lead in bone. IV. Distribution of lead in the human skeleton. *Arch. Environ. Health* **43**, 381–391.

Woodard, J. C., Shields, R. P., Aldrich, H. C., and Carter, R. L. (1982). Calcium phosphate deposition disease in great danes. *Vet. Pathol.* **19**, 464–485.

Woodard, J. C., Poulos, P. W., Jr., Parker, R. B., Jackson, R. I., Jr., and Eurell, J. C. (1985). Canine diffuse idiopathic skeletal hyperostosis. *Vet. Pathol.* **22**, 317–326.

Wronski, T. J., and Morey, E. R. (1983). Inhibition of cortical and trabecular bone formation in the long bones of immobilized monkeys. *Clin. Orthop. Relat. Res.* **181**, 269–276.

Wuthier, R. E., and Register, T. C. (1984). Role of alkaline phosphatase, a polyfunctional enzyme, in mineralizing tissues. *Proc. In. Conf. Chem. Bio. Miner. Tissues, 2nd,* 111–124, Sept. 9–14, 1984.

Xu, Y., Cruz, T. F., and Pritzker, K. P. H. (1991). Alkaline phosphatase dissolves calcium pyrophosphatase dihydrate crystals. *J. Rheumatol.* **18**, 1606–1610.

Xu, Y., Pritzker, K. Ph. H., and Cruz, T. F. (1994). Characterization of chondrocyte alkaline phosphatase as a mediator in the dissolution of calcium pyrophosphate dihydrate crystals. *J. Rheumatol.* **21**, 912–919.

Yamaguchi, A., Kohno, Y., Yamazaki, T., Takahashi, N., Shinki, T., Horiuchi, N., Suda, T., Koizumi, H., Tanioka, Y., and Yoshiki, S. (1986). Bone in the marmoset: A resemblance to vitamin D-dependent rickets, Type II. *Calcif. Tissue Int.* **39**, 22–27.

Yamauchi, M., Young, D. R., Chandler, G. S., and Mechanic, G. L. (1988). Cross-linking and new bone collagen synthesis in immobilized and recovering primate osteoporosis. *Bone* **9**, 415–418.

Yen, P. K.-J., and Shaw, J. H. (1957). Effects of repeated oral doses of demechlochortetracycline on bones and dentin of young rhesus monkeys. *J. Dent. Res.* **54**, 358.

Yen, P. K.-J., and Shaw, J. H. (1974). Effects of tetracyclines on membranous bone growth and dentin apposition in young rhesus monkeys. *J. Dent. Res.* **53**, 897.

Yen, P. K.-J., Shaw, J. H., and Hong, Y. C. (1972). Preliminary study of inhibitory effects of tetracyclines on membranous bone growth in rhesus monkeys. *J. Dent. Res.* **51**, 1651.

Yoo, T. C., Stuart, J. M., Takeda, T., Sudo, N., Floyd, R. A., Ishibe, T., Olson, G., Ortchik, D., Shea, J. J., and Kang, A. H. (1986). Induction of type II collagen autoimmune arthritis and ear disease in monkeys. *In* "Autoimmunity: Experimental and Clinical Aspects" (R. S. Schwartz and N. R. Rose, eds.), p. 341. New York Academy of Sciences, New York.

Yoo, T. J., Kim, S.-Y., Stuart, J. M., Floyd, R. A., Olson, G. A., Cremer, M. A., and Kang, A. H. (1988). Induction of arthritis in monkeys by immunization with type II collagen. *J. Exp. Med.* **168**, 777–782.

Yoshida, T. (1993). Measurement of bone mineral density (BMD) in primate species employing a dual energy X-ray absorptiometry. *Tsukuba Primate Cent. Med. Sci. News* **12**, 7–8.

Yosipovitch, Z. H., and Glimcher, M. J. (1972). Articular chondrocalcinosis, hydroxyapatite deposition disease, in adult mature rabbits. *J. Bone J. Surg. Am. Vol.* **54-A**, 841–853.

Young, D. R., and Schneider, V. S. (1981). Radiographic evidence of disuse osteoporosis in the monkey (*M. nemestrina*). *Calcif. Tissue Int.* **33**, 631–639.

Young, D. R., Niklowitz, W. J., and Steele, C. R. (1983). Tibial changes in experimental disuse osteoporosis in the monkey. *Calcif. Tissue Int.* **35**, 304–308.

Young, D. R., Niklowitz, W. J., Brown, R. J., and Jee, W. S. (1986). Immobilization-associated osteoporosis in primates. *Bone* **7**, 109–117.

Zeman, D. H., Roberts, E. D., Henk, W. G., and Watson, E. (1989). Macroscopic, microscopic and ultrastructural findings in experimental haemarthrosis of rhesus monkeys. *J. Comp. Pathol.* **101**, 117–129.

Zeman, D. H., Roberts, E. D., Shoji, H., and Miwa, T. (1991). Experimental haemarthrosis in rhesus monkeys: Morphometric, biochemical and metabolic analyses. *J. Comp. Pathol.* **104**, 129–139.

Zerath, E., Malouvier, A., Martin, F., Holy, X., Malecki, H., and Marie, P. J. (1994). Monkey bone studies after 16 days of chair restraint: A first step in an integrated feasibility study for a future space flight. *Trav. Sci. Chercheurs Serv. Sante Armees* **15**, 153–154.

Zook, B. C., and Paasch, L. H. (1980). Lead poisoning in zoo primates: Environmental sources and neuropathologic findings. *In* "The Comparative Pathology of Zoo Animals" (R. J. Montali and G. Migaki, eds.), p. 143. Smithsonian Institution Press, Washington, DC.

Zook, B. C., Eisenberg, J. F., and McLanahan, E. (1973). Some factors affecting the occurrence of lead poisoning in captive primates. *J. Med. Primatol.* **2**, 206.

Zucker, H., Flurer, C. I., Hennes, U., and Rambeck, W. A. (1988). 25(OH)D-3, but not 1,25(OH)-2D-3 cures osteomalacia in marmoset monkeys. *Workshop Vitam. D, 7th, 1988,* pp. 450–451 (abstr.).

Zvaifler, N. J. (1995). Rheumatoid arthritis. The multiple pathways to chronic synovitis. *Lab. Invest.* **73**, 307–310.

Chapter 12

Nervous System

P. K. Cusick and S. J. Morgan

I. INTRODUCTION

The nervous system is one of the most heterogeneous of the body's many organs. Its structural complexity is equaled, if not exceeded, by its functional diversity. Familiarity with structure is important, in many cases essential, to any hope of coming to terms with the clinical presentation of function/dysfunction concepts. The variety of nonhuman primates discussed in this volume allows only a very generic presentation of the rudiments of neuroanatomy; however, more extensive texts are available (Clark, 1975; Truex and Carpenter, 1969). Reviews of basic neuropathologic processes are organized according to the major cellular element involved. With this background of basic neuropathology in hand, specific conditions not presented in the etiology-based chapters are covered. The chapter finishes with a consideration of prominent nonhuman primate models of some of the more significant human neurologic diseases.

II. OVERVIEW OF NEUROANATOMY

The most primitive neural systems, exemplified by aquatic coelenterates such as the hydra, function as little more than monodimensional sensory nerve nets in which neurons and bidirectional synapses can be identified. The next level in the phylogenetic history of development of the nervous system is characterized by centralization and cephalization. Plathyhelminthes (flatworms), such as *Planaria,* typify this stage by development of a head with a brain and sense organs, a third germ layer (mesoderm) between the outside ectoderm and the inside endoderm, a bilaterally symmetrical body, and rudimentary organ systems. A further notch up the sophistication scale is the development of simple reflexes that can be coordinated both intrasegmentally and intersegmentally, as in the common earthworm. Evolution continued to refine this rudimentary system from invertebrates to vertebrates by providing a centralized area for integration of input and processing/organization of output designed to appropriately service a more complex network of sensory and motor components. Indeed, the primate nervous system, arguably the penultimate expression, is made up of a central portion, the brain and spinal cord, a peripheral portion, the cranial and spinal nerves, and an autonomic (involuntary) portion.

The spinal cord forms the "backbone" of the central nervous system. It will be sufficient for our purposes to think of the spinal cord as the conduit for communication between the brain and the rest of the body. On external gross examination the segmental organization of the cord and spinal nerves is obvious. Even with the unaided eye the characteristic arrangement of H-shaped central gray matter surrounded by white matter can be appreciated in cross sections. Gray matter is composed primarily of neurons with associated nonmyelinated fibers, neuroglia, and capillaries. The anterior "quadrants" of the "H," commonly called the anterior horns, contain the large cell bodies of efferent neurons that send axons peripherally through ventral nerve roots and spinal nerves to ultimately innervate skeletal muscles. These neurons are frequently referred to as "lower motor neurons." The posterior gray matter quadrants, the posterior horns, contain smaller neurons whose axons are confined to the central nervous system. Posterior horn cells communicate with incoming (afferent) fibers from the dorsal nerve root and serve a relay function for this information. The thick rim of white matter around the "H" appears so because it is composed predominantly of myelinated nerve fibers. Traditional thinking holds that these axons are "bundled" in an organized manner allowing identification of areas, or "tracts," that subserve

specific functions. The most rudimentary identification system divides tracts into two types: ascending, or sensory, and descending, or motor.

The spinal nerves enter and exit the spinal cord at regular intervals. Each spinal nerve is formed by the union of two roots: a dorsal sensory root and a ventral motor root. Immediately before the conjunction of the nerve roots, the dorsal root swells, forming the spinal ganglion, which contains the neurons of origin of the sensory nerve fibers.

The most cephalic portion of the central nervous system is the brain, where major structures such as the cerebral hemispheres, cerebellum, medulla, pons, and midbrain are easily identified. In the early embryo, the neural tube area from which the brain derives is divided into three primary regions: the prosencephalon (forebrain), the mesencephalon (midbrain), and the rhombencephalon (hindbrain). With further maturation, the prosencephalon develops into the telencephalon (cerebral hemispheres) and diencephalon (thalamus and hypothalamus) and the rhombencephalon develops into the cerebellum, pons, and medulla.

The brain stem, composed of the medulla, pons, midbrain, and diencephalon, is made up of ascending, descending, and decussating (crossing-over) fiber tracts; the origins of cranial nerves III through XII; other important neuronal clusters (nuclei), such as the red nucleus, substantia nigra, and thalamic nuclei; and the diffuse reticular formation. The numerous and complex interconnections of tracts and nuclei within brain stem subdivisions and between the brain stem and the cerebral hemispheres or cerebellum are important for coordination and movement, control of muscle tone, and the integration of sensory pathways. The diffuse reticular formation is an anatomically poorly defined neuronal network that is often referred to as the reticular activating system (RAS). It plays an important role in mediating states of consciousness. In the medulla, the reticular formation is thought to function in the synchronization of rhythmic vital reflexes, such as respiration and heartbeat, and protective reflexes, such as coughing and vomiting. In short, the brain stem is a "bottleneck" through which a considerable amount of information must funnel and in which a remarkable interaction takes place.

The cerebellum is positioned behind and below the cerebral hemispheres and covers the brain stem. It consists of a midline portion, the vermis, bounded on each side by the cerebellar hemispheres. The surface of the cerebellum appears as multiple leaves or folds compressed together. These slender convolutions are called folia and the crevices between them are sulci. Unlike the arrangement seen in the spinal cord, the internal organization of the cerebellum is such that each folia is composed of an outer rim of gray matter that covers an inner core of white matter. Embedded in the deeper white matter are neuronal clusters, the deep cerebellar nuclei. The cerebellum is connected to the brain stem by white matter pillars, the cerebellar peduncles. The cerebellum has no primary motor neurons nor does it form any direct connections with lower motor neurons in the spinal cord. Thus, although it does not function at a conscious level to initiate motor activity, it does significantly influence the unconscious interaction of muscle activity, muscle tone, and equilibrium. An intact cerebellum is necessary for the successful coordination of the activities of the diverse muscle groups needed for proper postural maintenance when sitting or standing and for effective walking or running. The coordination of motor actions requiring fine and accurate movements, such as picking up small objects, is also heavily dependent on proper cerebellar function.

At the "junction," so to speak, of the brain stem and cerebral hemispheres lies the diencephalon. The most prominent components of this part of the brain stem are the thalamus and the hypothalamus. The thalamus, a large gray matter structure, may be subdivided into various nuclei. While in humans it is generally agreed that all sensory impulses, with the exception of olfactory ones, enter the thalamus and are subsequently relayed to specific cerebral cortical areas, the thalamic nuclei should not be thought of as mere relay centers. Instead they are also thought to play a significant role in the two types of sensation: discriminative and affective. Discriminative sensation compares stimuli with respect to intensity, locality, and relative position in time and space. Affective sensation, sometimes considered synonymous with "emotion," deals with the pleasantness or unpleasantness of sensory stimuli. The hypothalamus, while small relative to the thalamus, directs a number of important functions: temperature regulation, water balance, activity on the anterior pituitary gland, appetite, and emotional expression.

The last portion of the brain to consider is the telencephalon, the cerebral hemispheres, which embodies the cerebral cortex, basal nuclei, limbic system, and rhinencephalon. The telencephalon encompasses the highest levels of sensory integration/ perception and motor control as well as memory, association, and personality. Like the cerebellum, the surface of the cerebrum presents a pattern of folds and grooves. The grooves are called sulci and the elevations are called gyri (not folia, as in the cerebellum). The complexity of the pattern of the gyri is a reflection of the neocortical development of the species and, hence, the capacity to think, communicate, remember, associate, and analyze input. The cortex can be roughly divided into four regions or lobes: frontal, parietal, temporal, and occipital. The rhinencephalon is concerned with olfactory process, i.e., the perception of odors. The limbic system is involved with emotional and behavioral patterns. The basal nuclei modulate motor activity.

During embryonic development, the entire substance of the central nervous system folds and forms itself around a central cavity. In the spinal cord this cavity is represented by the central canal. Moving cranially, the central canal widens in the brain stem and forms the fourth ventricle in the medulla and pons. At the level of the midbrain the cavity narrows again and is called the cerebral aqueduct of Sylvius or, simply, the cerebral aqueduct. Beyond the aqueduct the cavity widens again to form a chamber, the third ventricle, which is encompassed by the diencephalon. The cerebral hemispheres surround similar cavities, the lateral ventricles, which communicate via the interventricular foramena of Monro. This entire contiguous space, all four ventricles and the central canal, is filled with cerebrospinal fluid. The bulk of the cerebrospinal fluid is formed by vascular structures, the choroid plexuses, in the lateral ventricles. Thus formed, cerebrospinal fluid drains from the lateral ventricles, through the foramena of Monro to the third ventricle. Flow continues through the cerebral aqueduct to the fourth ventricle where two lateral apertures, the foramina of Luschka, permit passage into the subarachnoid space. Once in the subarachnoid space, cerebrospinal fluid may circulate cranially or caudally but will eventually return to the vascular system from whence it came via arachnoid villi. The most obvious function of the cerebrospinal fluid is that of a liquid cushion for the soft central nervous system tissues. Less obvious, perhaps, is its function as a fluid that modulates the fluctuations of pressure that occur.

The brain and spinal cord are covered by three layers of sheet-like connective tissue called the meninges. The innermost layer, the pia mater, is the most delicate of the three layers. It closely covers all surfaces of the central nervous system, even the walls of the deep sulci of the cerebral hemispheres. The outermost layer is a bilaminar structure called the dura mater. It is the toughest of the three layers. The dura mater forms two important connective tissue septae, which help to support the brain within the skull. One is the falx cerebri, which extends deep into the fissure between the left and the right cerebral hemispheres. The other is the tentorium cerebelli, which extends, somewhat at right angles to the falx, into the space between the cerebrum and the cerebellum. In so doing, the tentorium forms, with some species variation, a collar of greater or lesser restrictiveness around the midbrain of the brain stem. The dura mater also houses endothelium-lined venous sinuses that play a major role in drainage of blood from cerebral and meningeal veins and circulation of the cerebrospinal fluid. The remaining meningeal layer, a delicate structure between the dura mater and the pia mater, is called the arachnoid mater. It is separated from the pia mater by the subarachnoid space through which the cerebrospinal fluid flows. Cerebral blood vessels course through this space as well, prior to dipping into the brain parenchyma. Specialized outpouchings, arachnoid villi, penetrate the dural venous sinuses to allow the passage of cerebrospinal fluid from the subarachnoid space back into the venous circulation. Collectively, the pia and arachnoid are referred to as the leptomeninges. The dura is also described as the pachymeninges.

III. NEURONS

The neuron is generally thought of as the primary cell in the nervous system. At birth, an animal is born with the maximum

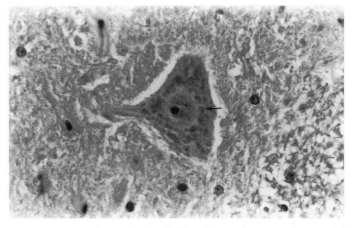

Fig. 1. Neuron from spinal cord. Note the prominent granular material known as Nissl substance (arrow). Hematoxylin and eosin stain.

number of neurons that it will ever have. With aging there is a slow but continual loss of neurons. Although neurons do not divide postnatally, there is some degree of differentiation and migration that occurs in the early perinatal period. The general function of the neuron is, stated simply, to provide for the generation and propagation of electrical impulses.

Although the brain makes up a relatively small percentage of the total mass of a primate, it accounts for approximately 20% of the total resting oxygen consumption. This tremendous oxygen consumption is considered to be related to the need to maintain ionic gradients across neuronal membranes. This, coupled with the fact that there is little storage of reserve energy within the neuron, makes it the most susceptible cell within the central nervous system to metabolic compromise, as by ischemia (Iversen, 1979).

By light microscopy, neurons vary considerably in size and shape, depending, in part, on their location within the brain. They are generally round to pyramidal and are relatively large in comparison to the remaining cells in the central nervous system. The most prominent component of the neuron is the cell body, which contains a centrally oriented nucleus with, most conspicuously in large neurons, a prominent central nucleolus and abundant lightly basophilic, slightly granular cytoplasm (Fig. 1). Processes of the neuron include dendrites, which tend to cluster as multiple short branching structures at one extremity of the cell and the axon, a single process that extends a variable distance from the cell body before branching. These processes are most readily visualized with special staining techniques, such as silver stains. The vast majority of axons are myelinated, with the myelin sheath being provided by the Schwann cell or the oligodendroglia in the peripheral and central nervous systems, respectively.

Ultrastructurally, a full complement of subcellular organelles can be seen within the neuronal cell body. The rough endoplasmic reticulum, involved with synthesis of protein destined

for export, i.e., extraneuronal use, may be aggregated in dense structures (Nissl substance) that can be visualized in standard hematoxylin and eosin (H&E)-stained histology preparations. Additional components include free ribosomes, a Golgi apparatus, lysosomes, smooth endoplasmic reticulum, mitochondria, neurofilaments, and microtubules. It is thought that proteins destined for internal use are synthesized by the free ribosomes (Hirano, 1991).

The term "neurofibril" has been used to refer to at least three different structures, including neurofilaments, microtubules, and microfilaments. Microfilaments are contractile by nature due to the presence of a contractile protein, actin. Microtubules (also known as neurotubules) are thought to play a major role in intraneuronal transport and maintenance of cell shape (Soifer, 1986). Neurofilaments are classified as "intermediate filaments" based on their size; they are unique to neurons. Although their function is not clear, they are thought to be a part of the cell cytoskeleton and possibly involved in intracellular transport (Hirano, 1991).

Neuron death or damage is marked by a variety of readily recognized morphologic changes. Ischemic cell change, for instance, is characterized by the presence of a shrunken, dense nucleus and a triangular to diamond-shaped cell body that, with H&E staining, is brightly eosinophilic (Fig. 2). Electron microscopic studies of neurons undergoing ischemic cell change include a wide spectrum of changes, varying from mild chromatin clumping, nucleolar condensation, and breakdown of polysomes to markedly shrunken neurons with electron-dense, nonidentifiable subcellular organelles. The number of neurons exhibiting the more severe ultrastructural changes varies with both the duration of ischemia and the location. It appears that 10–15 min of complete cerebral ischemia is followed by considerable neuronal injury. The "selectively vulnerable" brain

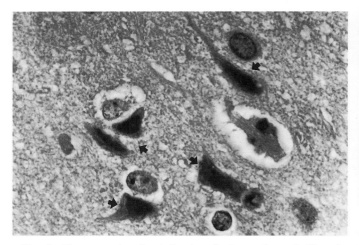

Fig. 2. Neurons undergoing ischemic cell change (arrows). Note the shrunken, condensed nucleus and the roughly triangular cytoplasm. Hematoxylin and eosin stain.

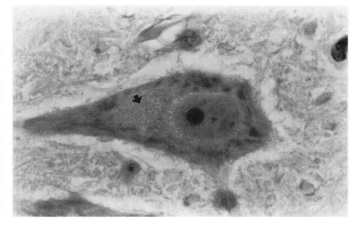

Fig. 3. Neuron from the spinal cord containing abundant intracytoplasmic lipofuscin granules (arrow). Hematoxylin and eosin stain.

regions include the cerebral cortex, particular regions of the hippocampus, and the Purkinje cells of the cerebellum. Although ischemic cell change is most commonly associated with primary ischemia, it is also frequently seen with certain metabolic disturbances and toxicities.

A number of neurochemical changes have been associated with neuronal damage/loss, including elevations in acetylcholine, arachidonic acid cascade products, catecholamine neurotransmitters (epinephrine and norepinephrine), monoamine neurotransmitters (dopamine), cytokines, and excitatory amino acids (glutamate and aspartate). Although it is beyond the scope of this chapter to cover the mechanisms of each of these in detail, excellent reviews of such material are available (Katsuki and Okuda, 1995; Yang *et al.,* 1995; McIntosh *et al.,* 1996).

Two major types of pigments may be found in the neuron: lipofuscin and neuromelanin. Lipofuscin granules, which stain yellow-brown with hematoxylin and eosin, are considered to be residual bodies derived from lysosomes (Schochet, 1972) (Fig. 3). Because there is not a turnover of neurons, as is the case with the majority of the other cells of the body, lipofuscin granules tend to increase with age. In addition, in both animals and humans, the amount of neuronal lipofuscin varies with the particular region of the central nervous system and with particular disease states, including Alzheimer's disease and amyotrophic lateral sclerosis in humans, and vitamin E deficiency in animals (Hirano, 1991). The question is unresolved as to whether lipofuscin accumulation, in and of itself, has any actual damaging effect on neurons. Neuromelanin granules stain dark brown with H&E and are argyrophilic (stain with a silver stain) (Hirano, 1991). Unlike lipofuscin, neuromelanin is prominent in only a few specific areas of the brain, such as the substantia nigra and the locus ceruleus.

Abnormal accumulations of cytoskeletal elements within the cytoplasm may be seen with a variety of naturally occurring and experimental conditions (Hirano, 1991). The classic example is

the "neurofibrillary tangle" seen in humans in cases of Alzheimer's disease. The tangles are most easily visualized with silver impregnation but may also be seen with routine H&E stains. Immunochemically, they react with tau, a neuron-specific microtubule-associated protein, and neurofilament-associated proteins. The axon terminals of affected neurons may participate in the formation of another degenerative change often associated with the presence of neurofibrillary tangles, the neuritic plaque (senile plaque) (Price *et al.,* 1985). In its most characteristic form, this structure consists of a cluster of abnormal axons and dendrites, largely synaptic connections, surrounding an amyloid core (Rewcastle, 1991). The pathologic significance of neurofibrillary tangles and neuritic plaques is not settled. True neurofibrillary tangles have not been found in nonhuman primates, whereas neuritic plaques similar to, but not identical with, those seen in humans have been described in aged nonhuman primates (Selkoe *et al.,* 1987; Cork *et al.,* 1987; Wisniewski *et al.,* 1973).

Numerous inclusions, both intranuclear and intracytoplasmic, have been described in neurons. Both eosinophilic and basophilic intranuclear inclusions have been identified in many encephalitides of viral etiology that, ultrastructurally, consist of viral particles (Hirano, 1991). In contrast, Negri bodies are intracytoplasmic inclusions seen in certain neurons (particularly pyramidal cells of the hippocampus or Purkinje cells) in cases of rabies. The inclusions are eosinophilic, round to oval, vary in size, and have a slight peripheral halo. Ultrastructurally, Negri bodies consist of tubular-shaped viral particles (Hirano, 1991). Another eosinophilic intracytoplasmic inclusion, a rodlike structure known as a Hirano body, is highly refractile in H&E preparations and ultrastructurally quite dissimilar from the Negri body, appearing as an organized array of interlacing filaments arranged in a herringbone pattern (Hirano, 1991). Hirano bodies may be seen in Sommer's sector of the hippocampus and adjacent areas and, in humans, have been described in Alzheimer's disease and Creutzfeldt–Jakob disease as well as a consequence of aging (Hirano, 1991). Identical structures have been reported in the cerebral cortex of aged primates and in kuru-infected chimpanzees (Wisniewski *et al.,* 1973; Hirano, 1991).

Transection of an axon is followed by complex sets of reactions, with degenerative changes in the distal stump known as Wallerian degeneration. The axon and associated nerve terminals are dependent on the cell body for a continual supply of nutrients. If this supply is disrupted, as by transection, the axon and terminals distal to the site of disruption undergo dissolution. The cause of this dissolution is multifactorial, with contributions from both intrinsic and extrinsic elements. In part, intrinsic factors include the interruption of axonal transport with loss of nutritive supply and activation of calcium-activated proteases (Griffin and Watson, 1988; Griffin, 1990). Extrinsic factors of importance include macrophage infiltration and subsequent mediator release (Lynn *et al.,* 1989). Soon after the initiation of axonal degeneration, myelin sheath degeneration begins; the myelin appearing as ovoid bodies on light microscopy. Although considerable controversy has existed as to the cell type(s) responsible for phagocytosis and removal of the myelin ovoids, studies indicate that the hematogenous macrophage is the primary myelin phagocyte of the nervous system (Stoll *et al.,* 1989). Although degenerative changes occurring in the central and peripheral nervous system are relatively similar, there are vast differences regarding the potential for regeneration following axonal severance.

In the central nervous system, effective axonal regeneration is not felt to occur following transection of nerve fibers (Griffin, 1990). In contrast, there is considerable potential for a successful regenerative response in the peripheral nervous system. In the peripheral nervous system, Schwann cells in the distal stump begin to proliferate a few days after axonal severance, with the formation of Schwann cell bands. Not only do these Schwann cell bands form a "tunnel" or pathway for the axonal regeneration, but the Schwann cells in the distal stump are thought to synthesize nerve growth factor, with resultant stimulation of axonal sprouts from the proximal stump (Tanichi *et al.,* 1988). Peripheral nerve axonal extension with reinnervation of tissues can be highly variable and is, at best, a relatively slow process. As growth occurs at the rate of only 1–3 mm/day, it may take considerable time for anatomical reinnervation, depending on the point at which the axon was severed. Additionally, functional reinnervation may not occur until some period after anatomical reinnervation, as synthesis and transport of proteins are shifted in favor of tubulin and actin (to promote motility of growth cones) as compared to neurotransmitters during the regenerative phase (Koo *et al.,* 1988).

Distal axonal degeneration differs from Wallerian degeneration in that it occurs in the distal regions of long large axons in the absence of mechanical severance of the axon. Cavanagh described this process in 1964 and coined the term "dying back" neuropathy. This condition is relatively commonly encountered in many metabolic, heritable, and toxic disorders (Griffin, 1990). Eventually, the more proximal aspects of the axon and smaller axons become affected. The pathogenesis is thought to be related to defects in axonal transport with a subsequent loss of trophic influence (Griffin and Watson, 1988).

In contrast to both Wallerian degeneration and distal axonal degeneration, demyelination refers to the loss of the myelin sheath with axonal preservation. The effect of myelin loss is the disruption of impulse conduction with a deficit in function that can be as severe as what would occur with axonal severance. Although there is potential for remyelination in both the central and the peripheral nervous system, remyelination in the central nervous system is generally less effective than in the peripheral nervous system. The less effective remyelination in the central nervous system is related to the differing characteristics of myelin-providing cells in the central (oligodendroglia) and peripheral (Schwann cell) nervous systems. A single oligodendroglial cell may provide myelin for as many as 30–40 different axons in contrast to the Schwann cell, which provides myelin for only one axon, thus complicating regenerative efforts in the central nervous system. A spatial difference also exists, as the dis-

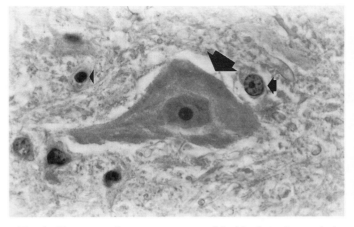

Fig. 4. Numerous cell types are represented in this photomicrograph, including a neuron (large arrow), an astrocyte (small arrow), and an oligodendroglia (arrowhead). Hematoxylin and eosin stain.

tance between an oligodendroglia and its associated axons may be considerably greater than the distance between a Schwann cell and its axon. Unlike distal axonal degeneration, in which toxins are a common etiology, demyelination is frequently associated with an immune-mediated or heritable condition (Griffin, 1990).

Chromatolysis, also known as the axon reaction, refers to changes that occur in the nerve cell body following axonal transection/disruption. By light microscopy, a chromatolytic neuron is characterized by an eccentrically located nucleus and abundant eosinophilic cytoplasm in which the Nissl substance appears to have "dissolved"—hence, chromatolysis or lysis of colored substance. It is characterized electron microscopically by dispersion of the stacks of granular endoplasmic reticulum (Nissl substance) (Price and Porter, 1970). Other electron microscopic alterations include an increase in size of the lysosomes and mitochondrial swelling. Biochemically, a chromatolytic neuron exhibits increased synthesis of proteins involved in axonal regeneration (including tubulin and actin) and a concurrent decrease in neurofilament synthesis (Hoffman *et al.,* 1985). Chromatolysis is a potentially reversible alteration.

IV. ASTROCYTES

The astrocyte is involved in a multitude of seemingly diverse, often poorly understood functions. In general, these functions can be grouped into development and maintenance of a stable neural environment and response to injury.

Astrocytes have rather characteristic anatomic features. Light microscopically, the astrocyte has a relatively large nucleus, small nucleolus, and numerous radiating processes (Fig. 4). It is these radiating processes, which are easily detected with metallic stains, such as Cajál's gold sublimate or Del Rio Hortega's silver carbonate techniques, that give the cell its classic "star" shape; thus, the name "astrocyte" (Blackwood, 1976). There are two distinct types of astrocytes, the fibrous type and the protoplasmic type, although they share numerous anatomic features. Although there is not an absolute locational separation, fibrous astrocytes predominate in the white matter whereas protoplasmic astrocytes predominate in the gray matter. As the name implies, protoplasmic astrocytes have more delicate processes than fibrous astrocytes.

Electron microscopic features common to astrocytes include an array of typical organelles such as mitochondria, Golgi apparatus, rough endoplasmic reticulum, and lysosomes. In addition, there are numerous characteristic rectilinear arrays of intramembranous particles known as orthogonal assemblies (Brightman and Tao-Cheng, 1988). These structures are especially numerous in those areas of the astrocyte that are adjacent to a capillary or pial surface, the astrocytic foot processes. However, the most characteristic constituent of the astrocyte is the presence of intermediate filaments known as glial fibrils, the major component of which is glial fibrillary acidic protein. Although not unique to astrocytes, the presence of this protein, is accompanied by vimentin synthesis, is interpreted as evidence of astrocytic differentiation (Hirano, 1991).

The maintenance of electrolyte balance in the region around the neuron, primarily with respect to potassium, is a major function of the astrocyte. The appropriate ionic composition is of paramount importance in the preservation of neuronal function because it is the balance, and resultant flow, of electrically charged molecules across the neuronal membrane that results in the production of an action potential and conduction of the nerve impulse. Astrocytes are thought to have a potassium scavenging function by which excess extracellular potassium, frequently generated by neuronal activity, is taken up and redistributed to regions of lesser concentration, thus preventing ionic imbalances and interference with normal initiation and propagation of the nerve impulse (Kimelberg and Norenberg, 1989).

Astrocytes play a critical role in synthesis by neurons of neurotransmitters, i.e., glutamate and γ-aminobutyric acid (GABA), whic are excitatory and inhibitory, respectively (Kimelberg and Norenberg, 1989). Astrocytes are frequently present at neuronal surfaces and synapses. Glutamine synthetase, an enzyme unique to astrocytes, catalyzes the reaction between glutamate and GABA, with resultant production of glutamine. Glutamine is then released from the astrocyte and taken up by the neuron, where it is thought to serve as the major precursor for remanufacture of GABA and glutamate. It has also been postulated that the astrocyte may serve some sort of insulating role at synapses. However, no synapses are completely surrounded by astrocytic foot processes and some synapses are completely devoid of astrocytes in their immediate vicinity (Hirano, 1991).

Astrocytes contribute significantly to the embryonic development of the brain. Primitive astrocytic cells known as radial astrocytes are thought to aid in the migration of neurons in the developing nervous system (Kimelberg and Norenberg, 1989). It is felt that the processes of these radial astrocytes provide a scaffolding, forming "migratory pathways" and thus guiding the movement of neurons and/or axonal processes from their embryonic to their final anatomical locations. For instance, in the monkey cerebellum, studies have shown that granule cells migrate inward from the outer layers, supported by fibers from radial astroglia. As another example, experiments in mice have indicated that the growth of axons from one side of the brain to the other, forming the corpus callosum, is supported by an astroglial "sling." In animals lacking the glial sling, the corpus callosum does not form. An additional developmental role for astrocytes relates to the formation of the blood–brain barrier. The sum and substance of the blood–brain barrier (as discussed in a subsequent section) are the result of the unique structural characteristics and properties of brain vascular endothelial cells. The presence and close association of astrocytes are apparently necessary for the induction of these features in the embryonic cerebrovascular endothelial cell.

Both intranuclear and intracytoplasmic inclusions have been described for astrocytes (Hirano, 1991). Astrocytic eosinophilic intranuclear inclusions may be seen with certain viral conditions, such as herpes encephalitis. Intracytoplasmic inclusions likely to occur are lipofuscin or tissue debris. The former occurs both with injury and as a normal function of aging. The latter may be seen following a variety of degenerative conditions, as astrocytes are known to be capable of a certain degree of phagocytic activity. Corpora amylacea, which are common inclusions in aged animals, including primates, are round basophilic, argyrophilic, periodic acid–Schiff (PAS)-positive structures. Electron microscopic findings indicate that these inclusions are found within astrocytic processes (Ramsey, 1965). Chemically, corpora amylacea are composed of a glycogen-like carbohydrate mixed with small amounts of protein (Austin and Sakai, 1972).

The presence of aberrant astrocytes with large, often kidney bean-shaped nuclei and relatively few fibers, known as Alzheimer's type II cells, has been described in instances of hepatic encephalopathy. Although the pathogenesis of such astrocytic damage is not completely understood, two basic theories exist. In hepatic encephalopathy, there are high blood levels of ammonia, short chain fatty acids, and mercaptans (Kimelberg and Norenberg, 1989). The ultrastructural astrocytic changes (increased numbers of mitochondria, elevated amounts of rough endoplasmic reticulum, and cytoplasmic glycogen) may be secondary to an increased metabolic activity directed at the detoxification of ammonia as glutamine synthetase and glutamate dehydrogenase, the enzymes primarily responsible for cerebral ammonia detoxification, are located within astrocytes (Martinez-Hernandez et al., 1977). Another possible pathogenesis is that the swelling may represent an abnormal accumulation of monovalent ions as astrocytes help maintain Na^+ and K^+ homeostasis in the central nervous system via a membrane-bound Na^+, K^+-activated ATPase pump (Benjamin et al., 1978).

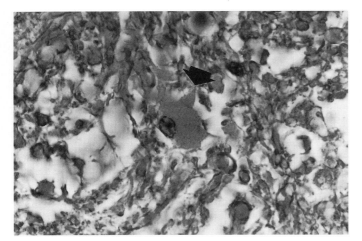

Fig. 5. Gemistocytic astrocyte (arrow) associated with an area of edema in the brain. Note the abundant cytoplasm and eccentrically located nucleus. Hematoxylin and eosin stain.

At high concentrations, ammonium ions have been shown to promote intracellular Na^+ and Cl^- and water accumulation in brain tissue. In any event, dysfunction of the astrocyte with resultant electrolyte and neurotransmitter imbalances is felt to be of major importance in the pathogenesis of hepatic encephalopathy.

The early reactions of astrocytes to injury can present readily identifiable morphologic changes (Hirano, 1991). Astrocytic swelling is a common and nonspecific initial response to injury. A variety of initiating factors, including hypoxia and a multitude of toxins, may be causes. By light microscopy, a swollen astrocyte appears to have a slightly vacuolated cytoplasm, whereas electron microscopic examination shows a dispersion of organelles with frequent presence of glycogen bodies. As astrocytic foot processes are in close contact with neuronal surfaces, marked astrocytic swelling may result in neuronal dysfunction. Subacutely, the common reaction to insults such as trauma, infarct, infection, or edema is astrocytic hypertrophy. The most pronounced presentation of this change is embodied by gemistocytic astrocytes or, simply, gemistocytes (Escourolle and Poirier, 1973). Gemistocytes have an abundant, homogenous, eosinophilic cytoplasm with an eccentric nucleus when viewed with a light microscope (Fig. 5). Ultrastructurally, the cytoplasm is crowded with organelles and abundant glial fibrils.

Chronic injury may lead to the development of fibrillary gliosis and an astrocytic scar (Fig. 6). Astrocytes increase in size and number, have more processes, and their entire cytoplasm becomes filled with glial filaments. While fibrillary gliosis can be appreciated with H&E staining, it is most clearly defined with special stains, such as the Holzer stain and Mallory's phosphotungstic acid hematoxylin (PTAH). The seeming motivation for this reaction appears to be an attempt to heal by "filling in" a defect. The process may be viewed as either a help or a hindrance, perhaps both (Kimelberg and Norenberg,

1989). On the one hand, the extensive cellularity and tangle of astrocytic processes might provide physical impediments to any attempts at successful reorganization of neuronal and oligodendroglial elements. On the other hand, the astrocytic processes might provide a helpful "scaffolding" to aid reorientation of tissue constituents, as previously discussed with respect to embryonic development. In addition, astrocytes are thought to be capable of releasing nerve growth factor, possibly promoting axonal growth in an area of injury.

Astrocytes are not indestructable—blithely swelling and/or proliferating in the face of injury and insult. With severe injury, an astrocyte may undergo swelling with a loss of its processes, referred to as clasmatodendrosis, and even die.

V. OLIGODENDROGLIA AND SCHWANN CELLS

Oligodendroglia were recognized as a separate and distinct glial entity in the early 1900s as a result of Del Rio-Hortega's (1918, 1921) development of a silver carbonate staining technique. The main functions of this cell, and the ones on which we will limit our focus, are the production and maintenance of myelin in the central nervous system. Similar functions in the peripheral nervous system are served by the Schwann cell, which cell type will also be considered here. The role of the Schwann cell in peripheral myelinogenesis was well known by the 1960s when a similar role for oligodendroglial cells in the central nervous system was proven (Bunge et al., 1962).

In routine paraffin sections, using H&E, oligodendroglia often present a typical "fried egg" appearance, particularly in white matter. That is to say, the nucleus appears dark and rounded within a circular clear space. The clear space is artifactual swelling of cytoplasm due to poor fixative penetration, a common problem with immersion techniques. Two types of

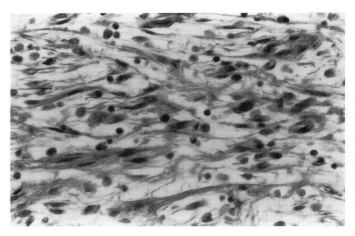

Fig. 6. Fibrillary astrocytosis associated with a chronic inflammatory process in the brain. Note the abundant fibrils associated with the astrocytes. Hematoxylin and eosin stain.

oligodendroglia can be recognized: satellite and interfascicular. Satellite oligodendroglia are found in the gray matter in close association with the cell bodies of large neurons. In contrast, interfascicular oligodendroglia are found in the white matter in close association with myelinated nerve fibers. In sections of white matter oriented to present the longitudinal plane of myelinated fibers, interfascicular oligondendroglia are frequently aligned in rows.

Ultrastructurally, satellite oligodendroglia are found to reside in small depressions on the surface of neuron cell bodies. It is tempting to presume some physiologically functional communication between these two cell types, perhaps via some specialized membrane junction, but no such evidence exists. In fact, it is most often the case that the oligodendroglial cell is separated from the neuron by an interposing astroglial cell process. The usual array of organelles can be identified within the cytoplasm: rough endoplasmic reticulum, free ribosomes, a prominent Golgi apparatus, mitochondria, and lysosomes (Peters *et al.,* 1976). A structure peculiar to the oligodendroglial cell is the dense body, thought to be a tertiary lysosome. Dense bodies are membrane bound and, in some planes, have a characteristic appearance that consists of a cap of amorphous-dense material resting atop a stack of parallel linear structures (Raine, 1991). Another feature of the oligodendroglia cytoplasm is the absence of intermediate filaments, despite the presence of numerous microtubules. This feature allows for the distinction between isolated processes from astrocytes and oligodendroglia in electron micrographs as astrocyte processes have both intermediate filaments and microtubules (Peters *et al.,* 1976).

With the exception of a denser cytoplasm, interfascicular oligodendroglial cells are virtually identical to satellite oligodendroglia on electron microscopic examination. In normal adult animals it is rare to find direct connections between the cell body and the myelin surrounding adjacent nerve fibers. It is clear, however, that myelin in the central nervous system is formed from processes extending from oligodendroglial cells (Bunge *et al.,* 1962).

Although much has been worked out regarding central nervous system myelinogenesis, it is a process that is far from understood (Raine, 1991). The myelin sheath is not a continuous covering along the entire length of an axon. At regular intervals there are short gaps in the myelin sheath that are called nodes of Ranvier. The segments of myelin between these nodes are called internodes. It is estimated that one interfascicular oligodendroglial cell may be responsible for between 30 and 50 internodes of myelin ensheathing several different axons. Internodal myelin is formed from flattened, shovel-shaped processes of oligodendroglial cells that have wrapped in a jelly roll fashion around axons. As the flattened process forms its multilayer wrapping, the cytoplasm is "squeezed" out and the inner surfaces of the cell membrane fuse forming the major dense line of the myelin sheath. The outer cell membrane surfaces of closely opposed adjacent turns of myelin do not fuse, but their close association forms the intraperiod line. The flattened oli-

godendroglial cell process that forms the myelin internode retains a thin rim of cytoplasm around its periphery. In cross section, the outer and inner rims are apparent and are known as the outer loop and inner loops, respectively. It is at these points that the intraperiod lines form a tight junction. On longitudinal section the rims at the sides of the flattened oligodendroglial process are apparent and form the lateral loops that flank the nodes of Ranvier.

In the peripheral nervous system, the role of the Schwann cell in myelinogenesis is analogous to that of the oligodendroglial cell. The situation is simplified in some respects because each Schwann cell is capable of forming only a single internode of myelin. The obvious implication, of course, is that the loss of one Schwann cell results in the loss of myelin from only one segment of an axon, but the loss of one oligodendroglial cell has the potential to produce a more widely scattered demyelinated lesion.

The substance of myelin, being essentially a cell membrane structure, is composed primarily of lipid and protein. The major lipid components are cholesterol, phosphoglycerides, galactolipids, and sphingomyelin (Raine, 1991). In myelin of adult animals, cholesterol is found only in the unesterified form. There are two main proteins in myelin: proteolipid protein (PLP) and myelin basic protein (MBP). Proteolipid protein is acidic and highly hydrophobic whereas MBP is basic and water soluble. Of the total structural proteins of central nervous system myelin, PLP makes up more than 50% and MBP accounts for about 30% (Raine, 1991).

Some of the unique biochemical characteristics of oligodendrocytes and myelin have been used to develop reliable immunocytochemical markers for the glial cell (Sternberger, 1984). Galactocerebroside is found in large amounts in oligodendroglial cells. Antisera to galactocerebroside used with an immunostaining technique will stain oligodendroglia but not other central nervous system cells (i.e., astrocytes, neurons, or microglia). Effective immunostaining procedures have also been developed using MBP, myelin-associated glycoprotein (MAG), and PLP. In addition, immunostaining based on specific enzyme activities has provided useful oligodendroglial determinants; 2',3'-cyclic nucleotide 3'-phosphohydrolase (CNP) and carbonic anhydrase (CA) being frequently used.

The pathology of the oligodendrocyte and Schwann Cell can be broadly considered in two categories (Raine, 1991). The first category addresses those conditions defined as demyelination. Demylination refers to the removal of apparently normal myelin from axons of the central nervous system and/or peripheral nervous system, usually against a background of perivascular infiltration by small lymphocytes, plasma cells, and large mononuclear cells. Multiple sclerosis, postinfectious/postvaccinal encephalomyelitis, progressive multifocal leukoencephalopathy, idiopathic polyneuritis, and diphtheritic neuropathy are included in this category. The reader is reminded of two things. First, this list is derived from human literature, not nonhuman primate literature. Second, this list will change as the progress

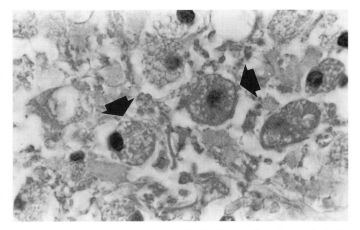

Fig. 7. Macrophages (arrows) associated with a region of necrosis in the central nervous system. Note the abundant intracytoplasmic vacuoles (lipid). Hematoxylin and eosin stain.

of research in this area further clarifies the process of demyelination. The second category involves a diverse group of conditions in which myelin loss follows parenchymal destruction as a sequela of damage to other tissue elements, such as blood vessels and axons. It can include ischemia, hemorrhage, trauma, neoplasia, necrosis, toxins, and genetic enzyme defects.

The physical aspects of demyelination appear to be similar in both the peripheral nervous system and the central nervous system (Raine, 1991; Compston *et al.,* 1991; Lampert, 1969). Macrophages of hematogenous origin surround myelin segments and phagocytize droplets of myelin. Ultrastructurally, processes from these macrophages can be seen between myelin layers, as if peeling away the outer portions of subsequent ingestion. Both immunoglobulin and complement have been implicated in the process of myelin breakdown and ingestion (Raine, 1991; Compston *et al.,* 1991).

Following demyelination it is only natural to focus attention on the reparative process of remyelination. Studies in humans and other animals have shown that remyelination occurs in both the peripheral nervous system and the central nervous system to a greater or lesser degree (Raine, 1991). The process is more clinically effective in the peripheral nervous system than in the central nervous system. Key to the process of remyelination is the ability of both Schwann cells and oligodendrocytes in areas of myelin destruction to proliferate and regenerate lost myelin sheaths (Johnson, 1991; Raine *et al.,* 1981; Ludwin and Bakker, 1988). This suggests one or both of the following: (1) during demyelination the myelin sheath is selectively targeted while the cell of origin (Schwann cell or oligodendrocyte) is spared or (2) subsequent to demyelination, new myelin-producing cells migrate into the affected area to regenerate the lost myelin. In the peripheral nervous system, there is evidence to support the sparing of Schwann cells with their subsequent replication and participation in the remyelination process (Lampert, 1969). In

the central nervous system, it also appears that oligodendrocytes proliferate in areas of demyelination and participate, albeit perhaps abortively, in a remyelination process, but the origin of such potentially regenerative cells is open to debate. One school of thought is that the mature oligodendrocyte, like the Schwann cell, is spared from destruction during the demyelination process. An alternative hypothesis holds that the proliferating oligodendrocytes seen in areas of demyelination arise, not from spared mature cells, but from an undifferentiated precursor cell pool, similar to the bipotential cells of the rat optic nerve that are capable of differentiating into either oligodendrocytes or astrocytes (Prineas *et al.,* 1989; Compston *et al.,* 1991). The generally ineffective outcome of central nervous system remyelination is ascribed to impediments such as a continuing inflammatory/immunologic process, physical barriers from reactive fibrillary astrogliosis, and/or the innately poor responsiveness to insult of oligodendrocytes and their possible precursors.

VI. MICROGLIA

The concept of the existence of microglial cells, a third type of glial cell distinct from astrocytes and oligodendrocytes, was introduced by Del Rio Hortega in 1919. Now, almost nine decades later, the existence of microglia is still a matter of extensive debate (Dickson *et al.,* 1991; Dolman, 1991). Scholarly discussions are well chronicled in the literature and will not be reprised here (Dolman, 1991; Jordan and Thomas, 1988; Perry and Gordon, 1988). Suffice it to say that one school of thought sees microglia as a resident population of central nervous system tissue macrophages that are derived from bone marrow precursor cells, monocytes. The opposing opinion denies the presence of any substantial population of resident macrophages; contending, instead, that any macrophages (microglia) in the central nervous system are a transient population of cells of hematogenous origin. Recognizing its tenuous nature, but to facilitate this presentation, we will opt for the existence of microglia. For the purposes of this discussion, the term "microglia" will refer to indigenous central nervous system cells that function, essentially, as microphages. The term "macrophage" will refer to a cell of the blood-derived mononuclear phagocytic system.

On the basis of morphology and function, microglia can be considered in two major subtypes: resting or ramified microglia and activated or ameboid microglia. Conversion from the resting to the activated form is thought to occur after tissue disruption, as by a pathologic process.

By light microscopy, resting microglia cannot be reliably identified using routine H&E staining; special techniques, classically Del Rio Hortega's silver carbonate method, must be used. With the appropriate special staining, resting microglia appear as unipolar to highly branched small cells distributed in nearly equal numbers throughout the white and gray matter. By electron microscopy, the microglial nucleus can be oval to elongated and irregular. Organelles are characteristically sparse; the presence of dense lysosomes is a prominent feature. There are no unique ultrastructural features that unequivocally identify resting microglia or their processes (Dolman, 1991).

Activated microglia are readily recognized on light microscopic examination of routine paraffin sections. Their appearance is that of a typical macrophage, having a rounded outline and containing phagocytized material such as lipid, hemosiderin, or other debris (Fig. 7). Understandably, the ultrastructural feature that most stands out is the presence of numerous membrane-bound phagosomes.

Microglia, as central nervous system tissue macrophages, share similar properties to those found in other tissue macrophages. The fundamental property of macrophages is phagocytosis, and abundant evidence, both morphologic and functional, shows that microglia are phagocytes. In their activated, but not their resting state, microglia demonstrate both ameboid mobility and adhesiveness. Macrophage colony-stimulating factor will promote microglial survival and differentiation (Frei *et al.,* 1987). Evidence suggests the existence of a cytokine-mediated microglia–astrocyte communication network analogous to that which exists outside the central nervous system between macrophages and lymphocytes (Frei *et al.,* 1987; Dickson *et al.,* 1991). Astrocytes can produce multispecific colony stimulating factor (IL-3), to which microglia will respond by proliferation. Microglia, however, can produce inflammatory cytokines, IL-1, and tumor necrosis factor, to which astrocytes will respond by proliferation.

Microglia are involved in a wide variety of pathologic conditions that share, as a common feature, the process of tissue breakdown. First and foremost among these is necrosis. The literature is replete with references to "foamy macrophages" and "fat granule cells" in such lesions carrying out their role as scavengers of necrotic tissue debris. Macrophage activity is a necessary part of the processes of demyelination and Wallerian degeneration.

In less overtly destructive conditions, such as some of the viral encephalitides, microglia have been described as "lamellar cells" and "rod cells" (Dolman, 1991). Lamellar cells, on light microscopy, do not appear to have abundant cytoplasm and their nuclei are crescent shaped and sometimes twisted. They collect around degenerating neurons to form what are called glial nodules. In rod cells, nuclei are sausage or rod shaped and sometimes, reportedly, of considerable length.

VII. BLOOD–BRAIN BARRIER

The brain requires a stable environment. The constant fluctuations in the physical and chemical environment that affect other organs of the body need to be minimized for the brain to function properly. The required constancy is affected by two very similar physicochemical barriers: the blood–brain barrier and the blood–cerebrospinal fluid barrier. These barriers provide direct control over nutritional and chemical factors by their ability to adjust the passage of molecules, such as glucose and amino acids, in and out of the central nervous system. In addition, they provide indirect control via the cerebrospinal and interstitial fluids over physical factors such as pressure and trauma.

The physical blood–brain barrier is determined by a distinctive anatomic feature of central nervous system capillaries. The endothelial cells of central nervous system capillaries are joined by tight junctions that form a continuous wall of cells in contradistinction to capillaries in general body organs where endothelia are fenestrated or otherwise compromised by transendothelial channels. Capillaries of the blood–brain barrier are surrounded by a basement membrane that is, in turn, virtually completely covered by foot processes from astrocytes. In fact, astrocytic foot processes were initially felt to constitute the major barrier effect of the blood–brain barrier. This hypothesis is now accepted as false. Astrocytic foot processes are now believed to have a significant inductive role that determines the unusual nature of central nervous system capillaries (Goldstein and Betz, 1986). Capillary endothelial cells in the central nervous system also contain a high density of mitochondria but few vesicles; features that relate to the chemical aspects of the blood–brain barrier.

Not all areas of the central nervous system have capillaries endowed with barrier-producing tight junctions (Betz *et al.,* 1989). Among those areas without blood–brain barriers are the pituitary gland, portions of the hypothalamus, and the pineal gland. The lack of a barrier likely relates to the needs of these tissues for ready access to circulating hormones.

The blood–cerebrospinal fluid barrier can, in some respects, be considered apart from the blood–brain barrier. Its barrier function does not consist of capillary endothelium tight junctions. The physical aspect of the blood–cerebrospinal fluid barrier is formed by the tight junctions that join choroid plexus epithelial cells at their apical surfaces (Nag, 1991). As with the capillary endothelium of the blood–brain barrier, the metabolic characteristics of the choroid plexus epithelium play a major role in creating and maintaining the blood–cerebrospinal fluid barrier.

There is no effective brain–cerebrospinal fluid barrier. The cerebrospinal fluid formed by the choroid plexuses and circulating through the ventricles and subarachnoid space is in continuity with, and similar to, brain extracellular fluid (Ramsay and Roberston, 1991; McComb and Davis, 1991). Ependymal cells lining the ventricles and the pia mater cells covering the central nervous system are not joined by tight junctions; thus, there is no significant restriction to free exchange of constituents between cerebrospinal fluid and extracellular fluid (Ramsay and Roberston, 1991).

Although tight junctions between cells provide the physical barrier, characteristics of the solute and carrier-mediated transport systems are vital for complete barrier function.

The solute characteristic of molecule size is a significant factor. Small molecules enter the brain more rapidly than large ones. Under normal conditions, large proteins and substances bound to serum proteins do not enter the cerebrospinal fluid or extracellular fluid. Another decisive solute property is lipid solubility. Diffusion is the primary mechanism whereby CO_2, O_2, volatile anesthetics, and other highly lipid-soluble compounds traverse the blood–brain barrier (Betz *et al.*, 1989). Diffusion is, simply, the process by which molecules in a solution move from an area of higher concentration to an area of lower concentration. The liquid-like bimolecular lipid layer structure of cell membranes is the key to this phenomenon. In essence, lipid-soluble molecules diffuse through the blood–brain barrier or the blood–cerebrospinal fluid barrier by "dissolving" in the cell membranes of barrier cells. However, many substances are not lipid soluble, such as glucose, amino acids, and ions (Na^+, K^+), that are essential for proper brain function. These substances make use of the complex system of specific carrier-mediated transport systems to enter the brain (Betz *et al.*, 1989; Goldstein and Betz, 1986).

Because glucose is the primary energy substrate for the brain, its transport system has been well studied. The glucose transporter in the capillary endothelial cell membranes of the blood–brain barrier is stereospecific in that it facilitates diffusion of the D-isomer of glucose, the biologically active form, and selectively rejects the L-isomer. A separate stereospecific transport system exists for pyruvate, ketones, and other monocarboxylic acids. Facilitated diffusion systems have also been identified for large essential amino acids: precursors for neurotransmitters synthesized in the brain. Transport systems for glucose and large neutral amino acids are considered symmetrical because they are found in the endothelial cell membrane facing the capillary lumen and in the endothelial cell membrane facing the brain; moving their target substance into, as well as out of, the brain. A variation of such transport systems that should be mentioned involves metabolic modification of the target substance after it has been transported into the endothelial cells. L-Dopa, which utilizes the large essential amino acid transport system, readily enters the endothelial cell from the blood or brain. Passage of L-Dopa out of the endothelial cell into the brain is regulated by its enzymatic modification to dopamine within the endothelial cell. This is possible because, although dopamine can pass from brain to endothelial cell via its own transport system, a transport mechanism in the opposite direction is not available. Asymmetric transport systems also exist. Characteristically, these systems are active, they require energy, and they are present on only one "side" of the endothelial cell. The systems that transport glycine and K^+ out of the brain, present only on the brain side of the endothelium, are examples of such asymmetric transport systems.

The end result of the regulatory efforts of the blood–brain barrier and the blood–cerebrospinal fluid barrier is the production and maintenance of a specialized and stable fluid environment. The fluid environment, represented by the cerebrospinal fluid and the extracellular fluid, functions to protect and support, maintain homeostasis, and eliminate metabolic wastes; any compromise has potentially widespread and devastating effects.

Vasogenic edema can be a significant and life-threatening consequence of blood–brain barrier breakdown. The edema is, simply, an increase in brain volume resulting from a localized or diffuse abnormal accumulation of water and sodium. In the vasogenic type of edema, defects in capillary endothelium tight junctions result in increased permeability and extravasation of fluid and plasma proteins. Extracellular fluid volume increases, brain volume increases, and, since expansion is limited by the cranial vault, intracranial pressure will eventually rise. If intracranial pressure increases sufficiently, cerebrovascular perfusion will be impaired, reducing the supply of necessary substrates such as oxygen and glucose to the brain. Another deleterious result of cerebral edema is that of herniation; predilection sites for herniation include the caudal lobe of the cerebellar vermis (protrudes over the medulla oblongata toward the foramen magnum), the rostral portion of the vermis (herniates into the brain stem), the median aspect of the occipital cortex (displaces beneath the tentorium cerebelli), and, in the case of unilateral cerebral edema, the cingulate gyrus (displaces beneath the falx cerebri) (Summers *et al.*, 1995).

The pathogenesis of cerebral edema is not limited to defects in the blood–brain barrier. Cellular, or cytotoxic, cerebral edema occurs when there is intracellular swelling of neurons, glia, and/or endothelial cells secondary to anoxia, hypoxia, or toxic insult. Initially, in contrast to vasogenic cerebral edema, the capillary permeability is normal and extracellular fluid volume is decreased. A third type of cerebral edema occurs in hydrocephalic conditions and is called interstitial edema. In this type of edema the extracellular fluid volume increases when cerebrospinal fluid migrates into the periventricular white matter secondarily to increased intraventricular pressure.

VIII. NATURALLY OCCURRING CONDITIONS

Spontaneous neurologic disease in the nonhuman primate is largely a consideration of infectious processes. There are, in addition, some uncommon and/or idiopathic conditions that deserve mention.

A. Infectious and Inflammatory Diseases

Numerous and sundry infectious agents have been reported in the central nervous system of nonhuman primates. Individual coverage is not within the scope of this chapter. Table I summarizes selected literature.

There are four principal routes by which infectious agents typically gain entry to the nervous system. Hematogenous spread is considered the most common route. A second route is direct implantation, which is usually secondary to trauma but could be iatrogenic from needle puncture during diagnostic or therapeutic procedures. Local extension from lesions adjacent to the central nervous system is a third route. Lastly, some infectious agents can gain access to the central nervous system by traveling along peripheral nerves.

The inflammatory reactions produced by infectious agents create a characteristic triad of histologic changes: perivascular cuffing, neuronophagia, and gliosis. Perivascular cuffing is the accumulation of leukocytes within the perivascular space in response to an inflammatory stimulus. With bacterial agents, neutrophils are the predominant cell type; hence, the common reference to suppurative meningitis/encephalitis. Viral etiologic agents typically generate nonsuppurative leukocyte infiltrates comprising lymphocytes admixed with small numbers of plasma cells and monocytes. When the monocyte/macrophage population assumes prominence, the process may be called granulomatous. Neuronophagia refers to the process of neuronal cell death and subsequent phagocytosis. It appears as a focal collection of macrophages/microglia surrounding the fragments of the dead neuron. Gliosis, the hypertrophy and/or hyperplasia of astrocytes in response to injurious stimuli, presents as localized to extensive hypercellularity. It generally reflects a degree of chronicity to the condition.

B. Progressive Multifocal Leukoencephalopathy

Progressive multifocal leukoencephalopathy (PML) is a demyelinating disease of the central nervous system recognized in humans as being associated with impaired immunological competence. It has been diagnosed with increasing frequency in acquired immunodeficiency syndrome (AIDS) patients (Holman *et al.*, 1991). It is the only chronic demyelinating disease of humans in which a virus (papovavirus) has consistently been demonstrated (Richardson, 1961; Weiner *et al.*, 1973). Macroscopically, multiple small gray foci are visible scattered about the subcortical white matter. Microscopically, these areas correspond to foci of demyelination. Bizarre astrocytes and oligodendroglia with enlarged nuclei are characteristic findings, and intranuclear inclusions are seen in both cell types. An inflammatory cell reaction is notably mild to absent (Leestma, 1991).

A spontaneously occurring disease with numerous similarities to PML has been described in eight macaques (Gribble *et al.*, 1975). Histologic changes consisting of demyelination accompanied by large, frequently bizarre astrocytes, oligodendroglia with enlarged nuclei, and intranuclear inclusions were reported. Additionally, electron microscopic examination revealed intranuclear inclusions in the macaque brain to be accumulations of papova-like virions. The viral agent is now felt to be simian virus 40 (King, 1993b).

Although immunologic competence was not assessed in these monkeys, some impairment could have been present as three of the eight were diagnosed with lymphoma and all were

TABLE I

INFECTIOUS AND INFLAMMATORY DISEASES

Organism	Reference
Bacterial	
Klebsiella pneumoniae	Fox *et al.* (1975)
Listeria monocytogenes	Anderson *et al.* (1993)
Streptococcus pneumoniae	Solleveld *et al.* (1984)
Viral	
Cytomegalovirus	Baskin (1987)
Herpes simplex virus	Hunt (1993)
Paramyxovirus	Steele *et al.* (1982)
Progressive multifocal leukoencephalopathy	King (1993b)
Simian immunodeficiency virus	King *et al* (1983)
Simian virus 40	King (1993b)
Protozoal	
Encephalitozoon cuniculi	Zeman *et al.* (1985)
Toxoplasma gondii	Wong *et al.* (1974)
Trypanosoma cruzi	Olsen *et al.* (1986)

being treated with isoniazid for prophylaxis of tuberculosis. Immune compromise secondary to simian immunodeficiency virus infection has been identified as the cause of reactivation of latent simian virus 40 infection in macaques (King, 1993b; King *et al.*, 1983).

C. Cytomegalovirus

It is likely that both humans and macaques are commonly asymptomatically infected with cytomegaloviruses and may shed the virus in urine, semen, breast milk, or other secretions. Under conditions of immunodeficiency, however, cytomegalovirus (CMV) infection can become a significant clinical problem in adult humans or monkeys, most notably in association with human immunodeficiency virus infection or simian immunodeficiency virus infection in the respective species (Leestma, 1991; Baskin, 1987).

Cytomegaloviruses are host-specific herpesviruses. Infection can take many forms, as the lung, liver, heart, intestine, kidney, salivary gland, and nervous system, among other tissues, can be affected. In the central nervous system, CMV produces a meningoencephalitis. Meningeal infiltration with neutrophils and macrophages can be severe and accompanied by edema and necrosis. Underlying brain or spinal cord shows perivascular cuffing, necrosis, and infiltration with inflammatory cells. A characteristic feature of CMV infections is the presence of cytomegaly and prominent intranuclear and intracytoplasmic inclusion bodies (Baskin, 1993).

D. Poliomyelitis

In humans, poliomyelitis is caused by an RNA virus from the *Enterovirus* genus of the Picornavirus family (Leestma, 1991).

Three serologically distinct strains have been identified. Effective polyvalent vaccines are widely available. The disease affects primarily those gray matter areas of the spinal cord, brain stem, and cerebral cortex subserving motor function. Initial clinical signs are stiffness of the neck and back, headache, and muscle spasms. Later changes include paralysis of one or more extremities, of the muscles of respiration, and, possibly, cranial nerve dysfunctions. Histopathologically, the changes seen include infiltration of the meninges and perivascular spaces by mononuclear inflammatory cells, neuronal cell swelling and chromatolysis, neuronophagia, and intranuclear inclusion bodies. Infectious virus is shed in the feces and enters the uninfected host by the oral route.

Although this disease is not common in nonhuman primates overall, chimpanzees, gorillas, and orangutans are the species most often associated with clinical cases of spontaneous poliomyelitis (Allmond et al., 1967; Suleman et al., 1984). Progressive paralysis of one or more of the extremities is the most obvious presenting nervous system sign. Lesions are most prominent in the anterior horns of the spinal cord with lesser involvement of the cranial nerve nuclei on the brain stem, the nuclear areas of the roof of the cerebellum, and the cerebral motor cortex. At the onset of central nervous system disease there is an infiltration by inflammatory cells that may be predominantly neutrophilic or be nonsuppurative and composed of lymphocytes and macrophages. Neuronal death and lysis are characteristic and are marked by neuronophagic nodules formed by focal accumulations of neutrophils early and mononuclear cells later. Surviving neurons may contain small, acidophilic intranuclear inclusions (Cowdry type B inclusions). Well-developed cases show lymphocytic perivascular cuffs, atrophy of affected gray matter areas with diminished numbers of large motor neurons, degeneration of related motor nerves, and atrophy of innervated muscles (Jortner and Percy, 1978). Serologic testing and/or necropsy evaluation can confirm the diagnosis. The introduction of the disease via a nonhuman or human primate carrier should be assessed. As in humans, preventive measures via vaccination can be instituted.

E. Traumatic Head Injury

Traumatic head injury in the nonhuman primate is most likely to result from falls, fighting, handling mishaps, or by experimental design. The subsequent damage to nervous tissue may take a number of forms (Hardman, 1991; Adams et al., 1983). Focal brain damage includes laceration, contusions, and intracranial hematoma. Diffuse brain damage can take the form of diffuse axonal injury or diffuse brain swelling.

Cerebral concussion is characterized by immediate and temporary loss of consciousness. It typically results from a blow to the head. It is important to realize, however, that an actual blow is not necessary to cause a concussion. The key occurrence is a jarring of the head, which may be accomplished by sudden acceleration/deceleration or rapid rotation of the head (Boll and

Barth, 1983). The duration of unconsciousness foretells the severity of injury (Adams et al., 1983; Gennarelli et al., 1982; Gennarelli, 1983).

A contusion is a bruise on the surface of the tissue. Contusions result when the brain shifts within the bony skull, coming into contact with the bony protuberances in the base of the skull or merely impacting the walls of the skull. An early concept of coup (contusions directly below the point of impact) and contrecoup (contusions on the side of the brain opposite the point of impact) injuries holds that frontal impacts usually produce coup lesions only, impacts to the back of the head usually produce both coup and contre-coup lesions, and impacts to the side of the head produce coup or contre-coup lesions with equal probability (Omaya et al., 1971). A more recent interpretation of coup/contre-coup phenomena says that coup lesions occur when the free mobile head is motionless at the moment of impact whereas contre-coup lesions occur when the free mobile head is accelerating and impacts against a stationary firm surface (Dawson et al., 1980).

A laceration is a mechanical tearing of tissue. It may occur if there is fracture or penetration of the bone surrounding the brain. However, if the brain, a jarring force of sufficient magnitude can produce lacerations without an accompanying skull fracture (Hardman, 1991).

Intracranial hematoma includes hemorrhage into the epidural space, the subdural space, and within the brain tissue (Hardman, 1991; Adams et al., 1983; Gennarelli, 1983). Not surprisingly, intracranial hemorrhage, to a greater or lesser degree, is found in association with lacerations and contusions. Epidural hemorrhage is generally the result of a skull fracture with the subsequent laceration of a meningeal artery. It may be localized or diffuse, slight to massive. Subdural hematoma occurs most commonly in association with a fall, i.e., impact to the nonstationary head. Subdural hematoma is the result of tearing of bridging veins, veins that traverse the space between the dura and the brain tissue.

Diffuse brain swelling is a somewhat enigmatic condition. There are two forms (Hardman, 1991). One form is attributable to brain edema which, in humans, is difficult to cope with clinically and often culminates in death. The second form of diffuse brain swelling appears to be the result of increased blood flow, i.e., hyperemia, and is generally treatable.

Diffuse axonal injury is an unlikely natural event for nonhuman primates as it is considered to be caused almost exclusively by vehicular mechanisms (Gennarelli, 1983). It is worthy of consideration, however, as experimental protocols creating this type of injury occur. In contrast to a fall, where there is short-term acceleration followed by sudden deceleration on impact with an unyielding surface, diffuse axonal injury results when acceleration is prolonged and deceleration is less than sudden. The deceleration may result from impact with a padded, or otherwise yielding, surface or may not involve impact at all (Gennarelli, 1983). Clinically, diffuse axonal injury is associated with prolonged unconsciousness. The neuropathology includes widespread axonal damage, presumably the result of shear forces created by acceleration–deceleration movements (Adams *et al.,* 1983; Gennarelli *et al.,* 1982; Boll and Barth, 1983).

F. Malformations

The incidence of congenital malformations of any type in nonhuman primates is not well documented. It follows then that the incidence of central nervous system malformations is equally poorly documented. The available literature, however, supports the presumption that the overall incidence of congenital malformations is low, on the order of 1%, making the incidence of central nervous system malformations even lower (Jerome, 1987; Wilson and Gavan, 1967; Wilson, 1978; Hendrickx and Binkerd, 1980, 1990; Hendrickx *et al.,* 1983; Hendrickx and Prahalada, 1986). Regardless, there are good reasons to be sensitive to the occurrence of central nervous system malformations. In terms of colony management, the possible genetic implications of some malformations may significantly impact the development and conduct of a breeding program. The increasing use of nonhuman primates in developmental and reproductive toxicity testing is making the maintenance of accurate colony historical incidence records highly desirable (Hendrickx and Binkerd, 1990; Korte *et al.,* 1987). Finally, there is the potential for the development of useful nonhuman models of human conditions (Hendrickx *et al.,* 1980; Hendrickx and Tarara, 1990; Tarara *et al.,* 1988).

The term "congenital malformation" means that the condition was present at birth. It does not imply a hereditary cause or any other cause. Malformations may be broadly classified as primary or secondary. Primary malformations are the result of an intrinsically abnormal developmental process. Secondary malformations are the result of an originally normal developmental process that has been perturbed by some outside influence. From another viewpoint, an etiologic classification of malformations might produce three major categories: malformations resulting from exogenous factors, such as infectious agents, radiation, chemicals, or drugs; malformations resulting from genetic or chromosomal factors; and malformations resulting from an interaction of both exogenous and genetic/chromosomal factors.

It is neither necessary nor desirable to produce a long listing of terms and definitions relating to nervous system malformations. There are readily available texts that provide such information (Escourolle and Poirier, 1973; Norman and Ludwin, 1991). There are also a number of references that detail the normal embryologic development of the nervous system in humans (Jacobsen, 1978; Purves and Lichtman, 1985). Unfortunately, literature regarding the neuroembryology of nonhuman primates is decidedly more fragmented (Hendrickx and Prahalada, 1986).

G. Epilepsy

Epilepsy is a condition of multiple and diverse etiologies that is characterized by attacks of unconsciousness, convulsions, or both and is sometimes associated with mental disturbances. An etiologic classification could include trauma, chemical toxicity, infectious agents, and genetic predisposition (spontaneous epilepsy). In humans, prevalence figures of 0.5–1.0% have been cited (Shorvon, 1992). Spontaneous generalized epilepsies are uncommon in the general population of subhuman primates, but the widely publicized condition in baboons is worthy of review. In addition, a seizure disorder originally referred to as amaurotic epilepsy is a good example of a chemical toxicity resulting from environmental contamination that has practical colony management/clinical implications. Seizures in nonhuman primates secondary to infectious disease to traumatic injury can be taken at face value and will not be considered in this discussion.

Primary generalized epilepsy in humans is characterized by diffuse rather than localized electroencephalogram (EEG) manifestations, likely genetic predisposition, and lack of a detectable structural central nervous system lesion. Light flickering at a frequency of about 15 flashes per second will precipitate a seizure in a substantial number of patients (Niedermeyer, 1990). The occurrence in an estimated 80–90% of Senegalese baboons (*Papio papio*) of a generalized seizure disorder precipitated by intermittent light stimulation was discovered in 1966 (Killam, 1979). This genetically transmitted disorder is an important model for the study of primary generalized epilepsy in humans. Since 1966, at least one other species of baboon (*P. cynocephalus*) has been reported to have a similar photosensitivity (Corcoran *et al.,* 1979). In *P. papio,* light flickering at frequencies of 20–25 Hz induces a characteristic set of EEG abnormalities associated with generalized tonic–clonic seizures (Killam, 1979; Wada and Naquet, 1986). Extensive study has shown that the degree of photosensitivity varies with sex and age (Wada and Naquet, 1986). Females are more often affected than males and no adverse responses to flickering light are expected before 5–6 months of age. It has also been reported that a small minority of *P. papio* have spontaneous recurrent seizures in the absence of predisposing intermittent light stimulation (Wada *et al.,* 1972). No anatomic or biochemical abnormality has been identified that would explain this photosensitive epilepsy in baboons.

In the 1930s, a disease called acute amaurotic epilepsy, characterized clinically by convulsions, blindness, and sudden death, was described in zoo-maintained nonhuman primates (Zook *et al.,* 1972a). Since that time there have been other reports of similar conditions and it is now known to be caused by lead poisoning. The clinical and histologic findings have been reviewed (Zook *et al.,* 1972a,b; Zook and Paasch, 1980). Briefly, clinical signs include convulsions, apparent blindness, and paralysis/paresis. Histologic findings include neuronal degeneration, gliosis, demyelination, and vascular degeneration. Additional diagnostic measures include analysis of blood and/or tissue lead levels. Blood levels that exceed 0.6 ppm and/or tissue levels from 1 to 10 mg/kg are considered to be indicative of lead toxicity (Galey *et al.,* 1990; Van Alstine *et al.,* 1993). It should be remembered that 70% of the lead in blood is adherent to red blood cells (Galey *et al.,* 1990); thus, whole blood rather than serum should be collected. Although fresh or frozen tissue is preferred, formalized tissue (liver and kidney) at times has proven useful in the evaluation of tissue lead levels (Hamir *et al.,* 1995). The source of lead is generally considered to be lead-containing paint on cages. In the past the incidence of lead poisoning in some zoo populations was estimated to be upward of 10% per year. This has likely diminished in the more prominent zoo facilities with increased awareness and recent changes in the percentage lead allowed in paints. In 1972, the maximum allowable percentage of lead in paint was reduced to 0.5%. In (1977) the maximum allowable level was decreased to 0.06% (Morgan *et al.,* 1991). In smaller, older, and/or poorly funded facilities it is a potential problem that should be considered when the appropriate clinical signs arise.

H. Periventricular Leukoencephalomalacia

Periventricular leukoencephalomalacia is relatively common in the human infant cerebrum, consisting of clusters of lipid-containing macrophages admixed with areas of necrosis and fewer numbers of lipid-laden cells with prominent processes. Despite its relatively frequent occurrence (40% of infants less than 1500 g), there is still considerable controversy concerning its pathogenesis (Perlman, 1994). Although previous research suggests that it is associated with perinatal/postnatal hypotension and ischemia, more recent evidence suggests that other factors, including excitotoxic neurotransmitter release, oxidant-induced injury (Perlman, 1994), or hypocarbia (Fujimoto *et al.,* 1994), may be important. One factor that makes evaluation of the condition in the human infant difficult is that the majority of tissues available for examination have variable degrees of autolytic changes.

To date, fetal and infant monkeys are the only animals, other than humans, in which a similar change has been described (Phillips, 1973; Sumi, 1974; Sumi *et al.,* 1973). In the monkey, lipid-laden cells identified electron microscopically include macrophages, immature glial cells, and, in some instances, astrocytes (Sumi, 1979). In studies that compared hypoxic brains of infant monkeys with brains of apparently normal infant monkeys, the brains considered to be hypoxic contained more macrophages and immature glial cells with lipid droplets and were the only brains in which lipid-laden astrocytes were found (Sumi, 1974, 1979). Thus, current evidence suggests that both the number and the cell type involved are of importance in determining the pathological significance of lipid-laden cells in the periventricular region.

I. Lysosomal Storage Disorders

Neuronal lysosomal storage disorders are rarely encountered in the nonhuman primate. However, as noted previously in this chapter, the pathologist/primatologist should be aware of potential storage diseases that may serve as valuable models of human disease. Lysosomal storage disorders, as defined in humans and many nonprimate animals, are many and varied (Jubb and

Palmer, 1993; Becker and Yates, 1991). The common characteristic in these various disorders is the failure of lysosomes to adequately carry out their function of catabolizing sequestered materials. Characteristically, such failure is the result of a genetically determined enzymatic defect that interrupts or otherwise impairs degradative pathways in the lysosome. The result is an accumulation/storage of undigested material within the lysosome. In nervous tissue (and be reminded that storage disorders are by no means restricted to nervous tissue) the classic morphologic presentation of a neuronal storage disorder is the large neuron swollen with accumulated material, reduced Nissl substance, and peripherally displaced nucleus. Ultrastructural changes are characteristic, but not necessarily specific, and include the presence of membranous cytoplasmic bodies (membrane-bound collections of electron-dense material often laminar in appearance).

Storage disorders can be categorized by their chemical nature into four large groups: lipidoses, mucopolysaccharidoses, mucolipidoses, and generalized glycogenoses (Becker and Yates, 1991). Among the lipidoses, a small group of disorders are called, collectively, ceroid lipofuscinosis. The stored material in these disorders is a heterogenous complex classified as a mix of ceroid and lipofuscin. Although intraneuronal lipofuscin is generally considered to be an age-related pigment (see previous section of this chapter), ceroid is generally regarded as a pathologically induced pigment (Hartroft and Porta, 1965). Ceroid lipofuscinosis has been subclassified in humans according to the age of clinical onset (Becker and Yates, 1991).

Ceroid lipofuscinosis is a neuronal storage disorder that has been described in a cynomolgus monkey (Jasty *et al.,* 1984). The estimated age of the monkey was 7 to 8 years. This monkey had been in a laboratory environment for at least 2 years. It was killed as part of its role as a control animal in an experiment. No clinical signs of illness were recorded. Histologically, a wide variety of tissue cells, including neurons in the central nervous system, epithelial cells of choroid plexus, and neuroglial cells in the optic nerve, contained numerous bright eosinophilic intracytoplasmic granules histochemically and ultrastructurally identified as ceroid.

IX. PROMINENT MODELS OF HUMAN DISEASES

A. Movement Disorders

Huntington's disease and Parkinson's disease represent opposite ends of the spectrum of movement disorders associated with basal ganglia dysfunction (DeLong, 1990). Parkinson's disease typifies the hypokinetic disorders that are characterized by difficulty in initiating movements, slowness of voluntary movements, muscular rigidity, and resting tremor. Huntington's disease exemplifies hyperkinetic disorders and is characterized by involuntary movements (dyskinesias) and varying degrees of hypotonia. Nonhuman primate models of movement disorders often have a singular advantage over other animal models in that, in addition to simply modeling the neuropathologic changes, they can present more of the clinical signs typically seen in humans. Thus, clinical improvement afforded by various therapeutic strategies and surgical procedures can be more relevantly assessed.

Huntington's disease, also commonly called Huntington's chorea, was first described by George Huntington in 1872 in a family from Long Island, NY (Rewcastle, 1991). It is a neurodegenerative disease of autosomal dominant inheritance. In 1993, the genetic defect responsible for this disease was identified as a trinucleotide expansion in a novel gene (Albin and Tagle, 1995). It is generally seen at 30 to 50 years of age but 5–10% of cases occur in children. The usual course of the disease is death in 15–20 years from pneumonia, myocardial infarction, or suicide. Clinical signs include progressive choreiform movements and dementia. Choreiform movements are sudden, involuntary muscle movements; quick, jerky, and purposeless. Dementia is a complex clinical syndrome of general mental deterioration. The neuropathology is characterized by neuronal loss and gliosis resulting in atrophy of the basal ganglia, most prominently the caudate nucleus and putamen; the thalamus and cortex are also affected, but to a lesser degree. The textbook presentation of Huntington's disease shows, in coronal sections of the brain, widening of the lateral ventricles from extensive caudate nucleus atrophy. Biochemically, the basal ganglia have reductions of GABA, glutamate, acetylcholine, and other assorted neurotransmitters. Glucose utilization in the caudate nucleus and cortex is reduced.

Primate models of Huntington's disease are based on the hypothesis that the characteristic neuropathology is related to the toxicity of excessive excitatory neurotransmitters, with glutamate being the most prevalent endogenous example. Numerous studies in nonhuman primates using glutamate and other excitatory amino acids, such as kainic acid, ibotenic acid, or quinolinic acid, have demonstrated morphologic, biochemical, and clinical changes similar to those described in humans (DiFiglia, 1990; DeLong 1990; Isacson et al., 1989). An extension of the excitotoxicity hypothesis proposes that the gene alteration associated with Huntington's disease produces a defect in oxidative phosphorylation that sensitizes neurons to the damaging effects of excitatory amino acids. Studies with 3-nitropropionic acid, an irreversible inhibitor of succinate dehydrogenase, show that it can produce striking similarities to the neuropathologic and neurochemical features of Huntington's disease in nonhuman primates (Beal, 1994).

It is worth emphasizing that a significant advantage in the baboon or macaque models of Huntington's disease over models in other species, such as the rat, lies with the ability to produce relevant clinical correlates; specifically, chorea, dystonia, postural asymmetries, and head/orofacial dyskinesias (DiFiglia, 1990).

Parkinson's disease was first described in 1817 (Rewcastle, 1991). The typical clinical presentation includes an expressionless face due to impairment of the facial muscles, general muscle rigidity, slowness in initiating and performing voluntary muscle movements, resting tremor (typified by "pill-rolling" movements of the fingers), preservation of the intellect, and a shuffling (festinating) gait. Onset is usually in the sixth decade. The cause of this disease is unknown, but a combination of genetic and environmental factors are believed to be involved. On gross examination the brain and spinal cord appear normal, but transverse sections through the midbrain show a distinctive loss of pigmentation in the substantia nigra. Microscopically, there is a loss of neuromelanin-pigmented neurons in areas of the brain where such neurons are normally found, such as the substantia nigra. In these areas of neuronal loss there is an astrocytic reaction and neuromelanin can be found lying free in the neuropil or within macrophages. Lewy bodies, seen in surviving neurons, are compact, neurofilamentous, cytoplasmic inclusions of unknown meaning. The classic biochemical alteration is a reduction in dopamine in affected areas, but norepinephrine and serotonin may also be reduced.

The literature contains numerous reviews on the use of 1-methyl-4-phenyl-1,2,3,6-tetrahydropyridine (MPTP) to produce nonhuman primate models of Parkinson's disease (Snyder and D'Amato, 1986; Kaakkola and Teravainen, 1990; Guttman, 1990; Bloem et al., 1990). The mechanism of MPTP neurotoxicity has also been reviewed (Singer and Ramsay, 1990; D'Amato et al., 1986). The first step in the process appears to be the oxidation of MPTP to 1-methyl-4-phenylpyridinium (MPP$^+$) by monoamine oxidase B within astrocytes. The MPP$^+$ is selectively transported into dopaminergic neurons, particularly in the substantia nigra, via the dopamine reuptake system. The accumulation and maintenance of toxic levels of MPP$^+$ are thought to be aided by the presence of neuromelanin, which binds MPP$^+$ and may serve as a depot. Intracellularly, MPP$^+$ is ultimately taken up by mitochondria. The final molecular target of MPP$^+$ is the inhibition of NADH dehydrogenase in the respiratory chain. Although it is true that a wide variety of animals, ranging from nonhuman primates to amphibians, are susceptible to the neurotoxic effects of MPTP, the nonhuman primate remains the only species in which a nearly complete presentation of the clinical, neuropathological, and biochemical features of Parkinson's disease can be consistently produced (Guttman, 1990; Bloem et al., 1990; Kopin and Markey, 1988).

B. Alzheimer's Disease

Alzheimer's disease is the most common cause of dementia in humans (Rewcastle, 1991). Dementia, perhaps contrary to popular belief, is not synonymous with old age. The clinical syndrome of dementia, albeit not always easily defined, consists principally of impairment of recent memory and a generalized decline in the ability to cope with the activities of daily living. It has been estimated that Alzheimer's disease affects about 5% of people over 65 years of age, with a slightly higher incidence in women than in men (Haltia, 1989; Rewcastle, 1991). The disease is insidious in onset; advanced cases are profoundly demented and often bedridden. Several histopathologic changes make up the characteristic constellation of lesions found in Alzheimer's disease: neurofibrillary tangles, neuritic plaques, granulovacuolar degeneration, Hirano bodies, and cerebrovascular amyloidosis (Cork *et al.,* 1987; Rewcastle, 1991; Kordower and Gash, 1986; Selkoe *et al.,* 1987). These changes are appreciated most easily in the cerebral cortex and hippocampus where, in addition, considerable loss of large pyramidal neurons is seen.

Biochemically, choline acetyltransferase and acetylcholinesterase are markedly reduced in the cortex and hippocampus of Alzheimer disease patients (Kordower and Gash, 1986; Price *et al.,* 1984).

Aged nonhuman primates, particularly macaques greater than 20 years of age, can provide structurally relevant, albeit not antigenically identical, models for such principal features of Alzheimer's disease as cerebrovascular amyloidosis and neuritic plaques (Cork *et al.,* 1987; Selkoe *et al.,* 1987; Fraser *et al.,* 1992). Behavioral studies in aged macaques are few, but deficits similar to those seen in Alzheimer patients have been reported (Davis, 1978). Neurochemical correlates to the choline acetyltransferase and acetylcholinesterase reductions, as well as other neurotransmitter abnormalities, seen in Alzheimer's disease are being actively pursued (Cork *et al.,* 1987; Kordower and Gash, 1986; Price *et al.,* 1984).

C. Radiation Myelopathy

It is well documented in the human medical literature that delayed deleterious effects on the central nervous system may be noted following exposure to radiation therapy (Schultheiss *et al.,* 1990; Lampert and Davis, 1964; Malamud *et al.,* 1954; Brown and Kagan, 1980). The incidence correlates positively with total radiation dose, dose per fraction, and length of spinal cord irradiated; it is approximately 1–10% following radiation therapy for nasopharyngeal carcinoma (Mesic, 1981; Tokar, 1979; Hung, 1968). The latent period or time between radiation therapy and onset of clinical signs is highly variable, extending from 3 to 48 months (Schultheiss *et al.,* 1990).

Despite the known sensitivity of the neuron to injury, the vast majority of the parenchymal loss in radiation myelopathy occurs in the white matter. Three basic changes have been identified and are known as type 1, type 2, and type 3 lesions. Type 1 lesions are characterized by white matter malacia and demyelination without significant evidence of vascular damage. Type 2 lesions, in contrast, appear to be primary vascular lesions (telangiectasia, fibrinoid necrosis, thrombosis, focal hemorrhage) with secondary malacia limited to the region with the vasculopathy. Type 3 lesions have features of both type 1 and type 2 lesions, as they are characterized by significant lesions in the vasculature coupled with disseminated white matter malacia and demyelination. Both human and nonhuman primates have a longer latency period with type 2 lesions as compared to type 1 and 3 lesions, suggesting that a similar pathogenesis may be involved in both species (Schultheiss *et al.,* 1988, 1990).

Although rodents and guinea pigs have been utilized extensively in studies on the mechanisms of radiation myelopathy, the longer life span and larger size of nonhuman primates offer several distinct advantages. Their longer life span not only allows studies involving retreatment, but also provides sufficient time for the detection of late manifestations of radiation injury that can be a major problem in the human (Schultheiss *et al.,* 1990). Additionally, the closer approximation of the monkey to the size of a human allows more reliable prediction of the dose response, as compared to smaller laboratory animals (Schultheiss *et al.,* 1990).

D. Transmissible Spongiform Encephalopathies

This group of chronic, progressive, fatal infections of the central nervous system of humans and animals is characterized by a prolonged incubation period—months to years (Gadjusek, 1990)—and the unique nature of the transmissible agent, dubbed the "prion" (a proteinaceous infectious particle without a nucleic acid component), to distinguish it from conventional viruses (Pruisner, 1982). These diseases are also known as "transmissible cerebral amyliodoses" as they are associated with modification of a host precursor protein into insoluble amyloid fibrils (Gajdusek, 1985). Naturally occurring transmissible spongiform encephalopathies in animals include scrapie of sheep and goats, transmissible mink encephalopathy, chronic wasting disease of captive mule deer and elk, and bovine spongiform encephalopathy (Palmer and Collinge, 1992).

Kuru is a prion disease of humans that is characterized by cerebellar ataxia and tremor that progresses to motor incapacity with dysarthria, loss of speech, and death, usually within 1 year after the onset of initial symptoms (Gajdusek, 1990). The incidence of the disease which is confined to New Guinea, was considerable at one time but, after epidemiologic studies traced its transmission to cannibalistic rituals, has markedly decreased (Gajdusek, 1990). Although the current incidence of the disease is extremely low, transmission and pathogenesis studies are still of interest as they can provide valuable information that may pertain to transmissible spongiform encephalopathies in general. Kuru can be transmitted to chimpanzees and New World and Old World monkeys via intracerebral, other parenteral, and oral routes (Gajdusek *et al.,* 1967; Beck *et al.,* 1975; Gibbs and Gadjusek, 1976; Comte-Devolx *et al.,* 1980; Gambarelli *et al.,* 1981). The time required for transmission varies both with the route and with the species of nonhuman primate involved. The basic histological features of neuronal vacuolization, severe astrocytic gliosis that appears to be out of proportion to the degree of nerve cell loss, and a lack of inflammatory response (hence, the designation of "encephalopathy" rather than "encephalitis) are common features between humans and nonhuman primates. However, the clinical signs in nonhuman primates may vary to some degree between species and in comparison with humans due to the varying topographic distribution of the predominant lesions. In humans, the most severe lesion is present in the cerebellum, whereas in monkeys, the most significant changes are present in the cerebrum and basal ganglia (Comte-Devolx *et al.,* 1980; Gambarelli *et al.,* 1981).

Creutzfeldt–Jakob disease (CJD) is another disease of humans that is classified as a transmissible spongiform encephalopathy. The primary feature is presenile dementia, with characteristic features including a rapidly progressive dementia, myoclonus, and marked progressive motor dysfunction with paroxysmal bursts of high-voltage slow waves on EEG (Gajdusek, 1990). The disease is usually fatal in less than 1 year (Brown *et al.,* 1984). Although worldwide in distribution, CJD is rare and, in some cases, has a familial pattern of inheritance. Despite its rarity, it is still cause for considerable concern as human-to-human transmission by various mechanisms has been suspected, including via corneal and dura mater grafts as well as by administration of pituitary-derived human growth hormone (Anonymous, 1987; Brown *et al.,* 1986; Duffy *et al.,* 1974). Additionally, there appears to be an unusually high incidence of CJD in patients who have undergone a previous craniotomy, raising the possibility that brain surgery either affords a mode of entry for the agent or precipitates the disease in patients already carrying a latent infection (Gajdusek, 1990). The latter is particularly concerning when one takes into account the resistance of prions to common methods of sterilization (they can pass through a 200-mm-diameter pore membrane filter, retain stability at temperature ranges of $-70°$ to $80°$ C, and, on lyophilization, are resistant to ultraviolet light, ionizing radiation, and ultrasonication and resist inactivation by formaldehyde, alcohol, ether, chloroform, acetone, hydrogen peroxide, glutaraldehyde, ethylene oxide, iodine, organic iodine disinfectants, quarternary ammonium salts, psoralens, and *cis*-diamine/dichloroplatinum compounds) (Gadjusek, 1990; Baringer *et al.,* 1980). Current recommended methods of inactivation include autoclaving and the use of sodium hydroxide or hypochlorite. Creutzfeldt–Jakob disease can be transmitted via various routes to chimpanzees and New World and Old World monkeys. In monkeys, lesions are predominantly gray matter, whereas in humans, both the gray and the white matter are affected. As is the case with the transmission of kuru, clinical signs vary with the specific anatomical site of the brain involved (Gibbs *et al.,* 1968; Tateishi *et al.,* 1981, 1983; Gadjusek and Gibbs, 1971, 1973; Gajdusek, 1990). At the cellular level, pathologic changes are indistinguishable from those in the natural disease or in experimental kuru.

Studies on nonhuman primates to elucidate the pathogenesis of transmissible spongiform encephalopathies are also of interest in the possible evaluation of some of the pathogenic mechanisms in Alzheimer's disease and aging. In both Alzheimer's disease and aging, amyloid fibrils are found that, although morphologically similar, are immunologically distinct from the amyloid fibrils found with the spongiform encephalopathies. Current research indicates that in the so-called nontransmissible cerebral amyloidoses (Alzheimer's disease and aging), the accumulation of amyloid is associated with interference with axonal transport and/or increased synthesis of precursor protein, whereas in the transmissible cerebral amyloidoses (kuru, CJD), there is release of a membrane-bound precursor into the extracellular space that is thought to be accelerated by defective plasma membranes which, in turn, is induced by prions (Lewis *et al.,* 1988; Lampert *et al.,* 1971).

E. Human Immunodeficiency Virus Encephalitis

It has been reported that as many as 80% of patients infected by the human immunodeficiency virus (HIV) and having acquired immunodeficiency syndrome (AIDS) have central nervous system disease at postmortem examination (Petito, 1988). A high percentage, about 50%, of rhesus monkeys experimentally infected with simian immunodeficiency virus (SIV) also develop a characteristic meningoencephalitis that is remarkably similar to that seen in humans with AIDS (King, 1993a). The availability of such a reliable model has clear benefits for investigations of basic mechanisms.

Simian immunodeficiency virus encephalitis comprises multifocal perivascular infiltrates of macrophages and characteristic multinuclear giant cells most commonly in the white matter and less often in the gray matter and leptomeninges. Lesions distribute throughout the cerebrum, cerebellum, brain stem, and spinal cord. Occasional infiltrates may include small numbers of neutrophils and lymphocytes. A mild loss of myelin may be found at the periphery of some lesions (King, 1993a; Letvin and King, 1990; Desrosiers, 1990; Sharer *et al.,* 1988).

There are several different SIV isolates from various species of nonhuman primates and all are classified in the subfamily Lentiviridae of the family Retroviridae similarly to HIV-2, the etiologic agent of human AIDS. Although the genomes of the various SIV isolates have considerable homology with HIV, not all consistently produce AIDS-like disease in all nonhuman primate species. Naturally occurring SIV infections have been reported in a number of African nonhuman primate species, but these are without clinically apparent disease. In Asian macaques, however, experimental SIV infection does produce an AIDS-like disease with SIV-inoculated rhesus monkeys being the most consistent model (King, 1993a).

REFERENCES

Adams, J. H., Graham, D. I., and Gennarelli, T. A. (1983). Head injury in man and experimental animals: Neuropathology. *Acta Neurochir. Suppl.* **32,** 15–30.

Albin, R. L., and Tagle, D. A. (1995). Genetics and molecular biology of Huntington's disease. *Trends Neurosci.* **18,** 11–14.

Allmond, B. W., Froeschle, J. E., and Guilloud, N. B. (1967). Paralytic poliomyelitis in large laboratory primates. *Am. J. Epidemiol.* **85,** 229–239.

Anderson, O. C. and McClure, H. M. (1993). Listeriosis. *In* "Nonhuman Primates. I. Monographs on the Pathology of Laboratory Animals" (T. C.

Jones, U. Mohr, and R. D. Hunt, eds.), pp. 135–141. Springer-Verlag, New York.

Anonymous (1987). Rapidly progressive dementia in a patient who received a cadaveric dura mater graft. *Morbid. Mortal. Wkly. Rep.* **36,** 49–50.

Austin, J. H., and Sakai, M. (1972). Corpora amylacea. *In* "Pathology of the Nervous System" (J. Minkler, ed.), Vol. 3, p. 2961. McGraw-Hill, New York.

Baringer, J. R., Gajdusek, D. C., Gibbs, C. J., Jr., Masters, C. L., Stern, W. E., and Terry, R. D. (1980). Transmissible dementias: Current problems in tissue handling. *Neurology* **30,** 302–303.

Baskin, G. B. (1987). Disseminated cytomegalovirus infection in immunodeficient rhesus monkeys. *Am. J. Pathol.* **129,** 345–352.

Baskin, G. B. (1993). Cytomegalovirus infection in nonhuman primates. *In* "Monographs on the Pathology of Laboratory Animals: Nonhuman Primates" (T. C. Jones, U. Mohr, and R. D. Hunt, eds.), Vol. 1, pp. 32–37. Springer-Verlag, New York.

Beal, M. F. (1994). Neurochemistry and toxin models in Huntington's disease. *Cur. Opin. Neurol.* **7,** 542–547.

Beck, E., Bak, I. J., Christ, J. F., Gajdusek, D. C., Gibbs, C. J., Jr., and Hassler, R. (1975). Experimental kuru in the spider monkey: Histopathological and ultrastructural studies of the brain during early stages of incubation. *Brain* **98,** 595–612.

Becker, L. E., and Yates, A. J. (1991). Inherited metabolic disease. *In* "Textbook of Neuropathology" (R. L. Davis and D. M. Robertson, eds.), 2nd ed. pp. 331–427. Williams & Wilkins, Baltimore.

Benjamin, A. M., Okamoto, K., and Quanstel, J. H. (1978). Effects of ammonium ions on spontaneous action potentials and on contents of sodium, potassium, ammonium and chloride ions in brain in vitro. *J. Neurochem.* **30,** 131.

Betz, A. L., Goldstein, G. W., and Katzmann, R. (1989). Blood-brain-cerebrospinal fluid barriers. *In* "Basic Neurochemistry: Molecular, Cellular, and Medical Aspects" (G. J. Siegel, ed.), 4th ed., pp. 591–606. Raven Press, New York.

Blackwood, W. (1976). Normal structure and general pathology of the nerve cell and neuroglia. *In* "Greenfield's Neuropathology" (W. Blackwood and J. A. N. Corsellis, eds.), pp. 1–42. Yearbook Medical Publ., Chicago.

Bloem, B. R., Irwin, I., Buruma, O. J., Haan, J., Roos, R. A., Tetrud, J. W., and Langston, J. W. (1990). The MPTP model: Versatile contributions to the treatment of idiopathic Parkinson's disease. *J. Neurol. Sci.* **97,** 273–293.

Boll, T. J., and Barth, J. A. (1983). Mild head injury. *Psychiat. Dev.* **3,** 263–275.

Brightman, M. W., and Tao-Cheng, J. H. (1988). Cell membrane interactions between astocytes and brain endothelium. *In* "The Biochemical Pathology of Astrocytes" (M. D. Norenberg, L. Hertz, and A. Schousboe, eds.), p. 21. Liss, New York.

Brown, P., Rodgers-Johnson, P., Gajdusek, D. C., and Gibbs, C. F., Jr. (1984). Creutzfeldt-Jakob disease of long duration: Clinical-pathological characteristics, transmissibility, and different diagnosis. *Ann. Neurol.* **16,** 295–304.

Brown, P., Cathala, F., Sadowsky, D., and Gajdusek, D. C. (1986). Creutzfeldt-Jakob disease in France: Clinical characteristics of 124 consecutive verified cases during the decade 1968–1977. *Ann. Neurol.* **6,** 547–551.

Brown, W. J., and Kagan, A. R. (1980). Comparison of myelopathy associated with megavoltage irradiation and remote cancer. *In* "Radiation Damage to the Nervous System" (H. A. Gilbert and A. R. Kagan, eds.), pp. 191–206. Raven Press, New York.

Bunge, M. B., Bunge, R. P., and Pappas, G. D. (1962). Electron microscopic demonstrations of connections between glia and myelin sheaths in the developing mammalian CNS. *J. Cell Biol.* **12,** 448–453.

Cavanagh, J. B. (1964). The significance of the "dying back" process in human and experimental neurological diseases. *Int. Rev. Exp. Pathol.* **3,** 219–267.

Clark, R. G. (1975). "Essentials of Clinical Neuroanatomy and Neurophysiology." Davis, Philadelphia.

Compston, A., Scolding, N., Wren, D., and Noble, M. (1991). The pathogenesis of demyelinating disease: Insights from cell biology. *Trends Neurosci.* **14,** 175–182.

Comte-Devolx, J., Vuillon-Cacciuttolo, G., Balzama, E., Bert., J., Gambarelli, D., de Micco, P., and Tamalet, J. (1980). Experimental kuru in the Rhesus monkey: A clinical study. *J. Med. Primatol.* **9,** 28–38.

Corcoran, M. E., Cain, D. P., and Wada, J. A. (1979). Photically induced seizures in the yellow baboon, *Papio cynocephalus. Can. J. Neurol. Sci.* **6,** 129–131.

Cork, L. C., Kitt, C. A., Struble, R. G., Griffin, J. W., and Price, D. L. (1987). Animal models of degenerative neurological disease. *Prog. Clin. Biol. Res.* **229,** 241–269.

D'Amato, R. J., Lipman, Z. P., and Snyder, S. H. (1986). Selectivity of the Parkinsonian neurotoxin MPTP: Toxic metabolite MPP$^+$ binds to neuromelanin. *Science* **231,** 987–989.

Davis, R. T. (1978). Old monkey behavior. *Exp. Gerontol.* **13,** 237–250.

Dawson, S. L., Hirsh, C. S., Lucas, F. V., and Sebek, B. A. (1980). The contrecoup phenomenon. Reappraisal of a classic problem. *Hum. Pathol.* **11,** 155–166.

DeLong, M. R. (1990). Primate models of movement disorders of basal ganglia origin. *Trends Neurosci.* **13,** 281–285.

Del Rio-Hortega, P. (1918). Noticia de neuvo y facil metodo para la coloracion de la neuroglia y del tijido conjunctivo. *Trab. Lab. Invest. Biol.* **15,** 367.

Del Rio-Hortega, P. (1919). El tercer elemento de los centros nerviosos. i. La microglia en estado normal. ii. Intervencion de la microglia en los procesos pathologicos. iii. Naruraleza probable de la microglia. *Bol. Soc. Es. Biol.* **9,** 69.

Del Rio-Hortega, P. (1921). La glia de escasas radiaciones (oligodendroglia). *Bo. R. Soc. Esp. His. Na.* **21,** 63.

Desrosiers, R. C. (1990). The simian immunodeficiency viruses. *Annu. Rev. Immunol.* **8,** 557–578.

Dickson, D. W., Mattiace, L. A., Kure, K., Hutchins, K., Lyman, W. B., and Brosnan, C. (1991). Microglia in human disease, with an emphasis on acquired immune deficiency syndrome. *Lab. Invest.* **64,** 135–156.

DiFiglia, M. (1990). Excitotoxic injury of the neostriatum: A model for Huntington's disease. *Trends Neurosci.* **13,** 286–289.

Dolman, C. L. (1991). Microglia. *In* "Textbook of Neuropathology" (R. L. Davis and D. M. Robertson, eds.), pp. 141–163. Williams & Wilkins, Baltimore.

Duffy, P., Wolf, J., Collins, G., DeVoe, A. G., Steeten, B., and Cowen, D. (1974). Possible person-to-person transmission of Creutzfeldt-Jakob disease. *N. Engl./J. Med.* **229,** 692–693.

Escourolle, R., and Poirier, J. (1973). "Manual of Basic Neuropathology." Saunders, Philadelphia.

Fox, J. G. and Rohovsley, M. W. (1975). Meningitis caused by *Klebsiella sp.* in two rhesus monkeys. *JAVMA* **167,** 634–636.

Fraser, P. E., Ngyuen, J. T., Inouye, H., Surewicz, W. K., Selkoe, D. J., Podlisny, M. B., and Kirschner, D. A. (1992). Fibril formation by primate, rodent, and Dutch-hemorrhagic analogues of Alzheimer amyloid β-protein. *Biochemistry* **31,** 10716–10723.

Frei, K., Bodmer, S., Schwerdel, C., and Fonatana, A. (1987). Astrocyte-derived interleukin 3 as a growth factor for microglia cells and peritoneal macrophages. *J. Immunol.* **137,** 3521–3527.

Fujimoto, S., Togari, H., Yamaguchi, N., Mizutani, F., Suzuki, S., and Sobajima, H. (1994). Hypocarbia an cystic periventricular leukomalacia in premature infants. *Arch. Dis. Child.* **71,** F107–F110.

Gadjusek, D. C. (1985). Hypothesis: Interference with axonal transport of neurofilament as a common pathogenetic mechanism in certain diseases of the central nervous system. *N. Engl. J. Med.* **312,** 714–719.

Gadjusek, D. C. (1990) Subacute spongiform encephalopathies: Transmissible cerebral amyloidoses caused by unconventional viruses. *In* "Virology" (N. F. Fields and D. M. Knipe, eds.), 2nd ed., pp. 2289–2324. Raven Press, New York.

Gadjusek, D. C., and Gibbs, C. J., Jr. (1971) Transmission of the two subacute spongiform encephalopathies of man (kuru and Creutzfeldt-Jakob disease) to New World monkeys. *Nature (London)* **230,** 588–591.

Gadjusek, D. C., and Gibbs, C. J., Jr. (1973). Subacute and chronic diseases caused by atypical infections with unconventional viruses in aberrant hosts. *Perspect. Virol.* **8**, 279–311.

Gajdusek, D. C., Gibbs, C. J., Jr., and Alpers, M. P. (1967). Transmission and passage of experimental "kuru" to chimpanzees. *Science* **155**, 212–214.

Galey, F. D., Slenning, B. D., Anderson, M. L., Breneman, P. C., Littlefield, E. S., Melton, L. A., and Tracy, M. L. (1990). Lead concentrations in blood and milk from periparturient dairy heifers seven months after an episode of acute lead toxicosis. *J. Vet. Diagn. Invest.* **2**, 222–226.

Gambarelli, D., Vuillon-Cacciuttolo, G., Toga, M., and Bert, J. (1981). Anatomical study of experimental kuru in the rhesus monkey. *Acta Neuropathol.* **53**, 337–341.

Gennarelli, T. A., (1983). Head injury in man and experimental animals: Clinical aspects. *Acta Neurochir. Suppl.* **32**. 1–13.

Gennarelli, T. A., Thibaultt, L. E., Adams, J. H., Graham, D. I., Thompson, C. J., and Marcincin, R. P. (1982). Diffuse axonal injury and traumatic coma in the primate. *Ann. Neurol.* **12**, 564–574.

Gibbs, C. J., Jr. and Gajdusek, D. C. (1976). Studies on the viruses of subacute spongiform encephalopathies using primates, their only available indicator. *In* "Inter-American Conference on Conservation and Utilization of American Non-human Primates in Biomedical Research," pp.83–109. Pan American Health Organization, Washington, DC.

Gibbs, C. J., Jr., Gajdusek, D. C., Asher, D. M., and Alpers, M. P. (1968). Creutzfelt-Jakob disease (subacute spongiform encephalopathy): Transmission to the chimpanzee. *Science* **161**, 388–389.

Goldstein, G. W., and Betz, L. A. (1986). The blood-brain barrier. *Sci. Am.,* September, pp. 74–83.

Gribble, D. H., Haden, C. C., Schwartz, L. W., and Henrickson, R. V. (1975). Spontaneous multifocal leukoencephalopathy (PML) in macaques. *Nature (London)* **254**, 602–604.

Griffin, J. W., (1990). Basic pathologic processes in the nervous system. *Toxicol. Pathol.* **18**, 83–88.

Griffin, J. W., and Watson, D. F. (1988). Axonal transport in neurological disease. *Ann. Neurol.* **23**, 3–13.

Guttman, M. (1990). MPTP-induced parkinsonism. *In* "Functional Imaging in Movement Disorders" (W. R. W. Martin, ed.), pp. 131–140. CRC Press, Boca Raton, FL.

Haltia, M. (1989). The hard core of Alzheimer's disease. *Ann. Med.* **21**, 67–68.

Hamir, A. N., Galligan, D. T., Ebel, J. G., Manzell, K. L., Niu, H. S., and Rupprecht, C. E. (1995). Lead concentrations in frozen and formalin-fixed tissues from raccoons (*Procyon lotor*) administered oral lead acetate. *J. Vet. Diagn. Invest.* **7**, 580–582.

Hardman, J. M. (1991). Cerebrospinal trauma. *In* "Textbook of Neuropathology" (R. L. Davis and D. M. Robertson, eds.), pp. 962–1003. Williams & Wilkins, Baltimore.

Hartroft, W. S., and Porta, E. A. (1965). Ceroid. *Am. J. Med. Sci.* **250**, 325–345.

Hendrickx, A. G. and Binkerd, P. E. (1980). Fetal deaths in non-human primates *In* "Embryonic and Fetal Death" (I. H. Porter and E. B. Hook, eds.), pp 45–69. Academic Press, New York.

Hendrickx, A. G., and Binkerd, P. E. (1990). Nonhuman primates and teratological research. *J. Med. Primatol.* **19**, 81–108.

Hendrickx, A. G., and Prahalada, S. (1986). Teratology and embryogenesis. *In* "Comparative Primate Biology" (W. R. Dukelow and J. Erwin, eds.), Vol. 3, pp. 333–362. Liss, New York.

Hendrickx, A. G., and Tarara, R. (1990). Triamcinolone acetonide induced meningocele and meningoencephalocele in rhesus monkeys. *Am. J. Pathol.* **136**, 725–727.

Hendrickx, A. G., Pellegrini, M., Tarara, R., Parker, R., Silverman, S., and Steffeck, A. J. (1980). Craniofacial and central nervous system malformations induced by triamcinolone acetonide in nonhuman primates. I. General teratogenicity. *Teratology* **22**, 103–114.

Hendrickx, A. G., Binkerd, P. E., and Rowland, J. M. (1983). Developmental toxicity and nonhuman primates: Interspecies comarisons. *In* "Issues and Reviews in Teratology" (H. Kalter, ed.), Vol. 1, pp. 149–180. Plenum, New York.

Hirano, A. (1991). Neurons and astrocytes. *In* "Textbook of Neuropathology" (R. L. Davis and D. M. Robertson, eds.), 2nd ed., pp. 1–94. Williams & Wilkins, Baltimore.

Hoffman, P. N., Thompson, G., Griffin, J. W., and Price, D. L. (1985). Changes in neurofilament transport coincide temporarily with alterations in the caliber of axons in regenerating motor fibers. *J. Cell Biol.* **101**, 1332–1340.

Holman, R. C., Janssen, R. S., Buehler, J. W., Zelasky, M. T., and Hooper, W. C. (1991). Epidemiology of progressive multifocal leukoencephalopathy in the United States: Analysis of national mortality and AIDS surveillance data. *Neurology* **41**, 1733–1736.

Hung, T. P. (1968). Myelopathy following radiotherapy of nasopharyngeal carcinoma. *Proc. Aust. Assoc. Neurol.* **5**, 421–428.

Hunt, R. D. (1993). *Herpes Simplex* infection. *In* "Nonhuman Primates. I. Monographs on the Pathology of Laboratory Animals" (T. C. Jones, U. Mohr, and R. D. Hunt, eds.) pp. 82–86. Springer-Verlag, New York.

Isacson, O., Riche, D., Hantraye, P., Sofroniew, M. V., and Maziere, M. (1989). A primate model of Huntington's disease: Cross-species implantation of striatal precursor cells to the excitotoxically lesioned baboon caudate-putamen. *Exp. Brain Res.* **75**, 213–220.

Iversen, L. L. (1979). The chemistry of the brain. *Sci. Am.,* September, pp. 134–149.

Jacobsen, M. (1978). "Developmental Neurobiology," 2nd ed., Plenum, New York.

Jasty, V., Kowalksi, R. L., Fonseca, E. H., Porter, M. C., Glemens, G. R., Bare, J. J., and Harnagel, R. E. (1984). An unusual case of generalized ceroid-lipofuscinosis in a cynomolgus monkey. *Vet. Pathol.* **21**, 46–50.

Jerome, C. P. (1987). Congenital malformations and twinning in abreeding colony of old world monkeys. *Lab. Anim. Sci.* **37**, 624–630.

Johnson, P. C. (1991). Peripheral nerve. *In* "Textbook of Neuropathology" (R. L. Davis and D. M. Robertson, eds.), 2nd ed., pp. 1004–1088. Williams & Wilkins, Baltimore.

Jordan, F. L., and Thomas, W. E. (1988). Brain macrophages: Questions of origin and interrelationships. *Brain Res. Rev.* **13**, 165–178.

Jortner, B. S., and Percy, D. H. (1978). The nervous system. *In* "Pathology of Laboratory Animals" (K. Benirschke, F. M. Garner, and T. C. Jones, eds.), Vol 1, pp. 344–347. Springer-Verlag, New York.

Jubb, K. V. F., and Palmer, N. (1993). The nervous system. *In* "Pathology of Domestic Animals" (K. V. F. Jubb, P. C. Kennedy, and N. Palmer, eds.), 4th ed., Vol. 1, pp. 267–440. Academic Press, San Diego, CA.

Kaakkola, S., and Teravainen, H. (1990) Animal models of parkinsonism. *Pharmacol. Toxicol.* **67**, 95–100.

Katsuki, H., and Okuda, S. (1995). Arachidonic acid as a neurotoxic and neurotrophic substance. *Prog. Neurobiol.* **46**, 607–636.

Killam, E. K. (1979). Photomyoclonic seizures in the baboon, *Papio papio. Fed Proc., Fed. Am. Soc. Exp. Biol.* **38**, 2429–2433.

Kimelberg, H. K., and Norenberg, M. D. (1989). Astrocytes. *Sci. Am.,* April, pp. 66–76.

King, N. W. (1993a). Simian immunodeficiency virus infection. *In* "Nonhuman Primates I. Monographs on the Pathology of Laboratory Animals" (T. C. Jones, U. Mohr, and R. D. Hunt, eds.), pp. 5–20. Springer-Verlag, New York.

King, N. W. (1993b). Simian virus 40 infection. *In* "Nonhuman Primates. I. Monographs on the Pathology of Laboratory Animals" (T. C. Jones, U. Mohr, and R. D. Hunt, eds.), pp. 37–42. Springer-Verlag, New York.

King, N. W., Hunt, R. D., and Letvin, N. L. (1983). Histopathologic changes in macaques with an acquired immunodeficiency syndrome (AIDS). *Am. J. Pathol.* **113**, 382–388.

Koo, E. H., Hoffman, P. N., and Price, D. L. (1988). Levels of neurotransmitter and cytoskeletal mRNAs during nerve regeneration in sympathetic ganglia. *Brain Res.* **449**, 361–363.

Kopin, I. J., and Markey, S. P. (1988). MPTP toxicity: Implications for research in Parkinson's disease. *Annu. Rev. Neurosci.* **11**, 81–96.

Kordower, J. H., and Gash, D. M. (1986). Animals and experimentation: An evaluation of animal models of Alzheimer's and Parkinson's disease. *Integr. Psychiatry* **4**, 64–80.

Korte, R., Vogel, F., and Osterburg, I. (1987). The primate as a model of hazard assessement of teratorgens in human. *Arch. Toxicol. Suppl.* **11**, 115–121.

Lampert, P. W. (1969). Mechanism of demyelination in experimental allergic neuritis. *Lab. Invest.* **20**, 127–138.

Lampert, P. W., and Davis, R. L. (1964). Delayed effects of radiation on the human central nervous system. *Neurology* **14**, 912–917.

Lampert, P. W., Hooks, J., Gibbs, C. J., Jr., and Gajdusek, D. C. (1971). Altered plasma membranes in experimental scrapie. *Acta Neuropathol.* **19**, 80–93.

Leestma, J. E. (1991). Viral infections of the nervous system. *In* "Textbook of Neuropathology" (R. L. Davis and D. M. Robertson, eds.), 2nd ed., pp. 804–903. Williams & Wilkins, Baltimore.

Letvin, N. L., and King, N. W. (1990). Immunologic and pathologic manifestations of the infection of rhesus monkeys with simian immunodeficiency virus of macaques. *J. Acquired Immune Defic. Syndr.* **3**, 1023–1040.

Lewis, D. A., Higgins, G. A., Young, W. G., Goldgaber, D., Gadjusek, D. C., Wilson, M. C., and Morrison, J. H. (1988). Distribution of precursor amyloid-beta-protein messenger RNA in human cerebral cortex: Relationship to neurofibrillary tangles and neuritic plaques. *Proc. Natl. Acad. Sci. U.S.A.* **85**, 1691–1695.

Ludwin, S. K., and Bakker, D. A. (1988). Can oligodendrocytes attached to myelin proliferate? *J. Neurosci.* **8**, 1239–1244.

Lynn, E. R., Perry, V. H., Brown, M. C., Rosen, H., and Gordon, S. (1989). Absence of Wallerian degeneration does not hinder regeneration in peripheral nerve. *Eur. J. Neurosci.* **1**, 27–33.

Malamud, N., Boldrey, E. B., Welch, W. K., and Fadell, E. J. (1954). Necrosis of brain and spinal cord following X ray therapy. *J. Neurosurg.* **11**, 353–362.

Martinez-Hernandez, A., Bell, K. P., and Norenberg, M. D. (1977). Glutamine synthetase: Glial localization in brain. *Science* **195**, 1356–1358.

McComb, J. D., and Davis, R. L. (1991). Choroid plexus, cerebrospinal fluid, hydrocephalus, cerebral edema, and herniation phenomena. *In* "Textbook of Neuropathology" (R. L. Davis and D. M. Robertson, eds.), 2nd ed., pp. 175–206. Williams & Wilkins, Baltimore.

McIntosh, T. K., Smith, D. H., Meaney, D. F., Kotapka, M. J., Gennarelli, T. A., and Graham, D. I. (1996). Neuropathological sequelae of traumatic brain injury: Relationship to neurochemical and biomechanical mechanisms. *Lab. Invest.* **74**, 315–342.

Mesic, J. B. (1981). Megavoltage radiation of epithelial tumors of the nasopharynx. *Int. J. Radia. Oncol. Biol. Phys.* **7**, 447–453.

Morgan, R. V., Moore, F. M., Pearce, L. K., and Rossi, T. (1991). Clinical and laboratory findings in small companion animals with lead poisoning: 347 cases (1977–1986). *J. Am. Vet. Med. Assoc.* **199**, 93–97.

Nag, S. (1991). The ependyma and choriod plexus. *In* "Textbook of Neuropathology" (R. L. Davis and D. M. Robertson, eds.), 2nd ed., pp. 95–114. Williams & Wilkins, Baltimore.

Niedermyer, E. (1990). "The Epilepsies" Urban and Schwarzenberg, Baltimore.

Norman, M. G., and Ludwin, S. K. (1991). Congenital malformations of the nervous system. *In* "Textbook of Neuropathology" (R. L. Davis and D. M. Robertson, eds.), 2nd ed., pp. 207–280. Williams & Wilkins, Baltimore.

Olson, L. C., Skinner, S. F., Palotay, J. L. and McGhee, G. E. (1986). Encephalitis associated with *Trypanosome cruzi* in a celebes black macaque. *Lab. Anim. Sci.* **36**, 667–670.

Omaya, A., Grubb, R. L., Jr., and Naumann, R. A. (1971). Coup and contrecoup injury: Observations on the mechanics of visible brain injuries in the rhesus monkey. *J. Neurosurg.* **35**, 503–516.

Palmer, M. S., and Collinge, J. (1992). Human prion diseases. *Curr. Opin. Neurol. Neurosurg.* **5**, 895–901.

Perlman, J. (1994). Periventricular leukomalacia in the premature infant: Is it preventable? *Ann. Neurol.* **94**, 531.

Perry, V. H., and Gordon, S. (1988). Macrophages and microglia in the nervous system. *Trends Neurosci.* **11**, 273–277.

Peters, A., Palay, S. L., and Webster, H. deF. (1976). "The Fine Structure of the Nervous System: The Neurons and Supporting Cells." Saunders, Philadelphia.

Petito, C. K. (1988). Review of central nervous system pathology in human immunodeficiency virus infection. *Ann. Neurol.* **23**, Suppl., S54–S57.

Phillips, D. E. (1973). An electron microscopic study of macroglia and microglia in the lateral funiculus of the developing spinal cord of the fetal monkey. *Z. Zellforsch. Mikrosk. Anat.* **140**, 145–167.

Price, D. I., Kitt, C. A., Struble, R. G., Whitehouse, P. J., Lehmann, J., Cork, L. C., Mitchell, S. J., and DeLong, M. R. (1984). The basal forebrain cholinergic system in the primate: Effects of aging and Alzheimer's disease. *In* "Alzheimer's Disease: Advances in Basic Research and Therapies" (R. J. Wurtman, S. H. Corkin, and J. H. Growdon, eds.). Center for Brain Sciences and Metabolism Charitable Trust, Cambridge.

Price, D. L., and Porter, K. L. (1970). Response of ventral horn neurons to axonal transection. *J. Cell Biol.* **53**, 24–37.

Price, D. L., Whitehouse, P. J., and Struble, R. G. (1985). Alzheimer's disease. *Annu. Rev. Med.* **36**, 349–356.

Prineas, J. W., Kwon, E. E., Goldenberg, P. Z., Ilyas, A. A., Quarles, R. H., Benjamin, J. A., and Sprinkle, T. J. (1989). Multiple sclerosis. Oligodendrocyte proliferation and differentiation in fresh lesions. *Lab. Invest.* **61**, 489–503.

Pruisner, S. B. (1982). Novel proteinaceous infectious particles cause scrapie. *Science* **216**, 136–144.

Purves, D., and Lichtman, J. W. (1985). "Principles of Neural Development." Sinauer, Sunderland, MA.

Raine, C. S. (1991). Oligodendrocytes and central nervous system myelin. *In* "Textbook of Neuropathology" (R. L. Davis and D. M. Robertson, eds.), 2nd ed., pp. 115–140. Williams & Wilkins, Baltimore.

Raine, C. S., Scheinberg, L., and Waltz, J. M. (1981). Multiple sclerosis. Oligodendrocyte survival and proliferation in an active established lesion. *Lab. Invest.* **45**, 534–546.

Ramsay, D. A., and Robertson, D. M. (1991). Meninges and their reaction to injury. *In* "Textbook of Neuropathology" (R. L. Davis and D. M. Robertson, eds.), 2nd ed., pp. 164–174. Williams & Wilkins, Baltimore.

Ramsey, H. J. (1965). Ultrastructure of corpora amylacea. *J. Neuropathol. Exp. Neurol.* **24**, 25–39.

Rewcastle, N. B. (1991). Degenerative diseases of the central nervous system. *In* "Textbook of Neuropathology" (R. L. Davis and D. M. Robertson, eds.), 2nd ed., pp. 904–961. Williams & Wilkins, Baltimore.

Richardson, E. P., Jr. (1961). Progressive multifocal leucoencephalopathy. *N. Engl. J. Med.* **265**, 815–823.

Schochet, S. S., Jr. (1972). Neuronal incusions. *In* "The Structure and Function of Nervous Tissue" (G. H. Bourne, ed.), Vol. 4, p. 129. Academic Press, New York.

Schultheiss, T. E., Stephens, L. C., and Maor, M. H. (1988). Analysis of the histopathology of radiation myelopathy. *Int. J. Radiat. Oncol. Biol. Phys.* **4**, 27–32.

Schultheiss, T. E., Stephens, C. L., Jiang, G., Ang, K. K., and Peters, L. J. (1990). Radiation myelopathy in primates treated with conventional fractionation. *Int. J. Radiat. Oncol. Biol. Phys.* **19**, 935–940.

Selkoe, D. J., Bell, D. S., Podlisny, M. B., Price, D. L., and Cork, L. C. (1987). Conservation of brain amyloid proteins in aged mammals and humans with Alzheimer's disease. *Science* **235**, 873–877.

Sharer, L. R., Baskin, G. B., Cho, E-S., Murphey-Corb, M., Blumberg, B. M., and Epstein, L. G. (1988). Comparison of simian immunodeficiency virus and human immunodeficiency virus encephalitides in the immature host. *Ann. Neurol.* **23**, Suppl., S108–S112.

Shorvon, S. D. (1992). Epidemiology and etiology of epilepsy. *In* "Diseases of the Nervous System. Clinical Neurobiology" (A. K. Asbury, G. M. McKhann, and W. I. McDonald, eds.), Vol 2, pp. 896–905. Saunders, Philadelphia.

Singer, T. P., and Ramsay, R. R. (1990). Mechanism of neurotoxicity of MPTP: An update. *FEBS Lett.* **274**, 1–8.

Snyder, S. H., and D'Amato, R. J. (1986). MPTP: A neurotoxin relevant to the pathophysiology of Parkinson's disease. *Neurology* **36**, 250–258.

Soifer, D. (1986). Factors regulating the presence of microtublues in cells. *Ann. N. Y. Acad. Sci.* **466**, 1–7.

Solleveld, H. A., van Zwietan, M. J., Heidt, P. J. and van Eerd, P. M. C. A. (1984). Clinicopathologic study of six cases of meningitis and meningencephalitis in chimpanzees. *Lab. Anim. Sci.* **34**, 86–90.

Steele, M. D., Giddens, W. E., Velerio, M., Sumi, S. M., and Stetzer, E. R. (1982). Spontaneous paramyxovival encephalitis in nonhuman primates (*Macaca mulatta* and *M. nemestrina*). *Vet. Pathol.* **19**, 132–139.

Sternberger, N. (1984). Patterns of oligodendrocyte function seen by immunocytochemistry. *Neurochem.* **5**, pp. 125–174.

Stoll, G., Trapp, B. D., and Griffin, J. W. (1989). Macrophage function during Wallerian degeneration of rat optic nerve: Clearance of degenerating myelin and la expression. *J. Neurosci.* **9**, 2327–2335.

Suleman, M. A., Johnson, B. J., Tarara, R., Sayer, P. D., Ochiegn, O. M., Muli, J. M., Mbete, E., Tukei, P. M., Ndirango, D., Kago, S., and Else, J. G. (1984). An outbreak of poliomyelitis causes by poliovirus type I in captive black and white colobus monkeys (*Colobus abyssinicus kikuyuensis*) in Kenya. *Trans. R. Soc. Trop. Med. Hyg.* **78**, 665–669.

Sumi, S. M. (1974). Periventricular leukoencephalopathy in the monkey. *Arch. Neurol. (Chicago)* **31**, 38–44.

Sumi, S. M. (1979). Sudanophilic lipid accumulation in astrocytes in periventricular leukoencephalomalacia in monkeys. *Acta Neuropathol.* **47**, 241–243.

Sumi, S. M., Leech, R. W., Alford, E. C., Jr., Eng, M., and Ureland, K. (1973). Sudanophilic lipids in the unmyelinated primate cerebral white matter after intrauterine hypoxia and acidosis. *Res. Publ. Assoc. Res. Nerv. Ment. Dis.* **51**, 176–197.

Summers, B. A., Cummings, J. F., and deLaHunta, A. (1995). Principles of neuropathology. *In* "Veterinary Neuropathology," pp. 36–39. Mosby, St. Louis, MO.

Tanichi, M., Clark, H. B., Schweitzer, J. B., and Johnson, E. M. (1988). Expression of nerve growth factor receptors by Schwann cells of axotomized peripheral nerves: Ultrastructural location, supression by axonal contact, and binding properties. *J. Neurosci.* **8**, 664–681.

Tarara, R. P., Wheeldon, E. B., and Hendrickx, A. G. (1988). Central nervous system malformations induced by triamcinolone acetonide in nonhuman primates: Pathogenesis. *Teratology* **38**, 259–270.

Tateishi, J., Koga, M., and Mori, R. (1981). Experimental transmission of Creutzfeldt-Jakob disease. *Acta Pathol. Jpn.* **31**, 943–951.

Tateishi, J., Sato, Y., and Ohta, M. (1983). Creutzfeldt-Jakob disease in humans and laboratory animals. *In* "Progress in Neuropathology" (H. M. Zimmerman, ed.), Vol. 5, pp. 195–221. Raven Press, New York.

Tokar, R. P. (1979). Carcinoma of the nasopharynx and optimization of radiotherapeutic management for tumor control and spinal cord injury. *Int. J. Radiat. Oncol. Biol. Phys.* **5**, 1741–1748.

Truex, R. A., and Carpenter, M. B. (1969). "Human Neuroanatomy," 6th ed. Williams & Wilkins, Baltimore.

Van Alstine, W. G., Wickliffe, L. W., Everson, R. J., and DeNicoloa, D. B. (1993). Acute lead toxicosis in a household of cats. *J. Vet. Diagn. Invest.* **5**, 496–498.

Wada, J. A., and Naquet, R. (1986). Experimental model in a primate predisposed to epilepsy. *In* "Intractable Epilepsy" (D. Schmidt and P. I. Morselli, eds.), pp. 39–59. Raven Press, New York.

Wada, J. A., Terao, A., and Booker, H. E. (1972). Longitudinal correlative analysis of epileptic baboon, *Papio papio. Neurology* **22**, 1272–1285.

Weiner, L. P., Johnson, R. T., and Herndon, R. M. (1973). Viral infections and demyelinating diseases. *N. Engl. J. Med.* **288**, 1103–1110.

Wilson, J. G. (1978). Developmental abnormalities: Nonhuman primates. *In* "Pathology of Laboratory Animals" (K. Benrischke, F. M. Garner, and T. C. Jones, eds.), Vol. 2, pp. 1911–1946. Springer-Verlag, New York.

Wilson, J. G., and Gavan, J. A. (1967). Congenital malformations in nonhuman primates: Spontaneous and experimentally induced. *Anat Rec.* **158**, 99–110.

Wisniewski, H. M., Ghetti, B., and Terry, R. D. (1973). Neuritic (senile) plaques and filamentous changes in aged rhesus monkeys. *J. Neuropathol. Exp. Neurol.* **32**, 566–584.

Wong, M. M., and Kozek, W. J. (1974). Spontaneous toxoplasmosis in macaques: A report of four cases. *Lab. Anim. Sci.* **24**, 273–278.

Yang, C., Tsai, P., Lin, N., Liu, L., and Kuo, J. (1995). Elevated extracellular glutamate levels increased the formation of hydroxyl radical in the striatum of anesthetized rat. *Free Radical Biol. Med.* **19**, 453–459.

Zeman, D. H. and Baskin, G. B. (1985). Encephalitozoonosis in squirrel monkeys. *Vet. Pathol.* **22**, 24–31.

Zook, B. C., and Paasch, L. H. (1980). Lead poisoning in zoo primates: Environmental sources and neuropathologic findings. *In* "The Comparative Pathology of Zoo Animals" (R. J. Montali and G. Migaki, eds.), pp. 143–152. Smithsonian Institution Press, Washington, DC.

Zook, B. C., Sauer, R. M., and Garner, F. M. (1972a). Acute amaurotic epilepsy caused by lead poisoning in nonhuman primates. *J. Am. Vet. Med. Assoc.* **161**, 683–686.

Zook, B. C., Sauer, R. M., and Garner, F. M. (1972b). Lead poisoning in captive wild animals. *J. Wildl. Dis.* **8**, 264–272.

Chapter 13

Behavioral Disorders

Kathryn Bayne and Melinda Novak

NONHUMAN PRIMATES IN BIOMEDICAL RESEARCH: DISEASES
ISBN 0-12-088665-0

I. INTRODUCTION

Primates in laboratory environments sometimes display abnormal patterns of behavior. In some cases, these behavior patterns are a symptom of other well-defined diseases or disorders (e.g., shivering and trembling during fever, hand tremors in aged macaques). In other cases, the etiology may relate to organic brain dysfunction and/or to certain environmental conditions. It is this latter kind of behavioral pathology that forms the basis for this chapter. This chapter first characterizes the nature and extent of abnormal behavior and then examines the possible physiological and environmental determinants of behavioral pathology in nonhuman primates. Finally, possible therapeutic interventions and preventative approaches are considered.

Terms such as "behavioral pathology" or "psychopathology" are often used to describe abnormal behavior in nonhuman primates. Because behavioral pathology implies that only the behavior is flawed, psychopathology is preferred because it acknowledges the role that the central nervous system may play in governing the development and maintenance of abnormal activity. However, one should be cautious not to use either of these terms indiscriminately. Abnormal behavior should be considered pathological if it is frequent (i.e., occupying a substantial part of the animal's time budget to the detriment of other activities), disruptive (interfering with biological functions, including eating, breeding, or parental care), or intense (i.e., producing irritation or tissue damage). There are other circumstances in which behavior may be pathological (i.e., if it occurs in an inappropriate context), but these cases may be much more difficult to identify.

Abnormal behavior appears to vary considerably in form and frequency across different primate species. Assessments of hundreds of monkeys at one regional primate research center have revealed that abnormal behavior is more prevalent in macaques than in squirrel monkeys (M. A. Novak, unpublished data). Within the macaque genus, rhesus and cynomolgus monkeys seem to have a greater predilection for developing abnormal behavior than pig-tailed monkeys (Sackett *et al.,* 1981). Abnormal behavior has also been reported in chimpanzees (Berkson and Mason, 1964; Fritz and Fritz, 1979). It should be noted, however, that comparisons of prevalence by species are invariably confounded with factors such as early rearing experiences, housing history, husbandry practices, age, and the frequency with which a given species is maintained in captivity. Inasmuch as both rhesus and cynomolgus macaques are among the most common primates in captivity, it is not surprising that much of what is known about psychopathology in nonhuman primates comes from studies and observations of macaques.

A. Behavioral Pathology: A Description

Abnormal behavior in nonhuman primates often takes the form of stereotypic behavior, i.e., a repetitive, frequently idio-

syncratic, highly ritualized action that does not serve any apparent biological purpose (Berkson, 1967; Ridley and Baker, 1982). Stereotypies can be further subdivided into whole body actions and fine motor movements. Whole body stereotypies include pacing, backflipping, and rocking. Fine motor stereotypies often involve the hands and/or face and include patterns such as eye salutes, ear or eye covering, and digit sucking. Most of these patterns are not dangerous to the monkeys displaying them and may even be adaptive under the existing environmental conditions or in the context of the physical state of the organism (Mason, 1991). For example, backflipping may be a replacement for species-typical locomotor activity that cannot be expressed fully in monkeys housed in individual cages (Draper and Bernstein, 1963). Digit sucking may emerge in some animals after weaning. It should be noted, however, that these patterns can become harmful if they constitute a major part of the daily activities of the animal or if they disrupt other functions such as parental care. Thus, the frequency of these activities and the disruption they create are relevant markers for pathology.

Nonhuman primates can also exhibit more intense and severe forms of abnormal behavior that can potentially yield tissue irritation or damage. The term "self-injurious behavior (SIB)" is used as a general descriptor for patterns such as hair plucking, head banging, and self-biting that are observed in a small percentage of captive nonhuman primates. Historically, this term originated in studies of humans and is still used today to describe the same patterns of destructive behavior in children and adults. Unlike the stereotypic patterns described previously, SIB is potentially dangerous, sometimes causing tissue damage and increased risk of infection. It is therefore difficult to conceive of these patterns as a normal adaptation to the environment. Instead, there is likely to be some organic or psychogenic origin.

B. Causes: The Interactionist View

If we are ever to understand psychopathology in nonhuman primates, its causes must be identified. A variety of factors have been proposed to account for the occurrence of abnormal behaviors in monkeys. These can be divided into environmental (extrinsic) determinants and central nervous system (CNS) (intrinsic) determinants. By far the most popular view is that abnormal behavior emerges as a result of certain laboratory conditions associated either with early rearing practices (e.g., rearing infants without mothers) or with later housing conditions (e.g., maintaining animals in individual cages). Indeed, as shown in later sections, there is support for this view. But it is also the case that abnormal behavior is sometimes associated with brain damage, painful disorders such as arthritis, and brain neurotransmitter dysfunction. Even in cases where the environment is assumed to play a major role, other factors may also be relevant. For example, although pathological behavior is more commonly observed in animals housed in individual cages than animals housed in social groups (Bayne *et al.,* 1992a), it is not seen in all, or even the majority of, individually housed animals. Thus, some animals may carry risk factors that make them vulnerable to this type of housing. Ultimately, the causes of psychopathology will be found in some interaction of extrinsic and intrinsic factors. Thus, both the consequences of individual cage housing and the risk factors that predispose some monkeys to develop psychopathology under these conditions must be studied.

II. HISTORICAL REVIEW OF ABNORMAL BEHAVIOR IN CAPTIVE NONHUMAN PRIMATES

A. Environmental Causes

The observance of abnormal behavior in captive primates dates back as early as 1928 when Tinklepaugh noted severe "self-mutilation" in a rhesus monkey named Cupid. Tinklepaugh concluded that the self-mutilation was related to a change in the social environment of the animal. Cupid had been housed with an older female for approximately 2 years when he was introduced to two new females. From the description of Tinklepaugh, it is clear that the introduction was unsuccessful and stressful to Cupid (he was observed "gnashing" his teeth). However, Tinklepaugh also suggested that he had contributed to the occurrence of Cupid's self-biting behavior. Cupid developed the habit of mouthing his feet and tail after Tinklepaugh trained him to somersault by bending the monkey's head down toward the genital region. The implications then from this informal report are that self-abusive behavior can be environmentally induced and learned.

Several methods of generating abnormal nonhuman primate behavior are found in the literature. Dr. Harry Harlow initiated the first systematic evaluation of psychological disorders in nonhuman primates in the 1960s. Harlow was able to consistently produce psychological disorders in infant monkeys that modeled anomalies observed in infant humans. Harlow and Novak (1973) categorized nonhuman primate behavioral pathology induced by various degrees of social isolation at different ages into three areas: (1) privation and deprivation syndromes, (2) fears and phobias, and (3) depression. Much can be learned from a reexamination of Harlow's research as some of the routine husbandry practices employed in laboratory animal facilities today mimic Harlow's conditions for experimentally induced psychopathology.

Harlow and colleagues induced different constellations of behavioral pathology by manipulating the degree of social isolation monkeys experienced during the vulnerable period of infancy. Two qualitatively different kinds of syndromes were observed depending on the timing of the isolation experience. Gewirtz (1961) defined these syndromes as (1) privation

wherein newborn organisms were isolated from all conspecifics at birth and not allowed to form an attachments and (2) deprivation wherein organisms were separated from others with whom they had formed attachments (mothers) and relationships (peers). These studies showed that privation induced bizarre stereotypic behaviors (e.g., self-clasping, self-orality, and repetitive locomotion), whereas deprivation resulted in emotional reactions (e.g., excessive aggression, fear, and vocalization). Both these syndromes of abnormal behavior were produced environmentally by deviations in the normal quality, quantity, and timing of social experience in infant monkeys.

B. Biological Causes

In addition to interest in environmental determinants, Harlow and colleagues examined the role of the CNS in the development of abnormal behavior. They studied the effects of lesions of various areas of the monkey brain and, in some circumstances, were able to compare the consequences of these lesions to human patients with certain kinds of brain damage. Although these studies were aimed primarily at understanding the cognitive impairments resulting from brain lesions, some lesions also produced changes in behavior. In the latter case, some of the behavioral consequences of lesioning were subtle and required context-specific situations for the abnormal behavior to be revealed.

Social testing in which a lesioned monkey was allowed to interact with a nonlesioned monkey proved to be a particularly sensitive means of detecting behavioral abnormalities. For example, bilateral amygdalectomy appeared to alter emotional responding such that lesioned animals responded with less fear to inanimate stimuli than normal controls, but with more fear to social stimuli (i.e., when the social stimulus was a normal control control animal; Thompson *et al.,* 1969). This study demonstrated that behavior may be abnormal because it has been either reduced in frequency (suppression) or increased in frequency (overreaction). The effects of bilateral lesions of the frontal granular cortex were studied in rhesus monkeys in order to better understand the consequences of frontal lobectomies on human personality and social behavior (Deets *et al.,* 1970). Nonhuman primates with frontal lesions were found to be "more withdrawn and distressed than control animals." Additionally, the lesioned animals did not approach other animals, did not explore the environment as frequently as control animals, and displayed excessive fear-related behaviors. Suomi *et al.* (1970) characterized the abnormalities in the frontal lobectomized monkeys using perference tests. When given a choice between another lobectomized or normal animal of the *opposite* sex, lesioned animals preferred another lobectomized animal. Unlike their normal control counterparts, however, when given a choice between a control animal of the *same* sex or a lesioned animal of the same sex, the lobectomized subject showed no preference (whereas normal control animals preferred a lobectomized animal of the same sex). These observations were note-worthy because they revealed subtle social differences between lesioned and control animals. Clearly, not all behavioral changes resulting from lesioning and mental disorders were overt.

C. Consideration of Psychological Disorders as a Disease Entity

Of the various abnormal behaviors exhibited by nonhuman primates, the self-injurious behavior that Tinklepaugh first noted has been studied most extensively and continues to be of interest to neuroscientists and behaviorists. The parallels between this nonhuman primate condition and the human situation are striking. The most robust common denominator between SIB in humans and nonhuman primates is the form of expression. Both humans and nonhuman primates bang their heads, slap or hit themselves, and bite or scratch their bodies with sufficient force to produce wounds. It should be noted, however, that self-injurious behavior in human beings is not a single disorder but rather a symptom for several different disorders.

Although the precise etiology for many abnormal behaviors has not been established, a biological cause appears to be responsible for some cases of human self-injurious behavior. Lesch-Nyhan disease (a deficiency in hypoxanthine–guanine phosphoribosyl transferase causing an overproduction of uric acid with a resulting central nervous system disorder) is often characterized by lip, finger, or tongue biting. It can be reversed with appropriate drug therapy (Lloyd *et al.,* 1981). Additionally, self-injurious behavior sometimes occurs in association with schizophrenia (de Lissovoy, 1963). Although a higher pain threshold in schizophrenics was initially proposed, this was later disproved. The inciting cause for self-mutilation in these patients has not been identified. However, it is likely to be an organic one. Otitis media has also been implicated as a cause of self-injury (specifically head banging), although it does not account for all instances of human head banging observed (Goldfarb, 1958).

Underlying physiological causes do not account completely for all behavioral pathology associated with known diseases. For example, self-mutilation (involving scratching and biting of fingers, lips, shoulders, and knees) is common in de Lange syndrome (a genetic disorder). In two human cases, the self-injurious behavior was eliminated with an operant conditioning program that included aversive stimulation (Carr, 1977). It has been argued that if a physiological cause was solely responsible for the self-inflicted wounding, then behavioral conditioning alone would not cure the patient.

There are many kinds of abnormal behavior, whether it be in monkeys or humans, that cannot be attributed to a specific biological or environmental cause. This problem arises, in part, because abnormal behavior is a symptom and not a disorder per se. In fact, the same kind of abnormal behavior may be linked to several different kinds of disorders that may have to be ruled out in turn. In addition, a variety of factors, both intrinsic and extrinsic to the organism, may interact to produce behavioral pathology. Because of these multiple, interacting causes of behavioral pathology, it has proven enormously difficult to identify successful treatment strategies.

III. ETIOLOGY OF PSYCHOLOGICAL DISORDERS

A. Experimental Rearing Environments and Their Effect on Behavior

It is now well established from the work of Harry Harlow that early rearing experiences can produce behavioral pathology in infant monkeys that continues throughout their lives. The extent and severity of the pathology are linked to the amount and quality of social stimulation an infant receives during early development. However, this relationship is not linear. Only the most severe forms of social privation produce behavioral abnormalities, whereas milder forms of social restriction can, in fact, yield nearly normal development. These findings are consistent with the biological concept of developmental homeostasis in which normal outcomes are often achieved despite earlier aberrant events. It is important to review Harlow's work because his research has major significance for how primates should be reared and maintained in captivity.

1. Total and Partial Isolation Rearing

The most severe form of social privation is total isolation, an experimental condition in which newborn rhesus monkeys are reared in chambers in which they cannot see, hear, or physically contact members of their own species. Partial isolation differs from total isolation in that rhesus monkeys are reared in mesh cages in which they can see and hear, but cannot contact other monkeys. Lack of physical contact appears to be the most important cause of behavioral pathology during early infancy because both partial and total isolation yield somewhat similar, negative outcomes. Whereas total isolation has always been an experimental procedure, partial isolation has been used both as an experimental procedure and as a "default" husbandry procedure arising in certain cases (e.g., mother rejects infant, infant has to be nursery reared, and there are no other animals in nursery). It is therefore important for colony managers to understand the consequences, both short and long term, of partial isolation rearing.

Monkeys reared in small isolation chambers or in mesh cages for the first 6–12 months of life develop profound behavioral and physiological abnormalities which, when taken together, comprise the *isolation syndrome* (Capitanio, 1986; Harlow and Harlow, 1962, 1965; Mitchell, 1968, 1970; Sackett, 1965,

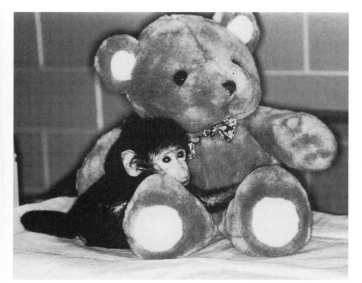

Fig. 1. Example of a simple inanimate surrogate.

1968). Symptoms of the isolation syndrome include (1) abnormal postures such as rocking or swaying, (2) motivational disturbances such as heightened fear or aggression, (3) inadequate coordination of motor patterns such as an inability to perform a double foot-clasp mount essential for mating behavior, and (4) deficits in communication and the development of social relationships (Mason, 1968). These abnormalities typically persist throughout the lifetime of the individual (Mitchell, 1968).

a. BEHAVIORAL EFFECTS.   Monkeys reared in partial or total social isolation develop a plethora of behavioral abnormalities, including rocking, huddling, self-clasping, and excessive self-orality (Cross and Harlow, 1965; Harlow and Harlow, 1965). Although infantile patterns of orality decrease markedly after the first year of life, they are usually replaced with stereotypic patterns (bizarre ritualized activities such as floating limb, hand salutes, eye pokes, backflips, head bobs, and hand weaving) and/or self-abusive behavior (as described by Tinklepaugh, 1928). These patterns have been observed to persist well beyond the 13th year of life (Fittinghoff *et al.,* 1974). Despite the appearance of gross behavioral abnormalities, isolation rearing appears to have little effect on growth and physical maturation (Kerr *et al.,* 1969).

Some of the early infantile abnormalities just described can be minimized if the infant monkeys are given access to an inanimate surrogate mother. These "mothers" consist of cylindrical wooden shapes covered with soft terry cloth and mounted angularly on a base. Infants invariable cling to surrogates, develop a strong attachment to them, and use them as a base of operations when exploring novel environments (see Fig. 1) (Harlow, 1958; Harlow and Suomi, 1970; Harlow and Zimmerman, 1959). Monkeys reared with surrogates in isolation still develop many, but not all, of the signs of the isolation syn-

drome. Some abnormal behavior is reduced (e.g., self-clasping). Alterations in other kinds of abnormal behavior have been shown to depend on the qualities of the surrogate. Infants exposed to swaying surrogates, for example, do not develop rocking behavior (Mason and Berkson, 1975). In all other respects, however, these monkeys are as deviant as monkeys reared in isolation without surrogates.

In addition to the profound behavioral disturbances just described, isolate-reared monkeys lack most basic social skills. When exposed to normal infants of the same age, isolates react with excessive fear (Mason and Green, 1962). They also fail to show appropriate social behavior (e.g., play and social contact) and are frequently attacked by the normal infants (Clark, 1968; Sackett, 1968). As juveniles, isolate-reared monkeys show unstable dominance interactions with frequent and prolonged fighting (Mason, 1961b). As adults, such monkeys are hyperaggressive in social situations and do not develop adequate social relationships with other monkeys (Anderson and Mason, 1974; Mason, 1961a). Isolate-reared monkeys are clearly inadequate as breeders. Males never acquire the appropriate sexual posture (Mason, 1960), and females are indifferent or abusive to their infants (especially male infants; Suomi, 1978). It should be noted that maternal responsiveness has been observed to improve in isolate-reared females on exposure to their second infant (Arling and Harlow, 1967). Isolate-reared monkeys are also defective in their patterns of communication. They show abnormalities in the production of clear calls that include temporal discontinuities and a lack of characteristic patterns of inflection (Newman and Symmes, 1974). Disturbances in visual communication (Brandt *et al.,* 1971) and in the development of expressive behavior (Mason, 1985) have also been recorded.

As a general rule, males appear to be more vulnerable to the effects of isolation than females. Males are more likely to exhibit grossly abnormal behavior (e.g., excessive self-biting) and fail to modify these behavior patterns with age or experience. Females, however, appear to be somewhat buffered from the effects of total isolation rearing and can modify their responses with experience, as in the case of maternal behavior cited earlier (Sackett, 1974). The effects of total isolation are usually more severe than those produced by partial isolation, with the difference largely being one of quantity rather than quality of abnormal behavior.

b. COGNITIVE EFFECTS.   Despite obvious behavioral pathology, isolation rearing does not appear to produce major cognitive deficits (Harlow *et al.,* 1969). When isolated and control monkeys were compared in discrimination learning, learning set, and oddity learning set, only two differences emerged. Monkeys reared in total isolation took a substantially longer period of time to habituate to the testing apparatus. Once habituated, however, isolated monkeys performed as well as controls on all tests except that of the oddity learning set (Gluck *et al.,* 1973).

c. PHYSIOLOGICAL EFFECTS.   Isolation rearing in rhesus monkeys appears to produce altered metabolism. Such mon-

TABLE I

OUTCOMES OF ISOLATION REARING IN THREE SPECIES OF MACAQUES [a]

Species	Level of self-directed activity	Level of exploration	Level of sociality
Macaca mulatta	High	Low	Low
M. nemestrina	Low	High	Low
M. fascicularis	High	High	High

[a]From Sackett *et al.* (1981).

keys have been shown to consume about 30% more food and fluid per meal than normally reared monkeys (Miller *et al.,* 1969, 1971). Despite this difference in food intake, isolate-reared monkeys are not significantly heavier than controls.

Neuroanatomical changes have also been linked to early isolation. Decreased dendritic branching has been reported in a variety of cell types both in cortical and in subcortical regions (Floeter and Greenough, 1979; Strubel and Riesen, 1978). In a study in which the brains of old isolate-reared monkeys and their matched controls were examined, major differences were found in the striatal patch matrix (Cork *et al.,* 1990). Fibers and terminals were missing in the striatal matrix of old isolate-reared monkeys, and striatal patches were reduced substantially.

Differences in hormone and neurotransmitter sensitivity have also been observed. Isolate-reared monkeys had higher basal levels of cortisol that control monkeys, although there was no difference in the amount of cortisol secretion in response to adrenocorticotropin (ACTH) stimulation (Sackett *et al.,* 1973) or to social separation (Champoux *et al.,* 1989). Early isolation experience also resulted in long-term alterations in dopamine receptor sensitivity (Lewis, *et al.,* 1990) and produced decreases in cell-mediated immunity and survival, particularly in male rhesus monkeys (Gluck *et al.,* 1989).

d. SPECIES EFFECTS. Many of the behavioral abnormalities that define the isolation syndrome (e.g., self-directed activity and inadequate social behavior) have also been observed in chimpanzees and squirrel monkeys following isolation rearing (Rogers and Davenport, 1969; Roy, 1981). However, major species differences in response to isolation rearing have emerged over time (Sackett *et al.,* 1976). In a comparative study of the effects of isolation on three species of macaques (rhesus macaques, pig-tailed macaques, and cynomolgus macaques), rhesus monkeys were clearly the most affected of the species studied (Sackett *et al.,* 1981; see Table I). Therefore, the extent of psychopathology produced by isolation rearing is clearly species dependent.

All of these studies reveal the devastating consequences of isolation rearing, particularly in the two most commonly used primates, rhesus and cynomolgus macaques, and emphasize the need for caution in rearing infants without any conspecific contact. Although partial isolation yields a somewhat milder syndrome than total isolation, the effects are nonetheless profound

and long-lasting. Animals reared in this manner display bizarre behavior, are difficult to socialize even under the best of circumstances, and cannot be used for breeding. Because of differences in physiology and brain development in comparison to normally reared monkeys, they may also be unsuitable for research.

2. Peer-Only Rearing

In contrast to early isolation rearing, monkeys separated from their mothers at birth and reared with other infants (peers) display only low levels of deviant behavior and develop many species-appropriate social responses (Harlow and Harlow, 1965). However, certain abnormalities are sometimes present. Peer-reared monkeys tend to cling and huddle together excessively and exhibit a delay in the development of play behavior. These differences are stronger in monkeys reared in pairs rather than trios or tetrads (Chamove *et al.,* 1973). Peer-reared monkeys also display more severe separation reactions than mother–peer-reared monkeys as indexed by higher rates of self-clasping and higher levels of cortisol, ACTH, and 3-methoxy-4-hydroxylphenylglycol (MHPG) (Higley *et al.,* 1991). In contrast to normally reared monkeys, peer-reared monkeys appear more emotional as juveniles (huddling and clinging to each other in response to novel stimuli). However, in adolescence, peer-reared monkeys are more aggressive than normally reared monkeys and show lower levels of 5-hydroxyindoleacetic acid (5–HIAA), a serotonin metabolite in the cerebrospinal fluid (CSF) (Higley and Suomi, 1989).

Occasional reproductive deficits have appeared with this rearing procedure. Some of the males failed to develop the appropriate sexual postures (double foot-clasp mount; Goy and Wallen, 1979; Goy *et al.,* 1974). This latter point is particularly noteworthy inasmuch as peer-only rearing was at one time a relatively common rearing procedure employed at several primate facilities. As was eventually discovered, some of these peer-only reared males proved unsuitable as replacements for old feral males in the breeding colony. However, peer-reared females show relatively normal maternal behavior (Champoux *et al.,* 1992).

Based on the information just presented, it is clear that peer-only rearing is a dramatically better rearing environment than partial isolation. Monkeys develop many forms of social behavior and show only some residual kinds of abnormal behavior. It is therefore strongly preferred to partial isolation as a rearing procedure.

3. Surrogate–Peer Rearing

However, even greater success has been achieved with surrogate–peer rearing, a variation on the peer-rearing procedure that produces nearly normal behavioral development. In this rearing condition, monkeys are reared with continuous access to inanimate surrogates and are provided with *brief* daily exposure to peers (e.g., 30–120 min per day). Such monkeys are nearly indistinguishable from monkeys reared with mothers and peers (Hansen, 1966; Rosenblum, 1961). Although surrogate–peer-reared monkeys tend to show somewhat higher levels of self-mouth and self-clasp than normal monkeys, they develop the full range of species-normative activity without any delay. Indeed, typical sex differences are apparent at the appropriate time points in development, reproductive and maternal behavior are normal, and complex patterns of social organization (e.g., matrilines) emerge (Novak *et al.,* 1994).

This outcome has been attributed to the restriction in peer contact (only for a short period every day), which appears to facilitate the formation of an attachment to the ever-present surrogate but not to the peers. Thus, surrogate–peer-reared infants cling to their surrogates, using them as a base of operations for their forays into the environment. Their peers become playmates rather than "attachment figures" and, as a result, they play extensively with each other during their brief periods of social interaction. Restriction of peer contact is apparently critical inasmuch as infants reared in the continuous presence of both inanimate surrogates and naive peers develop and behave in the same way as peer-only-reared monkeys (S. J. Suomi, personal communication).

4. Contraspecific Rearing

Although there have been relatively few attempts to rear rhesus monkeys with nonprimate mammals, Dr. William Mason and co-workers have examined the influence of mongrel dogs as surrogate mothers on the development of rhesus macaque infants. In a first set of studies, monkeys, whether socially experienced or not, were observed to develop attachments to dogs (Mason and Kenney, 1974). In subsequent studies comparing infants reared with dogs, dog-reared monkeys displayed lower levels of self-directed activity (Wood *et al.,* 1979) and were "more attuned to and better able to anticipate their partner's behavior" (Capitanio, 1984). However, dog-reared monkeys were clearly deficient in their social interactions, showing very little affiliative response to other monkeys (Capitanio, 1984).

5. Mother–Only Rearing

Although it has been assumed that mothers provide both necessary and sufficient stimuli for normative development in rhesus monkey infants, infants reared only with a mother during the first 6–12 months of life behaved somewhat differently than infants reared with mothers and peers. Mother–only-reared infants showed some tendency toward hyperaggressiveness in their interactions with peers, and this pattern of aggression persisted into adulthood and was manifested in a variety of situation (Alexander, 1966).

6. Conclusions

There is now no doubt that early social contact with conspecifics is critically important for the development of normal behavior and for the establishment and maintenance of normal social relationships in nonhuman primates. However, the relationship between the amount of early experience and the quality of subsequent behavior is not linear. Instead, a threshold phenomenon exists in that only the most severe forms of social privation (e.g., total and partial social isolation) appear to be associated with a severe loss of social functioning and the onset of obvious psychopathology. Indeed, as long as there is some conspecific contact (even with naive peers only), rhesus monkeys can acquire a broad range of species-normative behavior. The work of Harlow provides a clear set of guidelines regarding the suitability of different early rearing environments for macaques that apply today. In that regard, although mother–peer/social group rearing is ideal, monkeys also develop mostly normal behavior when raised with peers or when reared with surrogates and given brief daily peer experience during the first year of life. In situations where the research protocol requires that infants be separated from their mothers at birth, every effort should be made to avoid partial isolation rearing unless absolutely essential.

B. Individual Housing of Adult Primates

It seems clear from the literature (Bayne *et al,* 1991a; Reinhardt *et al.,* 1987) that maintaining some species of adult nonhuman primates for an extended period of time in individual housing (though this time period has not been precisely defined) can elicit abnormal behavior. It should be noted that these animals had been reared normally and had not displayed such behavior in social settings. In addition to these behavioral anomalies, some physiological measures appear to be abnormally elevated in individually housed animals as compared to their socially housed age/sex cohorts (Kaplan *et al.,* 1982; Line *et al.,* 1990).

The reasons for the development of behavioral pathology in monkeys housed in single cages after infancy remain unclear. Individually housed monkeys can usually see, hear, and smell other animals in the holding room. Occasionally, monkeys even touch each other to a limited degree by reaching through the cage. Thus, the term "individual" housing may be considered somewhat of an overstatement. It seems likely that the lack of more extensive *physical* contact with conspecifics contributes in a significant way to the induction of abnormal behavior. However, other factors may also play a role. For example, in the single cage setting, the animal typically has limited space to move in, has a restricted visual field, cannot escape any conflict situations between animals in the room, experiences little diversity in its environment, and has minimum control over its own environment. The impact of these factors on behavioral pathology probably varies with the species, age, sex, and rearing history of the animal and may even differ between individuals of the same age/sex group. An understanding of the natural social order of the animal in a free-ranging situation can serve as a useful guide in determining the appropriate housing conditions for a particular species.

TABLE II
BEHAVIORAL ASSESSMENT SCALE FOR ABNORMAL BEHAVIORS
IN RHESUS MONKEYS

Category[a]	Behavior
1	Behaviors that are locomotory in nature and repetitive (e.g., circle, rock, spin, pace, swing, somersault, bounce), yet can be arrested with appropriate diversionary stimuli
2	Behaviors that are environmentally oriented and stereotypic (e.g., cage manipulation)
3	Behaviors that are self-oriented and stereotypic[b] (e.g., autoerotic, coprophagia, huddle/withdrawal, self-clasping, self-suck, etc.) as these represent a dissociation from the environment
4	Behaviors that impair biologic function (e.g., result in an inability to reproduce or rear offspring, such as misdirected mounting, or result in decreased time spent eating to the degree that the animal weighs less than is typical for his/her weight range, such as locomotion from which the animal cannot be distracted)
5	Behaviors that are apparently painful (e.g., hair plucking, excessive pulling on appendages) as they result in a distress vocalization
6	Behaviors that compromise the physical health of the animal or result in physical harm (e.g., self-biting, head banging)

[a] Least detrimental (1) to most detrimental (6).
[b] A repetitive, non-goal-oriented activity.

IV. CLINICAL SIGNS OF PSYCHOLOGICAL DISORDERS

Since Congress amended the Animal Welfare Act in 1985, it has been incumbent on the biomedical, scientific, and veterinary communities to better understand the psychological attributes of nonhuman primates. New legislation and subsequent regulations from the United States Department of Agriculture mandate the provision of environments that promote the "psychological well-being" of all captive nonhuman primates. Within the last decade, researchers, veterinarians, and regulators have grappled with the concept of psychological well-being and it has proven enormously difficult to define in precise terms. However, there is little difficulty in recognizing the converse, ill-being.

A. Criteria for Assessing Well-Being

As with any physical disease process, standards for evaluating the behavioral health of nonhuman primates serve as the framework within which pathology is identified. Despite the difficulties associated with defining psychological well-being, criteria have been developed to assess the psychological status of nonhuman primates (Novak and Suomi, 1988). According to these criteria, animals should (1) exhibit adequate physical health based on their age (assessed by various physical signs

and clinical test results), (2) show a substantial range of species-typical behavior or, if individually housed, not exhibit excessive levels of deviant behavior (assessed by observational scoring procedures), (3) react appropriately to environmental challenges such as cage removal (assessed by observation), and (4) not be chronically distressed (assessed by clinical signs and hormone assays, if necessary) (see Selyé 1974 for a discussion of eustress and distress). Not all of these criteria need to be rated in order to evaluate psychological well-being, and other criteria may be applicable as well.

B. Measures of Psychological Disorders

Perhaps one of the most common means of determining if a nonhuman primate is afflicted with a psychological disorder involves monitoring the behavioral repertoire of that animal (the range of normal behaviors exhibited by a species) for the occurrence of potentially maladaptive patterns. Some abnormal behaviors are classified as stereotypies that consist of whole body actions such as pacing, backflipping, spinning, swaying, and rocking or fine motor patterns directed to the animal's own body such as eye saluting, hair pulling, biting, digit sucking, tail chewing, clasping, head banging, and face slapping. Most of these behaviors are considered abnormal because they are qualitatively or quantitatively different from the species behavioral norm (Erwin and Deni, 1979). Thus, although locomotion is usually considered a normal activity, repetitive and apparently non-goal-oriented pacing/circling in a cage, for example, would be considered abnormal as it occurs at a greatly increased frequency and is qualitatively modified by having no end point. The point at which an abnormal behavior must be regarded as maladaptive or pathological varies with the behavior under consideration. A behavior such as digit sucking, while considered a qualitatively abnormal behavior, is certainly not life threatening to the animal. However, self-biting can become quite severe, resulting in the infliction of wounds, and must be treated as a psychological disorder requiring immediate attention. Abnormal behavior may become pathological if it is (1) excessively frequent to the detriment of many other normal activities, (2) disruptive such that it interferes with basic biological functions, and/or (3) dangerous, producing tissue damage and possible infection. These three criteria are not mutually exclusive.

Not all pathology is reflected in odd or bizarre behavior. Monkeys can also exhibit emotional reactions, which, if extreme enough, might constitute some pathological state. Monkeys that cower in the back of their cage, hyperventilate, and fear grimace excessively are exhibiting distress (see Morton and Griffiths, 1985). Conversely, pathology may be present if monkeys show frequent and repetitive bouts of attack behavior (lunging against the cage, vocalizing, and threatening) to many different social stimuli with no evidence of habituation.

Although behavioral indices are clearly important in the identification of psychopathology, a more complete assessment of the mental health status of the the animal can be obtained if other measures, such as physiological and immunological indices, are also used to complement the behavioral recordings. Although plasma cortisol values can change rapidly with low-level intervention of the nonhuman primate (e.g., restraint), this serological measurement is used frequently to determine if an animal is distressed (Hennessy *et al.,* 1982; Line *et al.,* 1989; Suomi *et al.,* 1989). Changes in heart rate have also been used to evaluate the stress level of the animal (Rasmussen and Suomi, 1989; Reite *et al.,* 1978). Indeed, it has been shown that animals living in social housing conditions have lower heart rates than animals living individually (Adams *et al.,* 1988). Additionally, various immune functions are suppressed during times of stress. Selyé (1950), in his description of the stress response, noted changes in eosinophil and lymphocyte function and thymolymphatic involution. In humans, the lymphocyte response to mitogen stimulation is also affected by stress (Reite *et al.,* 1981). The mitogen stimulation test described for humans has been replicated in squirrel monkeys (Coe *et al.,* 1989). As with the human findings, lymphocytes taken from juvenile monkeys separated from their mothers showed significant reductions in proliferation when stimulated by concanavalin A (CONA) and pokeweed mitogen (PWM). Coe *et al.* (1985) have similarly shown that a stress response in squirrel monkeys (induced by maternal separation studies) includes a significant decrease in the complement proteins, C3 and C4, by 7 days after separation and a significant reduction in serum levels of immunoglobulins (IgG, IgM, and IgA) that resulted in a functional impairment to antigen challenge.

V. DIAGNOSIS OF PSYCHOLOGICAL DISORDERS

A. Ruling Out the Obvious

As with any other disease condition, behavioral pathology must be considered as only one differential diagnosis on a list of "rule outs" for abnormal behavior or for the occurrence of physiological measures outside the normal range. For example, urine drinking in macaques is frequently considered an aberrant behavior occurring in individually housed monkeys with *ad libitum* access to water. However, glucosuria resulting from diabetes should also be considered (see Levanduski *et al.,* 1992), and a urine dipstick test can readily be performed to eliminate this endocrinological disorder from the differential diagnosis list. Severe hair loss is another manifestation of a physical disorder (e.g., hypothyroidism, Sertoli cell tumor, hyperadrenocorticism) or a behavioral disorder (hair pulling by the animal). Similarly, a peripheral neuropathy should be considered, as well as the manifestation of a behavioral disorder, when self-mutilation of the extremities is noted.

A knowledge of the rearing history of the animal, the clinical history of the animal, and in particular the previous studies in which the animal has been used may assist in the differential diagnosis of an apparent behavioral problem. For example, a nonhuman primate used in certain pharmacological investigations, such as cocaine studies, can manifest tremors and "floating limbs." If the experimental history of the animal was not examined, these behaviors might be attributed to fear and withdrawal rather than to the effects of the drug, and an inaccurate diagnosis could be made. In such a case, the behavioral therapy typically used for fearful and withdrawn animals would be inappropriate.

B. Determining the Severity of the Problem

One question facing those who encounter abnormal behavior is "how serious is the problem?" Abnormal behavior clearly varies in severity, and what is needed is some "yardstick" by which monkeys can be evaluated objectively. One proposed ranking of abnormal behaviors is provided in Table II. In Table II, behaviors for which there is no conclusive proof that the activity is detrimental to the animal (categories 1–3), such as pacing, and for which there may, in fact, be some benefit accrued by the animal (e.g., the physiological benefits of exercise) are rated as the least problematic. In contrast, abnormal behaviors that may compromise the health of the animal are considered the most problematic (categories 4–6 on the scale). This scale is proposed as one possible way in which to standardize the assessment of the atypical components of the behavioral profile of an animal.

A behavioral assessment scale may prove useful to scientists, veterinarians, facility managers, and animal care personnel as a standardized means of assessing the behavioral profile of their nonhuman primates. For example, animals that have been classified at a rating of 6 should receive prompt medical attention and behavioral therapy. Animals that are rated at lower levels should receive attention at a correspondingly appropriate level.

VI. THERAPEUTIC STRATEGIES FOR REVERSING PSYCHOPATHOLOGY

Although it is not difficult to recognize abnormal behavior in nonhuman primates, the alleviation or eradication of such behavior has proven to be very problematic. The failure to identify specific therapeutic strategies that are effective in reducing or eliminating most forms of pathological behavior can be attributed to two factors. First, little is known about the etiology of behavioral pathology in individual nonhuman primates. Animals are usually identified in the colony as showing pathological behavior, and then retrospective analyses must be used in an attempt to understand what might have caused the problem. Second, deviant behavior is a symptom and not necessarily a disorder per se. In fact, the same deviant behavior may be a symptom of several different disorders.

However, in cases of experimentally induced psychopathology (e.g., isolation rearing in infant macaques), the picture is somewhat different. Not only is the precipitating cause known, but a variety of therapies have been tried, and some have been surprisingly successful. It is worth reviewing the rehabilitation efforts of Harlow and colleagues because they may provide guidance in the development of therapies for spontaneously occurring psychopathology in laboratory monkeys.

A. Social Recovery in Nonhuman Primates

As discussed previously, monkeys reared in total or partial isolation develop profound deficits in social behavior and show markedly deviant and bizarre behavior. These deficits can be attributed to a lack of physical contact experienced during the early formative months of life. Failure to receive conspecific contact during early development may have a number of different biological consequences (Sackett et al., 1982). (1) The neural structures/connections involved in the expression of normal behavior may atrophy in the absence of contact. This *neural deterioration hypothesis* has been confirmed for vision (cf Riesen, 1960, for visual deterioration in the absence of visual input). (2) The neural structures/connections may fail to mature properly if the relevant physical contact is not provided at a certain point in development. This is referred to as the *sensitive period hypothesis* (Fox, 1966). (3) Monkeys may fail to display relevant social behaviors because they have not had the opportunity to acquire them through experience (*learning deficit hypothesis;* Novak and Harlow, 1975). (4) Monkeys may possess all the relevant behavior patterns but may fail to express them in some situations because of heightened emotional arousal after removal from isolation. The *emergence stress hypothesis* suggests that normal behavior in isolated monkeys is masked by those abnormal behaviors associated with severe stress (Fuller, 1967). It should be noted that these hypotheses are not necessarily mutually exclusive.

For many years, Harlow and his colleagues attempted to rehabilitate rhesus monkeys that had been reared in isolation. Their efforts were designed to reduce stress or to provide a learning environment in which normal behavior could be acquired. Some of these attempts were disappointing, but others yielded surprising success, both in terms of reducing abnormal behavior and in eliciting and promoting appropriate social behavior.

1. Simple Adaptation to Alleviate Stress

It is clear that isolate-reared monkeys experience some kind of emergence stress when they are removed from isolation and placed in new situations. Abnormal and bizarre behavior increased dramatically in contrast to the levels observed in isolation, and the animals showed withdrawal and clutching (Clark, 1968). These effects occurred even when the monkeys were

moved from one individual cage to another (Novak and Harlow, 1975) and were heightened when the environment was markedly different or when other animals were present. In an effort to determine whether stress-related responses were masking normal behavior, some isolate-reared monkeys were given gradual and extensive familiarization with the physical aspects of these new environments. However, even the most intensive efforts at adaptation proved to be only partially effective (Clark, 1968). There was a reduction in the incidence of some kinds of abnormal behavior but only to levels observed when the animals were in isolation. Furthermore, isolate-reared monkeys did not exhibit species-appropriate social behavior when paired with other monkeys.

2. Exposure to Normally Reared Monkeys of the Same Age

It has been argued that isolate-reared monkeys fail to show species-appropriate behavior because they lack the opportunity to acquire such behavior through interactions with conspecifics. In another set of studies, Harlow and colleagues examined the therapeutic benefit of exposing isolate-reared monkeys to normally reared monkeys of the same age. As it turned out, this procedure had no positive effect and in fact was harmful to isolate-reared monkeys. Normally reared monkeys would approach and investigate the isolates, touching and pulling on parts of their bodies. When these actions failed to elicit the appropriate social response, the normal monkeys responded with threats and aggression (Capitanio, 1984; Clark, 1968; Cross and Harlow, 1965; Mason, 1960, 1961b; Mitchell, et al., 1966). Although isolated infant monkeys could be paired with one another without producing heightened aggression, no significant benefit in terms of a reduction in abnormal behavior or an increase in social behavior was derived from such contact (Suomi, 1973).

3. Exposure to Younger Monkeys

The failure of isolate-reared monkeys to "acquire" social responses from normally reared monkeys might be attributed to different levels of social sophistication. Even at 6 months of age, infant monkeys reared with mothers and peers were already highly developed, socially sophisticated organisms whose level of social interaction clearly outstripped isolated monkeys of the same age. Thus, it was still possible that isolate-reared monkeys might be rehabilitated if presented with less socially sophisticated partners. It was with this in mind that younger monkey therapy was instituted.

Exposure of 6- or 12-month-old totally isolated monkeys to younger monkeys of 3–4 months of age resulted in very dramatic changes in behavior (Novak and Harlow, 1975; Suomi and Harlow, 1972). Instead of threatening and attacking the isolates, the younger monkey therapists repeatedly attempted to contact, cling to, and play with the isolate-reared subjects. Initially, these overtures were rebuffed. However, the isolated animals eventually began to reciprocate these interactions. By the end of several months of therapy, isolated monkeys showed substantial rehabilitation. They exhibited a marked decline in abnormal behavior and showed a corresponding increase in social contact, exploration, and play (Novak and Harlow, 1975; Suomi and Harlow, 1972). As noted in a follow-up study, these improvements continued through adolescence (Novak, 1979).

Despite the remarkable success of younger monkey therapy, rehabilitated monkeys were not completely normal. Rehabilitated isolates were less affiliative than normally reared monkeys and showed deficits in sexual behavior. Males failed to develop the appropriate sexual postures required for copulation. This latter pattern, the double foot-clasp mount, appears to be particularly sensitive to rearing treatment, and isolated monkeys never acquired this pattern of behavior regardless of therapeutic intervention.

Overall, these studies support a learning deficit and emergence stress view of the isolation syndrome. However, the failure to see species-appropriate sexual postures suggests that the corresponding brain control elements may have atrophied or remained immature. This finding is consistent with some of the physiological anomalies that are know to be associated with isolation rearing.

4. Strategies for Adult Monkeys

The treatment of behavioral pathology in adult animals typically has variable results. In part, this variability is no doubt correlated with the chronicity of the condition. Cases in which animals have manifested aberrancies for shorter periods of time tend to resolve faster and with fewer interventions by facility staff. The benefits of social housing are extant. Safety, food finding, and reproductive skills are all enhanced by group living. Additionally, Boccia et al. (1989) have shown that receiving grooming from another monkey significantly reduced the heart rate of that animal, a finding that is interpreted as "tension reduction." Clearly this is an advantage that many individually housed primates do not share, which may contribute to their increased stress levels.

Two methods of social recovery are possible for adult nonhuman primates: (1) pair housing the target animal with a compatible socially experienced animal or (2) placing the target animal in a compatible group of conspecific animals. In either case, the social experience can be on a full-time or part-time basis.

Our understanding of an appropriate means of establishing compatible pairs of nonhuman primates has been greatly expanded. Pairs of monkeys of different age and sex classes have been successfully formed with no negative effect on the body weight or behavior of the animals (Reinhardt, 1988; Reinhardt et al., 1988a,b). Pairs of animals have also been formed between closely related species of primates (e.g., rhesus monkeys and cynomolgus monkeys) where visual signals are interpreted in a similar manner for both species. For example, a "grin" is interpreted by macaque species as a fear grimace. However, to another animal such as a chimpanzee, a "grin" is a friendly greeting and not a sign of fear or distress. Thus, although different species of macaques can live compatibly, more divergent

species (such as a chimpanzee and a macaque) may not be compatible due to misinterpretation of visual cues. Finally, compatible pairs of rhesus monkeys equipped with implantable devices have been established with no resulting damage to the experimental equipment (Reinhardt, et al., 1989; C. McCully, personal communication, 1991).

Group formation of some species of primates is a relatively simple matter (e.g., squirrel monkeys), whereas for other species it presents certain challenges. Bernstein et al. (1974) demonstrated that one of the major obstacles to group formation in macaques is the aggression that can occur between coalitions of previously formed subgroups of animals. For this reason, they recommend that unfamiliar animals be placed together in the new holding area at the same time. The benefits of group housing for monkeys exhibiting behavioral pathology have not yet been fully investigated.

B. Nonsocial Recovery in Nonhuman Primates

Harlow (1958) initially recognized the attachment between infant primates and inanimate "surrogate" mothers. The nature of the surrogate has taken many shapes and forms—from a simple diaper to a heated, rocking, cloth-covered apparatus with a rudimentary face, a bottle strapped onto it, and tilted at an angle that mimics the position of the infant on a natural mother (Harlow et al., 1971; Mason and Berkson, 1975). As indicated earlier, infants reared with inanimate surrogates cling to and seek comfort from these objects. Certain behaviors associated with distress, such as rocking, can be reduced with the appropriate type of inanimate surrogate. Suomi (1973) also noted that isolates exposed to surrogates at 6 months of age exhibited significantly more locomotion and exploration than isolates not exposed to surrogates. The exposure to the surrogate also appears to serve as a bridge for more normal contact with peers when the isolates were allowed social contact.

Similarly, experience with the treatment of behavioral pathology in adult primates with nonsocial, or environmental enrichment, devices has proven surprisingly successful. Hard rubber toys are used to reduce the incidence of self-biting in monkeys, artificial shearling mounted on plexiglass boards outside the cage can decrease the incidence of self-plucking (Bayne et al., 1991a), and foraging devices can interrupt the hyperactive repetitive locomotion patterns of some monkeys (Bayne et al., 1993). In this way, different pathologies are targeted with different enrichment therapies, as no single enrichment technique will ameliorate all conditions.

C. Genetic Influences on the Development of Behavioral Pathology

Evidence suggests that the incidence of behavioral pathology is not entirely attributable to the rearing history of the primate, but may be in part due to genetic factors. Suomi (1991) has identified differences in the way rhesus monkeys respond to stimulation. Some monkeys are "laid back" (nonreactive) and respond at an appropriate level to the stimulation. Others are "uptight" (or reactive) and overreact to the stimulus. The tendency to be reactive or nonreactive appears to be inherited. Suomi (1991) estimates that approximately 20% of the rhesus population is reactive. A possible consequence of these findings is that reactive monkeys may not benefit in the same way as nonreactors to changes in their environment that are designed to be enriching. Also, a reactive animal may not fare well in highly visible places in the room (e.g., near the door) where the constant flow of daily activities disturbs the animal. Routine and predictable husbandry and experimental schedules may be the best methods of reducing the disturbance profile of the reactive animal.

VII. PREVENTION OF BEHAVIORAL PATHOLOGY

A. Husbandry Decisions for Infant Primates

The development of normal behavior in nonhuman primates is critically dependent on how a primate is reared during infancy. The optimal rearing environment is probably one in which infants are raised in species-typical social groups. For rhesus monkeys, such groups would consist of mothers, other adults, adolescents, juveniles, and infants of both sexes. However, normal behavioral outcomes can also be achieved by rearing infants in social groups containing mothers and other young. The mother–peer condition is considered an ideal regimen for raising infant rhesus monkeys in the laboratory. For the biomedical researcher or the veterinarian, however, several other options are also available.

For research requiring continued direct access to infants or for veterinary reasons (i.e., mother has rejected an infant at birth) or for facility operations (mother–peer groups are not possible), two other rearing conditions may be relevant. These are peer-only rearing and surrogate–peer rearing (see Sections II,A,3 and II,A,4 for descriptions). Although species-normative patterns of behavior develop in both rearing conditions, surrogate–peer-related animals are not as fearful as peer-only reared animals (Chamove et al., 1973).

Surrogate–peer rearing may be particularly desirable for those studies in which infants must be accessed individually on a regular basis. Because surrogate–peer-reared infants form their primary attachment to an inanimate surrogate and not to the peers they are exposed to for several hours per day, the infants can be studied without distress during a nonsocial period. Infants can readily be removed from the cage while still clinging to their surrogates, and various manipulations (e.g., blood drawing, injections) typically can be performed with infants still clinging to their surrogates (e.g., infants can be trained to extend a leg for blood sampling while holding onto their

surrogate). Surrogate–peer rearing requires that infants be housed alone for portions of the day and that they be given intermittent contact (from 1 to 2 hr) with other naive infants. If infants are given continuous access to both inanimate surrogates and peers, they will develop their primary attachment to the other infants and resemble peer-only reared infants. Although peer-only reared infants can be accessed individually, separation from peers produces more powerful reactions than removal of mother-reared infants from their mother (Higley et al., 1991).

The single most important guideline to follow in rearing infant primates is to provide them with some sort of conspecific physical contact during early development, whether it be with a mother and peers, with peers only, or with a mother only, unless, of course, the research is focused on isolation rearing. Failure to do so will result in socially deficient, behaviorally bizarre monkeys that may compromise both the research operation and the husbandry practices of the facility. Given that primates are long-lived, early rearing regimens will have profound long-term consequences for caregivers and researchers alike.

B. Husbandry Decisions for Adult Primates

Strategies for designing adult primate holding areas that minimize the occurrence of psychological disorders will vary with the species of concern. A large part of the decision-making process will be based on the natural social structure of the animal. Thus, optimizing the well-being of a monogamous species will, in all likelihood, include pair housing. Where possible, solitary animals should be provided an environment in which they have the opportunity to visually remove themselves (or "hide") from other animals in the room (e.g., a privacy panel, see Reinhardt, 1990). Primates that live in social groups in free-ranging situations can be provided the same quality of lifestyle in the laboratory without impending the conduct of research (Rasmussen, 1991; Gordan, 1990). In the appropriate social setting, the primate expresses a broader range of species-typical behaviors and hones its coping skills as it adapts to different social challenges on a daily basis (e.g., Bayne et al., 1991b). Social living in a laboratory environment is clearly not a stress-free environment, but more closely approximates the quality and quantity of stress that is normal for the species. As each animal has an activity budget that is limited by the number of waking hours in a 24-hr period, the more time an animal spends engaged in normative activities, there is less time available for the display of pathological behaviors.

The lives of both solitary and social species can also simulate a free-ranging existence by allowing these types of animals to engage in nonsocial behaviors that occupy large portions of the activity budget. For example, in many species, foraging activities can occupy as much as 70% of the activity budget (Herbers, 1981; Malik and Southwick, 1988; Marriott, 1988; Milton, 1980; O'Neill et al., 1989; Strier, 1987). Such an important component of the behavior profile can be accommodated by providing food puzzles (Line and Houghton, 1987), foraging boards (Bayne *et al.,* 1991a, 1992b, 1993), or food treats distributed by facility personnel as an addition to the daily diet. Such foraging opportunities may help prevent abnormal appetitive behaviors (e.g., coprophagy). Providing objects to manipulate or groom can also satisfy other common behaviors exhibited by nonhuman primates, thereby preventing excessive self-directed behaviors. Finally, accommodating species-typical postures and locomotion patterns will further expand the behavioral repertoire the captive primate can express (Dexter and Bayne, 1994; Bayne *et al.,* 1989).

VIII. SUMMARY

The field of biomedical research is rapidly becoming more dependent on sophisticated techniques to answer the scientific questions of today. A consequence of this increase in technology is the need for refined animal models to assist in finding solutions to these questions. The role of the veterinarian in this area is a critical one, as it becomes his/her responsibility to keep the research animal healthy. Although the majority of the training and education of the veterinarian relates to the physical health of the animal, it is imperative that the entire well-being of the animal be addressed and cared for. Psychological disorders are a preventable and treatable condition that impairs the nonhuman primate research model. Moral, scientific, and regulatory reasons mandate action for eliminating psychological disorders from our primate colonies utilizing the many techniques available today.

There is a range of pathology associated with the various abnormal behaviors recorded in laboratory primates (for a listing of these behaviors, see Bayne *et al.,* 1991a). Some behaviors, such as self-mutilation, have an obvious impact on the health of the animal (Bayne *et al.,* 1995) and the research being conducted. The effect(s) on the long-term health of the animal and on the research objectives by more subtle behavioral abnormalities remains mostly undertermined. As biomedical research addresses more sophisticated and technical health-related questions, more refined animal models will become increasingly important. Accordingly, identifying methods of detecting and correcting stress factors adversely affecting the laboratory primate become particularly relevant to the overall health care of the animal and the success of the research project.

ACKNOWLEDGMENT

The authors thank Ms. Sandra Dexter for assistance with the preparation of this manuscript.

REFERENCES

Adams, M. R., Kaplan, J. R., Manuck, S. B., Uberseder, B., and Larkin, K. T. (1988). Persistent sympathetic nervous system arousal associated with tethering in cynomolgus macaques. *Lab. Anim. Sci.* **38,** 279–281.

Alexander, B. K. (1966). The effects of early peer deprivation on juvenile behavior of rhesus monkeys. Doctoral Dissertation, University of Wisconsin, Madison.

Anderson, C. O., and Mason, W. A. (1974). Early experience and complexity of social organization in groups of young rhesus monkeys (*Macaca mulatta*). *J. Comp. Physiol. Psychol.* **87,** 681–690.

Arling, G. L., and Harlow, H. F. (1967). Effects of social deprivation of maternal behavior of rhesus monkeys. *J. Comp. Physiol. Psychol.* **64,** 371–378.

Bayne, K., Suomi, S., and Brown, B. (1989). A new monkey swing. *Laboratory Primate Newsletter* **28**(4), 16–17.

Bayne, K., Mainzer, H., Dexter, S., Campbell, G., Yamada, F., and Suomi, S. (1991a). The reduction of abnormal behaviors in individually housed rhesus monkeys (*Macaca mulatta*) with a foraging/grooming board. *Am. J. Primatol.* **23,** 23–35.

Bayne, K., Dexter, S., and Suomi, S. (1991b). Ameliorating behavioral pathology in *Cebus apella* monkeys with social housing. *Lab. Primate Newsl.* **30**(2), 9–12.

Bayne, K., Dexter, S., and Suomi, S. J. (1992a). A preliminary survey of the incidence of abnormal behavior in rhesus monkeys (*Macaca mulatta*) relative to housing condition. *Lab. Anim.* **22,** 38–44.

Bayne, K., Dexter, S., Mainzer, H., McCully, C., Campbell, G., and Yamada, F. (1992b). The use of artificial turf as a foraging substrate for individually housed rhesus monkeys (*Macaca mulatta*). *Anim. Welfare* **1**(1), 39–53.

Bayne, K., Dexter, S., and Strange, G. (1993). The effect of food treat provisioning and human interaction on the behavioral well-being of rhesus monkeys (*Macaca mulatta*). *Contemp. Top. Lab. Anim. Sci.* **32**(2), 6–9.

Bayne, K., Haines, M., Dexter, S., Woodman, D., and Evans, C. (1995). A retrospective analysis of the wounding incidence of nonhuman primates housed in different social conditions. *Lab. Anim.* **24**(4), 40–44.

Berkson, G. (1967). Abnormal stereotyped motor acts. *In* "Comparative Psychopathology: Animal and Human" (J. Zubin and H. F. Hunt, eds.), pp. 76–94. Grune & Stratton, New York.

Berkson, G., and Mason, W. A. (1964). Stereotyped behaviors of chimpanzees: Relation to general arousal and other activities. *Percept. Mot. Skills* **19,** 635–652.

Bernstein, I. S., Gordan, T. P., and Rose, R. M. (1974). Factors influencing the expression of aggression during introduction to rhesus monkey groups. *In* "Primate Aggression, Territoriality, and Xenophobia" (R. L. Holloway, ed.), pp. 211–240. Academic Press, New York.

Boccia, M. L., Reite, M., and Laudenslager, M. (1989). On the physiology of grooming in a pigtail macaque. *Physiol. Behav.* **45,** 667–670.

Brandt, E. M., Stevens, C. W., and Mitchell, G. (1971). Visual social communication in adult male isolate-reared monkeys (*Macaca mulatta*). *Primates* **12,** 105–112.

Capitanio, J. P. (1984). Early experience and social processes in rhesus macaques (*Macaca mulatta*): I. Dyadic social interaction. *J. Comp. Psychol.* **1,** 35–44.

Capitanio, J. P. (1986). Behavioral pathology. *In* "Primate Biology: Behavior, Conservation, and Ecology" (G. Mitchell and J. Erwin, eds.), pp. 411–454. Liss, New York.

Carr, E. G. (1977). The motivation of self-injurious behavior: a review of some hypotheses. *Psychol. Bull.* **84**(4), 800–816.

Chamove, A. S., Rosenblum, L. A., and Harlow, H. F. (1973). Monkeys (*Macaca mulatta*) raised only with peers. A pilot study. *Anim. Behav.* **21,** 316–325.

Champoux, M., Coe, C. L., Schanberg, S. M., Kuhn, C. M., and Suomi, S. J. (1989). Hormonal effects of early rearing conditions in the infant rhesus monkey. *Am. J. Primatol.* **19,** 111–117.

Champoux, M., Byrne, E., Delizio, R., and Suomi, S. J. (1992). Motherless-mothers revisited: Rhesus maternal behavior and rearing history. *Primates* **33**, 251–255.

Clark, D. L. (1968). Immediate and delayed effects of early intermediate, and late social isolation in the rhesus monkey. Doctoral Dissertation, University of Wisconsin, Madison.

Coe, C. L., Wiener, S. G., Rosenberg, L. T., and Levine, S. (1985). Endocrine and immune responses to separation and maternal loss in nonhuman primates. *In* "The Psychobiology of Attachment and Separation," pp. 163–199. Academic Press, New York.

Coe, C. L., Lubach, G., and Ershler, W. B. (1989). Immunological consequences of maternal separation in infant primates. *In* "Infant Stress and Coping" (M. Lewis and J. Worobey, eds.), pp. 65–91. Jossey-Bass, San Francisco.

Cork, L. C., Martin, L. J., Lewis, M. H., and Gluck, J. F. (1990). Early social restriction of rhesus monkeys alters chemoarchitecture in the striatum but not in the bed nucleus-amygdala complex. *Soc. Neurosci. Abstr.* **16**, 442.

Cross, H. A., and Harlow, H. F. (1965). Prolonged and progressive effects of partial isolation on the behavior of macaque monkeys. *J. Exp. Res. Personality* **1**, 39–49.

Deets, A. C., Harlow, H. F., Singh, S. D., and Bloomquist, A. J. (1970). Effects of bilateral lesions of the frontal granular cortex on the social behavior of rhesus monkeys. *J. Comp. Physiol. Psychol.* **72**(3), 452–461.

de Lissovoy, V. (1963). Head banging in early childhood: A suggested cause. *J. Genet. Psychol.* **102**, 109–114.

Dexter, S., and Bayne, K. (1994). Results of providing swings to individually housed rhesus monkeys (*Macaca mulatta*). *Lab. Primate Newsl.* **33**(2), 9–12.

Draper, W. A., and Bernstein, I. W. (1963). Stereotyped behavior and cage size. *Percept. Mot. Skills* **16**, 231–234.

Erwin, J., and Deni, R. (1979). Strangers in a strange land: Abnormal behaviors or abnormal environments? *In* "Captivity and Behavior" (J. Erwin, T. Maple, and G. Mitchell, eds.), pp. 1–28. Van Nostrand-Reinhold, New York.

Fittinghoff, N. A., Jr., Lindburg, D. G., Gomber, J., and Mitchell, G. (1974). Consistency and variability in the behavior of mature, isolation-reared, male rhesus macaques. *Primates* **14**, 111–139.

Floeter, M. K., and Greenough, W. T. (1979). Cerebellar plasticity: Modification of purkinje cell structure by differential rearing in rhesus monkeys. *Science* **206**, 227–229.

Fox, M. W. (1966). Neuro-behavior ontogeny: A synthesis of ethological and neurophysiological concept. *Brain Res.* **2**, 3–20.

Fritz, P., and Fritz, J. (1979). Resocialization of captive chimpanzees: Ten years of experience at the Primate Foundation of Arizona. *J. Med. Primatol.* **8**, 202–221.

Fuller, J. L. (1967). Experimental deprivation and later behavior. *Science* **158**, 1645–1652.

Gewirtz, S. L. (1961). A learning analysis of the effects of normal stimulation, privation, and deprivation on the acquisition of social motivation and attachment. In (B. M. Foss, ed.) Determinants of Infant Behavior, New York, Wiley, pp. 213–290.

Gluck, J. P., Harlow, H. F., and Schiltz, K. A. (1973). Differential effect of early enrichment and deprivation on learning in the rhesus monkey (*Macaca mulatta*). *J. Comp. Physiol. Psychol.* **84**, 598–604.

Gluck, J. P., Ozer, H., Hensley, L. L., Beauchamp, A., Mailman, R. B., and Lewis, M. H. (1989). Early social isolation in rhesus monkeys: Long-term effects on survival and cell mediated immunity. *Soc. Neurosci. Abstr.* **15**, 297.

Goldfarb, W. (1958). Pain reactions in a group of institutionalized schizophrenic children. *Am. J. Orthopsychiatry* **28**, 777–785.

Gordan, T. (1990). Biomedical research on corral-housed primates. *In* "Monkey Behavior and Laboratory Issues Workshop, 1990." National Institutes of Health, Bethesda, MD.

Goy, R. W., and Wallen, K. (1979). Experiential variables influencing play, foot-clasp mounting and adult sexual competence in male rhesus monkeys. *Psychoneuroendocrinology* **4**, 1–12.

Goy, R. W., Wallen, K., and Goldfoot, D. A. (1974). Social factors affecting the development of mounting behavior in male rhesus monkeys. *In* "Reproductive Behavior" (W. Montagna and W. A. Sadler, eds.). Plenum, New York.

Hansen, E. W. (1966). The development of maternal and infant behavior in the rhesus monkey. *Behaviour* **27**, 107–149.

Harlow, H. F. (1958). The nature of love. *Am. Psychol.* **13**, 673–685.

Harlow, H. F., and Harlow, M. K. (1962). The effects of rearing conditions on behavior. *Bull. Menninger Clin.* **26**, 213–224.

Harlow, H. F., and Harlow, M. K. (1965). The effectional system. *In* "Behavior of Nonhuman Primates" (A. M. Schrier, H. F. Harlow, and S. Stollnitz, eds.), Vol. 2, pp. 287–334. Academic Press, New York.

Harlow, H. F., and Novak, M. A. (1973). Psychopathological perspectives. *Perspec. Biol. Med.* **16**, 461–478.

Harlow, H. F., and Suomi, S. J. (1970). The nature of love simplified. *Am. Psychol.* **25**, 161–168.

Harlow, H. F., and Zimmerman, R. R. (1959). Affectional responses in the infant monkey. *Science* **130**, 421–432.

Harlow, H. F., Schlitz, K. A., and Harlow, M. K. (1969). Effects of social isolation on the learning performance of rhesus monkeys. *Proc. Int. Congr. Primatol., 2nd,* Atlanta, *1968,* Vol. 1, pp. 178–185.

Harlow, H. F., Harlow, M. K., and Suomi, S. J. (1971). From thought to therapy: Lessons from a primate laboratory. *Am. Sci.* **59**, 538–549.

Hennessy, M. B., Mendoza, S. P., and Kaplan, J. N. (1982). Behavior and plasma cortisol following brief peer separation in juvenile squirrel monkeys. *Am. J. Primatol.* **3**, 143–151.

Herbers, J. M. (1981). Time resources and laziness in animals. *Oecologia* **49**, 252–262.

Higley, J. D., and Suomi, S. J. (1989). Temperamental reactivity in nonhuman primates. *In* "Handbook of Temperament in Children" (G. A. Kohnstamm, J. E. Bates, and M. K. Rothbard, eds.), pp. 153–167. Wiley, New York.

Higley, J. D., Suomi, S. J., and Linnoila, M. (1991). CSF monamine metabolite concentrations vary according to age, rearing, and sex, and are influenced by the stressor of social separation in rhesus monkeys. *Psychopharmacology* **103**, 551–556.

Kaplan, J. R., Adams, M. R., and Clarkson, T. B. (1982). Social status, environment and atherosclerosis in cynomolgus monkeys. *Arteriosclerosis (Dallas)* **2**, 359–368.

Kerr, G. R., Chamove, A. S., and Harlow, H. F. (1969). Environmental deprivation: Its effect on the growth of infant monkeys. *J. Pediatr.* **75**, 833–837.

Levanduski, S., Bayne, K., and Dexter, S. (1992). Use of behavioral observations in the detection of diabetes mellitus. *Lab. Primate Newsl.* **31**(1), 14–15.

Lewis, M. H., Gluck, J. P., Beauchamp, A. J., Keresztury, M. F., and Mailman, R. B. (1990). Long-term effects of early social isolation in *Macaca mulatta:* Changes in dopamine receptor function following apomorphine challenge. *Brain Res.* **513**, 67–73.

Line, S. W., and Houghton, P. (1987). Influence of an environmental enrichment device on general behavior and appetite in rhesus macaques. *Lab. Anim. Sci.* **37**(4), 508.

Line, S. W., Morgan, K. N., Markowitz, H., and Strong, S. (1989). Heart rate and activity of rhesus monkeys in response to routine events. *Lab. Primate Newsl.* **28**(2), 9–12.

Line, S. W., Morgan, K. N., Roberts, J. A., and Markowitz, H. (1990). Preliminary comments on resocialization of aged rhesus macaques. *Lab. Primate Newsl.* **29**(1), 8–12.

Lloyd, K. G., Hornykiewicz, O., Davidson, L., Shannak, K., Farley, I., Goldstein, M., Shibuya, M., Kelley, W. N., and Fox, I. H. (1981). Biochemical evidence of dysfunction of brain neurotransmitters in the Lesch-Nyhan syndrome. *N. Engl. J. Med.* **305**(19), 1106–1111.

Malik, I., and Southwick, C. H. (1988). Feeding behavior and activity patterns of rhesus monkeys (*Macaca mulatta*) at Tughlaqabad, India. *In* "Ecology and Behavior of Food-enhanced Primate Groups" (J. E. Fa and C. H. Southwick, eds.), pp. 95–111. Liss, New York.

Marriott, B. M. (1988). Time budgets of rhesus monkeys (*Macaca mulatta*) in a forest habitat in Nepal and on Cayo Santiago. *In* "Ecology and Behavior of Food-Enhanced Primate Groups" (J. E. Fa and C. H. Southwick, eds.), pp. 125–149. Liss, New York.

Mason, G. (1991). Stereotypies: A critical review. *Anim. Behav.* **41**, 1015–1037.

Mason, W. A. (1960). The effects of social restriction on the behavior of rhesus monkeys: I. Free social behavior. *J. Comp. Physiol. Psychol.* **53**, 583–589.

Mason, W. A. (1961a). The effects of social restriction on the behavior of rhesus monkeys: II. Tests of gregariousness. *J. Comp. Physiol. Psychol.* **54**, 287–290.

Mason, W. A. (1961b). The effects of social restriction on the behavior of rhesus monkeys: III. Dominance tests. *J. Comp. Physiol. Psychol.* **54**, 694–699.

Mason, W. A. (1968). Early social deprivation in the nonhuman primates: Implication for human behavior. *In* "Environmental Influences" (D. C. Glass, ed.), pp. 70–100. Rockefeller University and Russell Sage, New York.

Mason, W. A. (1985). Experimental influences on the development of expressive behaviors in rhesus monkeys. *In* "The Development of Expressive Behavior: Biology-Environment Interactions" (G. Ziven, ed.), pp. 117–152. Academic Press, New York.

Mason, W. A., and Berkson, G. (1975). Effects of maternal mobility on the development of rocking and other behaviors in rhesus monkeys: A study with artificial mothers. *Dev. Psychobiol.* **8**(3), 197–211.

Mason, W. A., and Green, P. C. (1962). The effects of social restriction on the behavior of rhesus monkeys: IV. Responses to a novel environment and alien species. *J. Comp. Physiol. Psychol.* **55**, 363–368.

Mason, W. T., and Kenney, M. D. (1974). Redirection of filial attachments in rhesus monkeys: Dogs as mother surrogates. *Science* **183**, 1209–1211.

Miller, R. E., Mirsky, I. A., Caul, W. F., and Sakata, T. (1969). Hyperphagia and polydipsia in socially-isolated rhesus monkeys. *Science* **165**, 1027–1028.

Miller, R. E., Caul, W. F., and Mirsky, I. A. (1971). Patterns of eating and drinking in socially-isolated rhesus monkeys. *Physiol. Behav.* **7**, 127–134.

Milton, K. (1980). "The Foraging Strategies of Howler Monkeys: A Study in Primate Economics." Columbia University Press, New York.

Mitchell, G. (1968). Persistent behavior pathology in rhesus monkeys following early social isolation. *Folia Primatol.* **8**, 132–147.

Mitchell, G. (1970). Abnormal behavior in primates. *In* "Primate Behavior: Developments in Field and Laboratory Research" (L. A. Rosenblum, ed.), Vol. 1, pp. 196–253. Academic Press, New York.

Mitchell, G. D., Raymond, E. J., Ruppenthal, G. C., and Harlow, H. F. (1966). Long-term effects of total isolation upon behavior of rhesus monkeys. *Psychol. Rep.* **18**, 567–580.

Morton, D. B., and Griffiths, P. H. M. (1985). Guidelines on the recognition of pain, distress, and discomfort in experimental animals and an hypothesis for assessment. *Vet. Rec.* **116**, 431–436.

Newman, J. D., and Symmes, D. (1974). Vocal pathology in socially deprived monkeys. *Dev. Psychobiol.* **7**, 351–358.

Novak, M. A. (1979). Social recovery of monkeys isolated for the first year of life: II. Long-term assessment. *Dev. Psychol.* **15**, 50–61.

Novak, M. A., and Harlow, H. F. (1975). Social recovery of monkeys isolated for the first year of life: I. Rehabilitation and therapy. *Dev. Psychol.* **11**, 453–465.

Novak, M. A., and Suomi, S. J. (1988). Psychological well-being of primates in captivity. *Am. Psychol.* **43**(10), 765–773.

Novak, M. A., O'Neill, P. L., Beckley, S. A., and Suomi, S. J. (1994). Naturalistic environments for captive primates. *In* "Indoor Naturalistic Habitats" (E. Gibbons, ed.), pp. 236–258. SUNY Press, Stony Brook, NY.

O'Neill, P., Price, C., and Suomi, S. (1989). Daily patterns in activity levels relative to age and sex in a free-ranging group of rhesus monkeys. *Am. Assoc. Lab. Anim. Sci. Meet.,* Little Rock, AR.

Rasmussen, K. L. R. (1991). Methodological considerations in research with socially living monkeys. *Lab. Anim. Sci.* **41**(4), 350–354.

Rasmussen, K. L. R., and Suomi, S. M. (1989). Heart rate and endocrine responses to stress in adolescent male rhesus monkeys on Cayo Santiago. *P. R. Health Sci. J.* **8**(1), 65–71.

Reinhardt, V. (1988). Preliminary comments on pairing unfamiliar adult male rhesus monkeys for the purpose of environmental enrichment. *Lab. Primate Newsl.* **27**(4), 1–3.

Reinhardt, V. (1990). A privacy panel for iso-sexual pairs of caged rhesus monkeys. *Am. J. Primatol.* **20**, 225–226.

Reinhardt, V., Houser, D., Cowley, D., Eisele, S., and Vertein, R. (1989). Alternatives to single caging of rhesus monkey (*Macaca mulatta*) used in research. 2. *Versuchstierkd.* **32**, 275–279.

Reinhardt, V., Cowley, D., Eisele, S., Vertein, R., and Houser, D. (1987). Preliminary comments on pairing unfamiliar female rhesus monkeys for the purpose of environmental enrichment. *Lab. Primate Newsl.* **26**(2), 5–8.

Reinhardt, V., Cowley, D., Eisele, S., Vertein, R., and Houser, D. (1988a). Pairing compatible female rhesus monkeys for cage enrichment has no negative impact on body weight. *Lab. Primate Newsl.* **27**(1), 13–15.

Reinhardt, V., Houser, D., Eisele, S., Cowley, D., and Vertein, R. (1988b). Behavioral responses of unrelated rhesus monkey females paired for the purpose of environmental enrichment. *Am. J. Primatol.* **14**, 135–140.

Reite, M., Short, R., Kaufman, I. C., Stynes, A. J., and Pauley, J. D. (1978). Heart rate and body temperature in separated monkey infants. *Biol. Psychiatry* **13**(1), 91–105.

Reite, M., Harbeck, R., and Hoffman, A. (1981). Altered cellular immune response following peer separation. *Life Sci.* **29**, 1133–1136.

Ridley, R. M., and Baker, H. F. (1982). Stereotypy in monkeys and humans. *Psychol. Med.* **12**, 61–72.

Riesen, A. H. (1960). Effects of stimulus deprivation on the development and atrophy of the visual sensory system. *Am. J. Orthopsychiatry* **30**, 23–26.

Rogers, C. M., and Davenport, R. K. (1969). Effects of restricted rearing on sexual behavior of chimpanzees. *Dev. Psychol.* **1**, 200–204.

Rosenblum, L. A. (1961). The development of social behavior in the rhesus monkey. Doctoral Dissertation, University of Wisconsin, Madison.

Roy, M. A. (1981). Abnormal behaviors in nursery-reared squirrel monkeys (*Saimiri sciureus*). *Am. J. Primatol.* **1**, 35–42.

Sackett, G. P. (1965). Effects of rearing conditions upon monkeys (*M. mulatta*). *Child Dev.* **36**, 855–868.

Sackett, G. P. (1968). The persistence of abnormal behavior in monkeys following isolation rearing. *In* "Ciba Foundation Symposium on the Role of Learning in Psychotherapy" (R. Porter, ed.), pp. 3–25. Churchill, London.

Sackett, G. P. (1974). Sex differences in rhesus monkeys following varied rearing experiences. *In* "Sex Differences in Behavior" (R. C. Friedman, R. M. Richert, and R. L. Vande Wiele, eds.), pp. 99–122. Wiley, New York.

Sackett, G. P., Bowman, R. E., Meyer, J. S., Tripp, R. L., and Grady, S. S. (1973). Adrenocortical and behavioral reactions by differentially raised rhesus monkeys. *Physiol. Psychol.* **1**, 209–212.

Sackett, G. P., Holm, R. A., and Ruppenthal, G. C. (1976). Social isolation rearing: Species differences in the behavior of macaque monkeys. *Dev. Psychol.* **12**, 283–288.

Sackett, G. P., Ruppenthal, G. C., Fahrenbruch, C. E., and Holm, R. A. (1981). Social isolation rearing effects in monkeys vary with genotype. *Dev. Psychol.* **17**, 313–318.

Sackett, G. P., Tripp, R., and Grady, S. (1982). Rhesus monkeys reared in isolation with added social, nonsocial, and electrical brain stimulation. *Ann. 1st. Super. Sanita* **18**, 203–214.

Selyé, H. (1950). "Stress." Acta, Inc., Montreal.

Selyé, H. (1974). "Stress without Distress." Lippincott, Philadelphia.

Strier, K. B. (1987). Activity budgets of woolly spider monkeys, or muriquis (*Brachyteles arachnoides*). *Am. J. Primatol.* **13**, 385–395.

Strubel, R. G., and Riesen, A. H. (1978). Changes in cortical dendritic branching subsequent to partial social isolation in stumptailed monkeys. *Dev. Psychobiol.* **11**, 479–486.

Suomi, S. J. (1973). Surrogate rehabilitation of monkeys reared in total social isolation. *J. Child Psychol. Psychiatry* **14**, 71–77.

Suomi, S. J. (1978). Maternal behavior by socially incompetent monkeys: Neglect and abuse of offspring. *J. Pediat. Psychol.* **3**, 28–34.

Suomi, S. J. (1991). Uptight and laid-back monkeys: Individual differences in the response to social challenges. *In* "Plasticity of Development" (S. Brauth, W. Hall, and R. Dooling, eds.). MIT Press, Cambridge, MA (in press).

Suomi, S. J., and Harlow, H. F. (1972). Social rehabilitation of isolate-reared monkeys. *Dev. Psychol.* **6,** 487–496.

Suomi, S. J., Harlow, H. F., and Lewis, J. K. (1970). Effect of bilateral frontal lobectomy on social preferences of rhesus monkeys. *J. Comp. Physiol. Psychol.* **70**(3), 448–453.

Suomi, S. J., Scanlan, J. M., Rasmussen, K. L. R., Davidson, M., Boinski, S., Higley, J. D., and Marriott, B. (1989). Pituitary-adrenal response to capture in Cayo Santiago-derived group M rhesus monkeys. *P. R. Health Sci. J.* **8**(1), 171–176.

Thompson, C. I. Schwartzbaum, J. S., and Harlow, H. F. (1969). Development of social fear after amygdalectomy in infant rhesus monkeys. *Physiol. Behav.* **4,** 249–254.

Tinklepaugh, O. L. (1928). The self-mutilation of a male *Macacus rhesus* monkey. *J. Mammal.* **9,** 293–300.

Wood, B. S., Mason, W. A., and Kenney, M. D. (1979). Contrasts in visual responsiveness and emotional arousal between rhesus monkeys raised with living and those raised with inanimate substitute mothers. *J. Comp. Physiol. Psychol.* **93,** 368–377.

Index

Entry followed by t or f denotes table or figure.